Physical Therapies in Sport and Exercise

For Churchill Livingstone:

Publishing Director: Mary Law
Project Manager: Gail Wright
Designer: Judith Wright
Illustrator: Ethan Danielson

Physical Therapies in Sport and Exercise

Edited by

Gregory S Kolt

BSc BAppSc(Phty) GradDipEd GradDipBehavHlthCare PhD
Professor of Health Science and Associate Dean (Research), Faculty of Health Studies, Auckland University of Technology, Auckland, New Zealand

Lynn Snyder-Mackler

BA CertPhysTher MS ScD
Professor, Department of Physical Therapy, Graduate Program in Biomechanics and Movement Sciences, University of Delaware, Newark, Delaware, USA

Foreword by

Per Renstrom

MD PhD
Professor of Sports Medicine, Section of Sports Medicine, Department of Surgical Sciences, Karolinska Institute, Stockholm, Sweden; Chairman, Swedish Sport Research Council; Member, Medical Commission of the International Olympic Committee (IOC) and IOC Publication Advisory Commission; Vice President, International Society of Arthroscopy, Knee Surgery and Orthopaedic Sports Medicine (ISAKOS); President, International Society of Medicine and Science in Tennis; Medical Director, ATP; Physician to the Swedish Davis Cup Team

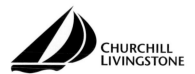

CHURCHILL
LIVINGSTONE

CHURCHILL LIVINGSTONE
An imprint of Elsevier Science Limited

First published 2003

ISBN 0 443 07154 3

British Library Cataloguing in Publication Data
A catalogue record for this book is available from the British Library

Library of Congress Cataloging in Publication Data
A catalog record for this book is available from the Library of Congress

Note
Medical knowledge is constantly changing. As new information becomes available, changes in treatment, procedures, equipment and the use of drugs become necessary. The editors, contributors and the publishers have taken care to ensure that the information given in this text is accurate and up to date. However, readers are strongly advised to confirm that the information, especially with regard to drug usage, complies with the latest legislation and standards of practice.

 ELSEVIER SCIENCE

your source for books, journals and multimedia in the health sciences

www.elsevierhealth.com

The publisher's policy is to use paper manufactured from sustainable forests

Printed in China by RDC Group Limited

Contents

Contributors

Michael J Axe MD
Clinical Professor, Department of Physical Therapy, University of Delaware; Orthopedic Surgeon, First State Orthopedics, Newark, Delaware, USA

Lizanne M Backe NP
Nurse Practitioner, Division of Sports Medicine, Children's Hospital, Boston, Massachusetts, USA

Lisa Casson Barkley MD FAAFP
Physician Specializing in Family Medicine, Education Faculty, Adolescent and Sports Medicine, Department of Internal Medicine, Christiana Care Health Services, Newark, Delaware, USA

Kim Bennell BAppSc(Physio) PhD
Associate Professor and Director of the Centre for Sports Medicine Research and Education, School of Physiotherapy, University of Melbourne, Melbourne, Victoria, Australia

Amy Brown MPT
Staff Therapist, Sports Medicine Department, Bayhealth Medical Center, Dover, Delaware, USA

David Butler MApp Sc PT
Lecturer, Neuro Orthopedic Institute, Adelaide, Australia

Terese L Chmielewski MA PT SCS
Doctoral Student, Biomechanics and Movement Science Program, Department of Physical Therapy, University of Delaware, Newark, Delaware, USA

Michael T Cibulka PT MHS OCS
Physical Therapist in Private Practice, Festus, Missouri; Clinical Instructor for Program in Physical Therapy,

Washington University, St Louis, Missouri; Clinical Faculty Member for Program in Physical Therapy, Creighton University, Omaha, Nebraska, USA

Jill Cook BAppSci PostGradDip PhD
Senior Lecturer, Musculoskeletal Research Centre, La Trobe University, Melbourne, Victoria, Australia

Andrew G Cresswell BEd MSc PhD
Associate Professor, Department of Neuroscience, Karolinska Institute, Stockholm, Sweden

Kay Crossley BAppSc(Physio) PostGradDip(Research) PhD
NHMRC Health Practitioner Fellow, Centre for Sports Medicine Research and Education, School of Physiotherapy, University of Melbourne, Melbourne, Victoria, Australia

Rafael Escamilla BS MS PhD MPT CSCS
Assistant Research Professor, Department of Surgery, Division of Orthopedic Surgery, Duke University Medical Center, Durham, North Carolina, USA

Andrew Garnham MBBS DipRACOG FACSP
Senior Lecturer (Sports Medicine), School of Health Sciences, Deakin University, Burwood, Victoria, Australia

Bruce Hamilton BPhEd MBChB DTM&H FACSP
Sports Physician, Australian Institute of Sport, Bruce, Australian Capital Territory, Australia

Paul W Hodges BPhty(Hons) PhD
NHMRC Research Fellow and Associate Professor, Department of Physiotherapy, University of Queensland, Brisbane, Australia

Zoë Hudson GradAssocPhys MCSP SRP
Private Physiotherapy Practitioner, Academic Associate,
Interdisciplinary Research Centre in Biomedical
Materials, Queen Mary, University of London, UK;
Physiotherapist for the Great Britain Paralympic Team

James J Irrgang PhD PT ATC
Assistant Professor Vice Chairman of Clinical Services,
Department of Physical Therapy, University of
Pittsburgh, Pittsburgh, Pennsylvania; Vice President for
Quality Improvement and Outcomes, Centers for
Rehabilitation Services, Pittsburgh, Pennsylvania, USA

Christopher AM Johnston BScH MD CCFP MSc DipSportsMed
(CASM)
Sports Medicine Fellow, Allan McGavin Sports Medicine
Centre, University of British Columbia,
Vancouver, British Columbia, Canada

Mark Jones BS MAppSc CertPhysTher GradDipAdvanManipPhysio
Senior Lecturer, Director, Graduate Programs in
Musculoskeletal and Sports Physiotherapy, International
Coordinator, School of Physiotherapy, Division of
Health Sciences, University of South Australia,
Adelaide, Australia

Pekka Kannus MD PhD
Professor of Injury Prevention, The UKK Institute, and
University and University Hospital of Tampere,
Tampere, Finland

Paul LaStayo PhD PT CHT
Assistant Professor, Department of Physical Therapy,
Northern Arizona University, Flagstaff, Arizona, USA

Rob Lloyd-Smith BA MDCM DipSportsMed(CASM)
Primary Care Physician, Allan McGavin Sports
Medicine Center, University of British Columbia,
Vancouver, British Columbia, Canada

Domhnall MacAuley MD FRCGP FFPHM FISM
Sports Medicine Specialist and General Practitioner,
Hillhead Family Practice and Department of
Epidemiology, Queen's University of Belfast, Belfast, UK

Jenny McConnell BAppSci(Phty) GradDipManTher MBiomedEng
Director, McConnell and Clements Physiotherapy,
Mosman, New South Wales, Australia

Peter J McNair PhD MNZCP
Professor, School of Physiotherapy, Auckland University
of Technology, Auckland, New Zealand

Mary E Magarey DipTechPhysio GradDipAdvanManipTher PhD
Senior Lecturer, Director, Graduate Programs in Sports
Physiotherapy, School of Physiotherapy, Division of
Health Sciences, University of South Australia,
Adelaide, Australia

Lyle J Micheli MD
Director, Division of Sports Medicine, Children's
Hospital, Boston, Massachusetts; Associate Clinical
Professor of Orthopedic Surgery, Harvard Medical
School, Boston, Massachusetts, USA

Susan Michlovitz PhD PT CHT
Professor, Department of Physical Therapy, Temple
University, Philadelphia, Pennsylvania, USA

Douglas Mintz MD
Assistant Professor, Weill Medical College of Cornell
University; Assistant Attending Radiologist, New York
Presbyterian Hospital and Hospital for Special Surgery,
New York, USA

Ryan L Mizner MPT
Doctoral Student, Biomechanics and Movement Sciences
Program, University of Delaware, Newark, Delaware,
USA

Robert J Nee MAppSc PT ATC
Assistant Professor, School of Physical Therapy, Pacific
University, Forest Grove, Oregon, USA

Gabriel Ng PhD MPhty ProfDipPhty
Associate Professor, Department of Rehabilitation
Sciences, The Hong Kong Polytechnic University,
Hong Kong

William J Padamonsky II MPT
Physical Therapy Sports Resident, Department of
Physical Therapy, University of Delaware, Newark,
Delaware, USA

Michael M Reinold PT
Physical Therapist, Healthsouth Sports Medicine and
Rehabilitation Center, Birmingham, Alabama, USA

Katherine Rudolph PhD PT
Assistant Professor, Department of Physical Therapy,
University of Delaware, Newark, Delaware, USA

Laura Schmitt MSPT SCS ATC
Associate Director, University of Delaware Physical
Therapy Clinic, Newark, Delaware, USA

Jennifer Stevens PhD MPT
Postdoctoral Fellow, Department of Physical Therapy,
University of Florida, Gainesville, Florida, USA

Jack Taunton MSc MD Dipl Sport Med (CASM)
Professor and Director, Allan McGavin Sports Medicine
Center, and Division of Sports Medicine, Department of
Family Practice, University of British Columbia,
Vancouver, British Columbia, Canada

Elly Trepman MD
Associate Professor, Section of Orthopaedic Surgery,
University of Manitoba, Winnipeg, Manitoba, Canada

Henry Wajswelner BAppSci(Physio) MPhysioapy(Research)
MManipulativePhysiotherapy
Private Practitioner and Sports Physiotherapist,
Australian Institute of Sport, Canberra, Australia

Amanda Weiss BA MD
Sports Medicine Fellow UCLA, Department of Family
Medicine, Division of Sports Medicine, University of
California Los Angeles, Los Angeles, California, USA

Suzanne Werner PhD PT ATC
Associate Professor, Division of Neurotechnology,
Department of Physical Therapy, and Division of
Surgical Sciences, Department of Sports Medicine,
Karolinska Institute, Stockholm, Sweden

Robbin Wickham MS PT SCS
Doctoral Fellow, Human Performance Laboratory, Ball
State University, Muncie, Indiana, USA

Kevin E Wilk
O/P Rehabilitation Center Healthsouth Sports Medicine
and Rehabilitation Center, Birmingham, Alabama, USA

DS Blaise Williams III PhD MPT
Assistant Professor, Department of Physical Therapy,
East Carolina University, Greenville, North Carolina,
USA

Wayne Woodzell BSc MPT
Sports Resident, Department of Physical Therapy,
University of Delaware, Newark, Delaware, USA

Preface

"To study the phenomena of disease without books is to sail an uncharted sea, while to study books without patients is not to go to sea at all"

— Sir William Osler

This book, *Physical Therapies in Sport and Exercise*, has evolved over the past two years to encompass not only rehabilitation from injury, but also prevention, recognition, and treatment of injuries in athletes and exercise participants of all ages. In echoes of Osler, the book is a map, but a map that needs to live in the real world of athletes with injuries. We have recently entered a new century. Most of the information contained in this volume would be foreign even to those who birthed the fitness revolution of the late twentieth century. While sciences such as anatomy have not changed, our knowledge of systems physiology is progressing almost from day to day. Concepts as simple as muscle fiber types have undergone enormous changes in our scientific lifetimes. Topics like motor control and psychology are crucial to the understanding of the care of athletes and other exercise participants in this era. New awareness of the importance of exercise and sport for all has given rise to the study of the special needs of older people, children, adolescents, and female athletes, as well as athletes with disabilities. In this book we have tried to contemporize all of the topics that comprise the area of physical therapy in sport and exercise. Authors from across the world, and in many sports medicine disciplines, have contributed in their expert areas. All the reader now needs to bring are the patients to sail the charted sea of physical therapy in sport and exercise.

Gregory S Kolt

Auckland and Delaware 2003   Lynn Snyder-Mackler

REFERENCE

Bean R B 1961 Sir William Osler: Aphorisms from his bedside teachings and writings. Charles C Thomas, Springfield, IL

Acknowledgements

A large number of people have contributed in a variety of ways to make this book a success. First, Mary Law, the Publishing Director who saw a place for a book like this and gave encouragement for the project to commence. As well, Gail Wright, our Project Manager is thanked for her efficiency, attention to detail, advice, and prompt responses to the many hundreds of emails that crossed the globe in making this book happen. I thank Kim Bennell who went well beyond contributing two chapters to this book, and was instrumental in developing the initial ideas and proposal and provided valuable advice throughout the project. Joanne Ryland and Salma Darwazeh were invaluable in the administration of the project – with 48 busy contributors from 8 countries, working on 30 chapters, this was no small task. Ruth Driver and Liesje Donkin undertook much of the time-consuming proofreading. Many of my colleagues at Auckland University of Technology and elsewhere have provided important information to add to this project. There are two people who have been very important to me in my professional life, and are indirectly responsible for me completing this project: my academic mentor, the late Professor Rob Kirkby, who provided an unparalleled enthusiasm for me to learn from; and David Zuker, one of the pioneers of sport physical therapy, who taught me so much. Last, but certainly not least, is my family. Emma, Daisy Chayne, and Satchel (and my parents, of course) have provided a balance in my life over this period, a great excuse to have time away from the book, and the encouragement and support to complete the project.

Gregory S Kolt

My doctoral students, sports PT residents, and colleagues in the Department of Physical Therapy, and Biomechanics and Movement Sciences program, at the University of Delaware contributed in tangible (many were contributors, read early drafts) and intangible ways. My family (Scott, Alexander, Noah, Moms, and Dads) and the army of people (especially Jill Heathcock) who keep our home life healthy during Scott's valiant fight with ALS inspire all I do. Sara Farquhar was academic publishing's loss and my gain, and provided invaluable editorial assistance.

Lynn Snyder-Mackler

Foreword

Based on extensive scientific evidence, it is clear that inactivity is definitely the largest risk factor for poor health and disease. Physical activity is, on the other hand, beneficial for health and this also has some scientific support. This message has been spread during the last 20–30 years to a large part of the world. People have started to become more active although they are not as active as they should be. There is a renewed interest in different types of physical activity and exercise, particularly for the elderly and young children of school age. The benefits of physical activity are obvious for the elderly as it strengthens bone mass and prevents hip fractures. For the young, there is not as much scientific support to show the benefits, however, it is important to try to get into the habit of carrying out some physical activity regularly from an early age. It is, nonetheless, never too late to start being physically active.

Many people enjoy watching top level sport in sport arenas and on television, and there is huge mass media interest in many aspects of sport. This puts increasing pressure on top level athletes: they have to practice harder, for longer periods of time, with higher intensity, and with less time to recover. Contact and collisions during games are getting rougher. All these factors increase the risk for injury. Athletes sustain injuries both of traumatic and overuse character, and overuse injuries, particularly, tend to increase both in frequency and in complexity. Unfortunately, there is not enough focus on prevention, which is a pity, as most overuse injuries can be prevented.

With the increasing awareness of the benefits of being physically active, the injury problem for the general population is also increasing among recreational athletes. Elderly people are tending to be more physically active today and this often generates some injury or pain problem. Active people often have a strong desire to recover as fast as possible after an injury.

There is increasing pressure to receive optimal injury management not only from physicians but also from physical therapists. The habit of including a physical therapist in the management team is gradually increasing and most people see much benefit from this. I have a physical therapist with me during all my clinics, which means that we can give every patient a rehabilitation program on the spot, and this is usually very much appreciated. This arrangement also makes sure that patients will see experts in the patients' specific injury, as the therapist can direct patients to where they need to go.

Physical therapy is a complex part of medicine and includes not only different aspects of exercises but also expertise on how different modalities can be used effectively. Rehabilitation exercises have been fairly extensively studied in the literature and they are well covered in this book in the first section, which describes management principles for musculo-skeletal tissues in physical therapy. This section provides major coverage on the structural biomechanics of the tissues in relation to the response of tissue injury to healing. The competition between healing and exercise is perhaps the most intriguing problem that the physical therapist faces. The therapist must introduce an exercise program to the injured person, which is as effective and extensive as possible without compromising healing of the tissue. There are very few objective ways of dosing the level of physical therapy exercises and therefore the skill and knowledge of the therapist is essential.

Modalities such as ultrasound, electrical stimulation and other types of heat treatment have historically played major roles in physical therapy. They are still used widely all around the world, mostly because people undergoing rehabilitation like them as they give a feeling of wellbeing. The problem is, however, that scientific support for the efficacy of the most common modalities is limited and this means that there is a great need for more

this area. This book, therefore, fills a gap, as it e evidence to support or refute the role of modalities in sports medicine.

It is also important for the physical therapist to be updated on what is new in the field. During the last few years there has been major interest in exercises that improve motor control and balance. There is also huge interest in why eccentric exercise is so effective in dealing with painful chronic tendinopathy and why a major overload seems to make the exercise even more effective. How effective is stretching? This book discusses these aspects as well.

As mentioned above, one of the problems that physical therapists face today is a lack of scientific study supporting the efficacy of different treatment techniques. It is therefore important to have a book like this, which outlines the available science of today and presents the current concepts of injury management. The physical therapist needs to know what to do. This is especially important today as most management in medicine must be evidence-based.

In sections 3 and 4 of the book, management of different regions, and management of different groups are described. People with special risk factors are discussed and this allows physical therapists to plan programs for a special group in detail. Towards the end of the book, there is a discussion about drugs, doping and other medical issues, which can be of benefit to some physical therapists active in sport.

This book will be a great addition to the existing literature for physical therapists active in sport, physical exercise and activity. It is very well-designed and well-planned and covers the whole field. The editors have managed to recruit some of the leading experts in the world, covering most of the important fields in sports physical therapy. Current concepts of injury management and the increasingly important role the physical therapist plays in the field of sports, physical exercise and activity, are described. The major advantage of this book is that the discussions are comprehensive and based on the scientific evidence available.

This is a high quality book in an increasingly important field. It is my sincere opinion that this book will not only be very beneficial but also enjoyable to read for everyone active in the field of physical therapy, sports, and physical activity.

Stockholm 2003   Per Renström

Abbreviations and acronyms

AAS	anabolic androgenic steroids	DJD	degenerative joint disease
AC	alternating current	DOMS	delayed onset muscle soreness
ACJ	acromioclavicular joint	DRG	dorsal root ganglion
ACL	anterior cruciate ligament	DRST	dynamic rotary stability test
ADL	activities of daily living	DRT	dynamic relocation test
ADR	autonomic dysreflexia	DRUJ	distal radioulnar joint
AIGS	abnormal impulse generating site	DSST	digit symbol substitution test
ALCL	accessory lateral collateral ligament	DXA	dual energy X-ray absorptiometry
ALL	anterior longitudinal ligament	EAT	eating attitudes test
APL	abductor pollicis longus	EBM	evidence-based medicine
ASIS	anterior superior iliac spine	EBP	evidence-based practice
ATLF	anterior talofibular ligament	ECG	electrocardiogram
ATP	adenosine triphosphate	ECRB	extensor carpi radialis brevis
ATPase	adenosine triphosphatase	ECRL	extensor carpi radialis longus
BMD	bone mineral density	ECU	extensor carpi ulnaris
CAL	coracoacromial ligament	EDC	extensor digitorum communis
CBT	cognitive-behavioral technique	EDI	eating disorders inventory
CDMP	cartilage derived morphogenic protein	EDNOS	eating disorders not otherwise specified
CECS	chronic exertional compartment syndrome	EEG	electroencephalogram
CHL	coracohumeral ligament	EIA	exercise-induced asthma
CIND	carpal instability non-dissociative	EIB	exercise-induced bronchospasm
CMC	carpometacarpal	EMG	electromyography
CNS	central nervous system	EPB	extensor pollicis brevis
CO	cardiac output	EPL	extensor pollicis longus
CP	cerebral palsy	ERT	estrogen replacement therapy
CPG	central pattern generators	ES	effect size
CSF	cerebrospinal fluid	FCU	flexor carpi ulnaris
CT	computed tomography	FDP	flexor digitorum profundus
CTS	carpal tunnel syndrome	FDS	flexor digitorum superficialis
DASH	Disabilities of the Arm, Shoulder and Hand Index	FEV1	forced expiratory volume in 1 s
		FOOSH	fall on outstretched hand
DC	direct current	FPL	flexor pollicis longus
DEXA	dual emission X-ray absorptiometry	FSH	follicle stimulating hormone
DHEA	dehydroepiandrosterone	GABA	gamma-aminobutyric acid
DHLNL	dihydroxylysinonorleucine	GAG	glycosaminoglycans
DHP	dihydropyridine	GDF	growth differentiation factor
DIP	distal phalangeal	GI	glycemic index

	onadotrophin releasing hormone	NSAID	non-steroidal anti-inflammatory drug
	round reaction forces	NSLBP	non-specific low back pain
GRI	ripping rotatory impaction test	OA	osteoarthritis
GTO	golgi tendon organ	OATS	osteochondral autograft transfer system
HALE	healthy active life expectancy	OCD	osteochondritis dissecans
HBV	hepatitis B	OCP	oral contraceptive pill
HCG	chorionic gonadotrophin	ORIF	open reduction with internal fixation
HCV	hepatitis C	PAES	popliteal artery entrapment syndrome
HHMD	histidinohydroxymerodesmosine	PAR-Q	Physical Activity Readiness Questionnaire
HIV	human immunodeficiency virus	PASS	pain anxiety symptoms scale
HLA	human leukocyte antigen	PCL	posterior collateral ligament
HLBS	high-load brief stress	PEFR	peak expiratory flow rate
HLNL	hydroxylysinonorleucine	PEMF	pulsed electromagnetic fields
HO	hyperbaric oxygen	PET	positron emission tomography
HOCM	hypertrophic obstructive cardiomyopathy	PFCA	patellofemoral congruence angle
HP	hydroxypyridinoline	PFJ	patellofemoral joint
HR	heart rate	PFPS	patellofemoral pain syndrome
HSV	herpes simplex virus	PIP	proximal interphalangeal
HVPC	high-volt pulsed current	PLL	posterior longitudinal ligament
HVTT	high velocity thrust technique	PNF	proprioceptive neuromuscular facilitation
IBSC	International Blind Sports Association		
IFT	interferential treatment	POL	posterior oblique ligament
IGHLC	inferior glenohumeral ligament complex	PPI	present pain intensity (scale)
IOC	International Olympic Committee	PRE	progressive resistance exercise
IP	interphalangeal	PRI	pain rating index
IPC	International Paralympic Committee	PROM	passive range of motion
IRRST	internal resistance strength test	PSIS	posterior superior iliac spine
ITP	interval throwing program	RCL	radial collateral ligament
IVF	intervertebral foramen	RCSP	resting calcaneal stance position
LBP	low back pain	rER	rough endoplasmic reticulum
LCL	lateral collateral ligament	RICE	rest, ice, compression and elevation
LF	ligamentum flavum	RM	repetition maximum
LH	luteinizing hormone	ROM	range of motion
LHB	long head of biceps	RSA	Roentgen stereophonogrammetric analysis
LLLD	low load, long duration	RSN	radial sensory nerve
LLPS	low-load prolonged stress	RYR	ryanodine receptor
LM	lumbar multifidus	SAID	specific adaptations to imposed demands
LOC	loss of consciousness	SCD	sudden cardiac death
LPD	lateral patellar displacement	SCFE	slipped capital femoral epiphysis
LPFA	lateral patellofemoral angle	SCI	spinal cord injury
LT	lunotriquetal	SCJ	sternoclavicular joint
LUCL	lateral ulnar collateral ligament	s.d.	standard deviation
MCL	medial collateral ligament	SEM	standard error of measurement
MCP	metacarpophalangeal	SFMPQ	Short Form McGill Pain Questionnaire
MDI	multidirectional instability	SGHL	superior glenohumeral ligament
MGL	middle glenohumeral ligament	SIJ	sacroiliac joint
MPQ	McGill Pain Questionnaire	SIP	sports inventory for pain
MRI	magnetic resonance imaging	SIRAS	Sport Injury Rehabilitation Adherence Scale
MTP	metatarsophalangeal	SIS	second impact syndrome
MVIC	maximum voluntary isometric contraction	SL	scapholunate
NCSP	neutral calcaneal stance position	SLAC	scapholonate advanced collapse
NCV	nerve conduction velocity	SLAP	superior labral anterior posterior
NMES	neuromuscular electrical stimulation	SMOC	Sports Medicine Observation Code
NRS	numerical rating scale	SMT	spinal manipulative therapy

SPECT	single photon emission computer tomography	URTI	upper respiratory tract infection
SRM	standardized response mean	US	ultrasound
STIR	short tau inversion recovery	USOC	United States Olympic Committee
STJ	scapulothoracic joint	VAS	visual analog scale
SV	stroke volume	VBI	vertebro-basilar insufficiency
TA	transverse abdominus	VL	vastus longus
TENS	transcutaneous electrical nerve stimulation	VML	vastus medialis longus
TERT	total end-range time	VMO	vastus medialis oblique
TFCC	triangular fibrocartilage complex	VRM	variable resistance machine
UCL	ulnar collateral ligament	VRS	verbal rating scale
		WADA	World Anti-Doping Agency

1

The role of the physical therapies in sport, exercise, and physical activity

Gregory S Kolt   Lynn Snyder-Mackler

INTRODUCTION

Sport, exercise, and physical activity pursuits are important in most societies. A result of participation in such activities, however, is the risk of injury. Not only does injury occur during competitive sport activities, but through preparation for such events, as well as during the general physical activities that an increasing number of people are becoming involved in.

The field of sports medicine has developed as a result of increased participation rates in sport, exercise, and physical activity, and the specific medical needs of participants (Matheson & Pipe 1996). Sports medicine is a multidisciplinary field that incorporates people from many professions. Brukner & Khan (2001) suggested that the ideal sports medicine team consists of the following:

- Family physician
- Sports physician
- Orthopedic surgeon
- Radiologist
- Physical therapist/physiotherapist
- Massage therapist
- Podiatrist
- Dietician/nutritionist
- Psychologist
- Athletic trainer/sports trainer
- A range of other professionals including osteopaths, chiropractors, exercise physiologists, biomechanists, nurses, occupational therapists, orthotists, optometrists
- Coach
- Fitness adviser.

Although this combination of professionals is ideal, in the majority of settings, sports medicine teams will be far smaller depending on the needs and demands of a particular sport and the availability of sports medicine practitioners.

People involved in sports medicine work towards several common goals. Two important goals are returning an individual to their preinjury level of functioning in the shortest possible time, and implementing strategies to avoid reinjury. Obviously there are several ways to rehabilitate each injury that an athlete presents with. Where possible, physical therapists should focus on techniques that have some level of proven efficacy. There are, however, a plethora of physical management methods that are being implemented on the basis of anecdotal evidence alone.

SPORTS REHABILITATION SPECIALISTS AND PHYSICAL THERAPISTS

In the context of this book, the terms 'sports rehabilitation specialist' and 'physical therapist' are used to describe the set of professions that use physical techniques and skills in the prevention, management, and rehabilitation of injury. For example, health professionals that would use these skills and techniques include physical therapists, physiotherapists, athletic trainers, athletic therapists, sports trainers, massage therapists, podiatrists, and sports physicians. Many of these professionals do not rely exclusively on physical methods to carry out their role, but usually combine such methods with other skills (e.g. psychological or behavioral techniques, pharmacological therapy, and electrophysical agents). The terms 'physical therapists' and 'sports rehabilitation specialists' will be used in a broad sense throughout this book.

Of the many professions listed above, several deal with issues that encompass more than sport and exercise alone. For example, physical therapy or physiotherapy is concerned with far reaching issues including cardiorespiratory problems, neurological conditions, physical developmental issues, and treatment of terminally ill people. Therefore, the aspect of those professions that deals with injury in sport and exercise is a specialized field that requires an expert knowledge, usually obtained through a combination of formal study and clinical experience. In the USA, a specialist certification process in sports physical therapy is possible through the American Physical Therapy Association. In Australia, postregistration university graduate programs in sports physiotherapy, in combination with other relevant experience, contribute to becoming a sports physiotherapist. In several other countries, a mixture of graduate study and clinical experience provide the skills to work in the area of sport and exercise physical therapy.

The role of physical therapists has changed dramatically over the past 30 years. Whereas traditionally, those involved in the physical therapies were required to work under the guidance and referral of a medical practitioner, many physical therapists are now considered primary contact practitioners. The ability to consult with and manage patients directly is different in each country. For example, in Australia, physiotherapists were granted primary contact status in the 1970s with other countries more recently following this lead. In the USA, direct access to physical therapists is controlled by the laws in each state; currently, over 30 individual states allow direct access. In many countries, the techniques that can be carried out by physical therapists are still somewhat restricted and guided by medical practitioners. In reading this book, therefore, physical therapists should be aware of their role in the health and medical system of the country they work in.

Not only are more physical therapists now working as primary contact practitioners, but the philosophy or approach to physical therapy has changed. Traditionally the main emphasis was on rehabilitation; however, more recently a major focus on preventive physical therapy has emerged for several reasons. In the cases of elite athletes, time out from sport due to injury can result in decreased performance rankings (individual and team), and in many cases, loss of earnings. In the cases of recreational or lower-level competitive athletes, time away from sport due to injury can result in a loss of enjoyment, reduced level of fitness, and loss of social opportunities. The older population is a new group that is increasingly involved in exercise and physical activity. The fitness and social rewards of their involvement can be affected when refraining from such activity due to injury or poor health. Thus, if effective preventive approaches to injury can be implemented, it is possible that injury rates may decline.

The medical needs of people involved in sport, exercise, and physical activity are best addressed through the team approach of sports medicine professionals. The various professions involved in the ideal sports medicine team have been listed above. It is apparent that individuals in the sports medicine team have a level of overlap in terms of their skills. In many situations, practitioners are required to be multiskilled. For example, if the sole practitioner with a sports team travelling overseas to a competition is a sports physician, it would be useful for that individual to be familiar with basic soft tissue techniques. Furthermore, physical therapists should be familiar with methods of creating orthotics for use with athletes when an orthotist is not available.

Traditionally, medical models have been biased towards a medical practitioner as the primary contact practitioner (Brukner & Khan 2001). The sports medicine model is based on a number of people as the possible primary contact practitioner (e.g. medical practitioner, physical therapist, podiatrist). This means that each member of the team should have a high-level of understanding of the role of other team members so that referral can be instigated where necessary, and so that collaborative treatment can be implemented.

An integral link in the modern day sports medicine team is the coach. Given that coaches are usually the individuals with the highest level of contact with the athlete, they form a vital link between the physical therapist and athlete. Coaches can be involved in the decision making process regarding time away from sport and return to activity. Also, they can play an important role in deciding on alternative activities that athletes can perform when restricted from sport-specific skills.

INJURY IN SPORT, EXERCISE, AND PHYSICAL ACTIVITY

Participation rates in sport and recreational activities have grown in recent times, giving rise to increased injury rates that have been described as a public health issue (Caine et al 1996). This increased participation is not surprising given the evidence of the physical (e.g. Malina 1994) and psychological (e.g. McAuley 1994) benefits of exercise. The costs involved in rehabilitation of people with such injuries, the loss of sport and work participation time, the risk of long-term injury, and the consequent reduced quality of life, are all major public health problems.

Sport and exercise injury rates vary from country to country. For example, in the UK, sport and exercise-related injuries accounted for 33% of all injuries reported in a population survey (Uitenbroek 1996). In the USA, of the estimated 17 million annual sport and recreation injuries, almost 2 million require hospital emergency room consultations (NEISS data highlights 1998).

Several aspects of participation can contribute to the incidence and severity of injury in sport. These include the nature of the activity, and the gender, age, and physical condition of the participant. Although most injuries in sport and exercise involve the musculoskeletal system, many other systems of the body can be involved (e.g. cardiorespiratory, neurological, etc.) In general, sport and exercise injury can be defined as any injury that is sports or physical activity related and results in keeping the individual out of practice, activity, or competition, or requires the individual to seek medical attention (Noyes et al 1988).

One of the contributing factors to the increasing number of injuries in sport is the changing sport and exercise population. That sport and exercise have been promoted as healthy activities means that a larger number of older people are participating in increased amounts of physical activity. Also, children and adolescents are participating in greater amounts of sport at younger ages (see Mafulli & Bruns 2001).

THE NEED FOR AN EVIDENCE BASE IN THE PHYSICAL THERAPIES

Optimal medical practice involves rational interpretation of research evidence and application of such evidence to clinical settings (Hart 2000). Physical therapy is an area that, until recently, was based on a small and often flawed body of research. We often rely on the journals that publish research to guide our clinical practice. We should be aware, however, that despite the best efforts, flawed research still sometimes appears in mainstream journals (Altman 1994). Evidence-based medicine (EBM) has been described as the conscientious, explicit, and judicious use of current best evidence in making decisions about the care of individual patients (Hart 2000). Several authors have written extensively on EBM (e.g. Sackett 1992, Sackett et al 1996, Sackett et al 1997). In sports medicine, the combination of clinical expertise and the best available evidence from systematic research can assist the practitioner in ensuring the most efficacious approach to patient management. The chapters of this book have, where possible, reported techniques and approaches to injury management that are supported by appropriate evidence. It is clear, however, that there are still several areas of the physical therapies in sport and exercise that lack sufficient evidence.

To address the dearth of evidence for clinical techniques in physical therapy, the American Physical Therapy Association developed a Clinical Research Agenda (Guccione et al 2000). The Clinical Research Agenda was developed to help guide the systematic progression of the scientific basis of the physical therapy profession. Many of the 72 research questions in the agenda can be related to the physical therapies as they apply to sport, exercise, and physical activity. Examples of research questions identified as important in the Clinical Research Agenda include:

- What are the reliability and validity of assessment and pronation of the foot in patients with knee pain?
- How can patient characteristics and environmental factors be used to predict adherence to home programs?
- What are the factors that motivate patients to adhere to a plan of care?
- Does immediate postoperative physical therapy intervention affect the rate of recovery of function in patients following orthopedic surgery, and, if so, how?

- What is the relative effectiveness of immobilization versus mobilization in patients with musculoskeletal impairments on tissue healing and recovery of function?
- What is the effect of various intensities and durations of interventions on the rate and degree of functional recovery after anterior cruciate ligament injury?

It is efforts like the Clinical Research Agenda that can help prioritize and guide research that will benefit the sports physical therapy profession.

A WALK THROUGH *PHYSICAL THERAPIES IN SPORT AND EXERCISE*

Sports physical therapy does not have a unitary model, and thus we have assembled a group of researchers and practitioners who represent the diversity of approaches in working with sport and exercise to contribute chapters to this book. The authors come from physical therapy, psychology, sports medicine, athletic training, orthopedic surgery, pediatrics, radiology, biomechanics, and nursing, and represent countries as diverse as the USA, Australia, New Zealand, Canada, Hong Kong, the UK, Finland, and Sweden. As previously mentioned, the chapters of this book have, where possible, reported techniques and approaches to injury management that are supported by appropriate evidence.

This book is divided into five sections:

Section 1: Management Principles for Musculoskeletal Tissue in the Physical Therapies. This section deals with five groups of body tissue: Muscle (Ch. 2), Tendon (Ch. 3), Ligament (Ch. 4), Bone (Ch. 5), and Nerves (Ch. 6). These chapters provide coverage of the basic structure and biomechanics of the tissues, the principles relating to the adaptation of the tissue to mechanical load, and the response of the tissue to injury and healing.

Section 2: Concepts in Managing Sport and Exercise Injuries. The chapters in this section provide general information that is important in the management of injuries from the various regions of the body. Chapter 7, Motor Control, covers the theory and application of motor control and motor relearning in the management of sport and exercise related injury. Chapter 8, Pain, outlines the mechanisms and theories of pain perception, and presents strategies to assess and manage pain from both a physical and cognitive-behavioral perspective. Chapter 9, Exercise-based Conditioning and Rehabilitation, outlines the evidence for the use of various forms of exercise in injury prevention and management. Chapter 10, Psychology of Injury and Rehabilitation, works through the psychological factors that affect the onset and rehabilitation of injury. Also, issues related to rehabilitation adherence and the role of physical therapists in applying basic cognitive-behavioral techniques are covered. Chapter 11, Screening for Sport and Exercise Participation, focuses on the principles and practical application of screening procedures that are used for sport and exercise participation. Issues related to general health, and sport-specific health and fitness are addressed. Chapter 12, Outcome Measures in Sport and Exercise Physical Therapies, covers a range of outcome measures that can be used in the sport and exercise physical therapies. This addresses both clinical measures and condition-specific functional measures. Chapter 13, Electrophysical Agents in Sport and Exercise Injury Management, evaluates, from a scientific perspective, various electrophysical agents commonly used by sport physical therapists. The emphasis is on outlining the evidence to support or refute the role of such modalities in sports medicine.

Section 3: Regional Sport and Exercise Injury Management. The 10 chapters in this section deal with the Spine (Ch. 14), Shoulder (Ch. 15), Elbow (Ch. 16), Wrist and Hand (Ch. 17), Pelvis, Hip, and Groin (Ch. 18), Thigh (Ch. 19), Knee (Ch. 20), Patellofemoral Joint (Ch. 21), Leg (Ch. 22), and Foot and Ankle (Ch. 23). In each of these chapters the content focuses on sport-specific applied anatomy, examination, and the management of common and less common sport and exercise related injuries to the region.

Section 4: The Role of Sport and Exercise Physical Therapies in Active Groups. Four groups of people are covered in this section: children and adolescents, older exercise participants, active females, and athletes with disability. Chapter 24, Children and Adolescents, outlines the assessment and management of conditions specific to this age group. In particular, injuries and conditions specific to the immature musculoskeletal system are highlighted. Chapter 25, Older Exercise Participants, focuses on the assessment and management of conditions specific to older people involved in sport and exercise. In particular, the impact of aging on the systems of the body is addressed, as well as the benefits that can be gained from participation in sport and exercise and guidelines for exercise participation. Chapter 26, The Active Female, focuses on conditions specific to women involved in sport and exercise. In particular, issues related to bone health are covered, as are the anatomical and physiological considerations for women. Other areas included are the menstrual cycle and performance, the female athlete triad, and exercise during pregnancy. Chapter 27, Athletes with Disability, presents information on the benefits of exercise and sport for people with disability, classification of athletes with disability, and injury management and assessment for a variety of disability groups in sport.

Section 5: Medical Considerations for Rehabilitation Practitioners in Sport and Exercise Settings. Section 5 has three chapters dealing with a variety of medical considerations for physical therapists working in sport and exercise. Chapter 28, Pharmacological Agents in Sport and Exercise, deals with therapeutic pharmacological agents and the impact they have on injury repair, exercise participation, and physical therapies management. The chapter also covers the effects of performance enhancing drugs on athlete health and well-being, and the International Olympic Committee Anti-Doping Code. Chapter 29, Medical Imaging of Injury, provides those working in the physical therapies with an understanding of the various imaging modalities used in diagnosing sport and exercise related injuries. Chapter 30, Medical Issues in Sport and Exercise, overviews common medical emergencies in sport and exercise including head injuries, cardiovascular conditions, and conditions related to environmental influences. The specific aim of this chapter is to outline the role of physical therapists in recognizing and providing first-aid management to athletes with medical conditions.

SUMMARY

Despite the many existing books that deal with sports physical therapy, the aim of this text is to provide a logical approach to the management of sport and exercise injuries that considers the available evidence for the efficacy of a variety of management approaches.

REFERENCES

Altman D G 1994 The scandal of poor medical research. British Medical Journal 308:283–284
Brukner P, Khan K 2001 Clinical sports medicine, 2nd edn. McGraw Hill, Sydney
Caine D J, Caine C G, Lindner K J 1996 Epidemiology of sports injuries. Human Kinetics, Champaign, IL
Guccione A A, Va A, Goldstein M, Elliott S 2000 Clinical research agenda for physical therapy. Physical Therapy 80:499–513
Hart L E 2000 Evidence-based sports medicine. In: Kumbhare D A, Basmajian J V (eds) Decision making and outcomes in sports rehabilitation. Churchill Livingstone, Edinburgh
Maffulli N, Bruns W 2001 Training and injuries in young athletes. In: Maffulli N, Chan K M, Macdonald R, et al (eds) Sports medicine for specific ages and abilities. Churchill Livingstone, Edinburgh
Malina R M 1994 Benefits of physical activity from a lifetime perspective. In: Quinney H A, Gauvin L, Wall A E T (eds) Toward active living: Proceedings of the International Conference on Physical, Activity, Fitness, and Health. Human Kinetics, Champaign, IL, p 47–53
McAuley E 1994 Enhancing psychological health through physical activity. In: Quinney H A, Gauvin L, Wall A E T (eds) Toward active living: Proceedings of the International Conference on Physical Activity, Fitness, and Health. Human Kinetics, Champaign, IL, p 83–90
Matheson G O, Pipe A L 1996 Twenty-five years of sports medicine in Canada: Thoughts on the road ahead. Clinical Journal of Sports Medicine 6:148–151
NEISS data highlights 1998 Consumer Product Safety Review 3(1):4–6
Noyes F E, Lindenfeld T N, Marshall M T 1988 What determines an athletic injury (definition)? Who determines an injury (occurrence)? American Journal of Sports Medicine 16 (1, suppl):65–68
Sackett D L 1992 Evidence-based medicine: A new approach to teaching the practice of medicine. Journal of the American Medical Association 268:2420–2425
Sackett D L, Rosenberg W M, Gray J A et al 1996 Evidence based medicine: What it is and what it isn't. British Medical Journal 312:71–72
Sackett D L, Richardson W S, Rosenberg W et al 1997 Evidence-based medicine. Churchill Livingstone, New York
Uitenbroek D G 1996 Sports, exercise, and other causes of injuries: Results of a population survey. Research Quarterly for Exercise and Sport 67:380–385

Management principles for musculoskeletal tissue in the physical therapies

2

Muscle

Peter J McNair   Andrew Creswell

INTRODUCTION

There are three types of muscle tissue within the body – skeletal muscle (striated voluntary), cardiac muscle (striated involuntary), and visceral (non-striated involuntary or smooth). This chapter will focus on skeletal muscle. Skeletal muscles develop force through contraction, which gives us the possibility of movement and interaction with our surroundings. In many pathological conditions muscle has been affected, either directly through injury or disease, or indirectly as a result of immobilization regimens. For the physical therapist to rehabilitate patients efficaciously, an understanding of muscle function is important. This chapter provides a foundation on which effective muscle training programs might be built. Its purpose is to examine the structure of muscle, its biomechanical characteristics, and how those characteristics influence its function. This chapter will focus on the factors that influence the force generation capacity of muscle. It will also describe the changes that occur when muscle is in states of injury and disuse. Although the focus is predominantly on muscle structure, we recognize the importance of neural activation in generating force. This area, however, is beyond the scope of this chapter (see Ch. 6).

GROSS STRUCTURE OF MUSCLE

FIBER STRUCTURE

To the naked eye, skeletal muscle is primarily made up of fibers. These fibers are grouped into bundles of approximately 10 to 20 fibers, each of which is called a fascicle. Each fascicle is surrounded by connective tissue (perimysium) that separates it from its neighboring fascicles. Muscle is built up from many such fascicles and is enclosed in a further thicker layer of connective tissue, the epimysium. Collagen fibers in all the layers of connective tissue are connected to the tendons at the end of the muscle. In this way, every individual muscle fiber is connected to the tendon and any force development from a muscle fiber will be exerted on the tendon.

At a microscopic level, each muscle fiber contains thousands of smaller units (myofibrils) which are responsible for contraction of the muscle (Fig. 2.1). A myofibril has a diameter of approximately 1 μm and is comprised of light and dark bands (striations) when viewed under a light microscope (Hess 1967). The striations result from the myofibrils comprising two types of filaments (proteins): a thicker and darker, highly refractory A-band representing the myosin filament (with a diameter of approximately 11 nm), and a thinner

(7 nm) lighter and less refractory I-band representing the actin filament (Huxley 1972). Both the myosin and actin filaments represent the smallest functional unit of the muscle. The myosin filaments are located centrally within a sarcomere and are held together at the M-region. The actin filaments make connections to the Z-disks, the boundary units between sarcomeres, where they receive partial structural support.

Close observation of the thicker myosin filament reveals that it has a head and tail configuration. The tail comprises two heavy molecular chains that are wound around each other. At one end of this chain are two globular heads. Attached to the myosin heads are two shorter and lighter amino acid chains. The function of these light chains is to partially stabilize the myosin head and partly to modulate the interaction of actin and myosin (McComas 1996).

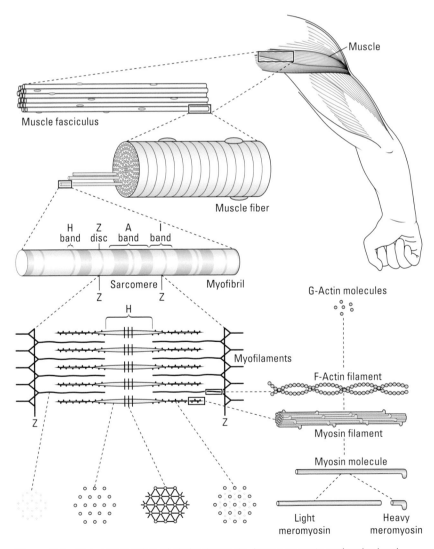

Figure 2.1　The organization of skeletal muscle, from a gross to molecular level. (Reproduced with permission from Guyton & Hall 2000.)

Actin is a globular protein that comprises approximately 300–400 actin molecules bound together in a chain approximately 1 µm long. Two such chains are twisted together to form a double-helical thin filament. Two other proteins, troponin and tropomyosin, are associated with the actin filament. Two strands of tropomyosin lie along the length of the actin filament, stiffening it. Troponin is a complex polypeptide and attaches to tropomyosin. One of the polypeptides, troponin T, attaches to tropomyosin, while troponin I binds to actin and indirectly prevents interaction with the myosin filament (Figs 2.2 and 2.3).

The sarcomere contains additional proteins other than actin and myosin to help organize the structure of the sarcomere. Proteins such as vimentin, desmin, and synemin develop myofibril stability while integrin may help connect myofibrils to surrounding connective tissues. The protein nebulin appears to maintain the lattice array of actin (Labeit et al 1991), while titin, one of the largest proteins, is seen as thin strands connecting the myosin

filament to the Z-disk (Trinick 1991). These strands are approximately 1 µm in length and are considered to be a longitudinal stabilizer for the myosin filament by keeping it centered within the sarcomere. They appear to additionally provide a degree of elasticity to the sarcomere when undergoing stretch, and also function as a template for the growth of the myosin filament.

FIBER TYPES

Not all muscle fibers look alike; some fibers appear redder than others. A deep red color comes mostly from a denser network of capillaries leading to an increased amount of myoglobin, a red pigment with oxygen binding capability. Using histological methods such as enzyme histochemistry, it can be seen that the redder fibers contain higher amounts of oxidative enzymes and mitochondria. Such fibers are termed type I fibers, and they have greater aerobic capacity. There is a gradual change of color to paler whiter fibers that are larger in diameter, have fewer mitochondria and oxidative enzymes, but greater amounts of glycolitic enzymes. These paler fibers are known as type II fibers and have a greater anaerobic capacity. Certain muscles have large percentages of type I or II fibers, for example, soleus or triceps brachii respectively, while most are generally more mixed in their composition.

The so-called 'speed' or rate of shortening of each fiber type is also different. The rate of shortening is dependent on the characteristics of the myosin (i.e. how quickly adenosine triphosphate [ATP] is broken down by the head of the myosin molecule, and how fast each cross-bridge cycle can be performed). In general, type I fibers are constituted of slow myosin and are often referred to as slow-twitch fibers, while type II fibers are made up of faster myosin and are called fast-twitch fibers. Fiber classification based on histochemical methods (i.e. typically staining for the enzymes myosin adenosine triphosphatase [ATPase], phosphorylase, succinate dehydrogenase, and malate) has determined that further classification of the type II fibers is possible: type IIA, type IIB (Gollnick et al 1972, Johnson et al 1973, Thorstensson 1976) and type IIC (Billeter et al 1980) are apparent. The difference between the type IIA and B fibers is related to their relative aerobic ability, with type IIA having greater aerobic potential. The IIC fibers are considered to have the foundation to form either type IIA or IIB fibers. More recently, the technique of immunocytochemistry has been able to identify an additional fiber type based on the properties of myosin heavy chain isoforms (Larsson et al 1991). This newly identified type IIX lies between IIA and IIB (Schiaffino & Reggiani 1994, Smerdu et al 1994), and it seems likely that in human skeletal muscle, the earlier classified type IIB fibers are actually of the type IIX.

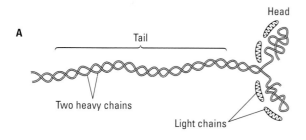

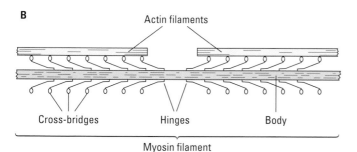

Figure 2.2A & B **A:** Myosin molecule. **B:** Many myosin molecules and their relationship to the actin filaments. (Reproduced with permission from Guyton & Hall 2000.)

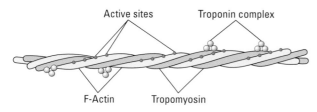

Figure 2.3   Actin filament, composed of two helical strands, together with troponin and tropomyosin. Attached to one end of each tropomyosin molecule is a troponin complex that initiates contraction. (Reproduced with permission from Guyton & Hall 2000.)

In general, the slow type I fibers are used continuously in the maintenance of posture while the faster type II fibers are used more intermittently for force development. When the force twitch of these fibers is recorded, and the interval between the onset of the twitch and the peak force is measured, the faster fiber types can have contraction times as low as 20 ms, while the slower fibers have times as protracted as 140 ms. In whole muscle, however, the muscle twitch depends on the fiber type proportions of the muscle. For example, the triceps surae has a high percentage of slow twitch fibers (approximately 80%, Gollnick et al 1974), and has a contraction time of approximately 120 ms (Sale et al 1982), while the biceps brachii has a higher percentage of fast twitch fibers (approximately 62%, Johnson et al 1973, Nygaard et al 1983) which results in a contraction time of only 65 ms (Bellemare et al 1983).

THE CONTRACTILE PROCESS

Force is generated in a muscle fiber when actin and myosin filaments interact. This event commences with action potentials spreading across the muscle fibers at approximately 3–5 m·s^{-1}. The potentials also spread deep within the fibers by way of the T-tubules (Peachey 1965a, Peachey 1965b), which have close contact with the terminal cisternae of the sarcoplasmic reticulum. The gap between these two structures is bridged by two proteins – a dihydropyridine (DHP) receptor and a ryanodin receptor (RYR). During rest, the ryanodin receptor channels are closed and Ca^{2+} remains within the sarcoplasmic reticulum. Depolarization of the T-tubules results in activation of the DHP receptors which in turn causes the RYR to open its Ca^{2+} channel and rapidly

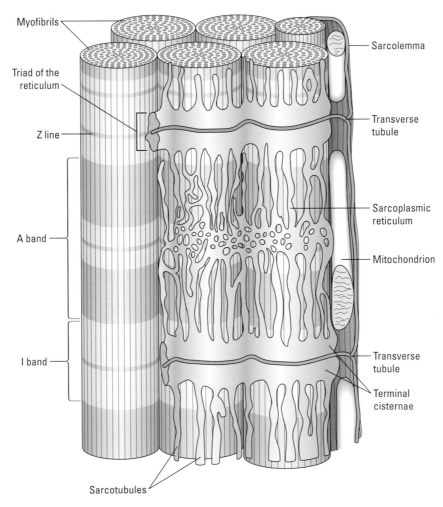

Figure 2.4 The transverse (T) tubule–sarcoplasmic reticulum system. This illustration was drawn from frog muscle, which has one T-tubule per sarcomere, located at the z-line. Mammalian skeletal muscle has two T-tubules per sarcomere, located at the A-I junction. (Reproduced with permission from Guyton & Hall 2000.)

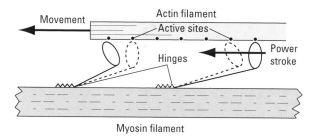

Figure 2.5 Cross-bridge formation and motion. (Reproduced with permission from Guyton & Hall 2000.)

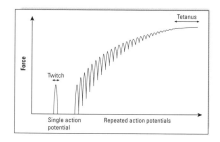

Figure 2.6 Force change associated with a single action potential, and the effect of repeated action potentials.

release Ca^{2+} along its concentration gradient out from the sarcoplasmic reticulum, thereby increasing cytostolic Ca^{2+} (Peachey 1965a, Peachey 1965b).

Figure 2.4 shows the transverse tubule–sarcoplasmic reticulum system. At rest, the binding sites for myosin on the actin filament are covered. However, with the release of Ca^{2+}, troponin undergoes a conformational change. This change lifts the tropomyosin molecule away from the actin filament and exposes sites on the actin filament for myosin head attachment, and allows the contraction to commence. Pumps in the sarcoplasmic reticulum continuously pump Ca^{2+} back into the sarcoplasmic reticulum. At rest, this event results in the concentration of Ca^{2+} in the sarcoplasmic reticulum being higher than that in the cytosol. When neural activation of a muscle ceases, Ca^{2+} is released from troponin and quickly pumped out of the cytosol. Tropomyosin then returns to its original position on actin and prevents any further binding of myosin to actin. Since the pump has to transport Ca^{2+} against its concentration gradient, adenosine triphosphate (ATP) is required to provide the necessary energy.

The force development is a result of the myosin heads, also called cross-bridges, bending while attached to the actin filament (Huxley & Simmons 1971, Narici 1999). After the cross-bridges have bent, they are released from actin, straighten, and then re-attach to a new actin site (Fig. 2.5). These events are termed cross-bridge cycling, and form the basis of the sliding filament theory (Huxley 1957, Huxley & Hanson 1954, Huxley & Simmons 1971). For their occurrence, energy is needed, and this is obtained by the splitting of ATP to adenosine diphosphate (ADP) and inorganic phosphate (P).

A single action potential that spreads over the fiber gives rise to a momentary increase in force that is called a muscle twitch (Huijing 1998). If rapidly repeated action potentials travel across the muscle fiber, Ca^{2+} cannot be pumped back into the sarcoplasmic reticulum before the next action potential arrives and the next release of Ca^{2+} takes place. This results in repeated cross-bridge cycling and a rapid summation of individual force twitches. If the action potentials arrive with a short inter-potential interval, individual twitches cannot be discerned from the force trace and the muscle is said to have reached tetanus. A muscle fiber generates its maximal force during tetanus (Fig. 2.6).

FACTORS INFLUENCING MAXIMUM FORCE GENERATION IN A MUSCLE

IN VITRO AND IN VIVO MEASUREMENTS OF MUSCLE FORCE

In vitro recordings of maximal forces can readily be gathered from either single muscle fibers or single muscles activated by electrical stimulation. It is difficult to study force development of single muscles in humans, primarily due to: tetanic stimulation of muscle being extremely painful to the subject, the spread of current to nearby muscles being difficult to control, and if the subject is operating the intensity control, it is not certain whether complete activation of the muscle has taken place (Herbert & Gandevia 1999, Westing et al 1990). Furthermore, it is not currently possible in humans to directly measure the force developed by the muscle. Methods for measurement of muscle forces have been developed for animal preparations, with buckle-type force transducers being used by several research groups (Gregor et al 1988, Walmsley et al 1978, Whiting et al 1984). This type of transducer is placed around the tendon of a freely moving animal, and gives a signal that is proportional to the muscular force. A similar type of buckle transducer has also been implanted with some success around the Achilles tendon in humans (Fukashiro et al 1995, Gregor et al 1991, Walmsley et al 1978), however, the transducer output gives Achilles tendon force and not the forces of the individual muscles of the triceps surae. Moreover, the difficulty of transducer calibration and discomfort to the subject have limited their extended use.

Less invasive measurements of muscle force usually involve voluntary muscle activation and the use of a load

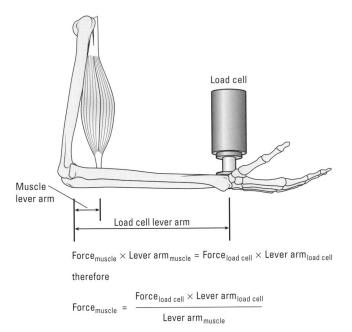

$$Force_{muscle} \times Lever\ arm_{muscle} = Force_{load\ cell} \times Lever\ arm_{load\ cell}$$

therefore

$$Force_{muscle} = \frac{Force_{load\ cell} \times Lever\ arm_{load\ cell}}{Lever\ arm_{muscle}}$$

Figure 2.7   The lever arms and forces associated with the calculation of torques.

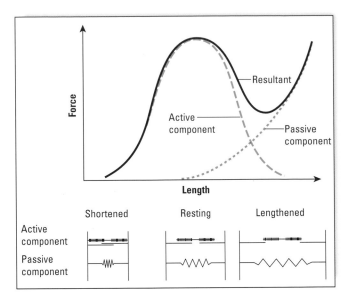

Figure 2.8   The force–length relationship, and the interaction of the contractile and passive elements.

cell or dynamometer. For their calculation, knowledge of two lever arm distances is also needed. The first is the lever arm between the force transducer and the center of rotation of the joint, and the second is the lever arm between the center of rotation of the joint and line of action of the muscle force (Fig. 2.7). These distances are particularly difficult to ascertain when the center of rotation of a joint shifts as the joint rotates through its range of motion. Traditionally, such measures have been obtained from cadavers (Spoor et al 1990), however, the recent use of magnetic resonance imaging (MRI) and ultrasonography has allowed more accurate and straight-forward estimation of in vivo joint-muscle lever arm lengths for the elbow (Fukunaga et al 2001), rotator cuff (Juul-Kristensen et al 2000a, Juul-Kristensen et al 2000b), spine (Tveit et al 1994), knee (Narici et al 1988, Spoor & van Leeuwen 1992), and ankle (Fukunaga et al 1996) joints.

The calculations presented in Figure 2.7 apply to muscle actions that are isometric. To measure muscle forces when a joint is in motion, knowledge of the moment of inertia of the moving limb and the angular acceleration of the joint is required. The moment of inertia is usually obtained from tables based on measurements taken on cadaveric specimens. Angular acceleration is usually acquired from recording the motion of interest with an electrogoniometer or by video.

FORCE–LENGTH RELATIONSHIP

The amount of force a muscle fiber can develop during maximal activation is dependent on the number of

established cross-bridges. This, in turn, means that the force that can be developed is dependent on the length of the muscle (Gordon et al 1966, Rack & Westbury 1969). During maximal activation, the greatest force development occurs with the muscle at its resting length (a sarcomere length of approximately 2.2 μm). At shorter lengths, the thin actin filaments begin to interfere with each other due to their overlap, cross-bridge formation is hindered, and force development is reduced. As the sarcomere becomes even shorter (below approximately 1.7 μm), the decrease in force is thought to be related to the forces that are required to deform the thicker myofilament. However, reduced Ca^{2+} release from the sarcoplasmic reticulum at shorter than optimal lengths (Rudel & Taylor 1971) may also be a contributing factor to the force reduction. At lengths above 2.2 μm, fewer binding sites are available for the myosin heads. This results in a reduction in active force production. To counter this loss of force, the stretch of passive tissues within the muscle (epimysium, perimysium, endomysium, titin, and nebulin) and tendon increases the passive force and hence total force is less affected (Fig. 2.8). The amount of force development by the passive tissues varies between muscles in accordance with differences in architecture and the amount of connective tissue (Woittiez et al 1983).

FORCE–VELOCITY RELATIONSHIP

A muscle can actively shorten if an external load generates less force than that being produced internally (often termed a concentric muscle action). The velocity of muscle shortening and its relationship to force development is well documented (Fenn & Marsh 1935, Hill 1938), with higher forces being generated at slower shortening velocities. As shortening velocity increases, the rate of cross-bridge cycling increases, the average force exerted by each cross-bridge decreases, and there may even be fewer cross-bridges attached. If a muscle is not working against a load, then it can reach maximal shortening velocities in the order of 10 muscle-lengths·s^{-1} (Edman 1979). Most muscles, however, have distinctly slower maximum shortening velocities, but are surprisingly constant over a large range of sarcomere lengths (Edman 1979).

If the force generated by an external load is greater than the force being produced internally, the muscle undergoes active lengthening (often termed an eccentric muscle action). Depending on the experimental techniques used, the maximal force recorded for a lengthening muscle action can be similar to or greater than that recorded for an isometric muscle activation. For isolated muscle preparations (in vitro), the force developed during lengthening increases rapidly above its isometric value, and at fast lengthening velocities can reach 1.8 times that developed isometrically (Abbott & Aubert 1951, Katz 1939). This large increase is probably due to the rate of cross-bridge detachment being slower than during lengthening actions at the same velocity. This would result in the cross-bridges remaining attached and being forcibly stretched until detachment finally takes place. Stretching beyond the normal range of cross-bridge attachment thereby results in utilization of elasticity within the cross-bridge and thus increased force development (Abbott & Aubert 1951, Edman 1979).

The advent of the isokinetic dynamometer has enabled the experimenter to record the net joint torque while moving the limb through a prescribed range of motion at a specified angular velocity. The in vivo relationship between muscle force and linear velocity of muscle shortening or lengthening is then inferred from the measurement of angle specific or peak joint torques recorded at various angular velocities. Several studies on the force–velocity relationship have been made in humans for the knee extensors (Harris & Dudley 1994, Perrine & Edgerton 1978, Thorstensson et al 1976, Westing et al 1988), elbow flexors (Hortobagyi & Katch 1990, Komi 1973, Pousson et al 1999), and plantar flexor muscles (Fugl-Meyer et al 1980, Gerdle & Langstrom 1987, Pinniger et al 2000).

Most data for shortening muscle action appears similar to that of isolated muscle. However, compared to isolated muscle, in vivo force measurements appear to plateau and be slightly lower as the velocity approaches zero (Perrine & Edgerton 1978). Isometric torques are, however, most often greater than the torques recorded during shortening muscle actions. During in vivo lengthening muscle action, the maximum joint torque generally fails

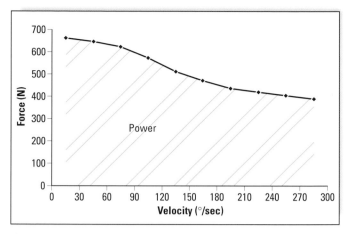

Figure 2.9 The force–velocity relationship.

to increase above the isometric value, regardless of lengthening velocity (Aagaard et al 1995, Dudley et al 1990, Westing et al 1991). However, there does appear to be some slight differences between muscle groups, and the level of training of the subjects under investigation (Aagaard et al 1996, Dudley et al 1990). For example, subjects who have been provided with practice sessions will often be able to generate higher forces. Thus, the inability to exceed forces produced isometrically, regardless of the angular velocity, may reflect a neural inhibitory process that limits voluntary torque production (Westing et al 1991, Westing et al 1990). Some support for this idea comes from comparing levels of voluntary muscle activation across velocities during lengthening, shortening, and isometric actions (Aagaard et al 2000, Westing et al 1991), as well as from data collected during in vivo torque measurements produced via percutaneous electrical stimulation (Dudley et al 1990, Westing et al 1991).

The power that a muscle can generate (the rate at which it can produce work) can be deduced from the force–velocity relationship (Hill 1938). Power can be measured as the product of force and velocity, and can be viewed as the area under the force–velocity curve (Fig. 2.9). It is zero when the muscle action is isometric, and when the muscle is not working against a load. Generally, it has been observed that maximum power is developed at velocities corresponding to 30–40% of the maximal shortening velocity of the muscle. This can readily be identified in cycling where changing gears results in load changes that allow the muscle to continuously work at its optimal shortening velocity (Sargeant et al 1981).

MUSCLE ARCHITECTURE

Muscle architecture cannot be overlooked when considering the maximal force that a muscle might generate.

The most commonly measured architectural features of muscle are related to volume, fiber length, and pennation angle. Until recently, such measurements have been difficult, or impossible to gather for living human muscle, and cadaver material has provided much of the available information (Wickiewicz et al 1983). The advent of MRI, and in particular ultrasound equipment, has now allowed in vivo measurements of muscle fiber architecture not only during rest, but also during active, isometric, shortening and lengthening muscle actions (Herbert & Gandevia 1995, Narici 1999, Rutherford & Jones 1992). Studies that have used such equipment have shown that pennation angle and fiber length, and thus physiological cross-sectional area, are dependent on joint position and the level of muscle activation (Herbert & Gandevia 1995). For example, for the medial gastrocnemius, pennation angle and fiber length decrease as the ankle joint angle increases, thereby resulting in an increase of the physiological cross-sectional area (Narici et al 1996). Increased voluntary activation of the medial gastrocnemius resulted in a 35% decrease in fiber length, and a 100% increase in pennation angle resulting in a 35% increase in physiological cross-sectional area (Narici et al 1996). Such findings cast some doubt on the calculations of cross-sectional area, and thus force potential that have previously been calculated using data gained from cadavers.

The theoretical force potential of a muscle can be calculated if the maximum force that can be generated per unit of cross-sectional area and the cross-sectional area of the muscle is known. The former variable appears to be at best 40 $N\cdot cm^{-2}$. However, this value, depending on the study, varies between 15 to 40 $N\cdot cm^{-2}$ (Edgerton et al 1990, Kanda & Hashizume 1992, Nygaard et al 1983). The wide range in these values may be attributed to differences in gender and muscle architecture. It is also evident that the maximum force per unit area is not dependent on muscle fiber type (Bottinelli et al 1996, Herbert & Gandevia 1995). Thus, the amount of total force produced by a muscle is directly related to its cross-sectional area. Although there are differences in the diameters of fibers within a muscle, the largest contributor to the different forces produced by different muscles is the absolute number of muscle fibers. Such numbers can range from approximately 4.0×10^4 for the first dorsal interossei to 1.0×10^6 for the medial gastrocnemius (Feinstein et al 1955).

The physiological cross-sectional area of muscle can be calculated with a knowledge of the mass and density $(1.056g/cm^3)$ of the muscle together with information related to fiber length. Mass and density are determinants of the muscle's volume, which are reflected in the different shapes of muscles in the body. The diversity in shape of each muscle often results in the line of pull of

individual fibers being quite different, and this can influence their force capability. Generally speaking, muscles are grouped according to the orientation of their fasciculi. These fasciculi are most often arranged either parallel or oblique to the final direction of pull at their insertion. Some muscles (e.g. sartorius) have fibers primarily parallel to the line of pull. Others (e.g. biceps brachii) can also have a similar arrangement in the belly of a fusiform muscle and the fibers converge to a tendon at either one or both ends of the muscle. Such muscles have longer muscle fibers and hence will have greater displacement potential, and are more effective at changing length quickly.

The length of a muscle fiber is determined by the number of sarcomeres in series. There are quite large differences in the number of sarcomeres per fiber, with long strap muscles like sartorius, which adducts and flexes the leg, having approximately 15.5×10^4 sarcomeres per fiber, while the shorter plantar flexors, soleus and medial gastrocnemius, have approximately 1.4×10^4 and 1.5×10^4 sarcomeres per fiber, respectively (Wickiewicz et al 1983). These numbers are often based on the premise that individual fibers run the full length of the muscle. However, in a number of instances, this is not the case. For example, several of the longer strap muscles (e.g. rectus abdominis) have discrete compartments, defined by fibrous bands. These compartments result in significantly shorter muscle fiber lengths with sarcomere numbers in the region of 5.5×10^4 (Chleboun et al 2001, McComas 1996). Such compartmentalization is likely to make force transmission throughout the muscle more complicated than if fibers extend the entire length of the muscle.

A limitation of muscles with longer muscle fibers is that they are less effective at generating force. The potential to generate force will be proportional to the number of sarcomeres in parallel. Fasciculi that are oblique to the line of pull are often described as being pennate (feather-like). Pennate muscles (e.g. gastrocnemius) typically have a long tendon running through the muscle to which short muscle fibers are attached at angles that generally range from 5 to 20°. The fiber organization of a pennate muscle ensures a relatively large physiological cross-sectional area since there can be many more fibers packed within the muscle. A larger cross-sectional area results in an increase in force potential even though the force contribution of each fiber is reduced due to its angle of pull. Pennate muscle fibers have significantly fewer sarcomeres in series than parallel fibered muscle. Therefore, for the same decrease in fiber length, the relative shortening per sarcomere length will be greater for a short fiber (Narici 1999). The muscle is therefore less suited to situations that demand long length changes or high velocity length changes.

STRUCTURES THAT INFLUENCE THE ELASTICITY OF MUSCLE

The connective tissues of muscle can be divided into three structures that are based on their position within muscle. Epimysium envelops the entire muscle, while perimysium surrounds bundles of muscle fibers, and endomysium provides a cover for the basement membrane of individual muscle fibers. Endomysium and perimysium are linked to one another, and these tissues are thought to provide a framework on which the muscle fibers attach and gain support. When muscle is stretched, it is thought that endomysium and perimysium are largely responsible for the passive tension generated in muscle at high sarcomere lengths. Purslow (1989) and Purslow & Trotter (1994) examined the morphology and mechanical properties of both endomysial and perimysial tissues. They noted that at resting muscle lengths the endomysial network was composed of wavy collagen fibrils arranged with a mean orientation to the muscle fibers of 60°. Perimysium was more organized with a cross-ply structural arrangement of crimped collagen fibers at a similar angle. Tensile stiffness was minimal at the resting length in both endomysial and perimysial tissues. When the muscle fibers were stretched to high sarcomere lengths, the angle of the collagen fibers to the muscle fibers in both endomysium and perimysium decreased, and the respective wavy and crimped appearance of these tissues was lost. Thus at high sarcomere lengths, Purslow (1989) and Purslow & Trotter (1994) suggested that both endomysium and perimysium may prevent overstretching of muscle.

It is also apparent that the contractile elements have elastic properties. Short-range stiffness is a term used to describe the ratio of change in force to change in length of the muscle fibers when stretched. When muscle fibers are activated, short-range stiffness is noted until fibers are stretched past approximately 1% of muscle length (Malamud et al 1996). Thereafter, a yielding of the fibers is noted and resistance in the tissues decreases. It has been shown that the short-range stiffness increases with muscle activation levels, and hence has been related to the number of cross-bridges formed between actin and myosin at the time of a rapid stretch (Ford et al 1981). It is has also been shown that type I muscle fibers are stiffer than type II fibers (Malamud et al 1996), and these findings have been related to the time course of the detachment and reattachment of cross-bridges.

Research (Huxley et al 1994) involving X-ray techniques has shown that elasticity lies within the myofilaments, and particularly within a protein named connectin (also termed titin) (Horowits et al 1986). Biochemical techniques have shown that individual filaments of connectin are attached from the z-line to the central region of the thick filament. Between the z-line and the myosin filament, the connectin is most elastic, whereas the section of connectin that is bound to the myosin filament is considerably less so (Higuchi 1996). Horowits (1992) has shown that much of the resting tension in sarcomeres is due to connectin, and that, at long sarcomere lengths, connectin becomes considerably more resistant to stretch. Connectin's role is also to center the thick myosin filament within the sarcomere, that is, prevent myosin from moving toward either z-line (Horowits et al 1986). This is particularly important when actin and myosin are interacting to generate force. In doing so, connectin will also keep sarcomere length relatively constant across the length of the muscle fiber during muscle activation.

INJURY AND DISUSE

It is apparent that when muscle is injured, the damage results in a decrease in the force generation capacity of muscle. Similarly, when joints are immobilized, muscles near to that joint are affected, and their capacity to generate force decreases. This section describes the changes that occur to muscle structure with injury and disuse. Due to ethical constraints, most experiments in muscle healing have been undertaken using animals, primarily rodents. Borisov (1999) recently examined how well these animals represent the processes occurring in humans. He stated that although there are similarities in the structure of the contractile mechanisms in skeletal muscles, there are distinct differences in the intensity and time course over which the restoration processes occur across species, and that the phylogenic age of the species is an important factor influencing the regenerative processes. Therefore, caution should be exercised when making inferences concerning the behavior of human tissues in response to injury and disuse.

THE MECHANISM OF INJURY

Two models are commonly used to induce an injury to muscle, and they supposedly simulate the contusion and strain injury paradigms. In the former, a mass (e.g. steel ball) is projected by a spring like device or by gravity to strike the tissue of interest. The shape of the mass and its momentum at impact will determine the magnitude of the injury. To simulate strain injuries, the animal's musculotendinous unit is exposed and one end is attached to an electromechanical device that lengthens the tissues at a particular rate. These rates range between 1–10 cm/min, which is relatively slow compared to the velocity of lengthening that can occur during functional activities. The resistance of tissue to stretching (force) is also often measured. Despite the uniformity of each of the procedures to create the injury, some authors (Minamoto et al 1999) have noted considerable variation in the extent of damage inflicted on different animals.

To assess the extent of damage that has occurred as a result of these insults, researchers will kill some of the animals immediately after the injury, dissect out the muscle of interest, and provide a qualitative description of the injury site using light or electron microscopy. The healing process can also be monitored by regular histology and immunohistochemistry (Kasemkjwattana et al 1998). These techniques might be used to monitor the expression of molecules such as desmin and vimentin, and thus provide measures of fiber regeneration and fibrosis respectively. Researchers may also electrically stimulate the muscle soon after injury, and describe the change in maximal force that the muscle can generate.

REGENERATION OF THE CONTRACTILE ELEMENTS

Although the mechanisms of injury are different for contusion and strain injuries, the regeneration of the contractile elements follows a similar pattern, and begins with the activation of satellite cells. Normally these cells are non-active in adults, and lie between the basal lamina and the sarcolemma of the muscle fiber (Mauro 1961). There is evidence that the number of satellite cells varies according to fiber type, with greater numbers observed in type I muscle fibers (Snow 1983). Contact with the basement membrane and the presence of various molecules is thought to inhibit their activity (Anderson 2000, Bischoff 1990). When the basal lamina of the muscle fiber is disrupted during injury, a number of events have been implicated in activating mitotic activity in the satellite cells. They include the shear forces as the injury occurs, hypercontraction of the myofibrils, retraction of the damaged fibers, and the release of human growth factors and chemicals such as nitric oxide (Anderson 2000). Thereafter, the satellite cells become less adherent to the basement membrane, become more active, and proliferate. The expression of genes and deoxyribonucleic acid (DNA) synthesis important to regeneration then commences.

Hurme et al (1991a) reported that, immediately after the trauma, muscle fibers that are ruptured retract and a gap is formed. At the ends of the retracted ruptured fibers, the intact sarcomeres have been observed to be hypercontracted immediately after the injury, and this activity is thought to block the inflow of inflammatory cells into the fiber and hence restrict their activity. Within hours, a membrane is formed that separates the intact

sarcomeres of a fiber from the injury site (Carpenter & Karpati 1989).

At the time of trauma, numerous blood vessels are also torn, and the gap between the retracted fibers is initially filled with blood. The release of cytokines at the time of injury attracts leukocytes and macrophages to the injury site (Robertson et al 1993). Within the first 2 days after injury, the macrophages become the dominant inflammatory cell at the injury site and their role is to remove necrotic tissue which includes cellular fragments and sarcoplasm from the damaged fibers (Grounds 1991). There is also some evidence to support their role in mediating satellite cell proliferation through chemotaxis (Kuschel et al 2000). Between 5–7 days after injury, the number of leukocytes and macrophages has decreased considerably. However, their numbers can be influenced by physical activity in the first few days after injury. In this respect, Lehto and colleagues (Lehto et al 1985) noted that 5 days after injury, there were few inflammatory cells observed in animals that had been immobilized. In contrast, significant numbers of these cells were still present in animals mobilized with a treadmill running program 2 days after injury.

It is apparent that the fibers tear in a manner that leaves remnants of the tube-like structure of the basal lamina intact but often with ragged ends (Hurme et al 1991a). The ragged edges of the basal lamina act as scaffolding for activated satellite cells, which are termed myoblasts. These fuse with one another to form a myotube within days of the injury (Fig. 2.10). Where this process occurs in the old basal lamina, it is more likely that the new myotubes will fuse with the capped off surviving fibers. These myotubes then take on the characteristics (fast or slow fiber types) of the muscle fiber to which they have joined (Zhang & Dhoot 1998). Zhang & Dhoot (1998) commented that perhaps specific myoblasts might only fuse with specific types of fibers. In most instances, the growth of the myotube is across the gap between the retracted fibers. Some authors (Järvinen & Lehto 1993) have described the new fiber as having a gradient of maturity, with areas closest to the original fiber displaying features more like undamaged muscle and the tip being the least developed.

Hurme et al (1991a) observed that at 7 days post injury, myotubes have grown within the damaged basal lamina and a new basal lamina was apparent. Once the myotube leaves the remnants of the old basal lamina and begins to traverse the central gap between fibers, it has been observed to split into multiple branches. It is thought that splitting may improve the chances of one branch being able to successfully pass through the collagen tissue of the central zone (Hurme et al 1991a). Lehto (1985) reported that the myotubes were more interlaced amongst the granulation tissue in rats that were immo-

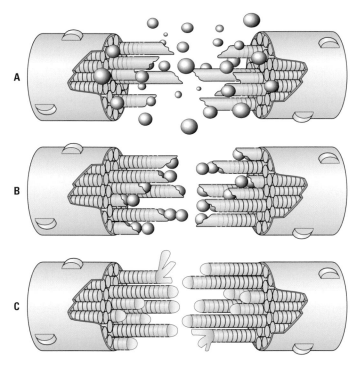

Figure 2.10A–C   **A**: The proliferation of satellite cells and subsequently myoblasts occurs in the first day after injury. **B**: Myoblasts are attracted to the ends of the surviving fibers. They subsequently fuse and growth begins. **C**: The new myotubes grow toward the central region from the periphery. Some myotubes split at their tips possibly to increase the chance of reuniting with the approaching myotubes from the other side of the injury site.

bilized immediately after injury compared to animals that had experienced early mobilization.

The stimulus for the myotubes to continue growing is not known, however, Hurme et al (1991a) suggested three factors that may be involved in the process. First, satellite cells may migrate along the new myotube to the tip. Second, the tip may grow from interactions with undifferentiated cells encountered in the central zone. Finally, there is also evidence of vesicular structures within the myotube that could supply essential materials to the tip. The maturation of myotubes into myofibers has been observed to occur after approximately 14 days (Kaariainen et al 1998). Whether the myofibers from each side of the injury site meet and subsequently fuse is questionable. Kaariainen et al (2000) suggested that the tip may adhere to the intervening scar tissues and form a 'mini musculotendinous junction'. While the scar tissue may decrease over months, and the tips become closer and interlaced, they may never actually fuse.

REGENERATION OF THE CONNECTIVE TISSUE ELEMENTS

Järvinen & Lehto (1993) suggested that there are two competitive processes occurring during muscle regenera-

tion after injury: regeneration of the myofibrils and the production of scar tissue. Like myofibril regeneration, there is a sequence of events that occurs to lay down collagen in the injured area. These events are linked to and are important for the successful regeneration of the myofibrils.

Within hours of the injury, fibronectin is observed at the injury site. This substance, which is derived from plasma, adheres to strands of fibrin and forms scaffolding on which fibroblasts attach in the next few days (Lehto et al 1985). The fibroblasts produce type I and III collagen, the latter being observed earlier. In rats, by 5 days, it has been observed (Lehto et al 1985) that connective tissue made up of type III collagen together with granulation tissue is seen extensively in the gap between the retracted fibers, and it provides the initial strength of the injured area. As the repair process continues, type I collagen becomes more predominant.

Lehto et al (1985) reported that a treadmill running program instigated 2 days after injury for rats led to a sustained presence of fibronectin and a fibrin clot in the damaged area. Interestingly, in the following weeks, these rats developed a dense network of scar tissue in the endomysial and perimysial structures. Furthermore, increased deposits of fat at the injury site were also observed. In contrast, animals that had been immobilized for 5 days had much greater resorption of scar tissue 8 weeks after injury. A ramification of excessive scar tissue is that the extensibility of the tissues is reduced. In this respect, Kaariainen et al (1998) reported that strain values remained at approximately 50% of control values at a 56-day follow-up of rat muscles that had sustained a laceration injury.

In respect to the strength of the tissues, stretching the muscle to failure has been shown to primarily occur at the site of injury during the first week after injury (Järvinen & Lehto 1993, Kaariainen et al 1998). Thereafter, the site of injury becomes increasingly more likely to be within the intact myofibers. Järvinen & Lehto (1993) suggested that this finding is due to the increased amount of scar tissue at the injury site, and Kaariainen et al (1998) commented that it may indicate that the strength of the adhesions of the myotubes to the newly laid connective tissue is greater than that of the atrophied muscle fibers. These authors (Kaariainen et al 1998) reported that although force to failure was significantly decreased (50% of control values from day 10 to 56 following injury), when the cross-sectional area of the tissue was accounted for, the injured muscle had recovered its strength by day 21.

Thus, in summary, it seems that there is a need to provide a period of rest soon after injury. In doing this, the amount of scar tissue laid down is limited and less dense, and the regenerating myofibrils can penetrate this tissue more easily. Also, it is speculated that normal muscle performance might be achieved. Alternatively, mobilizing the muscle early after the injury will strengthen the tissue more quickly; however, the density of connective tissue may act as a physical barrier that prevents the myofibrils from joining. Intuitively, this barrier might affect muscle activation patterns, and the additional junction caused by the scarring may predispose the area to recurring injury in the future. Furthermore, it is apparent that the scar tissue can affect the extensibility of the tissues. Muscle atrophy can be a source of structural weakness in the muscle; therefore, while the rehabilitation process may require a short period of immobilization, it should not be prolonged. The question is: how long? The answer, regrettably, is not known for the human model. In the rat, it appears to be between 3–5 days.

When muscle is damaged by a contusion type injury, it is apparent that damage occurs not only to the muscle fibers, but also to the nerves supplying those fibers. This damage can extend from minor disruption of myelin to complete rupture of the intramuscular nerves depending on the location of the injury and the forces involved. Hurme et al (1991b) noted that in the first 1–2 days following damage, phagocytic cells were present in the perineurial sheath. The depolarization of the nerves was affected with spontaneous action potentials being observed intermittently from 5 days after injury. These potentials were not present at 14 days and these authors suggested that this provided evidence that reinnervation was occurring at this time.

THE EFFECT OF IMMOBILIZATION ON MUSCLE

After many injuries, a joint is placed in an immobilized state and muscle activity about that joint decreases. While the muscles may not be damaged, an inactive muscle undergoes rapid changes in structure, and consequently function. The most obvious change is muscle atrophy. Normally, a balance between protein synthesis and degradation maintains the mass of the contractile elements. Within hours of immobilization, protein synthesis decreases, and, over a day, protein degradation increases. The magnitude and the rate of change in these processes differ across muscles and individual animals (Booth & Seider 1979, Goldspink 1977). Goldspink (1977) reported that over a 3-day period of immobilization with the muscle in a shortened state, the net weight of the animals' muscles decreased by 30%. Nicks et al (1989) examined whether such changes reflected modifications to either fiber size or fiber number. These researchers observed that following immobilization for 8 weeks, the fiber area of a rat's triceps brachii was decreased by 42%, whereas fiber numbers were unchanged. The position in which a muscle is immobilized influences the magnitude of atrophy considerably. Muscles that are immobilized in a shortened position are most affected. When muscles are immobilized in a lengthened state, they may increase in weight, for instance, Goldspink (1977) noted a 10% increase in muscle weight in the extensor digitorum muscle after 3 days of immobilization.

Related to these changes in muscle mass is a modification in the number of sarcomeres in series. In the early 1970s, Tabary et al (1972) reported that immobilization of a cat's soleus muscles in a plaster cast for 4 weeks in a shortened position led to a 40% decrease in sarcomeres in series. Tabary et al also noted that when these muscles were immobilized in a lengthened position, a 20% increase in sarcomeres in series occurred. Goldspink et al (1974) explored whether these changes were affected by denervation of the muscle. These researchers noted that sarcomere numbers did not appear to be under neural control, and they suggested that the mechanism was a local response to altered tension in the muscle.

The ultra structural changes that occur following immobilization of muscles in a shortened position involve segmental necrosis, predominantly though not exclusively at the ends of the muscle fibers as compared to the mid-region of the muscle. The work of Baker & Matsumoto (1988) provides an excellent description of this process. These authors immobilized the ankle joints of rats in maximal plantarflexion for up to 4 weeks. Within 2 days of immobilization, swelling of the mitochondria and sarcoplasmic reticulum had occurred, and by 5 days, the structure of the sarcomeres was breaking down and in many areas appeared kinked. By 7 days, fibers had lost their striated appearance with sarcomere structure being lost completely. These changes continued for approximately 2 weeks. By 4 weeks, although still immobilized, many fibers appeared to be regenerating. Normal sarcoplasmic structure was observed and, although the regenerating myofibrils were thinner than normal, they exhibited defined I- and Z-bands, and hence a distinctive sarcomere structure. Thus, the segmental necrosis at the ends of the fibers allows the length of the fiber to be adjusted. This in turn will affect the muscle mechanics (e.g. the length–tension relationship of the muscle). A muscle after immobilization in a shortened state, when stimulated electrically at different muscle lengths, will exhibit lesser peak force, and that force will be at a shorter muscle length compared to pre-immobilization (Williams & Goldspink 1978) (Fig. 2.11).

It has been of interest whether a particular fiber type is more affected by immobilization in a shortened position. The findings generally indicate that type I fibers undergo

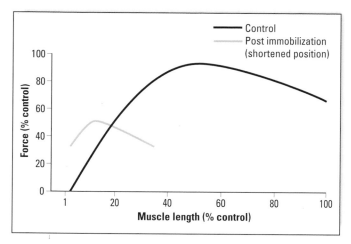

Figure 2.11 The force–length relationship in normal muscle, and muscle that has been immobilized in a shortened position. Note the shift in the position of peak forces towards shorter muscle lengths and the decreases in force able to be generated.

greater changes than type II fibers. However, Lieber et al (1988) have challenged these findings. These authors have argued that many studies have compared slow and fast muscles without due consideration for the normal activity level of the muscles and the subsequent change in use that occurs with immobilization; and also, that these muscles are often immobilized at different lengths, which will influence the magnitude of atrophy. This will be most apparent when muscles with different fiber lengths, and fiber length to muscle length ratios, are compared. Finally, the number of joints that a muscle spans might also affect the magnitude of the atrophic response. In a study that controlled for these factors, Lieber et al (1988) concluded that the type of muscle to be affected most by the immobilization process was a single joint muscle containing a relatively large proportion of type I fibers.

Together with structural changes, one might expect electromyographic activity in muscle immobilized in a shortened position to decrease. Fournier et al (1983) observed decreases in activation levels to approximately 50% of control values in animal muscles (soleus and medial gastrocnemius) immobilized in a shortened position for 4 weeks. These authors noted that there was a trend for a greater decrease in activity in the soleus compared to medial gastrocnemius muscle. Hnik et al (1985) also commented on large decreases in electromyographic (EMG) activity after 10 days of immobilization, but only in the soleus muscle. The tibialis anterior, which is a more phasic type muscle, was not affected by immobilization in a shortened position. A consistent finding across these studies is that EMG activity was least affected when the muscle was immobilized in a lengthened position. The findings of these studies also indicated that EMG activity was not a major factor influencing the degree of atrophy observed in the muscles during the immobilization process.

A common finding associated with immobilization is an increase in the connective tissue (endomysial, perimysial, and epimysial) relative to the muscle's contractile tissues. Williams & Goldspink (1984) reported increases in perimysial tissue within 2 days of immobilization, whereas changes in endomysial tissues took approximately a week to become apparent. The magnitude of the changes can be substantial. For example, Jozsa et al (1990) immobilized rat calf muscles in a shortened position for 3 weeks. Normal volume density of connective tissue of the soleus and gastrocnemius was 2–3%. After 1 week of immobilization, this had increased to 10% and 12% respectively. After three weeks, the amount was 30% in both muscles (Fig. 2.12). Williams & Goldspink (1984) reported that the connective tissue laid down during immobilization was less aligned in respect to the muscle fibers. These changes in the size and structure of connective tissue are likely to be responsible for the increased stiffness of muscle immobilized in a shortened position (Tabary et al 1972), and for decreased range of motion (Williams 1988). Järvinen et al (1992) has also shown that after 7 and 21 days of immobilization, elongation at the point of failure was decreased by 21% and 36% respectively.

Interestingly, Williams & Goldspink (1984) observed that increases in collagen content preceded any significant loss of sarcomeres in series. This finding would imply that early stiffness changes are associated with increased collagen within the muscle. Later work by Williams et al (1988) showed that these connective tissue changes can be modified by muscle activation. In this study, Williams et al (1988) electrically stimulated muscles immobilized in a shortened position, and noted that they lost more sarcomeres in series than unstimulated muscles, however, increases in collagen content within the muscle were not observed. Thus, it seems that either maintaining the immobilized muscle in a lengthened state or applying electrical stimulation can regulate collagen content. An important question is whether or not intermittent lengthening can minimize the loss of sarcomeres in series when muscle is immobilized in an shortened position. Williams also addressed this question in two studies (Williams 1988, Williams 1990). In the first study, Williams (1988) showed that 15 min of passive stretching every second day over 10 days was sufficient to prevent an increase in connective tissue within the muscle, however, fiber lengths and hence range of motion remained significantly decreased. In the second study (Williams 1990), where animals were immobilized for 2 weeks, sarcomeres decreased by 19% and range of motion was reduced by 41% in animals that were not stretched.

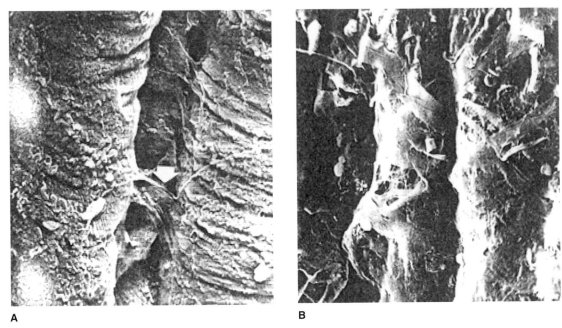

A   B

Figure 2.12A&B   A microscopic view of normal muscle fibers (A) and fibers that have been immobilized (B). Note the increased amount of connective tissue adhesions. (Reproduced with permission from Jozsa et al 1990.)

However, Williams reported that 30 min of stretching per day was sufficient to prevent a loss of sarcomeres in series, and maintain range of motion at control levels.

Recently, there has been considerable interest in the effect of lengthening normal muscle tissue. This work has been stimulated by studies that showed that leg lengthening procedures were at times unsuccessful because patients were often encumbered with muscle contractures and subsequently a loss of joint range of motion (Simpson et al 1996). It was suspected that the rate of stretching might be a factor influencing the poor results, and, to investigate this problem, rabbits underwent osteotomies and had their tibias lengthened at different rates until 20% increase in tibial length had occurred (Simpson et al 1996, Williams et al 1999). The main findings of these studies were that if rates were too high, then significant increases in connective tissue were observed, muscle fibers were damaged, and sarcomeres were not added in series. At medium rates of lengthening, sarcomeres were added to the muscle fibers; however, moderate increases in connective tissue were observed. At low levels of lengthening, sarcomeres were added to the muscle fibers as would be expected, and increases in connective tissue were minimal. Thus, it would appear that low rates of stretch are needed to attain optimal adaptations in both the contractile and passive elements of the muscle when it is stretched.

SUMMARY

Muscle is a complex structure, and we are continuing to discover new knowledge concerning its structure and function. For effective control of motion, it is important that our muscles function correctly. In many tasks, we are required to activate our muscles to high levels. The force potential of muscle is governed by its structure, architecture, and neural activation. Injury, disease, and disuse can be particularly detrimental to this potential. An understanding of muscle function, and its reaction to pathology, is important when designing and implementing effective training programs to limit and correct decreased muscle performance.

Acknowledgements

The authors would like to thank Jill Kerr for her advice concerning the structure of the chapter, and Stephen Stanley for his advice and technical expertise in drawing the figures.

REFERENCES

Aagaard P, Simonsen E B, Trolle M et al 1995 Isokinetic hamstring/quadriceps strength ratio: influence from joint angular velocity, gravity correction and contraction mode. Acta Physiologica Scandinavica 154:421–427

Aagaard P, Simonsen E B, Trolle M et al 1996 Specificity of training velocity and training load on gains in isokinetic knee joint strength. Acta Physiologica Scandinavica 156:123–129

Aagaard P, Simonsen E B, Andersen J L et al 2000 Neural inhibition during maximal eccentric and concentric quadriceps contraction: effects of resistance training. Journal of Applied Physiology 89:2249–2257

Abbott B C, Aubert X M 1951 Changes of energy in a muscle during very slow stretches. Proceedings of the Royal Society of London 139(B):104–117

Anderson J E 2000 A role for nitric oxide in muscle repair: nitric oxide-mediated activation of muscle satellite cells. Molecular Biology of the Cell 11:1859–1874

Baker J, Matsumoto D 1988 Adaptation of skeletal muscle to immobilisation in a shortened position. Muscle and Nerve 11:231–244

Bellemare F, Woods J J, Johansson R et al 1983 Motor-unit discharge rates in maximal voluntary contractions of three human muscles. Journal of Neurophysiology 50:1380–1392

Billeter R, Weber H, Lutz H et al 1980 Myosin types in human skeletal muscle fibers. Histochemistry 65:249–259

Bischoff R 1990 Interaction between satellite cells and skeletal muscle fibers. Development 109:943–952

Booth F, Seider M 1979 Early change in skeletal muscle protein synthesis after limb immobilisation of rats. Journal of Applied Physiology: Respiratory Environmental and Exercise Physiology 47:974–977

Borisov A 1999 Regeneration of skeletal and cardiac muscle in mammals: do nonprimate models resemble human pathology? Wound Repair and Regeneration 7:26–35

Bottinelli R, Canepari M, Pellegrino M A et al 1996 Force-velocity properties of human skeletal muscle fibres: myosin heavy chain isoform and temperature dependence. Journal of Physiology 495:573–586

Carpenter S, Karpati G 1989 Segmental necrosis and its demarcation in experimental micropuncture injury in skeletal muscle. Journal of Neuropathology and Experimental Neurology 48:154–170

Chleboun G, France A, Crill M et al 2001 In vivo measurement of fascicle length and pennation angle of the human biceps femoris muscle. Cells Tissues Organs 169:401–409

Dudley G A, Harris R T, Duvoisin M R et al 1990 Effect of voluntary vs. artificial activation on the relationship of muscle torque to speed. Journal of Applied Physiology 69:2215–2221

Edgerton V R, Apor P, Roy R R 1990 Specific tension of human elbow flexor muscles. Acta Physiologica Hungarica 75:205–216

Edman K A 1979 The velocity of unloaded shortening and its relation to sarcomere length and isometric force in vertebrate muscle fibres. Journal of Physiology 291:143–159

Feinstein N, Lindegard B, Nyman E et al 1955 Morphological studies of motor units in normal human muscles. Acta Anatomica 23:127–142

Fenn W O, Marsh B S 1935 Muscular force at different speeds of shortening. Journal of Physiology 85:277–297

Ford L, Huxley A, Simmons R 1981 The relation between stiffness and filament overlap in stimulated frog fibres. Journal of Physiology 311:219–249

Fournier M, Roy R R, Perham H et al 1983 Is limb immobilisation a model of muscle disuse? Experimental Neurology 80:147–156

Fugl-Meyer A R, Gustafsson L, Burstedt Y 1980 Isokinetic and static plantar flexion characteristics. European Journal of Applied Physiology and Occupational Physiology 45:221–234

Fukashiro S, Komi P V, Järvinen M et al 1995 In vivo achilles tendon loading during jumping in humans. European Journal of Applied Physiology and Occupational Physiology 71:453–458

Fukunaga T, Roy R R, Shellock F G et al 1996 Specific tension of human plantar flexors and dorsiflexors. Journal of Applied Physiology 80:158–165

Fukunaga T, Miyatani M, Tachi M et al 2001 Muscle volume is a major determinant of joint torque in humans. Acta Physiologica Scandinavica 172:249–255

Gerdle B, Langstrom M 1987 Repeated isokinetic plantar flexions at different angular velocities. Acta Physiologica Scandinavica 130:495–500

Goldspink D 1977 The influence of immobilisation and stretch on protein turnover of rat skeletal muscle. Journal of Physiology 264:267–282

Goldspink D, Tabary J, Tabary C et al 1974 Effect of denervation on the adaptation of sarcomere number and muscle extensibility to the functional length of the muscle. Journal of Physiology 236:733–742

Gollnick P, Armstrong R, Saubert C et al 1972 Enzyme activity and fibre composition in skeletal muscle of untrained and trained men. Journal of Applied Physiology 33:312–319

Gollnick P D, Sjodin B, Karlsson J et al 1974 Human soleus muscle: a comparison of fiber composition and enzyme activities with other leg muscles. Pflugers Archiv – European Journal of Physiology 348:247–255

Gordon A M, Huxley A F, Julian F J 1966 The variation in isometric tension with sarcomere length in vertebrate muscle fibres. Journal of Physiology 184:170–192

Gregor R J, Roy R R, Whiting W C et al 1988 Mechanical output of the cat soleus during treadmill locomotion: in vivo vs in situ characteristics. Journal of Biomechanics 21:721–732

Gregor R J, Komi P V, Browning R C et al 1991 A comparison of the triceps surae and residual muscle moments at the ankle during cycling. Journal of Biomechanics 24:287–297

Grounds M 1991 Towards understanding skeletal muscle regeneration. Pathology Research and Practice 187:1–22

Guyton A C, Hall J E 2000 Textbook of medical physiology, 10th edn. WB Saunders, Philadelphia, PA, p 68, 70, 71, 72, 84

Harris R T, Dudley G A 1994 Factors limiting force during slow, shortening actions of the quadriceps femoris muscle group in vivo. Acta Physiologica Scandinavica 152:63–71

Herbert R D, Gandevia S C 1995 Changes in pennation with joint angle and muscle torque: in vivo measurements in human brachialis muscle. Journal of Physiology 484:523–532

Herbert R D, Gandevia S C 1999 Twitch interpolation in human muscles: mechanisms and implications for measurement of voluntary activation. Journal of Neurophysiology 82:2271–2283

Hess A 1967 The structure of vertebrate slow and twitch muscle fibers. Investigative Ophthalmology 6:217–228

Higuchi H 1996 Viscoelasticity and function of connectin/titin filaments in skinned muscle fibres. Advances in Biophysics 33:159–171

Hill A V 1938 The heat of shortening and the dynamic constants of muscle. Proceedings of the Royal Society Series B 126:136–195

Hnik P, Vejsada R, Goldspink D et al 1985 Quantitative evaluation of electromyogram activity in rat extensor and flexor muscles immobilised at different lengths. Experimental Neurology 88:515–528

Horowits R 1992 Passive force generation and titin isoforms in mammalian skeletal muscle. Biophysical Journal 61:392–398

Horowits R, Kempner E, Bisher M et al 1986 A physiological role for titin and nebulin in skeletal muscle. Nature 323:160–164

Hortobagyi T, Katch F I 1990 Eccentric and concentric torque-velocity relationships during arm flexion and extension. Influence of strength level. European Journal of Applied Physiology and Occupational Physiology 60:395–401

Huijing P A 1998 Muscle, the motor of movement: properties in function, experiment and modelling. Journal of Electromyography and Kinesiology 8:61–77

Hurme T, Kalimo H, Lehto M et al 1991a Healing of skeletal muscle injury: an ultastructural and immunohistochemical study. Medicine and Science in Sports and Exercise 23:801–810

Hurme T, Lehto M, Falck B et al 1991b Electromyography and

morphology during regeneration of muscle injury in rats. Acta Physiologica Scandinavica 142:443–456

Huxley A, Stewart A, Sosa H et al 1994 X-ray diffraction measurements of the extensibility of actin and mysosin filaments in contracting muscle. Biophysical Journal 67:2411–2421

Huxley A F 1957 Muscle structure and theories of contraction. Progress in Biophysics and Chemistry 7:255–318

Huxley A F, Simmons R M 1971 Proposed mechanism of force generation in striated muscle. Nature 233:533–538

Huxley H E 1972 Molecular basis of contraction in cross-striated muscle. In: Bourne G (ed) Molecular basis of contraction in cross-striated muscle. Academic Press, New York, p 302–387

Huxley H E, Hanson J 1954 Changes in the cross-striations of muscle during contraction and stretch and their structural interpretation. Nature 173:973

Järvinen M, Lehto M 1993 The effects of early mobilisation and immobilisation on the healing process following muscle injuries. Sports Medicine 15:78–89

Järvinen M, Einola S, Virtanen E 1992 Effect of the position of immobilisation upon the tensile properties of the rat gastrocnemius muscle. Archives of Physical Medicine and Rehabilitation 73:253–257

Johnson A, Polgar J, Weightman P et al 1973 Data on the distribution of fibre types in thirty six human muscles. Journal of the Neurological Sciences 18:111–129

Jozsa L, Kannus P, Thoring J et al 1990 The effect of tenotomy and immobilisation on intramuscular connective tissue. Journal of Bone and Joint Surgery (Br) 72B:293–297

Juul-Kristensen B, Bojsen-Moller F, Finsen L et al 2000a Muscle sizes and moment arms of rotator cuff muscles determined by magnetic resonance imaging. Cells Tissues Organs 167:214–222

Juul-Kristensen B, Bojsen-Moller F, Holst E et al 2000b Comparison of muscle sizes and moment arms of two rotator cuff muscles measured by ultrasonography and magnetic resonance imaging. European Journal of Ultrasound 11:161–173

Kaariainen M, Kaariainen J, Järvinen T et al 1998 Correlation between biomechanical and structural changes during the regeneration of skeletal muscle after laceration injury. Journal of Orthopedic Research 16:197–206

Kaariainen M, Järvinen T, Järvinen M et al 2000 Relation between myofibers and connective tissue during muscle injury repair. Scandinavian Journal of Medicine and Science in Sports 10:332–337

Kanda K, Hashizume K 1992 Factors causing difference in force output among motor units in the rat medial gastrocnemius muscle. Journal of Physiology 448:677–695

Kasemkjwattana C, Menetrey J, Somogyl G et al 1998 Development of approaches to improve the healing following muscle contusion. Cell Transplant 7:585–598

Katz B 1939 The relations between force and speed in muscular contraction. Journal of Physiology 96:45–64

Komi P V 1973 Measurement of the force-velocity relationship in human muscle under concentric and eccentric actions. Medicine and Sport 8:224–229

Kuschel R, Deininger M, Meyermann R et al 2000 Allograft Inflammatory Factor-1 is expressed by macrophages in injured skeletal muscle and abrogates proliferation and differentiation of satellite cells. Journal of Neuropathology and Experimental Neurology 59:323–332

Labeit S, Gibson T, Lakey A et al 1991 Evidence that nebulin is a protein-ruler in muscle thin filaments. FEBS Letters 282:313–316

Larsson L, Edstrom L, Lindegren B et al 1991 MHC composition and enzyme-histochemical and physiological properties of a novel fast-twitch motor unit type. American Journal of Physiology 261:C93–101

Lehto M, Duance V, Restall D 1985 Collagen and fibronectin in a healing skeletal muscle injury. Journal of Bone and Joint Surgery (Br) 67B:820–828

Lieber R, Friden J, Hargens A et al 1988 Differential response of the dog quadriceps muscle to external skeletal fixation of the knee. Muscle and Nerve 11:193–201

McComas A J 1996 Skeletal muscle form and function. Human Kinetics, Champaign IL

Malamud J, Godt R, Nichols R 1996 Relationship between short range stiffness and yielding in type-identified chemically skinned muscle fibers from the cat triceps surae muscles. Journal of Neurophysiology 76:2280–2289

Mauro A 1961 Satellite cells of skeletal muscle fibers. Journal of Biophysics Biochemistry and Cytology 87:225–251

Minamoto V, Grazziano C, De Fatima Salvino T 1999 Effect of single and periodic contusion on the rat soleus muscle at different stages of regeneration. The Anatomical Record 254:281–287

Narici M 1999 Human skeletal muscle architecture studied in vivo by non-invasive imaging techniques: functional significance and applications. Journal of Electromyography and Kinesiology 9:97–103

Narici M V, Roi G S, Landoni L 1988 Force of knee extensor and flexor muscles and cross-sectional area determined by nuclear magnetic resonance imaging. European Journal of Applied Physiology and Occupational Physiology 57:39–44

Narici M V, Binzoni T, Hiltbrand E et al 1996 In vivo human gastrocnemius architecture with changing joint angle at rest and during graded isometric contraction. Journal of Physiology 496:287–297

Nicks D, Beneke W, Key R et al 1989 Muscle fibre size and number following immobilisation atrophy. Journal of Anatomy 163:1–5

Nygaard E, Houston M, Suzuki Y et al 1983 Morphology of the brachial biceps muscle and elbow flexion in man. Acta Physiologica Scandinavica 117:287–292

Peachey L D 1965a The sarcoplasmic reticulum and transverse tubules of the frog's sartorius. Journal of Cell Biology 25(suppl):209–231

Peachey L D 1965b Transverse tubules in excitation-contraction coupling. Federation Proceedings 24:1124–1134

Perrine J J, Edgerton V R 1978 Muscle force velocity relationships under isokinetic loading. Medicine and Science in Sports and Exercise 10:159–166

Pinniger G J, Steele J R, Thorstensson A et al 2000 Tension regulation during lengthening and shortening actions of the human soleus muscle. European Journal of Applied Physiology 81:375–383

Pousson M, Amiridis I G, Cometti G et al 1999 Velocity-specific training in elbow flexors. European Journal of Applied Physiology and Occupational Physiology 80:367–372

Purslow P 1989 Strain induced reorientation of an intramuscular connective tissues network: implications for passive muscle elasticity. Journal of Biomechanics 22:21–31

Purslow P, Trotter J 1994 The morphology and mechanical properties of endomysium in series-fibred muscles: Variations with muscle length. Journal of Muscle Research and Cellular Motility 15:299–308

Rack P M, Westbury D R 1969 The effects of length and stimulus rate on tension in the isometric cat soleus muscle. Journal of Physiology 204:443–460

Robertson T, Maley M, Grounds M et al 1993 The role of macrophages in skeletal muscle regeneration with particular reference to chemotaxis. Experimental Cell Research 207:321–331

Rudel R, Taylor S R 1971 Striated muscle fibers: facilitation of contraction at short lengths by caffeine. Science 172:387–389

Rutherford O M, Jones D A 1992 Measurement of fibre pennation using ultrasound in the human quadriceps in vivo. European Journal of Applied Physiology and Occupational Physiology 65:433–437

Sale D, Quinlan J, Marsh E et al 1982 Influence of joint position on ankle plantarflexion in humans. Journal of Applied Physiology: Respiratory, Environmental and Exercise Physiology 52:1636–1642

Sargeant A J, Hoinville E, Young A 1981 Maximum leg force and power output during short-term dynamic exercise. Journal of Applied Physiology: Respiratory, Environmental and Exercise Physiology 51:1175–1182

Schiaffino S, Reggiani C 1994 Myosin isoforms in mammalian skeletal muscle. Journal of Applied Physiology 77:493–501

Simpson A, Williams P, Kyberd P et al 1996 The response of muscle to leg lengthening. Journal of Bone and Joint Surgery (Br) 77B:630–636

Smerdu V, Karsch-Mizrachi I, Campione M et al 1994 Type IIx myosin heavy chain transcripts are expressed in type IIb fibers of human skeletal muscle. American Journal of Physiology 267:C1723–1728

Snow M 1983 A quantitative ultrastructural analysis of satellite cells in denervated fast and slow muscles of the rat. The Anatomical Record 207:593–604

Spoor C W, van Leeuwen J L 1992 Knee muscle moment arms from MRI and from tendon travel. Journal of Biomechanics 25:201–206

Spoor C W, van Leeuwen J L, Meskers C G et al 1990 Estimation of instantaneous moment arms of lower-leg muscles. Journal of Biomechanics 23:1247–1259

Tabary J, Tabary C, Tardieu C et al 1972 Physiological and structural changes in the cat's soleus muscle due to immobilisation at different lengths by plaster casts. Journal of Physiology 224:231–244

Thorstensson 1976 Muscle strength, fibre types and enzyme activities in man. Acta Physiologica Scandinavica Supplementum 443:1–45

Thorstensson A, Grimby G, Karlsson J 1976 Force-velocity relations and fibre composition in human knee extensor muscles. Journal of Applied Physiology 40:12–16

Trinick J 1991 Elastic filaments and giant proteins in muscle. Current Opinion in Cell Biology 3:112–119

Tveit P, Daggfeldt K, Hetland S et al 1994 Erector spinae lever arm length variations with changes in spinal curvature. Spine 19:199–204

Walmsley B, Hodgson J A, Burke R E 1978 Forces produced by medial gastrocnemius and soleus muscles during locomotion in freely moving cats. Journal of Neurophysiology 41:1203–1216

Westing S H, Seger J Y, Karlson E et al 1988 Eccentric and concentric torque-velocity characteristics of the quadriceps femoris in man. European Journal of Applied Physiology and Occupational Physiology 58:100–104

Westing S H, Seger J Y, Thorstensson A 1990 Effects of electrical stimulation on eccentric and concentric torque-velocity relationships during knee extension in man. Acta Physiologica Scandinavica 140:17–22

Westing S H, Cresswell A G, Thorstensson A 1991 Muscle activation during maximal voluntary eccentric and concentric knee extension. European Journal of Applied Physiology and Occupational Physiology 62:104–108

Whiting W C, Gregor R J, Roy R R et al 1984 A technique for estimating mechanical work of individual muscles in the cat during treadmill locomotion. Journal of Biomechanics 17:685–694

Wickiewicz T, Roy R, Powell P et al 1983 Muscle architecture of the lower limb. Clinical Orthopaedics and Related Research 179:275–283

Williams P 1988 Effect of intermittent stretch on immobilised muscle. Annals of the Rheumatic Diseases 47:1014–1016

Williams P 1990 Use of intermittent stretch in the prevention of serial sarcomere loss in immobilised muscle. Annals of the Rheumatic Diseases 49:316–317

Williams P, Goldspink D 1978 Changes in sarcomere length and physiological properties in immobilised muscle. Journal of Anatomy 127:459–468

Williams P, Goldspink D 1984 Connective tissue changes in immobilised muscle. Journal of Anatomy 138:343–350

Williams P, Catanese T, Lucey E et al 1988 The importance of stretch and contractile activity in the prevention of connective tissue accumulation in muscle. Journal of Anatomy 158:109–114

Williams P, Simpson A, Kyberd P et al 1999 Effect of rate of distraction on loss of range of joint movement, muscle stiffness, and intramuscular connective tissue content during surgical limb-lengthening: a study in the rabbit. The Anatomical Record 255:78–83

Woittiez R D, Huijing P A, Rozendal R H 1983 Influence of muscle architecture on the length-force diagram of mammalian muscle. Pflugers Archiv – European Journal of Physiology 399:275–279

Zhang J, Dhoot G 1998 Localized and limited changes in the expression of myosin heavy chains in injured skeletal muscle fibers being repaired. Muscle and Nerve 21(4): 469–481

3

Tendon

Jill Cook

INTRODUCTION

Tendon is a continuum of connective tissue that simply and effectively transfers force produced by contractile cells of muscles to their target, which is usually bone. They usually cross, and attach close to, a joint which permits rapid joint movement (Benjamin & Ralphs 1996).

Tendons have several functions other than directing muscle contraction. They act proprioceptively, and as both shock absorbers and energy storage sites (Benjamin & Ralphs 1995). In sport, these features are critical, as they enhance athletic function.

Tendons vary in length and size throughout the body. They can be long, broad, flat, round or aponeurotic, they may wind around bony pulleys, enclose sesamoids or fit into small areas (e.g. the carpal tunnel).

The peritendinous structures of tendons vary as much as the tendons themselves. Very organized and highly structured peritendon is present in the long finger flexors and extensors, contrasting with negligible peritendon in the tendons of the hip adductors and knee extensors.

Tendon injury affects individuals in the sporting and industrial population more than the general population. The prevalence of tendon injury varies between studies, depending on the tendon studied and the diagnostic criteria used. In the workplace, tendon injuries represent between 15% and 30% of medical cases, and in the sporting population, the prevalence is reported to be up to 50% in such conditions as tennis elbow in tennis players (Gross 1992).

Although tendon injury is a disabling and recurrent condition that is resistant to treatment, there are still many limitations on our understanding of the nature of tendon injury, repair, and treatment. Almekinders & Temple (1998) concluded that much of the pathology and etiology of tendinitis remains unclear and that currently used treatment methods may not significantly affect the natural history of the condition.

All tendons have similarities in microanatomy, histology, and pathology. This chapter will outline the anatomical structure and biomechanical properties of tendon tissue in both the normal and pathological state.

TENDONS – ANATOMY AND HISTOLOGY

As tendons come under the umbrella term of 'connective tissue', their structure is characteristic of this genre: a small cellular component that builds and maintains a much larger extracellular matrix. Macroscopically, healthy tendons are glistening and white, firm to touch but pliable (Józsa & Kannus 1997). Microscopically, the main components of tendon are the cells (tenocytes) and the extracellular matrix (collagen, elastin, and ground substance).

TENOCYTES

Tenocytes are the cellular components of tendon tissue that manufacture all the extracellular components of tendon. Consequently, tenocytes are rich in the organelles responsible for protein synthesis and transport, such as rough endoplasmic reticulum (rER) and Golgi apparatus. Despite this critical function, tenocytes are reported as being sparse in tendon (Khan et al 1999a) with a low respiratory quotient that indicates a low metabolic rate (O'Brien 1997).

Tenocytes are spindle-shaped longitudinally and stellate in cross-section with numerous cell processes extending between the collagen fibers (Kraushaar & Nirschl 1999, O'Brien 1997). Both epitenon cells and tenocytes communicate via these cell processes.

Tenocytes are not regulated from a central source but react to local stimuli (Leadbetter 1992). Tenocytes are deformed by, and respond to, mechanical load (Banes et al 1995), and change shape, function and composition in response to this load (Frank & Hart 1990). Tenocytes also communicate with each other in response to load (Shirakura et al 1995).

EXTRACELLULAR MATRIX

The extracellular matrix comprises the majority of tendon volume, and provides the strength and flexibility inherent in tendon. The components of the extracellular matrix are collagen, ground substance, elastin, connective tissue, and tenascin-C. The collagen and ground substance are the most important components of the matrix.

Collagen

Collagen, which endows tendon with its impressive tensile strength, is present in tendons as tightly packed fibers. Normal tendons consist mainly of type I collagen and small amounts of type III collagen found only in the endotendon of normal tendon (Williams et al 1984). Type I collagen has a large diameter (40–60 nm) and links together to form tight fiber bundles. Type III collagen is smaller in diameter (10–20 nm) and forms looser, more reticular bundles.

Collagen comprises 30% wet tendon weight and 80% dry weight. Collagen gives a tendon stiffness, rigidity, and strength when loaded, and flexibility when bent, compressed, twisted, or sheared.

The majority of collagen fibers run in the direction of stress (Frost 1990) with a spiral component, but some fibrils run perpendicular to the line of stress (Józsa et al 1991). The ratio of axial to non-axial fibers is between 10:1 and 26:1 (Józsa et al 1991). The larger diameter (> 1500 Å) fibers in longer tendons do not extend along the full length of the tendon (Benjamin & Ralphs 1995), but smaller diameter fibers may (Kirkendall & Garrett 1997).

Collagen fibers are formed in tendon cells and have a specific hierarchical order. In normal tendon, this structural order of collagen has five different levels (Robins 1988) and is described from microscopic to macroscopic structure (Fig. 3.1).

Level 1

Procollagen is formed in the rough endoplasmic reticulum of tenocytes as three polypeptide chains. Each procollagen chain consists of 1500 amino acid residues. Two of these chains are α-1 chains and the third is an α-2 chain with a different amino acid sequence. In the Golgi apparatus, procollagen forms a helix and is then transported to, and excreted from, the cell membrane in vacuoles via the cellular skeletal system of microtubules and microfilaments (O'Brien 1997). Procollagen is converted to insoluble tropocollagen in the extracellular matrix.

Level 2

Five tropocollagen molecules aggregate spontaneously to form collagen fibrils. There is an ordered overlap of one quarter of each tropocollagen molecule in fibrils which is responsible for the striated appearance of collagen on electron microscopy (Gross 1992). This overlap reinforces the collagen and leaves no weak transverse point where stress could cause disruption (O'Brien 1997, Robins 1988, Scott 1995).

Level 3

Fibrils, which are visible on electron microscopy, aggregate into bundles, forming fibers that are visible on light microscopy.

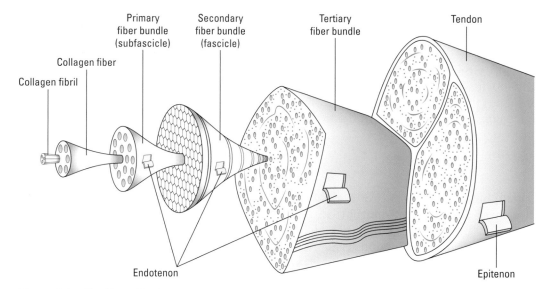

Figure 3.1 The hierarchical organization of tendon structure. (Reproduced from Khan et al 1999a, with the permission of Adis Press.)

Level 4

Fibers collect into fiber bundles hexagonal in shape and up to a third of a square mm in size.

Level 5

Fiber bundles group into fascicles surrounded by endotendon (O'Brien 1997). Fascicles are the longitudinal striations seen on ultrasonographic examination.

There is a regular sinusoidal pattern or 'crimp' in the extracellular matrix due to the tertiary structure of collagen, which is maintained in part by elastic fibers. This crimp has a periodicity of 100–200 µm (Robins 1988). Crimp facilitates shock absorption and allows tendon to stretch and recover fully. The so-called 'toe' area on the stress/strain curve represents crimp stretch.

The bonds between collagen helices are called cross-links. They are essential for the tensile strength of tendon and assist in maintaining tendon shape. The tendon strength gained from cross-links is reinforced by interaction between collagen and the proteoglycans in the ground substance.

Ground substance

Ground substance is found between collagen fibers and contributes to the viscoelastic properties of tendons. Although inconspicuous in normal tendon, ground substance still plays a very important role in the structure of the extracellular matrix of tendon. Ground substance organizes connective tissue by orientating and ordering collagen fibrils, and thus determines the ultimate tissue and organism shape (Scott 1995).

Ground substance attaches to, and surrounds, collagen fibril glycoproteins (Vogel et al 1984), helping collagen fibrils adhere to and slide past each other (Selvanetti et al 1997). Water, which comprises 60–80% of the weight of ground substance, allows gas and nutrient diffusion and cellular communication (O'Brien 1997, Scott 1988).

Ground substance is formed by an association between a proteoglycan and glycosaminoglycan (amino sugar) chains. Decorin constitutes most of the proteoglycan in tendon. This hydrophilic proteoglycan forms a tadpole-like ground substance that constitutes 90% of adult tendon. Aggregan, a large proteoglycan, and biglycan, both usually associated with cartilage, contribute to the other 10% of mature tendon (Vogel & Meyers 1999). In the area of tendon under anatomical compression, the amount of these alternate proteoglycans are significantly increased (Vogel et al 1993).

The bulbous proteoglycan part binds to specific sites of the collagen fiber (the D band) and the glycosamino-glycan chains associate and hold the protein parts, and hence the collagen, a specified distance apart. Most proteoglycans are oriented at 90° to the collagen fiber, while others are randomly arranged or lie parallel to the fiber (Scott 1988).

It is important for the tissue and the organism that collagen reaches a finite diameter in tissue and does not expand indefinitely. It appears that final collagen fibril diameter may be partly limited by the collagen structure itself, as well as being limited by ground substance (Rosenberg et al 1989, Scott 1988, Vogel et al 1984).

Tendons are subject to tensile loading, and both collagen and proteoglycans resist and transmit these tensile forces (Cribb & Scott 1995). Biological movement also causes compression and shearing of tissue, and tendons have weak resistance to these forces (Selvanetti et al 1997). Tendons that consistently undergo these forces have a higher amount of, and larger, proteoglycans, as proteoglycans resist the compressive forces on tendons (Giori et al 1993, Scott 1988). It appears that the compression of the tenocytes stimulates this proteoglycan response. Tendons may also have increased fibrocartilage in the loaded part of the tendon.

Elastin

Elastin is a small, but important part of normal tendon (2% of the dry mass of tendon) responsible in part for tendon flexibility (O'Brien 1997), but it has also been reported to be absent in normal tendon tissue (Józsa & Kannus 1997). Elastin is an insoluble, highly stable protein, which is rich in hydrophobic amino acids, and which lies closely related to the tenocyte.

Connective tissue

All bundles of collagen fibers and fascicles are surrounded by connective tissue called endotendon. The endotendon carries the blood vessels, nerves, and lymphatic vessels into and through the tendon. It appears to be the most important conduit of blood supply to the tendon (Ahmed et al 1998, Clancy 1990). The endotendon allows some movement between collagen bundles while still binding the collagen fibrils together (Józsa et al 1991).

Fascicle bundles aggregate to form a tendon and they are surrounded by peritendon. The peritendon contains two layers of connective tissue, the paratenon and the epitenon, which allow glide relative to surrounding tissue (Fig. 3.2). The epitenon and paratenon consist of a dense network of meshed collagen fibrils (Józsa et al 1991).

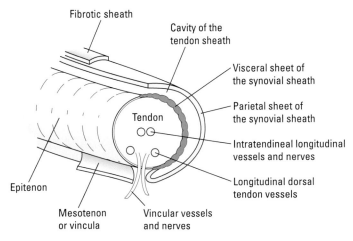

Figure 3.2 The structure of the tendon sheath. The peritendon comprises all the layers of connective tissue around the tendon. (Reproduced with permission from Józsa and Kannus 1997.)

The peritendinous structures vary in tendons depending on mechanical stress on the tendon and friction from surrounding structures. The paratenon can vary from a simple structure with loose, fatty areolar tissue to a complex, double-layered sheath lined with synovial cells (Clancy 1990). Paratenon with synovial cells is called tenosynovium, and a double-layered sheath without synovial cells is termed a tenovagium. All tendon connective tissue is continuous within the tendon, and in parts, continuous with muscle and bone connective tissue.

Tenascin-C

Tenascin-C is a protein found in tendon around the cells and collagen fibers. It appears in greater quantities at the junctional areas of the tendon: the bone–tendon and muscle–tendon junctions. It may be regulated by the amount of mechanical strain placed on the tenocytes. It is found in greater quantities after injury than in normal tendon. Tenascin-C is highly elastic and may provide some of the bonds between components of the extracellular matrix (Järvinen et al 2000).

BLOOD AND NERVE SUPPLY TO TENDON

BLOOD SUPPLY

Tendon is a relatively avascular structure compared to tissue such as muscle or skin, but for the metabolic demands that it has, tendon is well-vascularized tissue (Benjamin & Ralphs 1995, Hess et al 1989, Kirkendall & Garrett 1997). Tendon blood supply is variable, and affected by compression, torsion and friction.

Vascular supply to the tendon can arise from three sites: the musculotendinous junction, the bone–tendon junction, and the vessels in the surrounding connective tissue (Schatzker & Branemark 1969). It appears that the most important vascular supply to the tendon is from, and through, the surrounding connective tissue, via the peritendinous vessels (Archambault et al 1995, O'Brien 1992).

The bone–tendon junction is not traversed by blood vessels, and the fibrocartilage is avascular (Benjamin & Ralphs 1995, O'Brien 1997). Vessels for this region extend from the periosteum to the peritendon. Low intratendinous blood flow at tendon insertions has been shown experimentally in normal Achilles tendon insertion to the calcaneus (Astrom & Westlin 1994a).

Similarly, Clancy (1990) indicated that vessels from muscle do not connect directly with the tendon. The perimysium to peritendon vessels are the only vascular connection at this junction. These vessels are nonnutritive muscle vessels, and blood flow is affected by changes in muscle blood flow and metabolism (Clark et al 2000). Thus an increase in blood flow to muscle during exercise may redirect blood flow to muscle in preference to tendon.

It is suggested that normal tendons have critical areas of poor vascularity due to vascular and tendon anatomy, and that these areas are consequently more likely to develop pathology (Archambault et al 1995). Critical areas are reported to exist in the tendons of tibialis posterior at the medial malleolus, the Achilles 3–4 cm above the calcaneus, and the supraspinatus at the junction of the middle and lateral third. In the supraspinatus tendon, however, authors have reported the same area to contain the hypertrophied blood vessels of tendon pathology (Brooks et al 1992, Chansky & Iannotti 1991).

There is also evidence that the vascular supply of the Achilles tendon is adequate throughout its length. In a study of cadaver Achilles tendons, there was no variation in the number of blood vessels at any point along the length of the tendon (Ahmed et al 1998). Similarly, the recorded blood flow at the midpoint, insertion, and musculotendinous junction of normal Achilles tendon showed good correlation of flow between sites (Astrom & Westlin 1994a). These studies suggest that the blood supply at rest is not compromised at a particular point of the Achilles tendon.

It is still unclear, however, if the metabolic demands of the tendon are met by the blood supply in the active state. It is assumed that the metabolic demands of tendon remain low in exercise, due to the low number of cells (Kjaer et al 2000). Animal studies have shown increased blood flow in tendons during exercise (Archambault et al 1995).

Peritendinous flow in humans has been shown to be affected by work of the attached muscle, with a 2.5- to 4-fold increase in blood flow in the Achilles peritendinous space during muscle exercise (Langberg et al 1998). This suggests that the blood supply in the Achilles tendon is increased in exercise, as the tendon takes most of its midtendinous supply from the peritendon. This is not supported by studies which showed a decrease in tendinous blood flow during exercise (Astrom & Westlin 1994a). There are several differences in experimental methodology between these studies (method of assessing blood flow, type of exercise) and further studies have indicated that the blood flow increases proportional to the intensity of exercise (Kjaer et al 2000).

Other changes seen in the peritendinous region of the Achilles during exercise include increased metabolic activity, increased prostaglandins and increased type I collagen formation (Kjaer et al 2000).

NERVE SUPPLY

Tendons have a rich, almost exclusively afferent nerve supply that mediates proprioception (O'Brien 1997). Encapsulated and non-encapsulated nerve endings in tendon include type I Ruffini corpuscles, pressure receptors (stretch-sensitive), type II Paccinian corpuscles, type III Golgi tendon organs (mechanoreceptors), and type IV free nerve endings (pain) (O'Brien 1997). Most afferent nerve endings are near the muscle tendon junction (Kirkendall & Garrett 1997). Hence, the nerve supply of the midtendon may be minimal and pain sensitivity to pathological processes may be compromised.

TENDON STRUCTURES

The enthesis and myotendinous junction are two important structures of tendon.

ENTHESIS

Tendon insertion into bone (the enthesis) is a point of change in tissue flexibility from tendon to bone. Two types of enthesis have been described: the fibrocartilaginous enthesis and the fibrous enthesis. Fibrous enthesis occurs when the superficial tendon inserts into the periosteum and this occurs in metaphyseal and diaphyseal attachments (Benjamin & Ralphs 1996).

The fibrocartilaginous enthesis is a transitional zone where tendon graduates to bone through the sequence of layers, from normal tendon to fibrocartilage, then to mineralized fibrocartilage and finally to bone. This transition occurs within a variable distance (200–400 µ to several mm) (Benjamin & Ralphs 1998) and the thickness may be related to the amount of movement and load that occurs between the bone and tendon. The unmineralized fibrocartilage region has rows of rounded cells between bundles of type II collagen. Unlike tendon cells, these cells do not have connective arms to other cells (Benjamin & Ralphs 1998), hence there is no communication between bone and tendon cells. A distinct border (the blue line) separates mineralized from unmineralized fibrocartilage (Ferretti et al 1985). The blue line is composed of densely packed, randomly oriented collagen of various diameters that are continuous with both the mineralized and unmineralized fibrocartilage (O'Brien 1997).

The enthesis allows a gradual change in mechanical properties from the flexible tendon to the rigid bone. The fibrocartilage controls bending of fibers and distributes force to the bone (Kraushaar & Nirschl 1999). The more bending of fibers that occurs in a tendon due to load, the

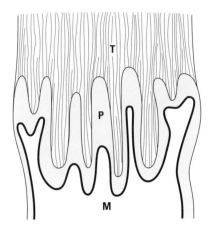

Figure 3.3 The myotendinous junction showing the high muscle to tendon ratio. T = Tendinous collagen fibrils. M = Muscle cell. P = Muscle processus. Closed arrowhead = Lamina densa of the muscular basement membrane. Open arrowhead = Lamina lucida of the muscular basement membrane. (Reproduced with permission from Józsa and Kannus 1997.)

more fibrocartilage is present at the enthesis. The enthesis also protects the tendon insertion from narrowing when the tendon is stretched, thus restricting the decrease in cross-sectional area (Benjamin & Ralphs 1998).

MYOTENDINOUS JUNCTION

The myotendinous junction is also a specialized anatomical area that allows transmission in force as well as the change in tissue flexibility and size. Because of these tissue changes, it is a common site of injury, usually termed a muscle strain (Clancy 1990). At this junction, the tendon bundles are invaginated, but separate from the muscle sarcomeres. Similar to the bone–tendon junction, the connective tissue of muscle and tendon blend together. As tendon collagen extends into the muscle at the musculotendinous junction, it provides more extensive attachment of tendon to muscle (O'Brien 1997) (Fig. 3.3). The amount of folding increases the surface area by 10-fold. There may be some structural differences in the myotendinous junctions between type 1 and type 2 muscle fibers (Kvist et al 1991).

BIOMECHANICAL PROPERTIES OF TENDONS

Tendons act as springs to store energy in locomotion and, as a result, the elastic properties of tendon are essential in athletic function. At the same time, tendons must transfer force efficiently to bone with minimal energy loss. Thus, the mechanical response of tendon to load is variable.

The mechanical properties of tendons can be expressed in terms of tensile stress and strain. Stress at any point in the tendon can be calculated by dividing the total tensile load of the tendon by the cross-sectional area at that point. Thus, the thinnest part of the tendon will be under the most stress. Strain is the amount the tendon stretches under load when compared to its unloaded length.

The relationship between stress and strain is well described by the stress–strain curve (Fig. 3.4). As illustrated, the initial load absorption is seen in the 'toe' region of the curve and represents tendon 'uncrimping'. The linear portion of the curve occurs between 2% and 4% strain and this slope represents the stiffness of the tendon. These two regions account for the normal physiological range of the tendon.

Pathological load on tendon begins at approximately 4% strain when collagen failure begins. Initially cross-links breakdown, but eventually fibers, fibrils and fascicles rupture, and this is represented by the plateau in the curve. At approximately 8–10% strain, the tendon fails completely. However, ultimate strain levels vary in tendons and individuals, and may occur between 8% and 30% strain (Gelberman et al 1988). The physiological magnitude of force produced by the muscle is normally well below that required to rupture a tendon unless it is weakened by other factors (Fyfe & Stanish 1992).

Tendon reacts differently depending on the amount and rate of load application. At low tensile loads, the tendon has high extensibility, while at higher tensile loads, this extensibility is reduced (Gelberman et al 1988). The rate of load application also influences tendon properties, with quicker load application resulting in both greater tendon stiffness and ability to withstand load

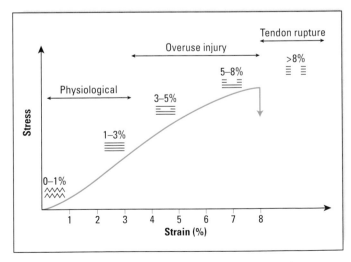

Figure 3.4 Stress–strain curve for tendon. (Reproduced from Khan et al 1998 Patellar tendinopathy: some aspects of basic science and clinical management. British Journal of Sports Medicine 32: 346–355, with permission from the BMJ Publishing Group.)

(Benjamin & Ralphs 1996). Larger tendons can withstand larger loads and longer tendons have greater absolute elongation before rupture (Fyfe & Stanish 1992).

Tendons are viscoelastic, mainly due to the presence of ground substance (Schatzmann et al 1998). Stress relaxation and creep are viscoelastic, time-dependent behaviors of normal tendons. Stress relaxation, the decrease in force needed to maintain tendon length over time, is important in sport when constant and repetitive loads are applied. Creep is the gradual lengthening of tendon under constant load. Hysteresis is the difference in the stress–strain curves after a tendon is stretched, and there is a release of heat from hysteresis.

Cyclic loading of tendon in athletic participation may cause creep, and thus may lead to failure of part or all of the tendon at lower loads (Selvanetti et al 1997). An alternative opinion is that cyclic loading in sports 'softens' the tendon and decreases the potential for fatigue failure (Woo & Tkach 1990). Both these reactions to loading are possible and the tendon response may depend on the rate of loading, the immediate biomechanical history of the tendon, and the condition of the tendon.

Tendons, therefore, resist tensile loads well, but only to a certain limit. This limit is determined by the size and shape of the tendon, and is affected by disease and non-tensile forces.

EFFECT OF EXERCISE

The effect of exercise on tendons has been investigated in animals. The animal models, the age of animals used, and the type of tendon studied vary in these studies. Some animal studies have shown that exercise increases the cross-sectional area, collagen fiber thickness, and cellularity of tendons in young animals, but results vary from species to species (Maffulli & King 1992). Adult animal tendons appear to respond to exercise by improving tensile strength and total weight of collagen, without the increase in tendon area (Kannus et al 1997, Maffulli & King 1992).

The effect of exercise on tendons in humans is unclear. Exercise may increase collagen synthesis, the size and number of fibrils, and consequently tensile strength (Kannus et al 1997, O'Brien 1997). Frost (1990) hypothesized that tendons increase in diameter with gradual load by adding collagen to increase cross-sectional diameter. Selvanetti et al (1997) suggested that exercise lowers crimp length and increases the strength of entheses.

Most effects of exercise on tendon appear to border on the pathological, with collagen fiber changes, tenocyte activation, and alterations in ground substance. It has been suggested that to effect a change in tendon strength, there must be a period of transient weakness (Archambault

et al 1995). This period provides a model for overuse tendinopathies, if load is reapplied before adaptation occurs. The time frame of transient weakness and adaptation to load is not known, making clinical application impossible.

There appears to be a fine line between load that stimulates positive cellular response and load that triggers a degrading response in tendons (Frank & Hart 1990). It has been suggested that the increase in inflammatory mediators in the peritendon during and after exercise is a stimulant to increased collagen formation along an undefined pathway (Kjaer et al 2000). The relationship between these changes in the peritendon and what occurs in the tendon itself are unclear, and demonstrating similar changes in the tendon remains experimentally difficult. Positron emission tomography may offer potential to further research in this area (Nuutila & Kalliokoski 2000).

TENDON PATHOLOGY

Knowledge and understanding of tendon pathology is improving as better technology allows more sophisticated research. Historically, inflammation was accepted as the pathology of both acute and overuse tendon injury, and the term for tendon inflammation was tendinitis. The histopathology of overuse tendon injury at end-stage disease, however, repeatedly shows little or no evidence of inflammation (Benazzo et al 1996, Ferretti et al 1983, Khan et al 1996).

There is a dearth of controlled, randomized, prospective studies on all aspects of tendon disease (Almekinders & Temple 1998), particularly those studies that examine the early stages of tendinopathy and the repair process of overuse tendinopathy.

NOMENCLATURE

Many different terms are used to describe chronic tendinopathy (Almekinders & Temple 1998, Astrom & Rausing 1995), even the spelling varies from author to author. More recent reviews have attempted to clarify the terms used when describing tendon pathology (Khan et al 1999a, Maffulli et al 1998), encompassing pathology states as well as clinical status.

The term tendinosis was first used in the 1970s (Puddu et al 1976) to describe the non-inflammatory tendon pathology reported at the end stage of the disease, and the term has been used interchangeably with the term degeneration. However, the terminology of degeneration suggests that a decrease in cellularity and function is involved (Leadbetter 1992). As tendinopathy is mainly hypercellular, and has an increase in tissue function, the term degeneration may not be the most applicable.

Failed healing response has also been used to describe the state of tendinopathy and this appears to be the most fitting concept. Clancy (1989) suggested that several factors may contribute to a tendon's failure to heal. These include diminished vascularity, decreased cellularity, lack of reparative cell migration, disease, and auto-immune or hereditary factors.

CAUSES OF TENDON INJURY

The amount, rate, frequency, and duration of load are all factors that affect the ability of the tendon to adapt to stress. Thus, tendon overload may occur if muscle tension is applied too quickly, repetitively or obliquely, or if sudden musculotendinous stretch occurs (Hess et al 1989). Tendons with anatomical pressures, such as those that abut a bony structure, or those that cross more than one joint, are also susceptible to overuse. Physio-logical susceptibility from poor vascularity also predisposes a tendon to damage (Kraushaar & Nirschl 1999).

There are several theories on the cause of tendon injury, including factors that influence either tendon load or the tendon repair process. Overload from repetitive submaximal loads (Hess et al 1989, Selvanetti et al 1997), too much load leading to, or resulting from, muscle weakness (El Hawary et al 1997, Frost 1990, Kannus 1997c, Molnar & Fox 1993), and impaired shock absorption (Kannus 1997c) have been considered in the literature. Direct load on the tendon causing impingement in the patellar tendon and supraspinatus tendon is also a possible mechanism, as tendons are susceptible to compressive load (Johnson et al 1996). Factors influencing tendon repair, such as insufficient time frames and accumulated microinjury (Hart et al 1995), are also thought to continue the cycle of tendon injury.

Acute tendon injuries such as partial or complete tears, are less common than overuse injuries in tendons and may be due to contusion as well as the tensile and compressive stresses discussed above. Acute tendon rup-ture is thought to occur only after the tendon is affected by other factors, such as degenerative changes (Kannus & Józsa 1991). Individual factors that set 'lower' levels of normal tendon function may also contribute to tendon injury (Hart et al 1995).

CAUSES OF PATHOLOGY

Just as the literature is unclear about the cause of tendon injury, there is also uncertainty about the intratendinous mechanism that initiates pathology. What happens in the tendon after an insult? There are three possible causes

of tendon pathology: vascular compromise, thermal damage, and biochemical irritation.

Vascular damage that affects the oxygen supply to the tendon is thought by many authors to be the most likely cause of tendinopathy (El Hawary et al 1997, Williams 1986). As there is no direct evidence of vascular compromise in human tendinopathy (Astrom & Westlin 1994b), the theory of impaired vascularity as a cause of tendinopathy has been challenged (Almekinders & Temple 1998, Leadbetter 1992).

Equine tendon studies indicate that thermal damage may also contribute to the onset of tendinopathy. Tenocyte death may result from exercise-induced hyper-thermia caused by intratendinous heat release from hysteresis (Wilson & Goodship 1992, Wilson & Goodship 1994) and limitations of intratendinous heat transfer (Hart et al 1995). Tenocyte death leaves the tendon with a diminished reparative ability.

Potential chemical damage to tendons comes from the inflammatory paradigm. Tendon injury may be caused by modulation of cellular activity (Leadbetter 1992) due to the release of free radicals, enzymes, or cytokines by inflammatory or intratendinous cells (Józsa & Kannus 1997).

NATURE OF TENDON PATHOLOGY

Although it is unclear what process initiates tendon pathology, the disease process is consistent and there are four aspects of tendinopathy that are found in most types of tendinopathy: changes in tenocyte function, collagen degradation, vascular ingrowth, and ground substance proliferation. All of these changes are critical components of tendon pathology and are discussed in the following section.

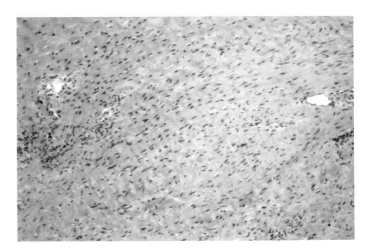

Figure 3.5 Proliferation of fibroblasts in an area of tendinopathy. The large number of cells in this area contrasts to normal tendon with sparse distribution of cells. (Reproduced with permission from Sally F. Bonar.)

TENOCYTES

In tendinopathy, there may be an increase or decrease in cell numbers and activity (Fig. 3.5). Tenocytes that are activated are stimulated into an active, blastic state by signals from the surrounding matrix, such as shear forces that stimulate mechanoreceptors on the cell surface, or from self-produced stimulants such as growth factors (Postlethwaite 1989). These cells become more rounded and the nucleus more prominent and numerous (Astrom & Rausing 1995).

Some areas of tendon are associated with tenocyte degeneration and death, not activation. The cell nucleus and organelles fail and the tenocyte is not capable of tendon repair (Józsa et al 1982).

EXTRACELLULAR MATRIX

Collagen

Collagen degradation is pivotal to the pathological process in tendons. It is described in all studies reporting tendon pathology and repair. The collagen is no longer tightly bundled and dense in network and loses its regular crimp, periodicity and birefringence under polarized light (Järvinen et al 1997, Jones et al 1996, Józsa et al 1984a, Józsa et al 1984b, Józsa et al 1990, Kannus & Józsa 1991, Khan et al 1996, Khan et al 1999a, Kraushaar & Nirschl 1999, Popp et al 1997, Scranton & Farrar 1992). These descriptions indicate there is a breakdown of the tightly packed collagen bundles of normal tendon, with a consequent loss of tissue and tendon strength. Apart from specific descriptions of transverse fiber disruption seen in tendon rupture, most descriptions of collagen changes allude to longitudinal disruption of the collagen.

Ground substance

The increase in ground substance is a central feature of tendinopathy and is the main component of the 'mucoid', 'cystic', and 'hyaline' appearance of pathology described in the literature (Astrom & Rausing 1995). The increase in ground substance has been suggested to be the primary response to mechanical overload, secondarily affecting the collagen formation and cross-links (Scott 1988). This is in contrast to the usual description of tendon reaction to overload, which is reported to have a primary effect on collagen.

Apart from an increase in ground substance, there may be a change in proteoglycans in the pathological state. The amount of aggregan is increased, changing the decorin to aggregan ratio. Aggregan forms chondroiten sulphate, which is the ground substance of cartilaginous tissue (Benazzo et al 1996).

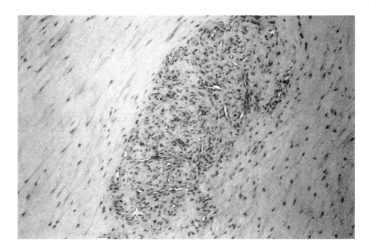

Figure 3.6 Vascular proliferation in an area of tendinopathy. The capillary infiltration is in contrast to normal tendon which is relatively hypovascular. (Reproduced with permission from Sally F. Bonar.)

Vascularity

Neovascularization has been well documented as an important component of tendon pathology (Fig. 3.6). It is closely related to collagen fiber degeneration and may be stimulated by hypoxia (Astrom & Rausing 1995). New vessels are generally considered to be an ingrowth of blood vessels, although Kraushaar and Nirschl (1999) believe they are the result of local metaplasia rather than ingrowth from an extrinsic source.

The new vessels in tendon pathology are thick-walled, with an irregular distribution (Astrom & Rausing 1995, Leadbetter 1992), and it appears that some may be compromised with obliterative and thrombotic vascular changes (Järvinen et al 1997, Kvist et al 1992, Leadbetter 1992). These immature and structurally incomplete vessels may result in poor vascular function (Kraushaar & Nirschl 1999). Consequently, the vascularity may not improve tendon oxygenation, and neovascularization does not appear to be associated with areas of improved repair (Kraushaar & Nirschl 1999).

However, direct measurement of vascularity in Achilles tendinopathy showed increased blood flow, with no evidence of local deficiency of vascular supply (Astrom & Westlin 1994b). Similarly, evidence of both arteriole and venous blood flow has been shown by Doppler ultrasound (US) in tendons diagnosed with tendinosis (Ohberg et al 2001)

OTHER PATHOLOGY

The previous section describes the histopathology of basic tendinopathy, however, it encompasses more than this simple entity. Variations in tendinopathy exist, with slight differences in histopathological appearance. These variations include all the vascular, cellular, collagen, and ground substance alterations as described in the previous section.

The names for these variations include hypoxic, mucoid, myxoid, lipoid, and calcific tendinopathy (Järvinen et al 1997, Józsa et al 1984c, Józsa et al 1982). It is unclear how or why tendon pathology varies in different tendons in the body and between individuals, and the causative factors underlying each type of pathology are unknown (Kannus 1997a).

All these types of tendon pathology may be found in the same tendon, even in close proximity to each other. They are all found in ruptured tendons and appear to have an etiological role in tendon weakness and rupture (Kannus & Józsa 1991). In a series of 891 tendon ruptures, hypoxic change was the most common histopathology (Kannus & Józsa 1991). In the same study, only one third of unruptured tendons in subjects of similar age and activity levels demonstrated histopathological changes.

Calcification in tendons is usually found in areas of pathology and is described as part of the process of tendon damage and repair. In the rotator cuff, however, acute calcifying tendinopathy can occur in areas of normal tendon. This process appears to be a cell-mediated response and is associated with specific human leukocyte antigens tissue (HLA) typing (A1) (Sengar et al 1987). This type of acute and often resolving tendinopathy has rarely been reported in other tendons. Sengar et al 1989 reported no association between this HLA typing and rotator cuff rupture.

Inflammation

Inflammation is the initial response of all tissues to injury, and is also the start of the reparative process. Thus, it is well accepted that inflammation occurs in a tendon after macrotrauma such as tenotomy and tendon rupture. The inflammatory response to tendon injury may be mediated by age, gender, disease, and individual, perhaps genetically determined, factors (Hart et al 1995).

There is a firm belief that an inflammatory process must occur to initiate tendon repair (Williams 1986). Kannus (1997a) stated that inflammation occurs acutely following injury, and may lead to tendon degeneration.

Histopathological studies at end-stage tendinopathy have demonstrated few inflammatory cells (Astrom & Rausing 1995, Khan et al 1996, Khan et al 1999a, Teitz et al 1997) and the concept of tendinosis without current or previous inflammation must be considered (Maffulli et al 1998). In overloaded rat tendon, Zamora and Marini (1988) demonstrated non-inflammatory overuse tendinopathy with activated tenocytes and disrupted collagen at 7 and 14 days after tendon overload.

However, inflammation in tendons may be apparent around intratendinous calcification and at the site of steroid injection (Leadbetter 1992, Selvanetti et al 1997). It is also apparent in rheumatoid arthritis, gout, seronegative arthropathies, and septic tendinopathies (Selvanetti et al 1997). Nirschl (1990) reported that inflammatory cells may be seen in tissues in close proximity to the tendon although absent from the tendon itself. There are no current scientific investigations that conclusively demonstrate inflammation in human overuse tendon pathology and more investigation is needed. Most investigators agree that inflammatory pathology affects peritendinous tissues (paratenonitis, peritendinitis, tenosynovitis, tenovaginitis) (Järvinen et al 1997, Józsa et al 1990).

STRUCTURAL CHANGES IN TENDON PATHOLOGY

Enthesopathies

Musculotendinous overuse affects the enthesis, as can metabolic, endocrine, and inflammatory disease (Benjamin & Ralphs 1996). All these stimulants cause the transitional bone–tendon zone to become abnormally organized. Pathology of the enthesis includes abnormalities in the fibrocartilage (thickening, mineralization, and myxomatosis) (Benjamin & Ralphs 1995, Ferretti et al 1985, Selvanetti et al 1997, Uhthoff & Matsumoto 2000), the mineralized fibrocartilage (cystic cavities) (Ferretti et al 1985), and the tendon (decreased cellularity, calcification) (Selvanetti et al 1997).

Although few authors mention inflammation as a component of enthesopathies, Kannus indicated that acute enthesopathies are inflammatory (Kannus 1997a). Occasional bony 'tug' lesions are seen at the enthesis in tendon injury, where a small fragment of bone is avulsed with the tendon, and this may enhance the repair as it may allow blood vessel ingrowth from the bone. This phenomenon provides the rationale for drilling bone in surgical procedures involving articular cartilage and enthesopathies.

Entheses may be prone to injury at a slower rate of load application compared with tendon (Fyfe & Stanish 1992). Enthesis failure often occurs at the subchondral bone, suggesting that the enthesis is not an area of weakness (Benjamin & Ralphs 1998). This is supported by studies of the mechanical properties of tendons that suggest the insertional regions of tendons withstand high strain without rupture (Wren et al 2001).

Paratenonitis

Paratenonitis commonly occurs where a tendon rubs over a bony protuberance or abuts another structure, but can occur anywhere along the length of a tendon. The term has been proposed as an umbrella term for the separate entities of peritendinitis, tenosynovitis, and tenovaginitis. Examples include paratenonitis of the abductor pollicis longus and extensor pollicis longus (De Quervain's disease), and of the flexor hallucis longus as it passes the medial malleolus of the tibia (Almekinders 1998, Józsa & Kannus 1997).

Paratenonitis is characterized clinically by acute edema and hyperemia of the paratenon with infiltration of inflammatory cells. Fibrinous exudate fills the tendon sheath after several hours to a few days, and causes the 'crepitus' that can be felt on clinical examination. In chronic paratenonitis, fibroblasts appear along with a perivascular lymphocytic infiltrate. Peritendinous tissue becomes macroscopically thickened and new connective tissue adhesions occur (Järvinen et al 1997). Myofibroblasts (cells with cytoplasmic myofilaments) also appear and make up about 20% of the non-inflammatory cells. These cells are capable of active contraction, indicating that scarring and shrinkage associated with paratenonitis is an active cell-mediated process (Järvinen et al 1997). Blood vessels proliferate, and marked inflammatory changes are seen in more than 20% of the arteries (Kvist et al 1992). Thus, inflammatory cells are found in both the cellular elements of the peritendon and the vascular ingrowth.

TENDON REPAIR

Soft tissue healing is usually sufficient to maintain function, however, repair of tendons is never complete (Frank et al 1999). Tendons appear to have the capacity to repair adequately, as both endogenous tenocytes and extrinsic cells originally from outside the tendon, can migrate to tendon damage and contribute to the repair process. There is some debate about the relative contributions of the intrinsic and extrinsic cells to tendon repair, and recent studies have indicated that the tendon is capable of healing without immigration of extrinsic cells (Kraushaar & Nirschl 1999). The type and site of the injury may determine which repair process is initiated (Gelberman et al 1988). Repair is influenced by age, tendon vascularity, gender, nutrition, hormones, activity, and disease (Hart et al 1995, Leadbetter 1992).

Clancy (1989) considers that the poor healing response in tendon is due in part to reparative cells failing to migrate to the site of injury. Alternatively, the poor healing response (Leadbetter 1992) may partly be explained by the inability of tenocytes to repair tendon quickly and adequately enough. There are, however, many chemotactic signals that stimulate the migration of cells to the injury site, including several that are produced without vascular damage. Tendon microtrauma should therefore produce a healing response with or without vascular disruption (Postlethwaite 1989).

Type III collagen is the collagen produced in repairing tendon after both acute and overuse tendon injury (Józsa et al 1990), and is considered by some authors to be a 'tendon patch' (Archambault et al 1995). It is smaller than type I collagen and forms a looser reticular network rather than the long thick bundles of type I (Józsa et al 1984b). This collagen was also more easily denatured experimentally, indicating that cross-links were weaker than in type I collagen. It has been hypothesized that this smaller diameter collagen may be, in part, responsible for the decrease in tendon strength associated with pathology (Archambault et al 1995, Williams et al 1984).

Post injury, type III collagen is reportedly replaced by type I collagen at a variable point in time and the tendon becomes stiffer and stronger as the replacing type I collagen matures (O'Brien 1997). Type III collagen comprised 20–30% of scarred equine tendon, and was still apparent up to 14 months after injury (Williams et al 1980, Williams et al 1984). The time frame for maturation and repair are unknown, and thus application to clinical practice is impossible.

MACROTRAUMATIC REPAIR

Tendon repair research has evaluated models of tendon rupture and experimental tenotomy (Hart et al 1995). These studies have indicated that tendon requires three stages for repair: cell proliferation, collagen synthesis, and collagen realignment (El Hawary et al 1997). The complete process includes inflammation, epitenon thickening, fibroblast proliferation, cell activation, vascular ingrowth, matrix, and collagen production and remodeling (Gelberman et al 1988, Leadbetter 1992).

In tenotomized rabbit Achilles tendon, inflammation and blood clotting are the primary processes until day 5, followed by an increase in ground substance and disorganized fibrils (day 7). The tendon remains very cellular until day 12 but by day 18, inflammatory cells are no longer present (Enwemeka 1989). As inflammation decreases post injury, so do both tendon cellularity and vascularity (Hart et al 1995).

Fibronectin in the ground substance, a major component of granulation tissue, may form a template for the reparative tendon (O'Brien 1997). It is apparent in equine tendon for 1 month post injury (Williams et al 1984).

MICROTRAUMATIC REPAIR

Overuse tendon injuries 'lack the ordered and timely triphased reparative response' of acute injury (Selvanetti et al 1997). Very little, however, has been written on the repair of overuse tendon injury especially in human tendons (Clancy 1989, El Hawary et al 1997), where experimental design and ethical considerations limit investigation.

There are several factors that contribute to the quality of tendon healing response, including the type and intensity of the injury, individual factors and treatment. Overloaded tendon has been called a tissue that has a failed healing response, defined as either an inadequate or extravagant inflammatory process response (Clancy 1989, Hart et al 1995). This may be associated with a failure of the alignment and cross-linking of collagen (Kraushaar & Nirschl 1999).

As has been postulated in Figure 3.7, there may be a cyclic relationship between normal tendon, pathology and repair. What is often reported as pathology may in fact represent tendon repair (Fredberg & Bolvig 1999). The distinction between repair and pathology may be important, as the presence of reparative signs such as type III collagen and tenocyte activity are a positive tendon response.

Do tendons repair completely and return to their original state? Although the theory of tendon repair describes the eventual replacement of type III collagen with type I collagen, it appears that there is less than perfect replacement, and consequently repair. Repaired tendons may only return to 70–80% of their original strength (Leadbetter 1993).

The future direction of tendon repair is to further explore critical factors in the tendons' response to injury. This includes investigation into tenocyte control systems, chemical signals for tendon maturation, and collagen stimulation (Kraushaar & Nirschl 1999). Similarly,

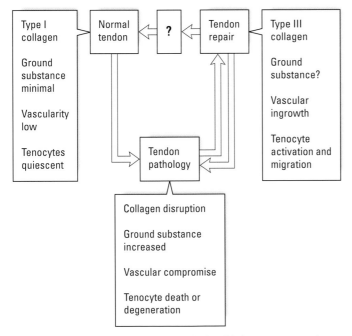

Figure 3.7 An hypothesized cyclic relationship between normal, pathological, and repairing tendon. Repair is an active state with tenocyte activity and extracellular matrix production. However, added strain on the tendon before completion of repair may push the tendon back into tendon pathology, with disruption of extracellular matrix and tenocyte destruction. It is unclear if complete tendon recovery occurs.

investigations in ligament tissue have suggested that altering the cellularity and altering cellular expression may offer improvement in the repair process (Frank et al 1999). This tissue engineering is in its embryonic stages, but may turn our current passive approach to tendon injury to more active interventions.

GROWTH FACTORS

A superfamily of growth, differentiation, and morphogenic factors exists in human cells, with each cell making and responding to some of these factors (Sanzone & Einhorn 1998). Growth factors are necessary for normal tissue repair, as load without growth factors may lead to cell death and matrix degradation (Banes et al 1995). Transforming growth factor-β (TGF-β) refers to several factors (TGF-β1 to TGF-β5) that may be released by platelets and initiate a repair cascade in soft tissue (Sporn & Roberts 1989).

Cells from both ligament and tendon have been shown to be responsive to several growth factors (Sanzone & Einhorn 1998). Growth factors act both embryogenically and as an intrinsic part of tissue repair, and have been shown to attract macrophages and tenoblasts to tissue injury (Jann et al 1999, Sporn & Roberts 1989), influence the differentiation of connective tissue cells into tendon forming cells (growth differentiation factors GDF-5 to GDF-7) (Sanzone & Einhorn 1998), and control extracellular matrix degradation (Robins 1988).

Bone morphogenic proteins have been shown to directly improve tendon repair (Aspenberg & Forslund 2000), with cartilage derived morphogenic proteins (CDMP) 1 and 2 increasing the strength of transected rat Achilles tendon and tendon cross-sectional area.

Growth factors offer an exciting potential therapy after tissue damage, and tendons in particular would benefit from agents that can facilitate repair.

TENDON PAIN

The source of pain in pathological tendon tissue is not clearly understood. Although the pain producing mechanisms are easy to explain if there is inflammation, the lack of inflammation in overuse tendinopathy leaves the source of pain unexplained. There are many theories about the cause of tendinopathic pain, and an increasing body of evidence that suggests a biochemical rather than structural cause of pain (Khan et al 2000).

If collagen disruption (either transverse or longitudinal) was the source of pain in the tendon, pain would accompany all forms of tendinopathy. However it is known that the removal of large chunks of collagen (e.g. in the harvesting of tendon tissue for ligament reconstruction) rarely results in tendon pain. Similarly, there is poor correlation between imaging changes after tendon surgery and symptoms (Khan et al 1999b). Both these observations suggest that collagen damage is not a source of pain.

The concept that intact collagen surrounding tendinopathy is overloaded and that it is the source of pain is also partly rebutted by the above discussion. This model suggests that tendons with greater areas of tendinopathy should be more painful, as there is less intact tissue sustaining greater load. Imaging studies have shown that there is little correlation between the amount of collagen disruption and pain, with large abnormal areas demonstrated as being asymptomatic on US, and tendons with normal imaging as having symptoms (Cook et al 2000, Cook et al 1998).

Although collagen disruption per se may not be the source of tendon pain, the tendon reaction to collagen damage may create a biochemical environment that stimulates nociceptors. There is a theoretical basis for this, as well as evidence to support it. Theoretically, hypoxia, cellular and extracellular debris, minor collagens, and proteoglycans have been suggested as the source of nociceptor stimulation. Glutamate (Alfredson et al 1999) and substance P (Gotoh et al 1998) have been shown to be associated with tendon pain, as have receptors to substance P (Ljung et al 1999). Other possible mechanisms for tendon pain include irritation of the surrounding (and usually well innervated) structures (e.g. fat pad in the knee, subacromial bursa in the shoulder) and increased intratendinous pressure (Johnson et al 1996). These remain theories only, and further investigation is required.

A clinical relationship between pain and tissue damage has been described (Fig. 3.8). This theoretical model allows clinical application of this complex relationship, however, research is required to validate the model.

The source of tendon pain is a clinically critical aspect of tendinopathy, as treatment for tendinopathy is primarily directed at decreasing pain. Further research in this area is underway, and pharmaceutical, not physical intervention may prove ideal.

ETIOLOGY OF TENDON INJURY

Risk factors contribute to the possibility of injury and may be considered intrinsic or extrinsic. Intrinsic factors are variations within the individual, such as anatomical, biomechanical, and genetic components, whereas extrinsic factors are those risks that come from outside the individual, such as environment and equipment. The following sections will consider each of the intrinsic categories of risk factors as they pertain to tendon.

INTRINSIC RISK FACTORS

How do the anatomy and biomechanics of each individual influence the load on tendons, and does this add potential for the subsequent breakdown of tendon tissue? Many factors such as age, disease, genetics and gender are hypothesized to influence either the onset of tendinopathy or the outcome of the condition.

Anatomical factors

Variations in anatomical structure have been suggested as predisposing factors in overuse tendon disease (Kannus 1997c), although studies linking anatomy to tendinopathy are rare. Well-designed studies showing a causative relationship between anatomy and tendon pathology are even less common (Almekinders & Temple 1998). More prospective studies (Witvrouw et al 2000) are required.

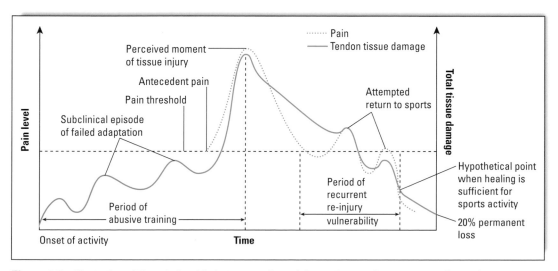

Figure 3.8 Illustration of the relationship between pain and tissue damage in overuse tendinopathy. (Reproduced from Khan et al 1999a with the permission of Adis Press.)

Factors linked to tendinopathy include leg length discrepancy, flexibility (increased or decreased), foot structure, valgum and varum joints, specific measurements (Q angle), limb rotation (femoral anteversion), and joint range of movement (Hess et al 1989, Neely 1998). Although some studies have reported a relationship between these factors and injury (often not specifically tendinopathy as stated above), just as many studies have found no relationship (Duri & Aichroth 1995, Ferretti et al 1983). Methods of assessment of anatomical factors and definition of injury are most likely to be the cause of these varying outcomes.

Age

Aging substantially reduces the ability of tendon to adapt to environmental stress (Leadbetter 1992, Tuite et al 1997) and causes the tendon to become stiffer, weaker, and less load-tolerant (Hess et al 1989). Increasing age negatively affects all components of the tendon – decreasing the rate of collagen turnover, the amount of ground substance, water content (Selvanetti et al 1997), vascularization, and the number of cells, their activity levels (Hess et al 1989, Leadbetter, 1992), and their organelle function (Clancy 1990). The amount of bone at insertion points is also reduced. Aging also increases collagen cross-linking and diameter (Maffulli & King 1992) and the width of the type II collagen-containing areas of fibrocartilage in the enthesis (Benjamin et al 1991).

It appears that age itself may not 'cause' tendinopathy; however, the disease process when initiated (probably at lower loads than in younger people) may be more severe in the older person. The severity of histopathologic changes and the prevalence of tendinopathy were associated with increasing age in a study that examined subjects with Achilles tendon symptoms (Astrom & Rausing 1995). Age has been implicated in many other studies, with the peak incidence of chronic tendon injuries occurring between 30 and 50 years (Almekinders & Temple 1998). However, cadaver tendons used as a control group (Khan et al 1996, Maffulli 1999) are often from an older subject and few tendons have pathology. Nirschl (1990) hypothesized that physiological age of the tissue may be more important than the chronological age of the subject, and the physiological age of tissue is increased by cumulative overuse.

Blood Group

There may be a link between an individual's blood group and tendon rupture. In a series of 891 tendon ruptures, individuals with blood type O were over-represented in tendon rupture, and blood type A individuals were under-represented, relative to the expected ratios in the population (Józsa et al 1989). The authors hypothesized

that N-acetylgalactosamine is a necessary component of connective tissue. This substance is lower in individuals with blood type O, and higher in blood type A individuals. The same over-representation of individuals with blood group O was found in subjects with Achilles tendon ruptures (Kujala et al 1992). Subsequently, also in Achilles tendon ruptures in Scotland, this association was not statistically demonstrated (Maffulli et al 2000), the authors hypothesizing that a different genetic population and distribution of ABO blood types were the possible cause of the different results.

Gender

The literature reports that several factors predispose females to the development of tendinopathy. The higher incidence of tendon and other overuse injuries in women reportedly occur because they are weaker musculoskeletally, have higher body fat, and less muscle mass and strength relative to males (Kannus 1997c). Anatomical and biomechanical factors specific to females, such as a wider pelvis, are also thought to contribute to tendinopathy. There are, however, several studies that demonstrate a lower rate of tendon injury in females. Although female military recruits had twice the rate of lower limb injury than males, tendinopathy at all sites in females was half (7%) that of males (15%) (Neely 1998). A lower rate of Achilles tendon ruptures in females has also been described (Järvinen 1992), despite the author suggesting that more females have overuse sports injuries.

A critical review of the literature provides support for the case that females have a lower prevalence of tendinopathy than males. Females are significantly under-represented in imaging, conservative treatment, and surgical treatment of tendinopathy especially in the lower limb. Likewise, several studies that recruited subjects without considering symptoms have indicated that females have less tendinopathy. Studies of 588 patellar tendons in two recent studies (Cook et al 2000, Cook et al 1998) revealed that females had half the prevalence of tendinopathy of males. In sports with a higher risk of tendinopathy (e.g. basketball), the prevalence rose in both genders, and the ratio of males to females remained at 2:1.

The reason for the difference in prevalence between genders is not known, although blood supply and hormonal factors have been suggested (Astrom & Westlin 1994a, Liu et al 1997). Although anatomical and physiological reasons are suspected, it is impossible to rule out sociological and environmental factors such as sports participation and competitiveness.

Blood flow in normal female Achilles tendons is higher than that of males (Astrom 1997). If reduced vascularity is a cause of tendinopathy, then females may have an inbuilt protective mechanism.

The role of estrogen in soft tissue injury and repair is unclear. Some authors suggest that estrogen may be protective for tendons (Leadbetter 1992). Nirschl (1990) stated that tendinosis in women has been attributed to a decrease in estrogen after menopause. Supporting these authors, in a study of 4000 Achilles tendon ruptures, the peak incidence of rupture in males was 30–39 years, compared to 80+ years in females, with a rising prevalence from 60 years (Maffulli et al 1999).

The role of estrogen in other collagen-based structures is variable. It is well known that estrogen offers a protective effect on bony tissue (Aloia 1982). The effect in ligament, structurally very similar to tendon, is less clear. Estrogen at physiological levels has been shown to decrease collagen synthesis and fibroblast proliferation in rabbit anterior cruciate ligaments (Liu et al 1997).

Clinically, the risk of an anterior cruciate ligament tear is significantly higher in females than males. The authors speculated that this may explain athletic ligament tears in females, as estrogen receptors are present in ligaments (Liu et al 1997). Other hormones and enzymes such as testosterone and insulin, as well as estrogen, are reported to increase collagen synthesis (O'Brien 1992). However, fluctuations in estrogen levels appear not to change ligament elasticity, as the menstrual cycle did not affect anterior cruciate ligament laxity (Karageanes et al 2000). Other intrinsic factors such as ligament size may be the reason behind this gender difference (Anderson et al 2001).

Systemic disease and genetics

Systemic diseases that have clinical manifestations in tendons include diabetes, sarcoidosis, systemic lupus erythematosis, hyperparathyroidism, and inflammatory arthropathies such as gout, rheumatoid arthritis, and psoriasis (David 1989, Järvinen et al 1997, Kaar et al 1993, Maddox & Garth 1986). Individuals with leukocyte antigen HLA B-27 appear to be vulnerable to Achilles tendinopathy (Järvinen et al 1997), independent of the antigen association with systemic diseases such as ankylosing spondylosis and psoriasis, conditions which can also present as an inflammatory enthesopathy.

Nirschl (1992) proposed a condition called mesenchymal syndrome, resulting in multiple sites of tendinopathy occurring in about 15% of patients with tendon disease. The etiology of this tendinopathy may be intrinsic to the individual and not caused by overuse. It is more common in females and it has more effect on the upper limb, but it also affects tendons in the lower limb. The condition remains undefined pathologically and genetically but it may be linked with the rheumatoid family of disorders or estrogen deficiency (Clancy 1989).

Tendons may be affected in genetic diseases that modify collagen. There are a number of inherited disorders that alter collagen and result in tissue fragility or hyperelasticity. These diseases include Marfan's syndrome, Ehlers-Danlos syndrome, and osteogenesis imperfecta (Cole 1993). Some subtypes of genetic disease have disorders of collagen cross-linking rather than of the collagen fiber itself (Eyre et al 1984). Most individuals with these inherited conditions have systemic manifestations of the disease, and tendon disorders are not a primary clinical problem.

Individual genetic profile may also contribute to the repair response. Some individuals produce exuberant scar tissue in ligament healing. There may also be an abnormal response in skin of type I collagen to transforming growth factor in subjects with scleroderma (Hart et al 1995). Clancy suggested that genetics may play a role in both the susceptibility to injury and the paucity of the healing response (Clancy 1989).

In other cases it is unclear if genetics play a role in the pathology and repair process of tendon disease. It has been reported that Achilles tendon ruptures occur in children of parents with a history of tendon rupture, and quadriceps tendon rupture has also been reported in one set of monozygotic twins (Kannus 1997b).

Nutrition

The effect of nutritional status on normal tendon and tendon injury and repair remains poorly investigated. The literature reports that lack of vitamin C, zinc, copper, iron, and manganese may affect tendons (Leadbetter 1992, O'Brien 1997). Copper deficiency affects the cross-links in collagen and elastin (Eyre et al 1984). The distinct lack of literature suggests an obvious further need for investigation in this area.

SUMMARY

Tendon injury, although common, has been the subject of limited investigation. Although recovery from acute tendon injury highlights the similarity of tendon repair to other tissue, it is evident from the resistant nature of overuse tendinopathy to treatment that direct application of this knowledge may not be appropriate. From this chapter it is evident that both the process of injury and the process of repair are poorly understood in overuse tendinopathy.

Physiotherapeutic intervention in tendinopathy is primarily based on clinical experience, and studies investigating the effect of treatment are lacking. Therefore, studies improving the understanding of the disease and repair process and the most effective treatment are needed.

REFERENCES

Ahmed I, Lagoloulos M, McConnell P et al 1998 Blood supply of the Achilles tendon. Journal of Orthopaedic Research 16(5):591–596

Alfredson H, Thorsen K, Lorentzon R 1999 In situ microdialysis in tendon tissue: high levels of glutamate, but not prostaglandin E_2 in chronic Achilles tendon pain. Knee Surgery, Sports Traumatology and Arthroscopy 7:378–381

Almekinders L C 1998 Tendonitis and other chronic tendonopathies. Journal of American Academy of Orthopaedic Surgery 6:157–164

Almekinders L C, Temple J 1998 Etiology, diagnosis, and treatment of tendonitis: an analysis of the literature. Medicine and Science in Sport and Exercise 30(8):1183–1190

Aloia J F 1982 Estrogen and exercise in prevention and treatment of osteoporosis. Geriatrics 37:81–85

Anderson A F, Dome D C, Gautam S et al 2001 Correlation of anthropometric measurements, strength, anterior cruciate ligament size, and intercondylar notch characteristics to sex differences in anterior cruciate ligament tear rates. American Journal of Sports Medicine 29(1):58–66

Archambault J M, Wiley J P, Bray R C 1995 Exercise loading of tendons and the development of overuse injuries: a review of the current literature. Sports Medicine 20(2):77–89

Aspenberg P, Forslund C 2000 Bone morphogenic proteins and tendon repair. Scandinavian Journal of Medicine and Science in Sports 10:372–375

Astrom M 1997 On the nature and etiology of chronic Achilles tendinopathy. Lund University, Sweden

Astrom M, Westlin N 1994a Blood flow in the normal Achilles tendon assessed by laser Doppler flowmetry. Journal Orthopaedic Research 12(2):246–252

Astrom M, Westlin N 1994b Blood flow in chronic Achilles tendinopathy. Clinical Orthopaedics 308:166–172

Astrom M, Rausing A 1995 Chronic Achilles tendinopathy: a survey of surgical and histopathologic findings. Clinical Orthopaedics 316:151–164

Banes A J, Hu P, Xiao H et al 1995 Tendon cells of the epitenon and internal tendon compartment communicate mechanical signals through gap junctions and respond differentially to mechanical load and growth factors. In: Gordon S L, Blair S J, Fine L J (eds) Repetitve motion disorders of the upper extremity. American Academy of Orthopaedic Surgeons, Park Ridge, IL

Benazzo F, Stennardo G, Valli M 1996 Achilles and patellar tendinopathies in athletes: pathogenesis and surgical treatment. Bull Hospital Joint Disease 54:236–240

Benjamin M, Ralphs J 1995 Functional and developmental anatomy of tendons and ligaments. In: Gordon S L, Blair S J, Fine L J (eds) Repetitive motion disorders of the upper extremity. American Academy of Orthopaedic Surgeons, Park Ridge, IL

Benjamin M, Ralphs J 1996 Tendons in health and disease. Manual Therapy 1(4):186–191

Benjamin M, Ralphs J R 1998 Fibrocartilage in tendons and ligaments – an adaption to compressive load. Journal of Anatomy 193:481–494

Benjamin M, Tyers R N S, Ralphs J R 1991 Age-related changes in tendon fibrocartilage. Journal of Anatomy 179:127–136

Brooks C H, Revell W J, Heatley F W 1992 A quantitative histological study of the vascularity of the rotator cuff tendon. Journal of Bone and Joint Surgery 74B:151–153

Chansky H A, Iannotti I P 1991 The vascularity of the rotator cuff. Clinics in Sports Medicine 10:807–822

Clancy W 1989 Failed healing responses. In: Leadbetter W, Buckwalter J A, Gordon S (eds) Sports-induced inflammation: clinical and basic science concepts. American Orthopedic Society for Sports Medicine, Park Ridge, IL

Clancy W G J 1990 Tendon trauma and overuse injuries. In: Leadbetter W B, Buckwalter J A, Gordon S L (eds) Sports-induced inflammation: Clinical and basic science concepts. American Academy of Orthopaedic Surgeons, Park Ridge, IL

Clark M, Clerk L, Newman J et al 2000 Interaction between metabolism and flow in tendon and muscle. Scandinavian Journal of Medicine and Science in Sports 10:338–345

Cole W G 1993 Genetics of connective tissue disease. Medical Journal of Australia 158:678–680

Cook J L, Khan K M, Harcourt P R et al 1998 Patellar tendon ultrasonography in asymptomatic active athletes reveals hypoechoic regions: a study of 320 tendons. Clinical Journal of Sports Medicine 8:73–77

Cook J, Coleman B, Khan K et al 2000 Patellar tendinosis in junior basketball players: a controlled clinical and ultrasonographic study of 268 tendons in players aged 14–18 years. Scandinavian Journal of Medicine and Science in Sports 10:216–220

Cribb A M, Scott J E 1995 Tendon response to tensile stress: an ultrastructural investigation of collagen: proteoglycan interactions in stressed tendon. Journal of Anatomy 187:423–428

David J M 1989 Jumper's knee. Journal of Orthopaedic and Sports Physical Therapy 11(4):137–141

Duri Z A, Aichroth P M 1995 Patellar tendonitis: clinical and literature review. Knee Surgery, Sports Traumatology and Arthroscopy 3:95–100

El Hawary R, Stanish W D, Curwin S L 1997 Rehabilitation of tendon injuries in sport. Sports Medicine 24:347–358

Enwemeka C S 1989 Inflammation, cellularity, and fibrillogenesis in regenerating tendon: implications for tendon rehabilitation. Physical Therapy 69:816–825

Eyre D R, Paz M A, Gallop P M 1984 Cross-linking in collagen and elastin. Annual Review of Biochemistry 53(7):717–748

Ferretti A, Ippolito E, Mariani P et al 1983 Jumper's knee. American Journal of Sports Medicine 11:58–62

Ferretti A, Puddu G, Mariani P et al 1985 The natural history of jumper's knee: patellar or quadriceps tendinitis. International Orthopaedics 8:239–242

Frank C B, Hart D A 1990 Cellular response to loading. In: Leadbetter W B, Buckwalter J A, Gordon S L (eds) Sports-induced inflammation: clinical and basic concepts. American Academy of Orthopaedic Surgeons, Park Ridge, IL

Frank C, Shrive N, Hiraoka H et al 1999 Optimisation of the biology of soft tissue repair. Journal of Science and Medicine in Sport 2(3):190–210

Fredberg U, Bolvig L 1999 Jumper's knee. Scandinavian Journal of Medicine and Science in Sports 9:66–73

Frost H M 1990 Skeletal structural adaptations to mechanical usage (SATMU): 4, Mechanical influences on intact fibrous tissue. The Anatomical Record 226:433–439

Fyfe I, Stanish W D 1992 The use of eccentric training and stretching in the treatment and prevention of tendon injuries. Clinics in Sports Medicine 11(3):601–624

Gelberman R, Goldberg V, An K-N et al 1988 Tendon. In: Woo S L-Y, Buckwalter J (eds) Injury and repair of the musculoskeletal soft tissues. American Academy of Orthopaedic Surgeons, Park Ridge, IL

Giori N J, Beaupre G S, Carter D R 1993 Cellular shape and pressure may mediate mechanical control of tissue composition in tendons. Journal of Bone and Joint Surgery 11:581–591

Gotoh M, Hamada K, Yamakawa H et al 1998 Increased substance P in subacromial bursa and shoulder pain in rotator cuff disease. Journal of Orthopaedic Research 16:618–621

Gross M T 1992 Chronic tendonitis: pathomechanics of injury, factors affecting the healing response, and treatment. Journal of Orthopaedic and Sports Physical Therapy 16(6):248–261

Hart D A, Frank C B, Bray R C 1995 Inflammatory processes in repetitive motion and overuse syndromes: potential role of neurogenic mechanisms in tendons and ligaments. In: Gordon S L, Blair S J, Fine L J (eds) Pathophysiology: connective tissue. American Academy of Orthopaedic Surgeons, Park Ridge, IL

Hess G P, Cappiello W K, Poole R M et al 1989 Prevention and treatment of overuse tendon injuries. Sports Medicine 8(6):371–384

Jann H, Stein L, Slater D 1999. In vitro effects of epidermal growth factor or insulin-like growth factor on tenoblast migration on absorbable suture material. Veterinary Surgery 28(4):268–278

Järvinen M 1992 Epidemiology of tendon injuries in sports. Clinics in Sports Medicine 11(3):493–504

Järvinen M, Jozsa L, Kannus P et al 1997 Histopathological findings in chronic tendon disorders. Scandinavian Journal of Medicine and Science in Sports 7:86–95

Järvinen T A H, Kannus P, Järvinen T L N et al 2000 Tenascin-C in the pathobiology and healing process of musculoskeletal tissue injury. Scandinavian Journal of Medicine and Science in Sports 10:376–382

Johnson D P, Wakeley C J, Watt I 1996 Magnetic resonance imaging of patellar tendonitis. Journal of Bone and Joint Surgery 78B (3):452–457

Jones A R, Lauder I, Findlay D B et al 1996 Chronic Achilles tendinitis: magnetic resonance imaging and histopathological correlation. Sports Exercise and Injury 2:172–175

Józsa L, Kannus P 1997 Human Tendons. Human Kinetics, Champaign, IL

Józsa L, Bálint B J, Demel Z 1982 Hypoxic alterations of tenocytes in degenerative tendonopathy. Archives of Orthopaedic and Traumatic Surgery 99:243–246

Józsa L, Bálint B J, Réffy A et al 1984a Fine structural alterations of collagen fibers in degenerative tendinopathy. Archives of Orthopaedic and Traumatic Surgery 103:47–51

Józsa L, Réffy A, Bálint B J 1984b Polarisation and electron microscope studies on the collagen of intact and ruptured human tendons. Acta Histochemica 74:209–215

Józsa L, Réffy A, Bálint J B 1984c The pathogenesis of tendolipomatosis. International Orthopaedics 7:251–255

Józsa L, Bálint J, Kannus P et al 1989 Distribution of blood groups in patients with tendon injury. Journal of Bone and Joint Surgery 71B:272–274

Józsa L, Réffy A, Kannus P et al 1990 Pathological alterations in human tendons. Archives of Orthopaedic and Trauma Surgery 110:15–21

Józsa L, Kannus P, Bálint J B et al 1991 Three-dimensional ultrastructure of human tendons. Acta Anatomica 142:306–312

Kaar T, O'Brien M, Murray P et al 1993 Bilateral quadriceps tendon rupture – a case report. Ireland Journal of Medicine and Science 162(12):502

Kannus P 1997a Tendon pathology: basic science and clinical applications. Sports Exercise and Injury 3:62–75

Kannus P 1997b Etiology and pathophysiology of tendon ruptures in sports. Scandinavian Journal of Medicine and Science in Sports 7(2):107–112

Kannus P 1997c Etiology and pathophysiology of chronic tendon disorders in sports. Scandinavian Journal of Science and Medicine in Sports 7:78–85

Kannus P, Jozsa L 1991 Histopathological changes preceding spontaneous rupture of a tendon. Journal of Bone and Joint Surgery 73A:1507–1525

Kannus P, Jozsa L, Natri A et al 1997 Effects of training, immobilization and remobilization on tendons. Scandinavian Journal of Medicine and Science in Sports 7:67–71

Karageanes S, Blackburn K, Vangelos Z 2000 The association of the menstrual cycle with the laxity of the anterior cruciate ligament in adolescent female athletes. Clinical Journal of Sport Medicine 10:162–168

Khan K M, Bonar F, Desmond P M et al 1996 Patellar tendinosis (Jumper's knee): findings at histopathologic examination, US and MR imaging. Radiology 200:821–827

Khan K M, Maffulli N, Coleman BD et al 1998 Patellar tendinopathy: some aspects of basic science and clinical management. British Journal of Sports Medicine 32:346–355

Khan K M, Bonar S F, Cook J L et al 1999a Histopathology of common overuse tendon conditions: update and implications for clinical management. Sports Medicine 6:393–408

Khan K M, Visentini P J, Kiss Z S et al 1999b Correlation of ultrasound and magnetic resonance imaging with clinical outcome after open patellar tenotomy: prospective and retrospective studies. Clinical Journal of Sports Medicine 9(3):129–137

Khan K, Cook J, Maffulli N et al 2000 Where is the pain coming from in tendinopathy? It may be biochemical, not only structural, in origin. British Journal of Sports Medicine 34(2):81–83

Kirkendall D T, Garrett W E 1997 Function and biomechanics of

tendons. Scandinavian Journal of Medicine and Science in Sports 7:62–66

Kjaer M, Langberg H, Skovgaard D et al 2000 In vivo studies of peritendinous tissue in exercise. Scandinavian Journal of Medicine and Science in Sports 10:326–331

Kraushaar B, Nirschl R 1999 Tendinosis of the elbow (tennis elbow). Clinical features and findings of histological, immunohistochemical, and electron microscopy studies. Journal of Bone and Joint Surgery America 81(2):259–278

Kujala U M, Järvinen M, Natri A et al 1992 ABO blood groups and musculoskeletal injuries. Injury 23(2):131–133

Kvist M, Józsa L, Kannus P et al 1991 Morphology and histochemistry of the myotendineal junction of the rat calf muscle. Acta Anatomica 141:199–205

Kvist M, Józsa L, Järvinen M 1992 Vascular changes in the ruptured Achilles tendon and its paratenon. International Orthopaedics 16:377–382

Langberg H, Bulow J, Kjaer M 1998 Blood flow in the peritendinous space of the human Achilles tendon during exercise. Acta Physiologica Scandinavia 163:149–153

Leadbetter W 1992 Cell matrix response in tendon injury. Clinics in Sports Medicine 11(3):533–578

Leadbetter W B 1993 Tendon overuse injuries: diagnosis and treatment. In: Renstrom P A F H (ed) Sports injuries. Basic principles of prevention and care. Oxford Press, London

Liu S H, Al-Shaikh R A, Panossian V et al 1997. Estrogen affects the cellular metabolism of the anterior cruciate ligament. A potential explanation for female athletic injury. American Journal of Sports Medicine 25(5):704–709

Ljung B, Forsgren S, Fridén J 1999 Substance P and calcitonin gene-related peptide expression at the extensor carpi radialis brevis muscle origin: implications for the etiology of tennis elbow. Journal of Orthopaedic Research 17(4):554–559

Maddox P A, Garth W P 1986 Tendinitis of the patellar ligament and quadriceps (Jumper's knee) as an initial presentation of hyperparathyroidism. Journal of Bone and Joint Surgery 68A:288–292

Maffulli N 1999 Achilles tendon ailments: clinical and biological aspects. Fifth IOC World Congress, Sydney

Maffulli N, King J B 1992 Effects of physical activity on some components of the skeletal system. Sports Medicine 13(6):393–407

Maffulli N, Khan K M, Puddu G 1998 Overuse tendon conditions. Time to change a confusing terminology. Arthroscopy 14:840–843

Maffulli N, Waterston W, Squair J et al 1999 Changing incidence of Achilles tendon rupture in Scotland: a 15 year study. Clinical Journal of Sports Medicine 9(3):157–160

Maffulli N, Reaper J A, Waterston S W et al 2000 ABO blood groups and Achilles tendon rupture in the Grampian region of Scotland. Clinical Journal of Sport Medicine 10(4):269–271

Molnar T, Fox J 1993 Overuse injuries of the knee in basketball. Clinics in Sports Medicine 12(2):349–362

Neely F 1998 Biomechanical risk factors for exercise-related lower limb injuries. Sports Medicine 26(6):395–413

Nirschl R P 1990 Patterns of failed healing in tendon injury. In: Leadbetter W B, Buckwalter J A, Gordon S L (eds) Sports-induced inflammation: clinical and basic concepts. American Academy of Orthopaedic Surgeons Park Ridge, IL

Nirschl R P 1992 Elbow tendonitis/tennis elbow. Clinics in Sports Medicine 11(4):851–870

Nuutila P, Kalliokoski K 2000 Use of positron emission tomography in the assessment of skeletal muscle and tendon metabolism and perfusion. Scandinavian Journal of Medicine and Science in Sports 10:346–350

O'Brien M 1992 Functional anatomy and physiology of tendons. Clinics in Sports Medicine 11(3):505–520

O'Brien M 1997 Structure and metabolism of tendons. Scandinavian Journal of Medicine and Science in Sports 7:55–61

Ohberg L, Lorentzon R, Alfredson H 2001 Neovascularisation in Achilles tendons with painful tendinosis but not in normal tendons: an ultrasonographic investigation. Knee Surgery, Sports Traumatology and Arthroscopy 9:233–238

Popp J E, Yu J S, Kaeding C C 1997 Recalcitrant patellar tendinitis. Magnetic resonance imaging, histologic evaluation and surgical treatment. American Journal of Sports Medicine 25(2):218–222

Postlethwaite A E 1989 Failed healing responses in connective tissue and a comparison of medical conditions. In: Leadbetter W B, Buckwalter J A, Gordon S L (eds) Sports-Induced Inflammation. American Academy for Orthopaedic Surgeons, Park Ridge, IL

Puddu G, Ippolito E, Postacchini F 1976 A classification of Achilles tendon disease. American Journal of Sports Medicine 4:145–150

Robins S P 1988 Functional properties of collagen and elastin. Baillière's Clinical Rheumatology 2(1):1–36

Rosenberg L, Choi H U, Neame P J et al 1989 Proteoglycans of soft connective tissue. In: Leadbetter W B, Buckwalter J A, Gordon S L (eds) Sports-Induced Inflammation. American Academy for Orthopaedic Surgeons, Park Ridge, IL

Sanzone A G, Einhorn T A 1998 The use of bone morphogenic proteins to heal fractures, articular cartilage defects, and ligament and tendon injuries. Sports Medicine and Arthroscopy Review 6:118–123

Schatzker J, Branemark P 1969 Intravital observation on the microvascular anatomy and microcirculation of the tendon. Acta Orthopaedica Scandinavia 126:S1–S23

Schatzmann L, Brunner P, Staubli H U 1998 Effect of cyclic preconditioning on the tensile properties of human quadriceps tendons and patellar ligaments. Knee Surgery, Sports Traumatology and Arthroscopy 6(1):56–61

Scott J E 1988 Proteoglycan-fibrillar collagen interactions. Journal of Biochemistry 252:313–323

Scott J E 1995 Extracellular matrix, supramolecular organisation and shape. Journal of Anatomy 187:250–269

Scranton P E, Farrar E L 1992 Mucoid degeneration of the patellar ligament in athletes. Journal of Bone and Joint Surgery 74A(3):435–437

Selvanetti A, Cippola M, Puddu G 1997 Overuse tendon injuries: basic science and classification. Operative Techniques in Sports Medicine 5(3):110–117

Sengar D P S, McKendry R J, Uhthoff H K 1989 Lack of association between HLA and rotator cuff rupture. Tissue Antigens 34(3):205–206

Sengar R J, McKendry R, Uhthoff H 1987 Increased frequency of HLA-A1 in calcifying tendinitis. Tissue Antigens 29(3):173–174

Shirakura K, Ciarelli M J, Arnoczky J H et al 1995 Deformation induced calcium signaling in tenocytes in situ. Combined Orthopaedic Research Societies Meeting, San Diego, California

Sporn M B, Roberts A B 1989 Transforming growth factor-β. Multiple actions and potential clinical applications. Journal American Medical Association 262(7):938–941

Teitz C C, Garrett W E, Miniaci A et al 1997 Tendon problems in athletic individuals. Journal of Bone and Joint Surgery 79A(1):138–152

Tuite D J, Renstrom P A F H, O'Brien M 1997 The aging tendon. Scandinavian Journal of Medicine and Science in Sports 7:72–77

Uhthoff H K, Matsumoto F 2000 Rotator cuff tendinopathy. Sports Medicine and Arthroscopy Review 8:56–68

Vogel K G, Paulsson M, Heinegard D 1984 Specific inhibition of type I and type II collagen fibrillogenesis by the small proteoglycan of tendon. Journal of Biochemistry 223:587–597

Vogel K G, Ordog A, Olah J 1993 Proteoglycans in the compressed region of human tibialis posterior tendon and in ligaments. Journal of Orthopaedic Research 11:68–77

Vogel K G, Meyers A B 1999 Proteins in the tensile region of adult bovine deep flexor tendon. Clinical Orthopaedics and Related Research 367 (Suppl.):344–355

Williams I F, Heaton A, McCullagh K G 1980 Cell morphology and collagen types in equine tendon scar. Research in Veterinary Science 28:302–310

Williams I F, McCullagh K G, Silver I A 1984 The distribution of types I and III collagen and fibronectin in the healing equine tendon. Connective Tissue Research 12:211–227

Williams J G 1986 Achilles tendon lesions in sport. Sports Medicine 3:114–135

Wilson A M, Goodship A E 1992 Hysteresis energy losses in the equine superficial digital flexor tendon during exercise produce a local temperature sufficient to damage fibroblasts in vitro. Transcripts of Orthopaedic Research Society 17:679

Wilson A M, Goodship A E 1994 Exercise-induced hyperthermia as a possible mechanism for tendon degeneration. Journal of Biomechanics 27:899–905

Witvrouw E, Lysens R, Bellemans J et al 2000 Intrinsic risk factors for the development of anterior knee pain in an athletic population. American Journal of Sports Medicine 28(4):480–489

Woo S-L Y, Tkach L V 1990 The cellular and matrix response of ligaments and tendons to mechanical injury. In: Leadbetter W B, Buckwalter J A, Gordon S L (eds) Sports-induced inflammation: clinical and basic concepts. American Academy of Orthopaedic Surgeons Park Ridge, IL

Wren T A L, Yerby S A, Beaupre G S et al 2001 Mechanical properties of the human Achilles tendon. Clinical Biomechanics 16:245–251

Zamora A J, Marini J F 1988 Tendon and myotendinous junction in an overloaded skeletal muscle of the rat. Anatomy and Embryology 179:89–96

4

Ligament

Gabriel Ng

INTRODUCTION

The musculoskeletal system of the human body provides the morphological framework and machinery of movement. Muscles and nerves are the power generators whereas bones, cartilage, joint capsules, and ligaments provide the structural strength to withstand forces imposed onto the body.

Injuries from sport or exercise often involve more than one structure and type of tissue. Understanding the organization and function of the body tissues can enhance the design of rehabilitation programs and help athletes return to their preinjury levels of sport performance and physical activity.

DEVELOPMENT OF BODY TISSUES

Human life begins from the instance when a sperm fertilizes an egg. The first 7 weeks of life is the embryonic stage, and then starting from week 8 until birth is the fetal stage (White et al 1991). At the beginning of week 4 of embryonic life, there is the formation of neural tissue and somite, which continue to develop into muscles and mesenchyme. Mesenchyme is the precursor of connective tissues, such as bones, cartilage, ligaments, etc.

Basically, the human body contains four distinct types of tissues: epithelial, nervous, muscle, and connective (Whiting & Zernicke 1998). Epithelial tissue is the lining of organs. It provides structural support for epithelia and constitutes a semipermeable barrier for the transport of materials between the epithelial and neighboring compartments. The nervous tissue is developed from the ectoderm that effects communications within the body by means of electrical signals. The third tissue type is the muscle, which exists in the three forms of skeletal, cardiac and smooth muscles, and which all contract in response to electrical stimulation. The final tissue type is the connective tissue, which exists as an aggregate of cells embedded in an extracellular matrix composed of 60% water by weight (Wheater et al 1991, Whiting & Zernicke 1998, Woodard & White 1986). Ligament is classified as a form of connective tissue.

STRUCTURE AND BIOCHEMISTRY OF LIGAMENT

The word 'ligament' is derived from a Latin word 'ligare' which means 'binding' (Dye & Dilworth Cannon 1988). As early as 3000 BC, in the Smith Papyrus, joint sprains began to be described and around 400 BC, Hippocrates described treatments for ligament injuries. Although in 100 BC, Hegator provided the first anatomical definition of ligament, the first correct description of ligament was provided by Galen in 130 AD (Snook 1983). Prior to this stage, ligaments were generally considered to be something similar to nerves but with a vague contractile function. In 1830, Schleiden & Schwann discovered cells and long fibers in dense connective tissues and then 20 years later, Rudinger & Hilton further discovered nerves in ligaments and postulated the ligament–muscle feedback system (Frank & Shrive 1994).

Ligament is classified as a form of dense regular connective tissue largely consisting of collagen (Whiting & Zernicke 1998). In general, there are at least two subgroups of ligaments: (1) skeletal ligaments in joints, and (2) suspensory ligaments in the abdominal organs (Frank et al 1985). The majority of skeletal ligaments are anatomically distinct, dense, relatively avascular, but homogeneous in appearance. At the microscopic level, ligaments comprise individual fibers running parallel to each other. Along the fibers are some scattered, long, thin fibroblasts that produce and maintain the surrounding matrix (Amiel et al 1984, Murray & Spector 1999).

According to Frank & Shrive (1994), the major functions of skeletal ligaments include:

- Attachment of articulating bones to one another across a joint
- guidance of joint movements
- maintenance of joint congruency
- action as position sensors for joints.

Traditionally, tendons and ligaments were considered to be similar structures and they were both regarded as dense parallel connective tissues (Copenhaver et al 1971, Ham 1974). Initially, the literature on 'ligaments' and 'tendons' used the terms synonymously (Clayton et al 1968, O'Donoghue et al 1961). However, biochemical

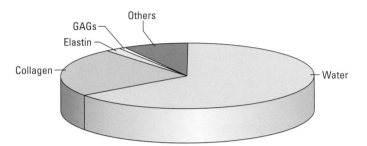

Figure 4.1 Approximate chemical composition of normal skeletal ligaments by weight. Collagen represents nearly three-quarters of their dry weight. Two-thirds of their total weight is made up of water.

analysis of ligaments and tendons by Amiel et al (1984) revealed strong similarities and yet subtle differences between these structures. Ligaments contain approximately two-thirds of water by weight. The remaining one-third of dry weight is a constituent of collagen, elastin, glycosaminoglycans (GAGs), fibroblasts, and other biochemical substances (Fig. 4.1) (Kasser 1996). In general, ligaments are more metabolically active than tendons. Ligaments have more protein but less total collagen content, and have a higher percentage of type III collagen and GAGs than do tendons.

COLLAGEN

Collagen is the major constituent of the extracellular matrix of all connective tissues, and makes up approximately 80% of the dry weight of ligaments (Amiel et al 1984, Woo et al 1994). Collagen is a form of secretory protein containing 3 α-chains entangled in a triple-helical manner, and the biosynthetic events are similar between all collagen polypeptides (Olsen 1991). The basic collagen molecule is the tropocollagen which aggregates into a collagen fibril in a specific quarter staggering pattern that has most mechanical and biochemical stability (Gross 1974, Hodge & Petruska 1963).

There are at least 18 types of collagen identified in the body. Each type differs from one another by the types of α-chains that make up the tropocollagen. In general, the amino acids that make up an α-chain follow the sequence of glycine-x-y, where in most cases, x is proline, y is hydroxyproline, and this sequence repeats itself. The number of each collagen type essentially reflects the chronological order in which they were discovered. Each type of collagen has its unique characteristics and location throughout the body. In general, collagen is involved in cell attachment and differentiation, chemotactic reaction, and immunopathological processes (Linsenmayer 1991).

Despite the different types of collagen in the body, types I, II and III may be regarded as most pertinent to sports physical therapists due to their abundance in the musculoskeletal system. Type I collagen constitutes about 90% of the total collagen in the body and is found in ligaments, tendons, bones, and fascia. Type II collagen is found in hyaline cartilage and nucleus pulposus of the intervertebral disk, and consists of fine fibrils that are dispersed in the ground substance. Type III collagen is mostly found in skin and blood vessels (Eyre 1980, Wheater et al 1991).

Collagen provides strength to the tissues. The ability to form covalent intramolecular and intermolecular cross-links is a key determination of the tensile strength and resistance to chemical enzymatic breakdown of collagen (Bailey et al 1974, Eyre 1980, Knott & Bailey 1998, Mechanic 1974, Patterson-Kane et al 1997, Tanzer 1973) (Fig. 4.2). Cross-links are formed by enzymatic reactions between the amino acids lysine and hydroxylysine (Amiel & Kleiner 1988). The most prevalent inter-molecular cross-links include hydroxylysinonorleucine (HLNL), dihydroxylysinonorleucine (DHLNL), and the more complex combinations of histidinohydroxymero-desmosine (HHMD). These are labeled as reducible cross-links due to the presence of a double bond. The relative concentrations of these cross-links can be expressed as ratios of DHLNL/HLNL or (DHLNL+HLNL)/HHMD. In some ligaments such as the anterior cruciate ligament (ACL), a very high ratio of DHLNL/HLNL has been reported (Amiel et al 1984). The HLNL is a more matured cross-link than DHLNL. The finding that the ACL contains a high proportion of DHLNL leads to the speculation that this ligament is endowed with a higher percentage of less matured cross-links to withstand a wide range of forces (Amiel et al 1990).

Besides reducible cross-links, there are also non-reducible cross-links that do not contain a double bond. In older people, less reducible cross-links are found in connective tissues, suggesting an age-related transformation of reducible to the more stable non-reducible cross-links (Tanzer 1976, Patterson-Kane et al 1997). Hydroxypyridinoline (HP) has been identified as a type of non-reducible cross-link (Fujimoto 1977, Fujimoto & Moriguchi 1978). Frank et al (1994) and Ng et al (1996a) have respectively demonstrated positive relationship between HP cross-link density and the mechanical strength of healing medial collateral ligament tissue and ACL graft in rabbits and goats.

PROTEOGLYCANS

Proteoglycans are important constituents of the extra-cellular matrix. Collagen fibrils resist tensile loading and proteoglycans resist compressive loading (Scott 1988). Proteoglycans are large molecules comprising a core protein, covalently linked to numerous GAG side chains that are polysaccharides of repeating disaccharide units. The GAGs contain a high density of negative charges that repel each other, thus enabling the proteoglycans to extend through a larger volume than they do when uncharged. These negatively charged GAG molecules interact electrostatically with a variety of positively

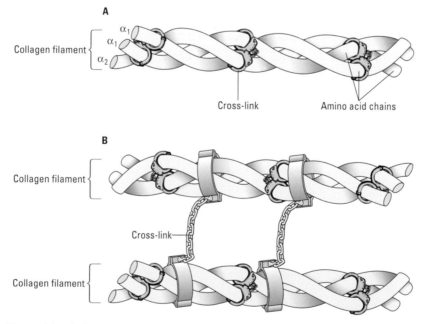

Figure 4.2 Collagen bonding increases tensile strength. **A**: Weak intramolecular cross-links form between amino acid chains within one collagen filament. **B**: Stronger intermolecular cross-links form from one collagen filament to another. (Reproduced from Hardy M A, The biology of scar formation, Physical Therapy, 1989, 69, 1014–1024, with permission of the American Physical Therapy Association.)

charged molecules such as water. The affinity of proteoglycans to water determines the viscosity of interstitial fluids and maintains the proper homeostatic environment for the cells and the surrounding matrix (Hardingham & Fosang 1992, Wight et al 1991).

Proteoglycans usually constitute about 1% of the ligament's dry weight (Amiel et al 1990, Frank & Shrive 1994). Studies of the relationships between proteoglycan and collagen reveal that some small size proteoglycans limit collagen fibrillogenesis through interaction between the proteoglycans' core protein and the surface of the collagen fibrils. Therefore, the size of collagen fibrils remain small when there are excessive small size proteoglycans (Pogany et al 1994, Vogel et al 1984, Vogel & Trotter 1987).

ELASTIN

Elastin is an extremely hydrophobic protein characterized by a high degree of reversible extensibility with small forces (Mecham & Heuser 1991). Most ligaments contain less than 5% of elastin by dry weight, but this may be important for the elasticity of the ligaments (Arnoczky et al 1993, Buckwalter & Cooper 1987). An exception is the ligamentum flavum in the spine which contains twice as much elastin than collagen, thus this ligament exhibits almost perfect elasticity when subject to loading (Kirby et al 1989, Nachemson & Evans 1968).

Other non-collagen proteins

There are some non-collagen proteins in the extracellular matrix that are present in small quantities but that are vital for wound healing should the tissue be injured. For example, thrombospondin is involved in the early organization of the extracellular matrix to initiate the healing process (Bornstein et al 2000, Chen et al 2000, Miller & McDevitt 1991, Raugi et al 1987). Tenascin induces cell migration so as to facilitate the deployment of fibroblasts to the wound site for collagen synthesis (Jones & Jones 2000, Koukoulis et al 1991, Sakakura & Kusano 1991). Fibronectin has the roles of chemattraction of fibroblasts, cell adhesion, and wound contraction (McDonald 1988, Tani et al 2001); laminin attracts neutrophils that are important for preventing bacterial infection (Gugssa et al 2000, Kleinman et al 1985). Therefore, these non-collagen proteins form the defense and repair network so as to enable the ligament to repair itself after injury and regain the normal functional strength.

LIGAMENT MORPHOLOGY

The structural arrangements of collagen in ligaments and tendons are very similar. The collagen of the midsubstance of these structures is hierarchically arranged in ascending orders of tropocollagen, microfibrils, subfibrils, fibrils, and fibers (Fig. 4.3). Tropocollagen molecules of about 1.5 nm in diameter are tightly packed in groups of five, forming microfibrils of approximately 3.5 nm in diameter. The microfibrils group into subfibrils, which aggregate to form fibrils of 50–500 nm. The fibrils further aggregate to form fibers of 50–300 microns in diameter, which become the smallest unit of collagen that can be seen using a light microscope (Frank & Shrive 1994).

When ligaments are viewed under a polarized light microscope, a distinct feature of accordion-like, wavy undulation of cells and matrix can be seen, which is known as ligament 'crimp' (Dale et al 1972, Dale & Baer 1974, Minns et al 1973, Murray & Spector 1999, Patterson-Kane et al 1997, Yahia & Drouin 1989). Crimp is a unique

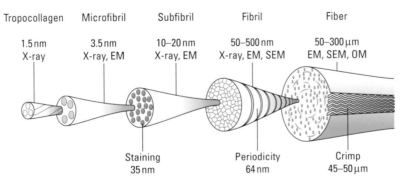

Figure 4.3 Schematic illustration depicting the hierarchical structure of collagen in ligament midsubstance. EM = electron microscope; SEM = scanning EM; OM = optical microscope. (Modified from Kastelic et al 1978 with the permission of Connective Tissue Research. Copyright 1978 from the Multicomposite Structure of Tendon by J Kastelic et al. Reproduced by permission of Taylor & Francis, Inc., http://www.routledge-ny.com)

feature in parallel arranged connective tissues. It provides a buffer against mechanical loading, such that any rapid external load will stretch out the wavy undulation of the ligament without damaging its fibers (Dale et al 1972, Diamant et al 1972, Oakes 1994, Viidik 1980).

The crimp patterns are tissue specific and relatively little is known about the factors that determine and maintain the collagen crimp. There are a number of hypotheses, however, suggesting the factors that maintain collagen crimp. Among these hypotheses, the collagen–proteoglycan interaction is most widely accepted (Viidik 1980). Shah et al (1977) demonstrated that elongation of crimp was due to straightening of the crimp period but the crimp angle remained constant. This finding suggests that the crimp junction, where collagen fibrils are acutely angulated to each other, is stiffer than the components that make up the crimp period.

The insertion of ligament to bone provides another mechanical buffer. An early study by Cooper & Misol (1970) reported that skeletal ligaments are not simply cemented to bones by Sharpey's fibers. Most ligaments insert to bones by gradual transition through layers of fibrocartilage and mineralized fibrocartilage. This layered arrangement of tissues with different mechanical strength can prevent stress concentrations so that the forces can be distributed over a large area.

At the ultrastructural level, Parry and co-workers (Parry & Craig 1977, 1979, Parry et al 1978a, 1978b) pioneered the analyses of connective tissues using transmission electron microscopy for different animal tissues at various ages. They quantified the collagen fibril diameter profiles of the tissues and, based on their findings, proposed an association between collagen fibril size and mechanical properties of the tissues.

More recently, a number of investigators have studied the ultrastructural morphology of both normal ligaments and tendons, and tissues under repair (Chapman 1989, Frank et al 1989, 1992, 1997, Matthew & Moore 1991, Neurath & Stofft 1992, Ng 1995, Postacchini & De Martino 1980). Findings confirmed that normal adult ligaments and tendons have bimodal distributions of collagen fibril diameter. For ligaments under repair, a more homogeneous distribution of small collagen fibrils exists in the early phase of repair, but the fibrils gradually enlarge over time (Frank et al 1992, 1997, Ng 1995, Oakes et al 2000, Postacchini & De Martino 1980), possibly due to the influence of mechanical loading to the healing tissues.

BIOMECHANICS

Ligaments are viscoelastic structures with unique mechanical properties. The ability of a ligament to withstand tensile loading often determines its level of competence (Woo et al 1990). Understanding the mechanical behavior of a ligament is important to determine its functional safety limit. Often, when a ligament is loaded to failure, the degree of damage is related to both the magnitude and rate that the load is applied (Nordin et al 2001).

Like other soft connective tissues, the biomechanical properties of ligaments can be considered from the structural and material perspectives. Structural properties are the physical properties of a ligament that are dependent on its size, shape and alignment to the external force. Material properties refer to the physical properties of the substances that make up the ligament per se, irrespective of their geometrical shapes or dimensions.

LOAD–DEFORMATION CHARACTERISTICS

A common way to analyze the biomechanical properties of ligaments is to subject a specimen to tensile loading under a constant rate of elongation with a material testing machine. The ligament is deformed until failure. The concomitant load and elongation data during the test will enable the construction of a load–deformation curve (Fig. 4.4). There are four typical regions in the curve that correspond to different geometrical alignment and integrity of the collagen fibers of the ligament.

The first region (I) is the toe-phase, which is characterized by a disproportionate increase in elongation with

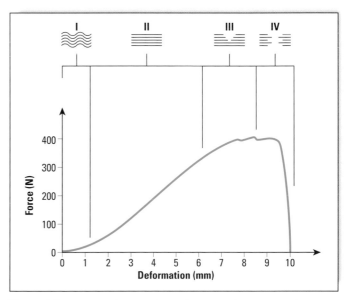

Figure 4.4 A typical force–deformation curve for ligament. I = toe region; II = linear region; III = region of microfailure; IV = failure region. At the top are schematic representations of fibers going from crimped (I) through recruitment (II) to progressive failure (III and IV). (From Frank C B, Shrive N G 1994 Ligament. In: Nigg B M, Herzog W [eds]. Biomechanics of the musculo-skeletal system. © 1994 John Wiley & Sons Limited. Reproduced with permission)

Table 4.1 Comparison of structural and material properties with different dimensions of the same tissue. By reducing the cross-sectional area to 50%, structural stiffness is halved but Young's modulus remains the same

Original size	Force	Stress	Elongation	Strain	Stiffness	Young's modulus
Length = l Area = A	F	$F/A = \sigma$	δl	$\delta l/l \times 100\% = \varepsilon$	$F/\delta l$	σ/ε
Length = l Area = 0.5A	F	$F/0.5A = 2\sigma$	$2\delta l$	$2\delta l/l \times 100\% = 2\varepsilon$	$F/2\delta l$	$2\sigma/2\varepsilon = \sigma/\varepsilon$

a small load. This is the region where the force is mostly absorbed by the collagen crimp. The wavy, crimp pattern will become straighter as the load progresses (Diamant et al 1972, Hirsch 1974, Viidik et al 1965). The other reason for the non-linear deformation is the heterogeneous distribution of the collagen fibers. Some fibers that are oriented parallel to the axis of loading may take up the load earlier than others, thus resulting in a stepwise recruitment of the collagen to withstand the load (Frank & Shrive 1994). The elongation is usually expressed as strain, which is defined as the percentage elongation over the original length. At the end of toe-phase, the strain has been reported to be approximately 4% (Diamant et al 1972, Haut & Little 1972, Viidik 1973), which is well within the functional safety limit of ligaments.

The second region (II) is the linear region in which the ligament follows more or less a linear fashion of elongation in response to loading. In this phase, the collagen fibers are stretched and become more parallel to each other. The slope in this region is defined as the stiffness (N/mm2), signifying the resistance of a ligament to elongating against tensile loading. Theoretically, if the load is removed in the linear region, the ligament should return to its original length without any permanent damage. Practically, however, towards the end of the linear region, some collagen fibers will fail (presumably those recruited first), resulting in pathological irreversible damage to the ligament. The severity of such damage is similar to a clinical grade 2 ligament tear where severe pain is evident and where an athlete cannot continue with a sporting activity (Oakes 1994).

When the linear region is surpassed, major disruption of collagen fiber bundles occurs (region III). The ligament loses stiffness unpredictably as more and more fiber bundles fail, and the force will be redistributed to the remaining fibers, thus increasing the likelihood of these fibers breaking. It only takes a little additional elongation before all the fibers fail, resulting in total rupture of the ligament (region IV) (Frank & Shrive 1994).

The highest point in the load–deformation curve is the ultimate tensile strength, and the area covered by the curve reflects the energy absorption capacity of the ligament. The tensile stiffness, ultimate tensile strength, and

energy absorption capacity are dependent on the physical size of the ligament. When a ligament is separated longitudinally into two halves, each half will only demonstrate 50% of its original stiffness and strength. In order to compare the mechanical properties of the materials that make up the ligament, the load needs to be converted to stress (MPa) by dividing it with the cross-sectional area of the ligament, and elongation converted to strain by dividing it with the original length. The resultant stress–strain curve represents the material properties of the ligament substance, and the slope of this curve represents the Young's modulus (Table 4.1).

From the functional perspective, it is of limited interest for clinicians to study the ultimate tensile strength or total energy absorption capacity of a ligament, because in most of our daily activities, we only use about 30% of the full potential strength of our ligaments (Viidik 1980). Furthermore, the upper limit of physiological strain to ligaments is in the vicinity of 5% or less (Fung 1981), which is well below the ultimate strain of most ligaments in the body.

VISCOELASTIC BEHAVIOR

Ligaments exhibit viscoelastic (time- or history-dependent) properties as a result of the complex interaction between the collagen fibers with its surrounding matrix (Nordin et al 2001). When a ligament is loaded and unloaded in successive manner, the load–deformation curve will shift to the right with each loading/unloading cycle instead of following the same path. This phenomenon is known as 'hysteresis' (Fig. 4.5), a process resulting from internal energy loss to heat during the loading/unloading cycles (Woo et al 1990). Hysteresis has important therapeutic implications such as during traction because the deformation is the desired effect of the treatment procedure. However, hysteresis can also be a manifestation of pathological deformation resulting from repetitive microtrauma (Garde 1988).

Ligament specimens that have been subjected to the freeze–thaw preparation procedure exhibit larger hysteresis than fresh specimens in the first few cycles of loading (Woo et al 1986). At a low temperature of testing,

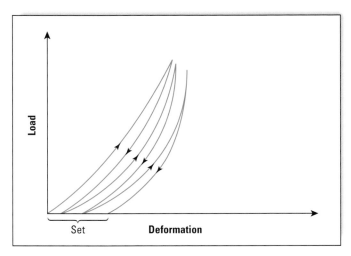

Figure 4.5   Schematic representation of hysteresis.

ligament specimens show a decrease in the area of the hysteresis loop (Woo et al 1987a). Another significant implication of hysteresis for physical therapists is that during ligament stress testing, it is important to precondition the ligament with a few trial tests so as to dissipate the energy of hysteresis and obtain more repeatable test results.

When a ligament is subject to a constant load over time, it exhibits 'creep' behavior such that the elongation increases gradually before reaching a plateau. Conversely, when a ligament is subject to constant elongation over time, it exhibits the 'load-relaxation' characteristic (Fig. 4.6) (Ng et al 1995, 1996b).

The significance of creep and load-relaxation for physical therapists is demonstrated during stretching. In order to stretch the joint effectively, the force must be sustained for a period of time in a constant manner so

that the ligaments and other soft tissues creep (Alter 1996). A study by Bandy & Irion (1994) demonstrated that stretching for 30 s produced the optimum results. No extra benefit was shown with longer than 30 s of stretch, probably because soft tissues creep most significantly in the initial 30 s of loading (Lee & Evans 1994).

With a stiff joint, pain will be elicited during stretching. If the joint is held at the end of the range and maintained in that position, the pain may decrease over time due to load-relaxation (Alter 1996, Etnyre & Abraham 1984). Such load-relaxation will render the stretching to be more tolerable by the patient before the therapist progresses further with larger stretching force.

Besides stretching, there are other clinical implications of the viscoelastic behavior of ligaments, in particular during exercises involving constant and repetitive ligamentous strains, such as jogging (Woo et al 1981, 1982). Cyclic load-relaxation will happen such that loading to joint tissues will decrease in order to protect the ligaments from over-load failure. The repetitive constant loading to the joint will lead to ligament creep, resulting in a temporary increase in ligament stress immediately after exercises (Sailor et al 1995). With adequate rest, creep disappears and the ligament will return to its original length (Badtke et al 1993, Eklund & Corlett 1984, Wilby et al 1987).

FACTORS AFFECTING LIGAMENT STRENGTH

Most ligaments in the body demonstrate the typical load–deformation curve discussed above. However, the exact biomechanical properties of each ligament are unique.

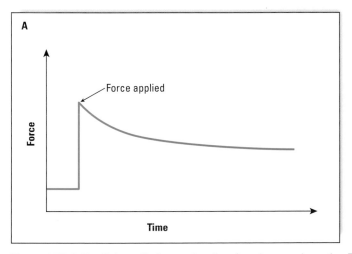

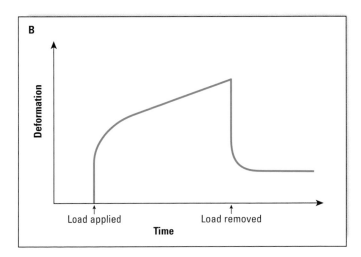

Figure 4.6A & B   Schematic force-relaxation **A** and creep-elongation **B** curve for ligaments. (From Frank C B, Shrive N G 1994 Ligament. In: Nigg B M, Herzog W [eds]. Biomechanics of the musculo-skeletal system. © 1994 John Wiley & Sons Limited. Reproduced with permission.)

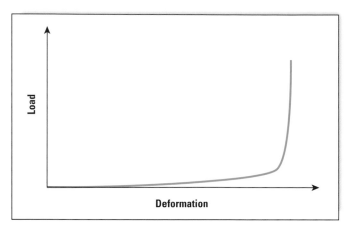

Figure 4.7   Load–deformation characteristics of ligamentum flavum.

There are certain internal and external factors affecting the strength of ligaments. These factors include structural components, the subject's age, strain rate, and loading direction. Each of these will be discussed in the following sections.

STRUCTURAL COMPONENTS

The strength of a ligament largely depends on the type and quantity of its collagen fibers. An anatomical study by Ramsey (1966) revealed that elastic fibers constitute more than two-thirds of the dry weight of ligamentum flavum. A later study by Nachemson & Evans (1968) demonstrated a very distinct biomechanical behavior of this ligament. It is almost perfectly elastic with an unusually high strain value of 70% before failure in young subjects (Fig. 4.7).

The decrease in electromyographic (EMG) activities of back muscles during trunk flexion movement was considered to be associated with energy stored in ligamentum flavum that provided passive support to the upper trunk (Kippers & Parker 1984, Ng & Walter 1995, Steventon & Ng 1995). Furthermore, the elastic nature of this ligament also has a protective function, such that it will not buckle into the spinal canal and impinge onto the spinal cord with trunk movements (Bogduk & Twomey 1987).

AGE

In considering the factor of age, the processes of maturation and aging should be considered separately. Oakes & Parker (1981) reported an increase in the mean collagen fibril diameter in rat ACL from birth to about 7 weeks and then a plateau afterwards. Larson & Parker (1982) found that the ultimate tensile strength of ACL changed in a similar pattern to the collagen fibril

diameter, demonstrating an increase from birth to maturity and then a leveling off. Woo et al (1990) compared the biomechanical properties of medial collateral ligament (MCL) in both skeletally immature and mature rabbits. They found that all skeletally immature specimens failed by tibial avulsion, whereas the mature specimens failed in the MCL substance regardless of the loading rate. These findings suggest that both the ligament substance and insertion site increased in strength with maturation, but the gain in strength is higher in the insertion than the ligament.

With aging however, Noyes & Grood (1976) found that the human femur–ACL–tibia complex from donors aged between 16–26 years had higher ultimate tensile strength and stiffness than donors aged between 48–86 years by a factor of 2 to 3. Similar findings have also been reported by Woo & Adams (1990) where the linear stiffness and ultimate tensile strength both decreased with aging independent of the direction of loading.

The change in biomechanical properties with age is likely to be mediated by the increase in quantity and quality of cross-links and collagen content with maturation, and the decrease of these with aging (Viidik et al 1982).

STRAIN RATE

Studies of the bone–ligament–bone complex have revealed that the structures responded differently at different strain rates. At load strain rates of less than 100% per s, most failures occurred in the insertions with bony avulsion, whereas at strain rates of 100% or higher per s, the failures occurred in the midsubstance of the ligaments (Crowninshield & Pope 1976, Haut 1983, Noyes et al 1974a). Besides the location of failure, the ultimate tensile strength and energy absorption capacity of the ligaments also increased with strain rate regardless of age of the subjects (Woo et al 1990).

LOADING DIRECTION

Ligament such as the ACL has its longitudinal axis oriented at an angle to the bones. Previous studies have shown that with loading applied along the longitudinal axis of tibia, the ultimate tensile strength of the ACL decreased with knee flexion, but when the load was applied along the ACL axis, no such change occurred (Figgie et al 1986, Woo et al 1987b).

Woo & Adams (1990) compared the direction of loading on 14 pairs of femur–ACL–tibia specimens with one leg tested along the tibial axis and the other tested along the ACL axis. They found higher ultimate strength and stiffness, but lower maximum strain to failure in the ACL when the load was applied along the ligament axis.

Table 4.2 Classification of ligament injury (Reproduced with permission from Leadbetter W B 1994. Soft tissue athletic injury. In: Fu F H, Stone D A [eds] Sports injuries: mechanisms, prevention, treatment. Williams and Wilkins, Baltimore, p733–780)

Grade	Severity	Degree	Structural involvement	Examination	Performance deficit
1	Mild	First	Negligible	No visible injury Locally tender only Joint stable	Minimal to a few days
2	Moderate	Second	Partial	Visible swelling Marked tenderness ± stability	Up to 6 weeks (may be modified by protective bracing)
3	Severe	Third	Complete	Gross swelling Marked tenderness Antalgic posture Unstable	Indefinite, minimum of 6–8 weeks

The mode of failure was also different such that midsubstance failure was produced with ACL axial loading but tibial insertion failure was produced with tibial axial loading. It was suggested that during tibial axial loading, the load was not evenly distributed to the collagen fiber bundles (Woo & Adams, 1990). Some fibers may take up more load than others, which tends to 'peel off' the insertion thus affecting the structural properties.

LIGAMENT INJURY AND REPAIR

The mechanisms of injury can be classified into seven categories (Leadbetter 1994):

1. Contact or direct trauma
2. Dynamic loading
3. Repetitive overuse
4. Structural vulnerability
5. Poor flexibility
6. Muscle imbalance
7. Rapid growth.

In sports medicine, the principal mechanism of injury is related to mechanical loading as characterized by the magnitude, location, direction, duration, frequency, variability, and rate of the load (Whiting & Zernicke 1998).

Injury to a ligament will compromise its joint stabilizing function and ability to control movements (Allen & Harner 1996, Kannus & Järvinen 1987, Parolie & Bergfeld 1986). Injury can also reduce the proprioceptive function of ligaments and lengthen the ligament–muscle reflex time (Beard et al 1994, Borsa et al 1997, Friden et al 1996, 1997, Lam et al in press, Wu et al 2001a, 2001b). Ligamentous injury can happen with a single dose of loading that surpasses the ligament's maximum

tolerance, or from cumulative overloads (repetitive sprains) with insufficient time to recover, such that these chronic insults can set the stage for an acute ligamentous rupture (DiGiovanni et al 2000, Griffith et al 2001).

Knowing the extent of injury is of paramount importance for sports physical therapists in determining the management of athletes' injuries. Minor ligament sprains may only cause some annoyances without functional loss, but if ignored and with repeated loading, these minor injuries can progress to more severe ones. Increasing the severity of sprains will cause more functional loss and require a longer time to heal. In the cases of total rupture of some ligaments, the results can be catastrophic or even fatal, such as rupturing the annular ligament of the alanto-axial joint in the cervical spine.

Every ligament injury is unique despite similarities in the biomechanical events and subsequent biological responses. Clinically, it is customary to grade the severity of ligament injury with some clinical classifications. The most typical is a three-level classification system that quantifies the structural involvement, signs, and functional loss (Leadbetter 1994) (Table 4.2).

Healing after injury is ligament-specific. Some ligaments, such as the MCL, have good healing potential, whereas others, such as the ACL, have a poor chance of healing in the case of total rupture without surgical intervention (Clancy et al 1988, Frank et al 1985, Hefti et al 1991, O'Donoghue et al 1971). Generally, the biological responses following ligamentous injury can be summarized into three phases: (1) bleeding and inflammation, (2) active repair with proliferation of bridging materials, and (3) remodeling (Frank 1996). The cellular activities and timing of each of these phases is depicted in Figure 4.8.

Oakes (1991) reviewed the literature on the clinical aspects of soft tissue repair and concluded that the acute management of a ligamentous injury will have a

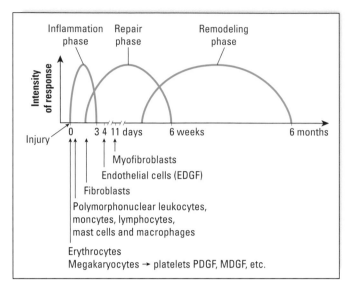

Figure 4.8 The three phases of healing and the cells involved. (From Oakes B W 1992 The classifications of injuries and mechanisms of injury repair and healing. In: Bloomfield J, Fricker P A, Fitch K D [eds]. Textbook of science and medicine in sport. p 201, 209 Blackwell Scientific Publications [www.blackwell-science.com], reproduced with permission.)

significant effect on the outcome of rehabilitation. If the injury is not managed appropriately in the early phase with adequate RICE (rest, ice, compression and elevation), the result will be uncontrolled bleeding and edema, causing abnormal arrangement of collagen fibers and a resultant scar that will become hypertrophic and painful (Fig. 4.9).

In the repair phase, water content remains high. The rate of collagen synthesis reaches its peak at about 3 weeks after injury (Amiel et al 1987). Studies incorporating quantitative collagen fibril analysis have indicated that early mobilization in the first 3 weeks could be detrimental to collagen orientation, but after this time frame, mobilization could increase the tensile strength of the repairing ligament (Oakes 1992).

The remodeling phase of ligament healing starts from week 6 and continues to week 26 or even up to 1 year. The water content of the ligament returns to normal while total collagen content remains slightly increased. The scar tissues continue to mature slowly and approximate the properties of the normal tissues. In a study of ACL repair in goat tissue with a 3-year follow-up period, Ng et al (1996b) induced a surgical transection injury to the posterolateral bundle of the ligament and kept the anteromedial bundle intact as an internal splint. It was found that the repair tissue attained 75% of the normal ultimate tensile strength at 1 year. At 3 years, the strength even surpassed that of the normal ligament by 28%. The structural stiffness of the ligament also improved with time and achieved 97% of the normal value at 3 years. The rate of improvement of Young's modulus, however,

did not parallel the stiffness as it only achieved 72% of the normal value at 3 years. Examination of the repair tissue with transmission electron microscopy, however, revealed that most of the collagen fibrils at 3 years were small at a size of less than 100 nm in diameter, with very few large fibrils scattered in the matrix. Furthermore, the cross-sectional area of the repair bundle increased by about 50% at 3 years (Ng 1995).

The research findings of Ng and his colleagues indicate two important points. First, under favorable conditions, such as a clean wound and an incomplete rupture with close approximation of the ruptured ends, healing of the ACL is possible. With enough time, the repair tissue can simulate the structural properties of a normal ligament. This has also been supported by other researchers using different animal models and ligaments (Chimich et al 1991, Hefti et al 1991). Second, the material properties of the repaired ACL remain inferior to the normal tissue even at 3 years. The good ultimate tensile strength and stiffness of the repair ligament is due to hypertrophy of the scar. Despite the hypertrophic scar increasing the structural strength, it will occupy more space, especially for intraarticular ligaments. It is possible that the large intra-articular scar tissue impinges on other structures of the joint, thus leading to degenerative changes in the longer term (Kannus & Järvinen 1987).

LIGAMENT GRAFTS

Ligament grafting, in particular, ACL grafts, have attracted much attention in clinical and basic science research in the past 2 decades. The following discussion will focus on the biological, biomechanical, and rehabilitation aspects of ACL autograft.

Since the first reported case of ACL graft by Hey Groves (1917), the surgical procedures, postoperative management, and rehabilitation have made significant advancement. Generally, ACL reconstruction will be the preferred choice of management for the following patient groups: (1) young and athletic people, (2) chronic cases with knee instability and episodes of giving way, and (3) combined ligamentous and meniscal injuries (Noyes & Barber-Westin 1997, Renstrom & Lynch 1998, Veltri & Warren 1994a, 1994b).

There is evidence in the literature to suggest that ACL reconstruction should not be performed in the acute phase due to increased risk of arthrofibrosis (Shelbourne et al 1991, Wasilewski et al 1993). The surgical repair should be delayed for 2–3 weeks, and during that period the patient should receive an aggressive rehabilitation program to improve the range of motion and resolve swelling. The success of an ACL graft depends on the

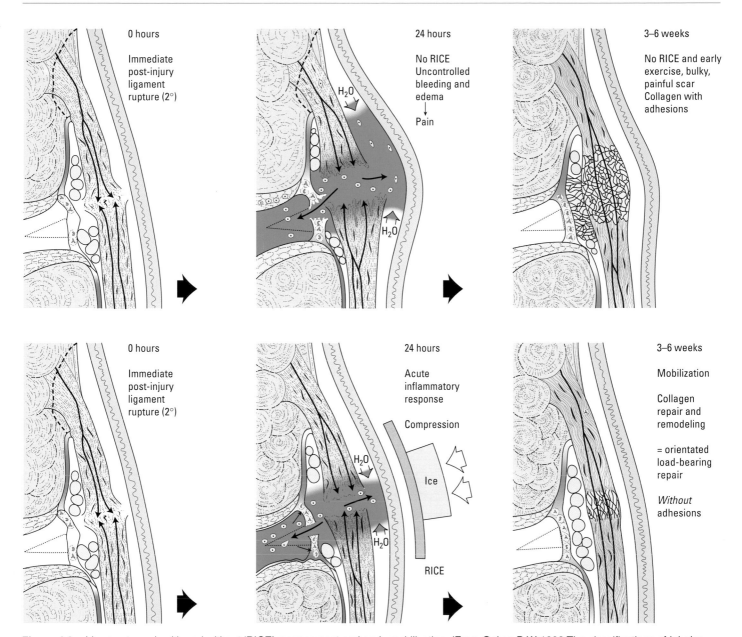

Figure 4.9 Ligament repair with and without 'RICE' management and early mobilization. (From Oakes B W 1992 The classifications of injuries and mechanisms of injury repair and healing. In: Bloomfield J, Fricker P A, Fitch K D [eds]. Textbook of science and medicine in sport. p 201, 209 Blackwell Scientific Publications [www.blackwell-science.com], reproduced with permission.)

mechanical response of the graft tissue and surgical procedures (Renstrom & Lynch 1998). The selection of graft has been a subject of interest for a long time. Currently, three main types of grafts are used:

1. Bone–patellar tendon–bone autograft
2. Quadrupled semitendinosus autograft
3. Bone–patellar tendon–bone allograft (Table 4.3).

Oakes (1988) studied the collagen remodeling mechanisms of ACL grafts in patients requiring arthroscopic intervention because of joint stiffness, meniscal, or cartilage problems at 9 months to 6 years postsurgery.

Biopsies were taken from the graft and analyzed with transmission electron microscopy. His results indicated a predominance of small diameter collagen fibrils not arranged in an orderly manner.

In a study of ACL–patella tendon autograft in goats (Ng 1995), it was found that most of the endogenous large collagen fibrils (greater than 100 nm diameter) in the original patellar tendon graft disappeared as early as 6 weeks after surgery. The collagen fibril sizes remained small throughout the first year. At 3 years, there were some large fibrils repopulating and scattering inside the graft, but the packing density and orientations of the

Table 4.3 Comparison of different ACL grafts

Graft type	Advantages	Disadvantages
Bone–PT–bone autograft	Good initial strength Does not trigger immune response	Disturbs extensor mechanism Predisposes to anterior knee pain
Quadrupled semitendinosus autograft	Does not affect knee extension mechanism Does not trigger immune response	Low ultimate tensile strength High failure rate reported May lead to hamstring weakness
Bone–PT–bone allograft	No risk of donor site morbidity Availability of larger grafts Shorter operation time and smaller incision with improved cosmesis	Potential risk of disease transmission Risk of immunological response of the recipient Higher cost

Bone–PT–bone – bone–patellar tendon–bone

collagen fibrils were still inferior to the normal tissues (Fig. 4.10).

Ng et al (1995, 1996a) studied the biomechanical strength and biochemical cross-link density of the ACL graft at different time intervals and found the rate of load-relaxation in the graft to be significantly faster than normal at less than 1 year. After the first year, however, the load-relaxation rate slowed down. The ultimate

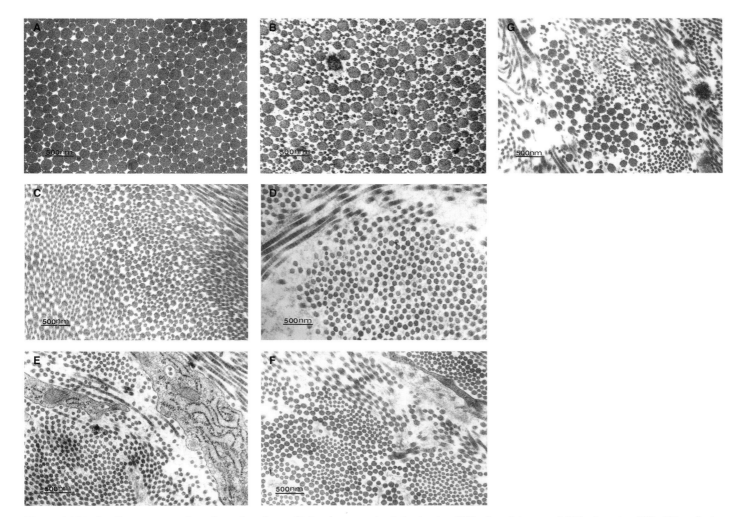

Figure 4.10A–G Transverse sections through collagen fibrils of **a** normal patellar tendon (PT) of goat; **b** normal ACL of goat; **c** ACL–PT graft at 6 weeks; **d** ACL–PT graft at 12 weeks; **e** ACL–PT graft at 24 weeks; **f** ACL–PT graft at 1 year; and **g** ACL–PT graft at 3 years. Magnification at ×20 000. The collagen fibril size remained small in the graft at all time points. Some large fibrils repopulated the graft at 3 years, but the orientation of the fibrils is still not parallel even at 3 years.

strength and stiffness of the graft dropped in the initial 3 months and then gradually improved, but only achieving 43% and 48% respectively of the normal values at 3 years. In these studies, there was a concomitant change in hydroxypyridinium cross-links density in the graft, which was significantly correlated with the Young's modulus of the graft.

The studies of ACL graft carried out by Ng and his colleagues (Ng et al 1995, 1996a) revealed that graft remodeling is a long and continuing process. Considering the long time (3 years) involved in these studies, and the persistent lower than normal biomechanical performance of the grafts in these time periods, the implication is that the grafts may never achieve the properties of normal tissues. The findings are in agreement with other animal studies that showed the ultimate tensile strength at 1 or 2 years after reconstruction was less than 50% of the normal value (Renstrom & Lynch 1998). In contrast, a biomechanical study with a human ACL graft revealed that the graft achieved 87% of ultimate tensile strength of the control value at 8 months after surgery (Beynnon et al 1997). The discrepancy between this human study and previous animal studies could be due to interspecies difference or success of the rehabilitation program in humans after ACL reconstruction. However, the Beynnon et al study only involved one subject and the strength of the normal ACL of that subject was 1015 N, which was substantially lower than the normal value of 1730 N to 2160 N reported in the literature (Noyes et al 1984, Woo et al 1991). Therefore, caution must be exercised in interpreting the result of that single case human study.

EFFECTS OF IMMOBILIZATION AND EXERCISE

Ligaments are sensitive to training and disuse. The original work in this area was carried out by Noyes et al (1974b) as a part of the US airforce experiments on the effect of long-term immobilization on ligaments. It was demonstrated that in primates, 8 weeks of cast immobilization of the lower limb resulted in substantial loss of strength in the ACL. With a reconditioning program, it took close to 1 year for the ligament to attain 91% ultimate tensile strength and 98% stiffness of the normal value.

From the metabolic perspective, Amiel et al (1983) analyzed the collagen turnover rate of rabbit MCL following 12 weeks of knee immobilization. They found that the collagen mass of MCL decreased by about 30% due to degradation of the collagen. In a later study, Amiel et al (1985) further demonstrated a close relationship

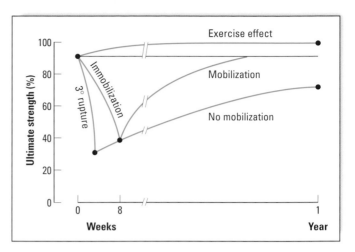

Figure 4.11 The effects of immobilization, remobilization and exercise on strength of ligament. After only 8 weeks of immobilization, ligament strength decreased substantially, and it takes months to recover. The rate of recovery is faster with mobilization than without mobilization. (Reproduced from Woo S L-Y, Gomez M A, Sites T J, Newton P O, Orlando C A, Akeson W H 1987 The biomechanical and morphological changes in the medial collateral ligament of the rabbit after immobilization and remobilization. Journal of Bone and Joint Surgery (Am) 69(A): 1200–1211. Copyright 1987 The Journal of Bone and Joint Surgery.)

between joint stiffness (as induced by immobilization) and decrease in GAGs of the joint tissues. Similar findings of ligament atrophy with immobilization were also reported by Woo et al (1987c). Woo and colleagues (1987c) demonstrated that an enforced exercise program could hasten the return of mechanical properties of the ligaments (Fig. 4.11).

The evidence in the literature clearly demonstrates that prolonged immobilization is detrimental to ligaments. The effects of immobilization are reversible but the effects of reconditioning took a longer time to show than that of immobilization. Exercise programs, however, can hasten the recovery following immobilization.

The beneficial effects of exercise on ligaments have been thoroughly investigated by several researchers (Andrews & O'Neill 1994, Cabaud et al 1980, Larsen & Parker 1982, Tipton et al 1970, 1975, Woo et al 2000). The early work of Tipton et al (1970) revealed that the MCL of dogs that had been subjected to 6 weeks of strenuous exercise training were significantly stronger and stiffer than those of the control group. Oakes & Parker (1981) studied the collagen fibril diameters of ACL and posterior cruciate ligaments of rats after 4 weeks of treadmill running and swimming. They found that the exercised rats had a higher number of collagen fibrils per unit area than the control rats. Interestingly, Oakes & Parker (1981) found a decrease in mean fibril diameter in the exercised rats, and they explained this phenomenon as related to the change in the type of GAGs in response to loading, which mediated the collagen fibril size.

Table 4.4 Means and (standard deviation) of anteroposterior laxity and stiffness of the knee joint of athletes in different sports measured by KT-2000 knee arthrometer (Reprinted from Physical Therapy in Sport, 2, Ng G Y F & Maitland M E Relationship of kinetic demands of athletic training and knee joint laxity, p 66–70, by permission of the publisher Churchill Livingstone.)

	Basketball	Running	Swimming	Control
Laxity (mm)	6.4 (2.29)	7.3 (2.08)	5.9 (2.30)	7.8 (2.40)
Stiffness (N/mm)	47.5 (23.09)	45.2 (23.09)	57.8 (32.37)	37.9 (15.90)

Andrews & O'Neill (1994) reported that pelvic exercise is useful in shortening the duration and lowering the intensity of ligament pain during pregnancy.

Ng & Maitland (2001) recently compared the anteroposterior laxity, stiffness and rate of change of stiffness, in the knee joints of athletes involved in basketball, running, swimming, and of sedentary control subjects during an instrumented KT-2000 anterior drawer test. It was found that swimmers had the lowest laxity and highest stiffness in their knees followed by the basketball athletes, runners, and then the control subjects (Table 4.4). This could be due to the different kinetic loading of these sports to the knees and to the response of the joint structures to loading. If this response also happens in ligaments under repair, it will have implications for the choice of rehabilitation exercises for subjects after ligament injuries.

Exercise may not always produce beneficial effects on ligaments. In the study by Burroughs & Dahners (1990), they examined the effect of the dosage of exercise on rats with differences of severity of injury to the MCL, ACL, and medial joint capsule. Burroughs & Dahners (1990) measured the tensile strength of the repairing ligaments and laxity of the knee joint, and found that exercise had a beneficial effect on the healing MCL that had no associated ACL injury. For the knee joints that demonstrated severe instability with combined injuries of the MCL, ACL, and the medial joint capsule, laxity in the joint deteriorated and no increase in tensile strength of the repairing ligaments was found with exercise training. Therefore, rehabilitation exercise programs should be carefully planned and monitored for athletes with severe joint instability.

SUMMARY

Ligaments are classified as dense connective tissue and the main organic constituent in most ligaments is collagen. The collagen determines the biomechanical strength and viscoelastic properties. Ligaments are important passive restraining structures for joints. Injuries to ligaments are common in sport and exercise and in the case of total rupture, the consequence can be debilitating if it is left untreated or mismanaged. Like many other body tissues, most ligaments are capable of repairing themselves after injury, but the whole process of remodeling for the repaired tissue may take 6–12 months, and the strength of the scar is persistently inferior to the normal tissue. For some ligaments, such as the ACL, active repair may not happen with total rupture, and surgical reconstruction is indicated.

Prolonged immobilization weakens ligament and it takes a considerable time of reconditioning exercise in order to regain the functional strength. Ligaments respond to mechanical loading by synthesizing collagen, and thus increase strength. Too much loading, however, is not beneficial to ligaments, particularly in an unstable joint. It is therefore important that rehabilitation exercise programs should be strategically designed in order to induce the appropriate amount of loading to ligament according to the stage and timing of repair.

REFERENCES

Allen A A, Harner C D 1996 When your patient injures the posterior cruciate ligament. Journal of Musculoskeletal Medicine 13:44–55
Alter M J 1996 Science of flexibility, 2nd edn. Human Kinetics, Champaign IL, p113–126
Amiel D, Kleiner J B 1988 Biochemistry of tendon and ligament. In: Nimni M E, Olsen B (eds) Collagen. Biotechnology, Vol III. CRC Press, Cleveland, p223–253
Amiel D, Akeson W H, Harwood F L et al 1983 Stress deprivation effect on the metabolic turnover of the medial collateral ligament collagen: a comparison between nine and 12–week immobilization. Clinical Orthopaedics and Related Research 172:265–270
Amiel D, Frank C B, Harwood F L et al 1984 Tendons and ligaments: a morphological and biochemical comparison. Journal of Orthopaedic Research 1:257–265
Amiel D, Frey C, Woo S L-Y et al 1985 Value of hyaluronic acid in the prevention of contracture formation. Clinical Orthopaedics and Related Research 196:306–311
Amiel D, Frank C B, Harwood F L et al 1987 Collagen alteration in medial collateral ligament healing in a rabbit model. Connective Tissue Research 16:357–366
Amiel D, Billings Jr E, Akeson W H 1990 Ligament structure, chemistry and physiology. In: Daniel D, Akeson W, O'Connor J (eds) Knee ligaments structure, function, injury, and repair. Raven Press, New York, p 77–91
Andrews C M, O'Neill L M 1994 Use of pelvic tilt exercise for ligament pain relief. Journal of Nurse-Midwifery 39:370–374
Arnoczky S P, Matyas J R, Buckwalter J A et al 1993 Anatomy of the anterior cruciate ligament. In: Jackson D W, Arnoczky S P, Frank C B et al (eds) The anterior cruciate ligament current and future concepts. Raven Press, New York, p 5–22

Badtke G, Bittmann F, Laxik D 1993 Changes in the vertebral column in the course of the day. International Journal of Sports Medicine 14:159

Bailey A J, Robins S P, Balian G 1974 Biological significance of the intermolecular cross-links of collagen. Nature 251:105–109

Bandy W D, Irion J M 1994 The effect of time on static stretch on the flexibility of the hamstring muscles. Physical Therapy 74:845–850

Beard D J, Kyberd P J, O'Connor J J et al 1994 Reflex hamstring contraction latency in anterior cruciate ligament deficiency. Journal of Orthopaedic Research 12:219–228

Beynnon B D, Risberg M A, Tjomsland O et al 1997 Evaluation of knee joint laxity and the structural properties of the anterior cruciate ligament graft in the human: a case report. American Journal of Sports Medicine 25:203–206

Bogduk N, Twomey L T 1987 Clinical anatomy of the lumbar spine. Churchill Livingstone, Melbourne, p 35–36

Bornstein P, Armstrong L C, Hankenson K D et al 2000 Thrombospondin 2, a matricellular protein with diverse function. Matrix Biology 19:557–568

Borsa P A, Lephart S M, Irrgang J J et al 1997 The effects of joint position and direction of joint motion on proprioceptive sensibility in anterior cruciate ligament – deficient athletes. American Journal of Sports Medicine 25:336–340

Buckwalter J A, Cooper R R 1987 The cells and matrices of skeletal connective tissues. In: Albright, Brand (eds) The scientific basis of Orthopaedics. Appleton and Lange, Norwalk, p 1–29

Burroughs P, Dahners L E 1990 The effect of enforced exercise on the healing of ligament injuries. American Journal of Sports Medicine 18:376–378

Cabaud H E, Chatty A, Gildengorin V et al 1980 Exercise effects on the strength of the rat anterior cruciate ligament. American Journal of Sports Medicine 8:79–84

Chapman J A 1989 The regulation of size and form in the asssembly of collagen fibrils in vivo. Biopolymers 28:1367–1382

Chen H, Herndon M E, Lawler J 2000 The cell biology of thrombospondin –1. Matrix Biology 19:597–614

Chimich D, Frank C, Shrive N et al 1991 The effects of initial end contact on medial collateral ligament healing: a morphological and biomechanical study in a rabbit model. Journal of Orthopaedic Research 9:37–47

Clancy W G, Ray J, Zoltan D 1988 Acute tear of the anterior cruciate ligament. Surgical versus conservative treatment. Journal of Bone and Joint Surgery 70A:1483–1488

Clayton M L, Miles J S, Abdulla M 1968 Experimental investigations of ligamentous healing. Clinical Orthopaedics and Related Research 61:146–153

Cooper R R, Misol S 1970 Tendon and ligament insertion. A light and electron microscopic study. Journal of Bone and Joint Surgery 52A:1–20

Copenhaver W M, Bunge R P, Bune M B 1971 Bailey's textbook of histology, 16th edn. Williams and Wilkins, Baltimore, p 125–127.

Crowninshield R D, Pope M H 1976 The strength and failure characteristics of rat medial collateral ligaments. Journal of Trauma 16:99–105

Dale W C, Baer E 1974 Fibre-buckling in composite systems: a model for the ultrastructure of uncalcified collagen tissues. Journal of Material Science 9:369–382

Dale W C, Baer E, Keller A et al 1972 On the ultrastructure of mammalian tendon. Experientia 28:1293–1295

Diamant J, Keller A, Baer E et al 1972 Collagen, ultrastructure and its relation to mechanical properties as a function of ageing. Proceedings of the Royal Society of London (Biology) 180:293–315

DiGiovanni B F, Fraga C J, Cohen B E et al 2000 Associated injuries found in chronic lateral ankle instability. Foot and Ankle International 21:809–815

Dye S F, Dilworth Cannon W D 1988 Anatomy and biomechanics of the anterior cruciate ligament. Clinics in Sports Medicine 7:715–725

Eklund J A E, Corlett E N 1984 Shrinkage as a measure of the effect of load on the spine. Spine 9:189–194

Etnyre B, Abraham L 1984 Effects of three stretching techniques on the motor pool excitability of the human soleus muscle. In: Roll W (ed) Abstracts of research papers 1984. American Alliance of Health, Physical Education, and Recreation. Reston, VA, p 90

Eyre D R 1980 Collagen: molecular diversity in the body's protein scaffold. Science 207:1315–1322

Figgie H E, Bahniuk E H, Heiple K G et al 1986 The effects of tibial-femoral angle on the failure mechanics of the canine anterior cruciate ligament. Journal of Biomechanics 19:89–91

Frank C B 1996 Ligament injuries: pathophysiology and healing. In: Zachazewski J E, Magee D J, Quillen W S (eds) Athletic injuries and rehabilitation. Saunders, Philadelphia, p 9–26

Frank C B, Shrive N G 1994 Ligament. In: Nigg B M, Herzog W (eds) Biomechanics of the musculo-skeletal system. John Wiley, Chichester, p 106–132

Frank C B, Amiel D, Woo S L-Y et al 1985 Normal ligament properties and ligament healing. Clinical Orthopaedics and Related Research 196:15–25

Frank C B, Bray D F, Rademaker A et al 1989 Electron microscopic quantification of collagen fibril diameters in the rabbit medial collateral ligament: A baseline for comparison. Connective Tissue Research 19:11–25

Frank C B, McDonald D, Bray D R et al 1992 Collagen fibril diameters in the healing adult rabbit medial collateral ligament. Connective Tissue Research 27:251–263

Frank C B, Eyre D, Shrive N 1994 Hydroxypyridinium cross-link deficiency in ligament scar. Transactions of the 40th Annual Meeting of Orthopaedics Research Society, New Orleans. 13:3

Frank C B, McDonald D, Shrive N 1997 Collagen fibril diameters in the rabbit medial collateral ligament scar: a longer term assessment. Connective Tissue Research 36:261–269

Friden T, Roberts D, Zatterstrom R et al 1996 Proprioception in the nearly extended knee. Measurements of position and movement in healthy individuals and in symptomatic anterior cruciate ligament injured patients. Knee Surgery, Sports Traumatology and Arthroscopy 4:217–224

Friden T, Roberts D, Zatterstrom R et al 1997 Proprioception after an acute knee ligament injury: a longitudinal study on 16 consecutive patients. Journal of Orthopaedic Research 15:637–644

Fujimoto D 1977 Isolation and characterization of a fluorescent material in bovine Achilles tendon collagen. Biochemical and Biophysical Research Communication 74:1124–1129

Fujimoto D, Moriguchi T 1978 Pyridinoline, a non-reducible cross-link of collagen. Journal of Biochemistry 83:863–867

Fung Y C B 1981 Biomechanics: mechanical properties of living tissues. Springer Verlag, New York, p 222

Garde R E 1988 Cervical traction: the neurophysiology of lordosis and the rheological characteristics of cervical curve rehabilitation. In: Harrison D D (ed) Chiropractic: the physics of spinal correction. Sunnyvale, CA, p 535–659

Griffith J F, Roebuck D J, Cheng J C et al 2001 Acute elbow trauma in children: spectrum of injury revealed by MR imaging not apparent on radiographs. American Journal of Roentgenology 176:53–60

Gross J 1974 Collagen biology: structure, degradation, and disease. Harvey Lecture 6(B):351–432

Gugssa A, Balan K V, Macias C et al 2000 Fibronectin/fibroblast growth factor/cell matrix signaling pathways and reciprocal membrane integration may be the regulators of cell growth and apoptosis in Trypanosoma musculi in co-cultures with fibroblasts. Journal of Submicroscopic Cytology and Pathology 32:281–296

Ham A W 1974 Histology, 6th edn. JB Lippincott, Philadelphia, p 374–377

Hardingham T E, Fosang A J 1992 Proteoglycans: many forms and many functions. FASEB Journal 6:861–870

Hardy M A 1989 The biology of scar formation. Physical Therapy 69:1014–1024

Haut R C 1983 Age-dependent influence of strain rate on the tensile failure of rat-tail tendon. Journal of Biomechanical Engineering 105:296–299

Haut R C, Little R W A 1972 A constitutive equation for collagen fibers. Journal of Biomechanics 5:423–430

Hefti F L, Kress A, Fasel J et al 1991 Healing of the transected anterior cruciate ligament in the rabbit. Journal of Bone and Joint Surgery 73A:373–383

Hey Groves E W 1917 Operation for the repair of the crucial ligaments. Lancet 2:674–675

Hirsch G 1974 Tensile properties during tendon healing. Acta Orthopaedica Scandinavica Supplementum153:1–145

Hodge A J, Petruska J A 1963 Recent studies with the electron microscope on ordered aggregates of the tropocollagen molecule. In: Ramachandran G (ed.) Aspects of protein structure. Academic Press, New York, p 289–301

Jones P L, Jones F S 2000 Tenascin-C in development and disease: gene regulation and cell formation. Matrix Biology 19:581–596

Kannus P, Järvinen M 1987 Conservatively treated tears of the anterior cruciate ligament: Long-term results. Journal of Bone and Joint Surgery 69A:1007–1012

Kasser J 1996 Orthopaedic knowledge update 5: home study syllabus. American Academy of Orthopaedic Surgeons, Park Ridge, IL

Kastelic J, Galeski A, Baer E 1978 The multicomposite structure of tendon. Connective Tissue Research 6:11–23

Kippers V, Parker A W 1984 Posture related to myoelectric silence of erectores spinae during trunk flexion. Spine 9:740–745

Kirby M C, Sikoryn T A, Hukins D W L et al 1989 Structure and mechanical properties of the longitudinal ligaments and ligamentum flavum of the spine. Journal of Biomedical Engineering 11:192–196

Kleinman J K, Cannon F B, Laurie G W et al 1985 Biological activities of laminin. Journal of Cell Biochemistry 27:235–242

Knott L, Bailey A J 1998 Collagen cross-links in mineralizing tissues: A review of their chemistry, function, and clinical relevance. Bone 22:181–187

Koukoulis G K, Gould V E, Bhattacharyya A et al 1991 Tenascin in normal, reactive, hyperplastic and neoplastic tissues: biologic and pathologic implications. Human Pathology 22:636–643

Lam R Y H, Ng G Y F, Chien E P in press Does wearing a functional knee brace affect hamstring reflex time on subjects with anterior cruciate ligament deficiency during muscle fatigue? Archives of Physical Medicine and Rehabilitation

Larson N, Parker A W 1982 Physical activity and its influence on the strength and elastic stiffness of knee ligaments. In: Howell M L, Parker A W (eds) Sports medicine: medical and scientific aspects of elitism in sport. Australian Sports Medicine Federation, Brisbane 8:63–73

Leadbetter W B 1994 Soft tissue athletic injury. In: Fu F H, Stone D A (eds) Sports injuries: Mechanisms, prevention, treatment. Williams and Wilkins, Baltimore, p 733–780

Lee R, Evans J 1994 Towards a better understanding of spinal posteroanterior mobilisation. Physiotherapy 80:68–73

Linsenmayer T F 1991 Collagen. In: Hay E D (ed) Cell biology of extracellular matrix, 2nd edn. Plenum Press, New York, p 7–44

McDonald J A 1988 Fibronectin: a primitive matrix. In: Clark R A F, Henson P M (eds) The molecular and cellular biology of wound repair. Plenum Press, New York, p 405–435

Matthew C A, Moore M J 1991 Regeneration of rat extensor digitorum longus tendon: the effect of a sequential partial tenotomy on collagen fibril formation. Matrix 11:259–268

Mecham R P, Heuser J E 1991 The elastic fiber. In: Hay E (ed) Cell biology of extracellular matrix, 2nd edn. Plenum Press, New York, p 79–109

Mechanic G L 1974 An automated scintillation counting system for continuous analysis: cross-links of (^{3}H)NaBH$_4$ reduced collagen. Analytical Biochemistry 61:349–354

Miller R R, McDevitt C A 1991 Thrombospondin in ligament, meniscus and intervertebral disc. Biochimica et Biophysica Acta 111:85–88

Minns R J, Soden P D, Jackson D S 1973 The role of the fibrous components and ground substance in the mechanical properties of biological tissues: a preliminary investigation. Journal of Biomechanics 6:153–165

Murray M M, Spector M 1999 Fibroblast distribution in the anteromedial bundle of the human anterior cruciate ligament: the presence of alpha-smooth muscle actin-positive cells. Journal of Orthopaedic Research 17:18–27

Nachemson A L, Evans J H 1968 Some mechanical properties of the third human lumbar interlaminar ligament (ligament flavum). Journal of Biomechanics 1:211–220

Neurath M F, Stofft E 1992 Collagen ultrastructure in ruptured cruciate ligaments. An electron microscopic investigation. Acta Orthopaedica Scandinavica 63:507–510

Ng G Y F 1995 A long term study of the biomechanical and biological changes of the ACL-PT autograft and ACL repair after hemi-transection injury in a goat model. Thesis, Department of Anatomy, Monash University, Australia

Ng G, Walter K 1995 Ageing does not affect flexion relaxation of erector spinae. Australian Journal of Physiotherapy 41:91–95

Ng G Y F, Maitland M E 2001 Relationship of kinetic demands of athletic training and knee joint laxity. Physical Therapy in Sport 2:66–70

Ng G Y, Oakes B W, Deacon O W et al 1995 Biomechanics of patellar tendon autograft for reconstruction of the anterior cruciate ligament in the goat: three-year study. Journal of Orthopaedic Research 13:602–608

Ng G Y F, Oakes B W, Deacon O W et al 1996a Long-term study of the biochemistry and biomechanics of anterior cruciate ligament-patellar tendon autografts in goats. Journal of Orthopaedic Research 14:851–856

Ng G Y F, Oakes B W, McLean I D et al 1996b The long-term biomechanical and viscoelastic performance of repairing anterior cruciate ligament after hemitransection injury in a goat model. American Journal of Sports Medicine 24:109–117

Nordin M, Lorenz T, Campello M 2001 Biomechanics of tendons and ligaments. In: Nordin M, Frankel V (eds) Basic biomechanics of the musculoskeletal system, 3rd edn. Lippincott Williams and Wilkins, Philadelphia, p 102–125

Noyes F R, Grood E S 1976 The strength of the anterior cruciate ligament in humans and rhesus monkeys: age-related and species-related changes. Journal of Bone and Joint Surgery 58A:1074–1082

Noyes F R, Barber-Westin S D 1997 A comparison of results in acute and chronic anterior cruciate ligament ruptures of arthroscopically assisted autogenous patellar tendon reconstruction. American Journal of Sports Medicine 25:460–471

Noyes F R, De Lucas J L, Torvik P J 1974a Biomechanics of anterior cruciate ligament failure: an analysis of strain rate sensitivity and mechanisms of failure in primates. Journal of Bone and Joint Surgery 56A:236–253

Noyes F R, Torvik P J, Hyde W B et al 1974b Biomechanics of ligament failure. 2. An analysis of immobilization, exercise and reconditioning effects in primates. Journal of Bone and Joint Surgery 56A:1406–1418

Noyes F R, Butler D L, Grood E et al 1984 Biomechanical analysis of human ligament grafts used in knee-ligament repairs and reconstructions. Journal of Bone and Joint Surgery 66A:344–352

Oakes B W 1988 Ultrastructural studies on knee joint ligaments: Quantitation of collagen fibre populations in exercised and control rat cruciate ligaments and in human anterior cruciate ligament grafts. In: Woo S L-Y, Buckwalter J (eds) Injury and repair of the musculoskeletal tissues, Section 2. American Academy of Orthopaedic Surgeons, Illinois, p 66–82

Oakes B W 1991 Clinical aspects of soft tissue repair. Sports Training, Medicine and Rehabilitation 2:279–283

Oakes B W 1992 The classification of injuries and mechanisms of injury, repair and healing. In: Bloomfield J, Fricker P A, Fitch K D (eds) Textbook of science and medicine in sport. Blackwell Scientific Publications, p 200–217

Oakes B W 1994 Tendon-ligament basic science. In: Harries M, Williams C, Stanish W D et al (eds) Oxford textbook of sports medicine. Oxford University Press, New York, p 493–511

Oakes B W, Parker A W 1981 Normal joint changes in collagen fibre populations in young rat cruciate ligaments in response to an intensive one month's exercise program. In: Russo P, Gass G (eds) Human adaptation. Cumberland College of Health Sciences, Sydney, p 223–230

Oakes B W, Deacon O W, Ng G Y et al 2000 Two biological determinants of anterior cruciate ligament graft strength. Book of abstract of 2000 Pre-Olympic Congress for International Congress on Sport Science, Sports Medicine and Physical Education, Brisbane, p 89–90

O'Donoghue D H, Rockwood C A, Zaricznyj B et al 1961 Repair of knee ligaments in dogs. I. The lateral collateral ligament. Journal of Bone and Joint Surgery 43A:1167–1178

O'Donoghue D H, Frank G R, Jeter G L et al 1971 Repair and reconstruction of the anterior cruciate ligament in dogs: factors influencing long term results. Journal of Bone and Joint Surgery 53A:710–718

Olsen B R 1991 Collagen Biosynthesis. In: Hay E (ed.) Cell biology of extracellular matrix, 2nd edn. Plenum Press, New York, p 177–220

Parolie J M, Bergfeld J A 1986 Long-term results of non-operative treatment of isolated posterior cruciate ligament injuries in the athlete. American Journal of Sports Medicine 14:35–38

Parry D A D, Craig A S 1977 Quantitative electron microscope observations of the collagen fibrils in rat-tail tendon. Biopolymers 16:1015–1031

Parry D A D, Craig A S 1979 Electron microscope evidence for an 80Å unit in collagen fibrils. Nature 282:213–214

Parry D A D, Craig A S, Barnes G R G 1978a Tendon and ligament from the horse: an ultrastructural study of collagen fibrils and elastic fibres as a function of age. Proceedings of Royal Society of London (Biology) 203:293–303

Parry D A D, Barnes G R G, Craig A S 1978b A comparison of the size distribution of collagen fibrils in connective tissues as a function of age and a possible relation between fibril size distribution and mechanical properties. Proceedings of Royal Society of London (Biology) 203:305–321

Patterson-Kane J C, Parry D A, Birch H L et al 1997 An age-related study of morphology and cross-link composition of collagen fibrils in the digital flexor tendons of young thoroughbred horses. Connective Tissue Research 36:253–260

Pogany G, Hernandez D J, Vogel K G 1994 The in vitro interaction of proteoglycans with type I collagen is modulated by phosphate. Archives of Biochemistry and Biophysics 313:102–111

Postacchini F, De Martino C 1980 Regeneration of rabbit calcaneal tendon maturation of collagen and elastic fibers following partial tenotomy. Connective Tissue Research 8:41–47

Ramsey R H 1966 The anatomy of the ligamenta falva. Clinical Orthopaedics and Related Research 44:129–140

Raugi G J, Olerud J E, Gown A M 1987 Thrombospondin in early human wound tissue. Journal of Investigative Dermatology 89:551–554

Renstrom Per A F H, Lynch S A 1998 An overview of anterior cruciate ligament management. In: Chan K M, Fu F, Maffulli N (eds) Controversies in orthopedic sports medicine. Williams and Wilkins, Hong Kong, p 5–22

Sailor M E, Keskula D R, Perrin D H 1995 Effect of running on anterior knee laxity in collegiate-level female athletes after anterior cruciate ligament reconstruction. Journal of Orthopaedic and Sports Physical Therapy 21:233–239

Sakakura T, Kusano I 1991 Tenascin in tissue perturbation repair. Acta Pathologica Japonica 41:247–258

Scott J E 1988 Proteoglycan-fibrillar collagen interactions. Biochemical Journal 252:313–323

Shah J S, Jayson M I V, Hampson W G J 1977 Low tension studies of collagen fibres from ligaments of the human spine. Annals of the Rheumatic Diseases 36:139–145

Shelbourne K D, Wickens J H, Mollabashy A et al 1991 Arthrofibrosis in acute anterior cruciate ligament reconstruction: the effect of timing of reconstruction and rehabilitation. American Journal of Sports Medicine 19:332–336

Snook G A 1983 A short history of the anterior cruciate ligament and the treatment of tears. Clinical Orthopaedics and Related Research 172:11–13

Steventon C, Ng G 1995 Effect of trunk flexion speed on flexion relaxation of erector spinae. Australian Journal of Physiotherapy 41:241–243

Tani N, Matsumoto K, Ota I et al 2001 Effects of fibronectin cleaved by neuropcin on cell adhesion and migration. Neuroscience Research 39:247–251

Tanzer M L 1973 Crosslinking of collagen. Science 180:561–566

Tanzer M L 1976 Cross-linking. In: Ramachandran G N, Reddi A H (eds) Biochemistry of collagen. Plenum Press, New York, p 137

Tipton C M, James S L, Mergner W et al 1970 Influence of exercise on the strength of the medial collateral knee ligament of dogs. American Journal of Physiology 218:894–902

Tipton C M, Matthes R D, Maynard J A et al 1975 The influence of physical activity on ligaments and tendons. Medicine and Science in Sports 7:165–175

Veltri D M, Warren R F 1994a Anatomy, biomechanics, and physical findings in posterolateral knee instability. Clinics in Sports Medicine 13:599–614

Veltri D M, Warren R F 1994b Operative treatment of posterolateral instability of the knee. Clinics in Sports Medicine 13:615–627

Viidik A 1973 Functional properties of collagenous tissues. International Review of Connective Tissue Research 6:127–215

Viidik A 1980 Interdependence between structure and function in collagenous tissues. In: Biology of collagen. Academic Press, New York, p 257–278

Viidik A, Sandqvist L, Magi M L 1965 Influence of postmortem storage on tensile strength characteristics and histology of rabbit ligaments. Acta Orthopaedica Scandinavica Supplementum 79:1–38

Viidik A, Danielsen C C, Oxlund H 1982 On fundamental and phenomenological models, structure and mechanical properties of collagen, elastic and glycosaminoglycan complexes. Biorheology 19:437–451

Vogel K G, Trotter J A 1987 The effect of proteoglycans on the morphology of collagen fibrils formed in vitro. Collagen Related Research 7:105–114

Vogel K G, Paulsson M, Heinegard D 1984 Specific inhibition of type I and type II collagen fibrillogenesis by the small proteoglycan of tendon. Biochemical Journal 223:587–597

Wasilewski S A, Covall D J, Cohen S 1993 Effect of surgical timing on recovery and associated injuries after anterior cruciate ligament reconstruction. American Journal of Sports Medicine 21:338–342

Wheater P R, Burkitt H G, Daniels V G 1991 Functional histology. A text and colour Atlas. Churchill Livingstone, Melbourne, p 52–57

White D R, Widdowson E M, Woodard H Q et al 1991 The composition of body tissues (II). Fetus to young adult. The British Journal of Radiology 64:149–159

Whiting W C, Zernicke R F 1998 Biomechanics of musculoskeletal injury. Human Kinetics, Champaign, IL, p 15–40, 87–136

Wight T N, Heinegard D K, Hascall V C 1991 Proteoglycans structure and function. In: Hay E (ed) Cell biology of extracellular matrix, 2nd edn. Plenum Press, New York, p 45–78

Wilby J, Linge K, Reilly T et al 1987 Spinal shrinkage in females: circadian variation and the effects of circuit weight-training. Ergonomics 30:47–54

Woo S L-Y, Adams D J 1990 The tensile properties of human anterior cruciate ligament (ACL) and ACL graft tissues. In: Daniel D, Akeson W, O'Connor J (eds) Knee ligaments structure, function, injury, and repair. Raven Press, New York, p 279–289

Woo S L-Y, Gomez M A, Akeson W H 1981 The time and history dependent viscoelastic properties of the canine medial collateral ligament. Journal of Biomechanical Engineering 103:293–298

Woo S L-Y, Gomex M A, Woo Y-K et al 1982 Mechanical properties of tendons and ligaments. I. Quasi-static and nonlinear viscoelastic properties. Biorheology 19:385–396

Woo S L-Y, Orlando C A, Camp J F et al 1986 Effects of postmortem storage by freezing on ligament tensile behavior. Journal of Biomechanics 19:399–404

Woo S L-Y, Lee T Q, Gomez M A et al 1987a Temperature dependent behavior of the canine medial collateral ligament. Journal of Biomechanical Engineering 109:68–71

Woo S L-Y, Hollis J M, Roux R D et al 1987b Effects of knee flexion on the structural properties of the rabbit femur-anterior cruciate ligament-tibia complex (FATC). Journal of Biomechanics 20:557–563

Woo S L-Y, Gomez M A, Sites T J et al 1987c The biomechanical and morphological changes in the medial collateral ligament of the rabbit after immobilization and remobilization. Journal of Bone and Joint Surgery 69A:1200–1211

Woo S L-Y, Young E P, Kwan M K 1990 Fundamental studies in knee ligament mechanics. In: Daniel D, Akeson W, O'Connor J (eds) Knee ligaments structure, function, injury, and repair. Raven Press, New York, p 115–134

Woo S L-Y, Hollis M, Adams D et al 1991 Tensile properties of the human femur-ACL-tibia complex. Effect of specimen age and orientation. American Journal of Sports Medicine 19:217–225

Woo SL-Y, An K N, Arnoczky S P et al 1994 Anatomy, biology, and biomechanics of tendon, ligament, and meniscus. In: Simon S R (ed) Orthopaedic basic science. American Academy of Orthopaedic Surgeons, Park Ridge, IL, p 89–126

Woo SL-Y, Vogrin T M, Abramowitch S D 2000 Healing and repair of ligament injuries in the knee. Journal of the American Academy of Orthopaedic Surgeons 8:364–372

Woodard H Q, White D R 1986 The composition of body tissues. The British Journal of Radiology 59:1209–1219

Wu G K H, Ng G Y F, Mak A F T 2001a Effects of knee bracing on the functional performance of patients with anterior cruciate ligament reconstruction. Archives of Physical Medicine and Rehabilitation 82:282–285

Wu G K H, Ng G Y F, Mak A F T 2001b Effects of knee bracing on the sensori-motor function of subjects with ACL reconstruction. American Journal of Sports Medicine 29(5): 641–645

Yahia L H, Drouin G 1989 Microscopical investigation of canine anterior cruciate ligament and patellar tendon: collagen fascicle morphology and architecture. Journal of Orthopaedic Research 7:243–251

5

Bone

Kim Bennell   Pekka Kannus

INTRODUCTION

Bone is a unique tissue with the principal responsibility of supporting loads that are imposed on it. Fractures occur when the load exceeds bone strength. Acute fractures result from a single injurious load, while stress fractures are due to the accumulation of microdamage with repeated loading. Osteoporotic fractures occur in bone that is weakened due to low bone mass and microarchitectural deterioration. Physical therapists working in the area of sport and exercise are often involved in the prevention, diagnosis, and rehabilitation of fractures. This chapter will firstly describe bone as an organ and tissue and then review how bone responds to mechanical loads. This will be followed by a discussion of the principles of prevention and treatment of acute, stress, and osteoporotic fractures and the role that physical therapists play in this area.

BONE ANATOMY

BONE CONSTITUENTS

Bone consists of an organic component (20–25% by weight), an inorganic component (70% by weight), and a water component (5% by weight).

Organic matrix

The organic matrix determines the structure and the mechanical and biochemical properties of bone. Ninety-eight percent of the organic matrix is made up of type I collagen and non-collagenous proteins, while the remaining 2% consists of cells (Einhorn 1996).

Collagen

Collagen is a protein that consists of three polypeptide

chains of about 1000 amino acids each and wound together in a helix pattern by cross-links of hydrogen bonding. Each molecule is aligned with the next in parallel order to form a collagen fibril. These fibrils are then grouped to form the collagen fiber (Einhorn 1996).

Non-collagenous proteins

Non-collagenous proteins make up only a small proportion of bone by weight but have great biological significance. Many of these proteins play a role in bone processes such as formation and resorption (Einhorn 1996).

Cells

Bone cells arise from different cell lines and carry out various functions. Osteoblasts are derived from local bone marrow mesenchymal cells and are located on all active bone surfaces. Their main function is to synthesize and secrete the organic matrix of bone. Once osteoblasts stop forming bone, they may either remain on the bone surface where they are known as bone-lining cells or they may surround themselves with matrix and become osteocytes. The main role of bone-lining cells is to contract and secrete enzymes that remove the thin layer of osteoid covering the mineralized matrix. This allows osteoclasts to attach to bone and begin resorption (Buckwalter et al 1995).

Osteocytes comprise more than 90% of the bone cells in the mature human skeleton. They are connected to other bone cells by numerous cytoplasmic projections that travel in channels (canaliculi) through mineralized matrix (Boivin et al 1990). These interconnections may allow the cells to sense deformation of bone by mechanical loads and to coordinate the remodeling process (described later).

Osteoclasts are derived from extraskeletal, hematopoietic stem cells. They are large, motile, multinucleated cells found on bone surfaces undergoing resorption. To resorb the bone matrix, osteoclasts bind to the bone surface and create an acidic environment by secreting protons and enzymes (Peck & Woods 1988). The acid environment digests the non-collagenous link between hydroxyapatite crystals and collagen (Khan et al 2001).

Inorganic component

The inorganic component of bone consists mainly of platelike crystals of hydroxyapatite (20–80 nm long and 2–5 mm thick) which itself is composed of calcium and phosphate. These crystals are found in and around collagen fibers and give bone its strength.

MACROSCOPIC AND MICROSCOPIC APPEARANCE

On the macroscopic level, the skeleton consists of two parts, the axial and the appendicular skeletons. The axial skeleton includes vertebrae, the pelvis, and other flat bones such as the skull and scapula. The appendicular skeleton includes all the long bones. Each long bone consists of two wider extremities (epiphyses), an essentially cylindrical shaft in the middle (diaphysis), and a zone between them (metaphysis) where remodeling of bone takes place during growth and development. In this way, bone can be described as an organ (Khan et al 2001).

Bone can also be described as tissue at the microscopic level. There are two types of bone tissue: woven bone and lamellar bone. Woven bone is considered immature bone with collagen arranged randomly. At birth, it makes up all the bone in the body; in later years it is found at sites of fracture healing or in response to extreme mechanical loads (Forwood & Burr 1993).

Lamellar bone is the name given to bone that eventually replaces woven bone. By the age of 4 years, most of the skeleton is lamellar bone. The collagen fibers arrange themselves along lines of principal force.

Anatomically, both woven and lamellar bone can be organized into compartments as either cortical or trabecular bone. Cortical bone forms the external part of long bones and is made up of dense, calcified tissue. The diaphysis of a long bone encloses the medullary cavity. Toward the metaphysis or epiphysis, cortical bone is thinner and the medullary cavity is replaced by cancellous or trabecular bone, which is characterized by an inner network of thin calcified trabeculae.

An important difference between cortical and trabecular bone is in the way the bone matrix and cellular elements are arranged. Calcium takes up 80–90% of cortical bone volume but only 15–25% of trabecular bone volume (Khan et al 2001). The trabecular arrangement permits bone marrow, blood vessels, and connective tissues to be in contact with bone. The main function of cortical bone is for structure and protection (Khan et al 2001).

Haversian bone is the most complex type of cortical bone. It consists of blood vessels that are circumferentially surrounded by lamellae of bone. This arrangement of cortical bone around a vessel is called an osteon. Osteons are usually aligned with the long axis of bone. They are the major structural units of cortical bone and are connected to one another by Volkmann's canals that run at right angles to the osteon (Buckwalter et al 1995).

BONE PHYSIOLOGY

It is well accepted that bone adapts its structure and

function to applied loads but can be injured if load exceeds strength. The areas of bone physiology that will be discussed include mechanotransduction (the mechanism whereby loading influences bone cell function) and the processes of modeling, remodeling, and fracture repair.

MECHANOTRANSDUCTION

It is not fully understood how bone responds to mechanical loads. It has been suggested that this response is controlled by a 'mechanostat' that endeavors to keep bone strain at an optimal level by adjusting bone structure (Frost 1983, Turner 1999). It is thought that bone strains resulting from mechanical loading are transduced into a cellular signal. Osteocytes have been proposed as the bone cells responsible for sensing strain and

transmitting signals (Aarden et al 1994). The cellular signals are then compared with the optimal strain for that region. If the signal falls within the optimal strain range, no adaptive response will occur and a state of remodeling or modeling equilibrium ensues. However, if the strains are above or below the optimal range, a state of overuse or disuse is perceived. This results in an appropriate response with net bone gain or loss in order to readjust bone strains (Fig. 5.1).

MODELING AND REMODELING

Bone modeling and remodeling are the processes that lead to changes in bone geometry and mass. Bone modeling is an organized bone cell activity that allows bone growth and adjusts bone strength through the strategically placed, non-adjacent activity of osteoblasts and osteoclasts (Frost 1990). Modeling improves bone strength not only by adding mass, but also by expanding the outer (periosteal) and inner (endocortical) diameters of bone (Khan et al 2001).

Remodeling is a continuous, sequential process of breakdown and repair of microscopic cavities in bone. Remodeling occurs on both periosteal and endosteal surfaces within cortical bone and on the surface of trabeculae. Both osteoclasts and osteoblasts are involved in remodeling, organized into discrete packets called basic multicellular units (Frost 1991).

Remodeling occurs in five stages: (i) quiescence, (ii) activation, (iii) resorption, (iv) reversal, and (v) formation (Parfitt 1988). A small area of bone surface is converted from rest to activity by an initiating stimulus, which may be hormonal, chemical, or physical. Osteoclast precursors are then recruited to the bone surface where they fuse to form multinucleated osteoclasts. These cells form a cavity by resorbing bone. A 1–2 week interval between termination of the resorptive processes and commencement of formation is known as the reversal phase. During this time, the bone site is weakened. Therefore continued mechanical loading during the reversal phase could result in microdamage accumulation and the beginning of a stress fracture (Brukner and Bennell 1997).

Repair of the resorption cavity is performed by osteoblasts and occurs in two stages: matrix synthesis and mineralization. First, a layer of type 1 collagen bone matrix, known as an osteoid seam, is deposited. After 5–10 days of maturation, the new matrix begins to mineralize with crystals of hydroxyapatite deposited within and between the collagen fibrils (Parfitt 1988).

A key feature of remodeling is that damaged tissue is replaced with an equal amount of new bone tissue in the healthy skeleton. In the aging and osteoporotic skeleton, however, the balance between the amount of bone resorbed and formed is shifted in favor of resorption, so

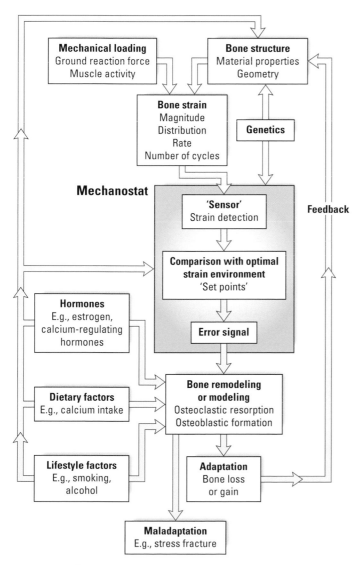

Figure 5.1 Schematic diagram of a mechanism for bone adaptation to mechanical loads.

that insufficient bone is formed to refill the resorption cavity (Parfitt 1988). A net loss of bone results, and eventually bone strength and integrity are compromised.

FRACTURE REPAIR

Unlike other tissues, bone repairs by regeneration. Primary bone healing occurs when there is direct and intimate contact between the bone ends. New bone grows directly across the bone ends to unite the fracture. The healing process involves osteoclastic bone resorption followed by osteoblastic new bone formation (Sheikh 2000a).

Secondary fracture healing represents mineralization and bony replacement of a cartilage matrix. The three main stages of fracture healing which may overlap include the inflammatory phase (10%), the reparative phase (40%), and the remodeling phase (70%) (Sheikh 2000a) (Table 5.1).

Inflammation is characterized by haematoma formation and the migration of inflammatory mediator cells to the injured site (Andrew et al 1994). These cells remove tissue debris and release growth factors and chemotactic agents which attract mesenchymal cells, fibroblasts, and endothelial cells to the site of injury (Einhorn 1998). These cells divide and differentiate to produce a connective tissue matrix into which neovascularization takes place (Glowacki 1998).

Reparation is performed by two cellular cascades. One is associated with chondrogenesis while the other is associated with osteogenesis. These two processes initially combine to form a bridge, known as the primary or provisional callus, which spans and surrounds the fracture site. The completion of this process results in clinical union. Following union, osteogenesis predominates with the cartilage formed during primary callus formation being replaced with new bone in a process of endochondral ossification (Einhorn 1998). The cartilage of the soft callus is invaded with blood vessels, chondroclasts, and osteoblasts. Chondroclasts degrade the cartilage matrix until only thin spicules of cartilage remain, forming cavities into which osteoblasts migrate. The osteoblasts line the cavities and begin producing new compact bone matrix rich in type I collagen. This results in the formation of the secondary or definitive callus and consolidation of the fracture clinically.

The final stage of bone repair is remodeling, performed by osteoclasts and osteoblasts. This stage may take months to years to complete. Remodeling functions to replace mineralized cartilage with cancellous bone, replace cancellous bone with new compact bone, replace callus between the ends of bone and remove any callus in the marrow cavity thereby restoring cavity continuity (Frost 1989).

BIOMECHANICS OF BONE

The key mechanical function of bone is to resist fracture. This depends on both its intrinsic material properties (mass, density, stiffness, and strength) and its gross geometric characteristics (size, shape, cortical thickness, cross-sectional area, and trabecular architecture) (Carter et al 1976, Currey 2001, Forwood 2001). Factors that affect skeletal strength and design include genetics, physical activity, hormones, and dietary factors (Khan et al 2001). Of these, the mechanical loading activity of bone is vitally important.

MATERIAL PROPERTIES OF BONE

The organic and inorganic components of bone (discussed previously) determine its material properties. The organic component, primarily type I collagen, provides tensile strength. Abnormal collagen matrix leaves bone brittle, irrespective of the amount of bone mineral present. The inorganic component, mineral, resists compressive forces. Functional tests under controlled conditions using a defined volume of bone can be used to measure the material behavior of bone as a tissue. When a load, or 'stress,' is applied, the bone is deformed. This deformation is referred to as 'strain'.

Stress and strain

Stress, the force applied per unit area, can be classified as tensile, compressive, torsional, or shear. Strain describes the deformation of a material without regard to its structural geometry and refers to the percentage change in bone length. Strain is greatest at the point of highest loading and dissipates along the length of the long bone (Nordin & Frankel 1989). For example, during walking or running, the highest measurable strain would occur at

Table 5.1 Stages of fracture healing

Healing phase	Duration	Events
Inflammatory	1–2 weeks	Formation of fracture hematoma Invasion by inflammatory cells
Reparative	Several months	Differentiation of mesenchymal cells Callus matrix laid down by chondroblasts and fibroblasts Mineralization of soft callus by osteoblasts to form woven bone
Remodeling	Months to years	Replacement of immature woven bone with mature lamellar bone by osteoclasts and osteoblasts Reforming of medullary cavity

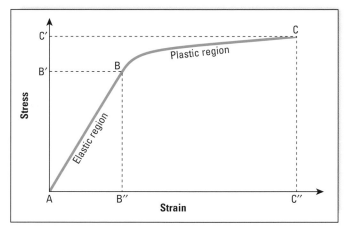

Figure 5.2 Stress–strain curve for a cortical bone sample tested in tension. Yield point (B): point past which some permanent deformation of bone sample occured. Yield stress (B′): load per unit area sustained by the bone sample before plastic deformation took place. Yield strain (B″): amount of deformation withstood by the sample before plastic deformation occurred. The strain at any point in the elastic region of the curve is proportional to the stress at that point. Ultimate failure point (C): the point past which failure of the sample occurred. Ultimate stress (C′): load per unit area sustained by the sample before failure. Ultimate strain (C″): amount of deformation sustained by the sample before failure. (Reproduced from Nordin M, Frankel V H 1989 Basic biomechanics of the musculoskeletal system, 2nd edn, Lea and Febiger with the permission of Lippincott Williams and Wilkins, copyright Lippincott Williams and Wilkins.)

the calcaneus and distal tibia. In addition, during locomotion, the greatest strain is generated at the cortex under compression.

The intrinsic material properties of bone include the concepts of stiffness and strength. The amount of force required to deform a structure is termed its stiffness and is represented by the slope of the stress–strain curve (see Fig. 5.2). The strength of the structure can be defined as the load at the yield or failure points, or as the ultimate load, depending on the circumstances. Strength is an intrinsic property of bone and is independent of its size (Khan et al 2001).

Bone mineral mass

Bone mass is a determinant of bone material properties; the distribution of bone mass and bone geometry are connected to bone strength and stiffness. Further, the strength and stiffness of bone is a function of density. Although bone mass is only one component of overall bone strength (Mosekilde 1993), it does explain more than 80% of that variable (Johnston & Slemenda 1993). Because bone mass is highly correlated with dual energy X-ray absorptiometry (DXA) results, this technique is used to measure bone mass and give an estimate of fracture risk in humans (Cummings et al 1993, Martin 1991). DXA technology and its clinical implications are discussed further in the section on osteoporosis.

STRUCTURAL PROPERTIES OF BONE

Geometric characteristics of bone include size, shape, cortical thickness, cross-sectional area, and trabecular architecture. Appendicular bone adapts to mechanical loads by endosteal resorption and periosteal apposition of bone tissue. This increases bone diameter, cortical thickness, or both, and thus provides greater resistance to loading.

For tension and compression loads, the strength of a bone is proportional to the bone cross-sectional area. Hence, a larger bone is more resistant to fracture as it distributes the internal forces over a larger surface area resulting in lower stresses (Hayes & Gerhart 1985). With respect to bending loads, both the cross-sectional area and the distribution of bone tissue around a neutral axis are important geometrical features. The area moment of inertia is the index that takes into account these two factors in bending. A larger area moment of inertia means that the bone tissue is distributed further away from the neutral axis (the axis where the stresses and strains are zero) and is more efficient in resisting bending (Fig. 5.3).

The length of a bone also influences its strength in bending. The longer the bone, the greater the magnitude of the bending moment caused by the application of a force. For this reason, the long bones of the lower extremity

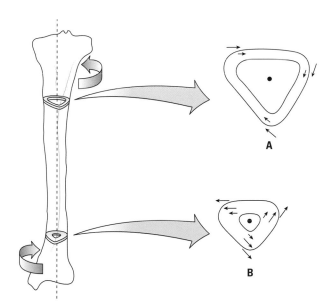

Figure 5.3 Distribution of shear stress in two cross-sections of a tibia subjeted to torsional loading. The proximal section (A) has a higher moment of inertia than does the distal section (B) because more bony material is distributed away from the neutral axis. (Reproduced from Nordin M, Frankel V H 1989 Basic biomechanics of the musculoskeletal system, 2nd edn, Lea and Febiger with the permission of Lippincott Williams and Wilkins, copyright Lippincott Williams and Wilkins.)

are subjected to high bending moments and hence high tensile and compressive stresses (Nordin & Frankel 1989).

The mechanical competence of whole bone can be characterized by the deformation it undergoes during loading. Deformation is characteristically measured and plotted as a load–deformation curve. This is similar to the stress–strain curve but it is used to assess whole bone. Generally, a linear relationship exists between the imposed load and the amount of bone deformation until the bone reaches its yield point. Prior to reaching this point, the bone is in its elastic region (if unloaded, it would return to its original shape). That is, applied forces in this region cause only temporary deformation. Beyond the yield point, the slope of the curve plateaus; the area beneath this part of the curve is called the plastic region. It marks the point at which permanent deformation occurs and, in extreme cases, the point at which local fractures or other damage may result. If the load continues to increase, failure load may be reached, and the structure may fail completely (Khan et al 2001).

HOW PHYSICAL ACTIVITY GENERATES LOAD ON BONES

The skeleton is subjected to forces produced by gravity (weightbearing), by muscles, and by other external factors. Bone tissue is an anisotropic material which means that its behavior varies depending on the direction of the applied load. In general, bone tissue can handle the greatest loads in a longitudinal direction (i.e. compressive forces), the direction of habitual loading, and

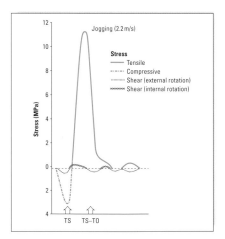

Figure 5.4 Calculated stresses on the anteromedial cortex of a human adult tibia during running. TS = toe-strike; TO = toe-off. (Reproduced from Nordin M, Frankel V H 1989 Basic biomechanics of the musculoskeletal system, 2nd edn, Lea and Febiger with the permission of Lippincott Williams and Wilkins, copyright Lippincott Williams and Wilkins.)

lesser loads when they are applied across the bone surface (i.e. bending, shear or impacting forces). None of this is straightforward, as the degree of anisotropy varies with the anatomical region (cortical or trabecular bone) and with the magnitude and direction of the mechanical load (Khan et al 2001).

During physical activity, contact with the ground generates forces within the body. Without muscle activity, ground reaction forces (GRF) are transmitted from the foot and along the lower limbs to the hips through a series of action–reaction forces (a system of three rigid links). However, forces applied to bone are primarily the result of muscular contraction. Therefore, with the additional influence of muscles and lever arms, GRFs vary. For example, running generates GRFs around 2–3 times body weight (Cavanagh & LaFortune 1980), whereas jumping and landing activities can be clearly higher at up to 12–22 times body weight (Heinonen et al 2001, McNitt-Gray 1991) (Fig. 5.4).

BONE'S RESPONSE TO LOCAL MECHANICAL LOADING

The skeleton's response to a load depends on the strain magnitude, rate, distribution, and cycles in the target bone (Khan et al 2001). Much of what we know about the influence of functional loads on bone comes from research with animal models where the applied load can be precisely controlled.

STRAIN MAGNITUDE

Strain magnitude can be defined as the amount of percentage change in bone length under mechanical loading. Early work using the turkey ulna clearly showed that bone formation increased with larger strain magnitudes (Rubin & Lanyon 1985). Activities that elicit high peak forces (or high strain magnitude) may have a greater effect on bone mass than activities associated with a large number of loading cycles (Whalen et al 1988).

STRAIN RATE

Strain rate, the rate at which strain develops and releases, determines bone's adaptive response. Higher strain rates are most effective for a maximal adaptive bone response (Turner et al 1995). Umemura et al (1995) compared jump training with running training in rats and found that jumping was associated with a higher strain rate and magnitude, and was more effective than running for eliciting a positive bone response.

STRAIN DISTRIBUTION

Strain distribution refers to the way strain is distributed across a section of bone. It has been hypothesized that unusual strains of uneven distribution are more likely to stimulate osteogenesis than repetitive strains that result from everyday activity (Lanyon 1984).

STRAIN CYCLES

Strain cycles denote the number of load repetitions that change bone dimensions at a given magnitude. Although a minimum number of loading cycles is required for a positive bone response, the number of strain cycles appears to be less important than strain magnitude or strain rate (Lanyon 1987, Rubin & Lanyon 1984, Umemura et al 1997).

CLINICAL BONE CONDITIONS

ACUTE FRACTURES

Acute fractures are caused either by direct trauma such as a car hitting a pedestrian or by indirect trauma such as a fall onto an outstretched hand resulting in a fracture of the humerus. The principles of fracture management involve:

1. Reduction – manipulating the bone to its correct anatomical position. Reduction may be achieved under anesthesia, by continuous traction (closed) or surgically (open).
2. Immobilization – holding the bone in the correct reduced position. Various devices are used to achieve different degrees of fixation including casts, external fixation, slings, plates, rods, screws, and pins.
3. Rehabilitation – returning the person to as full function as possible after the trauma

Physical therapy is important in the rehabilitation of patients with fractures and commences as soon as the fracture has been reduced. The main consideration affecting treatment is the stage of healing and thus it is important that the therapist liaises with the patient's medical practitioner (Atkinson et al 1999).

Healing times

Healing times vary depending on the location and severity of the fracture, associated injuries, and patient characteristics such as age, smoking status, and medical conditions (Sheikh 2000b). There are two major time-

Table 5.2 Approximate union and consolidation times in normal adult bone (reproduced with permission from Atkinson et al 1999)

Fracture site	Union time (weeks)	Consolidation time (weeks)
Proximal third of humerus	3	6
Distal third of radius/ulna	6	12
Proximal third of femur	4–6	8–12
Distal third of femur	6	12
Proximal third of tibia	6–8	12–16
Distal third of tibia	8–10	16–20

points relevant to fracture healing and it is important to establish where along the continuum of fracture healing the patient lies as this will influence rehabilitation:

1. Union – the partial repair of bone when the initial callus forms around the bone ends so that there is minimal movement. On X-ray, the fracture line will still be visible. Full bone maturity has not been reached so full weightbearing cannot be undertaken and some form of external support is usually still needed. This can be reduced as healing moves from union to consolidation (Atkinson et al 1999).
2. Consolidation – the bone is fully repaired and there is no movement at the fracture site. No fracture line can be seen on X-ray and bone trabeculae cross where the fracture previously was. Full function can now commence (Atkinson et al 1999).

The approximate union and consolidation times in normal adult bone are shown in Table 5.2. Healing times for children are generally half that of adults.

Rehabilitation of acute fractures

Physical therapy in fracture rehabilitation is dictated by a number of factors including the stage of fracture healing, the type of fracture, the immobilization device used, and the patient's weightbearing status. Following initial fracture management, the physical therapist must ensure that the patient understands the rehabilitation process and is educated as to steps to reduce the risk of complications. Exercises can be given to maintain the range of motion of joints that are not immobilized and techniques employed to reduce swelling and minimize pain.

When the fracture is stable and united, mild over-pressures can be applied to joints next to the fracture site, and exercises can be commenced to regain the range of motion at joints proximal and distal to the fracture site and to strengthen muscles that attach to the injured bone. The amount of resistance and weightbearing can be progressively increased. It is important that at all times, the patient does not experience pain at the actual fracture site (Atkinson et al 1999).

STRESS FRACTURES

Stress fractures are overuse bone injuries that result from the accumulation of microdamage that is not adequately repaired by the remodeling process. This section will provide a general overview of the assessment and treatment of stress fractures.

Diagnosis

When assessing the patient presenting with a possible stress fracture, there are four questions that need to be answered:

1. Is the pain bony in origin?
2. If so, which bone is involved?
3. At what stage in the continuum of bone stress is this injury?
4. What factors have predisposed this individual to a stress fracture?

To obtain an answer to these questions a thorough history, precise examination, and appropriate use of imaging techniques are used.

History

The patient generally reports a history of insidious onset of activity-related pain. Initially the pain will usually be described as a mild ache occurring with exercise, but the pain may well become more severe or occur at an earlier stage of exercise if the patient continues. The pattern of pain differs from that of overuse soft tissue injuries, as it tends to get worse with exercise rather than decreasing after a period of warm-up.

The presence of predisposing factors needs to be determined from the history (Table 5.3). Therefore a training or activity history is essential. In particular, note should be taken of recent changes in activity level such as increased quantity of training, increased intensity of training, changes in surface, equipment (especially shoes), and technique. A full dietary history should be taken and particular attention paid to the possible presence of eating disorders. Females should be asked about their menstrual history, including age of menarche and subsequent menstrual status.

A history of previous similar injury or any other musculoskeletal injury should be obtained. It is essential to obtain a brief history of the patient's general health and medication usage to ensure that there are no factors that may influence bone health. It is also important to obtain an understanding of the patient's work and sporting commitments (Brukner et al 1999).

Table 5.3 Risk factor assessment in a patient presenting with a stress fracture

Risk factor	Variables
Training	Type Volume Intensity Surface Changes in training
Footwear	Type Age of shoe Use of insoles
Lower limb alignment	Foot type Tibial torsion Knee varus/valgus Femoral anteversion Leg length
Muscle length and joint range	Flexibility of calf, hamstrings, hip flexors Range of ankle dorsiflexion, hip internal/external rotation
Menstrual status	Current and past menstrual patterns Use of the oral contraceptive pill Sex hormonal levels if irregular
Bone density – dual energy X-ray absorptiometry (DXA)	If amenorrheic or multiple stress fracture history
Dietary intake	Calcium Energy Other nutrients influencing absorption of calcium or bone health (e.g. protein, fiber) Presence of eating disorder

Physical examination

On physical examination, the most obvious feature is localized bony tenderness. This is easier to determine in bones that are relatively superficial, but may be absent in stress fractures of the shaft or neck of femur. Occasionally, redness and swelling may be present at the site of the stress fracture. There may also be palpable periosteal thickening, especially in a long-standing fracture. Percussion of long bones may result in the production of pain at a point distant from the percussion.

Joint range of motion is usually unaffected except in situations where the stress fracture is close to the joint surface, such as a stress fracture of the neck of femur. Specific stress fractures may be associated with specific clinical tests. Examples of these are the hop test for stress fractures in the groin region (Brukner et al 1999) and hip extension while standing on the contralateral leg used in the diagnosis of stress fractures of the pars interarticularis of the spine (Brukner et al 1999).

The physical examination must also take into account the potential predisposing factors, and in all stress fractures involving the lower limb a full biomechanical examination must be performed. Any evidence of leg length discrepancy, malalignment (especially excessive subtalar pronation), muscle imbalance, weakness, or lack of flexibility should be noted (Brukner et al 1999) (Table 5.3).

Imaging

Imaging plays an important role in supplementing clinical examination of stress fractures. In many cases a clinical diagnosis of stress fracture is sufficient. However, if the diagnosis is uncertain, or in the case of serious or elite athletes who wish to continue training if at all possible and require more specific knowledge of their condition, there are various imaging techniques available.

Radiography. Radiography has poor sensitivity but high specificity in the diagnosis of stress fractures. The classic radiographic abnormalities seen in a stress fracture are new periosteal bone formation, a visible area of sclerosis, the presence of callus or a visible fracture line. If any of these radiographic signs are present, the diagnosis of stress fracture can be confirmed (Santi et al 1989).

Unfortunately, in the majority of stress fractures there is no obvious radiographic abnormality. The abnormalities on radiography are unlikely to be seen unless symptoms have been present for at least 2–3 weeks. In certain cases, they may not become evident for up to 3 months, and in a percentage of cases, never become abnormal (Meurman & Elfving 1980).

Isotopic bone scan (scintigraphy). The triple phase bone scan is highly sensitive for diagnosing stress fractures (Prather et al 1977) and changes may be seen as early as 7 h after bone injury. A stress fracture appears as a sharply marginated or fusiform area of increased uptake involving one cortex, or occasionally extending the width of the bone in the third phase of the bone scan (Roub et al 1979) (Fig. 5.5). However, bone scintigraphy lacks specificity because other non-traumatic lesions such as tumor (especially osteoid osteoma) can also produce localized increased uptake. It is therefore vitally important to correlate the bone scan appearance with the clinical features.

The sensitivity of bone scintigraphy can be further increased by the use of single photon emission computer tomography (SPECT). Bone SPECT is most helpful in complex areas of the skeleton with overlapping structures that may obscure pathology such as the skull, pelvis and spine. It is particularly useful in the detection of stress fractures of the pars interarticularis in the spine.

Computerized tomography. Computerized tomography (CT) may be useful in differentiating those conditions with increased uptake on bone scan that may mimic stress fracture. CT scans are particularly valuable in

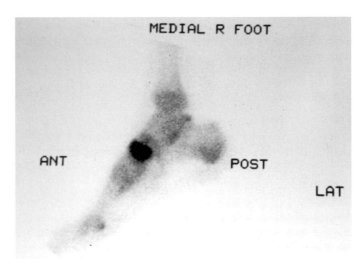

Figure 5.5 The typical bone scan appearance of a stress fracture.

imaging fractures where this may be important in treatment such as the navicular bone (Kiss et al 1993). CT scanning may also be valuable in detecting fracture lines as evidence of stress fracture in long bones (e.g. metatarsal and tibia) where plain radiography is normal and isotope bone scan shows increased uptake. CT scanning will enable the clinician to differentiate between a stress fracture that will be visible on CT scan and a stress reaction. Particularly in elite athletes, this may considerably affect their rehabilitation program and their forthcoming competition program (Fig. 5.6).

Magnetic resonance imaging. Magnetic resonance imaging (MRI), while not imaging cortical bone as well as CT scan, has certain advantages in the imaging of stress fractures. Specific MRI characteristics of stress fracture include new bone formation and fracture lines, and marrow and periosteal hemorrhage and edema. These changes are best seen if the MRI is performed within 3 weeks of symptoms (Lee & Yao 1988). Although CT scan

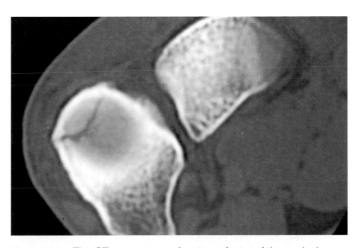

Figure 5.6 The CT appearance of a stress factor of the navicular.

visualizes bone detail, another advantage of MR imaging is in distinguishing stress fractures from a suspected bone tumor or infectious process.

Treatment

The actual time from diagnosis of a stress fracture to full return to sport or physical activity depends on a number of factors including the site of the fracture, the length of the symptoms, and the severity of the lesion (stage in the spectrum of bone stress). Most stress fractures with a relatively brief history of symptoms will heal without complication or delay and permit return to sport within the 4–8 week range. However there is a group of stress fractures that require additional treatment and special consideration. These are listed separately, later in the chapter.

While there are many subtleties involved in the treatment of stress fractures, the primary treatment is modified (most frequently reduced) activity. During the phase of modified activity, a number of important issues are attended to, including modification of risk factors, maintenance of muscular strength and fitness, pain management, investigation of bone health, and prescription of orthotic devices. The treatment of stress fractures can be divided into two phases: Phase I is the early treatment using modified activity and Phase II is the period from the reintroduction of physical activity to full return to sport.

Phase I

Pain management. Pain is seldom severe but can be a problem even with normal walking. Mild analgesics can be used as well as physical therapy modalities (e.g. ice, interferential, electrical stimulation). Practitioners often suggest non-steroidal anti-inflammatory drugs (NSAIDs) but there is some speculation that the mode of action of some may slow or prevent repair of the stress fracture as they reduce the bone remodeling process (Burr 2001). In some cases where activities of daily living are painful, it may be necessary for the patient with a stress fracture to be non-weightbearing or partial weightbearing on crutches for a period of up to 10 days.

Muscle strengthening. Skeletal muscle plays an important role in stress fracture development. At some regions, bone load is increased by muscular force while at others, it is reduced as muscles absorb energy (Scott & Winter 1990). In endurance sports, it is possible that even low levels of muscular fatigue can affect the total impact load to bone, particularly in the lower extremity. Following fatiguing exercise, bone strain, particularly strain rate, has been shown to increase (Fyhrie et al 1998, Yoshikawa et al 1994). Some studies have shown that reduced muscle strength (Hoffman et al 1999) and smaller muscle size (Bennell et al 1996, Milgrom 1989) predispose to stress fractures in athletes and military recruits. While there are no studies that have evaluated the role of muscle strengthening in the treatment of stress fractures, it is logical to include a specific strengthening program because of the important role of muscles in shock absorption, and to help counteract the effects of detraining. Muscle strengthening programs are usually prescribed for a period of 6–12 weeks and can begin immediately after diagnosis of the stress fracture. However, it is important that the exercises do not cause pain at the stress fracture site.

Maintaining fitness. Maintenance of fitness during periods of forced inactivity due to injury is a major concern to coaches and athletes. Inactivity has marked detrimental effects on the cardiovascular system as well as the metabolic and morphological characteristics of skeletal muscle.

Non-loading activities that maintain fitness are those that use as many large muscle groups as possible without over-loading the bone. The most common methods of maintaining fitness are cycling, swimming, deep water running, rowing, and stairmaster. For muscular strength, upper and lower body weight programs can usually be prescribed without risk. These work-outs should as much as possible mimic the athlete's normal training program in both duration and intensity.

Modification of risk factors. As with any overuse injury, it is not sufficient to merely treat the stress fracture itself. Stress fractures represent the result of incremental overload. Subtle adjustments to the modifiable factors that contribute to the total load are an essential component of the management of an athlete with a stress fracture. However, it should be pointed out that there have been few controlled trials to evaluate the effectiveness of risk factor modification in reducing stress fracture development or recurrence.

Training. Controlled trials in the military showed that the reduction of high impact activities, such as running and jumping, was associated with a decrease in stress fracture incidence, whereas the reduction of marching distance had no effect (Giladi et al 1985a, Scully & Besterman 1982). Other studies have shown that training interventions, such as the inclusion of rest periods (Scully & Besterman 1982, Worthen & Yanklowitz 1978), elimination of running and marching on concrete (Greaney et al 1983, Reinker & Ozburne 1979), and pre-entry physical conditioning (Milgrom et al 2000, Shaffer et al 1999), may also reduce stress fracture risk in the military.

While there are few data relating to athletes, it is imperative to obtain a detailed training history to try and identify any training parameters that may have contributed to an individual's stress fracture. Athletes should be encouraged to keep an accurate training log book and to monitor responses to training. Coaches need to be reminded that training regimens for athletes should be individualized.

Footwear and insoles. A recent Cochrane review concluded that the use of insoles inside the boots of military recruits during their initial training appears to reduce the number of stress fractures and/or stress reactions of bone by over 50% (Gillespie & Grant 2000). Whether the results can be generalized to the sporting population is not clear.

Another important contributing factor to stress fracture development may be inadequate training shoes. These shoes may be inappropriate for the particular foot type of the individual, may have general inadequate support/shock absorption or may be worn out. In a randomized trial, training in basketball shoes compared with normal military boots was associated with a significant reduction in the incidence of stress fractures in the foot but not in overall stress fractures (Milgrom et al 1992).

Biomechanical abnormalities. Intrinsic biomechanical abnormalities are thought to contribute to the development of overuse injuries in general and stress fractures in particular. The structure of the foot will partly determine how much force is absorbed by the bones in the foot and how much force is transferred to proximal bones during ground contact. The high arched (pes cavus) foot is more rigid and may be less able to absorb shock, resulting in more force passing to the tibia and femur. The low arched (pes planus) foot is more flexible, allowing stress to be absorbed by the musculoskeletal structures of the foot. It is also often associated with prolonged pronation or hyperpronation, which can induce a great amount of torsion on the tibia and may exacerbate muscle fatigue as the muscles have to work harder to control the excessive motion, especially at toe-off. Theoretically, either foot type could predispose to a stress fracture but results of studies have been conflicting (Brosh & Arcan 1994, Giladi et al 1985b, Montgomery et al 1989, Simkin et al 1989).

Since there is evidence to show that a leg length discrepancy increases the likelihood of stress fractures in both military (Friberg 1982) and athletic (Bennell et al 1996, Brunet et al 1990) populations, a heel raise should be provided if necessary. Other alignment features to be investigated include the presence of genu varum, valgum, or recurvatum, Q angle, and tibial torsion. Of these, only an increased Q angle has been found in association with stress fractures (Cowan et al 1996) although this is not a universal finding (Montgomery et al 1989, Winfield et al 1997).

A thorough biomechanical assessment is an essential part of both treatment and prevention of stress fractures. Until the contribution of biomechanical abnormalities to stress fracture risk is clarified through scientific research,

correction of such abnormalities should be attempted, if possible.

Muscle flexibility and joint range of motion. The role of flexibility is difficult to evaluate as flexibility encompasses a number of characteristics including active joint mobility, ligamentous laxity, and muscle length. Of the numerous variables that have been assessed in relation to stress fractures (Bennell et al 1996, Ekenman et al 1996, Giladi et al 1987, Hughes 1985, Milgrom et al 1994, Montgomery et al 1989, Winfield et al 1997), only increased range of hip external rotation (Giladi et al 1991, Giladi et al 1987, Milgrom et al 1994) and decreased range of ankle dorsiflexion (Hughes 1985) have been associated with stress fracture development and even these findings have been inconsistent.

The difficulty in assessing the role of muscle and joint flexibility in stress fractures may relate to a number of factors including the relatively imprecise methods of measurement, the heterogeneity of these variables, and the fact that both increased and decreased flexibility may be contributory. Until better evidence is available to the contrary, it is worth prescribing stretches if muscle flexibility and joint range are found to be restricted in the athlete who presents with a stress fracture.

Menstrual status. Women with stress fractures should be questioned about their current and past menstrual status. There is evidence to show that menstrual disturbances increase the risk of stress fracture (Barrow & Saha 1988, Bennell et al 1996, Carbon et al 1990, Tomten 1996, Winfield et al 1997) and lead to premature bone loss particularly at trabecular sites (Gremion et al 2001, Hetland et al 1993, Jonnavithula et al 1993, Myburgh et al 1993, Robinson et al 1995). Lower bone density in women may be associated with a greater risk of stress fractures although results from studies are mixed (Bennell et al 1995, 1996, Carbon et al 1990, Cline et al 1998, Frusztajer et al 1990, Girrbach et al 2001, Grimston et al 1991, Lauder et al 2000, Myburgh et al 1990). If menstrual disturbances are present, the athlete should be referred to a medical practitioner for review.

Dietary intake. Dietary surveys of various sporting groups often reveal inadequate intakes of nutrients that are important for skeletal health (Ronsen et al 1999, Ziegler et al 1999). However, there is currently little evidence to support low calcium intake as a risk factor for stress fractures in otherwise healthy athletic (Bennell et al 1996, Carbon et al 1990, Frusztajer et al 1990, Grimston et al 1991, Kadel et al 1992, Warren et al 1991) or military (Cline et al 1998) populations. In the only controlled trial, calcium supplementation of 500 mg daily had no significant effect on stress fracture incidence in male military recruits (Schwellnus & Jordaan 1992).

Athletes report a greater frequency of disordered eating patterns than the general population, especially those in sports emphasizing leanness and/or those competing at higher levels (Picard 1999). Low caloric intake has been hypothesized as one of the mechanisms for menstrual disturbances in sportswomen (Zanker & Swaine 1998). Disordered eating, amenorrhea, and osteopenia often occur simultaneously in athletic females, a syndrome that has been referred to as the 'female athlete triad' (Otis et al 1997). Abnormal and restrictive eating behaviors do seem to increase the likelihood of fracture in women (Bennell et al 1995, Bennell et al 1996, Frusztajer et al 1990, Nattiv et al 1997).

Healthy eating habits should be promoted in all individuals. If one is concerned about dietary intake in those presenting with a stress fracture, nutritional counseling should be recommended.

Bracing. The use of a pneumatic air brace may assist with stress fracture healing in the leg and reduce the time taken to return to sport (Batt et al 2001, Dickson & Kichline 1987, Gillespie & Grant 2000, Slayter 1995, Swenson et al 1997, Whitelaw et al 1991). It has been proposed that the brace may act by shifting a portion of the weightbearing load from the tibia to the soft tissue, which results in less impact loading (Swenson et al 1997). It is also suggested that the brace facilitates healing at the fracture site by compressing the soft tissue, thereby increasing the intravascular hydrostatic pressure and shifting fluid and electrolytes from the capillary space to the interstitial space (Swenson et al 1997). This theoretically enhances the piezoelectric effect and enhances osteoblastic bone formation.

Phase II

When normal, day-to-day ambulation is pain free, then resumption of the impact loading activities can begin. The rate of resumption of activity is individual and should be modified according to symptoms and physical findings. The time to return to sport is variable depending on a number of factors such as the site of stress fracture, the person's age, competitive level, and time to diagnosis (Benazzo et al 1992).

There are no studies that have compared different return-to-sport programs. However, since healing bone is weaker, a progressive increase in load is needed so that the bone will adapt with increases in strength. For lower limb stress fractures where running is the aggravating activity, a program that involves initial brisk walking increased by 5–10 min per day up to a length of 45 min is recommended (Brukner et al 1999). Once this is achieved without pain, slow jogging for increasing periods within the 45-min walk is recommended. Once the 45-min goal is achieved, the pace can be increased, initially at half pace then gradually increasing to full pace striding. Once full sprinting is achieved free of pain, functional activities such as hopping, skipping, jumping, twisting, and turning can be introduced gradually. A typical program for an uncomplicated lower limb stress fracture resuming activity after a period of initial rest and activities of daily living is shown in Table 5.4. This pattern of reintroduction of activity can be followed for other sports.

It is not uncommon for the patient to experience pain at some point during the reintroduction of activity. This is, by no means, an indication of a return of the stress fracture. In each instance, the activity should be discontinued, followed by several days of modified rest, and then training should resume at a level lower than that at which the pain occurred. Progress should be monitored clinically by the presence or absence of symptoms and local signs. It is not necessary to monitor progress by radiography, scintigraphy, CT, or MRI since radiological healing often lags behind clinical healing.

Table 5.4 Activity program following uncomplicated lower limb stress fracture following period of rest and ADL. (Taken from Brukner P, Bennell K, Matheson G 1999 Stress fractures. Blackwell Science, p.101, with permission)

	Day 1 (min)	Day 2 (min)	Day 3 (min)	Day 4 (min)	Day 5 (min)	Day 6 (min)	Day 7 (min)
Week 1	Walk 5	Walk 20	Walk 25	Walk 30	Walk 35	Walk 40	Walk 45
Week 2	Walk 20 Jog 5 Walk15	Walk 15 Jog 15 Walk 15	Walk 15 Jog 20 Walk 15	Walk 10 Jog 25 Walk 10	Walk 5 Jog 30 Walk 10	Walk 5 Jog 35 Walk 5	Jog 45
Week 3	Jog 45 Stride 10	Jog 45 Stride 10	Jog 45 Stride 15	Jog 45 Stride 15	Jog 45 Sprint 0	Jog 45 Sprint 10	Jog 45 Sprint 15
Week 4			Add functional activities Gradually increase all week				
Week 5			RESUME FULL TRAINING				

Box 5.1   Stress fractures that require specific treatment

Neck of femur
Pars interarticularis of the spine
Patella
Anterior cortex, mid-shaft tibia
Medial malleolus
Talus
Navicular
5th metatarsal
2nd metatarsal (base)
Sesamoid

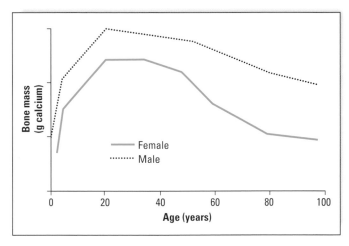

Figure 5.7   Changes in bone density with age in men and women. (Reproduced with permission from Bennell et al 2000.)

When training resumes it is important to allow adequate recovery time after hard sessions or hard weeks of training. This can be accommodated by developing micro- and macrocycles. Alternating hard and easy training sessions is a microcycle adjustment but graduating the volume of work or alternating harder and easier sessions can also be done weekly or monthly. In view of the history of stress fracture, it is advisable that some form of cross training (e.g. swimming and cycling for a runner), be introduced to reduce the stress on the previously injured area and reduce the likelihood of a recurrence (Brukner et al 1999).

Surgery. Surgery is virtually never required in the management of the routine stress fracture. However, in the case of a displaced stress fracture (e.g. neck of femur) or established non-union (e.g. anterior cortex of tibia, navicular, sesamoids, 5th metatarsal) surgery may be required.

Stress fractures requiring specific treatment. While the majority of stress fractures will heal without complications in a relatively short time frame with relative rest, there are a number of stress fractures with a tendency to develop complications, such as delayed or non-union, and which require specific additional treatment, such as cast immobilization or surgery. These are shown in Box 5.1. While it is beyond the scope of this chapter to cover the treatment of these in detail, readers are referred to other reviews in this area (Brukner et al 1999, Brukner & Bennell 1997, Egol & Frankel 2001).

OSTEOPOROSIS AND ASSOCIATED FACTORS

Osteoporosis is a metabolic bone disorder characterized by low bone mass and microarchitectural deterioration leading to skeletal fragility and increased fracture risk (Consensus Develoment Conference 1993). Physical therapists have a role to play in this condition through exercise prescription, education, and strategies to maximize function, reduce the risk of falls, and manage pain.

Bone mineral density (BMD) and falls are two major determinants of the risk of fracture (Lespessailles et al

1998, Petersen et al 1996). An individual's peak bone mass is reached around the late teens and early 20s (Bailey 1997, Young et al 1995). A slow rate of bone loss then starts in both sexes, and superimposed on this is an accelerated loss of bone in women at the menopause when estrogen production ceases (Fig. 5.7).

Approximately 60–80% of peak bone mass is determined by genes (Zmuda et al 1999). Other determinants include hormones, mechanical loading, nutrition, body composition, and lifestyle factors such as smoking and alcohol intake. Physical therapists need to be aware of risk factors for osteoporosis as well as medical conditions and pharmacological agents that predispose to secondary osteoporosis (Box 5.2).

A greater propensity to falling will increase the risk of fracture (Parkkari et al 1999). Many risk factors for fall initiation have been identified. These can be classified into intrinsic factors, for example, poor eyesight, reduced balance, and reduced lower limb strength, and extrinsic factors, such as home hazards, multiple drug use, and inappropriate footwear (Lord et al 1991, Lord et al 1994).

Measurement of bone mineral density

Dual energy X-ray absorptiometry (DXA) is currently the technique of choice to measure bone density and diagnose osteoporosis (Blake & Fogelman 1998). It has excellent measurement precision, is relatively inexpensive, widely available and uses only a small amount of radiation.

Physical therapists need to be able to interpret DXA scans as the results can guide patient management (Fig. 5.8). The most useful BMD scores are the Z- and T-scores. The Z-score compares the person's BMD with that of an age-matched group (calculated as the deviation from the mean result for the age- and sex-matched group

Box 5.2 Risk factors for osteoporosis and medical conditions predisposing to secondary osteoporosis. (Reproduced with permission from Bennell et al 2000.)

Risk factors for osteoporosis
- A family history of osteoporosis/hip fracture
- Postmenopausal without hormone replacement therapy
- Late onset of menstrual periods
- A sedentary lifestyle
- Inadequate calcium and Vitamin D intake
- Cigarette smoking
- Excessive alcohol
- High caffeine intake
- Amenorrhea – loss of menstrual periods
- Thin body type
- Caucasian or Asian race

Medical conditions predisposing to secondary osteoporosis
- Anorexia nervosa
- Rheumatological conditions (e.g. rheumatoid arthritis, ankylosing spondylitis)
- Endocrine disorders (e.g. Cushing's syndrome, primary hyperparathyroidism, thyrotoxicosis)
- Malignancy
- Gastrointestinal disorders (malabsorption, liver disease, partial gastrectomy)
- Certain drugs (corticosteroids, heparin)
- Immobilization (paralysis, prolonged bed rest, functional impairment)
- Congenital disorders (Turner's syndrome, Kleinfelter's syndrome)

Table 5.5 Diagnostic criteria for osteoporosis (reproduced from Bennell et al 2000)

Classification	DXA result
Normal	BMD greater than 1 s.d. below the mean of young adults (T-score above –1)
Osteopenia	BMD between 1 and 2.5 s.d. below the mean of young adults (T-score –1 to –2.5)
Osteoporosis	BMD more than 2.5 s.d. below the mean of young adults (T-score below –2.5)
Severe or established osteoporosis	BMD more than 2.5 s.d. below the mean of young adults plus one or more fragility fractures

s.d. – standard deviation

divided by the standard deviation of the group). This score indicates whether one is losing bone more rapidly than one's peers. The T-score is similarly defined but uses the deviation from the mean peak bone density of a young, healthy sex-matched group. The World Health Organization has defined bone mass clinically based on T-scores (World Health Organization 1994) and has categorized it into normal, osteopenia, osteoporosis and established osteoporosis (Table 5.5). DXA derived BMD scores have been shown clinically to predict fracture risk relatively well (Cummings et al 1993).

Signs and symptoms of osteoporosis

Low bone density per se is asymptomatic and many individuals are unaware that they have osteopenia or osteoporosis until a fracture occurs. The common fracture sites are the hip, vertebrae, and wrist and less commonly the ribs, pelvis, ankle, and upper arm (Sanders et al 1999). Vertebral compression fractures can cause loss of height and this may occur suddenly or gradually over time. A common clinical sign of advanced spinal osteoporosis is thoracic kyphosis or the 'dowager's hump'. This is due to anterior wedge fractures of the vertebral bodies (Ensrud et al 1997) but muscle weakness and pain may contribute (Cutler et al 1993). Postural changes may cause patients

to complain of a 'pot belly' with a bulging stomach and concertina-like skin folds. These changes also result in less space within the thorax and abdominal region and increased intra-abdominal pressure. This can cause shortness of breath and reduced exercise tolerance, hiatus hernia, indigestion, heartburn, and stress incontinence (Larsen 1998). Some patients complain of spinal pain due to fractures but not all fractures are symptomatic (Ross 1997).

Physical therapy assessment

A complete subjective and objective assessment is needed but the choice of questions and procedures depends on several factors including the age of the patient, severity of the condition, DXA results, co-existing pathologies, functional status, and reasons for consultation. Specific questioning for osteoporosis is shown in Table 5.6. There are a number of reliable and standardized measurement tools that can be used to gain a more accurate assessment of the patient's needs. These are summarized in Table 5.7.

Physical therapy management

Physiotherapy management will vary depending on assessment findings particularly the patient's age, DXA results, and functional status. The aims of treatment should be clearly established so that appropriate management can be instigated.

Exercise prescription for bone loading

While exercise influences bone material and structural properties, it is not known whether exercise reduces fracture rates which is the ultimate goal. The fact that there are no randomized, controlled trials to answer this question reflects inherent methodological difficulties.

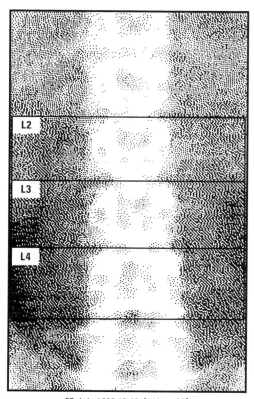

27 July 1999 15:40 [119 × 106]
Hologic QDR–1000/W (S/N 822)
Lumbar spine V4.62

Total BMD CV for L1–L4 1.0%			
CF	0.999	1.063	1.000
Region	**Area (cm²)**	**BMC (g)**	**BMD (g/cm²)**
L2	12.31	7.87	0.639
L3	14.21	9.76	0.687
L4	17.70	13.26	0.749
Total	44.23	30.90	0.699

Region	BMD	T (30.0)		Z	
N/A					
L2	0.639	−3.53	62%	−2.18	73%
L3	0.687	−3.61	63%	−2.19	74%
L4	0.749	−3.33	67%	−1.87	78%
L2–L4	0.699	−3.46	65%	−2.05	76%

♦ Age and sex matched
T = peak bone mass
Z = age matched

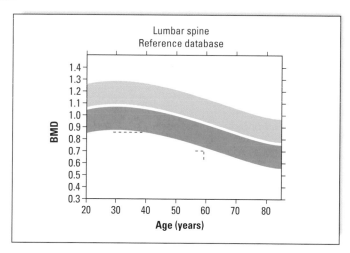

BMD(L2–L4) = 0.699 g/cm²

Figure 5.8 Results from a DXA scan of the lumbar spine of a 59-year-old woman showing the absolute bone density as well as T- and Z-scores. Since she has a T-score of -3.46 for the L2–4 she is considered to have osteoporosis at this site. A Z-score of -2.05 indicates that she also has lower bone density compared with her peers.

Table 5.6 Relevant questions for subjective assessment in the area of bone health (reproduced with permission from Bennell et al 2000)

Category	Specific questions
DXA results	Date performed T- and Z-scores Amount of change with serial scans
Family history of osteoporosis	Which family member? Which sites?
Fracture status	Site When? Related to minimal trauma?
Falls history	Number of falls in past year Mechanism of falls Associated injuries Risk factors (e.g. eyesight, home hazards)
Medical history	Particularly with relation to risk factors including ovariectomy, eating disorder, endocrine disorder
Medication	Current or past, especially long-term steroids, hormone replacement therapy, bisphosphonates
Menstrual history	Age of onset of periods Ever had ≤ 8 periods per year and number of years? Menopausal status including age at menopause and number of years since menopause
Smoking habits	Number of cigarettes per day and number of years smoked currently or in past
Diet	Dietary restrictions, such as vegetarianism, low fat Sources of daily calcium – yoghurt, cheese, milk Calcium supplementation – type and daily dose Amount of caffeine Number of glasses of alcohol per week
Exercise status	Amount and type of activity during youth Current exercise – type, intensity, duration, frequency Interests and motivational factors Exercise tolerance and shortness of breath
Posture	Noticed any loss of height? Difficulty lying flat in bed? Number of pillows needed Any activities encouraging bad posture?
Musculoskeletal problems and functional status	Pain, weakness, poor balance, incontinence Functional limitations
Social history	Occupation – full time/part time Hobbies Family

However, large-scale epidemiological studies suggest that physical activity is associated with a lower risk of fracture in both men and women (Joakimsen et al 1999, Kujala et al 2000, Paganini-Hill et al 1991).

The skeletal effects of exercise at different ages. It is presently thought that exercise in childhood and adolescence produces much higher gains in bone mass than does exercise in adulthood (Bass et al 1998, Bradney et al 1998, Conroy et al 1993, Heinonen et al 2000, McKay et al 2000, Morris et al 1997). In addition, it appears that childhood exercise stimulates the bone modeling process, expanding the bone size to produce a larger, possibly stronger bone (Bradney et al 1998, Haapasalo et al 1996). This phenomenon is generally not possible once growth has ceased.

Exercise in adulthood is important to conserve bone and to minimize bone loss with age (Kelley et al 2000, Wolff et al 1999). In adulthood, exercise must be continued in order to maintain exercise-induced BMD levels (Dalsky et al 1988). Attrition rates from exercise are high, even in supervised clinical trials (Bassey & Ramsdale 1994, Kerschan et al 1998). This reinforces the importance of developing strategies to improve compliance and encourage life-long participation in physical activity.

Table 5.7 Summary of outcome measurements that can be used to design and evaluate physical therapy programs for the prevention and treatment of osteoporosis

Variable	Measurement
Pain	• 10 cm visual analog scale • McGill Pain Questionnaire (Melzack 1975) • Daily analgesic use
Function and aerobic capacity	• Timed up and go (Podsiadlo & Richardson 1991) Time taken to rise from a chair, walk a distance of 3 m and return to sit down • Timed 6 m walk test (Hageman & Blanke 1986), time taken to walk 6 m at normal walking pace • Adapted shuttle walk (Singh et al 1994)
Self reported function and Health related quality of life	• SF-36 questionnaire (Ware & Sherbourne 1992) • Osteoporosis Functional Disability Questionnaire (Helmes et al 1995) • Quality of Life questionnaire of the European Foundation for Osteoporosis (QUALEFFO) (Lips et al 1999)
Balance	• Balancing on one leg or in stride standing – eyes open/closed, on hard surface/foam (Shumway-Cook & Horak 1986) Longest duration that the person can balance • Step test (Hill et al 1996) Number of times that the person can place the foot onto and off a step (7.5 cm or 15 cm high) in 15 s • Functional reach (Duncan et al 1990) Measure the distance that the person can reach forward in standing with the arm outstretched
Muscle strength	• Main muscles of interest include the quadriceps, ankle dorsiflexors, scapula retractors, trunk extensors, hip extensors and abdominals • Isometric, isotonic or isokinetic methods • Often assess 1 or 3 repetition maximum (1 or 3 RM) Determine the heaviest weight that the person can lift on one or three occasions • Grip strength using a hand held dynamometer
Posture and range of motion	• Measuring the distance of the tragus of the ear to the wall with the patient standing back against the wall to determine thoracic and cervical posture • Range of shoulder elevation

What types of exercise are best for improving bone strength? In humans, high impact exercises which generate ground reaction forces greater than twice body weight are more osteogenic than low-impact exercises (Bassey & Ramsdale 1994, Heinonen et al 1996, 1998).

Since lean mass (Flicker et al 1995, Young et al 1995) and muscle strength (Madsen et al 1993) are positively correlated with bone density, weight-training has been advocated for skeletal health (Gleeson et al 1990, Hartard et al 1996, Lohmann et al 1995, Snow-Harter et al 1992). Loss of muscle mass and strength with age is well documented (Harries & Bassey 1990, Rutherford & Jones 1992). Progressive weight-training even in the frail elderly can lead to large strength gains (Fiatarone et al 1990). In a unilateral exercise study, Kerr et al (1996) compared two strength-training regimens that differed in the number of repetitions and the weight lifted. The strength program (high loads, low repetitions) signifi-

cantly increased bone density at the hip and forearm sites whereas the endurance program (low loads, high repetitions) had no effect. Walking is frequently recommended in clinical practice to maintain skeletal integrity but generally the results of walking trials have not demonstrated significant effects on densitometry-derived bone density (Ebrahim et al 1997, Hatori et al 1993, Humphries et al 2000, Martin & Notelovitz 1993). This may relate to the fact that walking imparts relatively low magnitude, repetitive, and customary strain to the skeleton. While walking has numerous health benefits, some of which may influence fracture risk, it should not be prescribed as the exercise of choice for skeletal loading in healthy ambulant individuals. Whether walking is effective in those with restricted mobility is yet to be researched.

Non-weightbearing activities such as cycling and swimming do not stimulate bone adaptation despite increases in muscle strength (Orwoll et al 1989, Rico et al

1993, Taaffe et al 1995). This suggests that these activities do not generate sufficient strain to reach the threshold for bone adaptation.

Exercise dosage. The exact exercise dose required for maximal skeletal effects is not yet known. For an elderly or previously sedentary population, exercise should be gradually introduced to minimize fatigue and prevent soreness (Forwood & Larsen 2000). Exercise should be performed 2–3 times per week. Animal studies suggest that this is as effective for bone as daily loading (Raab-Cullen et al 1994).

For aerobic exercise, sessions should last between 15–60 min. The average conditioning intensity recommended for adults without fragility fractures is between 70 and 80% of their functional capacity. Individuals with a low functional capacity may initiate a program at 40 to 60% (Forwood & Larsen 2000).

Adults commencing a weight-training program may perform a few weeks of familiarization (Kerr et al 1996) followed by a single set of 8–10 repetitions at an intensity of 40–60% of 1 repetition maximum (RM). This can be progressed to 80%, even in the very elderly (American College of Sports Medicine 1998, Fiatarone et al 1994). Programs should include 8–10 exercises involving the major muscle groups. Supervision, particularly in the beginning, and attention to safe lifting technique is paramount.

Periodic progression of exercise dosage is needed, otherwise bone adaptation will cease. Increasing the intensity or weightbearing is more effective than increasing the duration of the exercise. A periodic increase in a step-like fashion may be better than progression in a linear fashion (Forwood & Larsen 2000). Nevertheless, there comes a point where gains in bone mass will slow and eventually plateau.

Clinical recommendations for exercise prescription. In children and adolescents, the goal is to maximize peak bone mass and strength. A variety of weightbearing, high-impact activities should be encouraged as part of the physical education curriculum in schools and during extracurricular sport and play. In the premenopausal adult years, the emphasis is on structured exercise to load bone. This could involve high-impact activities and weight-training. A healthy lifestyle should be promoted and, in females, attention paid to regular menstrual cycles. In the older adult years, a variety of exercise modes are needed to target clinically relevant hip, spine and forearm sites. Progressive weight-training and low-impact exercise are appropriate given that high-impact loading may be injurious. Other activities for balance, posture, and aerobic fitness could include a fast walking program, cycling, swimming, and specific exercises.

While exercise should be directed at improving or maintaining bone strength, in osteoporotic and older patients, the exercise focus shifts from specifically loading bone to preventing falls and improving function. Factors that will influence the choice of exercise program include bone density levels, patient's age, previous fractures, co-morbid musculoskeletal or medical conditions, lifestyle, interests, and current fitness level. Exercises to avoid in osteoporotic patients include high-impact loading, abrupt or explosive movements, trunk flexion, twisting movements, and dynamic abdominal exercises.

Posture and flexibility

In patients with osteopenia or osteoporosis, treatment should aim to minimize the flexion load on the spine, promote extended posture, and improve chest expansion. Land or water exercises can be designed to encourage diaphragmatic breathing, strengthen the hip, back and neck extensors and scapula retractors, and stretch the major upper and lower limb muscles (Bravo et al 1997, Chartered Society of Physiotherapy 1999). Postural re-education and dynamic stabilization for the trunk and limb girdles are particularly important to normalize mechanical forces (Figs 5.9 and 5.10). Stronger back extensors have been shown to be related to smaller thoracic kyphosis (Sinaki et al 1996). Patients can be advised to spend time lying in a prone or prone-on-elbows position to stimulate thoracic extension. Postural taping (Fig. 5.11) or bracing may be required to assist with maintenance of correct posture and for pain relief. Advice can be given about correct ways to lift as well as correct posture during standing, lying, sitting and bending.

Falls reduction

In elderly individuals or where falls risk factors have been identified, treatment should be directed towards reducing falls and their consequences. Patients who report multiple falls may benefit from referral to a falls clinic or to medical specialists for further evaluation and multi-faceted interventions (McMurdo et al 2000, Tinetti et al 1994). Exercise programs can address functional

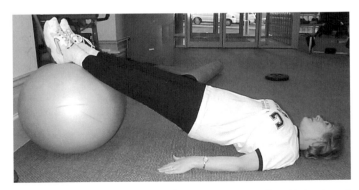

Figure 5.9 Hip extension exercises using a ball assist with trunk and pelvic stability. (Reproduced with permission from Bennell et al 2000.)

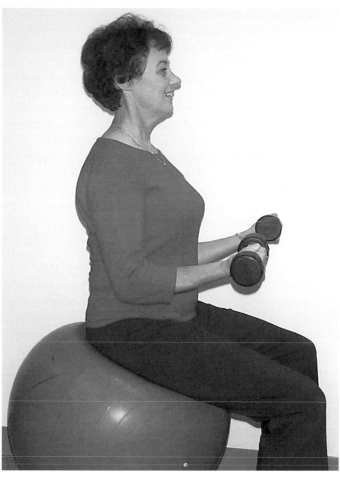

Figure 5.10   Upper limb exercises can be performed while sitting on a ball to increase dynamic stability and trunk control. (Reproduced with permission from Bennell et al 2000.)

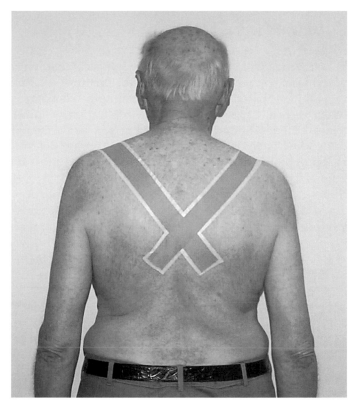

Figure 5.11   Taping may be used to facilitate thoracic extension and improve posture. (Reproduced with permission from Bennell et al 2000.)

impairments in elderly individuals (Bravo et al 1997, Kronhed & Moller 1998, Lord 1996, McMurdo & Rennie 1993, Morganti et al 1995, Nelson et al 1994, Simmons & Hansen 1996) and there is evidence that regular strength and balance training can reduce the risk of falling (Carter et al 2001). Consideration should also be given to home hazard modification and, in appropriate patients, prescription of gait aids and external hip protectors (Kannus et al 2000, Parkkari et al 1995, 1997).

Pain relieving techniques

Exercise has been shown to reduce back pain and improve psychological wellbeing in postmenopausal women with osteopenia (Bravo et al 1996, Preisinger et al 1996) and with established osteoporosis (Malmros et al 1998).

Hydrotherapy may be beneficial due to the heat and unloading effects (Bravo et al 1997), and is particularly useful for building patient confidence prior to com-

mencing a land-based exercise program. Other pain-relieving techniques include ice, hot packs, soft tissue massage, transcutaneous electrical nerve stimulation (TENS), interferential therapy, and shortwave diathermy. Gentle spinal mobilization can be performed even in patients with osteoporosis and osteopenia, provided care is taken and techniques that are well short of end range used. However, forceful joint manipulation is contraindicated. To deal more positively with chronic pain, cognitive and behavioral strategies or relaxation techniques may be employed by the physical therapist (see Ch. 8).

Education

A large part of the physical therapist's role is to provide osteoporosis education and to empower the individual to take control of the condition. In many cases, patients may be anxious and require reassurance and advice about safe activities. Physical therapists should continually update their knowledge about self-help groups, community programs, and reputable gymnasiums and exercise classes in the local area. Osteoporosis organizations are found in many countries and provide a range of useful services and resources.

SUMMARY

Bone injuries will be encountered by physical therapists working in a variety of settings. Acute fractures are due to a single load that exceeds bone strength while stress fractures result from the repeated application of lower loads. Osteoporotic fractures occur in a bone weakened due to low bone density and microarchitectural deterioration. Rehabilitation following acute fractures must be guided by a number of factors including the stage of healing, the type of fracture, the method of fixation, associated injuries and the age of the patient. Stress fracture management involves modified rest, pain relief, lower limb strengthening, attention to risk factors and a program of graduated return to activity. Prevention of stress fractures is an additional aim of physical therapists working with athletes. Identified risk factors in women include low bone density, a later than usual age of menarche, less lean mass, disordered patterns of eating, and leg length discrepancy. From a physical therapy perspective, prevention of osteoporotic fractures focuses on regular weightbearing activity that is commenced in childhood and continued throughout life. Management of the older individual with osteoporosis includes education, pain-relieving techniques (if appropriate) and exercises designed to improve posture, balance, range of motion, and lower limb strength.

REFERENCES

Aarden E M, Burger E H, Nijweide P J 1994 Function of osteocytes in bone. Journal of Cell Biochemistry 55:287–299

American College of Sports Medicine 1998 Position stand on exercise and physical activity for older adults. Medicine and Science for Sports and Exercise 30:992–1008

Andrew J G, Andrew S M, Freemont A J et al 1994 Inflammatory cells in normal human fracture healing. Acta Orthopaedica Scandinavica 65:462–466

Atkinson K, Coutts F, Hassenkamp A 1999 Physiotherapy in orthopaedics. Churchill Livingstone, Edinburgh

Bailey D A 1997 The Saskatchewan pediatric bone mineral accrual study – bone mineral acquisition during the growing years. International Journal of Sports Medicine 18:S191–194

Barrow G W, Saha S 1988 Menstrual irregularity and stress fractures in collegiate female distance runners. American Journal of Sports Medicine 16:209–216

Bass S, Pearce G, Bradney M et al 1998 Exercise before puberty may confer residual benefits in bone density in adulthood: studies in active prepubertal and retired female gymnasts. Journal of Bone and Mineral Research 13:500–507

Bassey E J, Ramsdale S J 1994 Increase in femoral bone density in young women following high impact exercise. Osteoporosis International 4:72–75

Batt M E, Kemp S, Kerslake R 2001 Delayed union stress fractures of the anterior tibia: conservative management. British Journal of Sports Medicine 35:74–77

Benazzo F, Barnabei G, Ferrario A et al 1992 Stress fractures in track and field athletes. Journal of Sports Traumatology and Related Research 14:51–65

Bennell K L, Malcolm S A, Thomas S A et al 1995 Risk factors for stress fractures in female track-and-field athletes: a retrospective analysis. Clinical Journal of Sports Medicine 5:229–235

Bennell K L, Malcolm S A, Thomas S A et al 1996 Risk factors for stress fractures in track and field athletes: a 12 month prospective study. American Journal of Sports Medicine 24:810–818

Bennell K, Khan K, McKay 2000 The role of physiotherapy in the prevention and treatment of osteoporosis. Manual Therapy 5:198–213

Blake G M, Fogelman I 1998 Applications of bone densitometry for osteoporosis. Endocrinology and Metabolism Clinics of North America 27:267–288

Boivin G, Anthoine-Terrier C, Obrant K J 1990 Transmission electron microscopy of bone tissue. Acta Orthopaedica Scandinavica 61:170–180

Bradney M, Pearce G, Naughton G et al 1998 Moderate exercise during growth in prepubertal boys – changes in bone mass, size, volumetric density, and bone strength – a controlled prospective study. Journal of Bone and Mineral Research 13:1814–1821

Bravo G, Gauthier P, Roy P M et al 1996 Impact of a 12-month exercise program on the physical and psychological health of osteopenic women. Journal of the American Geriatrics Society 44:756–62

Bravo G, Gauthier P, Roy P et al 1997 A weight-bearing, water-based exercise program for osteopenic women: its impact on bone, functional fitness, and well-being. Archives of Physical Medicine and Rehabilitation 78:1375–1380

Brosh T, Arcan M 1994 Toward early detection of the tendency to stress fractures. Clinical Biomechanics 9:111–116

Brukner P D, Bennell K L 1997 Stress fractures. Critical Reviews in Physical and Rehabilitation Medicine 9:151–190

Brukner P, Bennell K, Matheson G 1999 Stress fractures. Blackwell Science Asia, Melbourne

Brunet M E, Cook S D, Briuker M R et al 1990 A survey of running injuries in 1505 competitive and recreational runners. The Journal of Sports Medicine and Physical Fitness 30:307–315

Buckwalter J A, Glimcher M J, Cooper R R, Recker R 1995 Bone biology. Journal of Bone and Joint Surgery 77(A):1256–1275

Burr D 2001 Pharmaceutical treatments that may prevent or delay the onset of stress fractures. In: Burr D B, Milgrom C (eds) Musculoskeletal fatigue and stress fractures. CRC Press, Boca Raton, p259–270

Carbon R, Sambrook P N, Deakin V et al 1990 Bone density of elite female athletes with stress fractures. Medical Journal of Australia 153:373–376

Carter D R, Hayes W C, Schurman D J 1976 Fatigue life of compact bone-11. Effects of microstructure and density. Journal of Biomechanics 9:211–218

Carter N, Kannus P, Khan K M 2001 Exercise in the prevention of falls in older people: a systematic literature review examining the rationale and the evidence. Sports Medicine 31:427–438

Cavanagh P R, LaFortune M A 1980 Ground reaction forces in distance running. Journal of Biomechanics 13:397–406

Chartered Society of Physiotherapy 1999 Physiotherapy guidelines for the management of osteoporosis. Chartered Society of Physiotherapy, London

Cline A D, Jansen G R, Melby C L 1998 Stress fractures in female army recruits – implications of bone density, calcium intake, and exercise. Journal of the American College of Nutrition 17:128–135

Conroy B P, Kraemer W J, Maresh C M et al 1993 Bone mineral density in elite junior olympic weight lifters. Medicine and Science in Sports and Exercise 25:1103–1109

Consensus Develoment Conference 1993 Diagnosis, prophylaxis and treatment of osteoporosis. American Journal of Medicine 94:646–650

Cowan D N, Jones B H, Frykman P N et al 1996 Lower limb morphology and risk of overuse injury among male infantry trainees. Medicine and Science in Sports and Exercise 28:945–952

Cummings SR, Black DM, Nevitt MC et al 1993 Bone density at various sites for prediction of hip fractures. Lancet 341:72–75

Currey J D 2001 Bone strength: what are we trying to measure? Calcified Tissue International 68:205–210

Cutler W B, Friedmann E, Genovese-Stone E 1993 Prevalence of kyphosis in a healthy sample of pre- and postmenopausal women. American Journal of Physical Medicine and Rehabilitation 72:219–225

Dalsky G P, Stocke K S, Ehansi A A et al 1988 Weight-bearing exercise training and lumbar bone mineral content in postmenopausal women. Annals of Internal Medicine 108:824–828

Dickson T B, Kichline P D 1987 Functional management of stress fractures in female athletes using a pneumatic leg brace. American Journal of Sports Medicine 15:86–89

Duncan P, Weiner K, Chandler J et al 1990 Functional reach: a new clinical measure of balance. Journal of Gerontology 45:M192–197

Ebrahim S, Thompson P, Baskaran V et al 1997 Randomized placebo-controlled trial of brisk walking in the prevention of postmenopausal osteoporosis. Age and Ageing 26:253–260

Egol K A, Frankel V H 2001 Problematic stress fracture. In: Burr D B, Milgrom C (eds) Musculoskeletal fatigue and stress fractures. CRC Press, Boca Raton, p305–319

Einhorn T A 1996 The bone organ system: form and function. In: Marcus R, Feldman D, Kelsey J (eds) Osteoporosis. Academic Press, San Diego, p3–22

Einhorn T A 1998 The cell and molecular biology of fracture healing. Clinical Orthopaedics and Related Research 355S:S7–S21

Ekenman I, Tsai-Fellander L, Westblad P et al 1996 A study of intrinsic factors in patients with stress fractures of the tibia. Foot and Ankle International 17:477–482

Ensrud K E, Black D M, Harris F et al 1997 Correlates of kyphosis in older women. Journal of the American Geriatrics Society 45:682–687

Fiatarone M, Marks E, Ryan N et al 1990 High-intensity training in nonagenarians. Journal of the American Medical Association 263:3029–3034

Fiatarone M A, O'Neill E F, Ryan N D et al 1994 Exercise training and nutritional supplementation for physical frailty in very elderly people. New England Journal of Medicine 330:1769–1775

Flicker L, Hopper J L, Rodgers L et al 1995 Bone density determinants in elderly women: a twin study. Journal of Bone and Mineral Research 10:1607–1613

Forwood M R 2001 Mechanical effects on the skeleton: are there clinical implications? Osteoporosis International 12:77–83

Forwood M R, Burr D B 1993 Physical activity and bone mass: exercises in futility? Bone and Mineral 21:89–112

Forwood M, Larsen J 2000 Exercise recommendations for osteoporosis: a position statement for the Australian and New Zealand Bone and Mineral Society. Australian Family Physician 29:761–764

Friberg O 1982 Leg length asymmetry in stress fractures. A clinical and radiological study. Journal of Sports Medicine 22:485–488

Frost H M 1983 A determinant of bone architecture. The minimum effective strain. Clinical Orthopaedics and Related Research 175:286–292

Frost H M 1989 The biology of fracture healing: an overview for clinicians. Part I. Clinical Orthopaedics and Related Research 248:283–293

Frost H M 1990 Structural adaptations to mechanical usage (SATMU): redefining Wolff's Law. Anatomical Records 226:403–422

Frost H M 1991 Some ABCs of skeletal pathophyiology. 6. The growth/modeling/remodeling distinction. Calcified Tissue International 49:301–302

Frusztajer N T, Dhuper S, Warren M P et al 1990 Nutrition and the incidence of stress fractures in ballet dancers. American Journal of Clinical Nutrition 51:779–783

Fyhrie D P, Milgrom C, Hoshaw S J et al 1998 Effect of fatiguing exercise on longitudinal bone strain as related to stress fracture in humans. Annals of Biomedical Engineering 26:660–665

Giladi M, Milgrom C, Danon Y et al 1985a The correlation between cumulative march training and stress fractures in soldiers. Military Medicine 150:600–601

Giladi M, Milgrom C, Stein M et al 1985b The low arch, a protective factor in stress fractures. A prospective study of 295 military recruits. Orthopaedic Review 14:709–712

Giladi M, Milgrom C, Stein M et al 1987 External rotation of the hip. A predictor of risk for stress fractures. Clinical Orthopaedics and Related Research 216:131–134

Giladi M, Milgrom C, Simkin A et al 1991 Stress fractures: identifiable risk factors. American Journal of Sports Medicine 19:647–652

Gillespie W J, Grant I 2000 Interventions for preventing and treating stress fractures and stress reactions of bone of the lower limbs in young adults (Cochrane review). In: The Cochrane Library, issue 2. Update Software, Oxford

Girrbach R T, Flynn T W, Browder D A et al 2001 Flexural wave propagation velocity and bone mineral density in females with and without tibial bone stress injuries. Journal of Orthopaedic and Sports Physical Therapy 31:54–62

Gleeson P, Protas E, LeBlanc A et al 1990 Effects of weight lifting on bone mineral density in premenopausal women. Journal of Bone and Mineral Research 5:153–158

Glowacki J 1998 Angiogenesis in fracture repair. Clinical Orthopaedics and Related Research 355S:S82–S89

Greaney R B, Gerber R H, Laughlin R L et al 1983 Distribution and natural history of stress fractures in US marine recruits. Radiology 146:339–346

Gremion G, Rizzoli R, Slosman D et al 2001 Oligo-amenorrheic long-distance runners may lose more bone in spine than in femur. Medicine and Science in Sports and Exercise 33:15–21

Grimston S K, Engsberg J R, Kloiber R et al 1991 Bone mass, external loads, and stress fractures in female runners. International Journal of Sport Biomechanics 7:293–302

Haapasalo H, Sievanen H, Kannus P et al 1996 Dimensions and estimated mechanical characteristics of the humerus after long-term tennis loading. Journal of Bone and Mineral Research 11:864–872

Hageman P, Blanke 1986 Comparison of gait of young women and elderly women. Physical Therapy 66:1382–1387

Harries U J, Bassey E J 1990 Torque-velocity relationships for the knee extensors in women in their 3rd and 7th decades. European Journal of Applied Physiology 60:187–190

Hartard M, Haber P, Ilieva D et al 1996 Systematic strength training as a model of therapeutic intervention. American Journal of Physical Medicine and Rehabilitation 75:21–28

Hatori M, Hasegawa A, Adachi H et al 1993 The effects of walking at the anaerobic threshold level on vertebral bone loss in postmenopausal women. Calcified Tissue International 52:411–414

Hayes W C, Gerhart T N 1985 Biomechanics of bone: applications for assessment of bone strength. Bone and Mineral Research 3:259–294

Heinonen A, Kannus P, Sievanen H et al 1996 Randomised, controlled trial of effect of high-impact exercise on selected risk factors for osteoporotic fractures. Lancet 348:1343–1347

Heinonen A, Oja P, Sievanen H et al 1998 Effect of two training regimens on bone mineral density in healthy perimenopausal women: a randomised, controlled trial. Journal of Bone and Mineral Research 13:483–490

Heinonen A, Sievanen H, Kannus P et al 2000 High-impact exercise and bones of growing girls: A 9-month controlled trial. Osteoporosis International 11:1010–1017

Heinonen A, Sievänen H, Kyröläinen H et al 2001 Mineral mass, size and estimated mechanical strength of the lower limb bones of triple jumpers. Bone 29:279–285

Helmes E, Hodsman A, Lazowski D et al 1995 A questionnaire to evaluate disability in osteoporotic patients with vertebral compression fractures. Journals of Gerontology Series A-Biological Sciences and Medical Sciences 50:M91–M98

Hetland M L, Haarbo J, Christiansen C et al 1993 Running induces menstrual disturbances but bone mass is unaffected, except in amenorrheic women. American Journal of Medicine 95:53–60

Hill K, Bernhardt J, McGann A et al 1996 A new test of dynamic standing balance for stroke patients: reliability, validity, and comparison with healthy elderly. Physiotherapy Canada 48:257–262

Hoffman J R, Chapnik L, Shamis A et al 1999 The effect of leg length on the incidence of lower extremity overuse injuries during military training. Military Medicine 164:153–156

Hughes L Y 1985 Biomechanical analysis of the foot and ankle for predisposition to developing stress fractures. Journal of Orthopaedic and Sports Physical Therapy 7:96–101

Humphries B, Newton R U, Bronks R et al 2000 Effect of exercise intensity on bone density, strength, and calcium turnover in older women. Medicine and Science in Sports and Exercise 32:1043–1050

Joakimsen R M, Fonnebo V, Magnus J H et al 1999 The Truomso study – physical activity and the incidence of fractures in a middle-aged population. Journal of Bone and Mineral Research 13:1149–1157

Johnston J, Slemenda C 1993 Determinants of peak bone mass. Osteoporosis International Supplement 1:S54–S55

Jonnavithula S, Warren M P, Fox R P et al 1993 Bone density is compromised in amenorrheic women despite return of menses: a 2-year study. Obstetrics and Gynecology 81:669–674

Kadel N J, Teitz C C, Kronmal R A 1992 Stress fractures in ballet dancers. American Journal of Sports Medicine 20:445–449

Kannus P, Parkkari J, Niemi S et al 2000 Prevention of hip fracture in elderly people with use of a hip protector. New England Journal of Medicine 343:1506–1513

Kelley G A, Kelley K S, Tran Z V 2000 Exercise and bone mineral density in men: a meta-analysis. Journal of Applied Physiology 88:1730–1736

Kerr D, Morton A, Dick I et al 1996 Exercise effects on bone mass in postmenopausal women are site-specific and load-dependent. Journal of Bone and Mineral Research 11:218–225

Kerschan K, Alacamlioglu Y, Kollmitzer J et al 1998 Functional impact of unvarying exercise program in women after menopause. American Journal of Physical Medicine and Rehabilitation 77:326–332

Khan K, McKay H, Kannus P et al 2001 Physical activity and bone health, Human Kinetics, Champaign, IL

Kiss Z A, Khan K M, Fuller P J 1993 Stress fractures of the tarsal navicular bone: CT findings in 55 cases. American Journal of Roentgenology 160:111–115

Kronhed A, Moller M 1998 Effects of physical exercise on bone mass, balance skill and aerobic capacity in women and men with low bone mineral density, after one year of training – a prospective study. Scandinavian Journal of Medicine and Science in Sports 8:290–298

Kujala U M, Kaprio J, Kannus P et al 2000 Physical activity and osteoporotic hip fracture risk in men. Archives of Internal Medicine 160:705–708

Lanyon L E 1984 Functional strain as a determinant for bone remodeling. Calcified Tissue International 36:S56–S61

Lanyon L E 1987 Functional strain in bone tissue as an objective, and controlling stimulus for adaptive bone remodelling. Journal of Biomechanics 20:1083–1093

Larsen J 1998 Osteoporosis. In: Sapsford R, Bullock-Saxton J, Markwell S (eds) Women's health. A textbook for physiotherapists. WB Saunders, London, p412–453

Lauder T D, Dixit S, Pezzin L E et al 2000 The relation between stress fractures and bone mineral density: evidence from active-duty army women. Archives of Physical Medicine and Rehabilitation 81:73–79

Lee J K, Yao L 1988 Stress fractures: MR imaging. Radiology 169:2217–220

Lespessailles E, Jullien A, Eynard E et al 1998 Biomechanical properties of human os calcanei: relationships with bone density and fractal evaluation of bone microarchitecture. Journal of Biomechanics 31:817–824

Lips P, Cooper C, Agnusdei D et al 1999 Quality of life in patients with vertebral fractures: validation fo the Quality of Life questionnaire of the European Foundation for Osteoporosis (QUALEFFO). Osteoporosis International 10:150–160

Lohmann T, Going S, Pamenter R et al 1995 Effects of resistance training on regional and total bone mineral density in premenopausal women: a randomized prospective study. Journal of Bone and Mineral Research 10:1015–1024

Lord S 1996 The effects of a community exercise program on fracture risk factors in older women. Osteoporosis International 6:361–367

Lord S R, Clark R D, Webster I W 1991 Physiological factors associated with falls in an elderly population. Journal of the Geriatrics Society 39:1194–1200

Lord S R, Sambrook P N, Gilbert C et al 1994 Postural stability, falls and fractures in the elderly: results from the Dubbo Osteoporosis Epidemiology Study. Medical Journal of Australia 160:684–691

McKay H A, Petit M A, Schutz R W et al 2000 Augmented trochanteric bone mineral density after modified physical education classes: a randomized school-based exercise intervention study in prepubescent and early pubescent children. Journal of Pediatrics 136:156–162

McMurdo M, Rennie L 1993 A controlled trial of exercise by residents of old people's homes. Age and Ageing 22:11–15

McMurdo M E T, Millar A M, Daly F 2000 A randomized controlled trial of fall prevention strategies in old peoples' homes. Gerontology 46:83–87

McNitt-Gray J 1991 Kinematics and impulse characteristics of drop landings from three heights. International Journal of Sports Biomechanics 7:201–223

Madsen O R, Schaadt O, Bliddal H et al 1993 Relationship between quadriceps strength and bone mineral density of the proximal tibia and distal forearm in women. Journal of Bone and Mineral Research 8:1439–1444

Malmros B, Mortenson L, Jensen M B et al 1998 Positive effects of physiotherapy on chronic pain and performance in osteoporosis. Osteoporosis International 8:215–221

Martin R B 1991 Determinants of the mechanical properties of bones. Journal of Biomechanics 24:79–88

Martin D, Notelovitz M 1993 Effects of aerobic training on bone mineral density of postmenopausal women. Journal of Bone and Mineral Research 8:931–936

Melzack R 1975 The McGill pain questionnaire: major properties and scoring methods. Pain 1:277–299

Meurman K O A, Elfving S 1980 Stress fracture in soliders: a multifocal bone disorder. Radiology 134:483–487

Milgrom C 1989 The Israeli elite infantry recruit: a model for understanding the biomechanics of stress fractures. The Journal of the Royal College of Surgeons Edinburgh 34:S18–S22

Milgrom C, Finestone A, Shlamkovitch N et al 1992 Prevention of overuse injuries of the foot by improved shoe shock attenuation. A randomized, prospective study. Clinical Orthopaedics 281:189–192

Milgrom C, Finestone A, Shlamkovitch N et al 1994 Youth is a risk factor for stress fracture. A study of 783 infantry recruits. Journal of Bone and Joint Surgery 76(B):20–22

Milgrom C, Simkin A, Eldad A et al 2000 Using bone's adaptation ability to lower the incidence of stress fractures. American Journal of Sports Medicine 28:245–251

Montgomery L C, Nelson F R T, Norton J P et al 1989 Orthopedic history and examination in the etiology of overuse injuries. Medicine and Science in Sports and Exercise 21:237–243

Morganti C M, Nelson M E, Fiatarone M A et al 1995 Strength improvements with 1 yr of progressive resistance training in older women. Medicine and Science in Sports and Exercise 27:906–912

Morris F L, Naughton G A, Gibbs J L et al 1997 Prospective ten-month exercise intervention in premenarcheal girls: positive effects on bone and lean mass. Journal of Bone and Mineral Research 12:1453–1462

Mosekilde L 1993 Vertebral structure and strength in vivo and in vitro. Calcified Tissue International 53:S121–S126

Myburgh K H, Hutchins J, Fataar A B et al 1990 Low bone density is an etiologic factor for stress fractures in athletes. Annals of Internal Medicine 113:754–759

Myburgh K H, Bachrach L K, Lewis B et al 1993 Low bone mineral density at axial and appendicular sites in amenorrheic athletes. Medicine and Science in Sports and Exercise 25:1197–1202

Nattiv A, Puffer J C, Green G A 1997 Lifestyles and health risks of collegiate athletes – a multi-center study. Clinical Journal of Sport Medicine 7:262–272

Nelson M, Fiatarone M, Morganti C et al 1994 Effects of high-intensity strength training on multiple risk factors for osteoporotic fractures: a randomized controlled trial. The Journal of the American Medical Association 272:1909–1914

Nordin M, Frankel V H 1989 Basic biomechanics of the musculoskeletal system. Lea and Febiger, Philadelphia

Orwoll E S, Ferar J, Oviatt S K et al 1989 The relationship of swimming exercise to bone mass in men and women. Archives of Internal Medicine 149:2197–2200

Otis C L, Drinkwater B, Johnson M et al 1997 American College of Sports Medicine position stand. The female athlete triad. Medicine and Science in Sports and Exercise 29:I–X

Paganini-Hill A, Chao A, Ross R K et al 1991 Exercise and other factors in the prevention of hip fracture: The Leisure World study. Epidemiology 2:16–25

Parfitt A M 1988 Bone remodeling: relationship to the amount and structure of bone, and the pathogenesis and prevention of fractures. In: Riggs B L, Melton III L J (eds) Osteoporosis: etiology, diagnosis, and management. Raven Press, New York

Parkkari J, Kannus P, Heikkila J et al 1995 Energy-shunting external hip protector attenuates the peak femoral impact force below the theoretical fracture threshold – an in vitro biomechanical study under falling conditions of the elderly. Journal of Bone and Mineral Research 10:1437–1442

Parkkari J, Kannus P, Heikkila J et al 1997 Impact experiments of an external hip protector in young volunteers. Calcified Tissue International 60:354–357

Parkkari J, Kannus P, Palvanen M et al 1999 Majority of hip fractures occur as a result of a fall and impact on the greater trochanter of the femur: a prospective controlled hip fracture study with 206 consecutive patients. Calcified Tissue International 65:183–187

Peck W A, Woods W L 1988 The cells of bone. In: Riggs B L, Melton III L J (eds) Osteoporosis: etiology, diagnosis, and management. Raven Press, New York

Petersen M M, Jensen N C, Gehrchen P M et al 1996 The relation between trabecular bone strength and bone mineral density assessed by dual photon and dual energy X-ray absorptiometry in the proximal tibia. Calcified Tissue International 59:311–314

Picard C L 1999 The level of competition as a factor for the development of eating disorders in female collegiate athletes. Journal of Youth and Adolescence 28:583–594

Podsiadlo D, Richardson S 1991 The timed 'up and go': a test of basic functional mobility for frail elderly persons. Journal of the American Geriatric Society 39:142–148

Prather J L, Nusynowitz M L, Snowdy H A et al 1977 Scintigraphic findings in stress fractures. Journal of Bone and Joint Surgery 59(A):869–874

Preisinger E, Alacamlioglu Y, Pils K et al 1996 Exercise therapy for osteoporosis: results of a randomised, controlled trial. British Journal of Sports Medicine 30:209–212

Raab-Cullen D M, Akhter M P, Kimmel D B et al 1994 Bone response to alternate-day mechanical loading of the rat tibia. Journal of Bone and Mineral Research 9:203–211

Reinker K A, Ozburne S 1979 A comparison of male and female orthopaedic pathology in basic training. Military Medicine Aug:532–536

Rico H, Revilla M, Hernandez E R et al 1993 Bone mineral content and body composition in postpubertal cyclist boys. Bone 14:93–95

Robinson T L, Snow-Harter C, Taaffe D R et al 1995 Gymnasts exhibit higher bone mass than runners despite similar prevalence of amenorrhea and oligomenorrhea. Journal of Bone and Mineral Research 10:26–35

Ronsen O, Sundgot-Borgen J, Maehlum S 1999 Supplement use and nutritional habits in Norwegian elite athletes. Scandinavian Journal of Medicine and Science in Sports 9:28–35

Ross P D 1997 Clinical consequences of vertebral fractures. Amercian Journal of Medicine 103:30S–43S

Roub L W, Gumerman L W, Hanley E N, Williams Clark M, Goodman M, Herbert D L 1979 Bone stress: a radionuclide imaging perspective. Radiology 132:431–438

Rubin C T, Lanyon L E 1984 Regulation of bone formation by applied dynamic loads. Journal of Bone and Joint Surgery 66(A):397–402

Rubin C T, Lanyon L E 1985 Regulation of bone mass by mechanical strain magnitude. Calcified Tissue International 37:411–417

Rutherford O M, Jones D A 1992 The relationship of muscle and bone loss and activity levels with age in women. Age and Ageing 21:286–293

Sanders K M, Nicholson G C, Ugoni A M et al 1999 Health burden of hip and other fractures in Australia beyond 2000 – projections based on the Geelong Osteoporosis Study. Medical Journal of Australia 170:467–470

Santi M, Sartoris D J, Resnick D 1989 Diagnostic imaging of tarsal and metatarsal stress fractures. Part 11. Orthopaedic Review 18:178–185

Schwellnus M P, Jordaan G 1992 Does calcium supplementation prevent bone stress injuries? A clinical trial. International Journal of Sport Nutrition 2:165–174

Scott S H, Winter D A 1990 Internal forces at chronic running injury sites. Medicine and Science in Sports and Exercise 22:357–369

Scully T J, Besterman G 1982 Stress fracture – a preventable training injury. Military Medicine 147:285–287

Shaffer R A, Brodine S K, Almeida S A et al 1999 Use of simple measures of physical activity to predict stress fractures in young men undergoing a rigorous physical training program. American Journal of Epidemiology 149:236–242

Sheikh B 2000a Bone healing. In: Hoppenfeld S, Murthy V (eds) Treatment and rehabilitation of fractures. Lippincott Williams and Wilkins, Philadelphia, p1–6

Sheikh B 2000b Determining when a fracture has healed. In: Hoppenfeld S, Murthy V L (eds) Treatment and rehabilitation of fractures. Lippincott Williams and Wilkins, Philadelphia, p7–10

Shumway-Cook A, Horak F 1986 Assessing the influence of sensory interaction on balance: suggestions from the field. Physical Therapy 66:1548–1550

Simkin A, Leichter I, Giladi M et al 1989 Combined effect of foot arch structure and an orthotic device on stress fractures. Foot and Ankle 10:25–29

Simmons V, Hansen P D 1996 Effectiveness of water exercise on postural mobility in the well elderly: an experimental study on balance enhancement. Journal of Gerontology 51A:M233–M238

Sinaki M, Ito E, Rogers J W et al 1996 Correlation of back extensor strength with thoracic hyphosis and lumbar lordosis in estrogen-deficient women. American Journal of Physical Medicine and Rehabilitation 75:370–374

Singh S J, Morgan S J, Hardman A E et al 1994 Comparison of oxygen uptake during a conventional treadmill test and the shuttle walking test in chronic airflow limitation. European Respiratory Journal 11:2016–2020

Slayter M 1995 Lower limb training injuries in an army recruit population. PhD thesis. University of Newcastle

Snow-Harter C, Bouxsein M L, Lewis B T et al 1992 Effects of resistance and endurance exercise on bone mineral status of young women: a randomized exercise intervention trial. Journal of Bone and Mineral Research 7:761–769

Swenson E J, DeHaven K E, Sebastianelli W J et al 1997 The effect of a pneumatic leg brace on return to play in athletes with tibial stress fractures. American Journal of Sports Medicine 25:322–328

Taaffe D R, Snow-Harter C, Connolly D A et al 1995 Differential effects of swimming versus weight-bearing activity on bone mineral status of eumenorrheic athletes. Journal of Bone and Mineral Research 10:586–593

Tinetti M, Baker D, McAvay G et al 1994 A multifactorial intervention to reduce the risk of falling among elderly people living in the community. New England Journal of Medicine 331:822–827

Tomten S E 1996 Prevalance of menstrual dysfunction in Norwegian long-distance runners participating in the Oslo marathon games. Scandinavian Journal of Medicine and Science in Sport 6:164–171

Turner C H 1999 Toward a mathematical description of bone biology: the principle of cellular accommodation. Calcified Tissue International 65:466–471

Turner C H, Owan I, Takano Y 1995 Mechanotransduction in bone: role of strain rate. American Journal of Physiology 269:E438–E442

Umemura Y, Ishiko T, Tsujimoto H et al 1995 Effects of jump training on bone hypertrophy in young and old rats. International Journal of Sports Medicine 16:364–367

Umemura Y, Ishiko T, Yamauchi T et al 1997 Five jumps per day increase bone mass and breaking force in rats. Journal of Bone and Mineral Research 12:1480–1485

Ware JE, Sherbourne CD 1992 The MOS 36-item short-form health survey (SF-36). I. Conceptional framework and item selection. Medical Care 30:473–483

Warren M P, Brooks-Gunn J, Fox R P et al 1991 Lack of bone accretion and amenorrhea: evidence for a relative osteopenia in weight bearing bones. Journal of Clinical Endocrinology and Metabolism 72:847–853

Whalen R T, Carter D R, Steele C R 1988 Influence of physical activity on the regulation of bone density. Journal of Biomechanics 21:825–837

Whitelaw G P, Wetzler M J et al 1991 A pneumatic leg brace for the treatment of tibial stress fractures. Clinical Orthopedic and Related Research 270:302–305

Winfield A C, Bracker M, Moore J et al 1997 Risk factors associated with stress reactions in female marines. Military Medicine 162:698–702

Wolff I, van Croonenborg J J, Kemper H C G et al 1999 The effect of exercise training programs on bone mass: a meta-analysis of published controlled trials in pre- and postmenopausal women. Osteoporosis International 9:1–12

World Health Organization 1994 The World Health Organization assessment of fracture risk and its application to screening for ostoeporosis. Report of WHO Study Group

Worthen B M, Yanklowitz B A D 1978 The pathophysiology and treatment of stress fractures in military personnel. Journal of the American Podiatric Medical Association 68:317–325

Yoshikawa T, Mori S, Santiesteban A J et al 1994 The effects of muscle fatigue on bone strain. Journal of Experimental Biology 188:217–233

Young D, Hopper J L, Nowson C A et al 1995 Determinants of bone mass in 10- to 26-year-old females: a twin study. Journal of Bone and Mineral Research 10:558–567

Zanker C L, Swaine I L 1998 Relation between bone turnover, oestradiol, and energy balance in women distance runners. British Journal of Sports Medicine 32:167–171

Ziegler P J, Nelson J A, Jonnalagadda S S 1999 Nutritional and physiological status of US national figure skaters. International Journal of Sport Nutrition 9:345–360

Zmuda J M, Cauley J A, Ferrell R E 1999 Recent progress in understanding the genetic susceptibility to osteoporosis. Genetic Epidemiology 16:356–367

6

Nerves

Robert J Nee   David Butler

INTRODUCTION

Nervous system function is often conceptualized in terms of the generation, transmission, and processing of impulses related to motor control and nociception (see Chs 7 and 8). Health care practitioners may less commonly appreciate how chemical communication enables the nervous system to monitor and influence the health of musculoskeletal tissues. Chemicals from the periphery are carried within afferent axons to dorsal root ganglia and inform cell bodies about the health of innervated structures. The cell bodies respond by producing neuropeptides that are transported back to the periphery to enhance tissue health (Butler 1991, Rempel et al 1999, Shacklock et al 1994). In situations where musculoskeletal tissues are injured, cell bodies manufacture different neuropeptides that contribute to the inflammatory response necessary for healing (i.e. neurogenic inflammation) (Butler 2000, Costigan & Woolf 2000, Sluka 1996, Weinstein 1991).

The length of an axon can be 10 000 to 15 000 times the diameter of the cell body (Rempel et al 1999). In more clinically conceivable terms, major sensory axons within the femoral nerve are about 0.5 m long (Schwartz 1995), and tibial nerve axons may be over 1 m in length as they course from the spine to terminal branches in the foot (Butler 2000). Because of this unique cellular structure, neural tissues possess biomechanical properties that facilitate maintenance of electrochemical communication as neurons bend, glide, and stretch in concert with body movement (Butler 2000, Rempel et al 1999, Shacklock 1995a). Electrochemical and biomechanical activities of the nervous system are interdependent, and their interaction in healthy and injured neural tissues has been referred to as neurodynamics and pathodynamics respectively (Shacklock 1995a).

Sometimes sport or exercise activities place excessive mechanical demands on neural tissues, leading to symptoms associated with injury to the connective tissue and impulse conducting tissue components of the nervous system (Asbury & Fields 1984, Baron 2000, Butler 2000, Greening & Lynn 1998, Hall & Elvey 1999, Rempel et al 1999). Consequently, this chapter describes how the nervous system normally adapts to mechanical loads (neurodynamics) and discusses processes involved in neural tissue injury (pathodynamics). An understanding of these concepts can assist those working in the physical therapies in providing appropriate exercise and rehabilitation for their clients.

RELEVANT NEUROANATOMY AND PHYSIOLOGY

PERIPHERAL NERVE TRUNKS

Axons within peripheral nerve trunks are arranged into bundles called fascicles. Each fascicle is surrounded by a perineurial sheath composed of 6–15 layers of connective tissue contingent upon the fascicular diameter (Lundborg 1988, Matloub & Yousif 1992, Sunderland 1990) (Fig. 6.1). Although the primary orientation of connective tissue fibers is longitudinal, the inclination changes slightly between successive layers of the perineurium (Butler 1991, Butler 2000, Matloub & Yousif 1992). The laminated architecture enables the perineurial sheath to function as a viscoelastic tube. Because of this viscoelasticity, the perineurial tube is able to change dimensions and maintain a constant pressure within the fascicle regardless of the length of the nerve (Kwan et al 1992, Millesi et al 1995, Sunderland 1990). Since the interior of a fascicle is labeled the endoneurial space (Millesi et al 1995), this intrafascicular pressure is referred to as endoneurial fluid pressure (Lundborg 1988).

Besides preserving a constant mechanical environment for enclosed nerve fibers, the perineurium controls the biochemical milieu within the fascicle. The innermost connective tissue lamellae of the perineurial sheath create a metabolically active diffusion barrier which permits only certain chemicals and ions to come in contact with neural tissues (Butler 1991, Butler 2000, Lundborg 1988, Lundborg & Dahlin 1992, Matloub & Yousif 1992, Rempel et al 1999). For example, chemicals associated with edema around a fascicle or infection around a nerve trunk do not come in contact with the intrafascicular environment (Butler 1991, Lundborg 1988). The perineurial diffusion barrier works bidirectionally. Therefore, if mechanical or chemical stimuli cause endoneurial inflammation followed by intrafascicular edema, the resultant increase in endoneurial fluid pressure persists because the perineurium does not allow the inflammatory exudate to escape (Butler 1991, Lundborg 1988, Lundborg & Dahlin 1992, Lundborg et al 1983, Murphy 1977). Function of the perineurial diffusion barrier is very resistant to mechanical trauma (Lundborg 1988). Mechanical perturbation from a surgical procedure such as intraneural neurolysis or from experimentally sustained compression does not alter perineurial permeability (Lundborg 1988).

Structures within the endoneurial space rely on the optimal mechanical and biochemical environment regulated by the perineurium. In addition to axons, the endoneurial space accommodates Schwann cells, blood vessels, interstitial fluid, and a connective tissue network known as the endoneurium (Matloub & Yousif 1992, Rempel et al 1999) (Fig. 6.1). Schwann cells are glial cells that contribute to impulse conduction and provide

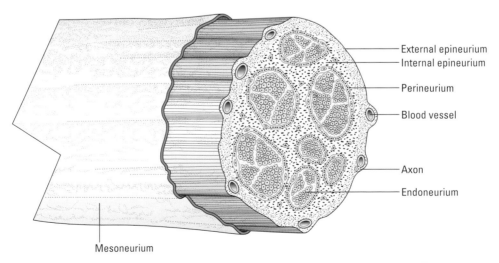

Figure 6.1 Peripheral neve connective tissue sheaths. (Reproduced with permission from Butler 1991.)

nutritional support for peripheral nerve fibers (Bear et al 2001, Matloub & Yousif 1992). A chain of Schwann cells envelops a single axon in a myelin sheath designed for high speed transmission of impulses. In the case of unmyelinated axons, a chain of Schwann cells surrounds several axons to insulate them from the endoneurial space (Bear et al 2001, Butler 1991, Matloub & Yousif 1992). Endoneurial connective tissue provides a scaffolding through which a capillary network courses to supply blood to nerve fibers and associated Schwann cells (Lundborg 1988). This connective tissue scaffolding becomes specialized to form an endoneurial tubule around each myelinated axon or group of unmyelinated axons (Butler 1991, Butler 2000).

Integrity of endoneurial tubules plays an important role in the movement capabilities of nerve fibers. Axons follow an undulated course within the endoneurium, and lengthening of a nerve trunk causes these undulations to straighten, effectively lengthening axons with minimal to no increase in endoneurial pressure (Millesi et al 1995, Sunderland 1990). Conversely, shortening of a nerve trunk causes the undulations to increase, enabling axons to adapt without being unduly compressed (Millesi et al 1995). This mechanism for accommodating change in length is lost when the endoneurial network is compromised, or when the perineurium is not able to function as a viscoelastic tube as previously discussed (Millesi et al 1995).

Just as axons follow an undulating path within the endoneurial space, each fascicle takes a tortuous course within the nerve trunk (Sunderland 1990). Fascicles repeatedly unite and divide along the length of a nerve to create fascicular plexuses. These plexuses enable the nerve trunk to adapt to changes in length, but also permit gliding between fascicles as nerves are twisted, compressed, or lengthened during joint movement (Kenneally et al 1988, Millesi et al 1995, Rempel et al 1999, Sunderland 1990). Fascicular gliding is possible due to the internal epineurium, a loose connective tissue incorporated between fascicles (Butler 1991, Butler 2000, Millesi et al 1995, Sunderland 1990) (Fig. 6.1). The internal epineurium also acts as a cushion to protect fascicles from compressive forces (Lundborg & Dahlin 1992, Sunderland 1990). Because they are adept at sheltering nerve fibers from mechanical loads, fascicular plexuses and internal epineurial tissues are well developed in portions of nerve trunks susceptible to injury (Butler 1991, Butler 2000, Lundborg & Dahlin 1992, Matloub & Yousif 1992, Rydevik et al 1984, Sunderland 1990). Examples of such locations include areas where nerves cross joints or pass through osseous (e.g. tarsal tunnel), osteoligamentous (e.g. carpal tunnel), or fibrous (e.g. arcade of Frohse) tunnels.

The external epineurium is the connective tissue layer wrapping around the internal epineurium and fascicles to separate them from neighboring structures (Butler 1991, Butler 2000, Matloub & Yousif 1992, Millesi et al 1995, Rempel et al 1999, Sunderland 1990) (Fig. 6.1). During limb movements, peripheral nerves exhibit a significant amount of sliding relative to surrounding tissues (Beith et al 1995, Hough et al 2000, McLellan & Swash 1976, Wilgis & Murphy 1986, Wright et al 1996, 2001). This excursion is facilitated by additional connective tissue enveloping the nerve trunk referred to as the mesoneurium or paraneurium (Butler 2000, Lundborg 1988, Millesi et al 1995, Sunderland 1990) (Fig. 6.1). If the mesoneurium becomes fibrotic, it can shrink and adhere to the external epineurium or adjacent non-neural structures, thereby impairing mobility of the nerve trunk (Millesi et al 1995).

NERVE ROOT COMPLEXES

Neural tissues undergo significant changes in connective tissue morphology and physiology as they pass through the intervertebral foramen (IVF) (Butler 1991, McCabe & Low 1969, Parke & Watanabe 1985, Rydevik et al 1984, Yoshizawa et al 1991). This area of transition is appropriately termed the nerve root complex (Rauschning 1997, Shacklock et al 1994). At the external aspect of the IVF, nerve fibers from the extremities are grouped into a ventral ramus while those from the posterior aspect of the spine and trunk are collected within a dorsal ramus. These rami merge to form a spinal nerve that enters the foramen and divides into sensory and motor roots. Nerve fibers in sensory and motor roots track proximally through the IVF and spinal canal to reach their destinations within the spinal cord (Bogduk 1997, Rydevik et al 1984). As they approach the spinal cord, sensory and motor nerve fibers display intradural connections between adjacent segments (Tanaka et al 2000), contradicting the common perception that nerve roots within each foramen are associated with a single spinal cord level. An enlargement of each sensory root contains the cell bodies of afferent nerve fibers passing through a particular IVF, and this enlargement is referred to as the dorsal root ganglion (DRG). The DRG has a variable location within each cervical or lumbar foramen (Jenis & An 2000, Kikuchi et al 1994, Tanaka et al 2000, Yabuki & Kikuchi 1996), and this structure warrants special mention as its mechanosensitivity and neurochemistry appear to play a significant role in radicular pain syndromes (Devor & Seltzer 1999, Hanai et al 1996, Hasue 1993, Nakamura & Myers 2000, Takebayashi et al 2001, Yabuki et al 2001). Additionally, connective tissue changes described below seem to take place just proximal to the DRG (McCabe & Low 1969, Olmarker & Rydevik 1991, Yoshizawa et al 1991).

Connective tissue layers of nerve trunks do not link exactly with meningeal layers of the spinal canal (Butler

1991, Murphy 1977, Olmarker & Rydevik 1991, Yoshizawa et al 1991). Peripheral nerve endoneurium encompasses nerve fibers in a connective tissue network that is continuous throughout the nerve root complex and eventually merges with pia mater (Butler 1991, Murphy 1977, Olmarker & Rydevik 1991, Sunderland 1974, Yoshizawa et al 1991). In contrast to nerve trunks, fascicles in sensory and motor roots run parallel to one another and are not enclosed in a durable perineurial sheath (Beel et al 1986, McCabe & Low 1969, Murphy 1977, Olmarker & Rydevik 1991, Yoshizawa et al 1991). A more delicate connective tissue derived from pia mater encircles each nerve root fascicle and has been labeled fascicular pia by Parke & Watanabe (1985). The same authors used the term radicular pia to describe the open mesh configuration of pial tissue that surrounds each nerve root (Fig. 6.2). The delicate and porous nature of these sheaths enables percolation of cerebrospinal fluid (CSF) to provide over 50% of the nutrition for sensory and motor roots (Rydevik et al 1990).

Since the perineurium is not present in sensory or motor roots, its structure must terminate somewhere in the region of the DRG. Perineurial tissue forms a tight capsule around each DRG (Murphy 1977, Olmarker & Rydevik 1991, Rydevik et al 1984, Rydevik et al 1989), contributing to the inherent mechanosensitivity of this structure (Butler 2000, Howe et al 1977, Sugawara et al 1996). However, proximal to the DRG, outer layers of perineurium merge with dura and arachnoid mater, while inner layers apparently meld with previously described fascicular and radicular pial sheaths (Butler 1991, Murphy 1977, Olmarker & Rydevik 1991, Yoshizawa et al 1991). This separation of perineurial layers facilitates transmission of mechanical loads to stronger dural tissues, sparing delicate nerve roots which exhibit 90% less tensile strength than peripheral nerves

(Beel et al 1986, Butler 1991). Concurrently, diffusion barrier mechanisms are maintained due to perineurial continuity with dura and arachnoid mater, preserving the biochemical environment of nerve root fascicles (Butler 1991).

Sensory and motor roots have minimal internal epineurium (Beel et al 1986, Murphy 1977, Rydevik et al 1984, Stodieck et al 1986, Sunderland 1990). This lack of fascicular cushioning, combined with the afore-mentioned parallel fascicular alignment and absence of perineurium, leads to concern that nerve roots are susceptible to mechanical injury (Murphy 1977, Rydevik et al 1984, Stodieck et al 1986, Sunderland 1990). However, under normal circumstances, anatomical features of the nerve root complex protect neural tissues from mechanical loads (Butler 1991, Sunderland 1974).

Nerve roots occupy only 30 to 40% of the space available within cervical and lumbar foramina (Jenis & An 2000, Sunderland 1974, Tanaka et al 2000), allowing ample room for adaptations to changes in foraminal dimensions known to occur with spinal movement (Fujiwara et al 2001, Muhle et al 2001, Yoo et al 1992). Adipose tissue and circulating CSF provide an additional safeguard against undesirable mechanical forces (Jenis & An 2000, Louis 1981, Rydevik et al 1984, Sunderland 1974). At the proximal portion of the IVF, the external epineurium links with arachnoid, dural, and epidural tissues to form a dural sleeve around each pair of sensory and motor roots (Bogduk 1997, Kenneally et al 1988, Olmarker & Rydevik 1991, Shacklock et al 1994, Sunderland 1974, Yoshizawa et al 1991). Neural tissues glide independently within the protective container of this dural sleeve as the entire nerve root complex moves within the IVF (Smith et al 1993, Sunderland 1974). These sleeves also shield enclosed nerve roots from tensile loads by acting as plugs when limb movement pulls

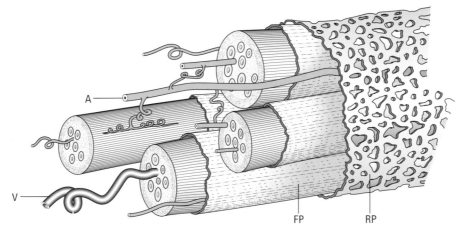

Figure 6.2 The intrinsic blood supply to a nerve root illustrating the coiled configuration of intraneural vessels. A = arteriole, FP = fascicular pia, RP = radicular pia, V = venule. (Reproduced with permission from Butler 1991.)

neural structures distal and lateral into the foramina (Butler 1991, Kenneally et al 1988, Smith et al 1993, Sunderland 1974). Attachments of dural sleeves to cervical and lumbar foramina assist this plugging mechanism in attenuating mechanical forces associated with nerve root movement (Grimes et al 2000, Moses & Carman 1996, Smith et al 1993). The previously described link between perineurium and dura is another anatomical element that deflects tensile forces away from fragile sensory and motor roots. Finally, major brachial and lumbosacral plexuses protect neural structures by preventing concentration of tensile loads at any single nerve root complex (Kleinrensink et al 2000).

NEUROMENINGEAL STRUCTURES

The length of the spinal canal is 5–9 cm longer in flexion than extension (Louis 1981, Rossitti 1993). Lateral flexion requires canal shortening on the concave side and lengthening on the convex side (Butler 1991, Butler 2000, Rossitti 1993, Shacklock et al 1994). Neuromeningeal structures must accommodate these changes. Since spinal cord tissues have six times less collagen content than mechanically delicate nerve roots (Stodieck et al 1986), durable connective tissue meninges and contained CSF offer requisite protection against mechanical forces produced by head, trunk, and limb movement.

The dura mater is the outermost meningeal layer and possesses the greatest mechanical strength (Butler 1991) (Figs 6.3, 6.4, and 6.5). Organization of collagen and elastin fibers changes between different layers of dural tissue. Inner layers appear to have a more longitudinal orientation, while outer layers exhibit a multidirectional arrangement to form a viscoelastic cylinder around the spinal cord and CSF (Nakagawa et al 1994, Runza et al 1999). In spite of differences between layers, the dominant fiber orientation is longitudinal, accounting for superior mechanical strength in this direction (Rossitti 1993, Runza et al 1999). Distribution of elastin within the dura correlates with mobility requirements. Compared to anterior dura, posterior dural tissue is further removed from the axis of motion for spinal flexion and extension. Consequently, posterior dura undergoes more displacement during sagittal plane movement and possesses more elastin to meet these mobility demands (Louis 1981,

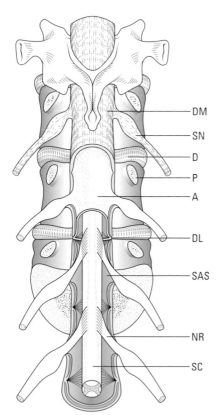

Figure 6.3 Diagram of the spinal canal, meninges, and spinal cord with the posterior vertebral arch removed. A = arachnoid, D = disk, DL = denticulate ligament, DM = dura mater, NR = nerve root complex, P = pedicle (cut), SAS = subarachnoid space, SC = spinal cord, SN = spinal nerve. (Reproduced with permission from Butler 1991.)

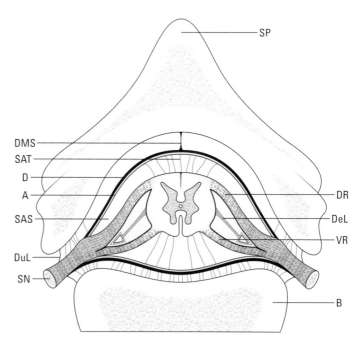

Figure 6.4 Diagrammatic cross-section of the cord and spinal canal illustrating intradural and extradural connections. A = arachnoid, B = body, D = dura, DuL = dural ligament, DeL = denticulate ligament, DMS = dorsomedian septum, DR = dorsal root, SAS = subarachnoid space, SAT = subarachnoid trabeculae, SN = spinal nerve, SP = spinous process, VR = ventral root. (Reproduced with permission from Butler 1991.)

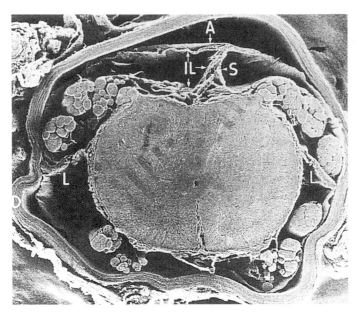

Figure 6.5 Scanning electron micrograph of the lumbar spinal cord of a 15-month-old child. L = denticulate ligaments, D = dura (note the layers), A = arachnoid, S = dorsal septum, IL = intermediate leptomeningeal layer. Note also the nerve root fascicles dispersed around the spinal cord. (Reproduced from Nicholas D S, Weller R O 1988 The fine anatomy of the human spinal meninges. Journal of Neurosurgery 69: 276–282 with the permission of the Journal of Neurosurgery.)

Nakagawa et al 1994, Rossitti 1993). The elastin content in posterior dural tissues is highest in the cervical and lumbar regions, because these portions of the vertebral canal have the most sagittal plane mobility (Louis 1981, Nakagawa et al 1994, Rossitti 1993).

Pia mater is the innermost meningeal layer consisting of a connective tissue mesh separating CSF from spinal cord tissues (Butler 1991, Butler 2000). A continuous lateral projection of pia mater forms the origin of a dentate ligament on each side of the spinal canal (Rossitti 1993). These ligaments become serrated to pierce the arachnoid and attach to the dura between the dural sleeves (Butler 1991, 2000, Rossitti 1993) (Fig. 6.3). Serrations of the dentate ligaments exhibit a superolateral orientation in the upper cervical spine, a transverse arrangement in the remainder of the cervical region, and a progressively inferolateral alignment in the thoracic and lumbar regions (Rossitti 1993).

The dura mater, pia mater, and dentate ligaments form a functional unit that shields the spinal cord from mechanical loads accompanying movement (Butler 1991, Rossitti 1993). Head, trunk, and limb motion create tension in the dura because of dural attachments to the skeleton at the cranial sutures, the foramen magnum, the coccyx via the filum terminale, the intervertebral foramina via the dural sleeves, and other margins of the spinal canal via meningovertebral ligaments and the

dorsomedian septum (Butler 1991, Butler 2000, Rossitti 1993, Shacklock et al 1994) (Fig. 6.4). These tensile forces are transmitted through serrations of the dentate ligaments to the pia mater for optimal positioning of the cord within the spinal canal (Rossitti 1993). Optimal positioning may involve any combination of axial, anteroposterior, or lateral displacement of the cord so it can follow the shortest path through the vertebral canal (Butler 1991, Louis 1981, Muhle et al 1998, Rossitti 1993). The varied orientation of dentate ligament attachments enables this mechanism of force transmission to move the spinal cord without generating significant mechanical stress within the delicate neural tissues (Butler 1991, Rossitti 1993). Similar events enable the spinal cord to adapt to mechanical loads imposed by limb movements (Kenneally et al 1988, Sunderland 1974).

Cerebrospinal fluid assists positioning of the cord within the spinal canal. The arachnoid mater is the intermediate meningeal layer that holds CSF within the subarachnoid space (Figs 6.4 and 6.5). CSF is contained under slight pressure to act as a hydraulic cushion protecting the spinal cord (Butler 1991, Louis 1981). Arachnoid trabeculae and an intermediate leptomeningeal layer are thought to optimize the cushioning effect of CSF by dampening any pressure waves caused by body movement (Nicholas & Weller 1988) (Fig. 6.5).

Spinal cord tissues possess intrinsic anatomical properties for adapting to movement of the vertebral column. In a neutral position, neurons and glia are arranged into folds and spirals, analogous to the undulating course of axons within the endoneurium of nerve trunks and nerve roots (Butler 2000, Murphy 1977, Rossitti 1993). These folds are increased posteriorly during spinal extension, enabling cord structures to adjust to a shorter vertebral canal. Conversely, with vertebral flexion these undulations unwind so cord tissues lengthen without detrimental increases in mechanical stress (Butler 2000, Louis 1981, Murphy 1977, Rossitti 1993) (Fig. 6.6). Different spinal cord tracts may also accommodate asymmetrical displacement associated with sagittal and frontal plane movements by sliding against each other (Louis 1981, Rossitti 1993, Yuan et al 1998), comparable to fascicular gliding in nerve trunks and nerve roots. These adaptive processes are most evident in the mobile cervical and lumbar regions (Louis 1981, Rossitti 1993).

INNERVATION OF NEURAL CONNECTIVE TISSUE

Considering the mechanical abilities of the nervous system, it follows that neural connective tissues should be innervated to enhance their capacity for protecting fragile nerve fibers.

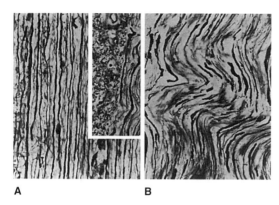

A   **B**

Figure 6.6 A & B   Strain behavior of a segment of human spinal cord taken from the area of the anterior median fissure and the anterior white commissure (× 525). **A**: No undulations are present when cord tissues are lengthened by spinal flexion. **B**: Nerve fibers fold on themselves as they shorten with spinal extension. (Reproduced from Brieg A 1978, with the permission of Almqvist and Wiskell International.)

Peripheral nerve connective tissue innervation

Endoneurial, perineurial, and epineurial connective tissues are innervated by local axon branches called nervi nervorum (Asbury & Fields 1984, Bove & Light 1997, Butler 1991, Hromada 1963). Autonomic fibers from nearby perivascular plexuses also innervate these connective tissue sheaths (Hromada 1963, Lincoln et al 1993, Thomas & Olsson 1984). Nervi nervorum possess nociceptive capabilities (Bove & Light 1997, Hromada 1963, Sauer et al 1999), and they contain neuropeptides that mediate the inflammatory response exhibited by nerve trunks exposed to irritating mechanical or chemical stimuli (Sauer et al 1999, Triano & Luttges 1982, Zochodne 1993).

Meningeal innervation

Studies addressing meningeal innervation have focused on the dura mater. Sinu-vertebral nerves innervate the ventral, lateral, and posterolateral aspects of the dura within the spinal canal, and they also innervate the dural sleeves of nerve root complexes (Cuatico et al 1988, Edgar & Nundy 1966, Groen et al 1988, Kallakuri et al 1998). These nerves originate from the ventral ramus just distal to the DRG, and they merge with sympathetic fibers from the gray ramus communicantes or sympathetic ganglion prior to entering the spinal canal through the intervertebral foramina (Butler 1991, Edgar & Nundy 1966). Once inside the spinal canal, sinu-vertebral nerves branch to span four or more spinal segments and form a plexus that innervates dural tissues (Butler 1991, Edgar & Nundy 1966, Groen et al 1988) (Fig. 6.7). Spinal dura innervation is most richly developed in the mobile

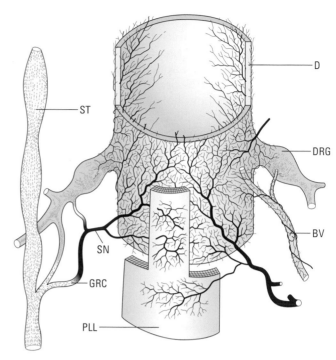

Figure 6.7   Diagram of the ventral aspect of the dura illustrating the sinu-vertebral nerve plexus. BV = blood vessel, D = dura, DRG = dorsal root ganglion, GRC = gray ramus communicantes, PLL = posterior longitudinal ligament, SN = sinu-vertebral nerve, ST = sympathetic trunk. (Reproduced with permission from Butler 1991.)

cervical and lumbar regions (Cuatico et al 1988), and although some controversy exists (Kumar et al 1996), it appears that this innervation has a nociceptive function (Kallakuri et al 1998).

The arachnoid and pia mater are collectively known as the leptomeninges (Butler 2000, Shacklock et al 1994). Their pattern of innervation is less clear, but authors have reported the presence of neural structures in these meningeal tissues (Bridge 1959, Jänig & Koltzenburg 1990). Additionally, mechanoreceptors located in pial ligaments that attach to the anterior spinal artery may provide a mechanism for detecting tensile forces (Parke & Whalen 1993).

NERVE JUICE AND BLOOD FLOW – THE LINK BETWEEN MECHANICS AND PHYSIOLOGY

Recalling the unique cellular architecture of neurons, a mechanism of intraneuronal communication must exist so that these cells can function within a mechanically dynamic setting. This cellular communication is accomplished through axoplasmic transport (Butler 1991, Dahlin & Lundborg 1990, Devor 1991, Lundborg 1988, Lundborg & Dahlin 1992, Rempel et al 1999). Retrograde axoplasmic transport provides the cell body with chemical feedback concerning the status of the axon and surrounding tissues. This feedback enables the genetic machinery of the cell body to produce neurotransmitters and other materials necessary for synaptic function, impulse transmission, and structural health of the axon (Butler 2000, Devor & Seltzer 1999, Lundborg 1988, Lundborg & Dahlin 1992, Rempel et al 1999, Shacklock et al 1994). The cell body also produces ion channels that are embedded in the cell membrane and determine neuron excitability (Bear et al 2001, Butler 2000, Costigan & Woolf 2000, Devor & Seltzer 1999, Koester & Siegelbaum 1995). Anterograde axoplasmic transport ferries all products from the cell body to appropriate destinations within the neuron (Bear et al 2001, Butler 2000, Dahlin & Lundborg 1990, Lundborg 1988, Lundborg & Dahlin 1992, Rempel et al 1999).

Axoplasm in mammals is five times more viscous than water (Haak et al 1976). Additionally, axoplasm exhibits thixotrophic properties, meaning it flows better when kept moving (Baker et al 1977, Butler 2000, Shacklock 1995a). Describing axoplasm as 'nerve juice' that needs movement can be a useful strategy in educating clients rehabilitating from neural tissue injuries (Butler 2000).

Bidirectional axoplasmic transport is a process that requires a continuous energy supply. Neural connective tissues also need nutritional support to maintain their viscoelastic properties. Therefore, vascular anatomy is designed to deliver adequate blood flow to meet the energy demands of the nervous system during all postures and movements (Lundborg 1988, Rempel et al 1999). External vascular systems feeding neural structures exhibit a coiled or pig-tailed configuration so that blood flow is not impaired during movement of peripheral nerve trunks or spinal nerve roots. This coiled architecture also exists within intraneural vessels so that normal fascicular gliding does not inhibit circulation (Dommisse 1994, Lundborg 1988, Parke & Watanabe 1985, Rempel et al 1999) (Fig. 6.2). In addition, intraneural vascular networks possess several anastomoses which allow the direction of blood flow to change in response to any local circulatory deficits imposed by mechanical loads associated with sport or exercise activities (Kobayashi et al 2000, Lundborg 1988, Parke & Watanabe 1985, Rempel et al 1999) (Fig. 6.8). Besides being mobile, intraneural vasculature protects neural tissues from harmful chemical stimuli. Endoneurial vessels possess a blood–nerve barrier that works in concert with the perineurial diffusion barrier to provide nerve fibers with an optimal chemical environment (Lundborg 1988, Rempel et al 1999).

Axoplasmic flow and intraneural circulation exemplify the theory of neurodynamics. These two physiological processes are vital to the physical health and function of neural tissues and, as will be discussed in subsequent sections, mechanical forces associated with daily or athletic activities can influence 'nerve juice' and blood flow.

NEURODYNAMICS

Shacklock (1995a) defined neurodynamics as the interaction between the mechanics and physiology of the nervous system. The following sections highlight some basic 'rules' of neurodynamics that have clinical relevance for examination and management of neural tissue injuries.

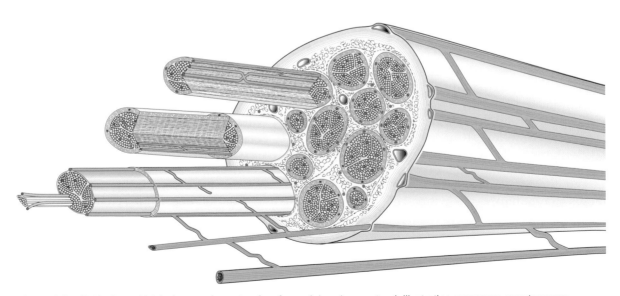

Figure 6.8 Extrinsic and intrinsic vascular networks of a peripheral nerve trunk illustrating numerous anastomoses between vessels. (Reproduced with permission from Butler 1991.)

THE NEURAL CONTAINER AND MECHANICAL INTERFACE

The concepts of a 'neural container' (Shacklock 1995a) and a 'mechanical interface' (Butler 1991) assist in understanding how body movements effect neural tissues. The body can be considered to be the container of the nervous system, and within this container musculoskeletal tissues form a mechanical interface with neural structures (Shacklock 1995a). Examples of interfacing tissues are the intervertebral foramina, the scalenes, the carpal tunnel, the anterior aspect of the sacroiliac joint (Atlihan et al 2000), the piriformis, the fibular head, and the tarsal tunnel. As the body or container moves, interfacing musculoskeletal tissues change dimensions and exert mechanical forces on neural structures (Shacklock 1995a). Consequently, management of neural tissue injuries should ensure that musculoskeletal structures of the neural container function at an optimal level, thereby minimizing physical forces on adjacent neural tissues (Butler 2000, Hall & Elvey 1999).

RELATIONSHIP OF NERVE STRUCTURES TO JOINT AXES

Neural tissue mobility during trunk and limb movement is dictated by the spatial relationship between nerve structures and the axes of joint motion (Beith et al 1995, Millesi et al 1995, Shacklock 1995a). Previous discussion in this chapter addressed how neuromeningeal structures are affected by sagittal and frontal plane motions of the spinal column. Neurodynamic tests biased toward various peripheral nerve trunks have evolved from clinical application of nerve geography. For example, the median nerve can be challenged mechanically by combining shoulder abduction, elbow extension, and wrist extension because it passes caudal to the glenohumeral joint and ventral to the axes of motion at the elbow and wrist (Kenneally et al 1988, Kleinrensink et al 2000, Kleinrensink et al 1995, Lewis et al 1998). In contrast, assessment of the movement capability of the ulnar nerve needs to incorporate elbow flexion with wrist extension since this structure courses dorsal to the axis of motion at the elbow and ventral to the wrist joint (Buehler & Thayer 1988, Butler 2000, Pechan 1973, Wright et al 2001). In the lower extremities, the tibial branch of the sciatic nerve is challenged by hip flexion, knee extension, and ankle dorsiflexion (Beith et al 1995, Troup 1981), while the peroneal branch can be loaded by ankle plantar flexion and inversion rather than dorsiflexion (Butler 2000, Mauhart 1990, Pahor & Toppenberg 1996).

Because of their three-dimensional structure, neural tissues are not displaced in a uniform manner during joint motion (Millesi et al 1995). With cervical flexion, the posterior portion of the cervical spinal cord is subjected to more displacement than the anterior portion (Yuan et al 1998). A peripheral nerve trunk may have a diameter of 1 cm or more, therefore, portions of the nerve at a greater perpendicular distance from the joint axis will be displaced more than parts nearer the axis of motion (Millesi et al 1995). As discussed previously, gliding between fascicles enables neural structures to adapt to asymmetrical displacement (Millesi et al 1995, Rossitti 1993).

STRAIN, EXCURSION, AND TENSILE STRESS

Neural containers in the spinal canal and extremities change in length during movement. Previous sections of this chapter have described how movement of the vertebral column alters the length of the spinal canal. Limb movement changes the length of neural containers surrounding peripheral nerve trunks. Zoch et al (1991) measured the container for the median nerve with the shoulder in 90° abduction. When comparing a position of elbow and wrist flexion to one of elbow and wrist extension, the distance from the upper border of the latissimus dorsi muscle to the wrist increased by approximately 10 cm. In the lower extremity, Beith et al (1995) found that combined motions of 90° hip flexion, 90° knee extension, and 20° ankle dorsiflexion increased the length of the neural container for the sciatic, tibial, and medial plantar nerves by 9–12 cm. Nerve structures adapt to these changes in the container with a mixture of strain, excursion, and tensile stress (Beith et al 1995, McLellan & Swash 1976, Millesi et al 1995, Shacklock 1995a, Smith et al 1993, Wilgis & Murphy 1986, Wright et al 1996, 2001).

Strain is defined as the percentage change in length of a structure relative to its original length (Rodgers & Cavanagh 1984). As discussed previously, axons take an undulatory course through all portions of the nervous system, folding and unfolding as neural tissues undergo strain (Louis 1981, Millesi et al 1995, Rossitti 1993, Sunderland 1990). This mechanism for adapting to length changes is dependent on the viscoelastic tubes created by the endoneurium, perineurium, and dura (Millesi et al 1995, Runza et al 1999). Nerve trunks and neuromeningeal structures are also able to fold and unfold at a macroscopic level (Fig. 6.9), because intraneural connective tissues facilitate gliding between fascicles (Louis 1981, Millesi et al 1995, Shacklock 1995a, Shacklock et al 1994, Sunderland 1990, Wright et al 1996). This macroscopic folding, or 'wrinkle effect' (Wright et al 1996), further contributes to the strain behavior of neural tissues, particularly when they need to shorten. Examples include folding of the neuromeningeal structures on the concave side of a laterally flexed spinal column (Shacklock et al

1994), and wrinkling of the median nerve at a flexed elbow (Wright et al 1996).

Once neural tissues have unfolded to the point where their undulations are eliminated, they respond to continued lengthening of the neural container by sliding (Shacklock 1995a). Excursion or sliding of neural tissues relative to interfacing structures has been documented within the spinal canal (Louis 1981, Rossitti 1993, Shacklock et al 1994), the intervertebral foramina (Kenneally et al 1988, Smith et al 1993, Sunderland 1974), and the extremities (Beith et al 1995, McLellan & Swash 1976, Millesi et al 1995, Wilgis & Murphy 1986, Wright et al 1996, 2001). Recalling previous sections on relevant neuroanatomy, this sliding is facilitated by mesoneurium surrounding peripheral nerve trunks.

Excursion does not only take place along the longitudinal axis of each neural structure. Neuromeningeal tissues slide in anteroposterior and lateral directions during movement of the spinal column (Shacklock et al 1994). Nerve root complexes move in a cephalocaudal direction within the intervertebral foramina during spinal (Shacklock et al 1994) (Fig. 6.9) and limb move-

ment (Kenneally et al 1988, Smith et al 1993, Sunderland 1974). Transverse sliding has also been observed in peripheral nerve trunks. Greening et al (1999) demonstrated that the median nerve moves radially and posteriorly within the carpal tunnel during wrist flexion. The superficial branch of the peroneal nerve exhibits a significant amount of transverse excursion when palpated on the dorsum of the foot (Butler 2000).

When sliding mechanisms have been exhausted, additional strain in neural tissues is associated with development of intraneural pressure or tensile stress (Kwan et al 1992, Millesi et al 1995, Shacklock 1995a). Tensile stress is defined as the force per unit area generated within a structure subjected to a tensile load (Rodgers & Cavanagh 1984). The viscoelastic behavior of biological tissues is often characterized by stress–strain curves. Nerve structures in situ appear capable of undergoing significant strain with development of relatively minimal tensile stress (Kwan et al 1992). One notable exception is the ulnar nerve at the elbow. During combined shoulder abduction, elbow flexion, and wrist extension, the ulnar nerve at the elbow undergoes at least 15% strain (Wright et al 2001), and develops a 4-fold increase in intraneural pressure (Pechan & Julis 1975). Viscoelastic capacities of nerve structures are due to the protective function of neural connective tissues (Sunderland 1990), but once these connective tissues become injured or fibrosed, viscoelasticity is compromised as the same amount of strain leads to detrimental increases in tensile stress or intraneural pressure (Beel et al 1984, Millesi et al 1995).

NON-UNIFORM MECHANICS AND ORDER OF MOVEMENT

Strain, excursion, and stress develop within neural tissues in a non-uniform fashion (Millesi et al 1995, Shacklock 1995a). For example, the median nerve accumulates more stress per unit of strain in areas where it has more branches (Millesi et al 1995). Flexion of the entire spinal column causes dural strain of 15% at L1–2, but approximately 30% at L5 (Louis 1981). The non-uniform mechanics of neural tissues are due to nerve branching, differences in fascicular plexuses and connective tissue content at different points along a nerve, variations in biomechanical function of each joint complex a nerve crosses, regional limitations in excursion because of attachments to the neural container, and exposure to a variety of forces from different interfacing structures such as bone, muscle, and fascia (Butler 2000, Shacklock 1995a).

As a result of their non-uniform mechanics, neural tissues are subjected to different mechanical loads depending upon the order of joint movement (Butler 2000, Shacklock 1995a). If the cervical spine is flexed in

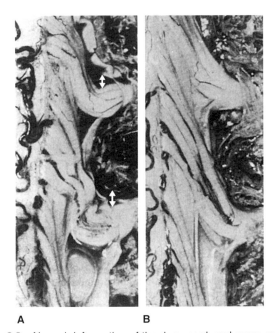

A   **B**

Figure 6.9 Normal deformation of the dura, cord, and nerve roots in the cervical canal in a cadaver due to sagittal plane movement of the cervical spine. A total laminectomy has been performed, and the dura opened and retracted although still able to transmit tensile forces. In **A** the cervical spine is in extension, the nervous system is slack, the root sleeves have lost contact with the pedicles (lower arrows), and the nerve roots have separated from the inner surfaces of the sleeves (upper arrows). In **B** the cervical spine has been flexed, and the nervous system including the dura has been stretched and moved in relation to surrounding structures. Note that the root sleeves have come in contact with the pedicles and the nerve roots now contact the inner surface of the sleeves. Note also the change in shape of blood vessels. (Reproduced from Brieg A 1978, with the permission of Almqvist & Wiskell International.)

isolation, neural structures in the lumbar region undergo cranial displacement relative to surrounding vertebrae (Butler 1991). However, when the entire spine is flexed, neural tissues in the upper lumbar region move in a caudal direction relative to corresponding vertebral segments (Louis 1981). Shoulder abduction from 90 to 110° causes proximal excursion of the median nerve at the elbow, while wrist extension from 0 to 60° causes the median nerve to slide distally within the cubital fossa (Wright et al 1996).

Health care practitioners have long noticed that the sequence of joint movement alters the symptom response and range of motion available during a neurodynamic test (Butler 2000). In 90° of shoulder abduction and external rotation, mimicking a base test for neural tissue mobility in the upper limb, Coppieters et al (2001) showed that elbow extension is significantly reduced when preceded by contralateral cervical side-bending and/or wrist extension. Johnson & Chiarello (1997) demonstrated that knee extension in a slump sit position is reduced when preceded by neck flexion, and further decreased when preceded by a combination of neck flexion, ankle dorsiflexion, and hip medial rotation.

There are two key points for clinical application of the above information. First, the greatest mechanical challenge for a segment of neural tissue occurs when the joint adjacent to the nerve is loaded first during the testing sequence. The development of strain, excursion, and tensile stress will spread to other portions of the neural tissue tract as more joint complexes participate in the movement (Shacklock 1995a). Second, neurodynamic examination should be modified to replicate the order of movement utilized by clients during symptomatic sport or exercise activities (Butler 2000).

THE MECHANICAL CONTINUUM

A fundamental principle of neurodynamics is appreciating that the nervous system forms a tissue continuum throughout the body, and this mechanical continuity should be evident from previous discussion on neuroanatomy. The most dramatic example of neural tissue continuity is the aforementioned ability of neck flexion to alter knee extension mobility in a slump sit position (Johnson & Chiarello 1997), but similar continuity exists in the extremities. Movement of the wrist and fingers affects median and ulnar neural tissues at the elbow and upper arm (Kleinrensink et al 1995, 2000, McLellan & Swash 1976, Wilgis & Murphy 1986, Wright et al 1996, 2001), and ankle dorsiflexion in a straight leg raise position affects lumbosacral nerve roots (Troup 1981). Ipsilateral straight leg raise can increase tensile stress in a median nerve already placed in a mechanically loaded position (Lewis et al 1998).

The implication of this tissue continuum is that mechanical events in one part of the nervous system will have an impact on remote areas along the neural tissue tract (Butler 2000, Shacklock 1995a). Loss of excursion in one segment of a nerve can cause detrimental increases in tensile stress or intraneural pressure in other areas (Wright et al 1996, 2001). Clinically, peripheral neurogenic syndromes in the carpal tunnel and tarsal tunnel may often be related to concomitant problems in the cervical and lumbar nerve roots (Mackinnon 1992, Sammarco et al 1993, Upton & McComas 1973). The hypothesis that injury in one site of a nerve can predispose remaining areas of the same nerve to injury is referred to as 'double or multiple crush' (Mackinnon 1992, Upton & McComas 1973). Animal models provide a pathophysiological explanation for 'double crush' by showing that impairment in axoplasmic flow at one site predisposes the remainder of the nerve to further entrapment injury (Mackinnon 1992). Pathological changes at each 'crush' site may be minor and localized to those fascicles affected most by injurious mechanical forces (Mackinnon 1992, Novak & Mackinnon 1998). These minor changes may not be detected electrodiagnostically (Mackinnon 1992, Novak & Mackinnon 1998), which may explain why electrodiagnostic studies have both denied (Bednarik et al 1999) and supported (Golovchinsky 1998) the 'double crush' hypothesis. In spite of somewhat conflicting information in the literature, physical therapists should be cognizant of the neural tissue continuum and examine along the entire tissue tract in clients with neural injuries (Butler 2000, Novak & Mackinnon 1998).

IMPACT ON PHYSIOLOGY

Mechanical forces from sport and exercise activities can alter intraneural circulation and axoplasmic flow. A clear relationship exists between nerve strain and intraneural circulation (Ogata & Naito 1986, Rempel et al 1999). Blood flow in peripheral nerves slows at 6 to 8% strain (Ogata & Naito 1986), and nerve conduction may also be compromised (Wall et al 1992). These values of strain occur in peripheral nerves during daily movement of extremity joints (Wright et al 1996, 2001), but anastomoses between intraneural vessels enable nerves to recover from temporary deficits in circulation and nerve conduction (Kobayashi et al 2000, Lundborg 1988, Parke & Watanabe 1985, Rempel et al 1999) (Fig. 6.8).

Neural tissues are also subjected to external compression by movement of interfacing structures. Extraneural pressure can be increased by events such as narrowing of the IVF, wrist motion that increases carpal tunnel pressure, or by muscle contraction (Farmer & Wisneski 1994, Fujiwara et al 2001, Mazurek & Shin 2001, Muhle et al 2001, Novak & Mackinnon 1998, Shacklock 1995a).

External compression alters nerve function in a direct dose–response relationship (Lundborg & Dahlin 1992, Novak & Mackinnon 1998, Rempel et al 1999), and extraneural pressures as low as 20 to 40 mmHg can impair axoplasmic transport, blood flow, and nerve conduction (Dahlin & McLean 1986, Rempel et al 1999, Rydevik et al 1981). As with the development of strain, these levels of compression occur during daily activities (Mackinnon 1992, Novak & Mackinnon 1998, Shacklock 1995a), but as long as the magnitude and duration of compression are not excessive, their effects on neural structures are completely reversible (Butler 1991, Dahlin & McLean 1986). Recall that anatomical features enable nerve root complexes and nerve trunks to recover from compressive loads. Adipose tissue, dural sleeves, and CSF safeguard nerve root complexes (Jenis & An 2000, Louis 1981, Rydevik et al 1984, Sunderland 1974), while fascicular plexuses and internal epineurium protect nerve trunks (Lundborg & Dahlin 1992, Sunderland 1990).

CLINICAL SIMULATION

Given the multiple forces imposed by interfacing structures, and the non-uniform mechanics of the neural tissue continuum, a series of base neurodynamic tests summarized by Butler (2000) have been proposed to examine the movement capabilities of the nervous system. These limb and trunk movements can simulate the tensile, compressive, and friction forces placed on neural tissues during sport or exercise activities. Sustained manual compression and isometric muscle contraction may be additional clinical methods for imparting mechanical loads onto neural structures (Mazurek & Shin 2001, Novak & Mackinnon 1998).

PATHODYNAMICS

Even though the nervous system is well designed to tolerate mechanical forces associated with body postures and movements, dynamic protective mechanisms in neural tissues sometimes break down, leading to symptoms of nerve injury (Novak & Mackinnon 1998, Shacklock 1995a) (Box 6.1).

VENOUS CONGESTION, INTRANEURAL EDEMA, FIBROSIS, AND MYELIN CHANGES

A summary of the processes related to the production of symptoms in neural tissue injury can be seen in Figure 6.10. Compromise in intraneural circulation appears to be the first step in the pathophysiological cascade of nerve injury. Compressive, tensile, friction, or

---

Box 6.1 Clinical features proposed as being associated with injury to nerve trunks or nerve root complexes. Any combination of features may occur in the clinical presentation of nerve injury (composed from information in Gifford & Butler 1997, Hall & Elvey 1999)

- Peripheral cutaneous or segmental distribution of symptoms
- Corresponding motor deficits
- Antalgic postures that correspond to unloading of sensitive neural tissues
- Active movement impairment
- Passive movement impairment that corresponds with active movement impairment
- Symptoms mechanically evoked by nerve compression and/or tension of appropriate neural structures that relate to active and passive movement impairments
- Made worse by negative emotional states
- Deep aching, cramping (i.e. nerve trunk pain)
- Superficial burning, stinging, and paresthesia
- In ongoing problems, often difficult to ease symptoms for any length of time with rest or medications
- In ongoing problems, pain may behave as if having 'a mind of its own' (i.e. spontaneous pain)

---

vibration stimuli that exceed the physical capacities of neural tissues will induce venous congestion, thereby impeding intraneural circulation and axoplasmic flow (Greening & Lynn 1998, Hasue 1993, Kobayashi et al 2000, Rempel et al 1999). Resulting hypoxia causes an inflammatory response in nerve trunks and DRGs, leading to subperineurial edema and increased endoneurial fluid pressure (Hasue 1993, Kobayashi et al 2000, Lundborg & Dahlin 1992, Novak & Mackinnon 1998, Olmarker & Rydevik 2001, Rempel et al 1999, Yabuki et al 2001). Endoneurial edema persists because, as discussed previously, the perineurial diffusion barrier does not allow the inflammatory exudate to escape.

Persistent endoneurial edema leads to intraneural fibrosis, decreasing the viscoelastic properties of neural connective tissues (Beel et al 1984, Millesi et al 1995, Novak & Mackinnon 1998, Rempel et al 1999). Bearing in mind the concept of a mechanical continuum, localized restrictions in nerve strain or sliding can cause detrimental increases in tensile stress at other segments of the neural tissue tract, potentially leading to additional injury (Bove & Light 1997, Hunter 1991, Wilgis & Murphy 1986, Wright et al 1996, 2001). The ability to tolerate external compression may also be decreased because of internal epineurial fibrosis and impairment of fascicular gliding. Additionally, fibrotic changes may effect the external epineurium and mesoneurium, further compromising nerve excursion and neural biomechanics (Bove & Light 1997, Greening & Lynn 1998, Millesi et al 1995). Studies have shown that longitudinal and transverse excursion of the median nerve is reduced in patients with carpal tunnel syndrome (Greening et al 1999, Valls-Sole et al 1995). Anatomical anomalies

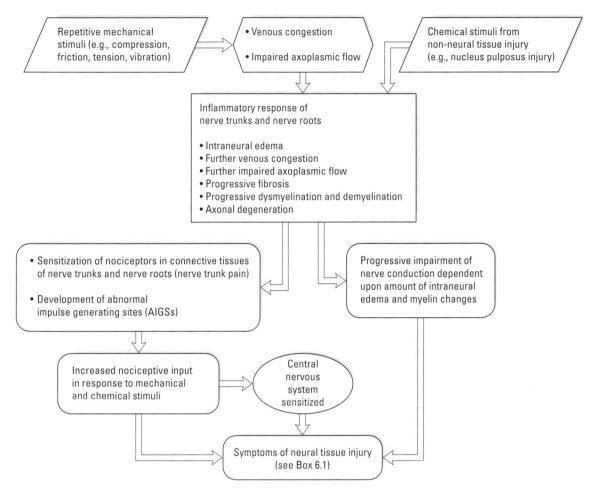

Figure 6.10 Summary of processes related to the production of symptoms of neural tissue injury. (Compiled from Hasue 1993, Bove & Light 1997, Greening & Lynn 1998, Gifford 2001.)

limiting excursion of the superficial peroneal nerve were found in a surgical study of eight patients with superficial peroneal neuralgia after ankle sprains (Johnston & Howell 1999).

After intraneural fibrosis, myelin and axon changes occur along a continuum. Initially, only thinning of myelin takes place, followed by segmental demyelination with progression to diffuse demyelination and axonal degeneration in more severe nerve injury (Hasue 1993, Novak & Mackinnon 1998, Rempel et al 1999). Greater amount and duration of endoneurial edema is directly correlated with more significant degradation in myelin content and axon structure (Rempel et al 1999). It has been hypothesized that these changes are related to impairment in bidirectional axoplasmic flow and altered function of the cell body (Dahlin et al 1987). The severity of impairment in nerve conduction measured by electrodiagnostic studies can indicate the amount of myelin and axon damage (Novak & Mackinnon 1998, Rempel et al 1999).

The inflammatory response exhibited by neural tissues does not have to be the result of direct mechanical over-load. Inflammatory processes in neighboring structures produce chemical stimuli that can induce an inflammatory reaction in nerve structures (Bove & Light 1997). A common example is that inflammatory processes associated with exposed nucleus pulposus produce chemical stimuli that inflame the nerve root complex, leading to radicular pain without mechanical compression (Gifford 2001, Olmarker & Rydevik 2001, Takebayashi et al 2001).

INCREASED MECHANOSENSITIVITY

It is important to remember that symptoms of neural tissue injury are not due solely to changes in nerve conduction (Box 6.1). Daily activities, clinical examination of the neural container, neurodynamic tests, and nerve palpation may evoke symptoms indicative of increased mechanosensitivity in injured neural tissues (Gifford & Butler 1997, Hall & Elvey 1999). Enhanced mechanosensitivity associated with nerve injury can be explained by increased nociceptive input from innervated connective tissues, and from abnormal impulse generating sites within impulse conducting tissues (Baron 2000, Devor & Seltzer 1999, Gifford & Butler 1997, Hall & Elvey 1999, Hasue 1993) (Fig. 6.10).

Innervated connective tissues

Nervi nervorum and sinu-vertebral nerves supplying nerve sheaths and dura have a nociceptive function (Bove & Light 1997, Hromada 1963, Kallakuri et al 1998, Sauer et al 1999). Once neural connective tissues are inflamed, these nociceptors become sensitized to mechanical or chemical stimuli, contributing to the enhanced mechanosensitivity observed in nerve injuries (Baron 2000, Bove & Light 1997, Devor & Seltzer 1999, Gifford & Butler 1997, Hall & Elvey 1999). When intraneural fibrosis has compromised the extensibility of neural connective tissues, already sensitized nociceptors will be subjected to more intense mechanical stimulation, because fibrotic connective tissues can no longer efficiently attenuate compressive, tensile, friction, and vibration loads associated with sport or exercise activities (Bove & Light 1997, Butler 2000). Consequently, normally asymptomatic movements may remain sensitive. Increased nociceptive activity from nervi nervorum has been referred to as nerve trunk pain (Asbury & Fields 1984), and this pain may be perceived as having a deep aching quality (Asbury & Fields 1984, Bove & Light 1997, Hall & Elvey 1999).

Abnormal impulse generating sites

An injured segment of peripheral nerve may develop the ability to repeatedly generate its own impulses (Devor & Seltzer 1999). These injured areas are referred to as abnormal impulse generating sites (AIGSs), because axons that normally just transmit impulses become capable of initiating them. The main features of AIGSs are mechanosensitivity and spontaneous firing (Butler 2000, Devor & Seltzer 1999).

Earlier discussion in this chapter alluded to the ensemble of ion channels that insert into the axon membrane and determine neuron excitability. Constant remodeling of ion channels normally occurs so that an afferent neuron maintains an appropriate level of sensitivity to surrounding stimuli (Bear et al 2001, Butler 2000, Costigan & Woolf 2000, Devor & Seltzer 1999, Koester & Siegelbaum 1995). Nerve injury alters the gene expression within the cell body (Baron 2000, Costigan & Woolf 2000). Consequently, the type and number of ion channels in the axon membrane changes so that neurons are more easily excited by mechanical and chemical input (Baron 2000, Devor & Seltzer 1999, Gifford 1998). Ion channels insert into areas of the axon membrane not covered by myelin, therefore, DRGs, areas of myelin thinning, and areas of segmental demyelination provide

opportunities for abnormal accumulation of mechanosensitive and chemosensitive ion channels (Amir & Devor 1993, Calvin et al 1982, Chen & Devor 1998, Devor & Seltzer 1999, England et al 1998, Liu et al 2000, Tal & Eliav 1996, Wall & Gutnick 1974). Presumably, ion channels are evenly spread along unmyelinated fibers.

With an abnormal accumulation of ion channels, the type and number of channels determines which stimuli will evoke symptoms. Normally innocuous lengthening, pinching, or friction forces become capable of eliciting symptoms in situations where concentrations of mechanosensitive channels are increased (Devor & Seltzer 1999, Gifford 1998, Gifford & Butler 1997). Nerve ischemia induced by repetitive movement or sustained positioning may create an exaggerated response from AIGSs packed with ischemosensitive channels (Devor & Seltzer 1999, Gifford 2001). Inflammatory chemicals from injured neural or non-neural tissues can stimulate chemosensitive channels (Butler 2000, Devor & Seltzer 1999).

Adrenaline (epinephrine) and noradrenaline (norepinephrine) also become capable of stimulating AIGSs (Baron 2000, Devor & Seltzer 1999, Greening & Lynn 1998, Hasue 1993, Shacklock 1995a). Presence of adrenosensitive channels provides a partial explanation for the observation that emotional stress can exacerbate symptoms of nerve injury (Butler 2000, Gifford 2001). Van Meeteren et al (1997) found that rats exposed to chronic intermittent stress recovered more slowly from sciatic nerve crush injury. Therefore, adrenoreceptors may influence healing of nerve tissues, and education that decreases patient apprehension may assist recovery (Butler 2000).

Abnormal impulse generating sites exhibit spontaneous activity, because the ensemble of ion channels places the axon membrane near the threshold for firing (Devor & Seltzer 1999). Therefore, patients experiencing nerve injuries may report that symptoms sometimes occur without any type of stimulus (Gifford 2001, Gifford & Butler 1997).

RECOVERY AND RELEVANCE OF NEURAL PATHOLOGY

Reports from animal studies of nerve injury state that neuropathic pain behavior and histological findings usually resolve in approximately 6–8 weeks (Lindenlaub & Sommer 2000). But when symptoms persist at 15 weeks, intraneural pathology is still present (Lindenlaub & Sommer 2000). Extraneural fibrosis adhering to interfacing structures may also be present 15 weeks after experimental nerve injury (Greening & Lynn 1998). Pathology does not always correlate with symptoms. Fifty percent of cadavers have neural connective tissue and nerve fiber changes, particularly at vulnerable sites such as the ulnar nerve at the elbow, but in life these subjects never complained of pain in these areas (Neary & Ochoa 1975).

A variety of issues contribute to the inconsistent relationship between neural pathology and pain. Pain is a complex biopsychosocial phenomenon that is only partly influenced by nerve injury (see Ch. 8). Additionally, increased nociceptive input from nerve injury causes changes in central nervous system processing (Baron 2000, Costigan & Woolf 2000, Devor & Seltzer 1999, Mannion & Woolf 2000). In neurogenic pain states, the central nervous system becomes sensitized and processes normally innocuous stimuli as painful (Doubell et al 1999, Mannion & Woolf 2000, Shacklock 1999, Zusman 1992) (Fig. 6.10). This sensitization results in potentially false positive responses to physical tests that place a mechanical load on neural tissues (Gifford 2001, Zusman 1992). Although the patient reports pain during the test, the neural tissues may be relatively normal. The pain response is simply due to altered processing in the central nervous system. Physical therapists need to consider these issues when interpreting symptomatic responses to neurodynamic and other physical examination tests (Gifford & Butler 1997, Shacklock 1999, Zusman 1992).

In spite of the inconsistent relationship between nerve pathology and pain, clinical studies have shown that neurogenic symptoms can be resolved by intervention directed at restoring normal neural biomechanics. Kornberg and Lew (1989) demonstrated that Australian football players recovered more quickly from grade one hamstring strains when slump mobilization was included as part of the rehabilitation program. Turl and George (1998) recently showed that persistent impairment in slump mobility is associated with repetitive hamstring injury, further supporting the findings of Kornberg and Lew (1989). Rozmaryn et al (1998) found that a program of exercises aimed at gliding flexor tendons and the median nerve reduced the rate of carpal tunnel surgery to 43%, compared to a surgical rate of 71% in patients who did not utilize the gliding exercises. Symptomatic improvement was maintained in the majority of cases over an average follow-up period of 23 months. A case study reported by Shacklock (1995b) described how neurodynamic intervention assisted in recovery from a 9-month history of heel pain.

SUMMARY

Neural tissues are well designed to tolerate mechanical forces associated with sport and exercise activities. When these mechanical forces exceed the physical capacities of the nervous system, symptoms of nerve injury occur. Neurogenic symptoms result from changes in neural connective tissues and impulse conducting tissues, as well as from changes in central nervous system processing (Fig. 6.10). Knowledge of neurodynamics and pathodynamics will enable clinicians to develop appropriate strategies for intervention when rehabilitating clients suffering from neural tissue injury.

REFERENCES

Amir R, Devor M 1993 Ongoing activity in neuroma afferents bearing retrograde sprouts. Brain Research 630:283–288

Asbury A K, Fields H L 1984 Pain due to peripheral nerve damage: an hypothesis. Neurology 34:1587–1590

Atlihan D, Tekdemir I, Ates Y et al 2000 Anatomy of the anterior sacroiliac joint with reference to lumbosacral nerves. Clinical Orthopaedics and Related Research 376:236–241

Baker P, Ladds M, Rubinson K 1977 Measurement of the flow properties of isolated axoplasm in a defined chemical environment. Journal of Physiology 269:10–11

Baron R 2000 Peripheral neuropathic pain: from mechanisms to symptoms. The Clinical Journal of Pain 16 (suppl):S12–S20

Bear M, Connors B, Paradiso M 2001 Neuroscience: exploring the brain. Lippincott Williams and Wilkins, Baltimore

Bednarik J, Kadanka Z, Vohanka S 1999 Median nerve neuropathy in spondylotic cervical myelopathy: double crush syndrome. Journal of Neurology 246:541–545

Beel J A, Groswald D E, Luttges M W 1984 Alterations in the mechanical properties of peripheral nerve following crush injury. Journal of Biomechanics 17:185–193

Beel J, Stodieck L, Luttges M 1986 Structural properties of spinal nerve roots: biomechanics. Experimental Neurology 91:30–40

Beith I D, Robins E J, Richards P R 1995 An assessment of the adaptive mechanisms within and surrounding the peripheral nervous system, during changes in nerve bed length resulting from underlying joint movement. In: Shacklock M O (ed) Moving in on pain. Butterworth-Heinemann, Australia

Bogduk N 1997 Clinical anatomy of the lumbar spine and sacrum. Churchill Livingstone, New York

Bove G M, Light A R 1997 The nervi nervorum: missing link for neuropathic pain? Pain Forum 6:181–190

Bridge C J 1959 Innervation of spinal meninges and epidural structures. Anatomical Record 133:533–561

Brieg A 1978 Adverse mechanical tension in the central nervous system. Almqvist and Wiskell, Stockholm

Buehler M J, Thayer D T 1988 The elbow flexion test. Clinical Orthopaedics and Related Research 233:213–216

Butler D S 1991 Mobilisation of the nervous system. Churchill Livingstone, Melbourne

Butler D S 2000 The sensitive nervous system. Noigroup, Adelaide

Calvin W H, Devor M, Howe J F 1982 Can neuralgias arise from minor demyelination? Spontaneous firing, mechanosensitivity, and afterdischarge from conduction axons. Experimental Neurology 75:755–763

Chen Y, Devor M 1998 Ectopic mechanosensitivity in injured sensory axons arises from the site of spontaneous electrogenesis. European Journal of Pain 2:165–178

Coppieters M, Stappaerts K, Everaert D et al 2001 Addition of test components during neurodynamic testing: effect on range of motion and sensory responses. Journal of Orthopaedic and Sports Physical Therapy 31(5):226–237

Costigan M, Woolf C 2000 Pain: molecular mechanisms. The Journal of Pain 1(3) (suppl 1):35–44

Cuatico W, Parker J C, Pappert E et al 1988 An anatomical and clinical investigation of spinal meningeal nerves. Acta Neurochirurgica 90:139–143

Dahlin L, McLean W G 1986 Effects of graded experimental compression on slow and fast axonal transport in rabbit vagus nerve. Journal of Neurological Science 72:19–30

Dahlin L, Lundborg G 1990 The neurone and its response to peripheral nerve compression. Journal of Hand Surgery 15B:5–10

Dahlin L, Nordborg C, Lundborg G 1987 Morphological changes in nerve cell bodies induced by experimental graded compression. Experimental Neurology 95:611–621

Devor M 1991 Neuropathic pain and injured nerve: peripheral mechanisms. British Medical Bulletin 47(3):619–630

Devor M, Seltzer Z 1999 Pathophysiology of damaged nerves in relation to chronic pain. In: Wall P D, Melzack R (eds) Textbook of pain, 4th edn. Churchill Livingstone, Edinburgh

Dommisse G F (ed) 1994 The blood supply of the spinal cord and the consequences of failure, 2nd edn. Churchill Livingstone, Edinburgh.

Doubell T P, Mannion R, Woolf C J 1999 The dorsal horn: state dependent sensory processing, plasticity and the generation of pain. In: Wall P D, Melzack R (eds) Textbook of pain, 4th edn. Churchill Livingstone, Edinburgh

Edgar M A, Nundy S 1966 Innervation of the spinal dura mater. Journal of Neurology, Neurosurgery, and Psychiatry 29:530–534

England J D, Happel L T, Liu Z P et al 1998 Abnormal distributions of potassium channels in human neuromas. Neuroscience Letters 255:37–40

Farmer J, Wisneski R 1994 Cervical spine nerve root compression: an analysis of neuroforaminal pressures with varying head and arm positions. Spine 19(16):1850–1855

Fujiwara A, An H, Lim T et al 2001 Morphologic changes in lumbar intervertebral foramen due to flexion-extension, lateral bending and axial rotation. Spine 26(8):876–882

Gifford L 1998 Pain. In: Pitt-Brooke J, Reid H, Lockwood J et al (eds) Rehabilitation of movement. WB Saunders, London

Gifford L 2001 Acute low cervical nerve root conditions: symptom presentations and pathobiological reasoning. Manual Therapy 6(2):106–115

Gifford L, Butler D 1997 The integration of pain sciences into clinical practice. The Journal of Hand Therapy 10:86–95

Golovchinsky V 1998 Double crush syndrome in lower extremities. Electromyography and Clinical Neurophysiology 38:115–120

Greening J, Lynn B 1998 Minor peripheral nerve injuries: an underestimated source of pain? Manual Therapy 3(4):187–194

Greening J, Smart S, Leary R et al 1999 Reduced movement of the median nerve in carpal tunnel during wrist flexion in patients with non specific arm pain. Lancet 354:217–218

Grimes P, Massie J, Garfin S 2000 Anatomic and biomechanical analysis of lower lumbar foraminal ligaments. Spine 25(16):2009–2014

Groen G J, Baljet B, Drukker J 1988 The innervation of the spinal dura mater: anatomy and clincial implications. Acta Neurochirurgica 92:39–46

Haak R A, Kleinhaus F W, Ochs S 1976 The viscosity of mammalian nerve axoplasm measured by electron spin resonance. Journal of Physiology 263:115–137

Hall T, Elvey R 1999 Nerve trunk pain: physical diagnosis and treatment. Manual Therapy 4(2):63–73

Hanai F, Matsui N, Hongo N 1996 Changes in responses of wide dynamic range neurons in the spinal dorsal horn after dorsal root or dorsal root ganglion compression. Spine 21:1408–1415

Hasue M 1993 Pain and the nerve root: an interdisciplinary approach. Spine 18(14):2053–2058

Hough A, Moore A, Jones M 2000 Measuring longitudinal nerve motion using ultrasonography. Manual Therapy 5(3):173–180

Howe J F, Loeser J D, Calvin W H 1977 Mechanosensitivity of dorsal root ganglia and chronically injured axons: a physiological basis for radicular pain of nerve root compression. Pain 3:25–41

Hromada J 1963 On the nerve supply of the connective tissue of some peripheral nervous system components. Acta Anatomica 55:343–351

Hunter J M 1991 Recurrent carpal tunnel syndrome, epineural fibrous fixation, and traction neuropathy. Hand Clinics 7(3):491–504

Jänig W, Koltzenburg M 1990 Receptive properties of pial afferents. Pain 45:300–309

Jenis L, An H 2000 Spine update: lumbar foraminal stenosis. Spine 25(3):389–394

Johnson E K, Chiarello C M 1997 The slump test: the effects of head and lower extremity position on knee extension. Journal of Orthopaedic and Sports Physical Therapy 26(6):310–317

Johnston E C, Howell S J 1999 Tension neuropathy of the superficial peroneal nerve: associated conditions and results of release. Foot and Ankle International 20:576–580

Kallakuri S, Cavanaugh J M, Blagoev D C 1998 An immunohistochemical study of innervation of lumbar spinal dura and longitudinal ligaments. Spine 23(4):403–411

Kenneally M, Rubenach H, Elvey R 1988 The upper limb tension test: the SLR of the arm. In: Grant R (ed) Physical therapy of the cervical and thoracic spine. Churchill Livingstone, New York

Kikuchi S, Sato K, Konno S et al 1994 Anatomic and radiographic study of dorsal root ganglia. Spine 19(1):6–11

Kleinrensink G J, Stoeckart R, Vleeming A et al 1995 Mechanical tension in the median nerve. The effects of joint positions. Clinical Biomechanics 10(5):240–244

Kleinrensink G J, Stoeckart R, Mulder P G H et al 2000 Upper limb tension tests as tools in the diagnosis of nerve and plexus lesions. Clinical Biomechanics 15:9–14

Kobayashi S, Yoshizawa H, Nakai S 2000 Experimental study on the dynamics of lumbosacral nerve root circulation. Spine 25(3):298–305

Koester J, Siegelbaum S 1995 Ion channels. In: Kandel E, Schwartz J, Jessell T (eds) Essentials of neural science and behavior. Appleton and Lange, Norwalk, CT

Kornberg C, Lew P 1989 The effect of stretching neural structures on grade one hamstring injuries. Journal of Orthopaedic and Sports Physical Therapy 13:481–487

Kumar R, Berger R, Dunsker S, Keller J 1996 Innervation of the spinal dura: myth or reality. Spine 21(1):18–26

Kwan M K, Wall E J, Massie J et al 1992 Strain, stress and stretch of peripheral nerve. Acta Orthopaedica Scandinavica 63(3):267–272

Lewis J, Ramot R, Green A 1998 Changes in mechanical tension in the median nerve: possible implications for the upper limb tension test. Physiotherapy 84(6):254–261

Lincoln J, Milner P, Appenzeller O et al 1993 Innervation of normal human sural and optic nerves by noradrenaline and peptide containing nervi vasorum and nervorum: effect of diabetes and alcoholism. Brain Research 632:48–56

Lindenlaub T, Sommer C 2000 Partial sciatic nerve transection as a model of neuropathic pain: a qualitative and quantitative neuropathological study. Pain 89:97–106

Liu X, Eschenfelder S, Blenk K H et al 2000 Spontaneous activity of axotomised afferent neurons after L5 spinal nerve injury in rats. Pain 84:309–318

Louis R 1981 Vertebroradicular and vertebromedullar dynamics. Anatomia Clinica 3:1–11

Lundborg G 1988 Intraneural microcirculation. Orthopedic Clinics of North America 19(1):1–12

Lundborg G, Dahlin L B 1992 The pathophysiology of nerve compression. Hand Clinics 8(2):215–227

Lundborg G, Myers R, Powell H 1983 Nerve compression injury and increased endoneurial fluid pressure: a 'miniature compartment syndrome'. Journal of Neurology, Neurosurgery and Psychiatry 46:1119–1124

McCabe J, Low F 1969 The subarachnoid angle: an area of transition in peripheral nerve. The Anatomical Record 164:15–34

Mackinnon S E 1992 Double and multiple 'crush' syndromes. Hand Clinics 8:369–390

McLellan D L, Swash M 1976 Longitudinal sliding of the median nerve during movements of the upper limb. Journal of Neurology, Neurosurgery, and Psychiatry 39:566–570

Mannion R, Woolf C 2000 Pain mechanisms and management: a central perspective. The Clinical Journal of Pain 16(suppl):S144–S156

Matloub H, Yousif N 1992 Peripheral nerve anatomy and innervation pattern. Hand Clinics 8(2):201–214

Mauhart D 1990 The effect of chronic ankle inversion sprains on the plantarflexion/inversion straight leg raise test. Australian Journal of Physiotherapy 36:277

Mazurek M, Shin A 2001 Upper extremity peripheral nerve anatomy. Clinical Orthopaedics and Related Research 383:7–20

Millesi H, Zoch G, Riehsner R 1995 Mechanical properties of peripheral nerves. Clinical Orthopaedics and Related Research 314:76–83

Moses A, Carman J 1996 Anatomy of the cervical spine: implications for the upper limb tension test. Australian Journal of Physiotherapy 42:31–35

Muhle C, Wiskirchen J, Weinert D et al 1998 Biomechanical aspects of the subarachnoid space and cervical cord in healthy individuals examined with kinematic magnetic resonance imaging. Spine 23:556–567

Muhle C, Resnick D, Ahn J et al 2001 In vivo changes in the neuroforaminal size at flexion-extension and axial rotation of the cervical spine in healthy persons examined using kinematic magnetic resonance imaging. Spine 26(13):E287–E293

Murphy R 1977 Nerve roots and spinal nerves in degenerative disk disease. Clinical Orthopaedics and Related Research 129:46–60

Nakagawa H, Mikawa Y, Watanabe R 1994 Elastin in the human posterior longitudinal ligament and spinal dura: a histologic and biochemical study. Spine 19(19):2164–2169

Nakamura S I, Myers R R 2000 Injury to dorsal root ganglia alters innervation of spinal cord dorsal horn lamina involved in nociception. Spine 25:537–542

Neary D, Ochoa R W 1975 Sub-clinical entrapment neuropathy in man. Journal of the Neurological Sciences 24:283–298

Nicholas D S, Weller R O 1988 The fine anatomy of the human spinal meninges. Journal of Neurosurgery 69:276–282

Novak C B, Mackinnon S E 1998 Nerve injury in repetitive motion disorders. Clinical Orthopaedics and Related Research 351:10–20

Ogata K, Naito M 1986 Blood flow of peripheral nerve: effects of dissection, stretching and compression. The Journal of Hand Surgery 11B:10–14

Olmarker K, Rydevik B 1991 Pathophysiology of sciatica. Orthopedic Clinics of North America 22(2):223–234

Olmarker K, Rydevik B 2001 Selective inhibition of tumor necrosis factor alpha prevents nucleus pulposus-induced thrombus formation, intraneural edema, and reduction of nerve conduction velocity. Spine 26(8):863–869

Pahor S, Toppenberg R 1996 An investigation of neural tissue involvement in ankle inversion sprains. Manual Therapy 1:192–197

Parke W W, Watanabe R 1985 The intrinsic vasculature of the lumbosacral spinal nerve roots. Spine 10(6):508–515

Parke W W, Whalen J L 1993 The pial ligaments of the anterior spinal artery and their stretch receptors. Spine 18(11):1542–1549

Pechan J 1973 Ulnar nerve manoeuvre as a diagnostic aid in pressure lesions in the cubital region. Ceskoslovenska Neurologie 36:13–19

Pechan J, Julis F 1975 The pressure measurement in the ulnar nerve: a contribution to the pathophysiology of cubital tunnel syndrome. Journal of Biomechanics 8:75–79

Rauschning W 1997 Anatomy and pathology of the cervical spine. In: Frymoyer J W (ed) The adult spine: principles and practice, 2nd edn. Lippincott-Raven, Philadelphia

Rempel D, Dahlin L, Lundborg G 1999 Pathophysiology of nerve compression syndromes: response of peripheral nerves to loading. Journal of Bone and Joint Surgery 81A:1600–1610

Rodgers M, Cavanagh P 1984 Glossary of biomechanical terms, concepts, and units. Physical Therapy 64(12):1886–1902

Rossitti S 1993 Biomechanics of the pons-cord tract and its enveloping structures: An overview. Acta Neurochirurgica 124:144–152

Rozmaryn L, Dovelle S, Rothman E et al 1998 Nerve and tendon gliding exercises and the conservative management of carpal tunnel syndrome. Journal of Hand Therapy 11:171–179

Runza M, Pietrabissa R, Mantero S et al 1999 Lumbar dura mater biomechanics: experimental characterization and scanning electron microscopy observations. Anesthesia and Analgesia 88:1317–1321

Rydevik B, Lundborg G, Bagge U 1981 Effects of graded compression on intraneural blood flow: an in-vivo study on rabbit tibial nerve. Journal of Hand Surgery 6:3–12

Rydevik B, Brown M, Lundborg G 1984 Pathoanatomy and

pathophysiology of nerve root compression. Spine 9(1):7–15

Rydevik B, Myers R, Powell H 1989 Pressure increase in the dorsal root ganglion following mechanical compression: closed compartment syndrome in nerve roots. Spine 14(6):574–576

Rydevik B, Holm S, Brown M et al 1990 Diffusion from cerebrospinal fluid as a nutritional pathway for spinal nerve roots. Acta Physiologica Scandinavica 138:247–248

Sammarco G J, Chalk D E, Feibel J H 1993 Tarsal tunnel syndrome and additional nerve lesions in the same limb. Foot and Ankle 14(2):71–77

Sauer S K, Bove G M, Averbeck B et al 1999 Rat peripheral nerve components release calcitonin gene-related peptide and prostaglandin E2 in response to noxious stimuli: evidence that the nervi nervorum are nociceptors. Neuroscience 92:319–325

Schwartz J 1995 The neuron. In: Kandel E, Schwartz J, Jessell T (eds) Essentials of neural science and behavior. Appleton and Lange, Norwalk, CT

Shacklock M O 1995a Neurodynamics. Physiotherapy 81(1):9–16

Shacklock M O 1995b Clinical application of neurodynamics. In: Shacklock M O (ed) Moving in on pain. Butterworth-Heinemann, Sydney

Shacklock M O 1999 Central pain mechanisms: a new horizon in manual therapy. Australian Journal of Physiotherapy 45:83–92

Shacklock M O, Butler D S, Slater H 1994 The dynamic nervous system: structure and clinical neurobiomechanics. In: Boyling J D, Palastanga N (eds) Grieve's modern manual therapy: the vertebral column, 2nd edn. Churchill Livingstone, Edinburgh

Sluka K 1996 Pain mechanisms involved in musculoskeletal disorders. Journal of Orthopaedic and Sports Physical Therapy 24(4):240–254

Smith S, Massie J, Chesnut R et al 1993 Straight leg raising: anatomical effects on the spinal nerve root without and with fusion. Spine 18(8):992–999

Stodieck L S, Beel J A, Lutges M W 1986 Structural properties of spinal nerve roots: protein composition. Experimental Neurology 91:41–51

Sugawara O, Atsuta Y, Iwahara T et al 1996 The effects of mechanical compression and hypoxia on nerve roots and dorsal root ganglia. Spine 21:2089–2094

Sunderland S 1974 Meningeal-neural relations in the intervertebral foramen. Journal of Neurosurgery 40:756–763

Sunderland S 1990 The anatomy and physiology of nerve injury. Muscle and Nerve 13(9):771–784

Takebayashi T, Cavanaugh J, Ozaktay A et al 2001 Effect of nucleus pulposus on the neural activity of dorsal root ganglion. Spine 26(8):940–945

Tal M, Eliav E 1996 Abnormal discharge originates at the site of nerve injury in experimental constriction neuropathy in the rat. Pain 64:511–518

Tanaka N, Fujimoto Y, An H et al 2000 The anatomic relation among the nerve roots, intervertebral foramina, and the intervertebral discs of the cervical spine. Spine 25(3):286–291

Thomas P K, Olsson Y 1984 Microscopic anatomy and function of the connective tissue components of peripheral nerve. In: Dyck P J, Thomas P K, Lambert E H et al (eds) Peripheral neuropathy, 2nd edn. Saunders, Philadelphia

Triano J, Luttges M 1982 Nerve irritation: a possible model of sciatic neuritis. Spine 7(2):129–136

Troup J D G 1981 Straight-leg-raising (SLR) and the qualifying tests for increased root tension: their predictive value after back and sciatic pain. Spine 6:526–527

Turl S E, George K P 1998 Adverse neural tension: a factor in repetitive hamstring strain? Journal of Orthopaedic and Sports Physical Therapy 27(1):16–21

Upton A R M, McComas A J 1973 The double crush in nerve entrapment syndromes. Lancet 18:359–361

Valls-Sole J, Alvarez R, Nunez M 1995 Limited longitudinal sliding of the median nerve in patients with carpal tunnel syndrome. Muscle and Nerve 18:761–767

van Meeteren N L, Brakee J H, Helders P J et al 1997 Functional recovery from sciatic nerve crush lesion in the rat correlates with individual differences in responses to chronic intermittent stress. Journal of Neuroscience Research 48:524–532

Wall E J, Massie J B, Kwan M K et al 1992 Experimental stretch neuropathy. Journal of Bone and Joint Surgery 74B:126–129

Wall P D, Gutnick M 1974 Ongoing activity in peripheral nerves: the physiology and pharmacology of impulses originating from a neuroma. Experimental Neurology 43:580–593

Weinstein J 1991 Neurogenic and nonneurogenic pain and inflammatory mediators. Orthopedic Clinics of North America 22(2):235–246

Wilgis E, Murphy R 1986 The significance of longitudinal excursion in peripheral nerves. Hand Clinics 2(r):761–766

Wright T W, Glowczewski F, Wheeler D et al 1996 Excursion and strain of the median nerve. Journal of Bone and Joint Surgery 78A:1897–1903

Wright T W, Glowczewski F, Cowin D et al 2001 Ulnar nerve excursion and strain at the elbow and wrist associated with upper extremity motion. Journal of Hand Surgery 26A(4):655–662

Yabuki S, Kikuchi S 1996 Positions of dorsal root ganglia in the cervical spine: an anatomic and clinic study. Spine 21(13):1513–1517

Yabuki S, Onda A, Kikuchi S et al 2001 Prevention of compartment syndrome in dorsal root ganglia caused by exposure to nucleus pulposus. Spine 29(8):870–875

Yoo J U, Zou D, Edward W T et al 1992 Effect of cervical spine motion on the neuroforaminal dimensions of human cervical spine. Spine 17:1131–1136

Yoshizawa H, Kobayashi S, Hachiya Y 1991 Blood supply of nerve roots and dorsal root ganglia. Orthopedic Clinics of North America 22(2):195–211

Yuan Q, Dougherty L, Margulies S S 1998 In vivo human spinal cord deformation and displacement in flexion. Spine 23:1677–1683

Zoch G, Reihsner R, Beer R et al 1991 Stress and strain in peripheral nerves. Neuro-Orthopedics 10:73–82

Zochodne D W 1993 Epineurial peptides: a role in neuropathic pain? Canadian Journal of Neurological Sciences 20:69–72

Zusman M 1992 Central nervous system contribution to mechanically produced motor and sensory responses. Australian Journal of Physiotherapy 38:245–253

Concepts in managing sport and exercise injuries

7

Motor control

Paul W Hodges

INTRODUCTION

Many factors influence movement of the body. These include not only the biomechanical properties of bone, articulations, and muscle, but also the controller, the system which must determine the requirements for movement and stability and generate appropriate strategies of muscle activity to effectively move the body and limbs, and control the relationship to the environment and between segments. An important consideration for sport and exercise is that injury and pain may affect the accuracy of the control system. Alternatively, inadequate function of the controller may contribute to the etiology of dysfunction and injury. The aim of this chapter is to consider the theory and application of motor control and motor learning as it applies to physical therapies for the management of sport and exercise related injury and pain, with reference to the elements of the neuromotor control system (receptors, controller), control strategies and how motor learning techniques can be used clinically to deal with changes in the control system when people have musculoskeletal pain.

FACTORS TO CONSIDER IN MOTOR CONTROL

In order to understand and develop strategies for application of motor learning to physical therapy management of sports and exercise-related injuries, it is essential to understand how movement is coordinated by the central nervous system (CNS). Performance of coordinated movement involves control of an appropriate sequence of movements of the limbs and trunk by an organized sequence of muscle activity. Furthermore, this coordinated pattern must be matched to environmental demands and be able to compensate for predictable or unpredictable disturbances that may interfere with the movement. For the CNS to meet the demands of sport and physical exercise, the coordination of these parameters must be streamlined. Numerous theories have been presented for the control of movement. This section will discuss the factors that must be addressed by the motor control system, provide a brief introduction to the major contemporary theories of motor control, and consider a specific example of motor control regarding postural and joint stability. Many theories of motor control have been presented in the literature, some from an anatomical basis and others from a behavioral point of view. This summary will focus on the behavioral approach.

CONTROL STRATEGIES

The CNS has a variety of strategies available for the control and coordination of movement. These strategies incorporate two basic systems of control that are derived from mechanical engineering. The first depends on sensory feedback (i.e. closed-loop strategies) and the second, controlled centrally, is largely independent of sensory feedback (i.e. open-loop strategies) (Fig. 7.1) (Schmidt & Lee, 1999). Each system requires a controller and effector organs (muscles). In both systems, the controller generates the movement command to drive the muscles for movement. In the closed-loop system, the control of the movement is continually updated and modified on the basis of feedback. In contrast, for open-loop control all aspects of the movement are preplanned and the movement is performed without consideration of feedback. This may occur because the feedback is not needed or is too slow to make adjustments to the movement.

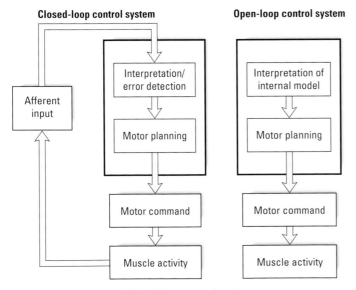

Figure 7.1   Open- and closed-loop control systems.

CLOSED-LOOP CONTROL – SENSORY CONTROL OF MOVEMENT

In a closed-loop system, the command to move is generated in a similar manner to an open-loop system (see below), however, the intended movement is compared against feedback regarding the status of the body and its relationship to the environment. If the feedback differs from the intended movement, an error command is generated to correct the movement performance. In this way, sensory feedback is used to mold and correct movement performance.

Clearly, this system requires effective systems for detecting the state of the environment, and the position and movements of the body segments. A variety of receptors are available including the visual system, auditory information, vestibular apparatus, and proprioceptors. The following section provides a review of the main receptor classes and their contribution to movement control.

Receptors

Endogenous information about movement and position of body segments is provided by a range of mechano-receptors ranging from free nerve endings to specialized receptor organs located in muscle, joints and skin (Fig. 7.2). Each of these receptor types provide afferent input that is useful for movement control.

Muscle spindles

Muscle spindles are the most complex of the mechano-receptors and consist of sensory and contractile components that lie parallel to muscle fibers so that they are stretched with the muscle. The sensory component has two main types of sensory endings, bag and chain fibers. These endings are sensitive to length and/or velocity of lengthening. The contractile component of the muscle spindle provides a mechanism for the CNS to control its sensitivity and to adapt the spindle to changes in muscle length. The contractile component of the muscle spindle is innervated by a special class of motorneurons, called

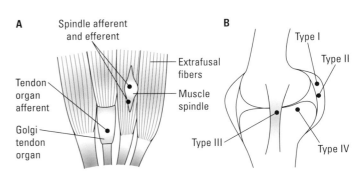

Figure 7.2   Location and types of muscle and joint receptors.

gamma-motorneurons. It is considered that alpha- and gamma-motorneurons are coactivated during muscle contraction. Many studies have confirmed that the input from muscle spindles is critical for the perception of movement, yet stimulation of single muscle afferents does not result in conscious perception.

Golgi tendon organs

Golgi tendon organs are located in series with the muscle fibers in the tendon. These receptors provide an inhibitory input to the alpha-motorneurons and were originally proposed to contribute only to strong contractions to prevent damage to the muscles. However, each receptor is attached to a small population of muscle fibers and is sensitive to small forces to provide discrete detection of tension in different parts of the muscle. Thus, these receptors are likely to provide an important contribution to feedback during movement.

Joint receptors

Joint receptors are encapsulated receptors (Ruffini endings and Pacinian corpuscles) situated in the joint capsule. The contribution of these receptors to perception of movement and movement control has often been considered to be limited. While some receptors are activated at specific ranges of motion, the majority fire at the end of range when the joint capsule is stretched. Other joint structures such as the ligaments also contain receptors which may contribute to proprioception. It is known that stimulation of receptors in the anterior cruciate ligament modulates activity of muscles surrounding the knee (Johansson et al 1991).

Skin receptors

There are several types of tactile receptors that are distributed in the layers of the skin. These receptors include Pacinican corpuscles, Mesiner corpuscles, Merkel cells and Ruffini endings and provide important tactile information. For example, input from the cutaneous receptors is important for the perception of movement of large and small joints such as those of the hand (Collins et al 2000). Furthermore, information derived from these receptors is critical for the coordination of grip force (Johansson et al 1991) and recent studies have shown a relationship between firing of afferent neurons and the motor-unit action potentials in the muscles of the wrist and hand (McNulty et al 1999).

Vestibular apparatus

The vestibular apparatus involves the saccule and utricle, which detect the position of the head with respect to gravity, and the semicircular canals, which provide information of acceleration of the head around the three major axes. The major function of the vestibular apparatus is to provide information about movements of the head. Integration of vestibular information and proprioceptive information from the neck and trunk allow the interpretation of the position of the body relative to gravity.

Visual system

The visual system provides information regarding the interaction between the body and environment or objects. As such, vision provides an important contribution to closed-loop control.

Auditory system

Although hearing does not play a major role in movement control, auditory information may provide useful feedback from environmental factors and issues such as success of performance. For instance, professional golfers can interpret the quality of a golf swing from the sound made when the ball is hit. There may also be more specific contributions such as feedback of the accuracy of movements involved in tasks, such as speech or foot contacts during running.

Closed-loop control mechanisms

Although the concept of closed-loop control may be considered in terms of higher information processing and consciousness, this system may operate at a variety of levels, from simple monosynaptic reflexes to complex, fine motor tasks involving coordinated finger movements. It is important to consider these different levels of control.

At the more basic end of the spectrum, closed-loop control may operate at the reflex level. The most basic of these is the monosynaptic stretch reflex. When muscle spindles are stretched, the afferent impulse from the receptor region of the spindles excite the alpha-motorneurons in the same muscle, resulting in contraction. This simple response is inflexible and represents a basic mechanism for the motor system to correct an error (i.e. to resist an imposed stretch). These responses are short in latency, and involve the time for transmission of the action potential along the afferent (sensory) and efferent (motor) nerves and a single synapse. In a sporting context, this aspect of movement control is likely to be important. For example, when the ankle is inverted, the body requires a rapid response of the peroneal muscles to overcome the inversion strain. However, even these most rapid responses may not be fast enough to prevent damage to joint structures.

More complex than the simple stretch reflex, are the long-loop reflexes that involve information processing at higher levels of the CNS, including transcortical mechanisms. These responses have a longer latency than the simple stretch reflex, are more flexible and can be modified voluntarily. Due to their flexibility, these responses are thought to have a greater role in error correction.

Another response group is the triggered responses. These responses are faster than a voluntary reaction time but involve a more complex and widespread response than is initiated via simple reflex mechanisms. For example, when the support surface on which a person is standing is rapidly moved, such as that which would occur when standing in a boat, a complex interplay of several body segments is initiated in order to maintain the equilibrium of the body. These responses have been shown to be too fast to be voluntary, but are task and context specific, and inconsistent with stretch reflexes.

The most complex level of closed-loop control is the fine control of long duration tasks that require accuracy. In these tasks, the sensory information may be used consciously to provide feedback of performance and to continually modulate movement performance. However, even during these conscious goal-directed tasks sensory information may be used at a subconscious level to modulate muscle activity.

Problems of closed-loop control

Even the fastest reflex responses involve a delay from stimulus to response. Thus, it has been argued that this system is unable to adequately meet the demands necessary to overcome the effects of external forces. For instance, the impact from a force applied to the posterior tibia is likely to be sufficient to injure the anterior cruciate ligament (ACL) before any reflex response could be initiated. More important is the consideration that the latency required to make corrections for an error involves delays in the order of hundreds of milliseconds to receive and interpret afferent information and then generate appropriate responses. Thus, with rapid movements there is little time to provide information, other than feedback that the movement has been completed and whether the goal has been achieved. On this basis it may be considered that closed-loop mechanisms are most appropriate for slow movements that need constant regulation for accuracy. Clearly, other mechanisms must exist.

OPEN-LOOP CONTROL – CENTRALLY CONTROLLED MOVEMENT

In contrast to the closed-loop control of movement, open-loop control implies that all aspects of the movement performance are preplanned by the CNS and that the movement occurs without modification by sensory feedback. Movements that are likely to fit into this category are ballistic and repetitive movements that are common in sport and exercise. Basic evidence that this type of control exists comes from studies of humans and animals with de-afferented limbs. In these cases, limb movement can occur that is almost indistinguishable from that of a limb with a full complement of sensory input, except for fine, controlled movements of the fingers that appear slightly clumsy (Taub & Berman 1968).

To reconcile these observations, theories have been developed about the mechanisms of generation of movement patterns. In animals, the presence of central pattern generators (CPG) has been confirmed (Grillner 1981). A CPG is a collection of neurons that may control a repetitive function such as locomotion or respiration. These neuron groups can control the alternating contraction of muscles to perform the movement, and while they can be modified by afferent feedback, they can function independently of feedback. The existence of CPGs has not been confirmed in humans.

Another organizational theory to explain the central control of movement is the concept of the motor program. The motor program theory involves a memory-based mechanism whereby a generalized motor program is stored as an abstract representation of a group of movements that are retrieved when a movement is performed (Schmidt & Lee 1999). This theory argues that the CNS stores details of invariant features of a movement (e.g. order of events, relative timing, relative force). This information is accessed, with selected task duration and muscles, when the movement is performed. While this theory is popular, there are several problems. One example is the issue of retention of the large amount of information that would need to be stored to cover the full complement of movement possibilities. Furthermore, there is the problem of the number of degrees of freedom. This issue was highlighted by Bernstein (1967) who argued that there are too many components that need to be controlled concurrently. For even the simplest movements of the hand, motion of each joint between the fingertip and the floor requires consideration. This is compounded when considering all of the muscles that are available to control each joint and the motor units within each muscle. As suggested by Bernstein, this is an enormous problem for the CNS in view of the resources required to individually control the large number of muscles and joints. A system is needed that can reduce processing demands, for instance, by grouping degrees of freedom together.

Another model of movement control has been presented to reconcile some of these difficulties in movement control: the dynamic pattern theory (Kelso 1984). The dynamic pattern theory argues that there is no central representation of all components of the movement; instead, the organization of the muscle contractions and joint movement is coordinated by environmental invariants and limb dynamics. Central to this theory is the idea that movements are attracted to steady-state behaviors, and movements follow the principles of non-linear dynamics. In other words, if a particular variable is changed systematically, the system may move between separate stable states. A familiar example to illustrate this point is the transition from walking to running. In the dynamic pattern theory, it is argued that at slower speeds the movements of the arm and legs are 'attracted' to a coordinated pattern that is walking, yet at faster speeds the pattern changes, in part for reasons of efficiency. Thus, coordinated movement is self-organized according to the characteristics of limb behavior and environmental constraints.

Thus, the contemporary theories of motor control vary in the level of emphasis placed on the different, centrally or environmentally driven aspects of movement performance. Currently, the debate continues regarding these two theories. Movement, in reality, may be coordinated by a hybrid of both possibilities.

MOVEMENT AND STABILITY – MOTOR CONTROL OF POSTURAL AND JOINT STABILITY

To this point, movement has been considered as a sequence of movements to achieve a goal, however, all movements are actually a complex interaction of movement and stability (Massion 1992). In reality, movement occurs in conjunction with a subtle background of postural adjustments. Movement perturbs stability as a result of the interaction between internal and external forces. These forces include the reactive moments from limb movements, changes in the influence of gravity on the body as a result of the modification of the position of the center mass with movement, and the interaction with objects and the environment (e.g. catching a ball). Even a simple action, such as a movement of a limb, changes the position of the center of mass, and is associated with reactive moments that are equal in amplitude but opposite in direction to the forces producing the moment. Thus, the CNS not only has to deal with coordination of muscle activity to perform the movement but must also counteract the disturbance to postural stability. Conversely, no posture is purely static. For example, even static posture involves some component of movement, of which at least one component is actively controlled. For example, breathing produces a cyclical movement of the trunk (Gurfinkel et al 1971). Although this perturbation presents a challenge to the

stability of the body, this movement is compensated by a coordinated sequence of movements of the trunk and lower limbs so that little, if any, movement is detected in forces recorded at the ground (Hodges et al 2002). It must be stated that there is considerable argument about which parts of a task are 'movement-related' and which are purely 'posture-related'. As many issues of relevance to sport and physical exercise relate to control of posture and joint stability, it is important to consider the normal control of these elements of movement control.

It should be noted that the perturbation to stability may affect the body at a number of different levels. First, it may affect the relationship between the body and the environment (i.e. postural equilibrium). Second, it may affect the relationship between adjacent regions of the body. Finally, it may result in shear of torsion forces at the intersegmental level (e.g. at the intervertebral level). Strategies must be available to control stability at each level and it is accepted that motor control strategies for each involve both closed- and open-loop processes, including reflex responses, and complex feedback mediated responses, such as triggered responses and feedforward strategies. In a basic sense, the division can be made between predictable and unpredictable perturbations.

Control of postural equilibrium

Reflexes have long been regarded as the cornerstones of postural control. While it is clear that short-latency stretch reflexes may help maintain postural stability by maintenance of muscle length, the situation is likely to be more complex. For example, when the floor is tilted to stretch the calf muscles, it would be expected that this would generate a stretch reflex in the homonymous muscles. However, if this was initiated, the response would tend to increase the perturbation and lead to a loss of balance. Instead, the response of the calf muscles is restricted and a more appropriate response is generated that involves multiple segments (Nashner 1977). Considerable research has been devoted to investigation of these 'triggered' responses, which involve multiple segments. Balance is perturbed in many of these studies by movement of the support surface. Two main strategies have been identified that involve either ankle movement ('ankle strategy') or hip movement ('hip strategy'), depending on the context and the support surface characteristics (Horak & Nashner, 1986).

What sensory information is used to initiate these triggered responses to maintain the equilibrium of the body? All sensory modalities including vestibular, somatosensory and visual information may be involved. On this basis, clinical assessment techniques have been developed with the aim of interpreting the specific contribution of each modality by removing or minimizing the input from one sensory modality or by providing conflicting information (Horak 1987). Recent studies have confirmed that vestibular input provides little contribution in quiet stance, as this system is not sensitive enough to detect small changes (Fitzpatrick et al 1996). Thus, in quiet stance, vision and proprioceptive information are the most critical.

However, the contribution of stretch reflexes to the maintenance of balance has also been considered in terms of maintaining muscle stiffness (Winter et al 1998). Muscle stiffness is the property of muscles to act like springs; in other words, it is the ratio of length change to force change. When a muscle is stiff, it takes large amounts of force for it to lengthen. Thus, if antagonist muscles on either side of a joint have high stiffness, then increased force is required to move the joint. In terms of postural control, the stiffness of the ankle muscles may resist falling. It is the stretch reflex, and the control of the gamma-motorneurons which control the sensitivity of the sensory component of the muscle spindles, that control this system.

Alternatively, if a perturbation is predictable, then the CNS has the opportunity to deal with the perturbation in advance of the movement. For instance, if a limb is moved, the CNS can predict the effect that this movement will have on the body and plan a sequence of muscle activity to overcome this perturbation. This type of strategy depends on the ability of the CNS to predict the interaction between body segments, and the body and its environment. Theoretically, this is thought to involve an 'Internal System of Body Dynamics' which is an abstract construct built up over a lifetime of movement experience (Gahéry & Massion 1981). Using this model, the CNS is able to determine how torques and inertias of adjacent and distant segments may interact, and how this will affect the external forces acting on the body. Several possibilities could explain the organization of the movement and postural parts of the task. In general, the postural activity could exist as a part of the motor command for movement or the postural part could be organized separately, but in parallel with the movement command. Several studies have investigated this question and are generally in support of the parallel process model (Massion 1992).

It is important to consider that both processes may act concurrently and the outcome of feedforward processes may be molded by later feedback mediated processes. In general, feedforward and feedback mediated responses closely match the demands of the task and are scaled to the amplitude of the perturbing forces and the context of the perturbation. As such, postural adjustments represent a finely tuned component of human movement.

Control of joint stability

Joint stability is dependent on multiple factors that include the passive, active and control systems. Although the passive structures that surround a joint provide support, particularly towards the end of range, a major contributor to joint control is the active/muscle system. Yet the active contribution that muscles provide to stability is dependent on the controller, the CNS (Panjabi 1992). All of the mechanisms described above for the control of postural equilibrium also apply to the control of joint stability, including the control of the relationship between adjacent segments and the fine tuning of control of torsion and shear forces at the intersegmental level. Both feedforward and feedback strategies exist. Reflex responses have been extensively investigated. For instance, studies have shown short-latency responses of the muscles of the trunk in response to the unexpected addition of a load, such as dropping a load in a bucket held in the hands (Wilder et al 1996). Similarly, the short-latency responses of the peroneal muscles have been identified as maintaining the position of the ankle in response to an inversion force (Hopper et al 1998). More complex triggered responses are also involved. For instance, activity of the neck and trunk muscles precedes movement of these segments when the support surface is moved. This suggests that these responses are triggered by distal afferent input (Keshner 1990). The reflex control of muscle stiffness (as outlined in the previous section) has also been implicated in the control of joint stability. Several authors have investigated this in biomechanical and in vivo experiments. These studies argue that reflex responses are too slow and that joint stability may be maintained by modulation of muscle stiffness. The stretch reflex may provide an important contribution to this control. Stiffness may also be affected by other sensory inputs; studies have shown that activity of the knee musculature may be affected by afferent input from the ACL (Johansson et al 1991).

Joint stability is also maintained in a feedforward manner. Two typical examples include the anticipatory reduction in activity of the biceps muscle when a person removes a mass from their own hand (Hugon et al 1982), and the activity of the trunk muscles in advance of the muscles responsible for movement of an upper or lower limb to overcome the perturbation to the trunk from limb movement (Fig. 7.3) (Hodges & Richardson, 1997). An additional finding from these trunk muscle studies was that the activity of the superficial muscles was linked to the direction of perturbation to the orientation of the spine. This suggests a contribution to control of the alignment of the spine, whereas the activity of the deep muscles occurred in a non-directional specific manner,

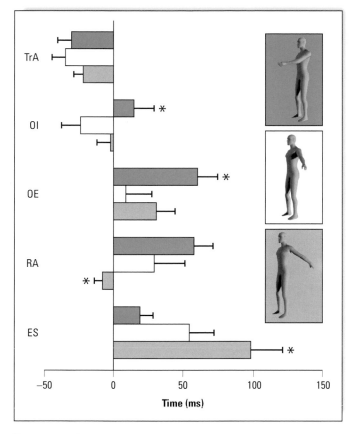

Figure 7.3   Feedforward control of trunk stability. Rapid arm movement is associated with a sequence of trunk muscle activity that varies between directions of limb movement. Data in this figure are presented relative to the onset of the deltoid muscle which flexes the arm. The onset of activity of many of the muscles varies between movement directions and is linked to the control of the alignment of the spine. The deep muscle, transversus abdominis, is controlled separately and does not vary with movement direction. It is thought that the CNS uses this muscle to control intersegmental motion. (Adapted from Hodges & Richardson 1996.)

which indicates a contribution to stiffening of the intervertbreal joints, i.e. intersegmental stability.

Problems for the control of postural equilibrium and joint stability

Although postural adjustments provide a precise compensation for perturbation to postural equilibrium and joint stability, their control requires special consideration. For example, postural adjustments themselves may perturb balance. For instance, the change in lower leg muscle activity that precedes arm movements would cause the person to fall over if it occurred too early. Thus, the temporal and spatial organization of the postural responses needs to be perfectly matched to the real or predicted perturbation. Another complication is that the requirements for control of joint stability and postural control may be contradictory. For example, the body may need to change the position of the spine in order to overcome a

challenge to equilibrium. Thus, the CNS must balance the requirements for stability and equilibrium, and it has been shown to achieve this goal effectively (Hodges et al 1999). A further complication is the fact that many muscles are required to perform multiple functions concurrently. For example, many trunk muscles are also involved in tasks such as respiration, and when posture is challenged the CNS needs to be able to integrate the postural and respiratory functions. Whether this integration occurs at spinal or higher centers has not been determined.

CHARACTERISTICS OF THE MUSCLE CONTROL SYSTEM

Another issue in motor control that requires consideration is the selection of muscles for movement and stability. To this point, discussion has focused on strategies for control of movement, but it is necessary to consider the selection of muscles. An important consideration is the redundancy in the muscle system (which contributes to the problem of degrees of freedom outlined above). Many muscles cross the joints and may be capable of performing similar functions, however, it has been proposed by several authors that there may be functional differentiation in the muscle system. A basic division is between muscles that perform functions based on their specific contribution to control of motion and stability (e.g. Bergmark 1989, Goff 1972, Janda 1978, Sahrman, 2002). Notably, Bergmark (1989) presented a model for the trunk that may be extrapolated to the other regions of the body. This model identified muscles as either 'local' or 'global', based on anatomical characteristics (Fig. 7.4). The local muscles are those that cross one or a few segment/s and that have limited moment arm to move the joint, but ideal anatomy to maintain joint stability. In contrast, the global muscles cross several joints, with a larger moment arm to generate torque at the

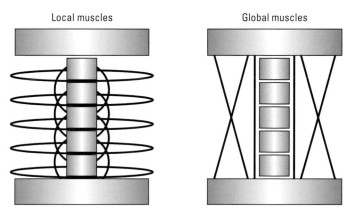

Figure 7.4   Local and global muscles. Local muscles cross few segments and control intersegmental motion. Global muscles cross several segments and have moment arms sufficient to generate torques. (Adapted from Bergmark 1989.)

joint. While simple division of muscles into groups is likely to oversimplify the complex control of spinal motion and stability, it provides a useful definition to consider clinically, as it contributes to our understanding of why the CNS uses different strategies to control the different muscle groups.

CHANGES IN MOTOR CONTROL IN MUSCULOSKELETAL INJURY AND PAIN

When pain and injury occur, the strategies used by the CNS to control movement and/or posture and stability may be compromised. The mechanism for these changes is poorly understood but may be due to changes at many levels of the CNS. This section will review some of the ways in which motor control may be affected by pain and injury, and consider possible mechanisms for these changes.

It is possible to consider the changes in motor control in view of the theories outlined in the previous section. Changes have been identified in both open- and closed-loop type components of movement control and in terms of both the 'stability' and 'movement' components of coordinated movement. Clearly, the implications of each of these will differ in terms of motor learning as a component of rehabilitation. The following section aims to present a variety of the motor control changes in relation to motor control theory.

CHANGES IN SENSORY CONTROL OF MOVEMENT – CLOSED-LOOP CONTROL PROBLEMS

Numerous deficits in the sensory control of movement have been identified, including changes in sensory feedback, abnormal reflex responses, and inaccurate coordination of movement. From behavioral studies of human movement, it is difficult to determine the exact component or components of the system that are responsible for the change in motor control. For instance, if the amplitude of activity of a muscle is increased during a pointing task, it is difficult to determine whether the change results from inaccurate feedback from the periphery, inaccurate interpretation of normal feedback or inability to initiate an appropriate command. The following sections deal with several specific instances in which changes in elements of the closed-loop system may be implicated.

Sensory deficits

The basis of closed-loop control is accurate feedback from movement. One of the most commonly identified motor

control deficits that has been identified in association with musculoskeletal pain and injury is the sensory deficit. This has been identified in two major ways: first, by measurement of the acuity or smallest perceptible stimulation, such as the smallest movement that can be accurately detected, and second, by the ability to accurately copy a position or return to a position of a limb after it has been demonstrated with the same or opposite limb. Using these methods, studies have identified the following: decreased acuity to spinal motion in low back pain (Taimela et al 1999); decreased acuity to ankle movement in the inversion/eversion direction (Garn & Newton 1988), but not plantarflexion or dorsiflexion following ankle sprain (Refshauge et al 2000); decreased acuity to shoulder motion with shoulder instability (Warner et al 1996); increased threshold to perception of vibration (indicating decreased sensory function) following ankle sprain (Bullock-Saxton 1994); and impaired ability to accurately reposition with low back pain (Brumagne et al 2000), ankle sprain, and knee osteoarthritis (Garsden & Bullock-Saxton 1999).

Due to the importance of sensory information to closed-loop control of movement, deficits such as those outlined above may lead to impaired movement control at a number of levels. For instance, decreased acuity may lead to delayed reflex responses as a result of increased time to reach the threshold for movement detection. More complex changes are also possible, such as impaired co-ordination during voluntary movement due to inaccurate feedback from movement. This inaccurate feedback may lead to faulty error detection and correction. Another possibility is that inaccurate feedback may lead to development of a faulty internal model of body dynamics. In this case, the CNS may generate commands that are inaccurate for performance of the required movement. An additional possibility is that the muscle spindle sensitivity may be altered by pain (Pedersen et al 1997).

The reason for sensory feedback to change with injury and pain may be multifactorial. For example, it may be due to injury to joint, muscle or cutaneous receptors. Alternatively, it may be due to changes in interpretation of the afferent input, such as the potential for afferent input to be misinterpreted as nociceptive in hyperalgesia. In addition, changes in muscle activity may affect sensory acuity. Muscle activity is known to augment acuity (Gandevia et al 1992); thus any change in activation may adversely affect movement sensation. Furthermore, many muscles, particularly deep muscles close to the joints, have extensive attachments to joint structures and contraction is likely to affect sensation. Finally, several studies have argued that sensory acuity may be reduced by fatigue (Carpenter et al 1998); thus decreased muscle endurance with injury or pain may lead to impaired sensory acuity.

Reflex changes

Changes in a variety of reflex responses have been identified in musculoskeletal pain syndromes. These changes include delayed reaction time of the peroneal muscle response to ankle inversion in ankle sprain (Lofvenberg et al 1995), delayed onset of activity of the erector spinae to trunk loading (Magnusson et al 1996), and delayed offset of activity of the oblique abdominal and thoracolumbar erector spinae muscles of the trunk in response to unloading in chronic low back pain (Fig. 7.5) (Radebold et al 2000). However, others have failed to find changes in reflex responses of the erector spinae, elicited by a muscle tap, with experimentally-induced pain.

Changes in reflex responses may be due to altered sensory acuity (see the section on Sensory Deficits above) and changes in motorneuron excitability may be the result of descending drive or spinal mechanisms (see the section on Changes in Motorneuron Excitability – Reflex Inhibition below). In addition, it has been suggested that reflex responses may be delayed by slowed conduction velocity in the motor axons (Kleinrensink et al 1994). This later mechanism is unlikely to be altered by motor learning.

Movement coordination

Although it is difficult to identify the exact site for changes in motor control from behavioral studies of human movement, several examples have been identified in the literature. For example, studies have identified decreased control of the trajectory of arm movement in a pointing task when vision is occluded in people with shoulder instability (Forwell & Carnahan 1996), and

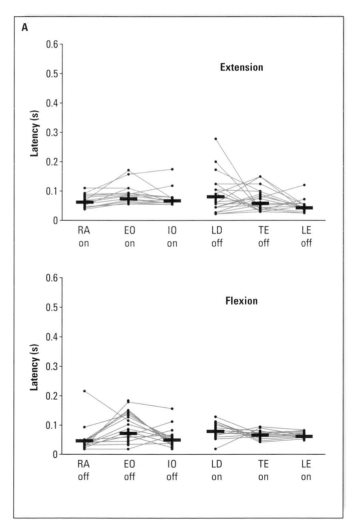
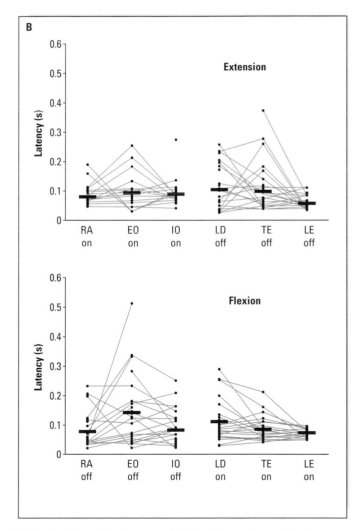

Figure 7.5 When a mass attached to the front (extension) or back (flexion) of the trunk is suddenly removed, the trunk muscles must reduce their activity to maintain the upright position of the trunk. When people have low back pain the offset of the external oblique abdominal and thoracic erector spinae muscles is delayed. **A**: Healthy controls. **B**: Low back pain patients. (Reproduced from Radebold et al 2000 with the permission of Lippincott Williams and Wilkins.)

changes in amplitude and time onset of muscle activity of serratus anterior and upper trapezius in shoulder impingement during arm elevation (Ludewig & Cook 2000). In addition, slow reaction time has been identified in low back pain (Luoto et al 1995), and has been associated with musculoskeletal injuries in a variety of sports (Taimela & Kujala 1992).

Many reasons could be hypothesized for these changes (Fig. 7.6). Again, sensory deficits may be responsible (see the section on Sensory Deficits above). In addition, authors have argued that changes may arise due to an inability to ignore unnecessary information, and the effect that this would have on limited attention resources (Luoto et al 1999). Alternatively, effects may be due to the direct or indirect influence of pain on planning of motor responses (see Derbyshire 1997). The effects may also occur as a result of fear or stress. Changes may also be due to alterations in cortical excitability (Valeriani et al 1999), motorneuron excitability (see the section on Changes in Motorneuron Excitability – Reflex Inhibition below), or delayed transmission in the CNS. Finally, motor control may be changed to reduce or limit motion to reduce pain provocation. This hypothesis has been refined as the pain adaptation model (Lund et al 1991) which argues that velocity and displacement is reduced by reduced agonist activity and increased antagonist activity.

Control of posture and joint stability

Joint stability

In addition to the numerous examples of changes in reflex responses of the erector spinae outlined above,

investigation of muscle activity during ongoing functional movements (i.e. closed-loop control) has lead to identification of changes in muscle recruitment thought to be associated with joint stability. For instance, changes in the time of activation of the medial and lateral vastii muscles has been identified during stair-stepping tasks in people with patellofemoral pain syndrome. While there has been much disagreement in the literature over whether or not impaired activity of the medial vastii (vastus medialis obliquus) leads to abnormal tracking of the patella and pain (Powers et al 1996), recent studies have identified delayed activity of this muscle in comparison to the lateral vastii, when stepping onto and off a step (Fig. 7.7) (Cowan et al 2001). In addition, reduced amplitude of multifidus (a muscle considered to provide a critical contribution to spinal stability) activity has been identified during functional tasks in people with low back pain (Lindgren et al 1993). While these changes imply impaired muscle activity, other studies provide evidence of augmented activity, such as sustained activity of the erector spinae muscles at the end of the range of spinal flexion, a point at which the erector spinae muscles are normally inactive, in people with low back pain (Shirado et al 1995). This has been replicated by experimental pain (Zedka et al 1999).

As outlined above, it has been argued that one response of the nervous system to pain is to reduce movement by a combination of augmentation or impairment of muscle activity. This somewhat simplistic view has gained some support in the literature. One interpretation of the results presented here is that the activation of the multisegmented global muscles, such as the erector

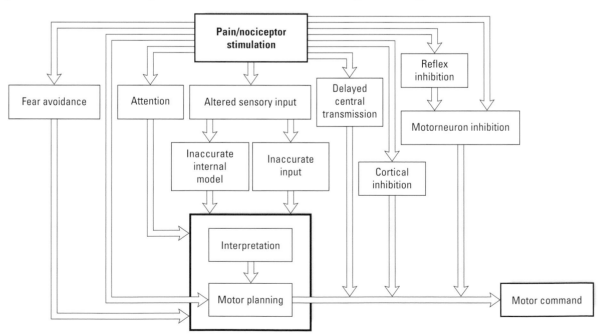

Figure 7.6   Proposed mechanisms for pain to affect motor control.

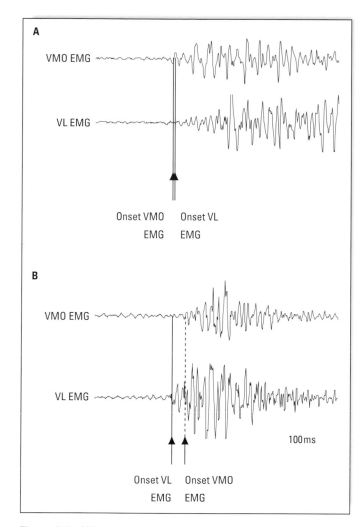

Figure 7.7   When people with no history of patellofemoral pain step up onto a step the onsets of the medial and lateral vastii occur simultaneously. However, when patellofemoral pain is present the onset of VMO occurs before that of VL. **A**: Control. **B**: Patellofemoral pain syndrome. (Adapted from Cowan et al 2001.)

spinae, may be modified to reduce the overall motion of the joints, by either reducing their activity as an agonist activation during movement, or by cocontraction to make a segment rigid. In contrast, a relatively consistent response of the system is to reduce the activation of the deep local muscles, which may compromise the fine-tuning of segmental control.

Postural control

Several studies have investigated parameters of ongoing closed-loop control of posture in people with low back pain. These studies have identified impairments of balance when standing on one (Luoto et al 1998) or two legs (Byl & Sinnott 1991) or sitting (Radebold et al 2001). Furthermore, an increased risk of low back pain or recurrence of pain has been identified for people with

poor performance in a test of standing balance (Takala & Viikari-Juntura 2000). Although it is not possible to determine the mechanism for these changes, they may be due to sensory deficits or changes in information processing or motor planning. These changes indicate a general reduction of the accuracy of the postural control system in these patients, hence, the relationship to increased risk of re-injury.

CHANGES IN MOTOR PLANNING – OPEN-LOOP CONTROL PROBLEMS

Feedforward strategies

The major factors that have implicated changes in the open-loop control of movement are changes in feed-forward strategies. As mentioned above, these strategies are preplanned by the nervous system and represent the pattern of muscle activity initiated by the CNS in advance of movement. Several studies have investigated onset of muscle activity in association with rapid limb movements. These studies have identified delayed onset of activity of the deep abdominal muscle, transversus abdominis, with arm and leg movements in people with chronic low back pain (Hodges & Richardson 1996). Furthermore, when people are given pain by the injection of hypertonic saline into the paraspinal muscles, similar changes are identified (Fig. 7.8) (Hodges et al 2001a). Further studies have challenged the coordination of these responses and suggest that the responses are a result of inappropriate motor planning, rather than changes in excitability or transmission of the command in the CNS (Hodges 2001). A similar change in the patterns of activation of the scapula muscles has been identified in association with shoulder movement (Wadsworth & Bullock-Saxton 1997).

The possible mechanisms for changes in feedforward responses are similar to those outlined above for changes in closed-loop control of movement. However, the changes must occur in motor planning as these responses are initiated in advance of movement. Despite the open-loop nature of the responses, they may be affected by sensory deficits if the internal model of body dynamics that is built up by movement experience, and that is used to generate the responses, is inaccurate.

CHANGES IN MOTORNEURON EXCITABILITY – REFLEX INHIBITION

A final factor that may influence motor control, and therefore the output of the motor system, irrespective of whether open- or closed-loop systems are involved, is changes in the excitability of the spinal motorneurons. One factor that may change motorneuron excitability is

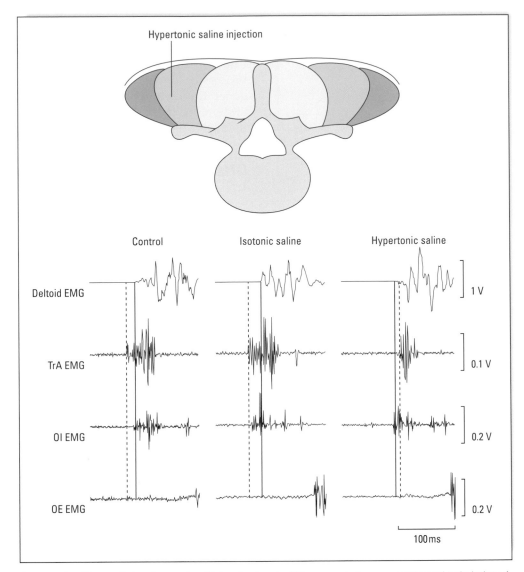

Figure 7.8 Change in trunk muscle with low back pain. When people have experimental pain induced by injection of hypertonic saline into the paraspinal muscles., the onset of EMG of transversus abdominis is delayed relative to the onset of the muscle responsible for arm movement when the arm is moved rapidly in response to a light. (Adapted from Hodges et al 2001a.)

reflex inhibition. The mechanism for reflex inhibition is generally considered to involve inhibition of the alpha-motorneuron as a result of afferent input from effusion (Stokes & Young 1984) or injury to joint structures (Ekholm et al 1960). For example, when effusion is present in the knee, the motorneuron excitability of quadriceps muscles is reduced (Spencer et al 1984). Furthermore, this affects certain muscles to different degrees, such as the oblique fibers of vastus medialis which become inhibited with lower volumes of effusion than others. Reflex inhibition has also been used as an argument to explain the rapid atrophy of multifidus in people with acute low back pain (Hides et al 1994), although this requires clarification.

PAIN OR CHANGES IN MOTOR CONTROL – WHICH COMES FIRST?

There is considerable debate in the literature regarding the sequence of changes in motor control and pain (Fig. 7.9). Numerous possibilities have been outlined above for injury and pain to affect motor control. Furthermore, several studies have indicated that many of the changes seen in clinical populations may be replicated in healthy subjects with experimentally-induced pain (Hodges et al 2001a, Zedka et al 1999). However, it is also possible that changes in motor control may lead to pain. Several authors have argued that poor control of a joint may lead to microtrauma and eventual injury (Farfan 1973, Panjabi

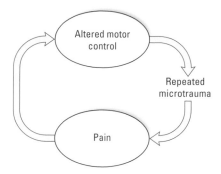

Figure 7.9 Possible cycle of pain, injury, and motor control changes.

1992), which may result from poor motor control. The events that might lead to initial changes in motor control require further investigation.

MOTOR LEARNING IN THE MANAGEMENT OF SPORTS-RELATED INJURIES

This section provides an overview of motor learning strategies that may be utilized to restore normal motor activity. The nervous system has considerable potential for plasticity and learning. In view of the evidence of changes in motor control in association with pain and injury as a result of sport and physical activity, motor learning forms an important component of the management of many conditions (including those outlined in the previous section). Motor learning refers to the acquisition and refinement of movement and coordination that leads to a permanent change in movement performance. Irrespective of the skill being trained, motor learning is characterized by several goals including improvement of motor performance (increased precision, decreased error), improved performance consistency (decreased variability), persistence of improvements (continued improvement over time leading to permanent improvement) and the adaptability of the skill to a variety of environments (novel contexts, decreased feedback, changes in physical or personal characteristics). Numerous motor learning strategies have been presented in the literature to achieve these goals. This section provides an overview of the stages of motor learning and several contemporary strategies for training specific motor skills that are applicable to the clinical situation for the management and prevention of injuries and pain. For a more comprehensive review, refer to Magill (2001), Schmidt & Lee (1999), and Shumway-Cooke & Woollacott (1995).

STAGES OF MOTOR LEARNING

Several authors have presented sequential models of the stages of motor learning. One popular model, first presented by Fitts & Posner (1967), considers that learning involves three main stages: the *cognitive, associative* and *autonomous* phases. In the *cognitive* phase, the focus is on cognitively oriented problems. All elements of the movement performance are organized consciously with attention to feedback, movement sequence, performance and instruction during repetition and practice. This phase is characterized by frequent, large errors and variability. Animal studies have identified increased size of the hand area of the sensory cortex during the cognitive phase of motor learning of a task involving interpretation of sensory information from the hand (Recanzone et al 1992). The second stage is the *associative* phase, in which the fundamentals of the movement have been acquired and the cognitive demands are reduced. The focus moves from simple elements of performance of the task to consistency of performance, success and refinement. Correspondingly, the frequency and size of errors are reduced. The final stage of motor learning, the *autonomous* stage, is achieved after considerable practice and experience. The task becomes habitual or automatic and the requirement for conscious intervention is reduced. Although the features of each stage are distinct, it is important to consider that there is a smooth transition between stages and it may not be obvious when a person moves between phases.

Other models of motor learning have similar features to this three-stage process with differences in the emphasis placed on elements of the progression of learning. Gentile (1987) divides learning into two phases based on the goal of the learner. In the first phase, the goal of the learner is to 'get the idea' of the task. The second phase involves fixation or diversification of the skill, that is, improved consistency in stable environments and improved transfer to new contexts. Irrespective of the specific features of each model the basic elements of motor learning are similar.

STRATEGIES FOR MOTOR LEARNING

Practice of parts and/or practice of the whole

There has been considerable debate in the literature regarding whether it is more optimal to train motor skills by practicing a whole movement, or with practice of essential components of the skill with later integration of the components into the complete skill. While both methods are likely to result in changes to skill performance, it is likely that specific types of skill are more amenable to each method. It has been argued that movements with simple organization (i.e. tasks composed of several elements that are independent) and high complexity (i.e. many elements) are amenable to practice of parts of the skill (Naylor & Briggs 1963). In contrast, movements with complex organization (i.e. tasks composed of a sequence of skills in which performance of one is dependent on performance of another) and low complexity (i.e. few elements) are best trained with practice of the whole task (Naylor & Briggs 1963).

In whole-task practice, it is possible to develop the spatial and temporal relationship of the independent elements of the task. However, when a skill is trained in parts, the attention demand is reduced to allow attention to be focused on a single element. At a later stage, it is important to perform the interdependent parts of a task together. This approach is ideal when there are a few discrete elements of a skilled task that are problematic and require training or refinement. Several techniques have been described for part-task training. These include *segmentation* and *simplification* (Magill 2001). In the *segmentation* approach, the task is broken up into smaller parts to be practiced as independent units, and then the practiced elements are integrated together progressively to practice the complete skill. In the *simplification* approach the movement or its parts are simplified to increase the ease of movement performance. *Simplification* may be achieved by changing parameters such as reduction of the attention demands, reduction of speed of the task or using additional strategies to augment the performance (Fig. 7.10) (e.g. application of tape over the

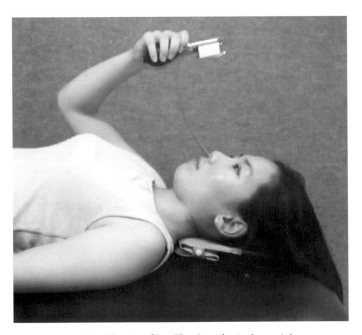

Figure 7.10 Simplification. Simplification of a task can take many forms. Here the performance of the control exercise for the upper cervical flexors in a patient with neck pain is simplified by modification of the position of the patient. In the supine position the gravitational load is reduced, making it easier for the subject to perform the task in a precise manner. Additional feedback of the task is provided with a pressure cuff placed under the cervical spine.

patella to change the timing of the vastii, reduction of swelling to reduce reflex inhibition, positioning to decrease load, improved sensory acuity to improve accuracy of feedback). Alternatively, a person can practice the whole task, but attend to a specific part of the task. In this way, a part practice environment can be integrated into whole practice. This latter approach may be facilitated by augmentation of the level of feedback (see below) of the movement element that is being addressed.

Instruction versus demonstration

Two major ways to teach a skill or part of a task are demonstration and instruction. The precise nature of instructions vary and may include: information of the goal, the steps in task performance or errors. Demonstration may involve visual information by showing the task or another form of feedback, such as kinesthetic information (e.g. moving the learner through a required range of motion or electrical stimulation of a muscle contraction). An essential component of both techniques is accurate analysis of the movement and identification of the elements to be trained or refined.

It has been argued that instruction or demonstration may lead to better improvement, depending on the task being performed. For example, it has been argued that demonstration is better for tasks in which a new pattern of coordination is being trained, rather than an adaptation of a pattern that has already been learnt (Magill & Schoenfelder-Zohndi 1996). The aim of demonstration fits with Gentile's goal for the first stage of motor learning to 'give the idea' of the task (Gentile 1987). If demonstration is selected as the technique for training a skill, this can be done either by demonstrating a skilled performance or allowing the learner to observe practice by an unskilled person. Additional improvement may be achieved if the learner is cued to the important elements of the skilled performance during the demonstration. Verbal instruction is one of the most common techniques for training a motor skill. Several important factors require consideration. First, the complexity of instruction needs to match the attention capacity of the learner; instruction will be most effective if the minimum instruction is given. Second, some types of information may hinder learning. Third, verbal instruction can be used for two purposes: to cue attention to a specific element, or to cue the patient to initiate an action.

Feedback

An important element of motor learning is the provision of augmented feedback. Feedback can be generally divided into two main types: knowledge of performance and knowledge of results. Put simply, feedback that provides knowledge of performance relates to ongoing sensory/perceptual information provided during the movement, whereas knowledge of results provides feedback of the outcome of the movement. Each of the sensory systems, including visual, auditory, proprioceptive and vestibular information, may be utilized to provide each form of feedback. This feedback may be intrinsic (naturally occurring) or augmented/enhanced in some way (e.g. electromyographic biofeedback or ultrasound imaging to increase awareness of muscle contraction, verbal feedback of quality of performance, video replay of performance). Thus, augmented feedback may be provided during the task or upon its completion and may be used to encourage and motivate achievement of the goal of a task or used to refine its performance. In general, feedback may be particularly important if the intrinsic information is not sufficient (e.g. when sensory acuity is impaired or due to lack of experience). If intrinsic information is sufficient, augmentation of the feedback may enhance the development of the skill.

Three issues require further consideration. First, should feedback of correct or incorrect aspects of performance be given? In general, feedback of errors leads to skill improvement, whereas feedback of correct elements is motivational; both may be beneficial. Second, should feedback provide qualitative or quantitative information? For example, qualitative information of speed of contraction or quantitative information of the number of seconds to complete the task could be provided. Although it may be assumed that quantitative feedback may be optimal, as it provides the most precise information, others argue that qualitative information provides an easier to interpret form of feedback in the early stages of learning. Third, there are several situations in which feedback may compromise motor learning, for instance, if a learner becomes dependent on the feedback that is not available during natural performance. This may occur if the intrinsic feedback is limited or complex. In this case, the learner may substitute the augmented feedback for the intrinsic feedback and may not learn to use the intrinsic feedback. In general, it is important to be certain that augmented feedback is accurate and that mechanisms are in place to ensure that learners will be able to progress to using available intrinsic feedback. It is generally accepted that it is better not to provide feedback on every trial to avoid dependence.

As mentioned earlier, augmented feedback may be provided in a variety of different ways. These include verbal feedback, providing descriptive information about an error or information on how to improve the performance, visual feedback using mirrors, video, etc, and enhanced kinesthetic information using biofeedback of muscle activity with electromyography (EMG) (Fig. 7.11),

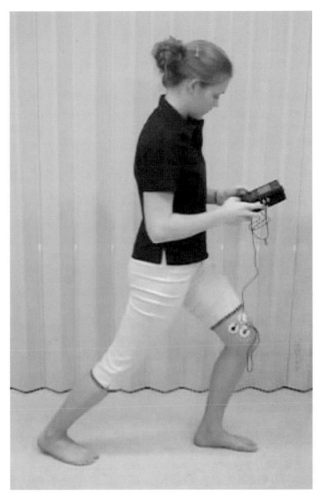

Figure 7.11 Augmented feedback. In order to provide additional feedback of contraction of vastus medialis obliquus, EMG biofeedback electrodes are placed over VMO of a patient with patellofemoral pain syndrome. Dual channel EMG could provide additional feedback of the relative activity of the medial and lateral vastii.

ultrasound or palpation of contraction, movement kinematics, or force output. All forms may be beneficial, but it is important to consider whether the learner is capable of using the selected feedback and the stage of learning.

Transfer of training

An important component of skill learning is that the performance of the skill can be transferred to different conditions in which the environment, personal characteristics or predictability are changed. In order to optimize transfer, it is considered essential to sequentially progress the task from easy to more complex situations. Transfer occurs when there are similarities in performance between tasks. In other words, specificity of practice is required to ensure transfer between environments. If the aim is to transfer a skilled movement to functional tasks, then it is necessary to progress to function. More specifically, it may be necessary to replicate sensory characteristics (e.g. limitation of visual feedback), environmental contexts (e.g. unstable surfaces, distractions) and personal contexts (e.g. anxiety, fatigue) to ensure that the elements of the skill can be transferred to specific contexts. A specific example of training transfer relates to bilateral transfer in which it is easier to learn a particular skill with one limb if it has already been learnt with the other (see Magill 2001).

Variability of practice

A goal of motor learning is that the trained task can be utilized under a variety of conditions. One method to facilitate this consistency of response is to vary environmental and personal contexts during practice (Schmidt & Lee 1999). Variability of practice aims to improve the performance of the task and enhance the ability to perform the task in novel environments. Progression may be provided by starting with practice in closed repeatable environments and progressing to complex open environments with increased levels of unpredictability.

Dosage

The ability of motor learning to change performance is influenced by the distribution of practice. Factors to consider are the frequency of training and the interval between practice sessions. Massed practice refers to few, longer sessions of practice, whereas distributed practice refers to more frequent, shorter sessions. In the literature, it is generally agreed that shorter practice sessions result in greater improvements in performance. Massed practice may lead to poorer retention and poorer performance outcome (Baddeley & Longman 1978). However, for short discrete tasks, massed practice may have additional benefits.

Mental practice

An additional tool that may lead to improvements in motor performance is mental practice. This strategy involves mental rehearsal of the task without actually moving. While it can lead to additional benefits, it is best when combined with physical practice.

Sensory learning

In addition to and in conjunction with training movement performance, strategies can be utilized to train sensation or the use of sensation to aid movement performance. A spectrum of strategies have been described in the literature that range from tasks aimed at improving sensory acuity (e.g. balance board training, joint repositioning) to training a learner to use visual or other sensory information to aid movement control. These strategies may be of critical importance when training an individual in the use of intrinsic feedback to guide movement as they would allow for accurate error detection and withdrawal of augmented feedback.

APPLICATION OF MOTOR CONTROL AND MOTOR LEARNING IN PHYSICAL THERAPY OF SPORTS AND EXERCISE-RELATED INJURIES – LOW BACK PAIN

This section will illustrate the implementation of motor learning strategies for musculoskeletal pain. One region of the body that has received extensive attention in relation to the motor control system and pain is lumbar spine pain. The spine is inherently unstable and is dependent on the contribution of muscle for its control. Obviously, the muscular contribution to stability is dependent on an efficient motor control system that can detect the status of stability and that is able to generate appropriate responses to maintain stability in the face of predictable and unpredictable challenges. It has been argued by several authors that changes in motor control may predispose to back pain, be caused by back pain and cause recurrence of back pain (Hodges & Richardson 1996, Panjabi 1992).

While there are many ways to investigate motor control of the spine, and many have been considered above, one aspect that has been investigated extensively is the problem of coordination of mobility and stability. To test this control, studies have investigated the control of the trunk muscles in association with rapid limb movements. This task provides a window to investigate one aspect of the motor control mechanism and is particularly relevant to sport as it involves a predictable and rapid limb movement. In this task, several studies have shown that there are changes in the pattern of muscle activity that is initiated prior to the onset of the movement (i.e. feedforward postural strategy) (Hodges & Richardson 1996). This change primarily involves a delay in the onset of activity of transversus abdominis, the deepest of the abdominal muscles, which has been shown to augment stability of the lumbar spine and sacroiliac joints (Hodges et al 2001b, Snijders et al 1995). On the basis of this and other evidence, clinical strategies have been developed that rely on the principles of motor learning to retrain motor control (see Richardson et al 1999).

The key element of this approach has been the identification of a specific element of motor control that is

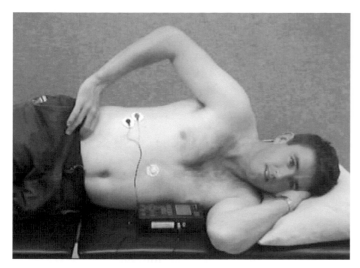

Figure 7.12 Simplification, segmentation, and augmented feedback are combined to optimize the performance of the coordinated contraction of the deep abdominal muscles in a patient with low back pain. Here the patient is performing a part task (deep muscle control) in preparation for functional training. The task is simplified by the position of the patient to reduce load. Feedback is augmented by use of tactile feedback of contraction from the fingers and EMG of the superficial abdominal muscles to reduce overactivity. The task is further simplified by having the patient perform a contraction of the pelvic floor muscle, which has been shown to trigger activation of the deep abdominal muscles.

visualization of contraction with ultrasound imaging. Part training is progressed by decreasing augmented feedback, training intrinsic feedback, improving performance and consistency, and changing the context of contraction by modifying body posture and environment. Once the performance of this movement element is improved, the program progresses to integrate other parts of the movement performance, such as the incorporation of the activation of other trunk muscles and the practice of a variety of functional tasks, including those that are pain provocative. This final stage of whole practice is progressed via practice in contexts of increasing complexity, such as exercise on unstable surfaces and open environments.

There is evidence from randomized controlled clinical trials that this approach is clinically beneficial (O'Sullivan et al 1997), and preliminary evidence that the clinical outcome is linked to the change in motor control strategy (Jull et al 1998). Thus, there is preliminary evidence that the motor relearning strategy can lead to changes in the preplanned postural component associated with movement of the limbs.

problematic (i.e. loss of tone, early activation of the deep intrinsic spinal muscles). In line with motor learning theory, outlined above, the training program involves segmentation and simplification (Fig. 7.12). First, movement is broken into parts and the deep muscle activation is trained as a *part* of the movement. Second, the performance of this maneuvre is simplified by positioning the patient to increase the ease of contraction of the muscle. Techniques to reduce or enhance activation of muscles involved in this task, and feedback of contraction, are augmented by palpation, observation or, in special cases,

SUMMARY

Motor control and motor learning are important elements in the management of pain and injury associated with sport and physical activity. Recent research has highlighted the incidence and extent of deficits in motor control that are present in the sporting population. Increasing numbers of clinical trails have been conducted to investigate the efficacy of motor learning techniques in the treatment of pain and reduction of injury recurrence. Future work is likely to lead to further developments in this field.

REFERENCES

Baddeley A D, Longman D J A 1978 The influence of length and frequency of training session on the rate of learning to type. Ergonomics 21:627–635

Bergmark A 1989 Stability of the lumbar spine. A study in mechanical engineering. Acta Orthopedica Scandinavica 60:1–54

Bernstein N 1967 The co-ordination and regulation of movements. Pergamon Press, Oxford

Brumagne S, Cordo P, Lysens R et al 2000 The role of paraspinal muscle spindles in lumbosacral position sense in individuals with and without low back pain. Spine 25:989–994

Bullock-Saxton J E 1994 Local sensation changes and altered hip muscle function following severe ankle sprain. Physical Therapy 74:17–28

Byl N N, Sinnott P L 1991 Variations in balance and body sway in middle-aged adults: subjects with healthy backs compared with subjects with low back dyfunction. Spine 16:325–330

Carpenter J E, Blasier R B, Pellizzon G G 1998 The effects of muscle fatigue on shoulder joint position sense. American Journal of Sports

Medicine 26:262–265

Collins D F, Refshauge K M, Gandevia S C 2000 Sensory integration in the perception of movements at the human metacarpophalangeal joint. Journal of Physiology 529:505–515

Cowan S, Bennell K, Hodges P et al 2001 Delayed onset of electromyographic activity of vastus medialis obliquus relative to vastus lateralis in subjects with patellofemoral pain syndrome. Archives of Physical Medicine and Rehabilitation 82:183–189

Derbyshire S W, Jones A K, Gyulai F et al 1997 Pain processing during three levels of noxious stimulation produces differential patterns of central activity. Pain 73:431–445

Ekholm J, Eklund G, Skoglund S 1960 On reflex effects from knee joint of cats. Acta Physiologica Scandinavica 50:167–174

Farfan H F 1973 Mechanical disorders of the low back. Lea and Febiger, Philadelphia, PA

Fitts P M, Posner M I 1967 Human performance. Brooks/Cole, Belmont, CA

Fitzpatrick R, Burke D, Gandevia S C 1996 Loop gain of reflexes controlling human standing measured with the use of postural and vestibular disturbances. Journal of Neurophysiology 76:3994–4008

Forwell L A, Carnahan H 1996 Proprioception during manual aiming in individuals with shoulder instability and controls. Journal of Orthopaedic and Sports Physical Therapy 23:111–119

Gahéry Y, Massion J 1981 Co-ordination between posture and movement. Trends in Neurosciences 4:119–202

Gandevia S C, McCloskey D I, Burke D 1992 Kinaesthetic signals and muscle contraction. Trends in Neurosciences 15:62–65

Garn S N, Newton R A 1988 Kinesthetic awareness in subjects with multiple ankle sprains. Physical Therapy 68:1667–1671

Garsden L R, Bullock-Saxton J E 1999 Joint reposition sense in subjects with unilateral osteoarthritis of the knee. Clinical Rehabilitation 13:148–155

Gentile A M 1987 Skill acquisition: action, movement and neuromuscular processes. In: Carr J H, Shephard R B, Gordon J et al (eds) Movement and science: foundations for physical therapy in rehabilitation. Aspen Publishers, Gaithersburg, MD

Goff B 1972 The application of recent advances in neurophysiology to Miss M. Rood's concept of neuromuscular facilitation. Physiotherapy 58:409–415

Grillner S 1981 Control of locomotion in bipeds, tetrapods, and fish. In: Brookhart M, Mountcastle V B (eds) Handbook of physiology – the nervous system. Motor control, vol ii, part 2. American Physiological Society, Washington, DC

Gurfinkel V S, Kots Y M, Paltsev E I et al 1971 The compensation of respiratory disturbances of erect posture of man as an example of the organisation of interarticular interaction. In Gelfard I M, Gurfinkel V S, Formin S V et al (eds) Models of the structural functional organisation of certain biological systems. MIT Press, Cambridge, MA

Hides J A, Stokes M J, Saide M et al 1994 Evidence of lumbar multifidus muscle wasting ipsilateral to symptoms in patients with acute/subacute low back pain. Spine 19:165–177

Hodges P 2001 Changes in motor planning of feedforward postural responses of the trunk muscles in low back pain. Experimental Brain Research 141:261–266

Hodges P W, Richardson C A 1996 Inefficient muscular stabilisation of the lumbar spine associated with low back pain: a motor control evaluation of transversus abdominis. Spine 21:2640–2650

Hodges P W, Richardson C A 1997 Feedforward contraction of transversus abdominis is not influenced by the direction of arm movement. Experimental Brain Research 114:362–370

Hodges P W, Cresswell A G, Thorstensson A 1999 Preparatory trunk motion accompanies rapid upper limb movement. Experimental Brain Research 124:69–79

Hodges P, Moseley G, Gabrielsson A et al 2001a Acute experimental pain changes postural recruitment of the trunk muscles in pain-free humans. Society for Neuroscience Abstracts 27 (304):13

Hodges P W, Eriksson A E M, Shirley D et al 2001b Lumbar spine stiffness is increased by elevation of intra-abdominal pressure. In: Proceedings of the International Society for Biomechanics. Zurich, Switzerland

Hodges P, Gurfinkel V S, Brumagne S et al 2002 Coexistence of stability and mobility in postural control: evidence from postural compensation for respiration. Experimental Brain Research, 144:293–302

Hopper D, Allison G, Fernandes N et al 1998 The reliability of the peroneal latency in normal ankles. Clinical Orthopaedics and Related Research 350:159–165

Horak F B 1987 Clinical measurement of postural control in adults. Physical Therapy 67:1881–1885

Horak F, Nashner L M 1986 Central programming of postural movements: adaptation to altered support-surface configurations. Journal of Neurophysiology 55:1369–1381

Hugon M, Massion J, Weisendanger M 1982 Anticipatory postural changes induced by active unloading and comparison with passive unloading in man. Pflügers Archives 393:292–296

Janda V 1978 Muscles, central nervous motor regulation and back problems. In: Korr I M (ed) The neurobiologic mechanisms in manipulative therapy. Plenum Press, New York

Johansson H, Sjolander P, Sojka P 1991 A sensory role for the cruciate ligaments. Clinical Orthopaedics and Related Research 268:161–178

Jull G A, Scott Q, Ricardson C et al 1998 New concepts for the control of pain in the lumbopelvic region. In: Vleeming A, Mooney V, Tilscher H et al (eds) Proceedings of the Third Interdisciplinary World Congress on Low Back and Pelvic Pain. Vienna, Austria

Kelso J A S 1984 Phase transitions and critical behaviour in human bimanual coordination. American Journal of Physiology: Regulatory, Integrative, and Comparative Physiology 15:R1000–1004

Keshner E A 1990 Controlling stability of a complex movement system. Physical Therapy 70:844–854

Kleinrensink G J, Stoeckart R, Meulstee J et al 1994 Lowered motor conduction velocity of the peroneal nerve after inversion trauma. Medicine and Science in Sports and Exercise 26:877–883

Lindgren K A, Sihvonen T, Leino E et al 1993 Exercise therapy effects on functional radiographic findings and segmental electromyographic activity in lumbar spine instability. Archives of Physical Medicine and Rehabilitation 74:933–939

Lofvenberg R, Karrholm J, Sundelin G et al 1995 Prolonged reaction time in patients with chronic lateral instability of the ankle. American Journal of Sports Medicine 23:414–417

Ludewig P M, Cook T M 2000 Alterations in shoulder kinematics and associated muscle activity in people with symptoms of shoulder impingement. Physical Therapy 80:276–291

Lund J P, Donga R, Widmer C G et al 1991 The pain-adaptation model: a discussion of the relationship between chronic musculoskeletal pain and motor activity. Canadian Journal of Physiology and Pharmacology 69:683–694

Luoto S, Hurri H, Alaranta H 1995 Reaction time in patients with chronic low back pain. European Journal of Physical Medicine and Rehabilitation 5:47–50

Luoto S, Aalto H, Taimela S et al 1998 One-footed and externally disturbed two-footed postural control in patients with chronic low back pain and healthy control subjects. A controlled study with follow-up. Spine 23:2081–2089

Luoto S, Taimela S, Hurri H et al 1999 Mechanisms explaining the association between low back trouble and deficits in information processing. A controlled study with follow-up. Spine 24:255–261

McNulty P A, Turker K S, Macefield V G 1999 Evidence for strong synaptic coupling between single tactile afferents and motoneurones supplying the human hand. Journal of Physiology 518:883–893

Magill R A 2001 Motor learning: concepts and applications. McGraw-Hill, New York

Magill R A, Schoenfelder-Zohndi B 1996 A visual model and knowledge of performance as sources of information for learning a rhythmic gymnastics skill. International Journal of Sport Psychology 27:7–22

Magnusson M, Aleksiev A, Wilder D et al 1996 Sudden load as an aetiologic factor in low back pain. European Journal of Physical Medicine and Rehabilitation 6:74–81

Massion J 1992 Movement, posture and equilibrium: interaction and coordination. Progress in Neurobiology 38:35–56

Nashner L M 1977 Fixed patterns of rapid postural responses among leg muscles during stance. Experimental Brain Research 30:13–24

Naylor J, Briggs G 1963 Effects of task complexity and task organisation on the relative efficiency of part and whole training methods. Journal of Experimental Psychology 65:217–244

O'Sullivan P B, Twomey L T, Allison G T 1997 Evaluation of specific stabilizing exercise in the treatment of chronic low back pain with radiologic diagnosis of spondylolysis or spondylolisthesis. Spine 22:2959–2967

Panjabi M M 1992 The stabilizing system of the spine. Part i. Function, dysfunction, adaptation, and enhancement. Journal of Spinal Disorders 5:383–389

Pedersen J, Sjolander P, Wenngren B I et al 1997 Increased intramuscular concentration of bradykinin increases the static fusimotor drive to muscle spindles in neck muscles of the cat. Pain 70:83–91

Powers C, Landel R, Perry J 1996 Timing and intensity of vastus muscle activity during functional activities in subjects with and without patellofemoral pain. Physical Therapy 76:946–955

Radebold A, Cholewicki J, Panjabi M M et al 2000 Muscle response pattern to sudden trunk loading in healthy individuals and in patients with chronic low back pain. Spine 25:947–954

Radebold A, Cholewicki J, Polzhofer G K et al 2001 Impaired postural control of the lumbar spine is associated with delayed muscle response times in patients with chronic idiopathic low back pain. Spine 26:724–730

Recanzone G H, Merzenich M M, Jenkins W M et al 1992 Topographic reorganization of the hand representation in cortical area 3b owl monkeys trained in a frequency-discrimination task. Journal of Neurophysiology 67:1031–1056

Refshauge K M, Kilbreath S L, Raymond J 2000 The effect of recurrent ankle inversion sprain and taping on proprioception at the ankle. Medicine and Science in Sports and Exercise 32:10–15

Richardson C A, Jull G A, Hodges P W et al 1999 Therapeutic exercise for spinal segmental stabilisation in low back pain: scientific basis and clinical approach. Churchill Livingstone, Edinburgh

Sahrman S 2002 Diagnosis and treatment of movement impairment syndromes. Mosby, St Louis MO

Schmidt R A, Lee T D 1999 Motor control and learning: a behavioural emphasis. Human Kinetics, Champaign, IL

Shirado O, Ito T, Kaneda K et al 1995 Flexion-relaxation phenomenon in the back muscles. A comparative study between healthy subjects and patients with chronic low back pain. American Journal of Physical Medicine and Rehabilitation 74:139–144

Shumway-Cooke A, Woollacott M H 1995 Motor control. Williams and Wilkins, Baltimore

Snijders C J, Vleeming A, Stoeckart R et al 1995 Biomechanical modelling of sacroiliac joint stability in different postures. Spine: State of the Art Reviews 9:419–432

Spencer J D, Hayes K C, Alexander I J 1984 Knee joint effusion and quadriceps reflex inhibition in man. Archives of Physical Medicine and Rehabilitation 65:171–177

Stokes M, Young A 1984 The contribution of reflex inhibition to arthrogenous muscle weakness. Clinical Science 67:7–14

Taimela S, Kujala U M 1992 Reaction times with reference to musculoskeletal complaints in adolescence. Perceptual and Motor Skills 75:1075–1082

Taimela S, Kankaanpaa M, Luoto S 1999 The effect of lumbar fatigue on the ability to sense a change in lumbar position. A controlled study. Spine 24:1322–1327

Takala E, Viikari-Juntura E 2000 Do functional tests predict low back pain? Spine 2:2126–2132

Taub E, Berman A J 1968 Movement and learning in the absence of sensory feedback. In: Freedman S J (ed) The neurophysiology of spatially oriented behaviour. Dorsey Press, Homewood, IL

Valeriani M, Restuccia D, Di Lazzaro V et al 1999 Inhibition of the human primary motor area by painful heat stimulation of the skin. Clinical Neurophysiology 110:1475–1480

Wadsworth D J, Bullock-Saxton J E 1997 Recruitment patterns of the scapular rotator muscles in freestyle swimmers with subacromial impingement. International Journal of Sports Medicine 18:618–624

Warner J J, Lephart S, Fu F H 1996 Role of proprioception in pathoetiology of shoulder instability. Clinical Orthopaedics 330:5–39

Wilder D G, Aleksiev A R, Magnusson M L et al 1996 Muscular response to sudden load. A tool to evaluate fatigue and rehabilitation. Spine 21:2628–2639

Winter D A, Patla A E, Prince F et al 1998 Stiffness control of balance in quiet standing. Journal of Neurophysiology 80:1211–1221

Zedka M, Prochazka A, Knight B et al 1999 Voluntary and reflex control of human back muscles during induced pain. Journal of Physiology 520:591–604

8

Pain

Gregory S Kolt

INTRODUCTION

Involvement in sport and exercise carries with it a risk of injury and resultant pain. More specifically, pain in sport can be associated with routine performance of sport skills (e.g. tackles in contact sports, or the extreme physical demands of endurance activities), minor postexercise soreness, sudden severe injury, chronic pathologies, or even some usual components of treatment and rehabilitation.

Pain is a debilitating and pervasive obstacle to effective injury rehabilitation in athletes (Taylor & Taylor 1998). As pain is so poorly understood, physical therapists tend to spend too little time educating athletes about pain and the myriad of ways it can affect them, and how they can manage it within the confines of their rehabilitation and training programs. Pain, and the physiological and psychological responses it evokes, can greatly inhibit rehabilitation progress if not dealt with adequately.

The experience of pain by athletes varies greatly, as does the way pain is communicated by behaviors. As a result, the measurement and quantification of pain is difficult, and at best, it can be relatively scaled, qualified or described. This difficulty in quantification makes the study of pain processes a challenge. However, an understanding of the biological and psychological mechanisms of the pain process and their interdependence is required.

Practitioners involved in the physical therapies as they relate to sport and exercise play an integral role in assisting athletes in coping with and managing pain. Therefore, a thorough knowledge of the biopsychology of pain, pain theories, the meaning of pain to athletes, and pain management strategies is essential for physical therapists in designing appropriate interventions.

This chapter will provide practitioners involved in the physical therapies with a background on the mechanisms of pain, theories of pain, methods used in the assessment of pain, and the management of pain. It should be noted that it is not the aim of this chapter to provide a detailed complex discussion of the neurophysiological aspects of pain.

MECHANISMS OF PAIN

The most common definition of pain in the musculo-skeletal literature has been the one adopted by the International Association for the Study of Pain (IASP), which is that pain is an unpleasant sensory and emotional experience associated with actual or potential tissue damage or described in terms of such damage (IASP 1986). This definition is widely accepted for research and clinical purposes, as it acknowledges that pain is a psychological, as well as physical, experience. The IASP (1986) definition will be used to describe the phenomenon of pain throughout this chapter.

NOCICEPTORS

The sensation, transmission, and perception of pain are the function of the nociceptive system of the nervous network. The process of nociception involves four processing components: transduction, transmission, modulation, and perception (Heil & Fine 1999). Transduction involves the translation of noxious stimuli into electrical activity at the sensory nerve endings. During transmission, the transduced electrical impulses are propagated throughout the sensory nervous system. Within the modulation phase, the nociceptive transmission is modified by several neural influences, including central, cortical, and peripheral sensory inputs. The fourth process, perception, describes the cognitive-emotional experience of pain from the resultant transduction, transmission, and modulation (Heil & Fine 1999).

The nociceptors usually have a threshold of excitation too high to be stimulated by normal innocuous stimuli, and their primary function is to monitor the body for noxious stimuli (Charman 1994). Their activation, and subsequent input of nociceptive impulses into the central nervous system (CNS), ensures rapid, non-conscious, aversive reflex responses. Noxious stimuli are carried predominantly by small myelinated alpha-delta (A-δ) fibers and unmyelinated C fibers.

There are three main types of nociceptors: unimodal, bimodal, and polymodal (Charman 1994). The unimodal nociceptors (predominantly A-δ) are mechanosensitive or thermosensitive, and respond to sharp mechanical pressure or tissue temperatures of 45°C or more respectively. The bimodal nociceptors (mainly A-δ mechano-heat receptors) also respond to mechanical and thermal stimulation, or a combination of both (Campbell & Meyer 1986). The majority of receptors are polymodal

(C fibers). These nociceptors react to mechanical, thermal, or chemical stimulation. These three categories of nociceptors apply at the cutaneous level and deeper levels (e.g. joint structures) (Charman 1994).

SPINAL CORD

The unmyelinated C fibers unite forming a single nerve fiber that enters the peripheral nerve sheath before reaching the dorsal root ganglion. The A-δ fibers travel as individual myelinated fibers to the dorsal root ganglion. As both of these fiber types enter the dorsal root of the spinal cord, they separate, with the myelinated fibers forming the dorsomedial bundle and the unmyelinated fibers forming the anterolateral bundle (Fig. 8.1) (Fitzgerald 1989).

There are several ascending nociceptive pathways or tracts that transmit pain sensations from the spinal cord to the brain (Smith 1976). In particular, the lateral and anterior spinothalamic tracts of the spinal cord receive the axons that have crossed into the grey commissure and transport the impulses to the thalamus where they terminate (Mehler 1962). The spinothalamic tract carries sharp, discriminatory, and spatial pain stimuli, predominantly of A-δ origin. There are also several more diffuse ascending pathways that carry multisynaptic unmyelinated and thinly myelinated fibers (Charman 1994).

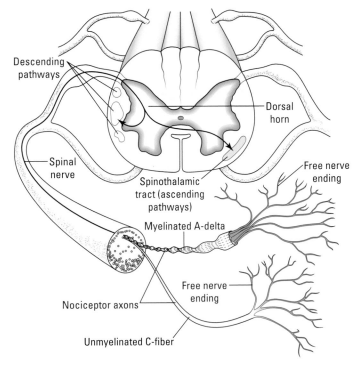

Figure 8.1   The spinal cord and peripheral nociceptors: Pain transmission fibers from the periphery enter the central nervous system via the dorsal root and synapse within the dorsal horns of the spinal cord. (Reproduced from Heil 1993 with the permission of Human Kinetics and Perry G Fine MD.)

THEORETICAL PERSPECTIVES OF PAIN

An understanding of the theoretical perspectives of pain is important in implementing pain management strategies. The two most widely accepted theoretical conceptualizations of pain and the role that psychological factors play in the experience of pain are the gate control theory of pain (Melzack & Wall 1965, Melzack 1986) and the parallel processing model of pain distress (Leventhal & Everhart 1979).

GATE CONTROL THEORY OF PAIN

The gate control theory of pain has been viewed as a breakthrough in neurophysiological approaches to understanding pain, and conceptually, it is still the most comprehensive and relevant of all pain theories for understanding the cognitive aspects of pain (Weisenberg 1999). The primary assumption in the gate control theory is that the substantia gelatinosa of the dorsal horns of the spinal cord contains a neural mechanism that acts as a pain gate (Melzack 1973, 1990, Melzack & Wall 1965). This gate can control (increase or decrease) the flow of nerve impulses from peripheral nerves of the CNS using the reciprocal activity of the large diameter A-β and the

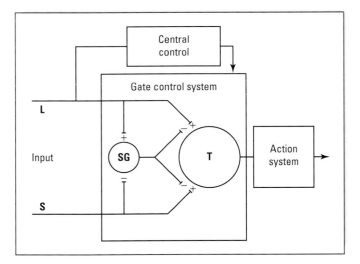

Figure 8.2 Schematic representation of the gate control theory of pain mechanisms: L = large diameter fibers; S = small diameter fibers; + = excitation; – = inhibition. The fibers project to the substantia gelatinosa (SG) and first central transmission (T) cells. The inhibitory effect exerted by the SG on the afferent fiber terminals is increased by activity in L fibers and decreased by activity in S fibers. The central control trigger is represented by a line running from the large fiber system to the central control mechanisms; these mechanisms, in turn, project back to the gate control system. The T cells project to the entry cells of the action system. (Reproduced with permission from Melzack R, Wall P D 1965 Pain mechanisms: A new theory. Science 150: 971–979. Copyright 1965 American Association for the Advancement of Science.)

small diameter A-δ and C fibers, and the influence from the cortex via the descending pyramidal and extrapyramidal tracts. When the amount of information that passes through the gate exceeds a critical level, the neural mechanisms responsible for pain experience and control are activated. The A-β fibers can depolarize the intermedullary afferent terminals and close the gate. Thus, the effectiveness of the excitatory synapses is lowered and the experience of pain is decreased (Fig. 8.2).

PARALLEL PROCESSING MODEL OF PAIN DISTRESS

The parallel processing model of pain distress suggests that pain can be processed along two pathways: informational or emotional, focusing on the psychosocial influences that affect the pain experience (Leventhal and Everhart 1979). The informational pathway focuses on issues such as location of pain, cause of pain, and the sensory characteristics of the pain. The emotional pathway in this model produces particular emotional responses to pain (e.g. distress, avoidance, fear) and a generalized state of arousal. It is apparent that, from their historical experiences of pain, individuals develop schemata that include both informational and emotional components of painful events. Thus, when subsequent episodes of pain occur, the experience of the pain will be determined by aspects of the pain schemata activated (Taylor & Taylor 1998). The main function of these schemata in the processing of pain is in the selection of what people attend to when experiencing pain (Leventhal & Everhart 1979). Their research showed that when people focus on informational elements of pain, they experience significantly less pain than when they focus on its emotional aspects. This information has important clinical implications for implementing pain management techniques.

EXPERIENCE OF PAIN

DESCRIPTIONS OF PAIN

It has been suggested that three different forms of pain can be distinguished on a temporal basis (Melzack & Dennis 1980), and that each of these is associated with distinct affective states (Craig 1994). These forms of pain are phasic, acute, and chronic. In addition, Crue (1983) described subacute pain and recurrent acute pain. It should be noted that pain is not always the immediate consequence of injury; in fact, substantial proportions of people report that pain emerged some time after the injury itself (Wall 1979).

Phasic pain

Phasic pain is of short duration and suggests an immediate impact of injury onset (Craig 1994). This usually involves reflexive withdrawal, protective movements, and non-verbal and expressive behaviors that are recognizable as pain to onlookers (Craig et al 1992). The main biological function of acute pain may be to trigger recuperative behavior rather than to indicate physical danger (Weisenberg 1999). This initial reaction to physical injury is subject to modulation dependent on the biological, physical, and social context in which it occurs.

Acute pain

Acute pain is caused by tissue damage and comprises of a phasic state as well as a continued tonic state that persists until healing takes place (Craig 1994). Acute pain is usually associated with a well-defined cause (Elton 1995). It has been suggested that acute pain, biochemically, is similar to an anxiety state, such that excessive activity of the sympathetic nervous system is evident, and feelings of anxiety and fear surface (Elton 1995). Weisenberg (1999) reported that the contradictory findings regarding the pain–anxiety relationship could be due to inconsistencies in pain definitions between studies, a variable response bias due to people's willingness to complain of pain when anxious, and the moderating role that attention has on both pain and anxiety (Crombez et al 1998). The other complicating factor in examining the pain–anxiety relationship is that of causality; that is, do high levels of anxiety impact on pain perception, or do pain levels affect anxiety?

From a clinical perspective, while physical therapists typically report anxiety to be linked to acute pain, it is also recognized as an integral part of the emotional reactions to chronic pain.

Chronic pain

In chronic pain, the tonic component that begins after the phasic component is over can persist long after healing of the injurious event. Heil (1993) summarized chronic pain well by describing it as long-lasting and constant, persisting long after the initial injury, and comprising physical, psychological, and social components. Some researchers and professional organizations have adopted a rather simplistic approach to describing chronic pain. The American Medical Association (1988) described chronic pain as a syndrome in which pain has persisted beyond the normal time of healing, while the IASP (1986) refers to chronic pain as one which is constant or recurring in nature, and that has endured for longer than 3 months. Despite semantic differences in definitions,

chronic pain involves a prolonged time course, with the likelihood of anxiety, depression, and social dysfunction increasing, the longer the pain persists (Craig 1994).

The difficulty in deciding when acute pain becomes chronic is a dilemma faced by all physical therapy practitioners. Although the term 'chronic pain' suggests an obligate temporal difference, more than just the length of time from onset distinguishes these two types of pain. It has been reported that acute pain can lead to CNS changes in the dorsal horn that outlast the nociceptive input from the periphery (Loeser 1996). The affective responses to perceived noxious stimuli may be related to individual genetics, past pain experiences, mood, or interpretation of the meaning of pain to generate and perpetuate long-term pain (Shipton 1999).

A particular aspect of chronic pain is depression, which may range from minor to clinical depression. Symptoms such as depressed mood, sleep disturbances, concentration difficulties, loss of interest, and appetite changes are common in chronic pain (Sullivan et al 1995). Despite attempts to explain the causal relationship between depression and pain, no definitive model is evident. Examples of suggested theoretical explanations include biomedical theories, psychodynamic theories, and those based on past experiences. For example, Eich et al (1990) suggested that pain, by increasing unpleasant effect, promotes access to memories and thoughts of previous unpleasant events. The negative cognitions, in turn, intensify the negative affect and perpetuate pain. Biomedical theories suggest that pain and depression share common biological systems (Magni 1987). From a psychodynamic perspective, patients with chronic pain and those who are depressed both have an inability to modulate or express intense unacceptable feelings (Beutler et al 1986).

Subacute pain

Subacute pain is similar to acute pain in relation to etiological and nociceptive mechanisms, and refers to pain that is evident regularly but not on a constant basis (e.g. daily pain for several weeks) (Crue 1983).

Recurrent acute pain

Recurrent acute pain has been described as the acute exacerbation of peripheral tissue pathology resulting from an underlying chronic pathology entity (e.g. degenerative joint or disk disease) (Crue 1983). Recurrent acute pain, unlike acute or chronic pain refers to discrete acute episodes that return over time. For example, daily pain for several weeks can be classified as subacute pain, whereas several time-limited pain episodes over months or years fits the description of recurrent acute pain (Thienhaus & Cole 1998). The reason for distinguishing between the various types of pain is to adopt the most beneficial management approach.

CLASSIFICATION OF PAIN

Due to the subjective nature of pain, and the wide variety of physical and psychological presentations, classifying pain is complex. However, without an accepted and commonly used method of classifying pain, communication between practitioners is difficult. The IASP (1986) developed a pain classification system based on descriptive lists of pain syndromes. In this classification system, a five-axis coding scheme is used to describe various aspects of pain:

- Axis I indicates the region of the pain (e.g. cervical region, lower limbs)
- Axis II indicates the organ system involved (e.g. musculoskeletal system and connective tissue; nervous system)
- Axis III indicates the temporal characteristics and pattern of occurrence of the pain (e.g. single episode, limited duration; continuous or nearly continuous, nonfluctuating)
- Axis IV relates to the patient's statement of pain intensity and duration since onset (e.g. mild with a duration of 1 month or less; medium with a duration of 1 month or less)
- Axis V indicates the presumed etiology (e.g. trauma, operation, burns, inflammatory)

Use of the IASP classification for chronic pain gives the practitioner vital information on the definition, anatomical location, main features, associated symptoms, laboratory findings, usual course, and potential complications for most pain problems. The system summarizes information on the physical and social disabilities, pathology, diagnostic criteria, and differential diagnoses for chronic pain conditions. Although the IASP system is detailed and provides specific definitions to encourage consistency of pain description, it is currently not in wide use (Thienhaus & Cole 1998). According to Thienhaus & Cole (1998), the IASP system has potential to be used more extensively over time because it is based on inclusion rather than exclusion criteria. Pain syndromes are diagnosed by signs and symptoms that are present, as opposed to those that are not present. Readers are referred to the original source (IASP 1986) for further information about the use of this complex pain classification system.

PAIN THRESHOLDS AND TOLERANCE

The way in which people experience pain is usually related to individual pain thresholds. There are several thresholds to pain, and distinguishing between them for clinical purposes is essential (Melzack & Wall 1996). *Sensation threshold* (or lower threshold) refers to the lowest stimulus value at which a sensation is reported. *Pain perception threshold* is the lowest stimulus at which a person reports that the stimulation feels painful. *Pain tolerance* (upper threshold) is the lowest stimulus level at which a person withdraws from the stimulus. *Encouraged pain tolerance* is the level at which the person withdraws from the stimulus after encouragement to tolerate higher levels of stimulation (Melzack & Wall 1996). According to Charman (1994) research has repeatedly shown that the majority of people have a uniform sensation threshold to recognize different stimuli. As stimulus intensity increases, most people will indicate that they initially perceive sensation at a common baseline level. It is the pain perception and pain tolerance thresholds that differ between people (Charman 1994).

The work of several researchers (e.g. Feuerstein & Beattie 1995, Melzack & Wall 1996) has led to the recognition that there is a multitude of factors (e.g. attention, anxiety, social reinforcement) that can influence an individual's perception of pain. Therefore, pain is more currently seen as consisting of sensory, affective, evaluative, cognitive, and behavioral elements (Sim & Waterfield 1997). This recognition helps explain the diversity of experiences and individual differences in pain severity.

Despite the large literature on the physical causes and treatment of injury in sport and exercise, there is a dearth of literature that has focused on the ability of athletes to tolerate and cope with the pain associated with injury and rehabilitation. Pain and discomfort are characteristics of most sport injury rehabilitation programs, and can interrupt, or in some cases terminate, treatment (Fisher & Hoisington 1993, Pen & Fisher 1994). As athletes differ in their ability to cope with pain (Gauron & Bowers 1986), their adherence to rehabilitation programs also differs. Being able to manage pain is, therefore, integral to successful completion of sport injury rehabilitation regimens. Meyers et al (2001), from a review of the literature, reported that a strong relationship between level of pain and physical/psychological dysfunction exists. Further to this, Jensen & Karoly (1991) reported that pain coping strategies were associated with the ability to function both physically and psychologically. It could be concluded, therefore, that an athlete's attitude towards pain, and the strategies used to cope with pain, will affect both sport performance and adherence to prescribed rehabilitation (Crossman 1997, Meyers et al 1993).

There is evidence that athletes have higher pain tolerance levels than non-athletes (Jaremko et al 1981, Scott & Gijsbers 1981, Tajet-Foxell & Rose 1995). Differences in pain tolerance have been found among different sports (Egan 1988). Tajet-Foxell & Rose (1995) compared pain and pain tolerance in professional ballet dancers and non-athlete control subjects using the Cold Pressor Test, a standard laboratory technique used to measure pain and pain tolerance. The most notable finding was that ballet dancers had significantly higher pain thresholds and pain tolerance thresholds than non-dancers. There are two general explanations for higher pain thresholds in athletes than non-athletes. First, compared to non-athletes, athletes have a greater exposure to physical training and increased fitness, resulting in higher levels of circulating endogenous opioids. The second explanation relates to psychological factors. As suggested by Tajet-Foxell & Rose (1995), athletes, as part of their physical training and performance, explore boundaries in relation to extreme physical activity and pain experience, giving a perception of control over the pain–physical activity interface.

Evidence also exists to show that male athletes demonstrate higher pain thresholds than do female athletes (Koltyn et al 1998, Tajet-Foxell & Rose 1995). When discussing pain tolerance, it is important to consider the sociocultural aspects of the sport and exercise environment. Wiese-Bjornstal & Shaffer (1999) referred to an attitude found commonly in sport that relates to 'acting tough' in the face of pain and injury and the unwillingness to seek out medical treatment for fear of being labeled 'weak'. In addition, the 'culture of risk' in sport (as described by Frey 1991) suggests that sport produces role pressures, and in some cases monetary inducements, to play with pain and injuries. Other cultural values inherent in sport link pain tolerance to the demonstration of masculine character, and view pain as being 'part of the game' and 'for the good of the team' (Frey 1991). These cultural values have also spread to the increasing number of females participating in competitive sport (Wiese-Bjornstal & Shaffer 1999).

Pain tolerance levels should be carefully considered when planning and implementing rehabilitation programs for athletes. Evidence exists for a positive association between pain tolerance and adherence to sport injury rehabilitation (Byerly et al 1994, Fields et al 1995, Fisher et al 1988); that is, those able to tolerate pain better tend to adhere more rigidly to their rehabilitation regimens.

From the practitioner's viewpoint, a study by Fisher et al (1993) reported that athletic trainers believed an injured athlete's ability to accept pain was important in treatment adherence.

It is also important to look more broadly than at the rehabilitation tasks themselves. Two recent studies focused on asking physical therapists what they believe differentiated athletes who cope successfully with injury from those who cope less successfully (Francis et al 2000, Ninedek & Kolt 2000). Interestingly, having a high pain tolerance was not perceived as important by physical therapists in either of the investigations (Francis et al

2000, Ninedek & Kolt 2000) or by professional athletes (Francis et al 2000) in coping with sport-related injury. It could be, that despite evidence summarized by Brewer (1998) indicating that adherence to injury rehabilitation is linked to pain tolerance levels, when the broader issues of coping with injury are considered, the impact of pain tolerance is diluted.

ASSESSMENT OF PAIN

There has been a plethora of pain assessment methods suggested in the literature, and several which are more commonly used in relation to sport and exercise injuries. Making pain tangible through the use of assessment tools ensures that pain is understood as important information that can facilitate rehabilitation (Taylor & Taylor 1998).

To effectively evaluate rehabilitation aimed at reducing pain is a challenge, as practitioners and researchers predominantly use patients' subjective interpretations of their pain to gauge or measure such changes (McDowell & Newell 1996). So that meaningful inferences can be drawn from pain measurement, the assessment on which pain measurements have been based must exhibit validity, reliability, and responsiveness (Sim & Arnell 1993). Validity refers to the ability of an instrument to measure what it purports to measure, thereby allowing meaningful information to be gained from the data. Reliability relates to the extent to which an instrument yields the same measurement on repeated uses, either by the same practitioner (intra-observer reliability), or by different practitioners (inter-observer reliability). Responsiveness refers to the capability of detecting small gradations of change that will be of clinical importance.

Measurement tools that assess the degree and quality of pain during rehabilitation include pain drawings (Ransford et al 1976), verbal rating scales, numerical rating scales, visual analog scales (Huskisson 1983), the McGill Pain Questionnaire (Melzack 1975), the Short-Form McGill Pain Questionnaire (Melzack 1987), the Sport Inventory for Pain (Meyers et al 1992), and the Pain Anxiety Symptoms Scale (McCracken et al 1992), just to mention a few. It is not the intent of this chapter to provide a review of each of these pain measures, but to highlight some of the more commonly used tools and their application to pain in sport.

VERBAL AND NUMERICAL RATING SCALES

The verbal rating scale (VRS) and numerical rating scale (NRS) are two of the more commonly used (Bolton & Wilkinson 1998) and extensively reviewed (Sim & Waterfield 1997) pain measures.

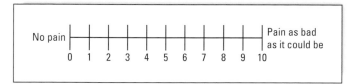

Figure 8.3 A numerical rating scale. The patient is instructed to mark the numbered vertical line as appropriate.

The VRS typically consists of a series of verbal pain descriptors that are ordered from least to most intense (e.g. no pain, mild, moderate, severe) (Jensen & Karoly 1991). This scale is scored by allocating a value of zero to the least intense descriptor, a value of 1 to the next intense descriptor word, etc. A problem in using this scale is that it lacks responsiveness (Sim & Waterfield 1997).

The NRS usually comprises a series of numbers (e.g. 0 to 10 or 0 to 100) anchored by words such as 'no pain' and 'extreme pain'. Patients choose the number that best reflects their intensity of pain (Fig. 8.3). Although this scale has the advantage of being simple, clear, and efficient, and therefore is easy to use in a clinical setting, it has been suggested that it lacks validity, as it represents only a single pain element (e.g. intensity) (Smith 1999).

The reliability of VRSs and NRSs has been demonstrated to be adequate (Melzack & Katz 1999). Responses given on measures like these do not reflect the complexity of the pain experience as well as multidimensional pain measures might.

VISUAL ANALOG SCALES

The visual analog scale (VAS) most commonly takes the form of a 10 cm horizontal line which is anchored at each end with terms representing the minimum score (e.g. 'no pain') on the left and the maximum score (e.g. 'worst ever pain') on the right (Fig. 8.4). Patients rate their pain by placing a vertical mark on the 10 cm line which corresponds to the level of pain intensity they are experiencing. A score is subsequently derived by measuring the distance in millimeters between this mark and the left-hand end of the scale. Although the reliability of the VAS has been shown to be high when repeatedly used on the same individual (Bowsher 1994), its content validity is questionable, mainly due to its ability to measure only a single aspect of pain (Sim & Waterfield 1997). As VASs

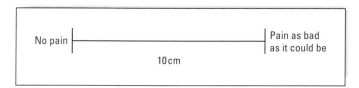

Figure 8.4 A visual analog scale for pain intensity.

have a large number of points that can be marked to reflect pain intensity, their responsiveness is high.

The advantages of using VASs include their favorable psychometric properties, ease and brevity of administration and scoring, minimal intrusiveness, and conceptual simplicity (Melzack & Katz 1999, Price et al 1983).

VASs have also been used to measure aspects of pain aside from simply intensity. For example, to measure pain affect, the patient could be asked to rate the unpleasantness of the pain experience with anchors of 'not bad at all' to 'the most unpleasant feeling imaginable' (Price et al 1987).

MCGILL PAIN QUESTIONNAIRE

The McGill Pain Questionnaire (MPQ) (Melzack 1975) is a multidimensional measure that has been recommended for its ability to describe the diverse dimensions of pain (McDowell & Newell 1996). It provides valuable information on the sensory, affective, and evaluative dimensions of pain experience and is able to discriminate among different pain problems (Reading 1984). The MPQ (Fig. 8.5) contains 20 subclasses of 78 adjectives divided among four dimensions: sensory, affective, evaluative, and miscellaneous. Patients choose one word in each category to describe their present pain. Separate scores can be obtained for each of these four dimensions in addition to a total score (Pain Rating Index [PRI]). In addition to the lists of pain descriptors, the MPQ contains line drawings of the body to record spatial distribution of the pain and words that describe the temporal properties of the pain. The final component of the MPQ is the Present Pain Intensity (PPI) scale, a number–word combination that provides an indication of the pain intensity at the time of completion of the questionnaire. The MPQ is designed to provide quantitative indices of the subjective pain experience. It is a widely used tool in both research and clinical settings and has been translated into several languages. The reliability and validity of the MPQ have been extensively researched and shown to be sound (see Melzack & Katz 1999). As the MPQ usually takes 5–10 minutes to administer (Melzack 1987), many practitioners and researchers have sought a shortened version for more regular use.

SHORT-FORM MCGILL PAIN QUESTIONNAIRE

The Short-Form McGill Pain Questionnaire (SF-MPQ) (Melzack 1987) was developed for use when the time taken to obtain information on pain is limited, and when more information than intensity is required. The SF-MPQ (Fig. 8.6) incorporates elements of the MPQ but allows for

McGill Pain Questionnaire

Patient's name _____ Date _____ Time _____ am/pm

PRI: S _____ A _____ E _____ M _____ PRI(T) _____ PPI _____
     (1–10)   (11–15)   (16)   (17–20)   (1–20)

1 FLICKERING __
  QUIVERING __
  PULSING __
  THROBBING __
  BEATING __
  POUNDING __

2 JUMPING __
  FLASHING __
  SHOOTING __

3 PRICKING __
  BORING __
  DRILLING __
  STABBING __
  LANCINATING __

4 SHARP __
  CUTTING __
  LACERATING __

5 PINCHING __
  PRESSING __
  GNAWING __
  CRAMPING __
  CRUSHING __

6 TUGGING __
  PULLING __
  WRENCHING __

7 HOT __
  BURNING __
  SCALDING __
  SEARING __

8 TINGLING __
  ITCHY __
  SMARTING __
  STINGING __

9 DULL __
  SORE __
  HURTING __
  ACHING __
  HEAVY __

10 TENDER __
  TAUT __
  RASPING __
  SPLITTING __

11 TIRING __
  EXHAUSTING __

12 SICKENING __
  SUFFOCATING __

13 FEARFUL __
  FRIGHTFUL __
  TERRIFYING __

14 PUNISHING __
  GRUELLING __
  CRUEL __
  VICIOUS __
  KILLING __

15 WRETCHED __
  BLINDING __

16 ANNOYING __
  TROUBLESOME __
  MISERABLE __
  INTENSE __
  UNBEARABLE __

17 SPREADING __
  RADIATING __
  PENETRATING __
  PIERCING __

18 TIGHT __
  NUMB __
  DRAWING __
  SQUEEZING __
  TEARING __

19 COOL __
  COLD __
  FREEZING __

20 NAGGING __
  NAUSEATING __
  AGONIZING __
  DREADFUL __
  TORTURING __

PPI
0 NO PAIN __
1 MILD __
2 DISCOMFORTING __
3 DISTRESSING __
4 HORRIBLE __
5 EXCRUCIATING __

BRIEF __	RHYTHMIC __	CONTINUOUS __
MOMENTARY __	PERIODIC __	STEADY __
TRANSIENT __	INTERMITTENT __	CONSTANT __

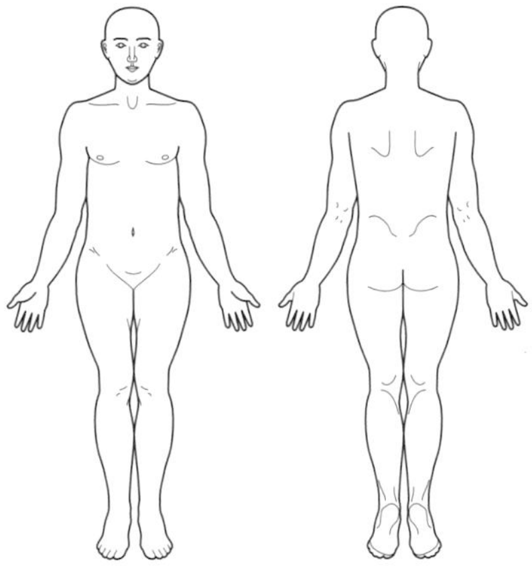

E = EXTERNAL

I = INTERNAL

COMMENTS:

Figure 8.5 McGill Pain Questionnaire. The descriptors fall into four major groups: sensory, 1–10; affective, 11–15; evaluative, 16; and miscellaneous, 17–20. The rank value for each descriptor is based on its position in the word set. The sum of the rank values is the pain rating index (PRI). The present pain intensity (PPI) is based on a scale of 0–5. (Reproduced with permission from Melzack 1975.)

Short-form McGill Pain Questionnaire
Ronald Melzack

Patient's name _____ Date _____

	NONE	MILD	MODERATE	SEVERE
THROBBING	0) _____	1) _____	2) _____	3) _____
SHOOTING	0) _____	1) _____	2) _____	3) _____
STABBING	0) _____	1) _____	2) _____	3) _____
SHARP	0) _____	1) _____	2) _____	3) _____
CRAMPING	0) _____	1) _____	2) _____	3) _____
GNAWING	0) _____	1) _____	2) _____	3) _____
HOT-BURNING	0) _____	1) _____	2) _____	3) _____
ACHING	0) _____	1) _____	2) _____	3) _____
HEAVY	0) _____	1) _____	2) _____	3) _____
TENDER	0) _____	1) _____	2) _____	3) _____
SPLITTING	0) _____	1) _____	2) _____	3) _____
TIRING-EXHAUSTING	0) _____	1) _____	2) _____	3) _____
SICKENING	0) _____	1) _____	2) _____	3) _____
FEARFUL	0) _____	1) _____	2) _____	3) _____
PUNISHING-CRUEL	0) _____	1) _____	2) _____	3) _____

No pain |————————————————————————————| Worst possible pain

PPI
0 NO PAIN   _____
1 MILD   _____
2 DISCOMFORTING   _____
3 DISTRESSING   _____
4 HORRIBLE   _____
5 EXCRUCIATING   _____

Figure 8.6   The Short-Form McGill Pain Questionnaire. The first descriptors represent the sensory dimension of pain experience and the last 3 represent the affective dimension. Each descriptor is ranked on an intensity scale of 0 = none, 1 = mild, 2 = moderate, 3 = severe. The present pain intensity (PPI) of the standard long-form McGill Pain Questionnaire and the visual analog scale are also included to provide overall pain intensity scores. (Reproduced with permission from Melzack 1987.)

a more rapid and simple acquisition of pain data. The SF-MPQ has three components: a descriptive component, the PPI, and a VAS. The main component of the SF-MPQ contains 15 descriptors (11 sensory and 4 affective) which are rated on an intensity scale where 0 = none, 1 = mild, 2 = moderate, and 3 = severe. The second component, the PPI is the same as that used in the MPQ. The third component is a VAS anchored by the terms 'no pain' and 'worst possible pain'. The PPI and VAS are included to provide indices of overall pain intensity.

Although there has been no evaluation of the reliability of the SF-MPQ, it has been shown to be correlated highly with the sensory, affective, and total PRI scores of the MPQ (Melzack 1987), and is highly sensitive to clinical changes brought about by various therapies (Melzack & Katz 1999). The SF-MPQ also has high content validity (Melzack & Katz 1992), and the inclusion of a VAS (not a component of the original MPQ) has been reported to enhance the test–retest reliability of the SF-MPQ beyond that of the MPQ (Bowsher 1994).

SPORT INVENTORY FOR PAIN

The pain assessment instruments discussed in this chapter have not been developed specifically for pain that is associated with sport and exercise injury. One questionnaire focused on sport is the Sport Inventory for Pain (SIP) (Meyers et al 1992). Although not aimed at pain intensity, the SIP was developed to identify and predict an athlete's ability to cope with pain. The SIP is a 25-item questionnaire comprising five pain subscales: coping (a measure of direct coping responses), cognitive strategies used in the face of pain, avoidance (the tendency to avoid pain-producing responses), catastrophizing (the tendency to be overwhelmed by pain), and body awareness (a measure of response style). The items are scored from 1 to 5 using a Likert-type scale anchored with 'strongly agree' and 'strongly disagree'. An example of an item from the coping scale is 'I see pain as a challenge, and it doesn't bother me', while one item from the catastrophizing scale asks athletes if they 'pray for the pain to stop'. Scores from individual items are summed up to obtain subscale scores. In addition, the first four subscales yield a composite score aimed at providing an overall index of the ability to perform athletically while in pain (Meyers et al 1992). It was reported that the SIP subscales demonstrated satisfactory test–retest reliability and internal consistency (Meyers et al 1992).

More recent research, however, challenged the integrity of the SIP. It was found that the SIP had an unstable factor structure (Bartholomew et al 1998b), and that the validity of the instrument and reliabilities of the individual subscales were poor (Bartholomew et al 1998a).

MANAGEMENT OF PAIN

The management of pain is complex and usually consists of several forms of therapy being used concurrently. Typically, approaches such as physical therapy, pharmacological therapy, and cognitive therapy are methods of choice. The complex nature of the pain experience, which can be moderated by various forms of psychosocial input, makes selection of appropriate modalities difficult. It is important, however, to focus more broadly than on the presenting signs and symptoms. Consideration of the impact of pain on the athlete, and the sport and non-sport aspects of their lives, is integral to successful rehabilitation.

Some guiding principles of management approaches to pain will be presented that focus on the physical, pharmacological, and cognitive therapies and their role in managing pain. Readers are referred to Weiner (1998a, 1998b) for a detailed account of pain management.

PHYSICAL REHABILITATION THERAPIES

The majority of patients that consult physical therapists do so, predominantly, because of a pain complaint. Rarely does a patient present complaining of poor biomechanics in their running technique. Rather, they will present with lower limb pain that, upon assessment, is linked to poor biomechanical sequencing. Thus, the physical therapist is required to attend to both the presenting pain, and the underlying cause of that pain.

There are several rehabilitation therapies that are used to manage pain. These include electrophysical agents, manual techniques, and interventions that change movement patterns thought to provoke pain.

Electrophysical agents

As outlined in Chapter 13, several electrophysical agents can provide an analgesic effect. Brukner & Khan (2001), in their review of the area, reported possible uses for transcutaneous electrical nerve stimulation (TENS), ultrasound, interferential stimulation, laser, cryotherapy, superficial heat, and high voltage galvanic stimulation in managing pain. It should be considered, however, that there is only limited evidence to support the use of these modalities in pain relief (Ellis 1998).

One of the electrophysical agents more commonly used to manage pain is TENS. When used for pain relief, TENS involves a high frequency current administered to the skin. This current selectively activates large-diameter, non-noxious fibers (A-β) and inhibits second order nociceptive transmission neurons within the CNS (Brukner & Khan 2001). Research on the efficacy of TENS in reducing pain of both an acute and chronic nature has produced conflicting findings (Ellis 1998). TENS can also be applied using high intensity, low frequency currents (acupuncture-like TENS). This form of TENS results in endorphin release within the CNS, and is often used to stimulate trigger points or acupuncture points. Research has shown that longer duration pain relief can be obtained from this form of TENS than when using the more traditional high frequency TENS (Johnson 1998).

The use of ultrasound therapy in managing pain is also common in physical therapy settings. The efficacy of ultrasound, when used for therapeutic purposes is still relatively unknown. Research that has addressed its effects has generally been poorly designed and has relied on small sample sizes, therefore making conclusions regarding efficacy difficult (van der Windt et al 1999). An adaptation of ultrasound therapy in physical therapy settings is phonophoresis, where a pharmacological agent (e.g. an analgesic) is used as a coupling medium and transferred to the superficial tissues via the thermal effect and acoustic streaming of the ultrasound (Baumert 1999). Baumert (1999) advocated that higher concentration pharmacological agents (e.g. 10% hydrocortisone) have been shown to produce the best results.

Interferential stimulation has also been suggested as a pain management therapy (Brukner & Khan 2001). Interferential stimulation involves two alternating medium frequency currents applied to the skin simultaneously. At the point where the two currents intersect, wave interference occurs, and it has an effect on pain similar to that of TENS. Little evidence exists on the efficacy of this type of electrical stimulation for pain management.

The use of laser has been increasing in physical therapy settings. It has been suggested that cold (or soft) lasers of varying intensity may, among other effects (e.g. elevation of blood cortisol levels), reduce pain. As for many electrophysical agents, the research investigating the efficacy of laser therapy has shown conflicting findings (see de Bie et al 1998).

Other modalities (although not classified as electrophysical agents) that are used extensively in physical therapy to manage pain are cryotherapy and superficial heat. Cryotherapy involves the application of ice or cold to the painful area, having the effect of decreasing conduction velocities of both motor and sensory nerves, reducing the rate of firing of muscle spindle afferents, and decreasing acetylcholine levels. These changes contribute to the reduction of pain and muscle spasm (Kaul & Herring 1994). The application of superficial heat, among other effects, can produce analgesia (Lehmann 1990).

Manual techniques

A major component of physical therapy management involves manual techniques. Such techniques involve various combinations of soft tissue massage, joint and soft tissue mobilization, and joint manipulation. Soft tissue massage is commonly used in pain management (Liston 1995) due to its effects of decreasing excessive tissue tension associated with activated mechanical nociceptors, and by aiding the removal of the chemical substances in soft tissue that activate chemical nociceptors (Brukner & Khan 2001). Soft tissue massage can also, according to the gate control theory of pain, reduce pain by stimulating the large, rapidly conducting nerve fibers through selectively closing the gate against the smaller pain fiber input (Arnheim & Prentice 2000).

Manual techniques that address myofascial trigger points are commonly used in pain management. The initial stimulation of trigger points results in impulses being sent to the CNS causing muscle contraction and vasoconstriction. The resulting increased vascular permeability and ischemia changes the extracellular environment and increases the sensitivity of nociceptors in the area (Travell & Simons 1983a). Treatment from a trigger point perspective should focus on all active and latent trigger points thought to contribute to the pain. It should also be noted that trigger points can develop secondary to the actual injurious event, simply as a result of the adaptive postures adopted (Travell & Simons 1983a). For a detailed approach to managing pain through myofascial trigger points, refer to Travell & Simons (1983a, 1983b).

Exercise

Exercise can play an important role in the management of long-term or chronic pain (Carabelli et al 1998). Several studies have shown that exercise reduces pain associated with conditions such as lumbar dysfunction and the arthritides (e.g. Silvermetz 1991). These findings are linked to suggestions that a low level of overall fitness is a contributing factor to the pathogenesis of chronic pain (Paris 1985). Carabelli et al (1998) suggested that exercise programs for pain management should include all major components of physical fitness: cardiorespiratory endurance, muscular strength, muscular endurance, flexibility, and body composition.

Exercise programs should initially address stretching, with chronic pain patients, to return muscles back to normal resting length (Carabelli et al 1998). Such stretches should focus on the muscles which, through postural changes during the pain episode, have become shortened. It should be remembered that painful stimuli could cause prolonged excitation of the spinal reflex causing continued muscle contraction (Carabelli et al 1998). In more recent times, aquatic therapy or hydrotherapy has been used as a medium to achieve many of the exercise program components. The buoyancy of the water aids the low-impact needs of many people with chronic pain. Exercise in suitably heated hydrotherapy facilities can also provide the additional benefits that superficial heat is capable of in terms of pain management (see above).

Not only does exercise provide physiological effects that can be beneficial to pain, but there may also be possible psychological mechanisms of exercise that assist pain. An early hypothesis by Bahrke & Morgan (1978) suggested that exercise distracts people from stressful stimuli (e.g. pain). Another hypothesis relates to self-efficacy theory; that is, people assess their self-efficacy in physical activities by using levels of fatigue, fitness, and pain. Therefore, as fitness increases through appropriate exercise, feelings of pain and fatigue will reduce, and self-efficacy should be increased resulting in a further desire to continue exercise (Petruzzello et al 1991). Other important effects of exercise in pain management include the reduction of stress that is so often associated with pain, and the promotion of relaxation (Shephard 1997).

PHARMACOLOGICAL AGENTS

Some form of pharmacological intervention is usually an integral and necessary component of pain management. While Chapter 28 provides details on the various forms of pharmacological agents that can reduce pain, this section will briefly describe some general principles of the use of such agents. The three common groups of drugs used in pain management in sport and exercise are analgesics, non-steroidal anti-inflammatory drugs (NSAIDs), and corticosteroids.

Analgesics are often used in the acute stage of soft tissue injuries to reduce pain. The most common forms of analgesics currently used are aspirin, paracetamol, and codeine. It should be noted, however, that the use of aspirin compounds in acute injuries is contraindicated due to their ability to inhibit platelet aggregation, which can therefore increase the bleeding associated with the injury. Paracetamol has no effect on inflammation and serves as an analgesic and antipyretic. Codeine is used in circumstances where a stronger analgesic is needed.

NSAIDs work to reduce inflammation by inhibiting cyclooxygenase and reducing the production of prostaglandins, thromboxane, and prostacyclins, all mediators of the inflammatory response (Buchanan 2000). In addition, NSAIDs have multiple other functions at a cellular level, including decreasing granulocyte and monocyte migration and phagocytosis, and displacing an endogenous anti-inflammatory peptide from plasma proteins (Buchanan 2000). Despite the widespread clinical use of NSAIDs for sport injuries, no convincing evidence exists for their efficacy in treating acute soft tissue injuries (Almekinders 1993).

Corticosteroids and their use in the treatment of sports injuries are controversial (Brukner & Khan 2001). They work by inhibiting both prostaglandin and leukotriene synthesis by blocking the action of phospholipase enzyme, which converts phospholipids in cell membranes to arachidonic acid (Buchanan 2000). Corticosteroids can be administered orally, by local injection, or by iontophoresis. The main concern with corticosteroids is with local injection and their effect on inhibiting collagen synthesis and tissue repair. Refer to Chapter 28 for an overview of the side effects and contraindications of corticosteroid use.

COGNITIVE THERAPIES

Physical therapists are becoming increasingly aware of psychosocial factors that influence injury, and are enhancing their management skills by adding a psychological dimension (Harding & Williams 1995). Due to the nature of their work, physical therapists are in an ideal situation to provide some form of basic psychological assistance to aid the injury rehabilitation process (Kolt 2000, Ninedek & Kolt 2000). Given that pain, and particularly chronic pain, has psychosocial elements, knowledge of managing pain from a cognitive perspective is imperative. Pain management approaches based on psychophysiology explore the relation between mental events and neuromuscular activity, whereby stress leads to autonomic arousal, muscle tension, and vascular changes, with a resultant influence on pain (Smith et al 2001).

The majority of psychological approaches to pain management focus around cognitive-behavioral techniques (CBTs), that is, techniques that address the patient's cognitions (thought processes) and behaviors. The techniques used include those that are aimed at reducing pain, those that address a patient's focus on their pain, and those that teach people to cope with pain. As will be evident in the following description of some relevant CBTs, there is a strong emphasis on educating patients about their pain and injury.

The cognitive-behavioral approach to managing pain is based around five assumptions (Turk & Okifuji 1999). First, individuals are active processors of information and not passive reactors. Second, thoughts can elicit and influence mood, affect physiological processes, can serve as an impetus for behavior, and can have social consequences; conversely, mood, physiological changes, environmental factors, and behavior can influence thought processes. Third, behavior is reciprocally determined by both the individual and environment factors. Fourth, individuals can learn more adaptive ways of thinking, feeling, and behaving. Finally, individuals should be active and collaborative in changing their maladaptive thoughts, feelings, and behaviors.

Taylor & Taylor (1998) categorized the non-physical and non-psychological pain management strategies as either pain reduction or pain focusing techniques. The pain reduction techniques are those that act on the nociceptive aspects of the pain, thus decreasing the amount of pain that is felt (e.g. muscle relaxation techniques). The pain focusing techniques are those that involve directing attention onto (association) or away from (dissociation) the pain as a way of reducing the pain (Taylor & Taylor 1998). Examples of pain focusing techniques include external focus, pleasant imagery, and hypnosis.

A brief summary follows of some CBTs and other psychological techniques that can be useful in the

management of pain; some techniques could fall into either category. Please note, however, that as suggested earlier in the chapter, the management of pain usually works best with several forms of therapy being used concurrently.

Reconceptualizing the pain

An essential feature of cognitive-behavioral treatment is for the patient to be able to reconceptualize the pain from being vague, undifferentiated, and overwhelming to being addressable, manageable, and controlled. This is achieved largely through education of the patient on the basis and causes of pain, and the treatment and rehabilitation program. Reconceptualization allows the patient to change their view of pain from one that is predominantly sensory in nature to a more multifaceted view with cognitive, affective, and socioenvironmental factors considered as contributors to the experience of pain (Turk & Okifuji 1999). The overall aim of this approach is to provide patients with better control over their lives, even if the pain itself cannot be completely ameliorated.

Relaxation

Several forms of relaxation exist that achieve their function by various means. Given that pain can elicit muscle tension that, in turn, restricts blood flow and further increases pain (Cousins & Phillips 1985), relaxation techniques that directly target muscle are indicated. The most common form of muscular relaxation is progressive relaxation (Jacobson 1938). Progressive relaxation involves systematically relaxing major skeletal muscle groups by firstly recognizing muscle tension present (initially achieved by contracting the muscles), then by relaxing those muscles. The role of muscle contraction before relaxation is proposed so that the patient can become sensitive to muscle tension, and therefore learn to recognize the sensations of relaxed muscle. As the patients become more familiar with the technique, they may merely relax muscle groups from whatever condition they are in at rest, rather than having to contract muscle groups first. It should be noted that divided opinion exists regarding the value of muscle contraction before relaxation (Lucic et al 1991, O'Bannon et al 1987, Payne 2000). In using progressive relaxation on patients with pain, it is important to monitor the level of muscle contraction used in the exercise so that it does not aggravate pain symptoms.

Another commonly used relaxation technique is Benson's Relaxation Response (Benson 1975). This technique is based on the proposal that there are four common elements underlying the elicitation of a relaxation response. The first element is a quiet environment, which allows for the reduction of external distractions. The second is the adoption of a comfortable position to reduce undue muscular tension. The third is an object to dwell on, such as the repetition of a word. The fourth element is a passive attitude that includes emptying all other thoughts from one's mind, and letting distracting thoughts that do return pass on while returning to a focused state. Practically speaking, the Relaxation Response is based around transcendental meditation and involves focus on breathing, repetition of a word in time with breathing, and in more recent adaptations, imagery that focuses on an object that moves in time with the patient's breathing (Kolt & McConville 2000). The Relaxation Response works by reducing the sympathetic nervous system activity that can accentuate pain (Wallace et al 1971). The Relaxation Response also serves as a distraction, drawing focus away from the pain and onto the more pleasant feeling of relaxation. It also provides a greater sense of control of pain and a reduction in the negative emotions associated with the pain and injury (Taylor & Taylor 1998).

For a more detailed account of relaxation techniques refer to Payne (2000).

Imagery

Different forms of imagery have been used in the management of pain. Imagery of pleasant situations, guided by either the practitioner or by the individual, is an internal dissociative strategy shown to be effective in reducing pain in medical and sport settings (Whitmarsh & Alderman 1993). In general, imagery involves individuals imagining themselves in a relaxing environment (i.e. an environment that has a relaxing meaning to the individual), and focusing on how it feels to be in that environment. This form of imagery aims to distract the individual from the feeling of pain. From clinical experience, the more complex the imagined scene is, and the more detail the individual is asked to attend to (i.e. using not just the sense of vision but other senses such as tactile, auditory etc.), the more they are distracted from their pain.

Specific types of imagery have also been developed. For example, in pain management imagery (Ievleva & Orlick 1999), individuals could imagine the pain being washed away or see cool colors soothing and reducing any inflammation and pain (e.g. seeing cool blue colors running through the painful area; imaging the pain leaving the body; imagining an ice-pack over the painful area). There is an increasing body of research suggesting that imagery can assist with pain and healing in athletes (Ievleva & Orlick 1999). For a more detailed discussion of the use of imagery, refer to Taylor & Taylor (1997, 1998), Ievleva & Orlick (1999), and Hall (2001).

Association and dissociation

Association involves patients focusing their attention on the pain. It has been suggested that such techniques allow patients to use the pain as important information about the extent to which they can exert themselves in rehabilitation and how far they can extend the physical limits (Taylor & Taylor 1998). Heil (1993) suggested that association methods heighten body awareness, increase perceptions of control over pain, and encourage a sense of emotional detachment by athletes. This emotional detachment, in turn, acts to separate the sensory aspects of pain from its physical manifestations. The initial association with the sensory aspects of pain produces an emotional dissociation, thereby diminishing the discomfort and perception of pain.

Dissociation, which involves directing a patient's attention away from the pain, can make pain more manageable (Fisher 1999). Such distractions could come from components of relaxation exercises, but could also come from activities like exercise, listening to music, or imagining doing other sport activities that demand deployment of attention. It has been reported that dissociation strategies are more effective for increasing pain threshold than are associative strategies (Fisher 1999). Fisher (1999) also suggested that dissociative strategies might be better in preparing athletes to cope with pain before its onset rather than after pain is present. The obvious clinical implication of this strategy is to prepare patients for painful aspects of rehabilitation.

Self-efficacy

Self-efficacy refers to the conviction that one has to successfully execute the behavior required to produce a certain outcome (Bandura 1977). For example, in an athlete with injury and pain, self-efficacy would relate to their belief that they can do something about the pain. In relation to pain, the encouragement of higher levels of self-efficacy by the physical therapist should be an underlying aspect of all communications with injured athletes during rehabilitation. As self-efficacy is an important component of sport injury rehabilitation, it will be covered in more detail in Chapter 10.

SUMMARY

Dealing with pain from sport and exercise injuries is complex. As pain is a subjective experience, two people with the same presenting injury could experience pain in very different ways. As evidence exists that athletes may have different pain sensitivities and pain tolerance levels than non-athletes, rehabilitation programs must be made specifically to cater for these differences. An understanding of the mechanisms of pain and how pain can influence adherence to rehabilitation are integral to successful rehabilitation.

The management of pain in sport and exercise goes beyond simply injury. There are aspects of normal sport participation that can evoke pain. Therefore, the pain management techniques outlined in this chapter have their place in the clinic, at home, on the training ground, and at competition. The predominant message from all the literature on pain management is that effective rehabilitation involves a combination of strategies utilizing both physical and psychosocial elements.

REFERENCES

Almekinders L C 1993 Anti-inflammatory treatment of muscular injuries in sports. Sports Medicine 15:139–145

American Medical Association 1988 Guides to the evaluation of permanent impairment, 3rd edn. American Medical Association, Washington

Arnheim D D, Prentice W E 2000 Principles of athletic training, 10th edn. McGraw Hill, New York

Bahrke M S, Morgan W P 1978 Anxiety reduction following exercise and meditation. Cognitive Therapy and Research 2:323–333

Bandura A 1977 Self-efficacy: toward a unifying theory of behavioral change. Psychological Review 84:191–215

Bartholomew J B, Brewer B W, Van Raalte J L et al 1998a A psychometric evaluation of the Sports Inventory for Pain. The Sport Psychologist 12:29–39

Bartholomew J B, Edwards S M, Brewer B W et al 1998b The Sports Inventory for Pain: a confirmatory factor analysis. Research Quarterly for Exercise and Sport 69:24–29

Baumert P W Jr 1999 Modalities in rehabilitation. In: Lillegard W A, Butcher J D, Rucker K S (eds) Handbook of sports medicine: a symptom-oriented approach, 2nd edn. Butterworth-Heinemann, Boston

Benson H 1975 The relaxation response. William Morrow, New York

Beutler L E, Engel D, Oro-Beutler M E et al 1986 Inability to express intense affect: a common link between depression and pain. Journal of Consulting and Clinical Psychology 54:652–759

Bolton J E, Wilkinson R A 1998 Responsiveness of pain scales; a comparison of three pain intensity measures in chiropractic patients. Journal of Manipulative and Physiological Therapeutics 21:1–7

Bowsher D 1994 Acute and chronic pain and assessment. In: Wells P E, Frampton V, Bowsher D (eds) Pain management by physiotherapy, 2nd edn. Butterworth-Heinemann, Oxford

Brewer B W 1998 Adherence to sport injury rehabilitation programs. Journal of Applied Sport Psychology 10:70–82

Brukner P, Khan K 2001 Clinical sports medicine, 2nd edn. McGraw Hill, Sydney

Buchanan W W 2000 Inflammation: its influences and consequences in athletes. In: Kumbhare D A, Basmajian J V (eds) Decision making and outcomes in sports rehabilitation. Churchill Livingstone, Edinburgh

Byerly P N, Worrell T, Gahimer J et al 1994 Rehabilitation compliance in an athletic training environment. Journal of Athletic Training 29:352–355

Campbell J N, Meyer R A 1986 Primary afferents and hyperalgesia. In: Yaksh T L (ed) Spinal afferent processing. Plenum Press, New York

Carabelli R A, Pertes S M, Koob K et al 1998 The role of exercise in the management of chronic pain. In: Weiner R S (ed) Pain management. A practical guide for clinicians (Vol 2), 5th edn. St. Lucie Press, Florida

Charman R A 1994 Pain and nociception: mechanisms and modulation in sensory context. In: Boyling J D, Palastanga N (eds) Grieve's modern manual therapy, 2nd edn. Churchill Livingstone, Edinburgh

Cousins M J, Phillips G D 1985 Acute pain management. Clinics in Critical Care Medicine 8:82–117

Craig K D 1994 Emotional aspects of pain. In: Wall P D, Melzack R (eds) Textbook of pain, 3rd edn. Churchill Livingstone, Edinburgh

Craig K D, Prkachin K M, Grunau R V E 1992 The facial expression of pain. In: Turk D C, Melzack R (eds) Handbook of pain assessment. Guilford Press, New York

Crombez G, Eccleston C, Baeyens F et al 1998 When somatic information threatens, catastrophic thinking enhances attentional interference. Pain 75:187–198

Crossman J 1997 Psychological rehabilitation from sports injuries. Sports Medicine 23:333–339

Crue B L 1983 The neurophysiology and taxonomy of pain. In: Brena S F, Chapman S L (eds) Management of patients with chronic pain. Spectrum, New York

de Bie R A, de Vet H C, Lenssen T F et al 1998 Low level laser therapy in ankle sprains: a randomized clinical trial. Archives of Physical Medicine and Rehabilitation 79:1415–1420

Egan S 1988 Acute pain tolerance amongst athletes. Physiotherapy in Sport 11(2):11–13

Eich E, Rachman S, Lopatka C 1990 Affect, pain, and autobiographic memory. Journal of Abnormal Psychology 99:174–178

Ellis B 1998 Transcutaneous electrical nerve stimulation for pain relief: recent research findings and implications for clinical use. Physical Therapy Reviews 3:3–8

Elton D 1995 Injury and pain. In: Zuluaga M, Briggs C, Carlisle J et al (eds) Sports physiotherapy. Applied science and practice. Churchill Livingstone, Edinburgh

Feuerstein M, Beattie P 1995 Biobehavioural factors affecting pain and disability in low back pain: mechanisms and assessment. Physical Therapy 75:267–280

Fields J, Murphey M, Horodyski M et al 1995 Factors associated with adherence to sport injury rehabilitation in college-age recreational athletes. Journal of Sport Rehabilitation 4:172–180

Fisher A C 1999 Counseling for improved rehabilitation adherence. In: Ray R, Wiese-Bjornstal D M (eds) Counseling in sport medicine. Human Kinetics, Champaign, IL

Fisher A C, Hoisington L L 1993 Injured athletes' attitudes and judgments toward rehabilitation adherence. Journal of the National Athletic Trainers Association 28:48–54

Fisher A C, Domm M A, Wuest D A 1988 Adherence to sports injury rehabilitation programs. Physician and Sportsmedicine 16 (7):47–51

Fisher A C, Mullins S A, Frye P A 1993 Athletic trainers' attitudes and judgements of injured athletes' rehabilitation adherence. Journal of Athletic Training 28:43–47

Fitzgerald M 1989 The course and termination of primary afferent fibres. In Wall P D, Melzack R (eds) Textbook of pain, 2nd edn. Churchill Livingstone, Edinburgh

Francis S R, Andersen M B, Maley P 2000 Physiotherapists' and male professional athletes' views on psychological skills for rehabilitation. Journal of Science and Medicine in Sport 3:17–29

Frey J H 1991 Social risk and the meaning of sport. Sociology of Sport Journal 8:136–145

Gauron E F, Bowers W A 1986 Pain control techniques in college-age athletes. Psychological Reports 59:1163–1169

Hall C R 2001 Imagery in sport and exercise. In: Singer R N, Hausenblas H A, Janelle C M (eds) Handbook of sport psychology, 2nd edn. John Wiley, New York

Harding V, Williams A C de C 1995 Extending physiotherapy skills using a psychological approach: cognitive-behavioural management of chronic pain. Physiotherapy 81:681–688

Heil J 1993 Psychology of sport injury. Human Kinetics, Champaign, IL

Heil J, Fine P G 1999 Pain in sport: A biopsychological perspective. In: Pargman D (ed) Psychological bases of sport injuries, 2nd edn. Fitness Information Technology, Morgantown, WV

Huskisson E C 1983 Visual analogue scales. In: Melzack R (ed) Pain measurement and assessment. Raven, New York

Ievleva L, Orlick T 1999 Mental paths to enhanced recovery from a sports injury. In: Pargman D (ed) Psychological bases of sport injuries, 2nd edn. Fitness Information Technology, Morgantown, WV

International Association for the Study of Pain (IASP) 1986 Classification of chronic pain: descriptions of chronic pain syndromes and definitions of pain terms. Pain 27:S1–S225

Jacobson E 1938 Progressive relaxation. University of Chicago Press, Chicago

Jaremko M E, Silbert L, Mann T 1981 The differential ability of athletes and nonathletes to cope with two types of pain: a radical behavioral model. The Psychological Record 31:265–275

Jensen M P, Karoly P 1991 Control beliefs, coping efforts, and adjustments to chronic pain. Journal of Consulting and Clinical Psychology 59:431–438

Johnson M I 1998 Acupuncture-like transcutaneous electrical nerve stimulation (AL-TENS) in the management of pain. Physical Therapy Reviews 3:73–93

Kaul M P, Herring S A 1994 Superficial heat and cold. How to maximise the benefits. Physician and Sportsmedicine 22:65–74

Kolt G S 2000 Doing sport psychology with injured athletes. In: Andersen M B (ed) Doing sport psychology. Human Kinetics, Champaign, IL

Kolt G S, McConville L C 2000 The effects of a Feldenkrais Awareness Through Movement program on state of anxiety. Journal of Bodywork and Movement Therapies 4:216–220

Koltyn K F, Focht B C, Ancker J M et al 1998 The effect of time of day and gender on pain perception and selected psychological responses. Medicine and Science in Sports and Exercise 30:S5

Lehmann J F 1990 Therapeutic heat and cold, 4th edn. Williams and Wilkins, Baltimore

Leventhal H, Everhart D 1979 Emotion, pain and physical illness. In: Izard C E (ed) Emotions in personality and psychopathology. Plenum, New York

Liston C B 1995 Massage. In: Zuluaga M, Briggs C, Carlisle J et al (eds) Sports physiotherapy. Applied science and practice. Churchill Livingstone, Edinburgh

Loeser J D 1996 Pain: concepts and management. 150 years on – a selection of papers presented at the 11th World Congress of Anaesthesiologists. Bridge, Rosebery, Australia

Lucic K S, Steffen J J, Harrigan J A et al 1991 Progressive relaxation training: muscle contraction before relaxation? Behavior Therapy 22:249–256

McCracken L M, Zayfert C, Gross R T 1992 The Pain Anxiety Symptoms Scale: development and validation of a scale to measure fear of pain. Pain 50:67–93

McDowell I, Newell C 1996 Measuring health: a guide to rating scales and questionnaires, 2nd edn. Oxford University Press, New York

Magni G 1987 On the relationship between chronic pain and depression when there is no organic lesion. Pain 31:1–21

Mehler W R 1962 The anatomy of the so-called 'pain tract' in man: an analysis of the course and distribution of the ascending fibres of the fasciculus anterolateralis. In: French J D, Porter R W (eds) Basic research in paraplegia. Thomas, Springfield, IL

Melzack R 1973 The puzzle of pain. Penguin, Harmondsworth

Melzack R 1975 The McGill Pain Questionnaire: major properties and scoring methods. Pain 1:227–299

Melzack R 1986 Neurophysiological foundations of pain. In: Sternbach R A (ed) The psychology of pain. Raven, New York

Melzack R 1987 The Short-Form McGill Pain Questionnaire. Pain 30:191–197

Melzack R 1990 The tragedy of needless pain. Scientific American 262:19–25

Melzack R, Wall P D 1965 Pain mechanisms: a new theory. Science 150:971–979

Melzack R, Dennis S G 1980 Phylogenic evolution of pain expression in animals. In: Kosterlitz H W, Terenius L Y (eds) Pain and society. Verlag Chemie, Weinheim

Melzack R, Katz J 1992 The McGill Pain Questionnaire: appraisal and current status. In: Turk D C, Melzack R (eds) The handbook of pain assessment. Raven Press, New York

Melzack R, Wall P D 1996 The challenge of pain, 2nd edn. Penguin, London

Melzack R, Katz J 1999 Pain measurement in persons with pain. In: Wall P D, Melzack R (eds) Textbook of pain, 4th edn. Churchill Livingstone, Edinburgh

Meyers M C, Bourgeois A E, Stewart S et al 1992 Predicting pain response in athletes: development and assessment of the Sports Inventory for Pain. Journal of Sport and Exercise Psychology 14:249–261

Meyers M C, Bourgeois A E, Murray N et al 1993 Comparison of psychological characteristics and skills of elite and sub-elite equestrian athletes. Medicine and Science in Sports and Exercise 25:S154

Meyers M C, Bourgeois A E, LeUnes A 2001 Pain coping response of collegiate athletes involved in high contact, high injury-potential sport. International Journal of Sport Psychology 32:29–42

Ninedek A, Kolt G S 2000 Sports physiotherapists' perceptions of psychological strategies in sport injury rehabilitation. Journal of Sport Rehabilitation 9:191–206

O'Bannon R M, Rickard H C, Runcie D 1987 Progressive relaxation as a function of procedural variations and anxiety level. International Journal of Psychophysiology 5:207–214

Paris S V 1985 The role of the physical therapist in pain control programs. Clinics in Anaesthesiology 13:155–167

Payne R A 2000 Relaxation techniques. A practical handbook for the health care professional, 2nd edn. Churchill Livingstone, Edinburgh

Pen L J, Fisher C A 1994 Athletes and pain tolerance. Sports Medicine 18:319–329

Petruzzello S J, Landers D M, Hatfield B D et al 1991 A meta-analysis of the anxiety reducing effects of acute and chronic exercise – outcomes and mechanisms. Sports Medicine 11:143–182

Price D D, McGrath P A, Rafii A et al 1983 The validation of visual analogue scales as ratio scale measures for chronic and experimental pain. Pain 17:45–56

Price D D, Harkins S W, Baker C 1987 Sensory-affective relationships among different types of clinical and experimental pain. Pain 28:297–307

Ransford A O, Cairns D, Mooney V 1976 The pain drawing as an aid to the psychologic evaluation of patients with low-back pain. Spine 1:127–134

Reading A E 1984 Testing pain mechanisms in persons with pain. In: Wall P D, Melzack R (eds) Textbook of pain. Churchill Livingstone, Edinburgh

Scott V, Gijsbers K 1981 Pain perception in competitive swimmers. British Medical Journal 283:91–93

Shephard R J 1997 Exercise and relaxation in health promotion. Sports Medicine 23:211–217

Shipton E A 1999 Pain. Acute and chronic, 2nd edn. Arnold, London

Silvermetz M A 1991 Clinical indications for developing a physical education and aerobic research center in a multidisciplinary pain management center. The Clinical Journal of Pain 7:37–40

Sim J, Arnell P 1993 Measurement and validity in physical therapy research. Physical Therapy 73:102–115

Sim J, Waterfield J 1997 Validity, reliability and responsiveness in the assessment of pain. Physiotherapy Theory and Practice 13:23–37

Smith A 1999 The effects of the Feldenkrais Method on pain and anxiety in people experiencing low back pain. Bachelor of Physiotherapy (Honours) thesis, La Trobe University, Melbourne, Australia

Smith A L, Kolt G S, McConville J C 2001 The effect of the Feldenkrais Method on pain and anxiety in people experiencing chronic low back pain. New Zealand Journal of Physiotherapy 29:6–14

Smith M C 1976 Retrograde cell changes in human spinal cord after anterolateral cordotomies: location and identification after different periods of survival. Advances in Pain Research and Therapy 1:91–98

Sullivan M J L, Bishop S R, Pivak J 1995 The pain catastrophizing scale: development and validation. Psychological Assessment 7:524–532

Tajet-Foxell B, Rose F D 1995 Pain and pain tolerance in professional ballet dancers. British Journal of Sports Medicine 29:31–34

Taylor J, Taylor S 1997 Psychological approaches to sports injury rehabilitation. Aspen Publishers, Gaithersburg, MD

Taylor J, Taylor S 1998 Pain education and management in the rehabilitation from sports injury. The Sport Psychologist 12:68–88

Thienhaus L, Cole B E 1998 The classification of pain. In: Weiner R S (ed) Pain management. A practical guide for clinicians (vol 1), 5th edn. St. Lucie Press, FL

Travell J G, Simons D G 1983a Myofascial pain and dysfunction. The trigger point manual. The upper extremities (vol 1). Williams and Wilkins, Baltimore

Travell J G, Simons D G 1983b Myofascial pain and dysfunction. The trigger point manual. The lower extremities (vol 2). Williams and Wilkins, Baltimore

Turk D C, Okifuji A 1999 A cognitive-behavioural approach to pain management. In: Wall P D, Melzack R (eds) Textbook of pain, 4th edn. Churchill Livingstone, London

van der Windt P A, van der Heijden G J, van der Berg S G et al 1999 Ultrasound therapy for musculoskeletal disorders: a systematic review. Pain 81:257–271

Wall P D 1979 On the relation of injury to pain. Pain 6:253–264

Wallace R K, Benson J, Wilson A F 1971 A wakeful hypometabolic physiologic state. American Journal of Physiology 221:795–799

Weiner R S (ed) 1998a Pain management; a practical guide for clinicians (vol 1), 5th edn. St. Lucie Press, FL

Weiner R S (ed) 1998b Pain management; a practical guide for clinicians (vol 2), 5th edn. St. Lucie Press, FL

Weisenberg M 1999 Cognitive aspects of pain. In: Wall P D, Melzack R (eds) Textbook of pain, 4th edn. Churchill Livingstone, London

Whitmarsh B G, Alderman R B 1993 Role of psychological skills training in increasing athletic pain tolerance. The Sport Psychologist 7:388–399

Wiese-Bjornstal D M, Shaffer S M 1999 Psychological dimensions of sport injury. In: Ray R, Wiese-Bjornstal D M (eds) Counseling in sports medicine. Human Kinetics, Champaign, IL

9

Exercise-based conditioning and rehabilitation

Rafael Escamilla   Robbin Wickham

INTRODUCTION

This chapter will present evidence for the use of exercise in injury prevention and rehabilitation. Specific areas covered will include strength and plyometrics training, interval training, endurance training, and stabilization training. Strength training has been shown to be effective in injury prevention and rehabilitation by increasing muscle, ligament, and tendon strength and size. Strength training can also increase bone strength and density, decrease the risk of osteoporosis, decrease risk of falling and subsequent injury, improve gait stability, walking speed, and efficiency, increase stair climbing and chair raising ability, and increase balance. Plyometric training is helpful in enhancing muscle strength and power, which decreases an athlete's injury risk by allowing muscles and connective tissue to absorb more energy. Interval training allows a greater volume of work to be performed compared to continuous training. Endurance training is important in enhancing the cardiovascular system, which improves overall function and enhances the rehabilitation process. Stabilization training is important in enhancing the core strength of the body.

STRENGTH TRAINING

In discussing strength training, it is important to consider the principles, types, and systems of strength training, physiological adaptations to strength training, and research evidence for employing strength training for injury prevention and rehabilitation. Strength training is an important component in sport and exercise for training, injury prevention, and rehabilitation. Research findings involving both males and females over a wide range of ages have shown that strength training, especially higher intensity training, is efficacious in minimizing injuries, maximizing performance, and

Table 9.1 Effects of strength training

Effect of strength training	Referenced evidence
Increase in muscle size, strength, and power	Bemben et al (2000) Hagerman et al (2000) Porter (2001)
Increase in neuromuscular function	Hakkinen et al (2000) Kraemer et al (1996) Taaffe et al (1999)
Increase in bone strength and density, and a decrease in osteoporosis	Granhed et al (1987) Kerr et al (2001) Weaver et al (2001)
Increase in ligament and tendon strength and thickness	Fleck & Falkel (1986) Kannus et al (1997) Zernicke & Loitz (1992)
Increase in balance, and decrease in risk of falling and subsequent injury	Gregg et al (2000) Ryushi et al (2000) Weiss et al (2000)
Increase in gait stability, walking speed, and efficiency	Carmeli et al (2000) Scandalis et al (2001) Schlicht et al (2001)
Increase in stair climbing and chair raising ability	Brill et al (1998) Chandler et al (1998) Weiss et al (2000)
Increase in hormonal adaptations	Borst et al (2001) Gorostiaga et al (1999) Kraemer et al (1999)
Decrease in blood pressure, glucose intolerance, and insulin resistance	Martel et al (1999) McLester et al (2000) Ryan et al (2001)
Decrease in body fat, an increase in fat free mass, and an increase in basal metabolic rate	Byrne & Wilmore (2001) Hagerman et al (2000) Lemmer et al (2001)
Increase in positive mood and a decrease in anxiety and tension	Beniamini et al (1997) Tsutsumi et al (1998) Tucker & Maxwell (1992)

enhancing rehabilitation. The large literature in this area has demonstrated benefits of strength training that span several different areas of human function (see Table 9.1).

PHYSIOLOGICAL ADAPTATIONS TO STRENGTH TRAINING

Research findings suggest that connective tissue growth is stimulated most effectively by moderate to higher intensity and volume (e.g. 3–5 sets of 8–12 repetitions) strength training (Stone 1988). This growth is further enhanced by using antigravity muscles and weight-bearing exercises (Stone 1988), especially for bone remodeling; however, overtraining should be avoided as it can adversely affect connective tissue rejuvenation. While connective tissue weakens with disuse, strength training increases the maximum tensile strength in connective tissue and the amount of energy that can be absorbed prior to failure (Stone 1988), thus minimizing injury risk.

Strength training can alter the mechanical principles of muscle fascia, tendons, ligaments, and bones by increasing both size and strength of these tissues (Zernicke & Loitz 1992). Several studies have shown that high intensity strength training increases bone strength by increasing bone mineral density, thereby reducing injury risk and providing protection against bone weakening processes such as osteoporosis (Kerr et al 2001, Weaver et al 2001). One study reported extremely high bone mineral content in the lumbar vertebrae in world-class powerlifters who lifted extremely heavy loads during weightbearing exercises (i.e. while performing squat and deadlift exercises) and who had very high annual training volumes (Granhed et al 1987). Although increases in bone strength occur at a much slower rate compared to increases in muscle strength (Conroy et al 1992), employing weightbearing exercises in a strength training program will maximize bone remodeling and strength gains (Stone 1988).

While optimal intensity for strengthening ligaments and tendons is not clear, studies have shown an increase in the strength and size of tendons and ligaments due to exercise (Michna & Hartmann 1989, Stone 1988). It is currently unknown if strength training has beneficial effects in increasing the thickness of articular cartilage, although weightbearing exercise has been shown to have this effect in articular cartilage tissue (Barneveld & van Weeren 1999). Since articular cartilage provides a cushion between bony surfaces of a joint, increasing articular cartilage thickness facilitates shock absorption, thereby decreasing injury potential (Barneveld & van Weeren 1999).

During the initial several weeks of a new strength training program, muscle strength is increased primarily by neural factors. These factors include increased efficiency in motor unit recruitment and synchronization, enhanced neural drive to muscles, increased neuromuscular coordination between muscles, decreased sensitivity in the golgi tendon organs (i.e. disinhibition), and motor learning effects (Hakkinen et al 2000, Kraemer et al 1996). Muscle hypertrophy and further strength increases occur sometime later (e.g. 6–8 weeks after a program begins).

PRINCIPLES OF STRENGTH TRAINING

When using overall strength training in sport and exercise, it is important to understand the principle of progressive overload, specificity, reversibility, fitness, and recovery.

Progressive overload principle

The basic premise of progressive overload is to progressively increase the load on the musculoskeletal system. Once muscles, tendons, ligaments, and bones adapt to a given stimuli, additional loads must be placed on these structures for further adaptation to occur. This is often done by small increases in load and keeping the repetitions the same, or by larger increases in load and at the same time decreasing the number of repetitions performed. The overload principle can be manipulated by varying several factors discussed below. They include exercise intensity, duration, volume, frequency, rest intervals, mode, and periodization.

Intensity

Training intensity is commonly synonymous with the amount of weight, load, or resistance being lifted or overcome; the higher the load lifted, the higher the training intensity. Intensity is most commonly expressed in terms of a percentage of an individual's one repetition maximum (1 RM). Training studies have shown that strength is maximized by employing heavy resistance between approximately 80–95% of an individual's 1 RM (Bemben et al 2000, Hagerman et al 2000, Kraemer 1997, Stone et al 1981), which equates to training between a 3 RM (heaviest weight performed for three consecutive repetitions) and 8 RM.

Training intensity can also be quantified and expressed as the power output generated while performing an exercise. Power is defined as work per unit time. Since Work = (Force)(Distance), and Speed = Distance/Time, then Power can be expressed as the product of force and speed as follows: Power = (Work/Time) = [(Force)(Distance)/Time] = (Force)(Speed). The highest power outputs recorded in sport activities occur in lifting maximum or near maximum loads during the snatch, and clean and jerk, exercises in weightlifting competitions (Garhammer 1993). These types of exercises are performed explosively, generating high force and power outputs. Explosive training with moderate to heavy loads produces maximum fast twitch fiber recruitment, which is important since the peak power output of fast twitch fibers is about four times as great as in slow twitch fibers (Faulkner et al 1986). Explosive power training, especially combined with strength training, also increases motor unit synchronization and the rate of force development (Hakkinen & Hakkinen 1995).

When using free weights or machine weights as resistance, the number of repetitions that relate to a given percentage of 1 RM is highly variable depending on the exercise employed, the muscle group being worked (smaller muscles produce fewer repetitions for a given percentage of 1 RM and larger muscles produce higher repetitions for a given percentage of 1 RM), and the training level (trained or untrained) of the individual (Kraemer 1997). Nevertheless, for trained athletes, the relationship between performing repetitions to failure and a percentage of one's 1 RM can be estimated as follows (Mayhew et al 1993):

10 RM $\approx$ 74–76% 1 RM
9 RM $\approx$ 76–78% 1 RM
8 RM $\approx$ 79–81% 1 RM
7 RM $\approx$ 81–83% 1 RM
6 RM $\approx$ 84–86% 1 RM
5 RM $\approx$ 86–88% 1 RM
4 RM $\approx$ 89–91% 1 RM
3 RM $\approx$ 92–94% 1 RM
2 RM $\approx$ 94–96% 1 RM

In addition, an individual's 1 RM can be estimated by dividing the load employed while performing a given number of repetitions to failure by the corresponding percentage of the 1 RM they are training at.

Volume

Training volume for any given exercise is determined by multiplying the total number of sets, repetitions, and load (or resistance); for example, performing 3 sets of 8 repetitions of bench press exercise with 100 kg has an exercise volume of 2400 kg (i.e. $3 \times 8 \times 100$). Typically, volume increases as intensity decreases, and volume decreases as intensity increases. For example, consider athletes who have a 150 kg 1 RM bench press; performing high intensity training for 4 sets of 4 repetitions at 90% of their 1 RM would yield an exercise volume of $(4)(4)[(0.90)(150)] = 2160$ kg. If the same athletes performed 4 sets of 8 repetitions at a lower intensity of 80% of their 1 RM, this would yield an exercise volume of (i.e. $4 \times 8 \times [0.80 \times 150]$) 3840 kg; in this example, the lower training intensity of 80% 1 RM produced 78% greater volume compared to the higher training intensity of 90% 1 RM. Since the weight is being moved through a given distance, training volume is also a measure of the total mechanical work performed during an exercise or training session.

Rest intervals and recovery

Rest intervals refer to the total rest time between repetitions, sets, and exercises for a given muscle group being worked. When training a specific muscle group, a 2–3 min rest interval between sets is common in strength training, often increasing with increasing intensities (e.g. a 4–5 min rest interval for >90% 1 RM training intensities) and decreasing with decreasing intensities (e.g. 1–2 min rest interval for 70–80% 1 RM training intensities, and a 30–60 s rest interval for 40–60% 1 RM training intensity). The increase in rest intervals with higher intensity training compared to lower intensity training is necessary in part due to the greater number of motor units recruited, a larger accumulation of lactate, and to allow complete recovery when training with near maximal loads. Also, multi-muscle, multi-joint exercises (e.g. squat, power clean, and bench press), which require a large energy expenditure, require longer rest times than single-muscle, single-joint exercises (e.g. leg extensions, leg curls, and arm curls), which have a much lower energy expenditure.

In some exercises, such as the barbell squat, it is not uncommon to rest several seconds between repetitions when training with near maximal loads, allowing the muscles to briefly rest so they will be able to contract with greater force during each repetition. This type of training allows maximum loads to be lifted for a greater number of repetitions than could otherwise be performed without the rest interval, increases the total work output accomplished during the set, and maximizes strength gains.

Rest intervals are also needed between exercise sessions in order to allow time for muscle and connective tissue to repair and regenerate from training (Pincivero et al 1997). Compared to low intensity training, high intensity training causes more muscle and connective tissue damage and requires greater time to repair and regenerate (Stone 1988). Typically, 48–72 h are needed between training sessions for muscle and connective tissue muscle to adequately recover (Stone 1988). Adequate rest and protein intake are two of the most common factors for muscle regeneration. Research has shown that a protein intake of 1.5–2 g/kg body mass is most effective in muscle regeneration after high intensity resistance training (Lemon 1998).

Larger muscles groups, such as the back and hip extensors, often require a longer rest period between training sessions compared to smaller muscle groups, especially those that move through a smaller range of motion (e.g. rectus abdominis, which may be trained daily with varying intensities and volume). A commonly employed rest interval protocol for any given muscle group is training on alternating days.

Duration

Training duration refers to the total quantity of time during resistance exercise, and will vary depending on the type of strength training that is being performed. As the number of exercises, repetitions, sets, and rest intervals increase within a session, training duration will also increase. A typical strength training session lasts between 20–60 min. Training duration also refers to the number of weeks or months a given strength training program is adhered to. A strength training program typically will last 6–12 weeks before intensity, duration, frequency or mode are modified, which is in accordance with a periodization model (Stone et al 1981, Stone 1990).

Frequency

Training frequency refers to how often an athlete engages in a strength training program. It is often expressed as total number of training sessions per week. Although strength training once per week can build or maintain strength (McLester et al 2000, Taaffe et al 1999), several studies have shown that strength gains are maximized when training consists of 2–3 sessions per week (DeMichele et al 1997, McLester et al 2000, Pollock et al 1993). Despite the evidence that performing multiple strength training sessions per week is superior in producing strength gains when compared to performing a single strength training session each week, it should be emphasized that single weekly sessions are still efficacious. The single weekly strength training session, therefore, may be preferred by individuals who have time constraints and whose goals are not to maximize strength gains.

Several studies have shown that strength gains can be maintained with as little as one strength training session per week (Taaffe et al 1999), or one training session every 2–4 weeks (Tucci et al 1992), as long as high intensity training to failure is employed. From these data it can be deduced that the intensity of training is more important than duration or frequency of training in maintaining strength gains.

For high level athletes and deconditioned individuals, it is not uncommon to split a large training session involving several muscle groups into multiple shorter training sessions throughout the week that involve only one or two muscle groups. This is referred to as split routine training. A large training session may also be split into multiple shorter training sessions throughout the day. An advantage of splitting a large training session into multiple shorter sessions is the decrease that occurs in physiological and psychological fatigue that accompanies long sessions. A split routine allows athletes to devote their full effort and intensity to each muscle group. The same principles are true for deconditioned individuals training the entire body by performing 3 sets of 8 exercises, three times per week. Individuals may elect to perform 4 upper body exercises in the morning, and the remaining 4 lower body exercises in the evening, or to perform 4 upper body exercises 1 day and the remaining 4 lower body exercises the following day.

Mode

The most common modes of strength training include resistance machines, free weights, body weight resistance, and resistance from elastic bands. There are several different types of machines now available, such as the commonly used variable resistance machines (VRM) (which often employ a cam to vary the lever arm

---

Box 9.1   Some advantages and disadvantages of machines

Advantages
- safe
- ease of use
- little knowledge of proper exercise form and technique is required
- a spotter for safety is not required
- little time to set up and change the weight is needed
- excellent muscle isolation

Disadvantages
- can be expensive
- often are heavy and bulky
- lack specificity to most movements that occur in sport due to largely single plane motion
- do not require balancing the weight while lifting through a range of motion
- do not allow for explosive training since many (e.g. the VRM) hinder acceleration
- may not offer an eccentric phase in the lift

Box 9.2   Free weights – advantages and disadvantages

Advantages
- relatively easy to use
- offer numerous multi-joint, multi-muscle exercises
- inexpensive
- take up little space (especially dumbbells)
- are more sport-specific than machines since they allow the weight to accelerate and move in multiple planes
- require more muscle activity from synergists and stabilizers in order to balance the weight, and have a large energy expenditure compared to machines
- allow both concentric and eccentric muscle movements
- allow counter movements similar to sport activities
- provide range of motions and muscle activation patterns similar to what occurs in sport
- provide endless exercise variations that can be performed
- elicit greater proprioception and coordination development compared to machines

Disadvantages
- require a greater knowledge of proper exercise form and technique than VRMs
- require more time to set up and change weights than VRMs
- are not as safe as machines
- may require a spotter for safety

---

throughout the range of motion) and several types of isokinetic machines. For a detailed discussion of the advantages and disadvantages of free weights and machines refer to Haff (2000). Some advantages and disadvantages of machines are shown in Box 9.1.

A potential advantage of the VRM is that it attempts to match muscle torques that are generated throughout a range of motion. For example, the muscle torques generated by the elbow flexor muscles during an arm curl exercise are small to begin with at full elbow extension (small muscle moment arms), progressively increase to a maximum torque of 90° elbow flexion (large muscle moment arms), and then progressively decrease as the elbow continues to flex. This is referred to as an ascending–descending muscle torque curve. The VRM attempts to match these curves by asymmetrically shaped cams in which the resistance moment arm varies throughout the range of motion. In effect, less resistance is offered at weaker joint positions and greater resistance is offered at stronger joint positions. However, studies have shown that some VRMs do not effectively match muscle torque curves of the body throughout a given range of motion (Harman 1983, Johnson et al 1990).

Free weights are also very common for strength training, and include both barbells and dumbbells. Some advantages and disadvantages of free weights can be seen in Box 9.2.

Periodization

When muscles and connective tissues are given the same stimuli for a prolonged period of time, the strength gains exhibited in these tissues begin diminishing. To continue to stimulate muscles and connective tissues, training intensities, volumes, and exercises must periodically be changed (Stone 1990). This is also important in preventing psychological staleness due to performing the same program for a prolonged period of time. Periodization is a system of training that varies training intensities and volumes throughout a year-long training cycle, referred to as a macrocycle (Stone et al 1981, Stone 1990). Periodized training has been shown to produce superior strength and power gains compared to single-set or multi-set training with a constant repetition scheme (Kraemer 1997, Kraemer et al 1997, Kraemer et al 2000, Marx et al 2001, Stone et al 2000), even when the training sets and repetitions employed have not been to failure (Kraemer et al 1997). In addition, periodization training has been shown to increase physical performance abilities in athletes (Kraemer et al 2000, Kraemer 1997).

A typical macrocycle is broken down into 3–4 mesocycles (each 3–4 months in duration), and each mesocycle can in turn be broken down into 3–4 microcycles (each 3–4 weeks in duration). A common periodization pattern for the strength athlete involves beginning a training microcycle with higher volume and lower intensities, and progressively increasing intensity and decreasing volume (Stone et al 1981). For example, consider a 4-month mesocycle comprising four microcycles of 4 weeks each. The initial 4-week microcycle could involve a higher training volume of 4 sets of 12 repetitions and a lower training intensity of 70% of 1 RM. This higher volume–lower intensity training microcycle, referred to as the preparatory phase (Stone et al 1981), will gradually allow the muscles and connective tissue to adapt to new stresses. Also, the first microcycle allows the athlete to adapt to performing new exercises that have not been performed recently, with an emphasis on proper lifting form and technique. As previously mentioned, the strength gains during this initial microcycle will primarily be due to neural factors. The second 4-week microcycle, referred to as the hypertrophy phase (Stone et al 1981), could involve training at 80% 1 RM intensity and decreasing the training volume to 4 sets of 8 repetitions. The emphasis of this cycle is on muscle hypertrophy, which research has shown to be effective when training occurs between approximately 8–10 RM (75–80% 1 RM) (Hakkinen et al 1998, Hurley et al 1995, McCall et al 1996, Narici et al 1996, Stone et al 1981). As muscles increase in size, their potential for strength also increases, since the force a muscle can generate is directly proportional to that muscle's physiological cross-sectional area (Brand et al 1986, Delp et al 2001). Compared to younger individuals beyond puberty, muscle hypertrophy occurs to a lesser extent in the elderly, who instead experience a greater period of strength gains due to neural factors (Welle et al 1996). The third 4-week microcycle, referred to as the strength phase (Stone et al 1981), could involve training at a 85–90% 1 RM intensity and decreasing the training volume to 4 sets of 4–6 repetitions. The emphasis of this cycle is on muscle strength. Upper and lower extremity, high intensity weight training studies, have demonstrated significant increases in muscle strength when training between 2–12 RM (Hagerman et al 2000, Kraemer et al 2001, Rhodes et al 2000, Taaffe et al 1999). However, many strength coaches believe that strength is maximized using multiple sets per session, multiple sessions per week, and an intensity between 2–6 RM (approximately 85–95% 1 RM). This approach is supported by data from several strength training studies (Kraemer 1997, Stone et al 1981). The final 4-week microcycle, referred to as the power phase (Stone et al 1981), could involve training at a 90–95% 1 RM intensity and decreasing the training volume to 3–5 sets of 2–3 repetitions. The emphasis of this cycle is muscle power, which research has shown is maximized in select explosive exercises (i.e. clean and jerk, power clean, snatch) while employing maximal or near maximal loads (Garhammer 1993).

Specificity principle

Muscles and connective tissue adapt specifically to the demands placed on them; this is known as the specific adaption to imposed demands (SAID) principle. For example, for muscles to hypertrophy, they have to be trained employing an optimal intensity for that specific adaptation, which as previously mentioned is approximately 70–80% 1 RM. Similarly, for muscles to maximally adapt to becoming stronger, a higher intensity should be employed (approximately 80–95% 1 RM), and for bones to increase in density and become stronger, weight-bearing exercises should be used.

In addition to applying the SAID principle to muscle and connective tissues, the SAID principle also applies to exercise selections for sport-specific movements. An example of this is the squat movement, which is specific to jumping in basketball. The squat is also sport-specific for American football, since it develops the largest and most powerful muscles of the body (i.e. gluteals, quadriceps, hamstrings, and erector spinae), which are important in both sprinting and jumping. In addition, an incline bench press follows a path that is more sport-specific to the shot-put in comparison to the flat bench press. Moreover, while the power clean is a sport-specific movement to several positions in American football, it is not a sport-specific movement for overhand throwing and hitting in baseball, and could potentially have deleterious effects.

Reversibility principle

Strength gains are transient and reversible with disuse, with further losses in strength due to disuse occurring at a greater rate than gains in strength due to training (Bloomfield 1997). However, as previously outlined, strength gains can be maintained with as little as one strength training session per week (Taaffe et al 1999) as long as high intensity training is employed.

Fitness principle

Unfit individuals achieve strength gains at a faster rate than trained individuals, but also lose strength due to disuse at a faster rate than trained individuals (Bloomfield 1997). As discussed previously, the initial strength gains experienced by unfit individuals are largely due to neural factors such as increased neuromuscular coordination between muscles and decreased sensitivity in the golgi tendon organs.

TYPES OF STRENGTH TRAINING

Isometric training

Isometric training occurs when tension develops in the muscle without a change in muscle length. Isometric training reached its peak popularity in the 1950s and 1960s largely due to the work of two Germans, Hettinger and Muller (Hettinger & Muller 1953). Several training studies (3–15 weeks in length) have shown moderate strength gains while performing multiple maximum isometric contractions 3–10 s in duration (Alway et al 1989, Carolan & Cafarelli 1992, Garfinkel & Cafarelli

1992). While isometric training is appropriate in rehabilitation settings in which joint movements are contraindicated, it is not such an effective form of strength training for athletes due to the static nature of the exercise compared to strength training through a range of motion that is more sport-specific. However, isometric training is valuable in some sports, such as competitive powerlifting, which require high levels of strength in static or near static positions. For example, while performing the 1 RM deadlift exercise during powerlifting competition, the most difficult part of the lift (known as the 'sticking point') is when the upward moving barbell just passes the knees with the knees flexed approximately 20° and the hips flexed approximately 60° (Escamilla et al 2000). The 'sticking point' is often where a lifter fails in an attempt at a successful lift. Since the barbell is very near a static position at the 'sticking point', isometric training with the body positioned in a similar manner may be helpful in developing the strength needed to move beyond the 'sticking point' and to have a successful lift.

Dynamic training

Dynamic training involves both concentric (muscle shortening) and eccentric (muscle lengthening) muscle contractions in which joint motion occurs. The two most common modes of dynamic training are free weights and machines (Figs 9.1A–H and 9.2A–F). The use of free weights is referred to as dynamic constant external resistance training since the weight remains constant throughout a range of motion. The use of many machines (e.g. the VRM) is referred to as dynamic variable resistance training since the cam system employed in machines varies the resistance throughout a range of motion in an attempt to match the torque generating capabilities of muscle. The advantages and disadvantages of free weights and machines have been previously discussed. Several upper and lower extremity training studies involving both free weights and machines have shown significant strength increases while performing approximately 3–4 sets of 2–10 RM for 3–4 days per week for 10–20 weeks (Hagerman et al 2000, Kraemer 1997, Kraemer et al 1997, Kraemer et al 2001, Marx et al 2001, Rhodes et al 2000, Taaffe et al 1999). While strength training studies using both machines (Smith & Melton 1981) and free weights (Wathen & Shutes 1982) have shown increases in sport-specific movements (e.g. short sprints and vertical jumps), free weights appear to offer more optimal sport-specific strength gains compared to machines (Haff 2000).

Other common forms of dynamic training involve elastic bands, manual resistance from a partner, and bodyweight exercises, such as push-ups, pull-ups, and sit-to-stand exercises. These exercises require no equipment to perform and can be done almost anywhere. It is common for children to start off with these exercises to build a strength base before advancing to machines and

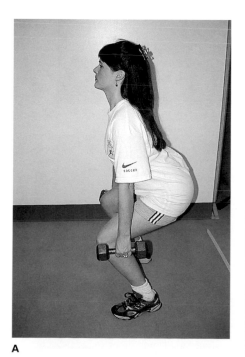
A

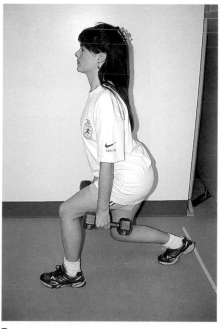
B

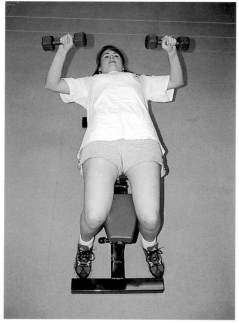
C

Figure 9.1A–H   Common free weight dumbbell exercises. **A**: Squat. **B**: Lunge. **C**: Bench press. **D**: Incline press. **E**: Shoulder press. **F**: Shoulder scaption. **G**: Bent over rows. **H**: Crunchies.

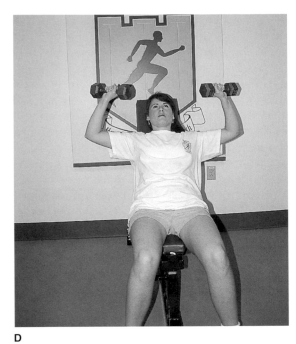

D

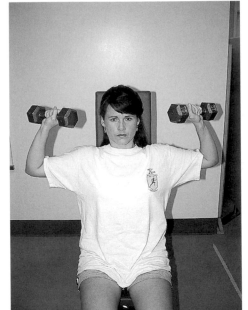

E

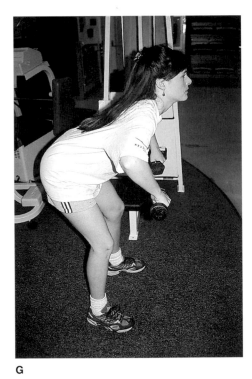

G

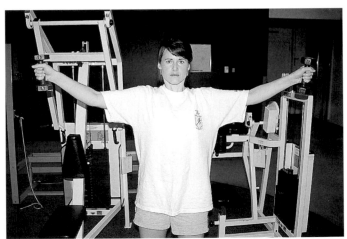

F

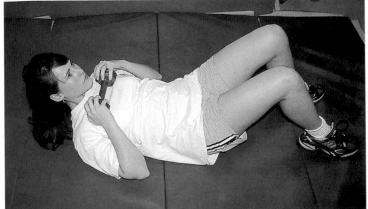

H

Figure 9.1A–H   (Cont'd)

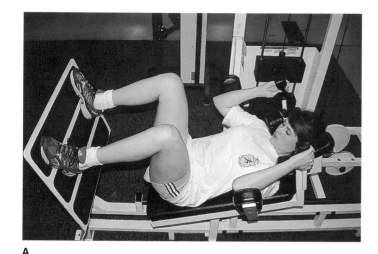

A

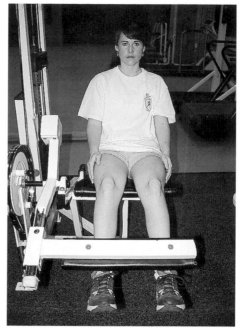

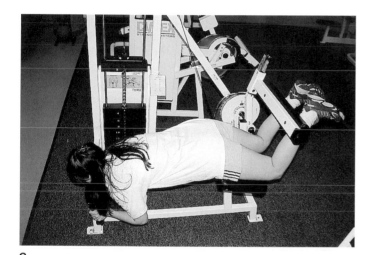

C

B

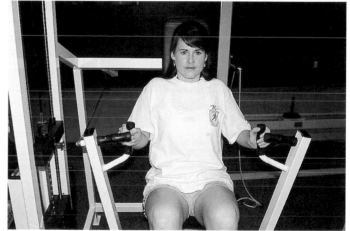

D

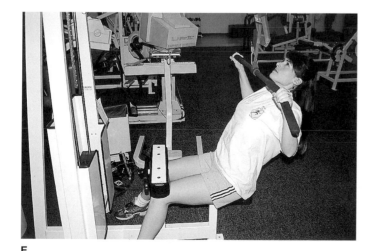

E

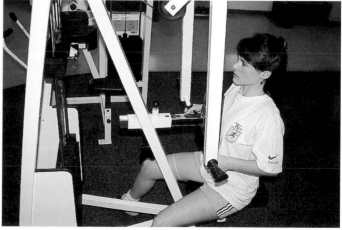

F

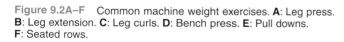

Figure 9.2A–F   Common machine weight exercises. **A**: Leg press.
B: Leg extension. **C**: Leg curls. **D**: Bench press. **E**: Pull downs.
F: Seated rows.

free weights. Bodyweight exercises, such as sit-to-stand, are appropriate during rehabilitation and strengthening, particularly for the elderly.

Eccentric training

Eccentric training, often referred to as negatives, involves eccentric muscle contractions only; for example, consider the bench press exercise. In dynamic training, concentric contractions from the pectoralis major, triceps brachii, and anterior deltoids result in the weight being pressed upward. During the downward phase of the bench press, these same muscles must now lengthen and contract eccentrically to control the descent rate as the weight is lowered. Due to differences in muscle mechanics, peak tension during eccentric contraction is much greater than peak tension generated during concentric contractions (Gohner 1994). Hence, a much greater amount of weight can be lowered at a given rate compared to the amount of weight that can be raised at that same rate. This allows an individual to lower a weight in a controlled manner that is well in excess of the 1 RM. Athletes will often use spotters to help lift the weight up, and then they will lower the weight eccentrically. This entire process is then repeated for multiple repetitions and sets. Research has shown that eccentric training does result in strength gains similar to the strength gains in isometric, concentric, and isokinetic training, and is most effective when used in combination with concentric contractions (Gohner 1994, Higbie et al 1996, Morrissey et al 1995, Tesch et al 1990). However, one undesirable effect of eccentric training is an excessive amount of muscle and connective tissue damage, which results in increased muscle soreness and an increased recovery period (Ebbeling & Clarkson 1989).

Isokinetic training

Isokinetic training involves moving through a range of motion at a constant speed. The harder an individual pushes or pulls against the machine, the greater the resistance that is accommodated by the machine, thereby producing an equal but opposite reaction force (torque) to the force or torque generated by the individual. This accommodation in resistance maintains a constant speed according to the speed setting on the machine. Most isokinetic machines generate speeds up to $300-500°/s$, allowing both concentric and eccentric contractions. Several isokinetic training studies have shown significant strength increases while performing approximately 1–5 sets of 5–15 repetitions between $60-120°/s$ for 3 days per week over 8–20 weeks (Mannion et al 1992, McCarrick & Kemp 2000, Narici et al 1996). A thorough review comparing the specificity and effectiveness of resistance training modes relative to different types of training (e.g. static versus dynamic, concentric versus eccentric, weight-training versus isokinetic) was written by Morrissey et al (1995).

Plyometrics

Eastern European athletes dominated power sports in the 1972 Olympic Games, spurring widespread interest in their training techniques. The alleged training regimen used by Valeri Borzov, a Russian track and field medalist, was jump training (Wilt 1975). In 1966, Yuri Verkhoshanski (Verkhoshanski 1966), a prominent Russian track and field coach, described a depth jump training program used in conjunction with traditional strength training to improve power in high caliber athletes. Wilt (1975) called the technique plyometric exercise, and specifically referred to activities using a quick stretch to facilitate force development in the subsequent shortening cycle. Thus, with little knowledge of how the new training augmented performance, the elite athletic world incorporated plyometric exercises (also called jump training, depth jump, or stretch-shortening exercises) into training programs for power sports.

All motion requires force production. The ability to generate force is a measure of strength. The ability to develop force rapidly is a measure of power. Since most activities (e.g. throwing a ball, putting the shot, sprinting) require rapid force development, rehabilitation programs must include techniques to improve power. Plyometric exercises are one training tool focusing on increased power production.

Theories of force augmentation

Three theories explain the augmented muscle force production observed in plyometric exercises. First, the rapid stretch of the agonist muscle activates the muscle spindle causing an increase in the firing rate of the Ia sensory neurons associated with the intrafusal nuclear chain and bag fibers (Swash & Fox 1972). Increased firing of the Ia neurons results in increased firing of the agonist and synergist alpha motor neurons via a monosynaptic spinal reflex leading to increased muscle contraction force (Asmussen & Bonde-Petersen 1974, Bosco et al 1986).

The second theory proposes a decrease in golgi tendon organ (GTO) sensitivity to stretch. The GTO, located in the muscle tendon, is activated by tension within the muscle. The GTO provides a protective mechanism by inhibiting agonist force production when tension reaches a level that could be damaging to the muscle. Plyometric training is thought to desensitize the GTO which would ultimately lead to enhanced force production by removing the inhibition of the agonist (Bosco & Komi 1979).

A third theory is based on neuromuscular adaptation. Motor learning literature states that acquisition of new skills progresses from cognitive to automatic (Higgins 1991). Performing jumping skills improves jumping as motor patterns are learned. With training, efficiency improves, leading to improved performance. Furthermore, with jump training, the time delay between the eccentric and concentric phases decreases, thereby enhancing the return of stored elastic energy (Voight 1992, Wilk et al 1993). This improved performance is seen after training even in the absence of changes in muscle cross-sectional area (Chu 1992, Voight 1992, Wilk et al 1993). Plyometric training has been shown to improve rebound time by minimizing the transition from eccentric to concentric contraction (Voight 1992), to decrease reaction time between the neural impulse and muscle contraction (Wilk et al 1993), and to recruit more motor units (Chu 1992).

Training program considerations

Before plyometric training is implemented, the athlete's age, body weight, strength relative to body weight, experience, and current strength and speed training regimen must be considered. Because of the risk of growth plate injuries, it is recommended that athletes younger than 16 do not perform drop jumps (LaChance 1995). Heavy athletes also should not perform drop jumps from a height greater than 18 inches due to the large impact forces associated with landing (Fowler et al 1997, Santos 1979). An adequate strength base assessed by squatting with 1.5–2.5 times body weight is necessary before the highest level of plyometric training (drop jumps and weighted drop jumps) is attempted (Wathen 1993). Also, the athlete should have 2–4 weeks of strength and sprint training as a base before beginning a plyometric training program (Santos 1979). Finally, inexperienced athletes will need to progress more slowly than elite athletes to allow proper skill acquisition (Chu 1992).

Like all training programs, the number of repetitions per training session, duration of the training session, and frequency of training must be regulated to minimize the risk of injury. The plyometric program should begin with low intensity vertical and horizontal jumps and progress to bounding, box jumps, and drop jumps (Fig. 9.3A–C). Weighted jumps are the highest level of plyometric exercise and are appropriate only for highly-trained athletes who demonstrate good technique on all other plyometric and weightlifting exercises. As intensity of the program increases, the duration and frequency of training sessions should decrease while recovery time between sets is increased. Forty-eight hours recovery between plyometric sessions is the minimum time recommended to promote complete recovery (Allerheiligen & Rogers 1995).

COMMON SYSTEMS OF STRENGTH TRAINING

Single-sets versus multi-sets

For a given exercise, single-set systems consist of performing a single-set of repetitions to failure, while multi-set systems consist of performing multiple sets of repetitions to failure. While maximum strength gains occur while employing single or multiple sets of near maximum loads between 2–6 repetitions (Stone et al 1981), significant strength and power gains have been reported in many training studies involving both single-set and multi-set training between approximately 2–12 repetitions (see Table 9.2). However, multi-set training involving both a constant and varied number of repetitions and sets has been shown to be superior to single-set training in maximizing strength and power gains (Table 9.2), especially in athletes training for sport and employing periodization techniques (Kraemer 1997, Kraemer et al 2000). This is contrary to previous beliefs (Carpinelli & Otto 1998, Feigenbaum & Pollock 1999) that single-set training is just as effective a multi-set training in producing strength gains. It should be emphasized

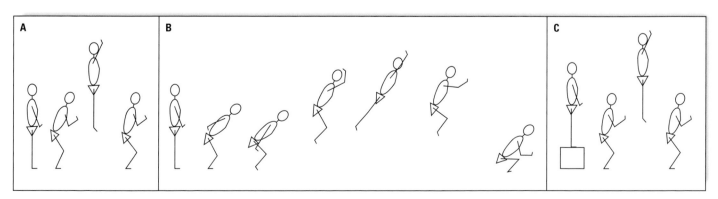

Figure 9.3A–C Plyometric exercises. **A**: vertical jump. **B**: broad jump. **C**: drop jump.

that there has never been a strength training study that has shown that single-set training produces superior strength gains compared to multi-set training, but several recent strength training studies have shown that multi-set training produces superior strength and power gains compared to single-set training (Table 9.2). This implies that athletes who desire to maximize strength gains should employ a multi-set system of training. However, since single-set systems are effective in maintaining or producing strength gains, single-set training systems are an effective alternative for those who have limited time for resistance training and whose goal is not to maximize strength gains but rather to build a functional strength base to enhance their activities of daily living (e.g. non-athletes, rehabilitation patients, and the elderly).

DeLorme – light to heavy

The DeLorme system of training is one in which the initial set starts out light, and progressively greater resistance is added in each subsequent set. The DeLorme system became popular in the 1950s and 1960s when DeLorme and colleagues reported significant strength gains during short-term training studies while performing 3 sets of 10 repetitions (DeLorme & Watkins 1948, DeLorme et al 1952). In the original DeLorme system, the resistances employed were equal to 50% of the lifter's 10 RM for the first set, 66% of 10 RM for the second set, and 100% of 10 RM for the third set. Variations of these training percentages may be employed when using the DeLorme system.

Oxford – heavy to light

The Oxford system of training is one in which the initial set starts out heavy, and progressively smaller resistance is employed in each subsequent set. Like the DeLorme system, the Oxford system became popular in the 1950s and 1960s. Several studies have reported significant strength gains using the Oxford Technique (Leighton et al 1967, McMorris & Elkins 1954, Zinovieff 1951). The resistances employed in the Oxford Technique are the same as in the DeLorme system but in reverse order: the resistance is equal to 100% of the lifter's 10 RM for the first set, 66% of 10 RM for the second set, and 50% of 10 RM for the third set. Variations of these training percentages may be employed when using the Oxford system.

Pyramid

The pyramid system combines the light-to-heavy and heavy-to-light systems, and is common both in power-lifting and weightlifting. A lifter can progress from light-to-heavy resistance on the way up the pyramid, and from heavy-to-light resistance on the way down the pyramid. Conversely, in an inverse pyramid, a lifter can progress from heavy-to-light resistance on the way down the pyramid, and from light-to-heavy resistance on the way up the pyramid. An early study of the pyramid type system of training has shown it to be effective in building leg and trunk strength, as well as elbow and extension strength (Leighton et al 1967). More recent literature evaluating this system is lacking. A typical example employing a pyramid system for strength training is as follows:

Set 1: 10 RM
Set 2: 8 RM
Set 3: 5 RM
Set 4: 3 RM
Set 5: 5 RM
Set 6: 8 RM
Set 7: 10 RM

Super-set

The super-set system (Leighton et al 1967) is typically performed in one of two ways. Using the first method, a super-set system involves performing one set each of multiple exercises (2–3) to work the same muscle group with little or no rest between exercises. In the second method, the super-set system involves performing one set of multiple exercises (2–3) that work muscle groups which have opposite muscle actions with little or no rest. Pairs of agonist–antagonist exercises are most common in this type of super-set system, which allows the agonist muscle group to rest while the antagonist muscle group works (and vice versa). Super-set systems are common in bodybuilding, and have been shown to increase muscle strength (Leighton et al 1967). Due to the large number of repetitions performed and high exercise volume, this type of training also produces a higher level of muscular endurance and has a high energy expenditure (Kraemer et al 1987).

Circuit

The circuit system of training consists of performing multiple exercises (typically 8–12) using higher repetitions (typically 12–20) and lower intensities (40-60% or 1 RM) with minimal rest intervals between exercises (10–20 s) (Beckham & Earnest 2000, Green et al 2001, Haennel et al 1991, Todd et al 1992). This type of training is most beneficial for those individuals whose primary aim is to increase their cardiovascular fitness and muscular endurance (Beckham & Earnest 2000, Green et al 2001, Haennel et al 1991, Todd et al 1992). This approach is useful for people who are deconditioned, have excess body fat and need to lose weight, and have cardiovascular issues (e.g. hypertension and cardiovascular

Table 9.2 Recent examples of strength and power gain comparisons between single-set (SS) versus multiple set (MSC and MSV) training studies

Authors	Group	Strength and power training protocol per workout session	Sex	No.	Age (years)	Frequency (days/week)	Duration (weeks)	Training sets × RM	Strength or power testing protocol	Mean % strength increase* for SS, MSC, and MSV	Result Difference between SS and MSC/MSV
(Borst et al 2001)	SS	7 MedX Ma circuit	M/F	11	35±7	3	25	1 × 8–12	1 RM Ma knee extension +	30% SS*	S
	MSC	7 MedX Ma circuit	M/F	11	41±7	3	25	3 × 8–12	1 RM Ma bench press	50% MSC*	S
(Hass et al 2001)	SS	9 MedX Ma circuit	M/F	21	40±6	3	13	1 × 8–12	1 RM Ma knee extension	13% SS*	NS
	MSC	9 MedX Ma circuit	M/F	21	39±7	3	13	3 × 8–12		12% MSC*	
									1 RM Ma leg curl	5% SS* / 10% MSC*	S
									1 RM Ma chest press	11% SS* / 10% MSC*	NS
									1 RM Ma overhead press	5% SS* / 15% MSC*	NS
									1 RM Ma biceps curls	10% SS* / 9% MSC*	NS
(Kraemer 1997)	SS	9 Universal and Marcy Ma circuit	M	17	C	3	14	1 × 8–12	1 RM FW hang cleans	3% SS / 20% MSV*	S
	MSV	7–9 Ma and FW exercises	M	17	C	3	14	2–5 × 1–10	1 RM Ma bench press	3% SS* / 11% MSV*	S
									Peak power from maximum effort vertical jump	3% SS / 17% MSV*	S
									Peak power from Wingate anaerobic cycle test	1% SS / 14% MSV*	S
(Kraemer 1997)	SS	10 Ma and FW exercises	M	22	C	3	24	1 × 8–12	1 RM Ma bench press	13% SS* / 29% MSV*	S
	MSV	8–13 Ma and FW exercises	M	22	C	4	24	2–4 × 3–15	1 RM Ma leg press	8% SS* / 20% MSV*	S
									Maximum effort vertical jump	7% SS* / 23% MSV*	S
									Peak power from Wingate anaerobic cycle test	5% SS* / 55% MSV*	S
(Kraemer et al 1997)	SS	4 Ma and FW exercises	M	16	C	3	14	1 × 8–12	1 RM FW squat	12% SS*	S[ss]
	MSC	4 Ma and FW exercises	M	14	C	3	14	3 × 10		26% MSC*	S[ss]
	MSV	4 Ma and FW exercises	M	13	C	3	14	1–3 × 2–10		22% MSV*	
(Kraemer 1997)	SS	10 Nautilus Ma circuit	M	20	C	3	10	1 × 8–12	1 RM Nautilus Ma bench press	4% SS / 13% MSC*	S
	MSC	10 Nautilus Ma circuit	M	20	C	3	10	3 × 8–12	1 RM Nautilus Ma leg press	3% SS / 19% MSC*	S

Table 9.2 (Cont'd)

Authors	Group	Strength and power training protocol per workout session	Sex	No.	Age (years)	Frequency (days/week)	Duration (weeks)	Training sets × RM	Strength or power testing protocol	Mean % strength increase* for SS, MSC, and MSV	Result Difference between SS and MSC/MSV
(Marx et al 2001)	SS	10 Ma exercise circuit	F	12	23±5	3	24	1 × 8–12	1 RM Ma bench press	12% SS* / 47% MSV*	S
	MSV	7–12 Ma and FW exercises	F	12	23±4	4	24	2–4 × 3–15	1 RM Ma leg press	11% SS* / 32% MSV*	S
									Maximum effort vertical jump	10% SS* / 40% MSV*	S
									40 yard dash	1% SS / 6% MSV*	S
									Peak power from Wingate anaerobic cycle test	4% SS / 27% MSV*	S
(Sanborn et al 2000)	SS	5 FW exercises	F	9	C	3	8	1 × 8–12	1 RM FW squat	24% SS* / 35% MSV*	NS
	MSV	5 FW exercises	F	8	C	3	8	3–5 × 2–10	Peak power from maximum effort vertical jump	0% SS / 11% MSV*	S
(Schlumberger et al 2001)	SS	7 Ma exercises	F	9	29±9	2	6	1 × 6–9	1 RM Ma bench press	4% SS / 10% MS*	S
	MSC	7 Ma exercises	F	9	24±3	2	6	3 × 6–9	1 RM Ma knee extension	7% SS* / 16% MS*	S
(Starkey et al 1996)	SS	MedX Dynamic Ma knee extension and flexion	M/F	18	34±10	3	14	1 × 8–12	MedX peak isometric knee extension	30% SS* / 27% MSC*	NS
	MSC	MedX Dynamic Ma knee extension and flexion	M/F	20	35±8	3	14	1 × 8–12	MedX peak isometric knee flexion	19% SS* / 18% MSC*	NS

SS = single-set; MSC = multiple sets using a constant number of repetitions and sets; MSV = multiple sets using a varied number of repetitions and sets
S = significant difference between SS and MSC or between SS and MSV; S^{ss} = significantly greater than SS; NS = non-significant difference between SS and MSC or between SS and MSV; * = significant increase in strength gain due to SS, MSC, or MSV training; C = college age; Ma = machine; FW = free weight

disease). However, studies have shown that strength increases also occur with circuit training, especially for the deconditioned (Sparling et al 1990, Stewart 1989). Circuit training is also effective for individuals who need a supervised, structured program and have limited time to work out.

The circuit is commonly set up so an individual moves from one exercise to another in a timed sequence, such as a 30 s exercise period followed by a 15 s rest interval. Following this format, a 12 exercise circuit would take approximately 10 min to perform. The circuit could be performed 2–3 times, thereby allowing 2–3 sets of each exercise to be performed in 20–30 min, which makes the circuit time efficient. A circuit is often set up to employ alternating upper and lower body exercises, or alternating muscle groups, thus allowing one muscle group to rest and recover while another muscle group is being worked. Also, multi-joint, multi-muscle exercises should comprise most of the exercises in the circuit, since they have a greater energy expenditure, and develop overall muscular strength and endurance to a greater extent compared to single-joint, single-muscle exercises (Beckham & Earnest 2000, Escamilla et al 2000). A circuit primarily consists of resistance machines rather than free weights since they are safer, easier to use, and take minimal time to change resistance.

INTERVAL TRAINING

Interval training typically involves moderate to high intensity exercise alternating with brief to moderate rest periods. In general, higher intensity training uses greater recovery periods and is more anaerobic, whereas lower intensity training uses shorter recovery periods and is more aerobic. Circuit training is an example of interval resistance training, consisting of approximately 30 s of exercise and 15 s of rest and recovery. Circuit training involves lower intensities of exercise followed by shorter rest intervals. A common higher intensity example of interval training involves sprinting a certain distance followed by walking or jogging that same distance. For example, consider an athlete who sprints 40–50 m followed by jogging slowly or walking back to the starting line; there is 5–10 s of higher intensity exercise followed by a 30–45 s recovery. This sequence is repeated multiple times. A primary advantage of interval training is that it allows a greater volume of work to be performed compared to continuous training. Interval training is more sport-specific for many athletic movements; for example, a running back in American football typically runs at high intensity for a few seconds followed by 30–45 s of rest.

ENDURANCE TRAINING

Endurance is the ability to perform sustained activity. Increased resistance to fatigue is gained through aerobic or endurance training. Although daily life requires fatigue resistance for optimal performance, the focus of this section will be on the training adaptations resulting from sustained exercise of 20 min or more.

MEASUREMENT OF AEROBIC FITNESS

An individual's endurance or aerobic fitness can be measured by several different techniques. The 12-min run and timed 1.5 mile run have been used for general screening of aerobic fitness (Cooper 1968). A more precise measurement of aerobic fitness is the treadmill or cycle ergometer test for maximal oxygen uptake (VO_2max) (Pollock et al 1976). VO_2max represents the maximum amount of oxygen used per unit time by the metabolically active tissues in the body. VO_2max is measured in liters of oxygen per minute (absolute VO_2max) or may be expressed relative to body weight (relative VO_2max). An individual's VO_2max is dependent on age (VO_2max declines from early adulthood to old age) (Paterson et al 1999, Trappe et al 1996), gender (males generally have a higher VO_2max than females) (Bouchard et al 1999), genetics (Bouchard et al 1999), and training status (aerobically fit individuals have a higher VO_2max than non-fit persons) (Ekblom et al 1968) (Table 9.3).

Maximal oxygen consumption or VO_2max is dependent on oxygen delivery to the cells and metabolic capacity of the tissues. This relationship is expressed in the Fick equation which relates oxygen uptake (VO_2) to cardiac output (CO) and arteriovenous oxygen difference (a-vO_2dif) as follows: $VO_2 = CO \times$ a-vO_2dif. To increase oxygen uptake, either CO, a-vO_2dif, or both must increase.

PHYSIOLOGICAL ADAPTATIONS TO ENDURANCE TRAINING

Cardiovascular

With endurance training, several physiological adaptations occur to enhance CO, the product of heart rate (HR)

Table 9.3 Maximal oxygen uptake for males

	Absolute VO_2max L·min^{-1}	Relative VO_2max mL·kg^{-1}·min^{-1}
Sedentary	2–2.5	< 30
Moderately trained	3–3.5	30–50
Well trained	4–4.5	50–70
Elite	> 5	> 70

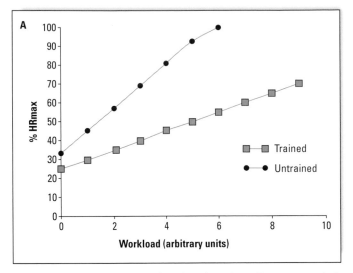
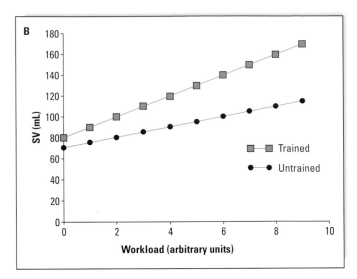

Figure 9.4A & B   Heart rate **A** and stroke volume **B** responses to increased workload in the trained and untrained state.

and stroke volume (SV). During exercise, HR increases as workload and intensity increase due in part to an increase in circulating noradrenaline (norepinephrine) from the sympathetic nervous system (Schwarz & Kindermann 1990). As intensity continues to increase, a maximum HR is achieved after which further increases in intensity produce no further increases in HR. With training, maximal HR is unchanged but occurs at a higher workload (Fig. 9.4A). Alternatively, HR at any submaximal intensity is lower after training (Wilmore et al 2001).

The second determinant of CO is SV. SV increases with increased workload due to an increase in myocardial contractility (force of contraction, inotropic effect) and an increase in venous return (Laughlin 1999) (Fig. 9.4B). Both contractility and venous return increase during exercise due to release of noradrenaline (norepinephrine) by the sympathetic nervous system (Schwarz & Kindermann 1990). Because contractility increases, more blood is ejected from the left ventricle during systole. Sympathetic stimulation also causes vasoconstriction of the peripheral vessels leading to greater blood return during diastole. Stretch of the myocardium enhances overlap of myosin and actin myofilaments and greater force is generated in the subsequent contraction (Starling's Law of the Heart). Increased HR and SV at maximal exercise produce the elevated CO.

Oxygen uptake at the tissue level is determined by oxygen delivery and tissue extraction. Due to elevated CO, blood flow to the metabolically active skeletal muscles is increased. Muscle blood flow is increased more in trained muscle than untrained muscle (Delp 1995). Not only is a greater percentage of the CO going to the active muscle but the blood also has a greater oxygen

carrying capacity as a result of increased red blood cell formation stimulated by erythropoietin (Bodary et al 1999). Adaptations in the muscle also provide improved oxygen extraction capacity at the tissue level (Roca et al 1992).

Muscle adaptations

Following endurance training, skeletal muscle undergoes characteristic changes. Progressive aerobic exercise leads to an increase in capillary density of the trained muscle mass (Gute et al 1996, Madsen & Holmskov 1995). The benefits of increased capillarity include decreased diffusion distance, increased red blood cell transit time, and improved blood distribution. Temperature elevation and decreased pH in the active muscle facilitate oxygen unloading from hemoglobin (the Bohr effect). The combined effect of increased capillarity and enhanced oxygen unloading results in an increase in the a-vO$_2$dif. Current theory holds that the increase in CO and increase in a-vO$_2$dif contribute equally to the increased VO$_2$max observed after training (Laughlin 1999).

Other changes in muscle tissue with training include an increase in the size and number of mitochondria (Holloszy 1967, Suter et al 1995), increased activity of enzymes associated with carbohydrate and fat oxidation (Mole et al 1971, Svedenhag et al 1983), and improved glucose uptake (Greiwe et al 2000, Houmard et al 1995). Increased mitochondrial density reduces oxygen diffusion distance and increases the surface area for oxidation. Fully oxidizing carbohydrate (yielding 38 adenosine triphosphate [ATP] per glucose molecule versus 2 ATP per glucose via glycolysis) has a glucose and glycogen sparing effect. Increased activity of enzymes involved in fat oxidation enhances breakdown of triglycerides, movement of fatty acids into mitochondria, and beta oxidation. Use of fats as an energy source also has a glucose/glycogen sparing effect. Additionally, endurance training decreases the expression of fast glycolytic (type IIb) muscle fiber type (O'Neill et al 1999). With endurance training VO_2max increases 15–20% in both young and older adults (Levy et al 1998).

The less fit a person is prior to the start of an endurance training program (thus having greater potential for improvement), the larger the increase in VO_2max. However, a physiological maximum for the individual does exist beyond which further training does not elicit further increases in VO_2max.

PRINCIPLES OF ENDURANCE TRAINING

The American College of Sports Medicine has established guidelines for exercise to improve aerobic fitness. These guidelines state that 30 min of daily activity at a HR greater than 60% of the predicted maximum HR (220 – age) at least three times per week promotes aerobic fitness and health gains (American College of Sports Medicine 2000).

Endurance training is associated with decreased risk of coronary artery disease, stroke, non-insulin dependent diabetes mellitus, hypertension, osteoporosis, and colon, breast, cervical, ovarian, and uterine cancers (American College of Sports Medicine 2000).

High-density lipoprotein cholesterol (the 'good' cholesterol) increases with endurance training while plasma triglyceride concentration decreases (Lindheim et al 1994, Schwartz et al 1992). Endurance training enhances insulin receptor sensitivity (Dela et al 1996, Houmard et al 1995) leading to improved glucose homeostasis. Systolic and diastolic blood pressure decreases with endurance training (Cononie et al 1991). Women participating in regular exercise, especially weightbearing exercise, maintain or possibly increase bone mineral density reducing the risk of osteoporotic fractures (Chow et al 1987, Smith et al 1989).

INJURY PREVENTION DURING ENDURANCE TRAINING

Whether the goal of aerobic training is to improve fitness, decrease body fat, or maximize athletic performance, certain training factors must be addressed to minimize the risk of injury. Common endurance training activities include swimming, cycling, rollerblading, cross country skiing, walking, and running (with running associated with the highest rate of overuse injuries). Training errors (inappropriate footwear, hard irregular terrain, excessive mileage, or rapid increase in mileage and speed) are responsible for a high percentage of injuries (Ballas et al

1997, Bovens et al 1989, Macera et al 1989). During the evaluation of an injured runner, it is important to assess the running shoes for signs of wear or breakdown as this will decrease the support and stability of the shoe. Likewise, total shoe mileage may provide insight into the cause of an injury. Runners should also be questioned about the surface on which they train. Hill running (Clement & Taunton 1981), running on concrete (Macera et al 1989), and running on crowded streets (Bovens et al 1989) all contribute to an increased risk of injury, but the strongest correlation with injury is weekly running frequency and distance (Bovens et al 1989, Macera et al 1989).

To minimize the risk of injury, Ballas et al (1997) recommended increasing mileage slowly (no more than a 10% increase per week), a weekly running mileage of less than 45 miles (72.5 km), running on a soft flat surface (rubber track, dirt path, etc.), alternating high intensity and low intensity workouts, and changing running shoes every 500 miles (800 km). Because shock absorption in running shoes is decreased by 50% after 300 miles (500 km) (Cook et al 1990), it may be necessary to replace shoes before 500 miles of wear. For all participants in aerobic conditioning programs, cross training is encouraged to balance muscle strength and flexibility as well as to reduce overuse injuries (Ballas et al 1997).

ENDURANCE TRAINING IN SPECIAL POPULATIONS

Children

Despite an increase in organized sports participation, the overall fitness level of youth in many developed countries is poor. Like adults, children who have a high daily level of activity show a higher VO_2max than do sedentary children. Using adult guidelines for frequency, intensity and duration, endurance training programs can lead to increased VO_2max in children (Mahon & Vaccaro 1989, Mandigout et al 2001) although the magnitude of the increase may be smaller (Mahon & Vaccaro 1989) and require higher training intensity to achieve (Rowland 1992). Endurance training appears to have no effect on blood lipid levels in children (Rowland et al 1996) but does enhance bone deposition (Eliakim et al 1997). Regular physical activity during childhood enhances skill acquisition, muscle strength and endurance, and weight management.

Older people

Many physiological changes occur with aging, nearly all of which contribute to a decrease in functional independence. Endurance training in older adults (including those

80+ years old) improves cardiovascular function measured by VO_2max (Buchner et al 1997, Steinhaus et al 1990), decreases resting HR, decreases systolic blood pressure, and results in fewer premature ventricular contractions (Steinhaus et al 1990). Participation in an endurance training program increases leg strength (Buchner et al 1997) and fat-free body mass (Wilmore et al 1999), while the percentage of body fat decreases (Wilmore et al 1999). Despite increased fat-free mass, resting metabolic rate is unchanged with regular participation in an endurance training program (Wilmore et al 1998).

Endurance training in the elderly has other benefits besides reduced disease risk. These benefits include improved balance, cognition, perception of self-efficacy, and decreased depression (American College of Sports Medicine 1998). Elderly clients should be encouraged to participate in moderate intensity exercise for at least 30 min, three or more times per week. Increased frequency, duration, and intensity lead to greater improvements in cardiorespiratory fitness. Individuals with orthopedic or balance disorders may find aquatic activities more suitable although the benefit of maintaining bone mass is lost due to the non-weightbearing nature of this activity.

STABILIZATION

Core strength and stability are vital in many activities. Yet in spite of the important role the trunk plays in force production by the extremities, it is often overlooked during training to the detriment of optimal athletic performance; as an example, consider the baseball pitcher. The pitcher does not merely draw the arm back and throw the ball; rather, a wind-up phase in which the leg is raised initiates the pitching sequence and force generated in the legs is transferred through the trunk to the throwing arm (Fleisig et al 1999). If core strength is lacking, the energy generated in the legs is lost and, instead, the pitcher has to rely solely on the musculature of the upper extremity. Over time, the stress placed on the shoulder and elbow musculature causes injuries. A strong core allows force to be transferred from the legs to the arm smoothly and efficiently (Gambetta & Clark 1999).

Training the core muscles involves more than general abdominal exercises and back extensions. Rather than focusing on individual muscle groups, core training emphasizes combined flexion, extension, and rotation movement patterns using sport-specific drills (Cook & Fields 1997). Training for maximum core stability is accomplished through daily workouts in which the

movements are varied. Proper technique is the primary focus and should not be sacrificed for increased resistance or repetitions. Core training begins with low intensity, low volume workouts and gradually progresses to higher difficulty routines. Training involves utilizing opposing muscle groups equally (e.g. back extensors and abdominals, anterior chest and scapular muscles, hip flexors and extensors). Rotational movements should be performed to both sides to reduce muscle imbalances. Finally, training movements should replicate the movements required for the actual sport and exercise activity (Hedrick 2000).

Progression of core stability training programs encourages continued adaptations. Progression is accomplished beginning with simple movements and advancing to complex exercises only when the basic movements have been mastered. Training should progress from a controlled environment to an environment with distractions (e.g. uneven surface, varied timing, etc.), from static to dynamic conditions, and from high level of support (lying) to low level of support (e.g. standing on one leg) (Gambetta & Clark 1999). For further discussion on core stability training, refer to Chapter 14.

SUMMARY

This chapter focuses on providing scientific rationale for the use of strength, plyometric, endurance, interval, and stabilization training in injury prevention and rehabilitation. Research supports the use of plyometric, interval, endurance, and stabilization training in injury prevention and rehabilitation. In addition, several research studies have reported that high intensity strength training results in several efficacious effects that enhance rehabilitation and prevent injuries. These include:

- An increase in muscle strength, size, and power
- An increase in neuromuscular function
- An increase in bone strength and density with a concomitant decrease in osteoporosis
- An increase in tendon and ligament strength and thickness
- An increase in balance and decrease in risk of falling and subsequent injury
- An increase in gait stability, walking speed, and efficiency
- An increase in chair rising and stair climbing
- An increase in hormonal adaptations
- A decrease in blood pressure, glucose intolerance, and insulin resistance
- A decrease in body fat, and an increase in fat free mass and basal metabolic rate.

REFERENCES

Allerheiligen B, Rogers R 1995 Plyometrics program design. Strength and Conditioning 17(4):26–31

Alway S E, MacDougall J D, Sale D G 1989 Contractile adaptations in the human triceps surae after isometric exercise. Journal of Applied Physiology 66(6):2725–2732

American College of Sports Medicine 1998 American College of Sports Medicine position stand. Exercise and physical activity for older adults. Medicine and Science in Sports and Exercise 30(6):992–1008

American College of Sports Medicine 2000 ACSM's guidelines for exercise testing and prescription. Lippincott Williams and Wilkins, Philadelphia

Asmussen E, Bonde-Petersen F 1974 Storage of elastic energy in skeletal muscles in man. Acta Physiologica Scandinavica 91:385–392

Ballas M T, Tytko J, Cookson D 1997 Common overuse running injuries: diagnosis and management. American Family Physician 55(7):2473–2484

Barneveld A, van Weeren P R 1999 Conclusions regarding the influence of exercise on the development of the equine musculoskeletal system with special reference to osteochondrosis. Equine Veterinary Journal (31):112–119

Beckham S G, Earnest C P 2000 Metabolic cost of free weight circuit weight training. Journal of Sports Medicine and Physical Fitness 40(2):118–125

Bemben D A, Fetters N L, Bemben M G et al 2000 Musculoskeletal responses to high- and low-intensity resistance training in early postmenopausal women. Medicine and Science in Sports and Exercise 32(11):1949–1957

Beniamini Y, Rubenstein J J, Zaichkowsky L D et al 1997 Effects of high-intensity strength training on quality-of-life parameters in cardiac rehabilitation patients. American Journal of Cardiology 80(7):841–846

Bloomfield S A 1997 Changes in musculoskeletal structure and function with prolonged bed rest. Medicine and Science in Sports and Exercise 29(2):197–206

Bodary P F, Pate R R, Wu Q F et al 1999 Effects of acute exercise on plasma erythropoietin levels in trained runners. Medicine and Science in Sports and Exercise 31(4):543–546

Borst S E, de Hoyos D V, Garzarella L et al 2001 Effects of resistance training on insulin-like growth factor-I and IGF binding proteins. Medicine and Science in Sports and Exercise 33(4):648–653

Bosco C, Komi P V 1979 Potentiation of the mechanical behavior of the human skeletal muscle through prestretching. Acta Physiologica Scandinavica 106:467–472

Bosco C, Tihanyi J, Latteri F et al 1986 The effect of fatigue on store and re-use of elastic energy in slow and fast types of human skeletal muscle. Acta Physiologica Scandinavica 128:109–117

Bouchard C, An P, Rice T et al 1999 Familial aggregation of VO2max response to exercise training: Results from the HERITAGE Family Study. Journal of Applied Physiology 87(3):1003–1008

Bovens A M, Janssen G M, Vermeer H G et al 1989 Occurrence of running injuries in adults following a supervised training program. International Journal of Sports Medicine 10:S186–S190

Brand R A, Pedersen D R, Friederich J A 1986 The sensitivity of muscle force predictions to changes in physiologic cross-sectional area. Journal of Biomechanics 19(8):589–596

Brill P A, Probst J C, Greenhouse D L et al 1998 Clinical feasibility of a free-weight strength-training program for older adults. Journal of the American Board of Family Practice 11(6):445–451

Buchner D M, Cress M E, de Lateur B J et al 1997 A comparison of the effects of three types of endurance training on balance and other fall risk factors in older adults. Aging 9(1–2):112–119

Byrne H K, Wilmore J H 2001 The effects of a 20-week exercise training program on resting metabolic rate in previously sedentary, moderately obese women. International Journal of Sport Nutrition and Exercise Metabolism 11(1):15–31

Carmeli E, Reznick A Z, Coleman R et al 2000 Muscle strength and mass of lower extremities in relation to functional abilities in elderly adults. Gerontology 46(5):249–257

Carolan B, Cafarelli E 1992 Adaptations in coactivation after isometric resistance training. Journal of Applied Physiology 73(3):911–917

Carpinelli R N, Otto R M 1998 Strength training. Single versus multiple sets. Sports Medicine 26(2):73–84

Chandler J M, Duncan P W, Kochersberger G et al 1998 Is lower extremity strength gain associated with improvement in physical performance and disability in frail, community-dwelling elders? Archives of Physical Medicine and Rehabilitation 79(1):24–30

Chow R, Harrison J, Notarius C 1987 Effect of two randomized exercise programmes on bone mass of healthy postmenopausal women. British Medical Journal 295:1441–1444

Chu D 1992 Jumping into plyometrics. Human Kinetics, Champaign, IL

Clement D B, Taunton J E 1981 A guide to the prevention of running injuries. Australian Family Physician 10:156–164

Cononie C C, Graves J E, Pollock M L et al 1991 Effect of exercise training on blood pressure in 70- to 79-yr-old men and women. Medicine and Science in Sports and Exercise 23(4):505–11

Conroy B P, Kraemer W J, Maresh C M et al 1992 Adaptive responses of bone to physical activity. Medicine, Exercise, Nutrition and Health 1:64–74

Cook G, Fields K 1997 Functional training for the torso. Strength and Conditioning 19(2):14–19

Cook S D, Brinker M R, Mahlon P 1990 Running shoes: their relation to running injuries. Sports Medicine 10:1–8

Cooper K H 1968 A means of assessing maximal oxygen intake. Journal of the American Medical Association 203:135–138

Dela F, Mikines K, Larsen J et al 1996 Training-induced enhancement of insulin action in human skeletal muscle: the influence of aging. Journal of Gerontology 51(4 suppl):B247–B252

DeLorme T L, Watkins A L 1948 Techniques of progressive resistance exercise. Archives of Physical Medicine 29:263–273

DeLorme T L, Ferris B G, Gallagher J R 1952 Effect of progressive exercise on muscular contraction time. Archives of Physical Medicine 33:86–97

Delp M D 1995 Effects of exercise training on endothelium-dependent peripheral vascular responsiveness. Medicine and Science in Sports and Exercise 27(8):1152–1157

Delp S L, Suryanarayanan S, Murray W M et al 2001 Architecture of the rectus abdominis, quadratus lumborum, and erector spinae. Journal of Biomechanics 34(3):371–375

DeMichele P L, Pollock M L, Graves J E et al 1997 Isometric torso rotation strength: effect of training frequency on its development. Archives of Physical Medicine and Rehabilitation 78(1):64–69

Ebbeling C B, Clarkson P M 1989 Exercise-induced muscle damage and adaptation. Sports Medicine 7(4):207–234

Ekblom B, Astrand P O, Saltin B et al 1968 Effect of training on circulatory response to exercise. Journal of Applied Physiology 24:518–528

Eliakim A, Raisz L G, Brasel J A et al 1997 Evidence for increased bone formation following a brief endurance-type training intervention in adolescent males. Journal of Bone Mineral Research 12(10):1708–1713

Escamilla R F, Francisco A C, Fleisig G S et al 2000 A three-dimensional biomechanical analysis of sumo and conventional style deadlifts. Medicine and Science in Sports and Exercise 32(7):1265-1275

Faulkner J A, Claflin D R, McCully K K 1986 Power output of fast and slow fibers from human skeletal muscle. In: Jones N L, McCartney N, McComas A J (eds) Human muscle power. Human Kinetics, Champaign, IL

Feigenbaum M S, Pollock M L 1999 Prescription of resistance training for health and disease. Medicine and Science in Sports and Exercise 31(1):38-45

Fleck S J, Falkel J E 1986 Value of resistance training for the reduction of sports injuries. Sports Medicine 3(1):61–68

Fleisig G S, Barrentine S W, Zheng N et al 1999 Kinematic and kinetic comparison of baseball pitching among various levels of development. Journal of Biomechanics 32(12):1371–1375

Fowler N E, Lees A, Reilly T 1997 Changes in stature following plyometric drop-jump and pendulum exercises. Ergonomics 40(12):1279–1286

Gambetta V, Clark M 1999 Hard core training. Training and conditioning 10(4):34–40

Garfinkel S, Cafarelli E 1992 Relative changes in maximal force, EMG, and muscle cross-sectional area after isometric training. Medicine and Science in Sports and Exercise 24(11):1220–1227

Garhammer J 1993 A review of power output studies of olympic and power lifting: methodology, performance prediction, and evaluation tests. Journal of Strength and Conditioning Research 7(2):76–89

Gohner U 1994 Experimental results on forced eccentric strength gains. International Journal of Sports Medicine 15 (1 suppl):S43–49

Gorostiaga E M, Izquierdo M, Iturralde P et al 1999 Effects of heavy resistance training on maximal and explosive force production, endurance and serum hormones in adolescent handball players. European Journal of Applied Physiology and Occupational Physiology 80(5):485–493

Granhed H, Jonson R, Hansson T 1987 The loads on the lumbar spine during extreme weight lifting. Spine 12(2):146–149

Green D J, Watts K, Maiorana A J et al 2001 A comparison of ambulatory oxygen consumption during circuit training and aerobic exercise in patients with chronic heart failure. Journal of Cardiopulmonary Rehabilitation 21(3):167–174

Gregg E W, Pereira M A, Caspersen C J 2000 Physical activity, falls, and fractures among older adults: a review of the epidemiologic evidence. Journal of the American Geriatrics Society 48(8):883–893

Greiwe J S, Holloszy J O, Semenkovich C F 2000 Exercise induces lipoprotein lipase and GLUT-4 protein in muscle independent of adrenergic-receptor signaling. Journal of Applied Physiology 89(1):176–181

Gute D, Fraga C, Laughlin M H et al 1996 Regional changes in capillary supply in skeletal muscle of high-intensity endurance-trained rats. Journal of Applied Physiology 81(2):619–626

Haennel R G, Quinney H A, Kappagoda C T 1991 Effects of hydraulic circuit training following coronary artery bypass surgery. Medicine and Science in Sports and Exercise 23(2):158–165

Haff G G 2000 Roundtable discussion: machines versus free weights. Strength and Conditioning 22(6):18–30

Hagerman F C, Walsh S J, Staron R S et al 2000 Effects of high-intensity resistance training on untrained older men: strength, cardiovascular, and metabolic responses. The Journals of Gerontology. Series A, Biological Sciences and Medical Sciences 55(7):B336–346

Hakkinen K, Hakkinen A 1995 Neuromuscular adaptations during intensive strength training in middle-aged and elderly males and females. Electromyography and Clinical Neurophysiology 35(3):137–147

Hakkinen K, Newton R U, Gordon S E et al 1998 Changes in muscle morphology, electromyographic activity, and force production characteristics during progressive strength training in young and older men. The Journals of Gerontology. Series A, Biological Sciences and Medical Sciences 53(6):B415–423

Hakkinen K, Alen M, Kallinen M et al 2000 Neuromuscular adaptation during prolonged strength training, detraining and re-strength-training in middle-aged and elderly people. European Journal of Applied Physiology 83(1):51–62

Harman E A 1983 Resistive torque analysis of 5 nautilus machines. Medicine and Science in Sports and Exercise 15(2):115

Hartmann S, Bung P 1999 Physical exercise during pregnancy-physiological considerations and recommendations. Journal of Perinatal Medicine 27(3):204–15

Hass C J, Garzarella L, de Hoyos D et al 2000 Single versus multiple sets in long-term recreational weightlifters. Medicine and Science in Sports and Exercise 32(1):235–242

Hedrick A 2000 Training the trunk for improved athletic performance. Strength and Conditioning 22(3):50–61

Hettinger R, Muller E 1953 Muskelleistung und Muskeltraining. Arbeits Physiologie 15:111–126

Higbie E J, Cureton K J, Warren G L et al 1996 Effects of concentric and eccentric training on muscle strength, cross-sectional area, and neural activation. Journal of Applied Physiology 81(5):2173–2181

Higgins S 1991 Motor skill acquisition. Physical Therapy 71(2):123–139

Holloszy J O 1967 Biochemical adaptations in muscle. Effects of exercise on mitochondrial oxygen uptake and respiratory enzyme activity in skeletal muscle. Journal of Biological Chemistry 242:2278–2282

Houmard J, Hickey M, Tyndall G et al 1995 Seven days of exercise increase GLUT-4 protein content in human skeletal muscle. Journal of Applied Physiology 79:1936–1938

Hurley B F, Redmond R A, Pratley R E et al 1995 Effects of strength training on muscle hypertrophy and muscle cell disruption in older men. International Journal of Sports Medicine 16(6):378–384

Johnson J H, Colodny S, Jackson D 1990 Human torque capability versus machine resistive torque for four Eagle resistive machines. Journal Applied Sport Science Research 4(3):83–87

Kannus P, Jozsa L, Natri A et al 1997 Effects of training, immobilization and remobilization on tendons. Scandinavian Journal of Medicine and Science in Sports 7(2):67–71

Kerr D, Ackland T, Maslen B et al 2001 Resistance training over 2 years increases bone mass in calcium-replete postmenopausal women. Journal of Bone Mineral Research 16(1):175–181

Kraemer W J 1997 A series of studies – the physiological basis for strength in American football: fact over philosophy. Journal of Strength and Conditioning Research 11(3):131–142

Kraemer W J, Noble B J, Clark M J et al 1987 Physiologic responses to heavy-resistance exercise with very short rest periods. International Journal of Sports Medicine 8(4):247–252

Kraemer W J, Fleck S J, Evans W J 1996 Strength and power training: physiological mechanisms of adaptation. Exercise and Sport Sciences Reviews 24:363–397

Kraemer W J, Stone M H, O'Bryant H S et al 1997 Effects of single vs. multiple sets of weight training: impact of volume, intensity, and variation. Journal of Strength and Conditioning Research 11(3):143–147

Kraemer W J, Hakkinen K, Newton R U et al 1999 Effects of heavy-resistance training on hormonal response patterns in younger vs. older men. Journal of Applied Physiology 87(3):982–992

Kraemer W J, Ratamess N, Fry A C et al 2000 Influence of resistance training volume and periodization on physiological and performance adaptations in collegiate women tennis players. American Journal of Sports Medicine 28(5):626–633

Kraemer W J, Mazzetti S A, Nindl B C et al 2001 Effect of resistance training on women's strength/power and occupational performances. Medicine and Science in Sports and Exercise 33(6):1011–1025

LaChance P 1995 Plyometric exercise. Strength and Conditioning 17(4):16–23

Laughlin M H 1999 Cardiovascular response to exercise. Advances in Physiology Education 22(1):S244–S259

Leighton J, Holmes D, Benson J et al 1967 A study of the effectiveness of ten different methods of progressive resistance exercise on the development of strength, flexibility, girth, and body weight. Journal of the Association for Physical and Mental Rehabilitation 21:78–81

Lemmer J T, Ivey F M, Ryan A S et al 2001 Effect of strength training on resting metabolic rate and physical activity: age and gender comparisons. Medicine and Science in Sports and Exercise 33(4):532–541

Lemon P W 1998 Effects of exercise on dietary protein requirements. International Journal of Sport Nutrition 8(4):426–447

Levy W C, Cerqueira M D, Harp G D et al 1998 Effect of endurance exercise training on heart rate variability at rest in healthy young and older men. American Journal of Cardiology 82(10):1236–1241

Lindheim S, Notelovitz M, Feldman E et al 1994 The independent effects of exercise and estrogen on lipids and lipoproteins in postmenopausal women. Obstetrics and Gynecology 83:167–172

McCall G E, Byrnes W C, Dickinson A et al 1996 Muscle fiber hypertrophy, hyperplasia, and capillary density in college men after resistance training. Journal of Applied Physiology 81(5):2004–2012

McCarrick M J, Kemp J G 2000 The effect of strength training and reduced training on rotator cuff musculature. Clinical Biomechanics 15(1 suppl):S42–45

McLester J R, Bishop P, Guilliams M E 2000 Comparison of 1 day and 3 days per week of equal-volume resistance training in experienced subjects. Journal of Strength and Conditioning Research 14(3):273–281

McMorris R O, Elkins E C 1954 A study of production and evaluation of muscular hypertrophy. Archives of Physical Medicine and Rehabilitation 35:420–426

Macera C A, Pate R R, Powell K E et al 1989 Predicting lower-extremity injuries among habitual runners. Archives of Internal Medicine 149:256–258

Madsen K, Holmskov U 1995 Capillary density measurements in skeletal muscle using immunohistochemical staining with anti-collagen type IV antibodies. European Journal of Applied Physiology and Occupational Physiology 71(5):472–474

Mahon A D, Vaccaro P 1989 Ventilatory threshold and VO₂max changes in children following endurance training. Medicine and Science in Sports and Exercise 21(4):425–431

Mandigout S, Lecoq A M, Courteix C et al 2001 Effect of gender in response to an aerobic training programme in prepubertal children. Acta Paediatrica 90(1):9–15

Mannion A F, Jakeman P M, Willan P L 1992 Effects of isokinetic training of the knee extensors on isometric strength and peak power output during cycling. European Journal of Applied Physiology and Occupational Physiology 65(4):370–375

Martel G F, Hurlbut D E, Lott M E et al 1999 Strength training normalizes resting blood pressure in 65- to 73-year-old men and women with high normal blood pressure. Journal of the American Geriatrics Society 47(10):1215–1221

Marx J O, Ratamess N A, Nindl B C et al 2001 Low-volume circuit versus high-volume periodized resistance training in women. Medicine and Science in Sports and Exercise 33(4):635–643

Mayhew J L, Ware J R, Prinster J L 1993 Using lift repetitions to predict muscular strength in adolescent males. National Strength and Conditioning Association Journal 15:35–38

Michna H, Hartmann G 1989 Adaptation of tendon collagen to exercise. International Orthopaedics 13(3):161–165

Mole P A, Oscai L B, Holloszy J O 1971 Adaptations of muscle to exercise. Increase in levels of palmityl-CoA synthase, carnitine palmityltransferase and palmityl CoA dehydrogenase and in the capacity to oxidize fatty acids. Journal of Clinical Investigation 50:2323–2330

Morrissey M C, Harman E A, Johnson M J 1995 Resistance training modes: specificity and effectiveness. Medicine and Science in Sports and Exercise 27(5):648–660

Narici M V, Hoppeler H, Kayser B et al 1996 Human quadriceps cross-sectional area, torque and neural activation during 6 months strength training. Acta Physiologica Scandinavica 157(2):175–186

O'Neill D S, Zheng D, Anderson W K et al 1999 Effect of endurance exercise on myosin heavy chain gene regulation in human skeletal muscle. American Journal of Physiology 276(45):R414–R419

Paterson D H, Cunningham D A, Koval J J et al 1999 Aerobic fitness in a population of independently living men and women aged 55–86 years. Medicine and Science in Sports and Exercise 31(12):1813–1820

Pincivero D M, Lephart S M, Karunakara R G 1997 Effects of rest interval on isokinetic strength and functional performance after short-term high intensity training. British Journal of Sports Medicine 31(3):229–234

Pollock M L, Bohannon R L, Cooper K H et al 1976 A comparative analysis of four protocols for maximal treadmill stress testing. American Heart Journal 92:39–46

Pollock M L, Graves J E, Bamman M M et al 1993 Frequency and volume of resistance training: effect on cervical extension strength. Archives of Physical Medicine and Rehabilitation 74(10):1080–1086

Porter M M 2001 The effects of strength training on sarcopenia. Canadian Journal of Applied Physiology 26(1):123–141

Roca J, Agusti A G, Alonso A et al 1992 Effects of training on muscle O₂ transport at VO₂max. Journal of Applied Physiology 73(3):1067–1076

Rhodes E C, Martin A D, Taunton J E et al 2000 Effects of one year of resistance training on the relation between muscular strength and bone density in elderly women. British Journal of Sports Medicine 34(1):18–22

Rowland T W 1992 Trainability of the cardiorespiratory system during childhood. Canadian Journal of Sport Science 17(4):259–263

Rowland T W, Martel L, Vanderburgh P et al 1996 The influence of short-term aerobic training on blood lipids in healthy 10–12 year old children. International Journal of Sports Medicine 17(7):487–492

Ryan A S, Hurlbut D E, Lott M E et al 2001 Insulin action after resistive training in insulin resistant older men and women. Journal of the American Geriatrics Society 49(3):247–253

Ryushi T, Kumagai K, Hayase H et al 2000 Effect of resistive knee extension training on postural control measures in middle aged and elderly persons. Journal of Physiological Anthropology and Applied Human Science 19(3):143–149

Sanborn K, Boros R, Hruby J et al 2000 Short-term performance effects of weight training with multiple sets not to failure vs. a single set to failure in women. Journal of Strength and Conditioning Research 14(3):328–331

Santos J 1979 Jump training for speed and neuromuscular development. Track and Field Quarterly Review 79(1):59

Scandalis T A, Bosak A, Berliner J C et al 2001 Resistance training and gait function in patients with Parkinson's disease. American Journal of Physical Medicine and Rehabilitation 80(1):38–43

Schlicht J, Camaione D N, Owen S V 2001 Effect of intense strength training on standing balance, walking speed, and sit-to-stand performance in older adults. The Journals of Gerontology. Series A, Biological Sciences and Medical Sciences 56(5):M281–286

Schlumberger A, Justyna S, Schlumberger D 2001 Single- vs. multiple-set strength training in women. Journal of Strength and Conditioning Research 15(3):284–289

Schwarz R, Kindermann W 1990 B-endorphin, adrenocorticotropin hormone, cortisol and catecholamines during aerobic and anaerobic exercise. European Journal of Applied Physiology 61:165–171

Smith E, Gilligan C, McAdam M et al 1989 Deterring bone loss by exercise. Calcified Tissue International 44:312–321

Smith M J, Melton P 1981 Isokinetic versus isotonic variable-resistance training. American Journal of Sports Medicine 9(4):275–279

Schwartz R S, Cain K C, Shuman W P et al 1992 Effect of intensive endurance training on lipoprotein profiles in young and older men. Metabolism 41:649–654

Sparling P B, Cantwell J D, Dolan C M et al 1990 Strength training in a cardiac rehabilitation program: a six-month follow-up. Archives of Physical Medicine and Rehabilitation 71(2):148–152

Starkey D B, Pollock M L, Ishida Y et al 1996 Effect of resistance training volume on strength and muscle thickness. Medicine and Science in Sports and Exercise 28(10):1311–1320

Steinhaus L A, Dustman R E, Ruhling R O et al 1990 Aerobic capacity of older adults: a training study. Journal of Sports Medicine and Physical Fitness 30(2):163–172

Stewart K J 1989 Resistive training effects on strength and cardiovascular endurance in cardiac and coronary prone patients. Medicine and Science in Sports and Exercise 21(6):678–682

Stone M H 1988 Implications for connective tissue and bone alterations resulting from resistance exercise training. Medicine and Science in Sports and Exercise 20(5 suppl):S162–168

Stone M H 1990 Muscle conditioning and muscle injuries. Medicine and Science in Sports and Exercise 22(4):457–462

Stone M H, O'Bryant H, Garhammer J 1981 A hypothetical model for strength training. Journal of Sports Medicine and Physical Fitness 21(4):342–351

Stone M H, Potteiger J A, Pierce K C et al 2000 Comparison of the effects of three different weight-training programs on the one-repetition maximum squat. Journal of Strength and Conditioning Research 14(3):332–337

Suter E, Hoppeler H, Claassen H et al 1995 Ultrastructural modification of human skeletal muscle tissue with 6-month moderate-intensity exercise training. International Journal of Sports Medicine 16(3):160–166

Svedenhag J, Henriksson J, Sylven C 1983 Dissociation of training effects on skeletal muscle mitochondrial enzymes and myoglobin in man. Acta Physiologica Scandinavica 117(2):213–218

Swash M, Fox K 1972 Muscle spindle innervation in man. Journal of Anatomy 112:61–80

Taaffe D R, Duret C, Wheeler S et al 1999 Once-weekly resistance exercise improves muscle strength and neuromuscular performance in older adults. Journal of the American Geriatrics Society 47(10):1208–1214

Tesch P A, Thorsson A, Colliander E B 1990 Effects of eccentric and concentric resistance training on skeletal muscle substrates, enzyme activities and capillary supply. Acta Physiologica Scandinavica 140(4):575–580

Todd I C, Wosornu D, Stewart I et al 1992 Cardiac rehabilitation following myocardial infarction. A practical approach. Sports Medicine 14(4):243–259

Trappe S W, Costill D L, Vukovich M D et al 1996 Aging among elite distance runners: a 22-yr longitudinal study. Journal of Applied Physiology 80(1):285–290

Tsutsumi T, Don B M, Zaichkowsky L D et al 1998 Comparison of high and moderate intensity of strength training on mood and anxiety in older adults. Perceptual and Motor Skills 87(3 Pt 1):1003–1011

Tucci J T, Carpenter D M, Pollock M L et al 1992 Effect of reduced frequency of training and detraining on lumbar extension strength. Spine 17(12):1497–1501

Tucker L A, Maxwell K 1992 Effects of weight training on the emotional well-being and body image of females: predictors of greatest benefit. American Journal of Health Promotion 6(5):338–344, 371

Verkhoshanski Y 1966 Perspectives in the improvement of speed-strength preparation of jumpers. Track and Field 9:11–12

Voight M L 1992 Stretch-strengthening: an introduction to plyometrics. Orthopedic Physical Therapy Clinics of North America 1(2):243–252

Wathen D 1993 NSCA position paper: explosive/plyometric exercises. National Strength and Conditioning Association Journal 15(3):16–19

Wathen D, Shutes M 1982 A comparison of the effects of selected isotonic and isokinetic modalities, and programs on the acquisition of strength and power in collegiate football players. National Strength and Conditioning Association Journal 4(1):40–42

Weaver C M, Teegarden D, Lyle R M et al 2001 Impact of exercise on bone health and contraindication of oral contraceptive use in young women. Medicine and Science in Sports and Exercise 33(6):873–880

Weiss A, Suzuki T, Bean J et al 2000 High intensity strength training improves strength and functional performance after stroke. American Journal of Physical Medicine and Rehabilitation 79(4):369–376

Welle S, Totterman S, Thornton C 1996 Effect of age on muscle hypertrophy induced by resistance training. The Journals of Gerontology. Series A, Biological Sciences and Medical Sciences 51(6):M270–275

Wilk K E, Voight M L, Keirns M A et al 1993 Stretch-shortening drills for the upper extremities: theory and clinical application. Journal of Orthopedic and Sports Physical Therapy 17(5):225–239

Wilmore J H, Stanforth P R, Hudspeth L A et al 1998 Alterations in resting metabolic rate as a consequence of 20 wk of endurance training: The HERITAGE Family Study. American Journal of Clinical Nutrition 68:66–71

Wilmore J H, Despres J P, Stanforth P R et al 1999 Alterations in body weight and composition consequent to 20 wk of endurance training: The HERITAGE Family Study. American Journal of Clinical Nutrition 70:346–352

Wilmore J H, Stanforth P R, Gagnon J et al 2001 Heart rate and blood pressure changes with endurance training: The HERITAGE Family Study. Medicine and Science in Sports and Exercise 33(1):107–116

Wilt F 1975 Plyometrics – What it is and how it works. Athletic Journal 55b:76–91

Zernicke R F, Loitz B J 1992 Exercise-related adaptations in connective tissue. In: Komi P V (ed) Strength and power in sport. Blackwell Scientific Publications, Oxford

Zinovieff A 1951 Heavy resistance exercise: the Oxford technique. British Journal of Physical Medicine 14:129–132

10

Psychology of injury and rehabilitation

Gregory S Kolt

INTRODUCTION

Participation in sport, exercise, and physical activity has dramatically increased in recent times, resulting in a greater potential for, and incidence of, physical injury. The costs involved in rehabilitating people injured through sport and exercise, the loss of sport and work participation time, interventions to reduce vulnerability, the risk of long-term injury, and the consequential reduced quality of life are all major public health concerns.

The extent of sport and exercise injuries varies across countries. For example, in Australia, 20% of child and adolescent and 18% of adult hospital emergency room consultations were related to sport injuries (Finch et al 1998). In the UK, sport and exercise-related injuries accounted for 33% of all injuries reported in a population survey (Uitenbroek 1996). In the USA, of the estimated 17 million annual sport and recreation injuries (see Brewer 2001), nearly 2 million require hospital emergency room consultations (NEISS data highlights 1998). Highlighting the problem further, Weaver et al (1999) suggested that in a single state in the USA, injuries sustained by high school athletes in 12 sports would produce medical costs of $10 million in the long term and a further $19 million of lost earnings.

The impact of sport and exercise injury is wide reaching. Not only are there the obviously detrimental effects on the financial, physical, and performance aspects of individuals in sport, but also a psychological impact is often apparent. In the past, a principal focus of sport injury rehabilitation has been to return individuals to their prior level of functioning by treating their overt physical problems. More current literature, however, highlights the increasing trend toward managing athletes more holistically, with a greater emphasis on addressing the psychological consequences of injury and rehabilitation (Brewer 2001, Francis et al 2000, Kolt 2000, Ninedek & Kolt 2000). The purpose of this chapter is to discuss the psychological precursors to injury, the psychological responses to injury, and the psychological factors that can influence rehabilitation from sport and exercise injury. The chapter will also focus on psychosocial approaches that can be used by physical therapists to complement their physical management programs.

PSYCHOLOGICAL PRECURSORS TO INJURY

An increasing body of research over the past few decades has focused on psychosocial variables and their influence on injury vulnerability and resiliency. This research has considered a wide range of psychosocial factors including stress, anxiety, self-confidence, locus of control, attention, cognitive mood states, coping mechanisms, motivation, and personality (Kirkby 1995, Williams & Andersen 1998).

Personality components were among the earlier variables researched in this area (e.g. Brown 1971, Govern & Koppenhaver 1965, Ogilvie and Tutko 1966), along with the stress caused by major life events (e.g. Bramwell et al 1975). Although this foundation work suggested that athletes' injuries were linked to factors such as life stress, fear of competition, hostility, masochism, and masculinity, no theoretical framework was offered to explain the relationships.

In response to the lack of an underpinning theoretical model, Andersen & Williams (1988) developed a multi-component theoretical model of stress and injury. This model suggested that most psychological variables, if they influence injury outcome, do so through a link with stress and a resulting stress response. The original stress–injury model was revised and refined over the following decade (Williams & Andersen 1998). This model (Fig. 10.1) is still viewed as the definitive explanation of the relationship between sports injury and psychological factors.

The majority of recent investigations into psychological variables and injury in sport have drawn upon the Williams & Andersen (1998) model of stress and athletic injury and its earlier version. Figure 10.1 shows that the model focuses on the stress response (the central portion of the model) and the three broad categories of variables hypothesized to influence this response: personality, history of stressors, and coping resources. Following the concepts of Folkman & Lazarus (1985), the stress response is viewed as the way in which the cognitive and physiological elements of stressful situations interact. That is, the impact of a stressor is likely to be a function of the individual's appraisal of the extent of the stressor, the coping processes used by the individual, and the perceptions of the resources that the individual has to manage the stressor. Applying this to a sports context, athletes continually appraise the demands of varying situations and their ability to meet those demands. When the demands of a particular situation outweigh the resources that the athlete has to respond to that situation, the stress response elevates.

The cognitive appraisal of demands and resources is connected bidirectionally to physiological and attentional responses (Williams & Andersen 1998). For example, a common somatic response to stress involves generalized muscle tension. This muscle tension can, in turn, lead to altered motor coordination and reduced flexibility, thus contributing to musculoskeletal injuries such as strains and sprains (Andersen & Williams 1988). Also relevant to this are the attentional changes related to stress. For example, narrowing of the visual field can occur during stress resulting in a failure to extract vital cues from the periphery and, thereby, increase the likelihood of injury (Andersen & Williams 1988). Also, under conditions of stress, attention can become distracted resulting in athletes attending to stimuli irrelevant to the task at hand and missing the more vital cues (Andersen & Williams 1988). In relation to the cognitive appraisal influence on the stress response, individuals will appraise the demands of a situation, the adequacy of their ability to meet those demands, and the potential consequences of success or failure (Williams & Andersen 1998). From a cognitive perspective, it is the level of match or mismatch between the demands, the ability to meet those demands, and the consequences of success or failure that will influence the stress response.

Three broad categories of variables influence the stress response: personality factors, history of stressors, and coping resources, as identified in Figure 10.1 (Williams & Andersen 1998). These variables can either act singly or

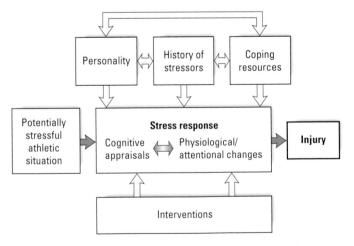

Figure 10.1 The stress and injury model. (Copyright 1998 from Psychosocial antecedents of sport injury: review and critique of the stress and injury model by Williams J M, Andersen M B. Reproduced by permission of Taylor and Francis, Inc., http://www.routledge-ny.com.)

in combination to influence the stress response, and ultimately, injury. The model indicates that an individual's history of stressors, personality factors, and coping resources can influence the stress response either directly or through a moderating influence on each other.

There is substantial evidence to support Andersen & Williams' (1988) assertion that an individual's history of stressors (i.e. major life events, chronic daily problems, and previous injuries) can have a substantial impact on the stress response and, thus, on injury. Reviews of the literature on life stress and injury provide excellent support for a relationship between these factors in a range of contact and non-contact sports (Williams & Roepke 1993, Williams & Andersen 1998). In fact, 27 of the 30 life stress studies published between 1970 and 1998 found some type of positive relationship between high life stress (both negative life stress, such as death of a close family member, or positive life stress, such as a competitive win at a major sports event) and injury in sport (e.g. Andersen & Williams 1999, Kolt & Kirkby 1996, Petrie 1993a, 1993b, Thompson & Morris 1994).

The history of stressors in the Williams & Andersen (1998) model includes daily hassles. The role of minor daily problems, irritations, and changes in influencing the stress response has been less researched than life stress, with less conclusive evidence available. While the early studies failed to show any positive relationship between daily hassles and injury (e.g. Blackwell & McCullagh 1990), a recent investigation found that athletes were more likely to incur an injury when they experienced significant increases in daily hassles in the week before and the week of the injury (Fawkner et al 1999).

The final type of stressor described in the Williams & Andersen (1998) model relates to past injuries. Previous injury can affect future injury when athletes have not recovered enough physically to return to sport, but do so anyway. Also, if athletes return to sport when physically, but not psychologically, prepared problems could arise from negative self-evaluations regarding their ability to perform, given their injury and reduced training schedule during the rehabilitation process. Furthermore, according to Williams & Andersen (1998), fear of reinjury can, in itself, be a substantial stressor, and thus can increase the likelihood of injury. This aspect of the model, however, has only received limited support (Lysens et al 1984).

The second category of variables thought to influence the stress response is components of personality (e.g. locus of control, competitive trait anxiety, hardiness, achievement motivation, and sensation seeking characteristics). Research of these variables has produced mixed findings and the literature in this area is too large to review in detail. However, it should be noted that positive links have been found to athletic injury for variables including locus of control, state anxiety, trait anxiety, negative state of mind, tough mindedness, and defensive pessimism (see Williams & Andersen 1998).

The final component of the model consists of coping resources, which are thought to influence the stress response. Coping resources can include social support, stress management skills, other psychological coping skills, and general coping behaviors, such as appropriate nutrition and sleep habits. There is significant evidence that coping resources are related to injury outcome or moderate the influence of life stress on injury vulnerability (Williams & Andersen 1998). For example, Andersen & Williams (1999) found that low levels of social support directly influenced stress responsivity, and hence injury vulnerability. Smith et al (1990a) also showed that coping resources can moderate the effect of stressors on psychological and physical outcomes.

Despite further research being required to verify certain aspects of the Williams & Andersen (1998) model of stress and injury, the evidence to date supports it as an explanation of injury occurrence that is useful in applied sport injury settings.

INTERVENTIONS TO REDUCE INJURY VULNERABILITY

Although previous focus on injury prevention has been on physical, rather than psychosocial dimensions (Petitpas & Danish 1995), more recently, those involved in sports medicine have become increasingly aware of psychosocial influences (Brewer et al 1994, Francis et al 2000, Ninedek & Kolt 2000). Based on the evidence available supporting the relationship between stress and injury vulnerability in sport, it is reasonable to assume that interventions to reduce stress levels or modify the stress response in athletes might decrease the risk of injury. Research in this area, however, has been sparse. A review of psychological interventions in sport injury prevention (Durso-Cupal 1998) found only four empirical studies that addressed this approach (Davis 1991, Kerr & Goss 1996, May & Brown 1989, Schomer 1990). A search of the literature post-1998 failed to identify any more recent studies.

In the earliest of the studies looking at sports injury prevention through psychological intervention, imagery, attention control, and other mental practice skills were used with US Olympic alpine skiers at the Calgary Olympic Games (May & Brown 1989). They reported a reduced injury rate, increased confidence, and enhanced self-control as a result of the intervention, however, they failed to employ a control group or statistical comparisons. A study where marathon runners were taught how to use appropriate attentional strategies (i.e. associative thought processes) over a 5-week period reported that heavy training could be facilitated without injury (Schomer 1990). However, this study did not use a control group either and did not use statistical procedures.

Two particular studies looked at the effect of stress management programs on injury prevention in athletes (Davis 1991, Kerr & Goss 1996). In the earlier of these, Davis (1991) used a program of imagery of sports skills and progressive muscular relaxation with collegiate swimmers and football players and found a 52% reduction in swimming injuries and a 33% reduction in football injuries. These findings, however, were based on a problematic methodology where no control group or statistical analyses were used.

The most comprehensive study looking at the role of stress management in injury prevention was that by Kerr & Goss (1996). In this study, Kerr & Goss provided a 16-session stress management program to 12 national and international level Canadian gymnasts over an 8-month period. The stress management program was based primarily on Meichenbaum's (1985) Stress Inoculation Training and included work on thought processes, self-talk, dealing with distractions, thought stopping, relaxation, imagery, and preparation for competition. A further 12 gymnasts, matched according to sex, age, and performance level, acted as a control group. It was found that the gymnasts who undertook the stress management intervention reported significantly lower levels of negative athletic stress from the mid-part of the season to the peak of the season. In relation to injury, although it appeared that the stress management group spent less time injured by the end of the 8-month intervention, the difference was not statistically significant. Notwithstanding this finding, Andersen & Stoove (1998), in commenting on the Kerr & Goss study, pointed out that Kerr & Goss probably showed a clinically significant effect in injury reduction from their stress management intervention, despite statistical significance not being achieved. That is, their failure to show a significant difference probably had more to do with the small sample size and resultant low power than the effectiveness of the intervention.

Sports medicine professionals have the perfect opportunity to teach athletes ways of handling stressful events, reaching goals, and identifying and overcoming barriers (Shaffer & Wiese-Bjornstal 1999). They further suggested that the role of various psychological techniques in reducing injury can 'psychologically strengthen' athletes and can have an effect on minimizing injury occurrence. The techniques commonly recommended in such interventions include the teaching of coping mechanisms, relaxation techniques, imagery or cognitive rehearsal, positive self-talk (including the minimization of negative thoughts), social support, and other general stress reduction methods (Ievleva & Orlick 1999, Shaffer & Wiese-Bjornstal 1999, Williams 2001). Smith et al (1990a)

proposed that, from an intervention perspective, resiliency to sport injuries could be increased by either increasing social support in athletes' lives or by instructing athletes in coping skills.

PSYCHOLOGY OF SPORT AND EXERCISE INJURY REHABILITATION

In addition to psychological factors playing a role in injury occurrence, more recent research has focused on the impact of psychological variables on the way athletes react to injury and the rehabilitation process that follows.

MODELS OF PSYCHOLOGICAL FACTORS IN INJURY REHABILITATION

To put into perspective the psychological responses athletes have to injury and the consequent rehabilitation process, it is important to consider appropriate theoretical models. Not only do such theoretical explanations allow better-grounded research to take place, but they also allow physical therapists to interpret psychological reactions displayed by athletes in a broader and more meaningful sense. Two types of models have been reported in the literature: the biopsychosocial model (Brewer et al 2001b) and psychological models.

Biopsychosocial model

Both the medical and psychological perspectives need to be considered in order to fully examine psychological factors within the overall context of sport injury rehabilitation (Brewer 2001). The most recent model of sport injury rehabilitation that has drawn on this combined structure is the biopsychosocial model of sport injury rehabilitation (Fig. 10.2) (Brewer et al 2001b). This model was developed by incorporating the frameworks of existing models of sport injury rehabilitation (Flint 1998, Leadbetter 1994, Wiese-Bjornstal et al 1998). The main components of the model are injury, sociodemographic factors, biological factors, psychological factors, social/contextual factors, intermediate biopsychological outcomes, and sport injury rehabilitation outcomes. In this theoretical explanation, the characteristics of injury (e.g. type, course, severity, location, and history) are proposed to influence the biological, psychological, and social/contextual factors. Also, sociodemographic factors (e.g. age, gender, race/ethnicity, and socioeconomic status) effect an influence on the biological, psychological, and social/contextual factors. The three categories of factors resulting from injury can influence the intermediate biopsychological outcomes (e.g. range of motion, strength,

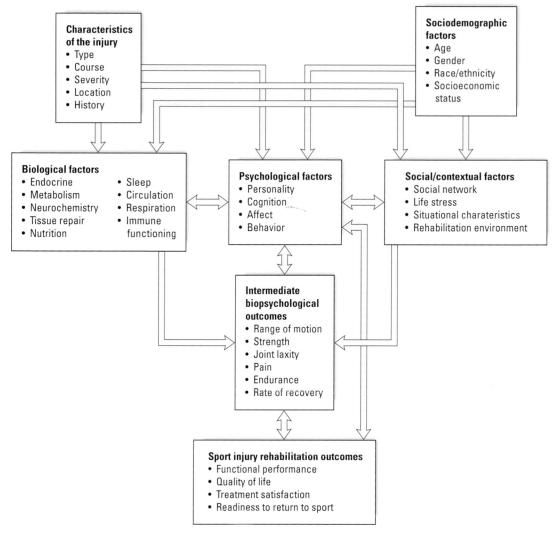

Figure 10.2   The biopsychosocial model of sport injury rehabilitation. (Reproduced from Brewer et al 2001b with the permission of Fitness Information Technology.)

joint laxity, pain, endurance, and recovery rate), and in turn impact on the rehabilitation outcomes. The psychological factors resulting from injury have a unique role in this model in that they have a direct bidirectional path to sport injury rehabilitation outcomes.

The biopsychosocial model described above has its advantage in proposing links between components of traditional psychological models and more medically focused models. However, by suggesting these links, it does not provide for the many interactions that can occur between specific psychological variables during the injury and rehabilitation process.

Psychological models

It is important to consider the many psychological models that have appeared in the literature. The grief response model and the cognitive appraisal model are two recognized models that can be applied to rehabilitation from a sport injury.

Grief response model

One of the commonly used models to explain psychological aspects of injury rehabilitation in sport and exercise is Kubler-Ross' (1969) grief response model. This model, initially developed to explain significant loss (e.g. death of a family member) suggests that individuals typically progress through five stages of grieving: denial, anger, bargaining, depression, and acceptance. This model has been applied to sport injury rehabilitation as a result of suggestions that injuries involve a loss of an aspect of the self (Gordon et al 1991, Macchi & Crossman 1996, Peretz 1970).

Table 10.1 Examples of typical thoughts and behaviors present at each stage of the grief response model as it relates to sport injury

Stage of reaction	Thoughts	Behaviors
1. Denial	'I can play my way through this injury It won't stop me'	Continue to play or train with an injury
2. Anger	'Why did the coach make me play this new position?' 'Just my luck to get injured before the finals'	Storm away from training or a team meeting
3. Bargaining	'If I do all my exercises at home, maybe I can begin playing a week earlier than the physical therapist said I could. They really don't know what athletes go through'	Failure to follow medical advice regarding rest and rehabilitation activities
4. Depression	'I'm not getting anywhere with this exercise program. Why should I even bother with going to rehabilitation?'	Lack of motivation Lethargy Withdrawal from sport involvement
5. Acceptance	'I can now see that the physical therapist was right. I should continue to follow the instructions'	Positive self-talk Displaying commitment to the rehabilitation program Adhering to rehabilitation advice

The grief response model indicates that each 'stage' is characterized by specific moods and behaviors, and that athletes will move through the various stages over the recovery and rehabilitation period. Initially, athletes may show *denial* of their injury, possibly rejecting the prognosis and refusing to accept the limitations placed upon them as a result of the injury. After denial, some athletes can experience *anger* and display extreme and abrupt emotional reactions (possible towards someone or something considered responsible for the injury); often, such responses are irrational. Following anger, athletes can enter a *bargaining* stage (e.g. bargaining with sports medicine providers over rehabilitation and return to sport guidelines). The fourth stage of the grief response model is that of *depression*. Athletes can show depressive symptoms when the full realization of the extent of an injury is recognized; this can result in diminished motivation for rehabilitation, and engagement in malproductive behaviors (Horsley 1995). *Acceptance* of the extent and implications of the injury characterize the final stage of this model. Table 10.1 shows examples of typical thoughts and behaviors present at each stage of the grief response model as it relates to sport injury.

Despite the early support for stage models such as the grief response model (Astle 1986, Lynch 1988), more recent evidence has indicated that athletes do not typically progress through the injury period in a structured and staged manner (Brewer 1994). Athletes vary considerably in the way they react to and deal with injury and are influenced by both personal and situational factors (Brewer 1994, Wiese-Bjornstal et al 1998). Consequently, models that consider such individual differences, whilst also recognizing staged responses to grief, have been developed (Evans & Hardy 1999).

Cognitive appraisal models

Cognitive appraisal models are those that are based around stress, coping, and emotional responsivity theories. In sport and exercise, several such theories have been proposed (e.g. Gordon 1986, Weiss & Troxel 1986). Weiss & Troxel (1986) reported a stress model based on the cognitive concept that people's experience of stress (i.e. that may arise from an injury) is a function of their thoughts about stressful situations. For example, a stressful situation (e.g. an injury) is cognitively appraised in relation to the situational and personal resources one has to deal with the situation, as well as the possible outcomes of the event. Then, an emotional response (comprising psychological and attentional components) follows the appraisal. The final stage of the stress process is the behavioral consequences that stem from the emotional responses. This stress process was summarized by Horsley (1995) (Fig. 10.3).

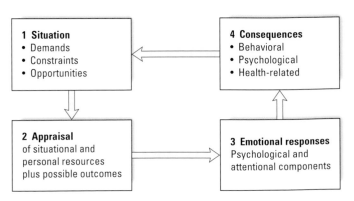

Figure 10.3 The stress process as an example of a cognitive appraisal model of response to sport injury. (Reproduced with permission from Horsley 1995.)

The most developed cognitive appraisal model to date is the Integrated Model of Psychological Response to the Sport Injury and Rehabilitation Process (Wiese-Bjornstal et al 1998). This model (Fig. 10.4) contends that an athlete's response to a sports injury is influenced by both preinjury variables (personality, history of stressors, coping resources, preventative interventions) and postinjury variables. In relation to postinjury variables, the cognitive

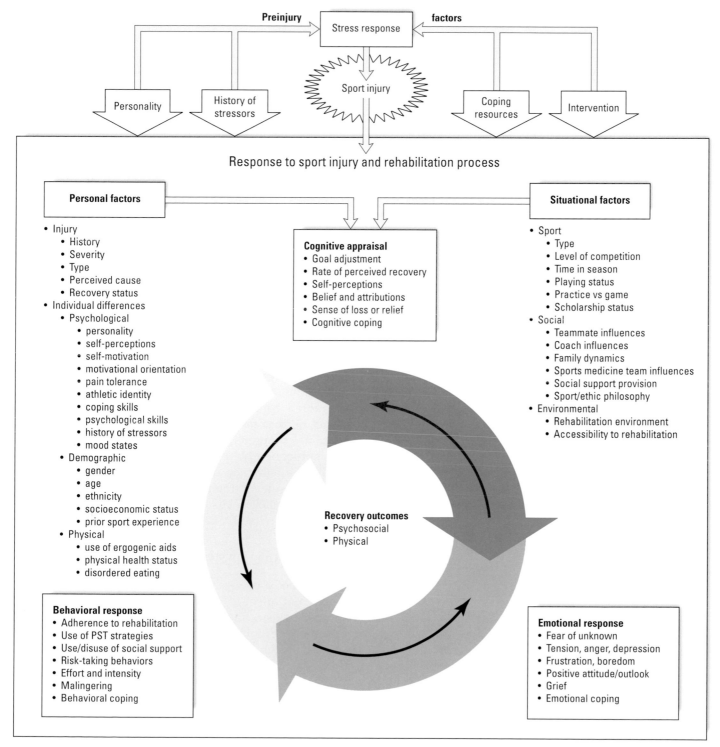

Figure 10.4   Integrated Model of Psychological Response to the Sport Injury and Rehabilitation Process. (Copyright 1998 from An integrated model of response to sport injury: psychological and sociological dimensions by Wiese-Bjornstal D M, Smith A M, Shaffer S M, Morrey M A. Reproduced by permission of Taylor and Francis, Inc., http://www.routledge-ny.com.)

appraisal of the injury is proposed to influence behavioral responses (e.g. adherence to rehabilitation), emotional responses (e.g. tension, anger, and depression), and the recovery outcomes (psychosocial and physical). The model indicates that both personal and situational factors can affect the cognitive appraisal or interpretation of the injurious event.

Although the interactional aspects of cognitive appraisal models have not been extensively researched, particular aspects of such models have been strongly supported (see review by Brewer 2001). Thus, cognitive appraisal models such as Wiese-Bjornstal et al's (1998) appear to be the best framework from which to view the psychological responses to sport injury and rehabilitation.

PSYCHOLOGICAL RESPONSES TO INJURY

Participants in sport and exercise can display a variety of psychological reactions to injury. These responses range from those that are productive and improve the chance for more efficacious rehabilitation to those that are unproductive, causing problems for effective rehabilitation and return to activity. Although the focus for rehabilitation should be on the productive responses to injury, an understanding of the unproductive or maladaptive reactions to the injury process is paramount to the physical therapist. An important feature of psychological responses to athletic injury is their transient nature. In general, the temporal pattern of psychological responses proceed from a negative to positive affect over time (McDonald & Hardy 1990, McGowan et al 1994, Smith et al 1990b, Smith et al 1993), although some support for oscillation between 'highs' and 'lows' during the rehabilitation period has been found (Pearson & Jones 1992).

In line with the cognitive appraisal explanations of the injury process described above, three categories of responses to injury will be discussed: cognitive responses, emotional responses, and behavioral responses.

COGNITIVE RESPONSES TO INJURY

Several cognitive responses have been linked with injury. These include changes in global and domain-specific self-esteem and self-confidence, and increases in negative thoughts and self-talk. Self-esteem appears to be the cognitive response that has been most extensively researched in relation to sport injury. Some studies have shown that global self-esteem decreases after injury (Leddy et al 1994) or differs as a result of injury status (i.e. injured or non-injured) (Kleiber & Brock 1992, Leddy et al

1994, McGowan et al 1994). Other studies have found no global self-esteem differences in relation to injury (Brewer & Petrie 1995, Smith et al 1993). When considering domain-specific self-esteem (i.e. self-esteem for particular sports activities), evidence exists that injured athletes report lower levels than non-injured athletes (Leddy et al 1994).

Some studies have looked at specific aspects of self-referent cognitive responses to injury (e.g. sport self-confidence and rehabilitation self-efficacy). For example, a recent study by Quinn & Fallon (1999) showed that sport self-confidence was high at the commencement of rehabilitation, decreased throughout rehabilitation, and increased again towards the end of the rehabilitation period for athletes with significant injuries (i.e. there was a mean recovery duration of 19.25 weeks). Also, the same group of athletes reported constant high levels of self-confidence in adhering to their rehabilitation programs. It is evident that domain-specific self-referent cognitions in response to injury are variable both between individuals and across periods of rehabilitation.

There appears to be three particular characteristics of the cognitive reactions of injured athletes: irrational and unrealistic beliefs, negative thought processes, and unwarranted worry about problems beyond their control. Relating irrational thoughts of injured athletes back to the early work of Beck (1976), athletes could exaggerate the meaning of the injury (e.g. catastrophize the situation), ignore important aspects of the injury (e.g. physical restrictions as a result of the injury), and rely on unwarranted conclusions when evidence is lacking (e.g. assuming that they will never play sport again). These irrational thoughts and beliefs can influence emotions and subsequently self-esteem and confidence (Horsley 1995). The tendency of injured athletes to worry about things outside of their control can have the effect of channeling their focus away from things that they can control (e.g. rehabilitation tasks).

EMOTIONAL RESPONSES TO INJURY

A large body of research has addressed the emotions, mood, and affect of injured athletes. Depression, anger, confusion, fear, and frustration appear to be common emotional responses to injury, particularly in the early phases of rehabilitation (Bianco et al 1999, Chan & Crossman 1988, Shelley & Sherman 1996, Smith et al 1990b, Udry et al 1997, Weiss & Troxel 1986). Qualitative studies have also shown that as rehabilitation is ending and return to sport is near, emotions related to fear of reinjury increase (Bianco et al 1999, Johnston & Carroll 1998). In relating these responses back to Wiese-Bjornstal et al's (1998) model, Brewer (2001) suggested it is important to consider that these emotional responses to injury seem to be influenced by several personal factors (e.g. previous injury experience) and situational factors (e.g. time of the season the injury occurred and rehabilitation progress).

Although it is usually considered that emotional disturbance linked to sport injury does not reach clinical levels (Heil 1993), epidemiological findings provide evidence that up to 24% of injured athletes do display clinically meaningful levels of emotional disturbance (Brewer 2001). At the extreme of the continuum, some athletes with severe depression consider attempting suicide (Smith & Milliner 1994). The majority of research indicates that, generally, negative emotions decrease and positive emotions increase as the rehabilitation period and recovery progress (Dawes & Roach 1997, Macchi & Crossman 1996, Miller 1998, Quinn & Fallon 1999). As mentioned earlier, however, negative emotions can increase again towards the end of the rehabilitation period with the prospect of returning to sporting activity and the associated fear of reinjury. This has been shown particularly with long-term rehabilitation from reconstructive knee surgery (Morrey et al 1999). More specifically, these two studies found that athletes who underwent reconstructive knee surgery showed high negative and low positive mood states around the time of the surgical intervention, which then progressed to more positive and less negative mood during the first few weeks post-surgery, returning to more negative and less positive as they were about to return to sporting activity.

BEHAVIORAL RESPONSES TO INJURY

Cognitive and emotional responses to injury impact on the behaviors displayed by athletes during the rehabilitation period. Some of the primary behavioral responses to injury are adherence to rehabilitation and the use of coping mechanisms. The behaviors related to rehabilitation adherence will be covered in a later section of this chapter. Coping mechanisms, due to the dynamic and changing nature of rehabilitation programs, can change over the course of rehabilitation (Udry 1997). Athletes utilize a broad range of coping behaviors. For example, a study of skiers who had sustained major injuries that precluded further participation for the remainder of a competitive season found that using social support, distraction, avoiding others and isolating oneself, and 'driving through' (e.g. working hard towards rehabilitation goals) were the predominant coping behaviors used (Gould et al 1997). Udry (1997) reported that athletes recovering from knee surgery used instrumental coping behaviors (i.e. those aimed at dealing directly with a stressor) most commonly. It is interesting to note that athletes tend to prefer active (i.e. behaviors that involve their own input) rather than passive

(i.e. behaviors that are reliant on others) coping strategies (Smith et al 1990b, Gould et al 1997).

A further behavioral response to injury involves malingering. Malingering behavior has been described by Rotella et al (1999) as an adjustment to negative circumstances that requires an external incentive for being injured. For example, athletes who are trying to avoid returning to sport after a significant injury may consciously exaggerate their symptoms. It has been suggested that athletes who repeatedly adopt this behavior might be doing so as a response to fear, requiring attention, or both (Rotella et al 1999). Reasons for malingering could include poor performance, an escape from the pressure of sport, personal realizations of limited ability, and rationalization of loss of place in a team. Physical therapists and other sports medicine practitioners should be aware of malingering as a behavior so that they can modify their approach to management accordingly.

POSITIVE RESPONSES TO INJURY

It should be noted, that on some occasions positive emotional benefits emerge from sport and exercise injuries. Udry et al (1997), based on interviews with injured elite athletes, reported an example of this. Of the athletes interviewed, 95% reported positive consequences of their injury that could be categorized into personal growth consequences, psychologically based performance enhancements, and physical-technical development opportunities. The athletes reported that they learnt to be more empathic toward other injured athletes and developed skills and interests outside of their sport. They also indicated that they became 'mentally tougher' and learned more about their psychological boundaries. Furthermore, they reported that they could spend time on the more physical and technical aspects of their sport.

The positive consequences of injury fit well with the Life Development Model (Danish et al 1995). According to the Life Development Model perspective, when people are faced with what are called 'critical life events' or 'turning points', they respond in several ways. Specifically, critical life events (e.g. major injuries) can lead to debilitation or decreased functioning, increased opportunities for growth, or in some individuals, no change at all.

It stands to reason that for rehabilitation practitioners and athletes to get the most out of the injury process, they should facilitate the positive consequences of such injuries. While recognizing that most athletes will not automatically derive such consequences from their injury, Udry (1999) suggested five particular recommendations for facilitating positive consequences from athletic injuries (Table 10.2).

Table 10.2 Summary of Udry's (1999) recommendations for facilitating positive consequences from athletic injuries

Recommendation for facilitating positive consequence from athletic injury	Comment
Recognize that deriving positive consequence takes effort	Injured athletes must not passively assume that positive consequences will occur; they will need to work on this
Recognize different problem-solving strategies can be used	A variety of techniques can be used. These include 'reversals' where a negative situation is converted to a positive one (or a less negative one) and 'extrications' where athletes voluntarily relinquish problematic roles
Recognize that reframing may not occur immediately	A considerable amount of time may be needed for athletes to counterbalance the negative aspects of their injuries
Avoid secondary victimization	Ensure that those who come into contact with injured athletes do not trivialize or minimize the experiences of the injured athlete
Acknowledge that positive consequences may extend beyond the individual athlete	Individuals whose lives are related to the injured athlete must often also work to counterbalance the negative impact of injury

ADHERENCE TO INJURY REHABILITATION

There are many aspects of rehabilitation that require adherence by athletes. These include attendance at rehabilitation appointments, adherence to advice given by physical therapists (e.g. regarding rest or activity restriction), home- and clinic-based rehabilitation exercises, cryotherapy usage, and adherence to advice given and changes made to rehabilitation during clinic appointments. Estimates of adherence to such rehabilitation behaviors range from 40–91% (Almekinders & Almekinders 1994, Daly et al 1995, Laubach et al 1996, Taylor and May 1996).

The assumption underlying most adherence research is that adherence to appropriate rehabilitation behaviors is related to rehabilitation outcome. Empirical support for this relationship, however, is limited. In fact, only a few studies have concluded that higher levels of adherence were related to a better sport injury rehabilitation outcome (Brewer et al 2000a, Derscheid & Feiring 1987, Shelbourne & Wilckens 1990, Treacy et al 1997).

MEASUREMENT OF REHABILITATION ADHERENCE

Given that adherence to sport injury rehabilitation involves a variety of behaviors over a number of settings, it is understandable that a range of adherence measures have been developed and used. Primarily, adherence measures have focused on attendance at clinic-based sessions, patient behavior during clinic sessions, and home-based rehabilitation components.

Attendance at rehabilitation

Several researchers have used attendance at rehabilitation sessions as a measure of adherence (Brewer et al 2000a, Byerly et al 1994, Daly et al 1995, Fields et al 1995, McEvoy & Kolt 1998, Udry 1997). Generally, attendance is calculated as a ratio of rehabilitation sessions attended to sessions scheduled. This simple measure, however, has been criticized on the basis that it only captures one aspect of rehabilitation and does not provide any information on what athletes do during rehabilitation sessions (Brewer 1998, Spetch & Kolt 2001). Also, attendance measures tend to be negatively skewed, as athletes usually attend the majority of scheduled rehabilitation appointments (Brewer 1998). Therefore, attendance measures should be used in conjunction with other adherence measures.

Adherence to clinic-based rehabilitation

Measuring patient behavior during rehabilitation sessions is important to physical therapists in their decision making regarding further rehabilitation. The Sport Injury Rehabilitation Adherence Scale (SIRAS) (Brewer et al 2000b) is the measure most commonly used in this area. The SIRAS can be used to rate the intensity with which participants complete rehabilitation exercises, the frequency of following practitioner instructions and advice, and the receptivity to changes in the rehabilitation program during that day's appointment (Fig. 10.5). The SIRAS has been used extensively and its psychometric properties have been well documented (Avondoglio et al 2000, Brewer et al 2000b, Brewer et al 2001a, Kolt et al 2001).

1. Circle the number that best indicates the intensity with which this patient completed the rehabilitation exercises during today's appointment:

minimum effort   1   2   3   4   5   maximum effort

2. During today's appointment, how frequently did this patient follow your instructions and advice?

never   1   2   3   4   5   always

3. How receptive was this patient to changes in the rehabilitation program during today's appointment?

very unreceptive   1   2   3   4   5   very receptive

Note: The Sport Injury Rehabilitation Adherence Scale can also be used with reference to adherence tendencies in general by using the present tense (without reference to "today's appointment")

Figure 10.5   Sport Injury Rehabilitation Adherence Scale. (Reproduced with permission from Brewer et al 2000b.)

The Sports Medicine Observation Code (SMOC) (Crossman & Roch 1991) is another instrument that can be used to measure clinic-based rehabilitation behavior. The SMOC allows practitioners to systematically code behavior into 13 categories (e.g. active rehabilitation, waiting, non-activity). These categories are grouped into productive behaviors (i.e. those behaviors which have a high probability of facilitating rehabilitation from injury), unproductive behaviors (i.e. those behaviors which have little or no potential of facilitating rehabilitation from injury), and concurrent behaviors (i.e. those behaviors which have a moderate potential of facilitating the rehabilitation process). Although not the original intent, the SMOC may be useful as a measure of adherence, as its productive behaviors score has been shown to correlate significantly with SIRAS scores (Kolt et al 2001).

Adherence to home-based rehabilitation

Measurement of adherence has also been applied to home-based rehabilitation (Almekinders & Almekinders 1994, Brewer 1998, Brewer et al 2000a, McEvoy & Kolt 1998, Spetch & Kolt 2001). This method of assessment usually involves self-reporting and has been criticized for that reason (Dunbar-Jacob et al 1993, Meichenbaum & Turk 1987), in that it can include biased, distorted, and inaccurate recall. Assessment of home-based rehabilitation can include single retrospective reports of adherence over the course of the home-based rehabilitation program or a daily home exercise adherence log or diary.

Researchers should focus on developing more objective assessment devices of home rehabilitation programs, as suggested by Brewer (1998). These could include, for example, home exercise programs administered by videotapes that contain electronic counters registering usage.

PREDICTORS OF SPORT INJURY REHABILITATION ADHERENCE

Personal factors, situational factors, and cognitive and emotional responses to injury can all affect adherence to rehabilitation (Brewer 2001). This suggestion fits well with Wiese-Bjornstal et al's (1998) integrated model of psychological response to sport injury and rehabilitation (Fig. 10.4). Several personal factors have been positively correlated with sport injury rehabilitation adherence. These include pain tolerance (Byerly et al 1994, Fields et al 1995, Fisher at al 1988) health locus of control (Murphy et al 1999), task involvement (Duda et al 1989), self-motivation (Brewer et al 2000a, Duda et al 1989, Fields et al 1995, Fisher et al 1988), and tough-mindedness (Wittig & Schurr 1994).

As well as personal variables, several situational variables have been identified as positively related to sport injury rehabilitation adherence. These include a belief in the efficacy of the treatment (Duda et al 1989, Taylor & May 1996), rehabilitation scheduling convenience (Fields et al 1995, Fisher et al 1988), the importance or value of the rehabilitation to the athlete (Taylor & May 1996), perceived injury severity (Taylor & May 1996), perceived exertion during rehabilitation (Fisher et al 1988), social support for rehabilitation (Byerly et al 1994, Duda et al 1989, Finnie 1999), and comfort of the clinical environment (Fields et al 1995, Fisher et al 1988).

Cognitive and emotional responses to injury can have an impact on adherence levels, in addition to personal and situational variables, which are linked to adherence. For example, athletes who show high rehabilitation self-efficacy are more likely to adhere to rehabilitation programs (Taylor & May 1996). Also, Daly et al (1995) reported that those athletes with a higher coping ability for their injuries tend to adhere better to rehabilitation regimens. Furthermore, Lampton et al (1993) indicated that athletes who attributed their recovery to stable and personally controllable factors, adhered to higher levels than their counterparts who attributed their recovery to unstable factors that were outside of their control.

ENHANCING SPORT INJURY REHABILITATION ADHERENCE

Several strategies have been suggested to enhance adherence to sport injury rehabilitation. Given the range of cognitive, emotional, and behavioral challenges faced by injured athletes (Kolt 2000), it is not surprising that a multi-faceted approach to rehabilitation adherence has been suggested. Fisher et al (1993a), based on surveys of athletic trainers and athletes (Fisher & Hoisington 1993, Fisher et al 1993b), suggested that the key components to enhance adherence should be education, communication and rapport, social support, goal setting, treatment efficacy and tailoring, threats and scare tactics, and athlete responsibility.

Education

Educating athletes on the nature of their injury, treatment rationale, realistic expectations, and injury management have been recommended (Weiss & Troxel 1986). Despite this ideal, however, Webborn et al (1997) reported that 77% of injured athletes they interviewed misunderstood some aspect of their rehabilitation, and only 14% were given any written instructions. Also, Schneiders et al (1998), in a randomized controlled study, reported that patients who were given written exercise instructions adhered to 77% of their home exercise program compared to 38.1% for those who received verbal exercise instructions only.

Communication and rapport

Although no studies have been found that specifically examined the relationship between adherence and communication and rapport between practitioner and patient, several investigators have suggested that athletes who feel that medical professionals are genuinely interested in their wellbeing, and who are aware of the psychological manifestations relating to their injury, may be more highly motivated to adhere to programs (Byerly et al 1994, Duda et al 1989, Ford & Gordon 1993).

Social support

Approaches such as peer modeling and injury support groups have been recommended for use in sport injury rehabilitation (Flint 1991, Wiese et al 1991). Peer modeling involves linking a currently injured athlete with an athlete who has successfully rehabilitated (preferably from a similar injury). Injury support groups are useful in providing a forum for athletes to regularly voice concerns about their injury and rehabilitation. Such groups can provide mutual understanding and support and can help to motivate injured athletes (Weiss & Troxel 1986). Modeling has been shown to improve adherence to post-surgical knee rehabilitation (Flint 1991).

Goal setting and attainment

Considerable research has focused on goal setting as a strategy to enhance adherence (Fisher 1999). The process

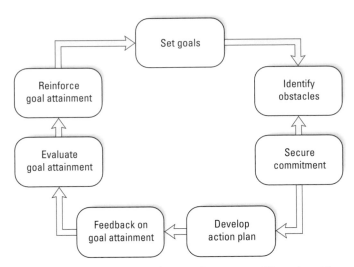

Figure 10.6   Goal setting implementation process. (Reproduced from Burton D, Naylor S, Holliday B 2001 Goal setting in sport: investigating the goal effectiveness paradox. In Singer R N, Hausenblas H A, Janelle C M (eds.) Handbook of sport psychology, 2nd edn. Copyright 2001 John Wiley & Sons, Inc. This material is used by permission of John Wiley and Sons, Inc.)

of goal setting for injured athletes contains three important elements. First, athletes and physical therapists should work together to establish challenging yet realistic and positive goals for rehabilitation; it is paramount that these goals are recorded and measurable (Wiese & Weiss 1987). Second, to enhance a sense of control by athletes, strategies for achieving these goals should be negotiated by the athlete and the practitioner. Third, the agreed goals should be closely monitored, periodically evaluated, and modified if necessary. See Figure 10.6.

Treatment efficacy and tailoring

An athlete's perception of treatment efficacy is important to their belief that rehabilitation goals will be met, therefore, rehabilitation programs should be tailored to the needs of individual athletes. Duda et al (1989) argued that perceived treatment efficacy can have an important impact on adherence behaviors. Therefore, in fostering perceptions of treatment efficacy, physical therapists should ensure that athletes are capable of performing their rehabilitation tasks and identifying the context of their rehabilitation as meaningful and worthwhile. Of interest, is that complex rehabilitation programs (e.g. those that contain skills beyond the abilities of the patient) can lead to lower levels of adherence (Sluijs et al 1993).

Athlete responsibility

Athletes need to feel responsible for their own rehabilitation (Fisher et al 1993a). By having a sense of control over their rehabilitation programs, athletes can increase commitment and adherence to the behaviors required for successful rehabilitation. This concept has been supported by Laubach et al (1996) who reported a positive relationship between personal control and rehabilitation adherence in a sample of athletes following knee surgery.

Threats and scare tactics

Increasing an athlete's perception of severity of an injury and susceptibility to poor rehabilitation, reinjury, or more serious debilitation can enhance their ability to adhere to appropriate rehabilitation guidelines (Taylor & May 1996). However, one must be careful in using such tactics, as by using threats or ultimatums, practitioners risk losing respect or harming rapport with athletes (Fisher et al 1993a). This approach would usually be used as a last resort to improve adherence.

There are several other cognitive-behavioral approaches that have been suggested for enhancing rehabilitation adherence but, like those described above, most have received little empirical support. These include imagery (Heil 1993, Weiss & Troxel 1986) and relaxation (Duda et al 1989, Weiss & Troxel 1986, Wiese & Weiss 1987).

ROLE OF PHYSICAL THERAPISTS IN PROVIDING PSYCHOLOGICAL SUPPORT FOR INJURED ATHLETES

Physical therapists are suited to provide some form of psychological assistance to injured athletes (Francis et al 2000, Gordon et al 1998, Kolt 2000, Ninedek & Kolt 2000, Pearson & Jones 1992). There are four main reasons for this suggestion (Kolt 2000). First, physical therapists are closely involved with injured athletes during rehabilitation and spend longer periods of time with athletes than most other health professionals. Athletes may be more likely, therefore, to raise psychological issues with them. Second, with the use of touch in physical therapy techniques (an integral aspect of physiotherapeutic skills), athletes are more likely to open up about psychosocial issues (Nathan 1999), making it beneficial to deal with them at the time, particularly if these issues are affecting recovery progress. Third, due to the psychological aftereffects of injury, it appears reasonable that such issues are discussed concurrently with the physical aspects of rehabilitation so as to maximally benefit the psychological and physical rehabilitation processes. Finally, according to some research reports (e.g. Pearson & Jones 1992), injured athletes feel that physical therapists are in an ideal position to provide them with basic counseling and psychological support.

If physical therapists are to incorporate basic psychological techniques into their rehabilitation, their willing-ness and ability to deliver appropriate services must be established. In recent surveys (Francis et al 2000, Ninedek & Kolt 2000), physical therapists reported that having knowledge about setting realistic goals, using a positive and sincere communication style, understanding individual motivation, understanding stress and anxiety, encouraging positive self-thoughts, encouraging self-confidence, and reducing depression were all important for them in dealing with injured athletes. Similar findings have been reported for athletic trainers (Wiese et al 1991).

Despite these findings, however, physical therapists have suggested that they were limited in their ability to deal with psychosocial aspects of the recovery process and desired further practical training in this area (Gordon et al 1991). A possible goal for future research and education involves developing a standardized educational framework for sport injury rehabilitation personnel (Gordon et al 1998). Further research efforts could examine the effects of physical therapists actively implementing basic psychological intervention strategies on the recovery of injured athletes.

There appears to be adequate justification for physical therapists to play a more active role in managing some of the basic psychological consequences of sport and exercise injuries. It should be emphasized, however, that where more severe psychological difficulties are experienced, athletes should be referred to other professionals (e.g. sport psychologists, psychiatrists) for further specialized intervention.

Clearly, qualified sport psychologists are the best-trained members of sports medicine teams to address athletes' post-injury emotional responses (Crossman 1997, Brewer et al 1991). However, access to a sport psychologist is often unavailable or limited in clinical settings (Gordon et al 1998, Larson et al 1996, Moulton et al 1997), and in circumstances where they are available, many athletes are reticent to accept formal psychological help (Pinkerton et al 1989). Some athletes view seeking psychological help as a sign of weakness and would rather endure the negative consequences of a problematic rehabilitation than request formal psychological assistance (Kolt 2000).

COGNITIVE-BEHAVIORAL INTERVENTIONS FOR INJURED ATHLETES

It is not the intent of this chapter to provide a detailed account of the many cognitive-behavioral techniques that can be of use to injured athletes during the rehabilitation program. Details on these techniques can be found in many sources (e.g. Heil 1993, Kolt 2000, Pargman 1991, Ray & Wiese-Bjornstal 1999, Taylor & Taylor 1997).

However, this chapter provides a brief outline of certain cognitive-behavioral techniques that are of use to the physical therapist in managing sport and exercise injuries.

RELAXATION TECHNIQUES

Several forms of relaxation exist that achieve their function by various means. Given that the stress and pain associated with injury can elicit muscle tension which, in turn, restricts blood flow and further increases pain (Cousins & Phillips 1985), relaxation techniques that directly target muscle are indicated in many circumstances. The most common form of muscular relaxation is progressive relaxation (Jacobson 1938). Progressive relaxation involves systematically relaxing major skeletal muscle groups by firstly recognizing muscle tension present (initially achieved by contracting the muscles), then by relaxing those muscles. The role of muscle contraction before relaxation is proposed in order to sensitize the individual to the recognition of muscle tension, so that the individual learns what the sensations of relaxed muscle are like. As the individual becomes more familiar with the technique, it may be possible to merely relax muscle groups from whatever condition they are in at rest, rather than having to contract muscle groups first. It should be noted that divided opinion exists regarding the value of muscle contraction before relaxation (Lucic et al 1991, O'Bannon et al 1987, Payne 2000). When using progressive relaxation on athletes with pain it is important to monitor that the level of muscle contraction used in the exercise does not aggravate pain symptoms.

Another commonly used relaxation technique is Benson's Relaxation Response (Benson 1975). As outlined in Chapter 8, this technique is based on the proposal that there are four common elements underlying the elicitation of a relaxation response. The first element is a quiet environment, which allows for the reduction of external distractions. The second is adopting a comfortable position to reduce undue muscular tension. The third is an object to dwell on, such as the repetition of a word. The fourth element is a passive attitude that includes emptying all other thoughts from one's mind, and letting distracting thoughts that do return pass on while returning to a focused state. Practically speaking, Benson's Relaxation Response is based around transcendental meditation and involves focus on breathing, repetition of a word in time with breathing, and in more recent adaptations, imagery that focuses on an object that moves in time with the patient's breathing (Kolt & McConville 2000). Benson's Relaxation Response works predominantly by distracting or drawing focus away from the stressors associated with injury and rehabilitation. As it is not uncommon for an injured athlete to

continually think about the negative consequences of their injury, Benson's Relaxation Response can distract them from this and allow a better focus on the rehabilitation activities. It also provides a greater sense of control over pain and a reduction in the negative emotions associated with the pain and injury (Taylor & Taylor 1998).

For a more detailed account of relaxation techniques refer to Payne (2000).

COGNITIVE REHEARSAL

The term cognitive rehearsal refers to cognitive-behavioral techniques such as mental rehearsal, visualization, mental practice, and imagery. The technique relates to practicing a skill in one's mind. As described by White & Hardy (1998), it involves a cognitive experience that mimics real experience. That is, it utilizes athletes' abilities to feel a movement, as well as hear the sounds and incorporate other senses in rehearsing an activity without actually experiencing the real thing.

Cognitive rehearsal is used by athletes for several reasons. Athletes typically use this skill to improve a variety of performance-related issues, including technique, mental preparation, tactics, and competitive performance (Vealey & Walter 1993). Only relatively recently, however, has cognitive rehearsal been considered as a tool to facilitate rehabilitation and return to sport following injury (Green 1992). Shaffer & Wiese-Bjornstal (1999) suggested using cognitive rehearsal as an adjunct to physical therapy so that athletes can achieve a specific mindset for maintaining a positive outlook, controlling stress, using positive and descriptive self-talk, and sustaining belief in the rehabilitation process. They also suggested that using cognitive rehearsal enables athletes to develop a sense of control over the injured body part. Other important benefits of cognitive rehearsal during rehabilitation include coping with pain and keeping physical skills from deteriorating during periods of no physical practice (Richardson & Latuda 1995).

As described in Chapter 8, different forms of imagery (or cognitive rehearsal) have been used in the management of pain. Imagery of pleasant situations, guided by either the practitioner or by the patient, is an internal dissociative strategy shown to be effective in reducing pain in sport and medical settings (Whitmarsh & Alderman 1993). In general, imagery involves patients imagining themselves in a relaxing environment (i.e. an environment that has a relaxing meaning to the patient), and focusing on how it feels to be in that environment. As is evident, this form of imagery aims to distract the patient from the feeling of pain or from the other stressors associated with injury and abstinence from training. From clinical experience, the more complex the scene to be imaged, and the more detail that patients are asked to attend to (i.e. using not just the visual sense but the tactile and auditory senses as well), the more they are distracted from their pain.

Specific types of imagery have also been developed. For example, in pain management imagery (Ievleva & Orlick 1999), patients could imagine the pain being washed away or see cool colors soothing and reducing any inflammation and pain (e.g. seeing cool blue colors running through the painful area; imaging the pain leaving the body; imagining an ice-pack over the painful area). In cognitive rehearsal based around sports skills, injured athletes can rehearse sport techniques to avoid skill level decline during rehabilitation (Hall 2001).

There is an increasing body of research suggesting that cognitive rehearsal can assist with pain and healing in athletes (Ievleva & Orlick 1999) and with many other aspects of rehabilitation (Green 1999, Hall 2001, Taylor & Taylor 1997).

SYSTEMATIC DESENSITIZATION

Systematic desensitization is the process of combining relaxation and imagery to overcome progressively stressful or fearful events (Shaffer & Wiese-Bjornstal 1999). For example, an athlete could image situations in which anxiety progressively heightens (e.g. attempting a sport skill in the rehabilitation clinic, returning for the first training session, returning to the first competitive event), and with each event being imaged (from least to most fear provoking), use relaxation to curb anxiety until it dissipates. This process is repeated until the list of anxiety producing situations has been dealt with. Despite the widespread use of this technique in sport settings, no research has investigated its use in rehabilitation.

COGNITIVE RESTRUCTURING

Cognitive restructuring involves athletes reframing negative and irrational thoughts into more positive, rational thoughts. This involves athletes firstly recognizing their negative self-talk, and then replacing it with positive or productive comments. Ievleva & Orlick (1991) reported that injured athletes who healed faster were more likely to use self-talk that was positive and encouraging compared to their counterparts who healed at a slower rate. Cognitive restructuring has been based on the behavior change work of Ellis (1967).

GOAL SETTING

Goal setting has been well recognized as an important part of rehabilitation (Shaffer & Wiese-Bjornstal 1999). As

this is a skill that many athletes are accustomed to using, adapting it to the rehabilitation setting should not be difficult. It has been suggested by Danish et al (1993) that teaching goal setting is a means of empowerment that encourages athletes to take greater responsibility for their return to sport following injury. General principles of goal setting have been covered earlier in the chapter in relation to enhancing rehabilitation adherence. The goal setting process (Fig. 10.6) has been well described by Burton et al (2001).

SOCIAL SUPPORT

The role of social support in injury rehabilitation has been widely investigated (Brewer 2001). In this context, social support refers to the quantity, quality, and type of interactions that athletes have with other people (Udry 1996). Richman et al (1993) described eight types of social support: listening support, emotional support, emotional challenge, task appreciation, task challenge, reality confirmation, material assistance, and personal assistance. Social support providers in sports injury rehabilitation can include physical therapists, medical personnel, coaches, team-mates, friends, family members, significant others, and sports administrators. Research has shown that, in general, injured athletes perceive family members and team-mates as better social support providers than medical professionals and coaches (although they do recognize that medical professionals and coaches are the most frequent providers of technical and informational support) (see review by Brewer 2001). It should be noted that the need for different types of social support changes throughout the rehabilitation period and it appears that the need for emotional support decreases as rehabilitation progresses, with a possible need for increased emotional support as the athlete returns to sport participation (Johnston & Carroll 1998).

SUMMARY

It is evident that research in the area of psychological aspects of injury and rehabilitation is growing. Models of the psychological predictors of injury have been developed and increasingly researched over the past 15 years. Findings have indicated a strong relationship between stress and injury in sport (Williams & Andersen 1998). A more recent area of research is that of the psychology of sport injury rehabilitation. Although athlete adherence to sport injury rehabilitation programs has been addressed both clinically and with empirical research, the use of cognitive-behavioral techniques in rehabilitation is based largely on anecdotal evidence. Extrapolating from research outside of sport, it stands to reason that such techniques are potentially valuable to injured athletes.

If physical therapists are to include basic psychological techniques in their rehabilitation programs, they must ensure that they seek appropriate training in these skills, and in how to combine a physical and psychological approach to rehabilitation.

REFERENCES

Almekinders L C, Almekinders S V 1994 Outcome in the treatment of chronic overuse sports injuries: a retrospective study. Journal of Orthopaedic and Sports Physical Therapy 19:157–161

Andersen M B, Williams J M 1988 A model of stress and athletic injury: prediction and prevention. Journal of Sport and Exercise Psychology 10:294–306

Andersen M B, Stoove M A 1998 The sanctity of $p < .05$ obfuscates good stuff: a comment on Kerr and Goss. Journal of Applied Sport Psychology 10:168–173

Andersen M B, Williams J M 1999 Athletic injury, psychosocial factors, and perceptual changes during stress. Journal of Sports Science 17:735–751

Astle S J 1986 The experience of loss in athletes. Journal of Sports Medicine and Physical Fitness 26:279–284

Avondoglio J B, Brewer B W, Cornelius A E et al 2000 Interrater reliability and construct validity of the Sport Injury Rehabilitation Adherence Scale. Paper presented at the annual meeting of the Association for the Advancement of Applied Sport Psychology, Nashville, TN

Beck A T 1976 Cognitive therapy and the emotional disorders. Penguin, London

Benson H 1975 The relaxation response. William Morrow, New York

Bianco T, Malo S, Orlick T 1999 Sport injury and illness: elite skiers describe their experiences. Research Quarterly for Exercise and Sport 70:157–169

Blackwell B, McCullagh P 1990 The relationship of athletic injury to life stress, competitive anxiety and coping resources. Athletic Training 25:23–27

Bramwell S T, Masuda M, Wagner N N et al 1975 Psychosocial factors in athletic injuries: development and application of the Social and Athletic Readjustment Rating Scale (SARRS). Journal of Human Stress 1:6–20

Brewer B W 1994 Review and critique of models of psychological adjustment to athletic injury. Journal of Applied Sport Psychology 6:87–100

Brewer B W 1998 Adherence to sport injury rehabilitation programs. Journal of Applied Sport Psychology 10:70–82

Brewer B W 2001 Psychology of sport injury rehabilitation. In: Singer R N, Hausenblas H A, Janelle C M (eds) Handbook of sport psychology, 2nd edn. John Wiley, New York

Brewer B W, Petrie T A 1995 A comparison between injured and uninjured football players on selected psychosocial variables. Academic Athletic Journal 10:11–18

Brewer B W, Van Raalte J L, Linder D E 1991 Role of the sport psychologist in treating injured athletes: a survey of sports medicine providers. Journal of Applied Sport Psychology 3:183–190

Brewer B W, Jeffers K E, Petitpas A J et al 1994 Perceptions of psychological interventions in the context of sport injury rehabilitation. The Sport Psychologist 8:176–188

Brewer B W, Van Raalte J L, Cornelius A E et al 2000a Psychological factors, rehabilitation adherence, and rehabilitation outcome following anterior cruciate ligament reconstruction. Rehabilitation Psychology 45:20–37

Brewer B W, Van Raalte J L, Petitpas A J et al 2000b Preliminary psychometric evaluation of a measure of adherence to clinic-based sport injury rehabilitation. Physical Therapy in Sport 1:68–74

Brewer B W, Cornelius A E, Van Raalte J L 2001a Clinical evaluation of the interrater agreement of the Sport Injury Rehabilitation Adherence Scale. In: Papaioannou A, Goudas M, Theodorakis Y (eds) Proceedings of the 10th World Congress of Sport Psychology (vol. 2). Christodoulidi, Thessaloniki, Greece, p 174–175

Brewer B W, Andersen M B, Van Raalte J L 2001b Psychological aspects of sport injury rehabilitation: toward a biopsychosocial approach. In: Mostofsky D I, Zaichkowsky L D (eds) Medical aspects of sport and exercise. Fitness Information Technology, Morgantown, WV

Brown R B 1971 Personality characteristics related to injury in football. Research Quarterly 42:133–138

Burton D, Naylor S, Holliday B 2001 Goal setting in sport: investigating the goal effectiveness paradox. In: Singer R N, Hausenblas H A, Janelle C M (eds) Handbook of sport psychology, 2nd edn. John Wiley, New York

Byerly P N, Worrell T, Gahimer J et al 1994 Rehabilitation compliance in an athletic training environment. Journal of Athletic Training 29:352–355

Chan C S, Crossman H Y 1988 Psychological effects of running loss on consistent runners. Perceptual and Motor Skills 66:875–883

Cousins M J, Phillips G D 1985 Acute pain management. Clinics in Critical Care Medicine 8:82–117

Crossman J 1997 Psychological rehabilitation from sports injuries. Sports Medicine 23:333–339

Crossman J, Roch J 1991 An observation instrument for use in sports medicine clinics. Journal of the Canadian Athletic Therapists Association April:10–13

Daly J M, Brewer B W, Van Raalte J L et al 1995 Cognitive appraisal, emotional adjustment, and adherence to rehabilitation following knee surgery. Journal of Sport Rehabilitation 4:23–30

Danish S J, Petitpas A J, Hale B D 1993 Life development interventions for athletes: life skills through sports. Counseling Psychologist 21:352–385

Danish S J, Petitpas A, Hale B D 1995 Psychological interventions: a life developmental model. In: Murphy S (ed) Sport psychology interventions. Human Kinetics, Champaign, IL

Davis J 1991 Sports injuries and stress management: an opportunity for research. The Sport Psychologist 5:175–182

Dawes H, Roach N K 1997 Emotional responses of athletes to injury and treatment. Physiotherapy 83:243–247

Derscheid G L, Feiring D C 1987 A statistical analysis to characterize treatment adherence of the 18 most common diagnoses seen at a sports medicine clinic. Journal of Orthopaedic and Sports Physical Therapy 9:40–46

Duda J L, Smart A E, Tappe M L 1989 Predictors of adherence in the rehabilitation of athletic injuries: an application of personal investment theory. Journal of Sport and Exercise Psychology 11:367–381

Dunbar-Jacob J, Dunning E J, Dwyer K 1993 Compliance research in pediatric and adolescent populations: two decades of research. In: Krasnegor N A, Epstein L, Johnson S B et al (eds) Developmental aspects of health compliance behavior. Erlbaum, Hillsdale, NJ

Durso-Cupal D 1998 Psychological interventions in sport injury prevention and rehabilitation. Journal of Applied Sport Psychology 10:103–123

Ellis A 1967 Rational-emotive psychotherapy. In: Arbuckle D S (ed) Counseling and psychotherapy: an overview. McGraw-Hill, New York

Evans L, Hardy L 1999 Psychological and emotional response to athletic injury: measurement issues. In: Pargman D (ed) Psychological bases of sport injury, 2nd edn. Fitness Information Technology, Morgantown, WV

Fawkner H J, McMurray N E, Summers J J 1999 Athletic injury and minor life events: a prospective study. Journal of Science and Medicine in Sport 2:117–124

Fields J, Murphey M, Horodyski M et al 1995 Factors associated with adherence to sport injury rehabilitation in college-age recreational athletes. Journal of Sport Rehabilitation 4:172–180

Finch C, Valuri G, Ozanne-Smith J 1998 Sport and active recreation injuries in Australia: evidence from emergency department presentations. British Journal of Sports Medicine 32:220–225

Finnie S B 1999 The rehabilitation support team: using social support to aid compliance to sports injury rehabilitation programs. Paper presented at the annual meeting of the Association for the Advancement of Applied Sport Psychology, Banff, Canada

Fisher A C 1999 Counseling for improved rehabilitation adherence. In: Ray R, Wiese-Bjornstal D M (eds) Counseling in sports medicine. Human Kinetics, Champaign, IL

Fisher A C, Hoisington L L 1993 Injured athletes' attitudes and judgments toward rehabilitation adherence. Journal of the National Athletic Trainers Association 28:48–54

Fisher A C, Domm M A, Wuest D A 1988 Adherence to sports injury rehabilitation programs. Physician and Sportsmedicine 16 (7):47–51

Fisher A C, Mullins S A, Frye P A 1993a Athletic trainers' attitudes and judgements of injured athletes' rehabilitation adherence. Journal of Athletic Training 28:43–47

Fisher A C, Scriber K C, Matheny M L et al 1993b Enhancing athletic injury rehabilitation adherence. Journal of Athletic Training 28:312–318

Flint F A 1991 The psychological effects of modeling in athletic injury rehabilitation. Unpublished doctoral dissertation, University of Oregon, Eugene

Flint F A 1998 Integrating sport psychology and sports medicine in research: the dilemmas. Journal of Applied Sport Psychology 10:83–102

Folkman S, Lazarus R S 1985 If it changes it must be a process: study of emotion and coping during three stages of a college examination. Journal of Personality and Social Psychology 48:150–170

Ford I W, Gordon S 1993 Social support and athletic injury: the perspective of sport physiotherapists. Australian Journal of Science and Medicine in Sport 25:17–25

Francis S R, Andersen M B, Maley P 2000 Physiotherapists' and male professional athletes' views on psychological skills for rehabilitation. Journal of Science and Medicine in Sport 3:17–29

Gordon S 1986 Sport psychology and the injured athlete: a cognitive-behavioral approach to injury response and injury rehabilitation. Science Periodical on Research and Technology in Sport March:1–10

Gordon S, Milios S, Grove J R 1991 Psychological aspects of the recovery process from sport injury: the perspective of sports physiotherapists. Australian Journal of Science and Medicine in Sport 23:53–60

Gordon S, Potter M, Ford I W 1998 Towards a psychoeducational curriculum for training sport-injury rehabilitation personnel. Journal of Applied Sport Psychology 10:140–156

Gould D, Udry E, Bridges D et al 1997 Stress sources encountered when rehabilitating from season-ending ski injuries. The Sport Psychologist 11:361–378

Govern J W, Koppenhaver R 1965 Attempt to predict athletic injuries. Medical Times 93:421–422

Green L 1992 The use of imagery in the rehabilitation of injured athletes. The Sport Psychologist 6:416–428

Green L B 1999 The use of imagery in the rehabilitation of injured athletes. In: Pargman D (ed) Psychological bases of sport injuries, 2nd edn. Fitness Information Technology, Morgantown, WV

Hall C R 2001 Imagery in sport and exercise. In: Singer R N, Hausenblas H A, Janelle C M (eds) Handbook of sport psychology, 2nd edn. John Wiley, New York

Heil J 1993 Psychology of sport injury. Human Kinetics, Champaign, IL

Horsley C 1995 Understanding and managing the injured athlete. In: Zuluaga M, Briggs C, Carlisle J et al (eds) Sports physiotherapy: applied science and practice. Churchill Livingstone, Melbourne Australia

Ievleva L, Orlick T 1991 Mental links to enhanced healing: an exploratory study. The Sport Psychologist 5:25–40

Ievleva L, Orlick T 1999 Mental paths to enhanced recovery from a sports injury. In: Pargman D (ed) Psychological bases of sport injuries, 2nd edn. Fitness Information Technology, Morgantown, WV

Jacobson E 1938 Progressive relaxation. University of Chicago Press, Chicago

Johnston L H, Carroll D 1998 The provision of social support to injured athletes: a qualitative analysis. Journal of Sport Rehabilitation 7:267–284

Kerr G, Goss J 1996 The effects of a stress management program on injuries and stress levels. Journal of Applied Sport Psychology 8:109–117

Kirkby R J 1995 Psychological factors in sport injuries. In: Morris T, Summers J (eds) Sport psychology. Theories, applications and issues. John Wiley, Milton, Australia

Kleiber D A, Brock S C 1992 The effect of career-ending injuries on the subsequent well-being of elite college athletes. Sociology of Sport Journal 9:70–75

Kolt G S 2000 Doing sport psychology with injured athletes. In: Andersen M B (ed) Doing sport psychology. Human Kinetics, Champaign, IL

Kolt G S, Kirkby R J 1996 Injury in Australian female competitive gymnasts: a psychological perspective. Australian Journal of Physiotherapy 42:121–126

Kolt G S, McConville L C 2000 The effects of a Feldenkrais Awareness Through Movement program on state anxiety. Journal of Bodywork and Movement Therapies 4:216–220

Kolt G S, Pizzari T, Schoo A M M et al 2001 The Sport Injury Rehabilitation Adherence Scale: a reliable and valid measure of clinic-based injury rehabilitation. In: Papaioannou A, Goudas M, Theodorakis Y (eds) Proceedings of the 10th World Congress of Sport Psychology (vol 4). Christodoulidi, Thessaloniki, Greece, p 144–146

Kubler-Ross E 1969 On death and dying. Macmillan, New York

Lampton C C, Lambert M E, Yost R 1993 The effects of psychological factors in sports medicine rehabilitation adherence. Journal of Sports Medicine and Physical Fitness 33:292–299

Larson G A, Starkey C, Zaichkowsky L D 1996 Psychological aspects of athletic injuries as perceived by athletic trainers. The Sport Psychologist 10:37–47

Laubach W J, Brewer B W, Van Raalte J L et al 1996 Attributions for recovery and adherence to sport injury rehabilitation. Australian Journal of Science and Medicine in Sport 28:30–34

Leadbetter W B 1994 Soft tissue athletic injury. In: Fu F H, Stone D A (eds) Sports injuries: mechanisms, prevention, and treatment. Williams and Wilkins, Baltimore, MD

Leddy M H, Lambert M J, Ogles B M 1994 Psychological consequences of athletic injury among high-level competitors. Research Quarterly for Exercise and Sport 65:347–354

Lucic K S, Steffen J J, Harrigan J A et al 1991 Progressive relaxation training: muscle contraction before relaxation? Behavior Therapy 22:249–256

Lynch G P 1988 Athletic injuries and the practicing sport psychologist: practical guidelines for assisting athletes. The Sport Psychologist 2:161–167

Lysens R, Steverlynk A, Vanden Auweele Y et al 1984 The predictability of sports injuries. Sports Medicine 1:6–10

McDonald S A, Hardy C J 1990 Affective response patterns of the injured athlete: an exploratory analysis. The Sport Psychologist 4:261–274

McEvoy J F, Kolt G S 1998 An investigation of adherence to rehabilitation programs in patients with low back pain. Paper presented at the Australian Conference of Science and Medicine in Sport, Adelaide Australia

McGowan R W, Pierce E F, Williams N et al 1994 Athletic injury and self-diminution. Journal of Sports Medicine and Physical Fitness 34:299–304

Macchi R, Crossman J 1996 After the fall: reflections of injured classical ballet dancers. Journal of Sport Behaviour 19:221–234

May J R, Brown L 1989 Delivery of psychological services to the U.S. alpine ski team prior to and during the Olympics in Calgary. The Sport Psychologist 3:320–329

Meichenbaum D 1985 Stress inoculation training. Pergamon, New York

Meichenbaum D, Turk D C 1987 Facilitating treatment adherence: a practitioner's guidebook. Plenum, New York

Miller W N 1998 Athletic injury: mood disturbances and hardiness of intercollegiate athletes [abstract]. Journal of Applied Sport Psychology 10 (Suppl.):S127–S128

Morrey M A, Stuart M J, Smith A M et al 1999 A longitudinal examination of athletes' emotional and cognitive responses to anterior cruciate ligament injury. Clinical Journal of Sport Medicine 9:63–69

Moulton M A, Molstad S, Turner A 1997 The role of athletic trainers in counseling collegiate athletes. Journal of Athletic Training 32:148–150

Murphy G C, Foreman P E, Simpson C A et al 1999 The development of a locus of control measure predictive of injured athletes' adherence to treatment. Journal of Science and Medicine in Sport 2:145–152

Nathan B 1999 Touch and emotion in manual therapy. Churchill Livingstone, London

NEISS data highlights 1998 Consumer Product Safety Review 3(1):4–6

Ninedek A, Kolt G S 2000 Sports physiotherapists' perceptions of psychological strategies in sport injury rehabilitation. Journal of Sport Rehabilitation 9:191–206

O'Bannon R M, Rickard H C, Runcie D 1987 Progressive relaxation as a function of procedural variations and anxiety level. International Journal of Psychophysiology 5:207–214

Ogilvie B C, Tutko T A 1966 Problem athletes and how to handle them. Pelham, London

Pargman D (ed) 1991 Psychological bases of sport injury, 2nd edn. Fitness Information Technology, Morgantown, WV

Payne R A 2000 Relaxation techniques. A practical handbook for the health care professional, 2nd edn. Churchill Livingstone, Edinburgh

Pearson L, Jones G 1992 Emotional effects of sports injuries: implications for physiotherapists. Physiotherapy 78:762–770

Peretz D 1970 Development, object-relationships, and loss. In: Schoenberg B, Carr A C, Peretz D et al (eds) Loss and grief: psychological management in medical practice. Columbia University Press, New York

Petitpas A, Danish S J 1995 Caring for injured athletes. In: Murphy S M (ed) Sport psychology interventions. Human Kinetics, Champaign, IL

Petrie T A 1993a The moderating effects of social support and playing status on the life stress-injury relationship. Journal of Applied Sport Psychology 5:1–16

Petrie T A 1993b Coping skills, competitive trait anxiety, and playing status: moderating effects of the life stress-injury relationship. Journal of Sport and Exercise Psychology 15:261–274

Pinkerton R S, Hinz L D, Borrow J C 1989 The college student athlete: psychological considerations and interventions. Journal of American College Health 37:218–225

Quinn A M, Fallon B J 1999 The changes in psychological characteristics and reactions of elite athletes from injury onset until full recovery. Journal of Applied Sport Psychology 11:210–229

Ray R, Wiese-Bjornstal (eds) 1999 Counseling in sports medicine. Human Kinetics, Champaign, IL

Richardson P A, Latuda L M 1995 Therapeutic imagery and athletic injuries. Journal of Athletic Training 30:10–12

Richman J M, Rosenfeld L B, Hardy C J 1993 The Social Support Survey: a validation study of a clinical measure of the social support process. Research on Social Work Practice 3:288–311

Rotella R J, Ogilvie B C, Perrin D H 1999 The malingering athlete: psychological considerations. In: Pargman D (ed) Psychological bases of sport injuries, 2nd edn. Fitness Information Technology, Morgantown, WV

Schneiders A G, Zusman G, Singer K P 1998 Exercise therapy compliance in acute low back pain patients. Manual Therapy 3:147–152

Schomer H H 1990 A cognitive strategy training programme for marathon runners: ten case studies. South African Journal of Research in Sport, Physical Education and Recreation 13:47–78

Shaffer S M, Wiese-Bjornstal D M 1999 Effective intervention strategies in sports medicine. In: Ray R, Wiese-Bjornstal D M (eds) Counseling in sports medicine. Human Kinetics, Champaign, IL

Shelbourne K D, Wilckens J H 1990 Current concepts in anterior cruciate ligament rehabilitation. Orthopedic Review 19:957–964

Shelley G A, Sherman C P 1996 The sport injury experience: a qualitative case study [abstract]. Journal of Applied Sport Psychology 8(suppl.):S164

Sluijs E M, Kok G J, van der Zee J 1993 Correlates of exercise compliance in physical therapy. Physical Therapy 73:771–786

Smith A M, Milliner E K 1994 Injured athletes and the risk of suicide. Journal of Athletic Training 29:337–341

Smith R E, Smoll F L, Ptacek J T 1990a Conjunctive moderator variables in vulnerability and resiliency research: life stress, social support and coping skills, and adolescent sport injuries. Journal of Personality and Social Psychology 58:360–369

Smith A M, Scott S G, O'Fallon W M et al 1990b Emotional responses of athletes to injury. Mayo Clinic Proceedings 65:38–50

Smith A M, Stuart M J, Wiese-Bjornstal D M et al 1993 Competitive athletes: preinjury and postinjury mood state and self-esteem. Mayo Clinic Proceedings 68:939–947

Spetch L A, Kolt G S 2001 Adherence to sport injury rehabilitation: implications for sports medicine providers and researchers. Physical Therapy in Sport 2:80–90

Taylor A H, May S 1996 Threat and coping appraisal as determinants of compliance with sports injury rehabilitation: an application of protection motivation theory. Journal of Sports Sciences 14:471–482

Taylor J, Taylor S 1997 Psychological approaches to sports injury rehabilitation. Aspen, Gaithersburg, MD

Taylor J, Taylor S 1998 Pain education and management in the rehabilitation from sports injury. The Sport Psychologist 12:68–88

Thompson N J, Morris R D 1994 Predicting injury risk in adolescent football players: the importance of psychological variables. Journal of Pediatric Psychology 19:415–429

Treacy S H, Barron O A, Brunet M E et al 1997 Assessing the need for extensive supervised rehabilitation following arthroscopic ACL reconstruction. American Journal of Orthopedics 26:25–29

Udry E 1996 Social support: exploring its role in the context of athletic injuries. Journal of Sport Rehabilitation 5:151–163

Udry E 1997 Coping and social support among injured athletes following surgery. Journal of Sport and Exercise Psychology 19:71–90

Udry E 1999 The paradox of injuries: unexpected positive consequences. In: Pargman D (ed) Psychological bases of sport injuries, 2nd edn. Fitness Information Technology, Morgantown, WV

Udry E, Gould D, Bridges D et al 1997 Down but not out: athlete responses to season-ending injuries. Journal of Sport and Exercise Psychology 19:229–248

Uitenbroek D G 1996 Sports, exercise, and other causes of injuries: results of a population survey. Research Quarterly for Exercise and Sport 67:380–385

Vealey R S, Walter S M 1993 Imagery training for performance enhancement and personal growth. In: Williams J M (ed) Applied sport psychology: personal growth to peak performance, 2nd edn. Mayfield, Mountain View, CA

Weaver N L, Marshall S W, Spicer R et al 1999 Cost of athletic injuries in 12 North Carolina high school sports [abstract]. Medicine and Science in Sports and Exercise 31(suppl.):S93

Webborn A D, Carbon R J, Miller B P 1997 Injury rehabilitation programs: what are we talking about? Journal of Sport Rehabilitation 6:54–61

Weiss M R, Troxel R K 1986 Psychology of the injured athlete. Athletic Training 21:104–109, 154

White A, Hardy L 1998 An in-depth analysis of the uses of imagery by high-level slalom canoeists and artistic gymnasts. The Sport Psychologist 12:387–403

Whitmarsh B G, Alderman R B 1993 Role of psychological skills training in increasing athletic pain tolerance. The Sport Psychologist 7:388–399

Wiese D M, Weiss M R 1987 Psychological rehabilitation and physical injury: implication for the sports medicine team. The Sport Psychologist 1:318–330

Wiese D M, Weiss M R, Yukelson D P 1991 Sport psychology in the training room: a survey of athletic trainers. The Sport Psychologist 5:15–24

Wiese-Bjornstal D M, Smith A M, Shaffer S M et al 1998 An integrated model of response to Sport Injury: Psychological and Sociological Dimensions. Journal of Applied Sport Psychology 10:46–69

Williams J M 2001 Psychology of injury risk and prevention. In: Singer R N, Hausenblas H A, Janelle C M (eds) Handbook of sport psychology, 2nd edn. John Wiley, New York

Williams J M, Roepke N 1993 Psychology of injury and injury rehabilitation. In: Singer R N, Murphey M, Tennant L K (eds) Handbook of research on sport psychology. Macmillan, New York

Williams J M, Andersen M B 1998 Psychosocial antecedents of sport injury: review and critique of the stress and injury model. Journal of Applied Sport Psychology 10:5–25

Wittig A F, Schurr K T 1994 Psychological characteristics of women volleyball players: relationships with injuries, rehabilitation, and team success. Personality and Social Psychology Bulletin 20:322–330

11

Screening for sport and exercise participation

Lisa Casson Barkley   Michael J Axe

INTRODUCTION

Every year, around the world, hundreds of thousands of athletes undergo preparticipation physical examinations or screenings prior to participating in organized sports and exercise. While their cost effectiveness as a screening tool has been debated (Bratton & Agerter 1995), these examinations fulfill several important functions. They help to detect medical conditions that may prevent the athlete from safe participation, screen for general health, and provide the opportunity for health education that can prevent future problems. A screening is an abbreviated preseason preparticipation physical examination designed to satisfy standards mandated in some countries, and to identify any significant health and medical problems. It includes reviewing the history, noting allergies, recording vital signs and cardiopulmonary status, and assessing the current condition of previous injuries. The major focus of this chapter is the medical aspects of preparticipation screening where evidence has shown a benefit (AAFP, AAP, AMSSM, AOSSM, AOASM 1997).

TARGET AUDIENCE

Preparticipation physical exams are most commonly performed on athletes involved in organized athletic programs or on older people entering physical activity programs. In some countries (e.g. the USA), middle school, high school, and college/university athletes are mandated to take such preseason examinations. In several other countries, these examinations are increasingly used, particularly at elite and professional levels of sport. The examination does, however, have a much broader target audience as athletic participation widens to all age groups. In the USA, for example, there has been a particularly significant increase in the number of athletes who participate at the youth level who are of preschool and elementary school age. As our world becomes more technologically advanced and less manual labor is required in our daily lives, medical professionals encourage participating in sport and exercise at a recreational level at all ages to maintain physical fitness and weight control. Furthermore, as medical advances allow individuals to live longer, more senior adults will be participating in sport and exercise pursuits.

GOALS AND OBJECTIVES OF SCREENING EXAMINATIONS

Preparticipation screening examinations can fulfill the following goals and objectives, which can be beneficial to people involved in sport and exercise (AAFP, AAP, AMSSM, AOSSM, AOASM 1997):

- To detect medical conditions that may place an athlete at risk for injury or death.
- To detect medical and musculoskeletal conditions that will limit or prevent an athlete from participating safely in a particular sport. A detailed history and focused physical examination is the best defense currently available to detect conditions that may lead to sudden death or increased morbidity or mortality from existing medical conditions. This allows for proper rehabilitation and/or use of protective equipment that can correct abnormalities that may otherwise endanger the athlete and their competitors.
- To define sport and exercise activities that an athlete can participate in safely. If an athlete cannot play a chosen sport for a medical reason, it is very important to provide alternative activities.
- Provide general health screening on a limited basis. The preparticipation screening examination is not designed to replace regular health examinations. The reality is, however, that is does, especially in adolescent athletes who are generally healthy and would not otherwise enter the health care system. It has been reported that over 78% of athletes use the preparticipation examination as the only health maintenance contact (Carek & Futrell 1999). It is therefore important to use this examination as an opportunity to address global health needs.
- Counsel and educate athletes on sport and health related issues. This is especially important in adolescent athletes who may be starting to engage in high-risk behaviors, which can adversely affect their current and future health. It also helps foster an open relationship between the athlete and the medical staff, making it easier to discuss any future concerns or problems.
- Fulfill legal and/or insurance requirements in certain sectors and countries. Identifying and addressing health problems of athletes involved in organized sports programs may provide some degree of protection from liability of the athlete and the institution that sponsors the activity. It may also lead to lower insurance rates for institutions (Mac 1998).

HOW ARE PREPARTICIPATION SCREENING EXAMINATIONS DONE?

WHEN TO CONDUCT EXAMINATIONS

Timing of examinations should allow for the opportunity to rehabilitate injuries that are discovered, and/or to perform diagnostic testing and evaluation. The generally recommended time is 6–8 weeks before the start of the preseason or the start of an exercise program. If the examination is done too close to the start of the preseason or the exercise program, valuable time needed to diagnose or rehabilitate would be lost from the participation time. If the examination is done too far in advance, new problems or injuries can occur by the time the activity starts.

The frequency of performing these examinations is not uniform. Different sports governing associations have varying requirements. Some countries have quite strong recommendations. For example, in the USA, the American Heart Association recommends a complete history and physical examination at the entrance to high school, with a repeat history and physical examination every 2 years (Maron et al 1996a). A screening to include a history review, blood pressure measurement, and injury assessment should occur in each intervening year. It has been suggested that college level and university athletes have a complete evaluation upon entrance to the school and a history screening and blood pressure measurement yearly during the next 3 to 4 years (Maron et al 1998).

PERFORMING THE EXAMINATION

There are two recognized ways to perform examinations: individually or station based. Both types of processing have advantages and disadvantages. Individual examinations are on a one-on-one basis with the athlete or exercise participant and the medical provider and physical therapist present. The advantages of this type of examination are: the personal attention, which facilitates the provision of health education and assessment of high-risk behavior; it allows for the development of a relationship between the athlete and the providers, which will lay the foundation for future communication;

and confidentiality and privacy are easier to maintain. The disadvantages are: whether or not the medical provider has specific knowledge relating to the specific needs of athletes, which can lead to varying degrees of injury assessment; these examinations are also time consuming.

In the USA, school-based health centers are another location where individual examinations can be performed. These centers are established in some high schools and middle schools to improve access to care for adolescents. The centers provide multidisciplinary health care providers such as physicians, nurse practitioners, dietitians, and social workers. The location in the school provides easier follow-up of identified problems, and helps establish relationships with the athletes.

Station-based examinations allow for more rapid processing of a large number of athletes. Athletes progress through several sites where different providers perform the different phases of the preparticipation examination. The advantages are that providers can be chosen for their expertise, improving the quality of that component of the examination. The typical stations include history review, vital signs, general medical evaluation, cardiopulmonary assessment, musculoskeletal evaluation, and determination of medical clearance by senior medical personnel. The disadvantage is that there is little privacy, making it difficult to establish relationships with athletes and to discuss sensitive issues. Also, the exam areas are often noisy making it difficult to listen for heart murmurs and to hear systolic and diastolic blood pressure readings (Esquivel & McCormick 1987).

PREPARTICIPATION HISTORY

The history, as in most areas of health care, is the most important component of the preparticipation examination. Most conditions that predispose athletes to injury or death during athletic participation, if they can be identified at all, are detected in the history rather than on physical examination. Rifat et al (1995) reviewed 2574 preparticipation physical examinations and reported that the history indicated 88% of abnormal findings and 57% of restrictions from sport.

Self-report history

Self-report history forms provide a very useful and consistent means of obtaining the pertinent history and can be reviewed rapidly for areas of concern and potential risk. For high school athletes and younger athletes, it is very important that parents or guardians help the athlete with the completion of the history form. This better ensures that all elements of the history are reported accurately.

Surgical history

The past surgical history is important. Athletes and exercise participants who have had previous surgery need the time to heal and to have proper rehabilitation before returning to play.

Medical history

The past medical history uncovers conditions such as asthma, bee sting allergies, and diabetes, which require special care to allow safe participation. It is often helpful to ask participants what is the sickest they have ever been. For most young athletes the answer is usually a viral illness, which is reassuring. Occasionally, this question will help uncover important but forgotten history.

Allergies should be noted on emergency cards that are carried with the team. Athletes often travel and may not be treated by medical personnel who are familiar with their history. Allergies to insects are important, especially in outdoor sports. If a serious allergy is known, such as respiratory distress or tongue swelling after an insect sting, an adrenaline (epinephrine) pen should be available at all times for the athlete. Food and environmental allergies should be noted since athletes may travel and be exposed to different environments. A small number of athletes will even experience urticaria or anaphylaxis related to exercise itself.

Medication history should include current prescription medications as well as any over-the-counter medications. Certain medications have side-effects that can affect athletic performance (see Ch. 28). For example, beta-blockers used to control hypertension can affect endurance, diuretics can affect hydration status, and the antibiotic tetracycline can increase risk of sunburn. Over-the-counter medications that may seem innocuous can also have unwanted side-effects that adversely affect athletic performance. For example, certain cold and cough medications containing sympathetomimetics may cause tachycardia.

It is also helpful to get an accurate history of any vitamin, herbal remedies, or supplements. It is useful to ask about these, specifically, as many athletes do not consider these preparations as medications. Often it will be necessary to actually look at the label to determine the components of the supplement as many contain several substances. Athletes are especially prone to taking these preparations if they believe it will improve athletic performance. Often, however, the efficacy and/or safety of these supplements are unknown. Some athletes take ergogenic substances to gain an advantage in athletic competition. It is advisable to inquire about such substances as anabolic steroids and growth hormone.

Some sports governing organizations, including the International Olympic Committee and the National Collegiate Athletic Association (in the USA), have lists of medications that are banned to their athletes (see Ch. 28 for further details). Failure to comply with these restrictions can have serious consequences. Of note is that some of the banned substances are over-the-counter medications. This point was highlighted during the Sydney Olympic Games in 2000 when a gymnast was stripped of her medal for taking a cold medication that was banned.

Cardiac history

The cardiac history is extremely important, as this is the best tool available at this time to detect medical conditions that would place an athlete or exercise participant at risk for sudden cardiac death (Mac 1998) (see Ch. 30). Sudden death in athletes is fortunately an uncommon occurrence, affecting about 0.2 to 0.5 young athletes per 100 000 per year (Maron et al 1996b). Unfortunately, many athletes with cardiac defects that lead to sudden death are asymptomatic until the fatal event occurs, which is usually a ventricular arrhythmia. Warning symptoms during exercise include syncope or near syncope, chest pain, irregular heart rhythms, and tachycardia. Athletes may also fatigue earlier than their peers. These symptoms need to be distinguished from deconditioning that usually occurs in the beginning of the season and resolves as the fitness level improves. Previous history of heart murmurs and diagnostic testing, high cholesterol, and hypertension should be obtained (Mac 1998).

In the under 35-year-old age group, congenital cardiac abnormalities are the most common cause of sudden cardiac death. A family history of cardiac problems that have lead to death before the age of 50 years will give clues toward familial heart disease. Maron et al (1996b) found the following breakdown of causes in 158 athletes in the USA from 1985 to 1995: hypertrophic cardiomyopathy in 36%, anomalous coronary arteries in 19%, increased cardiac mass in 10%, ruptured aorta in 5%, tunneled left anterior descending coronary artery in 5%, aortic stenosis in 4%, myocarditis in 3%, dilated cardiomyopathy in 3%, arrhythomogenic right ventricular dysplasia in 3%, mitral valve prolapse in 2%, coronary artery disease in 2%, and other causes in 5%.

The most common cause of sudden death in young athletes, hypertrophic cardiomyopathy, is an asymmetrical hypertrophy of the left ventricle that can lead to outflow obstruction and fatal arrhythmias. Symptoms may include syncope, chest pain, palpitations, or dyspnea with exertion or a heart murmur. Often, however, the athlete is asymptomatic. Although it appears more common in males and African Americans, a recent study from the Centers for Disease Control and Prevention showed a higher incidence in females than previously suspected. The rates of sudden cardiac death increased 30% in females from 1989 to 1996 (Zheng et al 2001).

Marfan's syndrome

Marfan's syndrome, a connective tissue disorder due to lack of fibrillin, should be asked about, specifically. Marfan's syndrome diagnosis is made on the presence of at least two of four major features of the disease. These are positive family history, and ocular, cardiac, and skeletal abnormalities. These athletes are at risk of sudden death from aortic rupture. If an athlete has any significant positive history responses, further evaluation should be pursued before clearance is given to participate (Cantwell 1986).

Coronary artery disease

In athletes older than 35 years, coronary artery disease is the most common cause of exercise related sudden death (Maron et al 1996b). Younger athletes with a personal or family history of coronary artery disease should also be assessed. Risk factors include age, family history of coronary artery disease in a first-degree relative, male gender, cigarette smoking, hypercholesterolemia, diabetes, hypertension, obesity, and sedentary lifestyle. Males over the age of 40 years and females over the age of 50 years with two or more risk factors should be considered for exercise stress testing prior to the start of an exercise program. Screening questions of symptoms such as those on the Physical Activity Readiness Questionnaire (PAR-Q) (Thomas et al 1992) are helpful in screening at risk athletes (Kenney 1995).

Heat related illness

Heat illness is important to note as previous heat related problems would increase risk of recurrent problems. Athletes at the extremes of age, obesity, poor physical fitness, not being acclimatized to the heat, and those taking certain medications such as diuretics, will increase the risk of heat related problems. Athletes should be educated during the preparticipation exam about proper hydration and encouraged to monitor their fluid status and take measures to acclimatize to the heat before the season starts. This type of education is also important for athletes travelling to competitions in hotter and more humid climates than they are used to. Fluid status can be monitored by observing the color of the athlete's urine. A well-hydrated athlete will have clear to light yellow urine whereas the dehydrated athlete will have dark yellow, concentrated urine. Another way to monitor hydration status is to weigh the athlete before and after a practice session. Most weight loss will be due to fluid losses and should be replaced before the athlete returns to play. This method allows for the determination of the individual athlete's sweat rate, which allows for accurate fluid replacement (Murray 1994).

Acclimatization is a process inducing physiological adaptations in response to the stress of exercising in the heat. The process takes 7 to 14 days to complete. This will help protect the athlete from heat illness by starting to sweat sooner, decreasing salt loss in sweat, increasing time to exhaustion, and improving cardiovascular responses to heat stress. Athletes should exercise in the heat for 60 to 90 min and increase the intensity of the workouts over a 2-week period to achieve these protective changes (Maughan & Shirreffs 1997).

Appropriate guidelines should be given to the athlete about hydration. Athletes should be advised to pre-hydrate about 2 h before an event with at least 17 ounces (0.5 L) of fluids. During the event, they should drink 4–8 ounces (0.12–0.25 L) of fluids every 20 min and after the event it is best to rehydrate within 2 h. Twenty-four ounces (0.7 L) of fluids should be consumed for every 1 pound (0.45 kg) of weight loss. Fluid breaks should be scheduled into the activity rather than taken as needed. Athletes have been found to replace only two thirds of their fluid loss by voluntary drinking alone (Coyle 1994). Also, by the time the athlete is thirsty, dehydration has already occurred. Sports drinks that contain 6–8% carbohydrates, sodium, and other electrolytes should be favored over water as the taste will encourage increased consumption, and it has been shown that athletes who drink these substances can perform longer with less fatigue (Coyle 1994).

Neurological history

Neurological history includes seizure disorders, history of burners or stingers, previous concussions, and loss of consciousness. Level of control of any seizure disorders should be determined. Burners or stingers are transient traction injuries of the brachial plexus of nerves. The history should include frequency of symptoms, residual weakness, and any lasting neurological deficits.

Concussions should be assessed for severity and residual symptoms. There are multiple guidelines available to assess and grade the severity of concussions (see Ch. 30). There is, however, very little evidence as to the validity of any of these guidelines. Table 11.1 shows the concussion assessment guidelines from the Brain Injury Association (Quality Standards Subcommittee of the American Academy of Neurology 1997).

Respiratory history

Respiratory history focuses on detection of exercise-induced bronchospasm (EIB). This condition involves airway obstruction that only occurs related to exercise. The usual symptoms are coughing, wheezing, chest tightness, or shortness of breath that occur during or after exercise. At times, the symptoms of EIB are mistaken for deconditioning. A previous history of asthma or allergic rhinitis is a risk factor for the development of EIB. EIB is also more pronounced during exercise in cold, low humidity environments and in the presence of environmental allergens (Storms 1999). Most athletes respond well to treatment with short acting bronchodilators, such as albuterol, taken 20–30 min before the start of exercise. Athletes can also induce a refractory period of reduced symptoms by warming up with an intense workout to invoke bronchospasm prior to the start of exercise. This

Table 11.1 Grading and management of concussion. (Modified from the Quality Standards Subcommittee of the American Academy of Neurology 1997.)

Grade	Confusion	Loss of consciousness (LOC)	Length of symptoms	Management
Grade 1	Transient	None	Less than 15 min	May return to play same day if no symptoms at rest and with exertion
Grade 2	Transient	None	More than 15 min	No return to play same day Re-examine next day Return to play after 1 week of no symptoms at rest and with exertion
Grade 3	Any amount	Brief or prolonged LOC	N/A	No return to play same day Transport to emergency room if indicated Brief LOC – return to play after 1 week of no symptoms at rest and with exertion. Prolonged LOC – return to play after 2 weeks of no symptoms at rest and with exertion

refractory period can last 30–90 min. Athletes with underlying asthma or allergic rhinitis should be treated for these conditions (Storms 1999).

Vision history

Vision history should determine if the athlete requires correction of visual acuity and whether glasses or contact lenses are used. Glasses should have lenses made of polycarbonate material that will not shatter if they are hit, to avoid eye injury. Previous eye injury or surgery should be noted. The risk of eye injury in sports is often overlooked. The American Academy of Ophthalmology recommends protective eyewear with polycarbonate lenses for all sports that are at high risk for eye injury. These sports include those that use a small ball or sticks (e.g. baseball, tennis, lacrosse), those with close contact (e.g. basketball), and those that cause intentional injury (e.g. boxing) (Vinger 2000).

Skin conditions

Skin conditions should be noted in the history to detect those that may be contagious, such as herpes, molluscum contagiosum, and tinea corporis. These are especially important in contact sports, such as wrestling.

Musculoskeletal history

Musculoskeletal history should focus on previous injuries and type of treatment given. Many athletes, especially at school level and younger, have not received adequate rehabilitation of previous injuries. The most important risk factor for a repeat injury is having a previous injury that was not completely rehabilitated (Bar-Or et al 1988). Previous surgery should be cleared for return to play by the surgeon who performed the procedure. Inquiry should also be made about the use of protective equipment such as knee or ankle braces.

Immunization

The preparticipation exam is an opportune time to review immunizations to make sure that they are up to date. This is especially important in team sports where communicable diseases are easily spread. Tetanus immunization booster is given in adolescence and updated every 5–10 years. Two measles, mumps and rubella vaccines are needed. Adolescents who have not had chicken pox need immunization, and meningococcal vaccine should be considered. Hepatitis B vaccine should be given to athletes who have not received the series and should be recommended to coaches. As discussed in Chapter 30, athletes involved in international travel should receive appropriate immunizations for the area (Centers for Disease Control and Prevention 1999).

Female athletes

Female athletes deserve special consideration during their examination to evaluate those at risk for the female athlete triad (see Ch. 26). The triad includes amenorrhea, which is the loss of menstruation in a female who previously had menstrual cycles, eating disorders, and osteoporosis. This triad of disorders has significant health consequences, which may affect the athlete for the rest of her life, especially with premature osteoporosis. Age at menarche and date of the first day of the last menstrual period should be noted.

Menarche

Menarche is the onset of menses and is often delayed in young athletes who are participating in strenuous activities. Menarche may be delayed by 5 months for every year of intense prepubertal training (Frisch et al 1981). The average age of menarche for non-athletic females has decreased over the years. The mean age for menarche is 12.88 years in Caucasians and 12.16 years in African Americans (Herman-Giddens et al 1997). The number of normal menstrual periods that occur yearly should be assessed. Secondary amenorrhea is defined as missing at least three consecutive menstrual cycles in a woman who has established menstrual cycles. The most common cause of secondary amenorrhea, even in athletes, is pregnancy and this should be ruled out before concluding that the amenorrhea is related to exercise. Prolonged amenorrhea can have negative effects on bone health, as estrogen is a necessary component to make adequate bone. If the amenorrhea persists for more than 3 years and occurs during the time of peak bone accretion, the effects are usually irreversible (Hobart & Smucker 2000). Athletes should be made aware that amenorrhea is not a normal occurrence and that it should be investigated if it persists. Often athletes and coaches feel that amenorrhea is a good sign of hard training.

Eating disorders

Eating disorders (see Ch. 26) include a spectrum from disordered eating which does not meet the energy requirements of the athlete, to frank eating disorders such as anorexia nervosa and bulimia nervosa. Anorexia nervosa has the following diagnostic criteria: weight less than 85% of ideal body weight, amenorrhea, distorted body image and intense fear of gaining weight. There are restricting anorexics that decrease intake of food to achieve weight loss and bulimic anorexics that regularly purge or binge eat (American Psychiatric Association 1994).

Bulimia nervosa is characterized by recurrent episodes of binge eating, which involve eating large amounts of food in 2-h time periods, and using a pathological method to get rid of the food to prevent weight gain. By definition, the binge eating and compensatory behaviors must occur at least twice a week for 3 months (American Psychiatric Association 1994). Bulimics have a distorted self-evaluation based on body shape and weight. There are two types of bulimics: the purging type who use methods such as vomiting, laxatives, diuretics, and diet pills to lose the weight; and the non-purging type who use other methods such as excessive exercise to lose weight (American Psychiatric Association 1994).

One approach to begin a discussion on eating behaviors is to inquire how the athlete feels about their current weight. The hallmark of eating disorders is a distorted self-image about weight; athletes with an eating disorder will feel that they are overweight even when they are not. Also ask about pathological weight control behaviors, which include vomiting, taking diet pills and laxatives, using saunas, or wearing heavy clothing to sweat and lose weight. Exercise to excess is often used as a way to purge calories, especially in adolescents with eating disorders. At times, it may be difficult to determine when this behavior is pathological as it may be perceived as a sign of being a good athlete. Inquire how much exercise is done in addition to that needed to meet the requirements of the sport. Eating disorder patients often fit in well in an athletic environment because they are typically compulsive in their behaviors and are perfectionists (Thompson & Sherman 1993). Certain sports are more at risk than others. These include sports that have weight classes (e.g. weightlifting, rowing, boxing), those in which appearance is important for judging (e.g. gymnastics, ballet, figure-skating), and endurance sports (Thompson & Sherman 1993).

Osteoporosis

Osteoporosis occurs in the triad due to the lack of the necessary substrates to keep bone formation above bone resorption. The dietary deficits in calcium and vitamin D as well as the low estrogen hormonal status can lead to premature osteoporosis. This usually manifests clinically as stress and other fractures and recurrent musculoskeletal injuries. Osteoporosis that occurs before menopause is very difficult to treat, and may be largely irreversible (Hobart & Smucker 2000). Hormonal replacement is controversial in its ability to reverse the problem (Taitel and Lippman 1995).

Adolescents

The preparticipation examination is also an opportune time to inquire about the general health of the athlete, especially adolescents. Adolescents are often an underserved population as they may not be evaluated by medical providers on a regular basis. It is also the time when risk-taking behaviors that will have adverse health consequences can begin. Talking to adolescent and young adults about high-risk behaviors requires some preliminary discussion about confidentiality and its limits. If adolescents reveal that they are engaging in high-risk behaviors, they need some reassurance as to what will be done with that information. If there is not an agreement about confidentiality, this information will most likely not be revealed. It is also useful to determine the social support systems available to the adolescent to deal with stressful situations. Teenagers who do not have social supports, have poor coping mechanisms to deal with stress, and who feel socially isolated, are more likely to develop high risk behaviors such as smoking, substance abuse, sexual activity and suicide (Goldenring & Cohen 1988). It is often useful to discuss less personal topics first and lead up to more sensitive issues. One mnemonic for this discussion is HEADSS (Goldenring & Cohen 1988). 'H' is for home environment: questions should focus on who lives in the home, who is a support person for the adolescent, and what type of environment is present in the home. 'E' is for education, vocational goals, and employment: adolescents who are failing in school or who are having behavior problems in school deserve further evaluation. 'A' is for activities in and out of school: this includes peer activities, hobbies, and religious involvement. 'D' is for drug, tobacco, and alcohol use by the teenager, peers, and family members. 'S' is for sexual activity, sexual orientation, contraception use, and sexually transmitted infection history. The other 'S' is for suicidal ideation and depression. Athletes engaging in high risk behaviors should be counseled for risk factor reduction by appropriate health care personnel and referred as necessary.

PREPARTICIPATION PHYSICAL

The physical examination is a screening examination to rule out pathology that will make athletic participation unsafe. Athletes should be dressed in clothes that will make it possible to visualize the anatomy (AAFP, AAP, AMSSM, AOSSM, AOASM 1997). It is important to be sensitive to exposure of the body in athletes during the examination. Young adolescents are particularly sensitive to the changes in their bodies so it is best to expose only the area that needs to be examined, to cover that area when finished, and then to expose the next area.

Vital signs

Vital signs include blood pressure, pulse, height, weight, and visual acuity. Blood pressure should be measured in

Table 11.2   Blood pressure measurements in male and female children and adolescents. If systolic or diastolic blood pressure is at or above the 95th percentile, the child may be hypertensive and warrant further observation and consideration of other risk. (Modified from the National High Blood Pressure Education Program 1996.)

Male 95th percentile blood pressure measurements by percentage of height for age

Age (years)	5th percentile height	50th percentile height	95th percentile height
6	109/72	114/74	117/76
7	110/74	115/76	119/78
8	111/75	116/77	120/80
9	113/76	117/79	121/81
10	114/77	119/80	123/82
11	116/78	121/80	125/83
12	119/79	123/81	127/83
13	121/79	126/82	130/84
14	124/80	128/82	132/85
15	127/81	131/83	135/86
16	129/83	134/85	138/87
17	132/85	136/87	140/89

Female 95th percentile blood pressure measurements by percentage of height for age

6	108/71	111/73	114/73
7	110/73	113/74	116/76
8	112/74	115/75	118/78
9	114/75	117/77	120/79
10	116/77	119/78	122/80
11	118/78	121/79	124/81
12	120/79	123/80	126/82
13	121/80	125/82	128/84
14	123/81	126/83	130/85
15	124/82	128/83	131/86
16	125/83	128/84	132/86
17	126/83	129/84	132/86

the right arm in the sitting position and the athlete should be sitting with the back and arm supported. If the blood pressure is found to be elevated, it is necessary to repeat the measurement again during the examination. Three consecutive elevated blood pressures on three different occasions are needed to diagnose hypertension. It is important to note in adolescent athletes and children that normal blood pressure levels are lower than in adult athletes (National High Blood Pressure Education Program 1996) (Table 11.2). Height and weight should be compared to standard charts. Body mass index or body fat measurements may also be included. This is especially important in sports that have weight limits. Athletes who are over- or underweight should have a dietary evaluation and underweight athletes should be screened for eating disorders, regardless of gender. Visual acuity should be tested using Snellen eye charts. Athletes should have vision that is correctable to 20/40 or better (AAFP, AAP, AMSSM, AOSSM, AOASM 1997, Vinger 2000).

The head, ears, eyes, nose, and throat

Examinations of the head, ears, eyes, nose, and throat should document the lack or presence of infection. The eyes should be checked for equal pupils. Any asymmetry such as anisocoria should be noted so that if the athlete should receive a head injury, the pupil asymmetry will not be attributed to the trauma. Nasal passages should be checked for symmetry and patent airflow. The pharynx should be checked for signs of infection. The condition of the teeth should be noted, especially for any loose or damaged teeth and dental erosions that may be the result of vomiting in eating disorder patients.

Lungs

Lung examination should assess for equal breath sounds and the presence of wheezing and other abnormal sounds. Athletes with exercise-induced bronchospasm should have normal lung examinations at rest. The presence of wheezing during the screening examination indicates baseline asthma or underlying respiratory infection (Storms 1999). These conditions should be treated appropriately.

Abdomen

Abdominal examination should check for hepato-splenomegaly, which may be the result of infections such as mononucleosis. Also check for other abdominal masses or tenderness that may require further evaluation.

Skin

Skin examination should check for infectious conditions as well as acne, abnormal lesions and signs of sun exposure. Acne may be exacerbated by helmets and sweating. Any evidence of a communicable skin disease should be treated prior to beginning team training in close contact sports. During the treatment phase, an individualized training schedule should be established for the affected athlete.

Genitourinary tract

Genitourinary examination and level of sexual development should be assessed in male athletes. This examination is not currently recommended in female athletes (AAFP, AAP, AMSSM, AOSSM, AOASM 1997). Testicular examination should check for abnormal lumps, varicocoeles, and bilateral descended testicles. Athletes should be given education in how to perform testicular self-examinations, as this form of cancer is more common in young males aged 20 to 35 years (Chan 2001). The presence of hernias should be ruled out. Sexual maturity rating should be done based on development of pubic hair, penis and testicular size. Traditionally, this information was used to help group males according to maturity rather than age in contact sports. It has not been shown, however, that such grouping will prevent injuries to less mature and smaller athletes (AAFP, AAP, AMSSM, AOSSM, AOASM 1997).

Cardiology

Cardiac examination is important in an attempt to detect cardiac abnormalities that could lead to sudden death. The American Heart Association recommendations include a minimum of auscultation of the heart for murmurs in at least the supine and standing positions, palpation of femoral artery pulses, and evaluation for physical examination findings of Marfan's syndrome. Heart size should be assessed clinically by palpating the point of maximal impulse on the precordium. Heart rate and rhythm should be assessed on auscultation.

The murmur of hypertrophic cardiomyopathy is louder when there is less blood in the heart, which increases outflow tract obstruction. It is therefore important to listen to the heart in different positions to accentuate this murmur. Getting the athlete to perform a Valsalva maneuver or to stand from a squatting position will increase the murmur of hypertrophic cardio-

myopathy, as these positions decrease the amount of blood in the left ventricle (Allen et al 1994).

Functional murmurs are a common finding on examination particularly in young athletes. These murmurs are typically louder in the supine position and the change in intensity of sound is reversed in comparison to the above maneuvers for hypertrophic cardiomyopathy.

Palpation of pulses in the upper and lower extremity is important to rule out coarctation of the aorta, which will result in diminished femoral pulses compared to upper extremity pulses (Allen et al 1994).

Marfan's syndrome

The physical examination findings of Marfan's syndrome include cardiac, ocular, musculoskeletal, and skin conditions. Cardiac abnormalities include mitral or aortic valve regurgitation murmurs, dilated aortic root, aortic dissection and dysrhythmias. Ocular findings include myopia, lens subluxations, and retinal detachment. Musculoskeletal findings include arm span longer than height, tall stature, pectus excavatum deformity of the anterior chest wall, scoliosis, flat feet, and hyperextensible joints. Skin findings include stria distensae. Inguinal hernias are more frequent. Athletes with a family history and physical examination findings suggestive of Marfan's syndrome should undergo further evaluation to confirm the diagnosis (Cantwell 1986).

Musculoskeletal

The musculoskeletal examination should be a screening for asymptomatic, at risk athletes and should include a joint-specific examination for previously injured athletes. The objectives are to compare symmetry, side-to-side laxity, and assess range of motion, gross strength, and neurological function. Any areas of abnormality should be further evaluated with a joint-specific examination. The *Preparticipation Monograph* recommends the following 14 point screening examination (AAFP, AAP, AMSSM, AOSSM, AOASM 1997) (Fig. 11.1): there is a general inspection of body habitus, neck range of motion, trapezius strength, deltoid strength, shoulder range of motion, elbow range of motion, hand and finger range of motion. Spine assessment begins with inspection with the back towards the examiner, back extension to assess for spondylolysis or spondylolisthesis and back flexion for scoliosis. Lower extremity examination focuses on the range of motion and laxity of the hips, knees and ankles, hamstring flexibility, and quadriceps contraction. Functional testing includes squat and duck walk for four steps. To successfully perform these tests, a functional range of motion, adequate strength of the hips, knees and

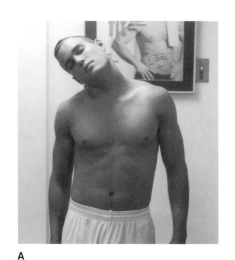

A

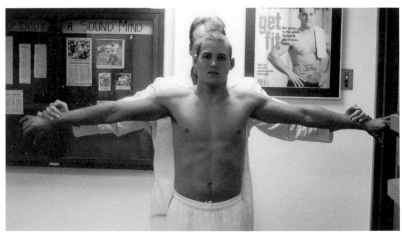

B

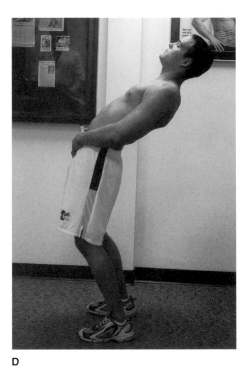

C

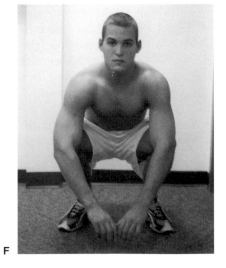

D

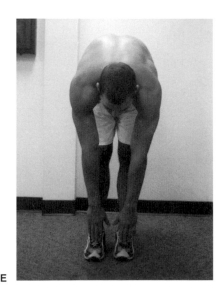

E

F

Figure 11.1A–F The preparticipation screening musculoskeletal exam. **A**: Inspection, neck range of motion. **B**: Resisted shoulder shrug and deltoid strength. **C**: Range of motion of shoulders, elbows, wrists, fingers. **D**: Inspection of back, hyperextention of back. **E**: Scoliosis check. **F**: Tighten quadriceps, stand on toes and heels, squat and duck walk four steps.

ankles, and balance are required. The lower extremity functional testing is completed by standing on the toes and heels to assess calf symmetry and strength (AAFP, AAP, AMSSM, AOSSM, AOASM 1997).

The joint-specific examination should be performed if there are abnormalities in the above screening examination or if there is a past history of musculoskeletal injury. This should also focus on joints relevant to participation in sports and exercise activities. The shoulder examination should consist of range of motion (particularly internal rotation) and strength testing of the rotator cuff. Instability and impingement testing should be performed. Assessment of neck range of motion, winging of the scapula, and evaluation of pulses with the arm in the high five position to assess for thoracic outlet syndrome complete the shoulder examination. Hip evaluation should rule out referred knee pain especially in the adolescent population. The knee examination consists of range of motion, strength testing, ligamentous, patellofemoral, and meniscus evaluations, and testing for the presence of a painful plica. The ankle examination also consists of range of motion and strength testing. Anterior drawer and talar tilt testing evaluate for lateral ankle laxity. The squeeze test and external rotation stress tests assess syndesmosis injuries and the Thompson's test is used to assess Achilles tendon continuity (AAFP, AAP, AMSSM, AOSSM, AOASM 1997).

SPORT-SPECIFIC EXAMINATION CONSIDERATIONS

During the preparticipation examination, it is important to consider the demands of the particular sport in which the athlete will be participating. This will help focus the examiner to look for physical findings that may correlate to specific injuries in playing that sport.

American football favors athletes who have power, speed, and explosive movements. Those athletes who have increased tightness with lateral cervical flexion may be at increased risk of developing stingers or burners (Michael et al 1996).

Basketball involves running, jumping, cutting, pivoting, and explosive movements. Injuries to the ankle, knee, and foot are the most common in this sport. Athletes who have decreased calf flexibility and decreased ankle eversion strength may be at increased risk of ankle sprains (Dombroski 1995).

Wrestling is an anaerobic sport that involves muscle endurance, strength, and flexibility. Injuries most often involve the knee, shoulder, ribs, elbow, and back. Athletes with lower abdominal weakness may be at risk for lumbar strain injuries (see Ch. 14).

Overhead sports, such as tennis and volleyball, involve flexibility, strength, and muscular endurance. Athletes

with scapular dyskinesis and loss of internal rotation may be at risk for ipsilateral shoulder impingement (Nicola 1997).

Swimming involves aerobic endurance, strength, and flexibility. Athletes with weak hip flexors may be at risk for contralateral shoulder impingement. Also, those with tight pectoralis minor muscles may be at risk for ipsilateral shoulder impingement (Hammer 1997).

Soccer involves running, cutting, pivoting, and explosive movements. Athletes with rectus femoris tightness may be at risk for quadriceps strains (Barkley 1997).

Fitness and performance testing is an optional component of preparticipation evaluations that can supply valuable extra information for the athlete and the coaching staff but it is often sacrificed due to time constraints and lack of personnel capable of performing the tests. These evaluations by athletic trainers, strength coaches, and rehabilitation specialists can be extensive and involve expensive equipment or can be performed in a more basic fashion. There are many options for taking measurements that can be adapted to the evaluation site and level of play. The areas of concern are usually flexibility, strength, endurance, power, speed, and agility (Bar-Or et al 1998).

Screening tests are not routinely recommended for asymptomatic athletes during the preparticipation examination. Urinalysis for protein and glucose has been recommended in the past but has not been shown to be cost effective in detecting renal abnormalities and diabetes (Peggs et al 1986). Much attention has been focused on screening large populations of athletes with echocardiogram or electrocardiogram to detect cardiac abnormalities that may lead to sudden death. These methods of evaluation as a screening tool again are not cost effective and the problem of detecting falsely positive abnormalities causes significant delay in clearance to play for asymptomatic athletes (Maron et al 1996a). Hemoglobin and hematocrit levels, especially in female athletes who are more prone to iron deficiency anemia from menstrual blood losses, should be considered in at risk athletes, but not routinely ordered (AAFP, AAP, AMSSM, AOSSM, AOASM 1997).

DETERMINING CLEARANCE

The vast majority of preparticipation examinations will result in clearance of the person to participate in the desired sport or exercise activity. Smith & Laskowski (1998) found that only 1.9% of 2739 athletes were disqualified from participation as a result of their examinations. When determining if a condition should disqualify an athlete from participating, the following questions should be considered (AAFP, AAP, AMSSM, AOSSM, AOASM 1997):

1. Will the problem place the athlete at increased risk of sudden death?
2. Will other athletes be placed at higher risk of injury?
3. Can this athlete safely play, with treatment (i.e. medication, protective equipment, rehabilitation)?

The level of competition and the age of the athlete are critical in making these decisions. If the increased risk of injury will have a long-lasting effect on the athlete's future health, the athlete should not be cleared for return to play. If clearance is denied for the chosen sport or exercise activity, it is very important to identify activities the person can safely participate in. The importance of participating in sport or exercise should not be under-estimated. Rifat et al (1995) found that adolescents rated not making the team as more devastating than their parents separating, the death of a close friend, or academic failure. It is also important to discuss these decisions with the athletes and their families to determine what they want to be communicated to the coaches and athletic staff. The medical provider has primary responsibility to abide by the athlete's wishes for disclosure of information, and proper permission should be obtained before sharing medical information with others. However, this may be problematic as coaches and athletic staff expect to be part of the communication process when problems are identified and evaluation is being performed (Mitten 1996).

Decisions about participation in a specific sport are made easier by classification of sports according to their physical requirements (Table 11.3).

There are only a few conditions in which participation is contraindicated. These are fever, carditis, and diarrhea that is more than mild (AAFP, AAP, AMSSM, AOSSM, AOASM 1997). Fever is generally defined as an oral temperature greater than 100.4°F (38°C). Fever increases heart rate and cardiovascular workload, which can lead to orthostatic hypotension, heat illness, and diminished performance. Carditis is an inflammation of the heart muscle or the surrounding myocardium, and is usually the result of a viral illness. This condition places the athlete at risk for sudden death with exertion; therefore, athletes should not participate for at least 6 months after the onset of the illness and have cardiac function evaluated before return to play. Moderate to severe diarrhea results in fluid loss that can lead to dehydration and heat illness in exercising individuals. Diarrhea is defined as the frequent passage of watery bowel movements. Participation should be postponed until the diarrhea resolves. There are several cardiac conditions that disallow competitive play. These are detailed in the 26th Bethesda Conference recommendations for determining eligibility in athletes with cardiovascular abnormalities (26th Bethesda Conference 1994). Hypertrophic

Table 11.3 Classification of sports by contact (reproduced with permission from the Preparticipation Physical Evaluation [monograph] Leawood, Kansas: American Academy of Family Physicians, American Academy of Pediatrics, American Medical Society for Sports Medicine, American Orthopaedic Society for Sports Medicine, American Osteopathic Academy of Sports Medicine 1996)

Contact/ collision sport	Limited contact sport	Non-contact sport
Basketball	Baseball	Archery
Boxing	Bicycling	Badminton
Diving	Cheerleading	Body building
Field hockey	Canoeing/kayaking (whitewater)	Canoeing/kayaking (flat water)
Football (flag and tackle)	Fencing	Crew/rowing
Ice hockey	Field (high jump and pole vault)	Curling
Lacrosse	Floor hockey	Dancing
Martial arts	Gymnastics	Field (discus, javelin, shot put)
Rodeo	Handball	Golf
Rugby	Horseback riding	Orienteering
Ski jumping	Racquetball	Power lifting
Soccer	Skating (ice, inline and roller)	Race walking
Team handball	Skiing (cross-country, downhill and water)	Riflery
Water polo	Softball	Rope jumping
Wrestling	Squash	Running
	Ultimate frisbee	Sailing
	Volleyball	Scuba diving
	Windsurfing/surfing	Strength training
		Swimming
		Table tennis
		Tennis
		Track
		Weight lifting

Table 11.4   Medical Conditions and Sports Participation. This table is designed to be understood by medical and non-medical personnel. In the 'Explanation' column, the words 'needs evaluation' mean that a physician with appropriate knowledge and experience should assess the safety of a given sport for an athlete with the listed medical condition. Unless otherwise noted, this is because of the variability of the severity of the disease or of the risk of injury among the specific sports, or both (reproduced with permission from the Preparticipation Physical Evaluation [monograph] Leawood, Kansas: American Academy of Family Physicians, American Academy of Pediatrics, American Medical Society for Sports Medicine, American Orthopaedic Society for Sports Medicine, American Osteopathic Academy of Sports Medicine 1997)

Condition	May participate	Explanation
Atlantoaxial instability (instability of the joint between cervical vertebrae 1 and 2)	Qualified yes	Athlete needs evaluation to assess risk of spinal cord injury during sports participation
Bleeding disorder	Qualified yes	Athlete needs evaluation
Carditis (inflammation of heart)	No	May result in sudden death with exertion
Hypertension (high blood pressure)	Qualified yes	Those with significant essential (unexplained) hypertension should avoid weight and power lifting, bodybuilding, and strength training. Those with secondary hypertension (caused by a previously identified disease) or severe essential hypertension need evaluation
Congenital heart disease (structural heart defects present at birth) Mild, moderate and severe congenital heart disease are defined in 26th Bethesda Conference: Recommendations for eligibility for competition in athletes with cardiovascular abnormalities. January 6–7, 1994. Med Sci Sports Exerc 1994; 26 (10 suppl): S246–253.	Qualified yes	Those with mild forms may participate fully; those with moderate or severe forms, or who have undergone surgery, need evaluation
Dysrhythmia (irregular heart rhythm)	Qualified yes	Athlete needs evaluation because some types require therapy or make certain sports dangerous or both
Mitral valve prolapse (abnormal heart valve)	Qualified yes	Those with symptoms (chest pain, symptoms of possible dysrhythmia) or evidence of mitral regurgitation (leaking) on physical exam need evaluation. All others may participate fully
Heart murmur	Qualified yes	If murmur is innocent (does not indicate heart disease), full participation is permitted. Otherwise, the athlete needs evaluation
Cerebral palsy	Qualified yes	Athlete needs evaluation
Diabetes mellitus (well controlled)	Yes	All sports can be played with proper attention to diet, hydration, and insulin therapy. Particular attention is needed for activities that last 30 min or more
Diarrhea (American Academy of Pediatrics recommendation)	Qualified no	Unless disease is mild, no participation is permitted, because diarrhea may increase the risk of dehydration and heat illness (see Fever below)
Eating disorders (anorexia nervosa, bulimia nervosa)	Qualified yes	These patients need both medical and psychiatric assessment before participation
Functionally one-eyed athlete, loss of an eye, detached retina, previous eye surgery or serious eye injury	Qualified yes	A functionally one-eyed athlete has a best corrected visual acuity of <20/40 in the worse eye. These athletes would suffer significant disability if the better eye was seriously injured as would those with loss of an eye. Some athletes who have previously undergone eye surgery or had a serious eye injury may have an increased risk of injury because of weakened eye tissue. Availability of eye guards approved by the American Society for Testing Materials (ASTM) and other protective equipment may allow participation in most sports, but this must be judged on an individual basis
Fever	No	Fever can increase cardiopulmonary effort, reduce maximum exercise capacity, make heat illness more likely, and increase orthostatic hypotension during exercise. Fever may rarely accompany myocarditis or other infections that may make exercise dangerous
Heat illness (history of)	Qualified yes	Because of the increased likelihood of recurrence, the athlete needs individual assessment to determine the presence of predisposing conditions and to arrange a prevention strategy

Table 11.4 *(Cont'd)*

Condition	May participate	Explanation
Human immunodeficiency virus (HIV) infection	Yes	Because of the apparent minimal risk to others, all sports may be played that the state of health allows. In all athletes, skin lesions should be properly covered, and athletic personnel should use universal precautions when handling blood or body fluids with visible blood
Kidney (absence of one)	Qualified yes	Athlete needs individual assessment for contact/collision and limited contact sports
Liver (enlarged)	Qualified yes	If the liver is acutely enlarged, participation should be avoided because of risk of rupture. If the liver is chronically enlarged, individual assessment is needed before contact/collision or limited contact sports are played
Malignancy	Qualified yes	Athlete needs individual assessment
Musculoskeletal disorders	Qualified yes	Athlete needs individual assessment
History of serious head or spine trauma, severe or repeated concussions, or craniotomy	Qualified yes	Athlete needs individual assessment for contact/collision or limited contact sports, and also for noncontact sports if there are deficits in judgment or cognition. Recent research supports a conservative approach to management of concussions
Convulsive disorder (well controlled)	Yes	Risk of convulsion during participation is minimal
Convulsive disorder (poorly controlled)	Qualified yes	Athlete needs individual assessment for contact/collision or limited contact sports. Avoid the following non-contact sports: archery, riflery, swimming, weight or power lifting, strength training, or sports involving heights. In these sports, occurrence of a convulsion may be a risk to self or others.
Obesity	Qualified yes	Because of the risk of heat illness, obese persons need careful acclimatization and hydration
Organ transplant recipient	Qualified yes	Athlete needs individual assessment
Ovary (absence of one)	Yes	Risk of severe injury to the remaining ovary is minimal
Pulmonary compromise including cystic fibrosis	Qualified yes	Athlete needs individual assessment, but generally all sports may be played if oxygenation remains satisfactory during a graded exercise test. Patients with cystic fibrosis need acclimatization and good hydration to reduce the risk of heat illness
Asthma	Yes	With proper medication and education, only athletes with the most severe asthma will have to modify their participation
Acute upper respiratory infection	Qualified yes	Upper respiratory obstruction may affect pulmonary function. Athlete needs individual assessment for all but mild disease (see Fever above)
Sickle cell disease	Qualified yes	It is unlikely that individuals with sickle cell trait (AS) have an increased risk of sudden death or other medical problems during athletic participation except under the most extreme conditions of heat, humidity, and possibly increased altitude. These individuals, like all athletes, should be carefully conditioned, acclimatized, and hydrated to reduce any possible risk
Skin (boils, herpes simplex, impetigo, scabies, molluscum contagiosum)	Qualified yes	While the patient is contagious, participation in gymnastics with mats, martial arts, wrestling, or other contact/collision or limited contact sports is not allowed. Herpes simplex virus probably is not transmitted via mats
Spleen (enlarged)	Qualified yes	Patients with acutely enlarged spleens should avoid all sports because of risk of rupture. Those with chronically enlarged spleens need individual assessment before playing contact/collision or limited contact sports
Testicle (absent or undescended)	Yes	Certain sports may require a protective cup

cardiomyopathy is a condition that will disqualify most athletes from all but the lowest intensity sport activities. Athletes with congenital coronary artery anomalies should generally not participate in competitive sports. Prolonged Q-T syndrome is also an electrical condition that will disallow athletic participation since these athletes are at risk for sudden death from ventricular arrthymias. Athletes with severe aortic regurgitation or stenosis, multivalvular disease, arrhythomogenic right ventricular dysplasia, pulmonary hypertension, or significant ventricular dysfunction should not participate in competitive sports. Individual assessment is needed by a cardiologist of all of these conditions.

For all other medical conditions listed in Table 11.4, participation is allowable based on individual circumstances and ability to use protective gear.

SUMMARY

The preparticipation evaluation is an important intervention for athletic populations. Although it involves many components, the examination can be performed efficiently and in a timely manner. Individual examinations allow for relationship building and education of athletes, whereas station-based examinations allow for screeners with specific areas of expertise. The medical history can be preprinted and reviewed with the athlete during the visit. Most information that will be of concern will be revealed in the history. The physical examination is a screening that includes all the major body systems with the exception of the genital area in females. The focus in the examination is on finding pathology that may affect athletic performance. Health education and assessment of high-risk behaviors is especially important in adolescents who may not undergo any other health maintenance examination. The information gained from the history and physical examination is utilized to make clearance decisions. Communication with all involved participants is necessary when abnormalities are discovered. Although little evidence exists as to the cost effectiveness of this evaluation, identification of cardiac abnormalities, medical conditions that can affect long-term health, and musculoskeletal injuries that can be rehabilitated, are very important health outcomes for athletes. Medical and health care personnel who care for athletes should be well versed in the components of this evaluation.

REFERENCES

Allen H D, Golinko R J, Williams R G 1994 Heart murmurs in children: when is a workup needed? Patient Care 28(7):123–151

American Academy of Family Physicians, American Academy of Pediatrics, American Medical Society for Sports Medicine, American Orthopaedic Society for Sports Medicine, American Osteopathic Academy of Sports Medicine (AAFP, AAP, AMSSM, AOSSM, AOASM) 1996 Preparticipation physical evaluation, 2nd edn. McGraw-Hill Healthcare, Minneapolis, MN

American Psychiatric Association 1994 Diagnostic and statistical manual of mental disorders 4th edn. American Psychiatric Association, Washington, DC, p 539–550

Barkley K L 1997 Soccer. In: Mellion M B, Walsh W M, Shelton G L (eds) The team physician's handbook 2nd edn. Hanley and Belfus, Philadelphia, PA, p 672–684

Bar-Or O, Lombardo J A, Rowland T W 1988 The preparticipation sports exam. Patient Care 22:75–102

Bratton R L, Agerter D C 1995 Preparticipation sports examinations efficient risk assessment in children and adolescents. Postgraduate Medicine 98(2):123–132

Cantwell J D 1986 Marfan's syndrome: detection and management. Physician and Sportsmedicine 14(7):51–55

Carek P J, Futrell M 1999 Athlete's view of the preparticipation physical examination attitudes toward certain health screening questions. Archives of Family Medicine 8:307–312

Centers for Disease Control and Prevention 1999 Vaccine-preventable diseases: improving vaccination coverage in children, adolescents, and adults. A report on recommendations from the Task Force on Community Preventive Services. Morbidity and Mortality Weekly Report 48(RR-8):1–15

Chan D 2001 Testicular cancer: an update on recognition and management. Family Practice Recertification 23 (12):27–34

Coyle E E 1994 Fluid and carbohydrate replacement during exercise: how much and what? Sports Science Exchange 7(3):1–10

Dombroski R T 1995 Wrestling. In: Baker C L (ed) The Hughston Clinic sports medicine book. Williams and Wilkins, Media, PA, p 677–670

Esquivel M T, McCormick D P 1987 Preparticipation sports evaluation, part 1: the station-method examination. Family Practice Recertification 9(1):41–58

Frish R E, Gotz-Welbergen A V, McArthur J W et al 1981 Delayed menarche and amenorrhea of college athletes in relation to age of onset of training. Journal of the American Medical Association 246(14):1559–1563

Goldenring J M, Cohen E 1988 Getting into adolescent HEADS. Contemporary Pediatrics 5:75

Hammer R W 1997 Swimming and diving. In: Mellion M B, Walsh W M, Shelton G L (eds) The team physician's handbook, 2nd edn. Hanley and Belfus, Philadelphia, PA, p 718–728.

Herman-Giddens M E, Slora E J, Wasserman R C et al 1997 Secondary sexual characteristics and menses in young girls seen in office practice: a study from the Pediatric Research in Office Settings Network. Pediatrics 99(4):505–512

Hobart J A, Smucker D R 2000 The female athlete triad. American Family Physician 61:3357–3364

Kenney W L (ed) 1995 Health screening and risk stratification American College of Sports Medicine's guidelines for exercise testing and prescription 5th edn. Williams and Wilkins, Media, PA

Mac M 1998 Managing the risks of school sports. The School Administrator 55(10):42–46

Maron B J, Thompson P D, Puffer J C et al 1996a Cardiovascular preparticipation screening of competitive athletes: a statement for health professionals from the sudden death committee and congenital cardiac defects committee, American Heart Association. Circulation 94:850–856

Maron B J, Shirani J, Poliac L C et al 1996b Sudden death in young competitive athletes: clinical, demographic, and pathological profiles. Journal of the American Medical Association 276(3):199–204

Maron B J, Thompson P D, Puffer J C et al 1998 Cardiovascular preparticipation screening of competitive athletes: Addendum. Circulation 97:2294

Maughan R J, Shirreffs S M 1997 Preparing athletes for competition in the heat: developing an effective acclimatization strategy. Sports Science Exchange 10(2):1–8

Michael D J, Moeller J L, Hough D O 1996 Basketball injuries. In: Sallis RE, Massimino F (eds) Essentials of sports medicine. American College of Sports Medicine, St. Louis, MO, p 558–570

Mitten M J 1996 When is disqualification from sports justified? Medical judgment vs patient's rights. Physician and Sportsmedicine 24(10):75–78

Murray B 1994 Fluid replacement: the American College of Sports Medicine position stand. Sports Science Exchange 7(3):1–10

National High Blood Pressure Education Program 1996 Update on the 1987 Task Force Report on High Blood Pressure in Children and Adolescents. Pediatrics 98(4):649–658

Nicola T L 1997 Tennis. In: Mellion M B, Walsh W M, Shelton G L (eds) The team physician's handbook, 2nd edn. Hanley and Belfus, Philadelphia, PA, p 816–827

Peggs J F, Reinhardt R W, O'Brien J M 1986 Proteinuria in adolescent sports physical examinations. Journal of Family Practice 22(1):80–81

Quality Standards Subcommittee of the American Academy of Neurology 1997 The management of concussion in sports (practice parameter). Neurology 48:581–585

Rifat S F, Ruffin M T IV, Gorenflo D W 1995 Disqualifying criteria in a preparticipation sports evaluation. Journal of Family Practice 41:42–50

Smith J, Laskowski E R 1998 The preparticipation physical examination: Mayo Clinic experience with 2739 examinations. Mayo Clinic Proceedings 73:419–429

Storms W 1999 Exercise induced asthma: diagnosis and treatment for the recreational athlete. Medicine and Science in Sports and Exercise 31(suppl):S33–S38

Taitel H F, Lippman J S 1995 Effects of oral contraceptives on bone mass: a review of the literature. Female Patient 20:30–47

Thomas S, Reading J, Shepard R J 1992 Revision of the Physical Activity Readiness Questionnaire (PAR-Q). Canadian Journal of Sport Science 17:338–345

Thompson R A, Sherman R T 1993 Helping athletes with eating disorders. Human Kinetics, Bloomington, p 45–65

26th Bethesda Conference 1994 Recommendations for determining eligibility for competition in athletes with cardiovascular abnormalities. Journal of the American College of Cardiology 24(4):845–899

Vinger P F 2000 A practical guide to sports eye protection. Physician and Sportsmedicine 28(6):49–67

Zheng Z, Menash G A, Croft J 2001 Sudden cardiac death in young people. Paper presented at American Heart Association's 41st Annual Conference on Cardiovascular Disease Epidemiology and Prevention 2001. Online. Available: http//www.cdc.gov/od/oc/media/pressrel/r010301.htm. 02 Aug 2001

12

Clinical outcomes in sport and exercise physical therapies

James J Irrgang

INTRODUCTION

Outcomes management is the process of data collection, analysis, and interpretation of the efficiency and effectiveness of patient treatment, with the intent of improving quality of care and lowering health care costs (Dobrzykowski 1997), and is an integral component of the process of care provided by physical therapists (American Physical Therapy Association 2001). Outcomes data can be used to make patient management decisions, assess clinician performance, assess organizational performance and to provide evidence for the effectiveness of interventions provided by physical therapists and other rehabilitation specialists. The validity of the inferences made from outcomes data is dependent on the outcome measures themselves and the circumstances under which the data was collected.

A framework for assessing outcomes of sports physical therapy is presented in Figure 12.1. Important outcomes of sports physical therapy include clinical outcomes, process outcomes, patient satisfaction, and costs (Irrgang 1996). Clinical outcomes are usually the primary interest when attempting to demonstrate effectiveness of rehabilitation and reflect the clinical status of the patient. Disablement schemes, such as the Nagi Disablement Model (Nagi 1991) and the recent International Classification of Functioning, Disability and Health (ICF) proposed by the World Health Organization (2001) provide a useful framework for identifying relevant clinical outcome measures and will be discussed in greater detail below.

Process outcomes represent the utilization of resources and include measures such as the duration of care, number of visits, and number and type of interventions provided to the patient. Evaluation of process outcomes can be used to answer the question 'Did the intervention provided to the patient match the patient's diagnosis (classification) based upon the findings of the examina-

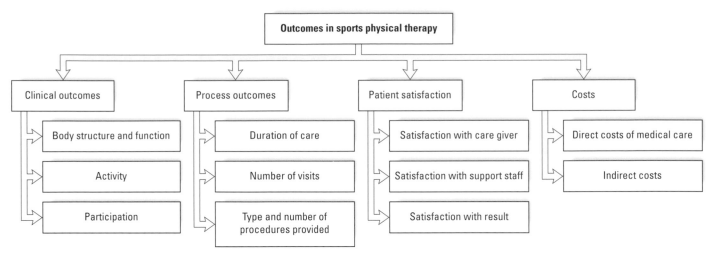

Figure 12.1   Framework for assessing outcomes of sport physical therapy.

tion?' Selection of the most appropriate intervention for a particular patient requires the ability of the clinician to examine, evaluate, and diagnose the condition in order to select the most appropriate form of intervention. Achieving optimal process outcomes requires application of the principles of evidence-based practice (see Ch. 1). Evaluation of process outcomes can be used to assess clinician and organizational performance. Expert clinicians would be expected to choose the most optimal interventions given a patient's diagnosis. Sources of process outcomes data may include scheduling and billing databases and patient records.

Patient satisfaction may also be an important outcome for sports physical therapy. Aspects of patient satisfaction include satisfaction with the caregiver, support staff, and the clinical result. Patient satisfaction is usually measured anonymously using a written survey. Domains of patient satisfaction that are commonly measured include satisfaction with access to care, physical environment, patient care, billing issues, and overall satisfaction with the experience during the episode of care. Patient satisfaction instruments commonly use Likert-type rating scales that reflect the degree of satisfaction or dissatisfaction on a 5 to 7 point scale. Most patient satisfaction instruments have been developed by the user and have not undergone psychometric testing; however, Goldstein et al (2000) developed and tested a 26-item patient satisfaction survey to measure the outcome of physical therapy intervention. Patient satisfaction data can be aggregated to compare the levels of patient satisfaction achieved by individual clinicians or facilities, and may be useful for quality improvement initiatives to identify opportunities for improvement. Development and use of a standardized patient satisfaction instrument to measure the outcomes of sports physical therapy would be valuable to permit benchmarking between providers and organizations.

The costs of care may also be an important outcome of sports physical therapy. The total costs to an individual due to an injury include the direct costs for medical care as well as indirect costs. The direct costs for medical care for an injury go beyond the costs for rehabilitation and include the costs for diagnosis, medical/surgical management, and any equipment that may be necessary to facilitate recovery. The indirect costs of an injury may be related to work time lost, decreased productivity, or cost related to assistance required to perform activities of daily living or household activities. When discussing costs, one must be careful to distinguish costs from charges. From the perspective of the provider of sports rehabilitation, costs are the costs of providing a service including costs related to manpower, space, equipment, and supplies. From the perspective of the patient or payer, costs are the charges for the services that are rendered. Charges are closely related to the services (i.e. the process outcomes) that are provided during the episode of care. Costs can be used to calculate the value of sports physical therapy, which is defined as the ratio of the benefit of care divided by the costs of providing that care. The aim of sports physical therapy should be to provide high value, which is of large benefit at a relatively low cost. An important question that needs to be answered is 'Does sports physical therapy reduce the total costs associated with an injury?' The answer to this question requires detailed analyses and the expertise of a medical economist.

While process outcomes, patient satisfaction, and cost are important outcomes of sports physical therapy to consider, the remainder of this chapter will focus on clinical outcomes. This will include a discussion of a framework for identifying important clinical outcomes, considerations for selecting outcome measures, and collecting, analyzing, and interpreting outcomes data.

FRAMEWORK FOR IDENTIFYING CLINICAL OUTCOMES

Disablement models provide a useful framework for identifying relevant clinical outcomes of sports physical therapy. Disablement models have been proposed by Nagi (Nagi 1965, 1991), the World Health Organization (1980, 2001), and the National Center for Medical Rehabilitation Research (National Institutes of Health 1992). Disablement is the impact of injury or illness on the function of specific body systems, on basic human performance, and on an individual's role in society (Jette 1994, Verbrugge & Jette 1994). While the terminology used by the models differs somewhat, each of the models defines disablement at the tissue/cellular level, organ/body system level, personal level, and societal level (Table 12.1).

The Nagi scheme is the model of disablement accepted in the Guide to Physical Therapist Practice (American Physical Therapy Association 2001). The Nagi disablement model includes active pathology, impairment, functional limitations, and disability. Active pathology may result from infection, trauma, metabolic imbalance, and/or degenerative disease conditions, and may interrupt or interfere with normal cellular processes. Active pathology includes the simultaneous efforts by the organism to regain homeostasis. Impairment is a loss or abnormality of an anatomical, mental, or emotional nature that results in loss or abnormal function at the organ or body system level. Functional limitations refer to the manifestations of pathology and impairment on the function of the individual as a whole and may include limitation in physical or psychological function. Disability refers to the function of the individual within society and is defined as 'the inability or limitation experienced by the individual in performing socially defined roles and tasks within the context of a sociocultural and physical environment' (Nagi 1991). Disability may affect family and other interpersonal interactions, work and other economic pursuits, education, recreation, and/or self-care.

Recently, the World Health Organization (WHO) introduced a revision of the International Classification of Impairments, Disabilities and Handicaps, the International Classification of Functioning, Disability and Health (ICF) (World Health Organization 2001). The ICF provides a unified and standard language and framework for the description of health and health-related states that can be used to measure health outcomes.

In the ICF, health domains are described from the body, individual, and societal perspectives in terms of (1) body structure and function and (2) activity and participation. In the ICF, functioning is an umbrella term that refers to all body functions, activities, and participation, while disability is the umbrella term for impairments, activity limitations, and participation restrictions. Body structures are the anatomical parts of the body, such as organs, limbs, and their components. Body function refers to the physiological functions of the body systems including psychological function. Impairments are problems in body structure or function. Activity is the execution of a task or action by an individual, while participation is involvement in life situations. Activity limitations are difficulties an individual may have in executing activities, and participation restrictions are problems an individual may experience in involvement in life situations. The ICF provides a detailed description of body structure and function, activity and participation. For example, the activity and participation domain includes learning and applying knowledge, general tasks and demands, communication, mobility, self-care, domestic life, interpersonal interactions and relationships, major life areas, and community, social and civic life.

The descriptions of body structure and function, activity and participation provided by the ICF can be used to identify important clinical outcomes of sports physical therapy. To illustrate this, consider an athlete with an acute knee sprain. Impairment of body structure may include disruption of the anterior cruciate ligament (ACL) or injury to the meniscus, articular cartilage, or subchondral bone. Clinical outcome measures to evaluate body structure may include radiographs and magnetic resonance imaging. Impairment of body function may include limited range of motion, weakness, or laxity of the knee. Measures of clinical outcome at the level of impairment of body function for this individual may include goniometry to measure the range of knee motion, isometric or isokinetic testing to measure quadriceps performance, or use of the KT-1000

Table 12.1 Comparison of disablement schemes

System	Tissue/cellular level	Organ/system level	Personal level	Societal level
Nagi	Active pathology	Impairment	Functional limitation	Disability
ICIHD	Disease	Impairment	Disability	Handicap
NCRMM	Pathophysiology	Impairment	Disability	Societal limitation
ICF	Impairment of body structure and function	Impairment of body structure and function	Active restriction	Participation restriction

(MedMetric, San Diego, CA) to measure anterior tibial laxity. Activity limitations experienced by this individual may include difficulty walking, climbing stairs, running, jumping, and landing or cutting and pivoting. The resulting participation restrictions may include the inability to participate in sports such as football, soccer, or basketball. Clinical outcome in terms of activity and participation can be measured by observing and rating the performance of the individual while executing a variety of activities, or by the use of standardized self-reports of activity limitations and participation restrictions. In summary, clinical outcome measures of body structure and function may include the results of diagnostic studies such as laboratory tests and imaging studies, as well as the findings from clinical examination of the involved structure or region. Clinical outcome measures of activity and participation may include observation of the individual or use of standardized self-reports of activity limitations and participation restrictions.

HEALTH-RELATED QUALITY OF LIFE

Health-related quality of life is an individual's perception of his or her health. Broadly, health-related quality of life encompasses an individual's perception of his or her physical, emotional, and social function. Health-related quality of life deals with what people perceive their health condition to be and the consequences of it; hence, it is the individual's subjective sense of wellbeing (World Health Organization 2001). Because health-related quality of life encompasses an individual's physical, emotional, and social function, it overlaps with the activity and participation domains of the ICF. As such, health-related quality of life measures can be used to measure the individual's perception of his or her activity and participation.

Several health-related quality of life measures have been developed. These can be classified as general or specific measures of health-related quality of life. General measures of health-related quality of life are designed to be applicable across a number of disease processes and interventions, and across demographic and cultural subgroups (McSweeney & Creer 1995). Health-related quality of life instruments are designed to give a comprehensive and general overview of health-related quality of life. General health-related quality of life measures are usually multidimensional and scores can be obtained for each dimension, or they can be combined to provide an overall measure. The most widely known and accepted general measure of health-related quality of life is the Medical Outcomes Study Short Form – 36 (McHorney et al 1993, McHorney et al 1994, Ware & Sherbourne 1992).

General measures of health-related quality of life permit comparisons across populations with different health conditions (Guyatt et al 1993, McSweeny & Creer 1995) and are more likely to detect unexpected effects of intervention (Kessler & Mroczek 1995, McSweeney & Creer 1995). An important limitation of general health-related quality of life measures is that they tend to be less responsive than specific measures of health-related quality of life, to changes in health status (Guyatt et al 1993). Therefore, use of general health-related quality of life measures might make it more difficult to detect the effects of an intervention for a specific condition. General measures of health-related quality of life are susceptible to ceiling effects. The presence of ceiling effects limits the ability to detect the effects of intervention, especially when used by young, healthy, high-level functioning individuals such as athletes. Because general measures of health-related quality of life measure a broad range of health including emotional function, the content may appear less relevant to patients and clinicians. Finally, general measures of health-related quality of life tend to be longer and more difficult to score.

Specific health-related quality of life measures are designed to focus on aspects of health that are specific to the primary condition or population of interest, with the intent of creating a more responsive measure (Guyatt et al 1993). Specific measures of health-related quality of life have been developed for specific diseases (e.g. osteoarthritis of the knee), specific populations of patients (e.g. the frail elderly), specific functions (e.g. physical function) or for a particular impairment (e.g. pain) (Guyatt et al 1993).

Specific measures of health-related quality of life are responsive to small changes and are easy to administer and interpret (McSweeney & Creer 1995). The increased responsiveness of specific measures of health-related quality of life stems from the fact that they include only those important aspects of health-related quality of life that are relevant to the condition or population being studied (Guyatt et al 1993). Specific health-related quality of life measures usually relate closely to areas commonly assessed by clinicians, therefore they are more likely to be accepted by clinicians for routine use. Since specific health-related quality of life measures relate more closely to a particular condition, they are also more likely to be accepted by patients. Disadvantages of specific measures of health-related quality of life are that they do not measure all aspects of health status and they do not allow for comparisons between different disease states and/or populations.

Specific health-related quality of life measures include disease-specific, region-specific, and patient-specific measures. Disease-specific measures of health-related quality of life are developed for a particular injury or illness. The content of disease-specific, health-related quality of life measures includes the symptoms, activity limitations, and participation restrictions commonly experienced by individuals with the injury or illness for which the instrument was developed. Examples of disease-specific health-related quality of life measures include the Lysholm Knee Score (Tegner & Lysholm 1985), the Cincinnati Knee Rating System (Noyes et al 1984, Barber-Westin et al 1999), and the Quality of Life Assessment in Anterior Cruciate Ligament Deficiency (Mohtadi 1998) for knee ligament injuries. Also, there is the Western Ontario and McMaster Universities Osteoarthritis Index (WOMAC) (Bellamy et al 1988) for osteoarthritis of the knee and hip, and the Western Ontario Shoulder Instability Index (Kirkley et al 1998) for shoulder instability.

Region-specific, health-related quality of life measures have been developed to determine the effects of a variety of pathologies and impairments affecting a particular region. The content of region-specific measures of health-related quality of life reflects the symptoms, activity limitations, and participation restrictions commonly experienced by individuals with impairment of the particular region for which the instrument was developed. Examples of region-specific measures of health-related quality of life include the following:

- Disabilities of the Arm Shoulder and Hand Index (DASH) (Beaton et al 2001a) for the upper extremity
- American Shoulder and Elbow Surgeons Patient Self-Evaluation Form (Richards et al 1994) for the shoulder
- Simple Shoulder Test (Lippitt et al 1993) for the shoulder
- Oswestry Low Back Pain Disability Questionnaire (Fairbank et al 1980) for the lumbar spine
- Quebec Back Pain Disability Scale (Kopek et al 1995) for the lumbar spine
- Lower Extremity Function Scale (Binkley et al 1999) for the lower extremity
- Knee Outcome Survey (Irrgang et al 1998) for the knee
- International Knee Documentation Committee Subjective Knee Form (Irrgang et al 2001) for the knee.

Patient-specific measures of health-related quality of life are defined by the patient. Patients are requested to provide a list of three to five relevant activities that they are either unable to do or have difficulty doing as a result of their problem, and then provide a rating of the difficulty they have doing each activity on an 11-point scale that ranges from 'unable to do' to 'able to do at preinjury level' (Stratford et al 1995, Westaway et al 1998). Patient-specific measures have been tested for the low back (Stratford et al 1995), knee (Chatman et al 1997), and cervical spine (Westaway et al 1998). Patient-specific measures of health-related quality of life are applicable to a large number of clinical conditions, efficient and easy to administer and record, and have been found to have adequate psychometric properties. While patient-specific measures of health-related quality of life are responsive to within subject change, between subjects comparisons are not possible because the content of each is determined by each patient.

CLINICAL OUTCOMES THAT SHOULD BE MEASURED

The most important clinical outcome of rehabilitation for athletes is whether they can return to their prior level of activity and participation with the same intensity, frequency, duration, and skill without symptoms and risk of reinjury. Furthermore, this outcome should be achieved in the shortest period of time possible. While on the surface this outcome appears easy to determine, it is difficult to quantify due to the varying demands of sports and levels of participation. Thus, function (i.e. the activity and participation) of the athlete is an important clinical outcome of sports physical therapy.

Using the ICF model of functioning and disability, the range of clinical outcome measures includes measures of body structure and function, activity, and participation. Whyte (1994) suggested that the level of outcome measurement should be at or higher than the level of intervention. For example, the aim of ACL reconstruction is to restore stability of the ACL deficient knee. Thus an appropriate clinical outcome measure of ACL reconstruction is anterior laxity of the knee. One would expect that if surgery was successful, it would reduce anterior tibial translation as measured with the KT-1000. Also, restoring stability of the knee should allow the athlete to return to running, jumping and landing, cutting and pivoting, and ultimately to sports such as football, soccer, or basketball. Thus, potential clinical outcome measures following ACL reconstruction include measurement at the levels of body structure and function, activity, and participation.

As another example, consider an athlete with a grade II posterior cruciate ligament injury with 6 to 10 mm of increased posterior tibial translation compared to the non-involved knee. Non-operative management for this individual may include quadriceps strengthening and a functional exercise progression. In this case, measurement of laxity would not be an appropriate outcome measure for this intervention because the intervention would not be expected to reduce posterior tibial translation. Appropriate clinical outcome measures for this case include strength testing of the quadriceps as well as the ability of the athlete to return to sports activities and participation. Therefore, clinical outcome measures should be thoughtfully selected and be appropriate for the intervention that was provided.

In the past it was believed that there was a direct link between impairment, functional limitations, and disability, however, there is a growing body of literature to the contrary. For example, Snyder-Mackler et al (1997) found no relationship between laxity measured with the KT-1000 and function and disability measured with the Knee Outcome Survey in ACL deficient copers and non-copers. Pantano et al (2001) obtained similar results 3–5 years after ACL reconstruction. Laxity, range of motion, and isokinetic quadriceps and hamstring strength were not significantly related to function and disability as measured with the Knee Outcome Survey. Thus, at least at the knee, there does not appear to be a direct relationship between impairment of body structure and function and the resulting activity limitations and participation restrictions.

This lack of a direct relationship between impairment of body structure and function and activity and participation limitations is inherent in the ICF model (Fig. 12.2). In this model, disability is the outcome of a complex interaction between the individual's health condition and contextual factors (World Health Organization 2001). Contextual factors include environmental and personal factors. Environmental factors are the make up of the physical, social, and attitudinal environment in which individuals live and conduct their lives. Personal factors include gender, race, age, other health conditions, fitness, lifestyle, habits, upbringing, coping styles, social background, education, profession, past and current experiences, overall behavior pattern and character style, individual psychological assets, and other characteristics, all or any of which may play a role in disability (World Health Organization 2001). Research is needed to explore these complex interactions between health conditions and contextual factors and the resulting disability.

The lack of a direct relationship between impairment of body structure and function and the resulting disability

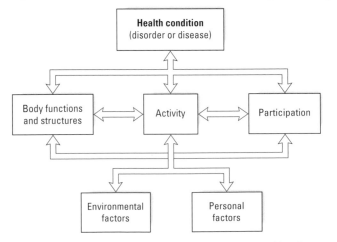

Figure 12.2 Model of functioning and disability proposed by the World Health Organization in the International Classification of Functioning Disability and Health. (Reproduced with permission from ICF – International Classification of Functional Disability and Health-2, World Health Organization 2001.)

(i.e. activity limitations and participation restrictions) implies that measures of impairment should not be combined with measures of disability into a single composite score. Rather, reports of clinical outcome should include separate summaries of relevant measures of impairment of body structure and function that are appropriate for the interventions that were provided and valid measures of disability. Furthermore, because the relationship between impairment and the resulting activity limitations and participation restrictions is not direct, and because activity limitations and participation restrictions are of the utmost concern to the athlete, the primary clinical outcome should be measures of activity limitation and participation restriction. Activity limitation and participation restriction may be measured either through direct observation of performance or by general or specific measures of health-related quality of life.

SELECTION OF CLINICAL OUTCOME MEASURES

When selecting clinical outcome measures, one must consider the purpose for which the information will be used as well as practical and psychometric considerations of the instrument. Kirshner & Guyatt (1985) classified health indices according to their purpose as discriminative, predictive, or evaluative measures of health. Discriminative health measures are those that distinguish individuals or groups of individuals on an underlying dimension when no external criterion is available for validating the measure. Predictive health indices are those which attempt to classify individuals into a set of predefined categories when an external criterion measure exists concurrently or in the future to determine if the individual has been correctly classified. Evaluative health indices are those that have been developed to measure change within an individual or of a group over time on the dimension of interest. To demonstrate the effects of sports physical therapy, one is interested in measuring change in body structure and function, activity, and participation over time. Thus, demonstration of clinical outcomes requires the use of evaluative health indices.

Practical considerations for selection of clinical outcome measures include ease of use, acceptance, and costs (McSweeney & Creer 1995). Self-administered health-related quality of life measures are attractive clinical outcome measures because they require minimal resources for administration, however, the reading level must be appropriate for the intended audience. Ease of use of self-administered health-related quality of life measures is determined by the time required for administration and scoring, as well as the effort required to interpret and use the data. Costs for administrating and scoring a measure of health-related quality of life will greatly influence its acceptance in clinical practice and research. Clinical outcome measures that require special expertise or equipment for administration, scoring, and interpretation are likely to be more costly and less readily accepted than self-administered health-related quality of life measures that can be scored manually (McSweeney & Creer 1995).

PSYCHOMETRIC CONSIDERATIONS FOR SELECTION OF A CLINICAL OUTCOME MEASURE

A number of authors have discussed psychometric considerations for selecting a clinical outcome measure (Guyatt et al 1993, Hoffman et al 1995, Kessler & Mroczek 1995, Kirshner & Guyatt 1985, Lohr et al 1996, McSweeney & Creer 1995, Testa & Nackley 1994, Testa & Simonson 1995). Important psychometric considerations when selecting an evaluative clinical outcome measure include reliability, validity, and responsiveness. According to contemporary validity theory, in which validity is defined as 'the degree to which empirical evidence and theoretical rationales support the adequacy and appropriateness of the inferences and actions based on the tests scores' (Messick 1989), these psychometric considerations all fall within the realm of validity. Knowledge of the psychometric characteristics of a clinical outcome measure allows one to interpret the appropriateness and usefulness of the inferences and actions that are based on the scores from the measure. Furthermore, the nature of the evidence that is required to interpret the appropriateness and usefulness of scores from a particular clinical outcome measure is dependent on the intended purpose and/or use of the measure (Kirshner & Guyatt 1985). When selecting a clinical outcome measure, one must consider the psychometric evidence to support the validity of the inferences that will be made and the actions that will be taken based upon the clinical outcome measure.

Validity evidence to support use and interpretation of a clinical outcome instrument to measure change should include evidence that: the items are all related to the construct being measured (i.e. the items are unidimensional), the score is related to other measures of the construct and not unduly related to other constructs (i.e. the score demonstrates convergent and divergent evidence of validity), the score remains stable when the underlying condition measured by the outcome instrument remains stable (i.e. the score demonstrates test re-test reliability), and the score changes with improvement or deterioration of the condition measured

by the instrument (i.e. the score is responsive). Among these, evidence for reliability and responsiveness is most important and will be discussed in greater detail below.

Reliability

Reliability of a clinical outcome measure implies consistency of measurement. Measures of reliability include internal consistency and test re-test reliability. Internal consistency is applicable to outcome measures such as measures of health-related quality of life that consist of multiple items. Internal consistency is the degree to which all items on the scale consistently measure the underlying condition and is concerned with measurement errors related to the sampling of items that are included on the instrument (Crocker & Algina 1986). Internal consistency is most commonly estimated with coefficient alpha.

Test re-test reliability is the degree to which scores remain stable when there is no change in the underlying construct that is being measured. Test re-test reliability for a clinical outcome measure is estimated by measuring individuals two or more times over a period of time when the individual's condition is expected to remain stable. The amount of time between repeat measurements is an important issue when determining test re-test reliability. The length of time should not be so short that memory or recall artificially inflates the test re-test reliability estimate. Conversely, the length of time between repeat administrations of the clinical outcome measure should not be too long to avoid change in the condition that is being measured. In general, the length of time between repeat administrations of the clinical outcome measure should be relatively short (e.g. 1–3 days) when the condition being measured is expected to change rapidly (e.g. patients within the first 4 weeks after ACL reconstruction). The time between repeat administrations of the clinical outcome measure should be longer (e.g. 4 weeks or more) when the condition is not expected to change (e.g. individuals who are 3 to 5 years status post ACL reconstruction). Given this, it is evident that test re-test reliability should not be considered a property of the instrument itself, but rather the degree of consistency of measurement when applied to certain populations under particular measurement conditions (Streiner & Norman 1995).

The type of reliability coefficient used to estimate test re-test reliability is dependent on the nature of the data. Percent agreement and Cohen's kappa statistic, which is the agreement above chance agreement, are recommended for nominal or ordinal level data, while the intraclass correlation coefficient (Shrout & Fleiss 1979) is recommended for interval or ratio level data. Because test re-test reliability is concerned not only with the relative standing of individuals on repeated measurement, but also the degree to which the repeated measurement yields the same score, the intraclass correlation coefficient is recommended over the Pearson correlation coefficient when estimating test re-test reliability for continuous data.

The standard error of measurement can be used to interpret estimates of internal consistency and test re-test reliability. The standard error of measurement (SEM) is defined as:

$$SEM = \sigma \sqrt{1 - r}$$

where σ is the standard deviation of the scores and r is the reliability coefficient. When coefficient alpha is used to determine the standard error of measurement, the interpretation should be limited to the error associated with a measure at a single point in time. If one is concerned with error over repeated measurements, the intraclass correlation coefficient should be used to determine the standard error of measurement. The standard error of measurement can be used to determine a confidence interval that can facilitate interpretation of a score. For example, coefficient alpha for the Activities of Daily Living Scale of the Knee Outcome Survey was found to be 0.92 in a sample of 397 patients presenting for outpatient physical therapy with a variety of knee impairments and the corresponding standard error of measurement was approximately 6 points on the Activities of Daily Living Scale (Irrgang et al 1998). Thus the 95% confidence interval (i.e. ±1.96 SEM) for an observed score of 70 ranges from 58 to 82. This means that if an individual has a true score of 70, 95% of the time the individual would have an observed score between 58 and 82.

When one is concerned about the magnitude of the expected difference between scores on re-testing, an intraclass correlation coefficient should be used to calculate the SEM. Furthermore, the standard error of measurement should be multiplied by the $\sqrt{2}$ to take into account that there is error associated with both the first and second scores (Streiner & Norman 1995). To illustrate this, consider test re-test reliability of the International Knee Documentation Committee Subjective Knee Score, which was found to be 0.94 when estimated over an average interval of 50 days in 33 individuals who were participating in long-term outcome studies following ACL reconstruction, meniscal replacement, or proximal and distal realignment of the knee extensor mechanism (Irrgang et al 2001). The standard deviation of the scores for this data was 18. Given this, the 95% confidence interval of the expected difference between the scores was ±12.2 points. Thus, a change in the score over a 4-week interval greater than 12.2 points represents a true change beyond measurement error, while a change less

than 12.2 points may occur due to chance alone because of measurement error at each point in time. The expected difference between scores due to error associated with re-testing is called the minimal detectable change and is interpreted as the amount of change that needs to be observed before it can be considered beyond the bounds of measurement error for an instrument in a particular application (Beaton 2000).

Responsiveness

Responsiveness is the degree to which a clinical outcome score changes as the underlying condition that is measured by the scale changes. A clinical outcome measure that is responsive will reflect improvement as an individual's condition improves and deterioration as the individual's condition worsens. Demonstration of responsiveness for a clinical outcome measure requires evidence that the measure accurately detects change when change has occurred. Studies to demonstrate responsiveness of a clinical outcome measure should link the amount of change in the outcome score to a construct of change. The construct of change is the way that was used to demonstrate that change has in fact occurred (Beaton 2000). Examples of a construct for change include change from before to after treatment of a known efficacy or change in those deemed to be better or worse, based on an external marker of change (Beaton 2000, Stratford et al 1996).

Factors that will affect the magnitude of change for a given instrument include the patient group under study, the type of treatment being studied, timing of the data collection, and the construct for change (Beaton 2000). For example, one would expect greater change over a similar time frame for those with an acute condition compared to those that have a chronic condition. The patient group, type of treatment, and timing of data collection must be comparable before the results of a responsiveness study can be applied to a particular clinical setting or used to judge the meaningfulness of a change score (Beaton 2000). The construct for change must also be considered when interpreting the results of a responsiveness study. The construct of change is defined by the answers to: (1) Who is the focus of the analysis?; (2) Which scores are being compared?; and (3) What kind of change or difference is being examined? (Beaton 2000, Beaton et al 2001b).

The focus of the analysis can be at the group or individual level. When the focus of the analysis is at the group level, summary statistics, such as the mean, standard deviation, median, and range or combinations of these statistics in the form of an effect size, standardized response mean or Guyatt's responsiveness index are reported for the entire group or the subgroup of individuals who improved (Beaton 2000). While these group statistics provide useful information about what should be expected for a group of individuals, they do not provide meaningful information that can be used to interpret change of a particular individual.

When the focus of analysis is at the individual level, receiver operating characteristic curves are used to determine the cutoff value for the change score that has the highest sensitivity and specificity for change (Beaton 2000). Sensitivity of change is the proportion of subjects that have improved according to a criterion of change that have a change score above the cutoff point. Specificity of change is the proportion of subjects that have not improved according to a criterion measure of change that has a change score below the cutoff point (Deyo & Centor 1986). When the focus of the analysis is at the individual level, the challenge is to select the cutoff point in the change score that best discriminates between those that have improved and those that have not improved. The results of a responsiveness study, where the focus of analysis has been at the individual level, can be used to determine if a particular individual has improved or not, given the similarities of other aspects of the responsiveness study (e.g. patient group, type of treatment, and timing of data collection) (Beaton 2000).

The construct of change for a responsiveness study is also defined by the scores that are being compared (Beaton 2000). Possibilities include comparison of scores within subjects, between subjects, or between group differences within subject change. A within-subjects comparison of scores is made over time by comparing before and after scores within an individual or group of individuals. A between-subjects comparison entails a comparison of health states between persons at a single point in time. Differences in the scores between pairs of subjects, one of whom states he or she is healthier than the other, can be used to determine minimally clinically important differences, however, it is doubtful that this construct for change is comparable to constructs that link responsiveness to longitudinal change over time (Beaton et al 2001b). A between-groups difference of within-subject change compares the within-group change over time between two or more groups. This comparison is concerned with the amount of change in one group over time compared to the amount of change over the same period of time in another group. An example of this is a clinical trial, in which the within-subject change in the experimental group is compared to the within-subject change in the control group. Demonstration of responsiveness would entail demonstrating that the within-subject change is greater in the experimental group than in the control group. In essence, this comparison is a combination of a within-subjects and between-subjects comparison.

The third determinant of the construct for change is what kind of change is being quantified in the study to provide evidence for responsiveness. The change that is being quantified can include: (1) change that is considered greater than measurement error; (2) change that is observed over time before and after a treatment; (3) change in those that have improved according to a criterion measure of change; or (4) change in those that have had a major improvement according to a criterion measure of change (Beaton 2000, Beaton et al 2001b).

The minimal detectable change is the amount of change that is considered to be greater than measurement error (Christensen & Mendoza 1986). It is calculated as the confidence interval for the standard error of measurement for the expected difference between before and after scores (see Reliability section above). Calculation of the standard error of measurement to determine the minimum detectable change requires the use of the test re-test reliability coefficient and multiplication by the $\sqrt{2}$ to correct for error associated with measurements made at two points in time. The minimum detectable change can be considered to be the lowest change score that can be confidently considered above measurement error. It provides an anchor for interpretation of a change score because only when a change score exceeds the minimum detectable change can the clinician be confident that the change score represents true change of the individual and not measurement error (Beaton 2000).

Observed change is the change that occurs in an individual before and after a treatment or over a period of time that is expected to result in improvement for most individuals (Beaton 2000, Beaton et al 2001b). No criterion measure of change is used to determine if individuals have truly changed. This type of change assumes that with treatment or the passage of time, most subjects will improve and the analysis is performed on all subjects being studied. The observed change provides information on how much change should be expected for individuals receiving a particular treatment or being observed for a similar period of time.

Estimated change utilizes a criterion measure of change to determine whether a change has occurred (Beaton 2000, Beaton et al 2001b). The criterion measure of change is used to separate a group of individuals into those that have improved and those that have not improved. Many different criterion measures of change have been proposed from different perspectives including the patient, clinician, payer, or society (Beaton 2000). The analysis involves contrasting the change score between those that have improved and those that have not improved. The estimated change provides an estimate of the magnitude of the change score in individuals who improve, and because a criterion measure of change is used, it provides an opportunity to determine the best change score to use as a threshold for improvement in similar individuals.

Important change is similar to estimated change; however, it implies that not only has changed occurred, but the change that has occurred is important to the patient, clinician, payer, or society (Beaton 2000, Beaton et al 2001b). Important change is often referred to as the minimum clinically important change. It is determined by using a criterion measure that determines that important change has occurred.

The above taxonomy developed by Beaton (Beaton 2000, Beaton et al 2001b) can be used when judging the usefulness of a clinical outcome to evaluate change over time. When selecting an outcome instrument to measure change, one should review the evidence to support its reliability and validity for a particular application.

Ideally, the evidence to support use of a clinical outcome measure should be determined under conditions that are similar to those under which the measure will be utilized. This requires careful analysis to determine if the patient group, type of treatment, timing of data collection, and construct of change that were used in the study to provide evidence for the usefulness of the clinical outcome measure matches the patient group, type of treatment, timing of data collection, and construct for change of the application for which the instrument will be used. To facilitate this, Beaton (2000) has provided guidelines for evaluating evidence to support the use and interpretation of a clinical outcome instrument to measure change (see Box 12.1).

Box 12.1 Guidelines for evaluating evidence to support use and interpretation of a clinical outcome instrument to measure change (reproduced with permission from Beaton D E 2000 Understanding the relevance of measured change through studies of responsiveness. Spine 25(24):3192–3199)

First, be clear about the type of information you need to know about. Define your patient group and type of change you need to understand. Second, appraise whether this study offers you the right kind of information by asking these questions:

1. Are the patients similar enough to my own?
   Yes
   No

2. Are they looking at a similar type of treatment?
   Yes
   No
   Time between treatment _____

3. What category of responsiveness is being studied?
   A. Who is the focus of the analysis and the results presented? Individuals or groups of patients?
      group level
      individual level
   B. Which data are being contrasted?
      over time (same patients, over time)
      one point in time (between persons)
      hybrid (between group differences of within person change)
   C. What type of change is being quantified?
      minimum change detectable given measurement error
      observed change in a given population
      observed change in those deemed to have changed (estimated change) – according to:
         patient
         clinician/researcher
         payer
         society
      observed change in those deemed to have had an important change – according to:
         patient
         clinician/researcher
         payer
         society

COLLECTING, ANALYZING AND INTERPRETING CLINICAL OUTCOME MEASURES

Outcomes management requires collection, analysis, and interpretation of data to improve the quality of care that is provided and to reduce health care costs. The ultimate aim of an outcomes management system should be to increase value, which is defined as the ratio of quality to costs. High value is achieved by maximizing improvements in quality while minimizing costs. Outcomes data can be used to make patient management decisions, and to provide evidence for the effectiveness of interventions provided by physical therapists and other rehabilitation specialists. When utilized as part of a quality improvement initiative, outcomes data can be used to assess performance of individual clinicians as well as of organizations as a whole. In addition to the quality of the outcome measures, validity of the inferences made from outcomes data is dependent on the circumstances under which the data was collected and interpreted.

COLLECTION OF OUTCOMES DATA

To minimize selection bias, outcomes data should be collected from all individuals with the condition of interest. If this is not possible, then outcomes data should be collected from a representative random sample of individuals. Selection bias in outcomes data can arise when the sample is not representative of the population of individuals that are of interest to the clinician. For example, excluding individuals from the analysis with incomplete follow-up data due to individuals terminating treatment before the course of care is complete may result in an overly favorable outcome. While it is acknowledged that collection of outcomes data from all individuals with the condition of interest or collection of data from a truly random sample may not be possible, attempts should be made to detect bias by determining if the sample of individuals for whom outcomes data is complete is different at the start of care from the sample of individuals with incomplete outcomes data. This requires consistent collection of outcomes data from all individuals at the start of care.

An important concept in the revised ICF classification system is that contextual factors interact with an individual's health condition to determine the individual's level of functioning (i.e. the individual's activity and participation) (World Health Organization 2001). Contextual factors include both personal and environmental factors. Personal factors include features of the individual that are not part of a health condition such as gender, race, other health conditions, fitness, lifestyle habits, upbringing, coping styles, social background, education, profession, past and current life experiences, character, and psychological status (World Health Organization 2001). Environmental factors include the individual's immediate environment, such as the home, workplace, or school, as well as services and systems in the community that can have an impact on the functioning of the individual. Because an individual's level of function and disability are the result of an interaction between the individual's health condition with personal and environmental contextual factors, attempts to describe the clinical outcome of care provided by the physical therapist should include collection of information that may mediate or modify the clinical outcome. Thus, an outcomes data collection system should attempt to capture personal and environmental factors that may impact on clinical outcome.

To make valid inferences, the outcomes data collection system should make use of valid (as broadly defined above) clinical outcome measures. When selecting an outcome measure, use of a 'common currency' will facilitate the ability to compare results between organizations as well as to data in the literature for benchmarking purposes. Linking the outcomes data collection system to scheduling and billing systems will facilitate incorporation of process and cost outcomes. Procedures should be established to facilitate systematic collection of outcomes data to allow for assessment of the individual over time. These procedures should minimize the burden on staff and patients required to collect the outcomes data. The use of computer technology can greatly facilitate this process.

Components of a comprehensive outcomes data collection system should include relevant clinical outcome measures. This should include both general and specific health-related quality of life measures to quantify disability in terms of activity limitations and participation restrictions. A general measure of health-related quality of life, such as the SF-36, should be included to provide a comprehensive assessment of health, including physical, emotional, and social functioning. Additionally, a general measure of health-related quality of life permits comparisons across populations with different health conditions (Guyatt et al 1993, McSweeney & Creer 1995) and is more likely to detect unexpected effects of intervention (Kessler & Mroczek 1995, McSweeny & Creer 1995). A specific measure of health status, such as the DASH for conditions affecting the upper extremity or the Oswestry Low Back Disability Questionnaire for conditions affecting the low back, should be included to enhance detecting the effects of intervention on an individual's level of function and disability.

As interventions provided by physical therapists are often directed at impaired body structure and function, a comprehensive outcomes data collection system may also include relevant measures of impairment. Inclusion of impairment measures will enable clinicians to determine if interventions directed at impairments were effective at alleviating the impairment and will allow for exploration of relationships between impairment, activity limitations, and participation restrictions. However, as noted above, because the relationship between impairment and disability is not direct, and as disability is of the utmost concern to the athlete, measures of impairment should not be the only clinical outcome measure included in the outcomes database.

To account for factors that may mediate or modify clinical outcome, contextual factors including characteristics of the individual as well as characteristics of the environment in which the individual must function should be included in a comprehensive outcomes data collection system. Examples of personal factors that may be included are gender, age, level of education, and comorbidities. Environmental factors that may be included in an outcomes data collection system are the nature and demands imposed by work or the type of sports activities in which the individual is able to participate. To describe process outcomes, the outcomes data collection system should include information regarding the duration of care, number of visits, and type of procedures provided to the individual. This information may be obtained from the scheduling and/or billing systems.

Systematic collection of outcomes data requires the development of forms that are either completed by the patient or clinician. These forms should be user-friendly and utilize a type font size that is easy to read. The forms should include clear instructions to facilitate accurate completion and to minimize the burden of administration. To minimize the burden of completing the form, the form should maximize the use of check boxes. The form should be organized to facilitate scoring and entry of data into a computerized database. Software programs, such as Teleforms (Cardiff Software Inc., San Marcus, CA) can be used to develop forms that can be scanned or faxed into a computerized database. Once in the database, routines can be written to automatically score the data and to store it for analysis at a later time. An alternative to the use of paper forms to collect outcomes data is the use of computers with user-friendly interfaces. Advances in computer technology including the use of touch screens, wireless networks, and the internet, have opened new avenues for collection of outcomes data.

Outcomes data should be collected at the initiation of care, at regular intervals during the course of care, and at the conclusion of care. Data that should be collected at the initiation of care include general and specific measures of health-related quality of life, as well as the personal and environmental factors that may mediate or moderate the outcome of care. To measure the response to intervention during the course of care, specific measures of health-related quality of life should be collected on a regular basis (e.g. every 1–2 weeks) during the course of care. Collection of specific measures of health-related quality of life at regular intervals during the course of care will also ensure that some follow-up outcomes data is available for analysis should an individual terminate care before the episode of care is completed. At the conclusion of care, general and specific measures of health-related quality of life, as well as a measure of patient satisfaction, should be collected. To assess the lasting effects of intervention after the course of care is completed, efforts should be made to collect follow-up data, including general and specific measures of health-related quality of life. Alternatives to having an individual return to the clinic to collect this data include the use of telephone or mailed surveys that may include the use of electronic mail and the world wide web.

ANALYZING AND INTERPRETING CLINICAL OUTCOMES DATA

Clinical outcomes data can be analyzed and interpreted at either the individual or group level. At the individual level, clinical outcomes data can be used to determine if a particular individual is better, worse, or unchanged as a result of intervention. This entails calculation of a change score, which is the difference in the clinical outcome measure from initiation of care to follow-up. To determine if the individual is better, worse, or unchanged, the change score can be compared to either the minimum detectable change or minimal clinically important difference. If the change score exceeds the minimal detectable change, then one can be confident that the amount of change as measured by the clinical outcome instrument exceeds the bounds of measurement error for the instrument in a particular application. If the change

score exceeds the minimal clinically important difference, then we can be confident that the change, as measured by the clinical outcome instrument, exceeds the amount of change described by others as being an important amount of change. The validity of the decisions made at the individual level is dependent on how well the evidence for interpretation of the change score matches the condition under which the decision is applied. As discussed in the above section on responsiveness, application of evidence supporting responsiveness of a clinical outcome measure should consider the degree to which the patient group, type of treatment, timing of data collection and construct for change used to provide evidence for responsiveness of the clinical outcome measure matches the patient group, type of treatment, timing of data collection and construct for change under which the evidence will be applied.

Measures of central tendency and dispersion are used to summarize data at the group level. Measures of central tendency include the mean, median, and mode. The mean is the average score for the group. The median is the middle score or the score at the 50th percentile. The most frequent score is the mode. When data are skewed, such as when there are a few extreme scores, the median will provide a better representation of the entire group than will the mean. This is because the few extreme scores affect the mean, while the median will not be affected as much.

Measures of dispersion include the range, standard deviation, and variance. The range is the distance between the highest and lowest score for the entire group. The standard deviation is the square root of the variance. The variance is equal to the average squared distance between each individual score and the group average as given by the following formula:

$$\sigma^2 = \frac{\sum_{i=1}^{n}(x_i - \bar{x})^2}{n}$$

In this formula σ^2 is the variance, x_i is the score of the ith individual from 1 to n, $\bar{x}$ is the group average and n is the number of individuals in the sample. Scores that are spread over a larger range will have a larger variance and standard deviation, while scores that are very closely distributed to the group mean will have a smaller variance and standard deviation.

A number of indices have been developed to summarize change in the clinical outcome measure over time. These include a change score, effect size, standardized response mean, and Guyatt's responsiveness index. A complete description and use of these statistics can be found in Stratford et al (1996), however, the effect size and standardized response mean deserve additional comment. The effect size (ES) is calculated as:

$$ES = \frac{\text{Average change}}{\text{Standard deviation of initial scores}}$$

and the standardized response mean (SRM) is calculated as:

$$SRM = \frac{\text{Average change}}{\text{Standard deviation of change scores}}$$

Both the ES and SRM relate the average change in the clinical outcome score from the initial to follow-up measure to the variability of the scores. The ES relates the average change to the variability of the initial measures, while the SRM relates the average change to the variability of the change scores. The resulting statistics interpret the magnitude of change in terms of the variability of the scores. For example, an ES of 0.5 is interpreted to mean that the average change from the initial to follow-up measure was equal to one-half of a standard deviation of the initial scores. Cohen (1969) provides guidelines for interpreting the ES: an ES greater than or equal to 0.8 is considered large, 0.5 is considered medium, and 0.2 is considered small.

Use of an ES to describe clinical outcomes data is described in Figure 12.3. This figure is a radar graph that displays the ES over the episode of care for patients with a variety of knee impairments. Each axis of the graph represents the ES for one of the 8 scales of the SF-36. Graphs such as this can be used to benchmark (i.e. compare) the performance of an individual or organization against data from an external organization. For example, in Figure 12.3, the effect of physical therapy intervention provided by a large, for profit, outpatient rehabilitation organization in the Pittsburgh PA, US region is compared to data published by Jette & Jette (1996). On average, the improvement in physical function achieved by the outpatient rehabilitation organization in Pittsburgh is approximately 0.1 of a standard deviation larger than that reported by Jette & Jette (1996), and the improvement in social function is approximately 0.3 of a standard deviation larger. While this implies that individuals with knee impairments treated in Pittsburgh may experience slightly better improvement from a course of physical therapy in health-related quality of life as measured by the SF-36, the results must be interpreted carefully because the validity of this inference is dependent on a number of factors including differences in patient and therapist characteristics, medical diagnosis, and length of care between the two samples.

Several statistics can be calculated to determine if the change over time, either within or between groups of

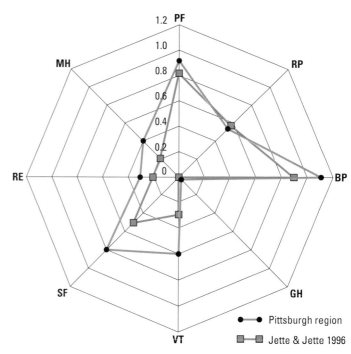

Figure 12.3 Radar graph of the effect size of each of the 8 scales of the SF-36 following a course of physical therapy in patients with a variety of knee impairments. Data from patients receiving physical therapy from a large multi-center non-profit outpatient physical therapy organization in the Pittsburgh, PA, US region is benchmarked against data reported by Jette (1996). Each of the axes represents a scale of the SF-36. PF = Physical Function Scale. RP = Role Limitations Due to Physical Function. BP = Bodily Pain. GH = General Health. VT = Vitality. SF = Social Function. RE = Role Limitations Due to Emotional Health. MH = Mental Health.

individuals, is statistically different from zero. The paired t-test can be used to answer the question 'Is the magnitude of change within a group over time significantly different from 0?', while the independent t-test of change scores can be used to answer the question 'Is the magnitude of change over time in one group larger than the magnitude of change for another group?' The statistical significance of these comparisons is largely dependent on the sample size. A large change may not be significant if the sample size is too small, and a small change may be statistically significant but not clinically meaningful if the sample size is large. Therefore, the significance of any statistical results must be interpreted clinically.

SUMMARY

Clinical outcomes data can be used to facilitate patient management decisions, assess clinician and organizational performance, and to provide evidence for the effectiveness of interventions provided by physical therapists and other rehabilitation specialists. The validity of the inferences made from outcomes data is dependent on the validity of the outcome measures themselves and the circumstances under which the data was collected, analyzed, and interpreted. Clinical outcomes may include measures of impairment of body structure and function, activity limitation, and participation restriction. However, because the relationship between impairment and the resulting activity limitation and participation restriction is not direct, and because activity limitations and participation restrictions are of the utmost concern to the athlete, the primary clinical outcome should be measures of activity limitation and participation restriction. Activity limitation and participation restriction may be measured either through direct observation of performance or by general or specific measures of health-related quality of life. Clinical outcomes data must be collected systematically to ensure valid inferences from the data.

REFERENCES

American Physical Therapy Association 2001 Guide to physical therapist practice – second edition. Physical Therapy 81:9–744

Barber-Westin S D, Noyes F R, McCloskey J W 1999 Rigorous statistical reliability, validity, and responsiveness testing of the Cincinnati knee rating system in 350 subjects with uninjured, injured, or anterior cruciate ligament-reconstructed knees. American Journal of Sports Medicine 27:402–416

Beaton D E 2000 Understanding the relevance of measured change through studies of responsiveness. Spine 25(24):3192–3199

Beaton D E, Katz J N, Fossel A H et al 2001a Measuring the whole or the parts? Validity, reliability, and responsiveness of the Disabilities of the Arm, Shoulder and Hand outcome measure in different regions of the upper extremity. Journal of Hand Therapy 14:128–146

Beaton D E, Bombardier C, Katz J N et al 2001b Looking for important change/differences in studies of responsiveness. Journal of Rheumatology 28:400–405

Bellamy N, Buchanan W W, Goldsmith C H et al 1988 Validation study of WOMAC: a health status instrument for measuring clinically important patient relevant outcomes to antirheumatic drug therapy in patients with osteoarthritis of the hip or knee. Journal of Rheumatology 15:1833–1840

Binkley J M, Stratford P W, Lott S A et al 1999 The Lower Extremity Functional Scale (LEFS): scale development, measurement properties, and clinical application. North American Orthopaedic Rehabilitation Research Network. Physical Therapy 79:371–383

Chatman A B, Hyams S P, Neel J M et al 1997 The patient-specific functional scale: measurement properties in patients with knee dysfunction. Physical Therapy 77:820–829

Christensen L, Mendoza J L 1986 A method of assessing change in a single subject: an alteration of the RC Index. Behavior Therapy 17:305–330

Cohen J 1969 Statistical power analysis for the behavioural sciences. Academic Press, New York

Crocker L, Algina J 1986 Introduction to classical and modern test theory. Jovanovich College Publishers, Harcourt Brace, Fort Worth, TX

Deyo R A, Center R M 1986 Assessing the responsiveness of functional scales to clinical change: an analogy to diagnostic test performance. Journal of Chronic Diseases 39:897–906

Dobrzykowski E A 1997 The methodology of outcomes measurement. Journal of Rehabilitation Outcomes 1(1):8–17

Fairbank J C, Couper J, Davies J B et al 1980 The Oswestry low back pain disability questionnaire. Physiotherapy 66:271–273

Goldstein M S, Elliott S D, Guccione A A 2000 The development of an instrument to measure satisfaction with physical therapy. Physical Therapy 81:1061–1062

Guyatt G H, Feeny D H, Patrick D L 1993 Measuring health-related quality of life. Annals of Internal Medicine 118:622–629

Hoffman L G, Rouse M W, Brin B N 1995 Quality of life: a review. Journal of the American Optometric Association 66:281–289

Irrgang J J 1996 Outcomes in sports medicine: classification schemes for physical impairments, functional limitations and disability. Project Focus 96. The Conference on Sports Related Injury. Presented by the Foundation for Physical Therapy. The American Physical Therapy Association, Alexandria, VA

Irrgang J J, Snyder-Mackler L, Wainner R S et al 1998 Development of a patient-reported measure of function of the knee. Journal of Bone and Joint Surgery (Am) 80A:1132–1145

Irrgang J J, Anderson A F, Boland A L et al 2001 Development and validation of the International Knee Documentation Committee Subjective Knee Form. American Journal of Sports Medicine 29:600–613

Jette A M 1994 Physical disablement concepts for physical therapy research and practice. Physical Therapy 74:380–386

Jette D U, Jette A M 1996 Physical therapy and health outcomes in patients with knee impairments. Physical Therapy 76:1178–1187

Kessler R C, Mroczek D K 1995 Measuring the effects of medical interventions. Medical Care 33(4):AS109–AS119

Kirkley A, Griffin S, McLintoch H et al 1998 The development and evaluation of a disease-specific quality of life measurement tool for shoulder instability. The Western Ontario Shoulder Instability Index (WOSI). American Journal of Sports Medicine 26:764–772

Kirshner B, Guyatt G 1985. A methodological framework for assessing health indices. Journal of Chronic Diseases 38:27–36

Kopec J A, Esdaile J M, Abrahamowicz M et al 1995 The Quebec Back Pain Disability Scale: measurement properties. Spine 20:341–352

Lippitt S B, Harryman D T II, Matsen F A III 1993 A practical tool for evaluation of function: the Simple Shoulder Test. In: Matsen F A III, Fu F H, Hawkins R J (eds) The shoulder: a balance of mobility and stability. The American Academy of Orthopaedic Surgeons, Rosemont

Lohr K N, Aaronson N K, Alonso J et al 1996 Evaluating quality-of-life and health status instruments: development of scientific review criteria. Clinical Therapeutics 18:979–992

McHorney C A, Ware J E Jr, Raczek A E 1993 The MOS 36-Item Short-Form Health Survey (SF-36): II psychometric and clinical tests of validity in measuring physical and mental health constructs. Medical Care 31:247–263

McHorney C A, Kosinski M, Ware J E Jr 1994 Comparisons of the costs and quality of norms for the SF-36 health survey collected by mail versus telephone interview: results from a national survey. Medical Care 32:551–567

McSweeny A J, Creer T L 1995 Health related quality-of-life assessment in medical care. Disease of the Month 41(1):6–71

Messick S 1989 Meaning and values in test validation: the science and ethics of assessment. Educational Researcher 18(2):5–11

Mohtadi N 1998 Development and validation of the quality of life outcome measure (questionnaire) for chronic anterior cruciate ligament deficiency. American Journal of Sports Medicine 26:350–359

Nagi S Z 1965 Some conceptual issues in disability and rehabilitation. In: Sussman M (ed) Sociology and rehabilitation. American Sociological Association, Washington, DC

Nagi S Z 1991 Disability concepts revisited: implication for prevention. In Pope A M, Tarlov A R (eds) Disability in America: toward a national agenda for prevention. National Academy Press, Washington, DC

National Institutes of Health 1992 National Advisory Board on Medical Rehabilitation Research, Draft V: report and plan for medical rehabilitation research. National Institutes of Health, Bethesda, MD

Noyes F R, McGinnis G H, Mooar L A 1984 Functional disability in the anterior cruciate insufficient knee syndrome: review of knee rating systems and projected risk factors in determining treatment. Sports Medicine 1:278–302

Pantano K J, Irrgang J J, Burdett R et al 2001 A pilot study on the relationship between physical impairment and activity restriction in persons with anterior cruciate ligament reconstruction at long-term follow-up. Knee Surgery, Sports Traumatology and Arthroscopy 9:369–378

Richards R R, An K N, Bigliani L U et al 1994 A standardized method for the assessment of shoulder function. Journal of Shoulder and Elbow Surgery 3:347–352

Shrout P E, Fleiss J L 1979 Intraclass correlation: uses in assessing rater reliability. Psychological Bulletin 86:420–428

Snyder-Mackler L, Fitzgerald G K, Bartolozzi A R et al 1997 The relationship between passive joint laxity and functional outcome after anterior cruciate ligament injury. American Journal of Sports Medicine 25:191–195

Stratford P W, Binkley J 1995 The Quebec Back Pain Disability Scale: measurement properties. Spine 20:2169–2170

Stratford P, Gill C, Westaway et al 1995 Assessing disability and change on individual patients: a report of a patient specific measure. Physiotherapy Canada 47(4):258–263

Stratford P W, Binkley J M, Riddle D L 1996 Health status measures: strategies and analytic methods for assessing change scores. Physical Therapy 76, 1109–1123

Streiner D L, Norman G R 1995 Health measurement scales: a practical guide to their development and use, 2nd edn. Oxford Medical Publications, New York

Tegner Y, Lysholm J 1985 Rating systems in the evaluation of knee ligament injuries. Clinical Orthopaedics and Related Research 198:43–49

Testa M A, Nackley J F 1994 Methods for quality-of-life studies. Annual Review of Public Health 15:535–559

Testa M A, Simonson D C 1996 Assessment of quality-of-life outcomes. New England Journal of Medicine 334:835–840

Verbrugge L, Jette A M 1994 The disablement process. Social Science and Medicine 38:1–14

Ware J E Jr, Sherbourne C D 1992 The MOS 36-item short-form health survey (SF-36). I. Conceptual framework and item selection. Medical Care 30:473–483

Westaway M D, Stratford P W, Binkley J M 1998 The Patient-Specific Functional Scale: validation of its use in persons with neck dysfunction. Journal of Orthopaedic and Sports Physical Therapy 27:331–338

Whyte J 1994 Toward a methodology for rehabilitation research. American Journal of Physical Medicine and Rehabilitation 73:428–435

World Health Organization 1980 International classification of impairments, disabilities, and handicaps. World Health Organization, Geneva

World Health Organization 2001 International classification of functioning, disability and health. World Health Organization, Geneva

13

Electrophysical agents in sport and exercise injury management

Lynn Snyder-Mackler   Laura Schmitt
Katherine Rudolph   Wayne Woodzell

INTRODUCTION

Rehabilitation of the injured athlete can be particularly challenging as return to a high level of function is expected. The clinician must make prudent decisions to achieve a speedy return-to-play without jeopardizing the wellbeing of the athlete. Athletic injury can be associated with tissue damage that can range from localized cellular damage to ruptured tendon or fracture. Injury is accompanied by inflammation, edema, and pain and can result in the loss of muscle strength and function due to disuse or immobilization. The use of electrophysical agents may help to facilitate more rapid healing of damaged tissues. This chapter presents the principles of electrophysical agents that are common in sports medicine and that clinicians may use in conjunction with other rehabilitation interventions.

TREATMENT OF INFLAMMATION AND EDEMA

CRYOTHERAPY

Cryotherapy is the use of ice and other cold modalities to reduce the harmful effects of tissue injury: hemorrhage, edema, muscle spasm, and pain, all of which can lead to loss of function. The application of the RICE principle (rest, ice, compression, and elevation) immediately after injury has been successful in minimizing tissue inflammation and edema (Green et al 2001) through a mechanism that involves blood vessel constriction and decreased cellular metabolism (Thorsson et al 1985, Karunakara et al 1999). Reduced circulation and cellular metabolism result in the release of fewer metabolic byproducts, thereby minimizing further tissue injury (Knight 1995). Commonly used application techniques are commercial cold packs, ice bags, ice massage, Cryo/Cuff (AirCast, Summit, NJ), and cold baths.

Temperature of the cold modality, duration of application, area of targeted tissues, and the physical makeup of the athlete all affect the depth of tissue cooling. Skin temperatures cool rapidly but may not be a good indicator of the intensity of cooling that occurs in deeper tissues. Palmer & Knight (1996) found greater than 20°C temperature reduction in human skin after the application of an ice pack for 20 min, however, Zemke et al (1998) found only a 4°C reduction at a depth of 1.7 cm in the human calf. Levy & Lintner (1997) found no significant temperature difference in the glenohumeral joint or subacromial space before and after a 90-min application of cold via a Cryo/Cuff (AirCast, Summit, NJ). During treatment, it is unlikely that cryotherapy will produce changes in tissue temperatures at depths greater than 2 cm.

Athletes will typically feel three phases before reaching analgesia: intense cold leading to burning followed by aching. The choice of cold application is dependent on the target tissue depth and size. Smaller target areas, such as the patellar tendon, can be treated with ice massage while larger areas should be treated with a cold whirlpool (Zemke et al 1998). Ice massage is the application of ice directly to the skin for 5–7 min while a cold bath involves immersion of the affected body part in water, typically 15°C (Eston & Peters 1999, Michlovitz 1996). Zemke et al (1998) demonstrated that while both ice massage and ice bags were effective in reducing intramuscular temperature, ice massage was more time efficient. In a busy physical therapy or athletic training facility, ice massage would be an effective and efficient way to reduce pain and inflammation if the area of the target tissue is small.

Cryotherapy is used post-surgically to reduce pain and swelling and improve range of motion. Ohkoshi et al (1999) investigated the effects of prolonged cooling with circulating cold water at 5 and 10°C after anterior cruciate ligament (ACL) reconstruction. The use of cryotherapy at 10°C decreased scores on an analog pain scale and the amount of pain medication administered. The study group who had treatment with the 5°C cooling demonstrated decreased blood loss but had no decrease in pain ratings (Ohkoshi et al 1999). It must be noted, that the applicability of this study may be limited due to the feasibility of applying extreme cold water continuously at such low temperatures for 48 h, but it demonstrates that the use of ice after surgery may be beneficial if the tissues can be cooled adequately.

Many athletes receive ice before or during a sporting event due to previous muscular trauma. Some clinicians may have concerns that the application of cold during athletic activity will decrease sensory perception, however, evidence to the contrary exists. Ingersoll et al found that a 20-min immersion in 1°C water did not affect the athlete's sensory perception of the ankle or foot (Ingersoll et al 1992). Evans et al (1995) demonstrated no significant difference in agility after immersion of the ankle in 1°C water for 20 min. These studies demonstrate that the application of ice does not significantly affect agility or perception, therefore the fear of returning an athlete to participation after icing does not seem warranted.

A treatment utilizing an ice bag or cold pack typically lasts 10–15 min. In contrast, an ice massage will only last 5–7 min. The goal of the treatment is to cool the affected area and ultimately produce the sensation of analgesia. Contraindications to the use of cold involve hypersensitivity, decreased sensation, and poor blood flow. The use of ice to treat athletic injuries is routine but it is not without risk. Application of ice can cause nerve injury to superficial nerves, particularly over the ulnar, peroneal, and femoral cutaneous nerves (Bassett et al 1992). When treating tissues over these areas, the athlete's sensation should be monitored closely to determine if treatment should be discontinued.

ELECTRICAL STIMULATION

General principles

Several forms of electrical stimulation are used to affect tissue edema but through very different mechanisms. Before discussing the specific electrical stimulation modalities, a brief overview of electrical stimulation principles will be presented. Electrical stimulation involves the use of electrical current for therapeutic purposes and may result in the activation of excitable tissues, changes in cellular function, or the transcutaneous delivery of medications to target tissues.

Two types of current are used, alternating current (AC) and direct current (DC) (Fig. 13.1). Alternating current involves the bidirectional flow of charged particles and can be applied continuously, in pulses or in bursts of current. Direct current is unidirectional and can be applied continuously or in the form of interrupted pulses. Continuous DC is used in applications including wound care and iontophoresis and has chemical effects that warrant special considerations, which will be discussed later. Interrupted DC and AC that are used therapeutically have no chemical effect because the pulse duration is well below the very long pulse durations of 50–300 ms that would result in electrochemical changes at the cellular level (Alon 1991). AC can be delivered continuously or in bursts. The shape of the waveforms can take many forms and can be modified by adjusting the amplitude and phase duration of each pulse. Physiologically, the most important characteristic of a

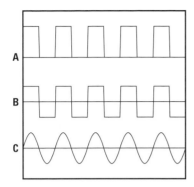

Figure 13.1 Illustrations of different waveforms. **A**: Interrupted direct current. **B**: Alternating current with a square wave configuration. **C**: Alternating current with a sine wave configuration.

waveform is the amount of electrical charge delivered to the tissues, called the phase charge, which is expressed in coulombs or microcoulombs (10^{-6} coulombs). Phase charge is the time integral of a single phase of current. In a square wave pulse, the phase charge is the pulse amplitude times the phase duration. When applying pulsed DC, increasing the pulse duration and/or amplitude of a waveform will recruit more neurons (Crago et al 1980). When using AC, decreasing the stimulation frequency will increase the phase charge.

The recruitment of neurons with electrical stimulation occurs differently than in volitional activation. When neurons are recruited volitionally they are activated according to the size principle whereby smaller diameter fibers are recruited before larger diameter fibers (Kandel et al 1995). When using electrical stimulation, the excitation of neurons follows the reverse order. With electrical stimulation, large diameter neurons, whose membrane resistance is lower, are activated before small diameter fibers, whose membrane resistance is higher. Physiologically, this means that the sensory neurons are recruited first, followed by motor neurons, and finally neurons that transmit noxious signals. In general, with clinical stimulators, selective activation of sensory neurons is achieved with short pulse durations, from 2–50 µs; activation of motor neurons is achieved with pulse durations of 200–600 µs; and pain fibers are activated with long pulse durations upwards of 1 ms.

Clinically, as stimulation intensity is increased, one will typically experience a tingling sensation, followed by a muscle twitch and then a painful sensation. It is important to understand that when applying current transcutaneously, the location of the neuron beneath the skin is also important. For example, when applying a waveform of a given phase charge, a small diameter neuron that is located close to the surface of the skin will experience higher current than a large diameter neuron at a deeper location, so the small diameter fiber may be activated before the neuron with a larger diameter. This

explains why in some applications in which the stimulating electrode is located over the motor point of the muscle whose motor neurons are very close to the skin, a motor response may precede a sensory response.

In addition to changing the phase charge, the frequency at which pulses or bursts are delivered affects the intensity of response. For example, when producing a motor response, increasing the frequency of stimulation will produce more summation of twitch forces and may result in a strong tetanic contraction if the frequency is sufficiently high. When AC is delivered in bursts, the carrier frequency refers to the frequency of stimulation within the burst, and the burst frequency is that which affects the force of the contractions. Size and spacing of electrodes need to be considered in order for a treatment to be more effective in effecting a desired response.

Electrical stimulation and tissue edema

Electrical stimulation has been used to lessen the formation of edema and to reduce existing edema. High-volt pulsed current (HVPC) involves the use of pulsed DC consisting of twin spikes of high amplitude (up to 500V), small pulse duration (50–200 µs) waveforms that are delivered at 1–120 twin spikes per second (Fig. 13.2).

HVPC is commonly used in wound care but it has also been used to prevent the formation of edema in animal models. Studies have shown that the application of HVPC within the first hour after injury can help prevent the formation of edema (Thornton et al 1998). Electrodes have been placed directly on skin overlying the injury or submerged in a water bath and the intensity of stimulation produces a strong sensory response (10% below motor threshold) (Taylor et al 1997, Taylor et al 1992, Thornton et al 1998). The evidence suggests that HVPC inhibits microvascular leakage that minimizes further tissue edema (Taylor et al 1997, Taylor et al 1992, Thornton et al 1998). These studies were performed in animal models so further research is needed to investi-

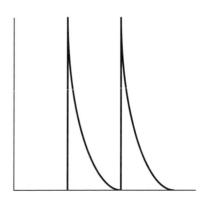

Figure 13.2 Twin-spikes of the high volt pulsed galvanic electrical stimulation.

gate the effects in humans. However, the benefits of early intervention with HVPC appear promising (Mendel & Fish 1993).

The use of electrical stimulation to reduce existing edema has proven less effective. Research has shown that motor level stimulation is no better at reducing tissue edema than compression boots, which mimic the effect of muscle pumping (Griffin et al 1990). Therefore, the added time and expense of using electrical stimulation in this manner appears unfounded. It could be, however, that motor level electrical stimulation might be useful in reducing existing edema when individuals cannot perform volitional contractions.

Iontophoresis

Iontophoresis is the transcutaneous delivery of medication by DC through the mechanism of electrostatic repulsion. Many drugs that are placed in a solution ionize into positively and negatively charged ions that will be affected by an electric field. Negatively charged ions are repelled from the negative electrode, while positively charged ions are repelled from the positive electrode. Electrodes used in iontophoresis include a delivery electrode that is designed to deliver the medication and dispersive electrode to complete the circuit. The delivery electrode is small so it will concentrate the current to deliver medication to a precise area of tissue. The dispersive electrode is larger with a lower density of current so the effect on the skin is minimized.

Due to the continuous nature of direct current, chemical burns at the electrode–skin interface are possible. When the delivery electrode is positive (anode), the chemical reaction on the skin involves the release of hydrogen ions that decreases the pH and results in an acidic reaction. Current density of the positive electrode should be held below $1.0 \, \text{mA/cm}^2$. When the delivery electrode is negative (cathode), sodium hydroxide ions are produced that increase the pH in an alkaline reaction. This reaction is more caustic to the skin and current density should not exceed $0.5 \, \text{mA/cm}^2$. Most clinical iontophoresis units limit the peak current to 4.0 mA. Commercial electrodes provide even current distribution and typically have buffering systems to help regulate pH minimizing chemical reactions (Schmidt 1993).

When choosing iontophoresis treatment parameters, the clinician must balance time efficiency with patient safety and comfort. Current dosage refers to the total amount of current used to deliver the medication taking into account both peak current and treatment duration. For example, if the treatment consisted of 2 mA delivered over 20 min, the dosage would be 40 mA/min. Dosages used for iontophoresis have ranged from 40–80 mA/min. In general, higher peak currents can lead to discomfort in some patients, however, it appears that greater treatment dosages are associated with greater success in treating pain and inflammation (Bertolucci 1982, Braun 1987, Delacerda 1982). Clinicians may choose to alter the treatment dosage by increasing the treatment duration in patients who are less tolerant of high peak currents.

Treatment principles

Prior to beginning the treatment, the skin should be thoroughly inspected. Skin abrasions reduce the resistance to current flow, thereby increasing the potential for skin irritation (Schmidt 1993). Clinicians should be aware that mild to moderate erythema under the delivery or dispersive electrode is a typical response to iontophoresis treatment (Japour et al 1999) and should resolve within several hours after treatment. Skin thickness and skin sensitivity must be considered when deciding on treatment parameters. Tissues that are close to the skin surface are more likely to receive the drug during iontophoresis. Treating areas with thick skin, such as on the palmar and plantar surfaces, can be difficult because of increased resistance to ion flow, so an alternative electrode location may be chosen. Electrophysical agents that increase blood flow, such as continuous ultrasound, may drive the drug away from targeted tissue; therefore use of heating agents in conjunction with iontophoresis is not recommended. Three to four treatments should be adequate to determine if iontophoresis is yielding positive results (Braun 1987, Harris 1982, Lark & Gangarosa 1990).

Medications

In sports medicine, the most common medications used for iontophoresis include anti-inflammatories and local anesthetics (Table 13.1) but other medications have been used. Acetic acid has been used to treat calcific tendinitis (Robinson & Snyder-Mackler 1995, Schmidt 1993) and potassium iodide or sodium chloride (2% solution) has been used to treat scar tissue (Schmidt, 1993).

Efficacy of iontophoresis

Heel pain is common in sports medicine. Acetic acid (5% solution) has been shown to provide relief of recalcitrant heel pain in 94% of patients who received an average of 5.7 treatments of iontophoresis at an intensity 30–60 mA/min with the delivery electrode placed over the heel (Japour et al 1999). In a controlled clinical trial, Myerson et al (1986) found that 0.4% dexamethasone sodium phosphate reduced heel pain in an average of 6 treatments administered over 2–3 weeks. In this trial, the treatment dose was 80 mA/min and the active electrode

Table 13.1 Medications used in iontophoresis

Drug	Indication	Effect	Delivery electrode
Dexamethasone sodium phosphate (4 mg/mL)	Inflammation	Anti-inflammatory	Negative
Lidocaine (lignocaine) HCL (4% solution with or without adrenaline [epinephrine])	Pain	Local anesthetic	Positive
Acetic Acid (2–5% solution)	Calcific tendinitis	May increase solubility of calcium deposits	Negative
Potassium iodide (10% solution)	Scar tissue	Help to break down collagen	Negative
Sodium chloride (2% solution)	Scar tissue	Help to break down collagen	Negative

was placed on the plantar aspect of the heel. After 6 treatments, the treatment group noted significantly greater improvement based on physical examination and completion of the Maryland Foot Score, which assesses both pain and function of the foot (Myerson et al 1986). Iontophoresis can be an effective modality to decrease inflammation, decrease pain, and treat calcifications and scar tissue.

ULTRASOUND

Ultrasound (US) is the application of high frequency sound waves, between 1–3 MHz, applied continuously or in pulses. Continuous US has thermal effects while pulsed ultrasound does not. The non-thermal effects of pulsed US include cavitation and mechanical and chemical changes that may effect cellular permeability and metabolism (Rivenburgh 1992). Cavitation is the vibrational effect of US on gas bubbles leading to changes in local pressure and improved membrane permeability.

Another manner in which US is used to affect tissue inflammation and edema is through phonophoresis. Phonophoresis is the use of continuous US to enhance the transcutaneous absorption of anti-inflammatory drugs to underlying tissue. Corticosteroid gel, methyl salicate cream, and betamethasone in US gel are some commonly used drugs that have demonstrated delivery rates at above 80% (Cameron & Monroe 1992). Because of the high water content of most tissues, an important characteristic of the medication is its affinity to water. The medium in which the drug is delivered must allow transmission by being hydrophilic. Many creams, such as hydrocortisone, are hydrophobic and do not transmit well (Cameron & Monroe 1992).

Studies have shown beneficial effects of phonophoresis in decreasing pain and inflammation. Ciccone et al (1991) demonstrated the use of trolamine salicyte phonophoresis decreased stiffness and pain greater than US alone. Shin & Choi (1997) applied indometacin to the temporo-mandibular joint and evaluated pain relief using a visual analog pain scale and pain threshold. They applied 1% indometacin cream at 1 MHz, 0.8 to 1.5 w/cm^2 continu-ous for 15 min to the temporomandibular joint and found decreased pain scale scores and a 14% increase in pain threshold. In contrast, Klaiman et al (1998) showed no significant decrease in tolerance to pressure pain as compared to US alone when using a 0.05% flucinonide gel on lateral epicondylitis.

Despite the beneficial effect of some phonophoresis applications, the effectiveness of phonophoresis has been questioned in the literature (Bare et al 1996, Benson et al 1989, Byl 1995, Oziomek et al 1991). Bare et al (1996) looked at the delivery of 10% hydrocortisone acetate gel using 1 MHz US at an intensity of 1w/cm^2 for 5 min and measured its transmission by determining the relative cortisol serum level in the bloodstream. They demonstrated no increase in blood cortisol levels as compared to US alone (Bare et al 1996). Similar studies by Oziomek et al (1991) and Benson et al (1989) on the absorption of salicylate and benzydamine have also found no enhancement of the absorption of the drug with US.

The benefits of phonophoresis appear to be specific to both the drug choice and depth of target tissue. The frequency of the ultrasonic waves is inversely proportional to the depth of tissue penetration. The depth of penetration for 1 MHz US is 2–5 cm while that of 3 MHz US is only 1–2 cm (Michlovitz 1996), so consideration of the depth of the target tissue is important.

TREATMENT OF PAIN

An important component to successful rehabilitation of the injured athlete is the treatment of pain for which many modalities can be a useful adjunct. As described in Chapter 8, two mechanisms by which pain is relieved are through the gate control mechanism and by the release of endogenous opiates. The gate control theory states that activity of the large diameter sensory fibers can modulate pain impulses from peripheral neurons thereby influencing the experience of pain. The opioid-mediated analgesic system blocks pain transmission through neural and/or hormonal mechanisms whereby endogenous opiates are released in response to painful stimuli. Of note is that the release of endogenous opiates is achieved through exercise as well (Surbey et al 1984).

HEAT AND COLD

Pain reduction has been demonstrated by the application of both heat and cold. Ohkoshi et al (1999) found reduced pain in individuals who received cryotherapy with 10°C circulating water after surgery. Cold can affect pain directly by decreasing nerve conduction velocities of both motor and sensory nerves, thereby interfering with the transmission of nerve signals. Extreme cold has also been found to reduce pain via the release of endogenous opiates (Washington et al 2000).

The application of superficial heat, among other effects, can also produce analgesia (Lehman & Delateur 1990). Heat should not be used in acute injury since it increases blood flow to the area (Greenberg 1972) and may increase edema. One should wait at least 48 h or until swelling has resolved to allow completion of the inflammatory phase.

Superficial heat is thought to reduce pain following the acute phase of injury by increasing tissue temperature and promoting relaxation, although the exact mechanism is not fully understood. Commonly used forms of heating modalities are hot packs or warm whirlpools. Researchers have speculated that reduction in pain and muscle spasm occurs through the increased blood flow and an elevation of the pain threshold (Rivenburgh 1992, Lehman et al 1958). The increased blood flow occurs by vasodilation of blood vessels, while the pain threshold is thought to increase through a thermal effect on free nerve endings (Rivenburgh 1992).

Lehman & Delateur (1990) found that circulation increased and muscle relaxed at 40–45°C. Achieving an elevated tissue temperature is greatly affected by the depth of the target tissue. Superficial heating techniques, such as hot packs and warm whirlpools, warm tissues to a depth of approximately 0.5 cm (Michlovitz 1996), so deeper structures may not benefit from superficial heating methods. Superficial heat is typically applied for 10–15 min.

Continuous US produces thermal effects that result from absorption of sound waves and is often used to heat deeper tissues. Thermal effects include increased soft tissue extensibility, increased blood flow, and decreased muscle spasm (Rivenburgh 1992), all of which can reduce a patient's experience of pain. Klaiman et al (1998) demonstrated decreased pain and increased pressure tolerance in response to an 8-min treatment (1 MHz continuous US at 1.5 w/cm²) to the elbow. The rise in tissue temperature is typically 2–3°C, which can cause a reduction in muscle spasm and pain relief (Draper &

Ricard 1995). Draper & Ricard (1995) demonstrated that a rise of 4°C occurs in 3–4 min when using a 3 MHz US frequency. When a frequency of 1 MHz was used, the rise in temperature took up to 6 min (Draper & Ricard 1995). The composition of the target tissue may influence the heating effect of US. Tissues that are high in collagen content, such as bone, absorb more US energy than tissues with high water content, so caution must be exercised when using continuous US on bony areas. Moving the US applicator more rapidly or reducing the intensity of the US may help improve patient tolerance and prevent tissue damage.

ELECTROANALGESIA

All manners of electrical stimulation (sensory, motor and noxious) are used in reducing pain associated with injury, although the mechanism of pain relief depends on the intensity of stimulation and the patient's subjective experience of the stimulus.

Sensory level stimulation

Two modes of sensory level electrical stimulation that are commonly used for pain relief are conventional transcutaneous electrical nerve stimulation (TENS) and interferential electrical stimulation. Both are thought to reduce pain through the gate control mechanism and are therefore only effective for the duration of the treatment. Although all methods of electrical stimulation used clinically are applied transcutaneously, transcutaneous electrical nerve stimulation (TENS) has become synonymous with a comfortable sensory level of stimulation. The term 'conventional TENS' is used here to differentiate the comfortable sensory sensation from the very intense, often unpleasant sensation associated with high intensity, 'acupuncture-like TENS' that is also used for pain relief.

Jensen et al (1985) studied pain level, amount of pain medication administered, and knee range of motion in 90 patients who had undergone arthroscopic knee surgery. The subjects were randomized into three groups: control, sham TENS, and TENS. The group that received TENS (pulse duration of 300 μs and pulse rate of 70 Hz) had significantly less pain, needed less pain medication and achieved greater joint range than the sham or control groups (Jensen et al 1985). Conventional TENS is thought to have effects in addition to analgesia including increased blood flow and skin temperature, however, research has yielded conflicting results. In a recent study, Cramp et al (2000) applied conventional TENS for 15 min at 4 Hz and 110 Hz (both at 200 μs) to a healthy population. Skin temperatures as well as blood perfusion levels were measured at 3-min intervals for 30 min. The results showed increased blood flow and skin temperature when 4 Hz TENS as compared to 110 Hz and the control was used (Cramp et al 2000). Neither high nor low frequency stimulation demonstrated any changes in skin temperature when compared to the control group, questioning the vasodilatory effects of conventional TENS (Cramp et al 2000).

When using conventional TENS, stimulation parameters usually include pulse durations ranging from 2–50 µs, stimulation frequency of 50–100 pulses per second (pps) and intensity levels such that a strong but comfortable tingling sensation is experienced. Because of adaptation to the tingling sensation, the intensity is increased throughout the treatment. Analgesic effects of conventional TENS occur only when the stimulation is applied for treatment durations ranging from 15–20 min up to hours.

Interferential current involves the application of two unique sinusoidal frequencies that are applied to the tissue simultaneously via two channels. The electrodes of these channels are positioned in the form of an 'X' such that the currents intersect over the painful area. The frequency of the currents typically ranges from 4000–4200 Hz, which intersect at deeper tissue layers (Bertoti 2000). Interferential current is purported to provide greater analgesic effects than other forms of electrical stimulation, however, research does not support this assertion. Interferential treatments have been found no better than placebo in decreasing pain (Taylor et al 1987), increasing blood flow (Indergand & Morgan 1995), or decreasing edema (Bertoti 2000, Christie & Willoughby 1990, Nussbaum et al 1990).

Motor and noxious electrical stimulation

Many procedures in rehabilitation are uncomfortable so clinicians often benefit from the opioid-mediated analgesic system. However, the release of endogenous opiates can be initiated intentionally with high intensity electrical stimulation and can be particularly useful in treating subacute and chronic pain. Unlike analgesia produced through the gate control mechanisms, analgesia associated with the release of endogenous opiates lasts several hours. Any stimulation parameters capable of producing a motor or noxious response are adequate to produce analgesia, thus, waveforms with longer pulse durations are usually required.

One type of high level electrical stimulation used to produce analgesia is sometimes referred to as strong low rate TENS or acupuncture-like TENS. With this technique, stimuli are delivered continuously at a low frequency (2–4 pps) with pulse durations over 150 µs to produce a rhythmic muscle contraction. Evidence suggests that stronger contractions are associated with greater pain relief (Picker 1988, Picker 1989). Sometimes the current is delivered at sites remote to the injury

corresponding to acupuncture points. Clinical observations indicate that tolerance to intense motor level contractions is limited, so clinicians may have more success when using sites remote to the injury or over areas with no muscle tissue.

High frequency (> 100 pps) stimuli have also been used to produce a noxious sensation that will elicit the release of endogenous opiates. Long pulse durations (1 ms, up to 1 s) are required to activate actual pain fibers (Robinson & Snyder-Mackler 1995); however, clinical stimulators rarely provide such long pulse durations. To compensate for the shorter than desired pulse durations, clinicians should use very small electrodes in order to produce high current density and deliver a stimulus producing a painful sensation. When using waveforms with large phase charges, sensory, motor and possibly pain fibers will be activated. Therefore, it is important to choose electrode placements that avoid areas of muscle tissue if motor level contractions are not desired.

Manal & Snyder-Mackler (1997) described a treatment that produces electroanalgesia with high intensity electrical stimulation using a current that is sometimes referred to as 'Russian current'. The stimulus characteristics are similar to those used by the Soviet researcher Yakov Kots to strengthen Soviet Olympic athletes (Kots et al 1977). Manal and Snyder-Mackler's protocol involves identifying a specific point of pain that is surrounded by small electrodes through which the current is delivered (Fig. 13.3). The current is a burst-modulated AC sine wave configuration and a 2500 Hz carrier frequency that is applied at 50 bursts/s. Within the burst, the 2500 Hz current is delivered with a duty cycle of 50% (10 ms on, 10 ms off) and the electrical stimulation is provided for 12 s on and 8 s off for a total of 12–15 min (Manal & Snyder-Mackler 1997). The amplitude of the current is

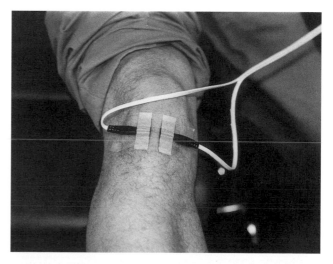

Figure 13.3 Electrode placement for electroanalgesia with high intensity electrical stimulation.

increased to maximal tolerance. The intensity is increased throughout the treatment as tolerance allows. Securing the electrodes with tape and replacing the electrodes frequently helps to maintain good electrode contact. This is important when delivering high current density to minimize the chance of electrical burns, which can sometimes occur with high intensity AC. Manal & Snyder-Mackler (1997) stated that this protocol often produces long lasting analgesia, well over the several hours that one would expect from an opioid-mediated response. The exact mechanism of its success is not fully understood, however, it appears to be an effective modality to treat palpable, painful, soft tissue structures.

When using any treatment for analgesia, objective documentation of pain relief is essential. Techniques to provoke the patient's signs of pain, as well as pain and functional status questionnaires, should be used to determine the effectiveness of treatment. If significant improvement in symptoms is not noted, another modality may be more appropriate (Manal & Snyder-Mackler 1997).

TREATMENT OF IMPAIRED MUSCLE FUNCTION

NEUROMUSCULAR ELECTRICAL STIMULATION FOR MUSCLE STRENGTHENING

As discussed previously, motor level electrical stimulation can be used for edema reduction in persons who are unable to activate their muscles volitionally and for pain relief. When using electrical stimulation for treating muscle weakness, some unique issues must be addressed. Rapid restoration of muscle strength, power, and endurance are vitally important in the rehabilitation of athletes. Training should target the specific muscles that are impaired and training should be sport-specific. The overload principle states that strength increases in proportion to the amount of overload that the muscle experiences during exercise (Hillebrandt & Houtz 1956). Overload can be applied to specific weakened muscles through the use of electrical stimulation providing that the peripheral nerve and the muscle are intact.

When using Neuromuscular Electrical Stimulation (NMES), the clinician must balance the need for high force production with the presence of rapid muscle fatigue. Stimulating muscle electrically differs from volitional activity in ways that lead to rapid fatigue. Because of the reversal of the order of motor unit recruitment with electrical stimulation, larger diameter motor neurons, associated with large fast fatigable motor

units are stimulated before smaller, slow twitch, fatigue-resistant motor units. In contrast to volitional contractions, when stimulating muscle electrically, motor units are activated synchronously and recover from fatigue only during the times when the stimulation is absent. During the application of NMES, muscle fatigue must be monitored and can be addressed by increasing the rest time between contractions.

Research into the benefits of NMES to strengthen muscle has produced conflicting results. For example, Delitto et al (1988) and Snyder-Mackler et al (1995) found that NMES is superior to volitional exercise in regaining strength after ACL reconstruction, while Paternostro-Sluga et al (1999) found no difference in the same population. Several methodological factors may account for the discrepancy in results. Delitto et al (1988) studied 20 patients who had undergone ACL reconstruction within 6 weeks of participation, half of whom received NMES with burst-modulated AC (2500 Hz, triangle wave form, 50 bursts per second [bps], 15 s on, 50 s off). The other half of the sample performed volitional exercise. Patients in both groups contracted their quadriceps femoris and hamstring muscles simultaneously during rehabilitation, 5 days a week for a 3-week period. Stimulation amplitude was increased to maximal tolerance but no net extension torque was generated due to the activity of the antagonist hamstrings. The voluntary exercise group also performed 15 cocontractions of their quadriceps and hamstrings at a maximal level with no net extension torque, holding for 15 s and resting for 50 s. The NMES group demonstrated greater isometric strength gains than the volitional exercise group, 6 weeks after surgery (Delitto et al 1988). Snyder-Mackler et al (1991) reported similar results in a group of patients following ACL reconstruction that received NMES and volitional exercise or performed volitional exercise alone. Following 4 weeks of treatment, the NMES with volitional exercise group demonstrated significant strength gains in the quadriceps (Snyder-Mackler et al 1991).

In contrast to the previous findings, Paternostro-Sluga et al (1999) studied the effect of NMES on quadriceps strength in persons who had undergone an ACL reconstruction or repair. Three groups were evaluated: group 1 – NMES and exercise; group 2 – TENS and exercise; group 3 – control group (exercise alone); and NMES was supplied by a battery-powered, portable muscle stimulator with rectangular, monophasic, square wave pulses, daily for 6 weeks. The regimen included two different sets of parameters: set 1 (30 Hz, 5 s on with a 1 s ramp, 15 s off time) was repeated four times and set 2 (50 Hz, 10 s on with a 2 s ramp, 50 s off) was repeated twice. The pulse duration was 200 μs and the amplitude was set to perform a 'strong muscle contraction'. Subjects performed 12 repetitions in each set. The TENS group received analgesic stimulation (biphasic rectangular wave form at 220 µs and 100 Hz, sensory perception, treatment time was 30 min). The results indicated no statistical significant difference between the three groups (Paternostro-Sluga et al 1999). Because a battery-operated portable stimulator was used, it is likely that an appropriate dose of electrical stimulation was not provided. Studies have shown that NMES induced contractions that are below 50% of the volitional force are inadequate to produce strength gains (Snyder-Mackler et al 1994) and portable muscle stimulators may be unable to produce muscle contractions in the quadriceps femoris muscles that are in a therapeutic range. Snyder-Mackler et al (1994) studied patients following ACL reconstruction who received NMES through clinical, line-powered stimulators and portable, battery-powered stimulators. They found that on average, the patients who used the portable stimulators did so with an average current output that was 89% of the capacity of the stimulator and experienced a greater number of contractions than those in the clinical stimulator group, but that the training intensity of contraction was only 8.9% of the volitional force. Those in the portable stimulator group showed no correlation between the current amplitude and strength gains suggesting that portable stimulators may not be appropriate for strengthening the quadriceps femoris muscles. Portable units may be effective, however, in generating adequate force in smaller muscles in which NMES is warranted (Snyder-Mackler et al 1994).

Clinically, NMES for quadriceps strengthening is performed with an isometric contraction of the leg. The parameters used to achieve maximal results include pulse duration of 400–600 µs, stimulation frequency of 50–100 Hz intensity, and at least 50% of the maximal volitional isometric contraction. Electrodes are placed over the vastus medialis oblique (VMO) and just distal to the anterior superior iliac spine (ASIS) on the rectus femoris and 10 contractions are elicited for 15 s on and with a 50 s rest period to achieve desired strength gains (Fig. 13.4). When using burst-modulated current, 400–600 µs pulse durations are achieved with a carrier frequency of approximately 1600–2500 Hz and the frequency is set to 50–100 bps.

Many investigations of NMES have involved the quadriceps femoris muscles, however, other muscles can benefit from NMES for strengthening. Starring (1991) showed subjective improvement in L5/S1 stability after 2 weeks of NMES with burst-modulated AC. The stimulation parameters were 2500 Hz AC with a burst frequency of 75 bps, 15 s on and 50 s off, and with the electrodes placed over the erector spinae. Kahanovitz et al (1987) performed a randomized, controlled, clinical trial to investigate strength gains of the low back musculature with electrical stimulation. One hundred

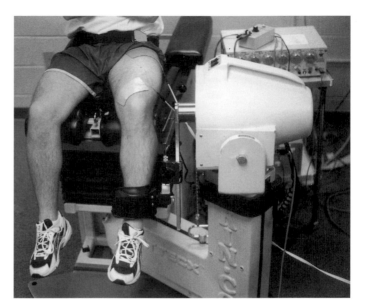

Figure 13.4 Electrode placement for neuromuscular electrical stimulation for strengthening the quadriceps femoris muscles.

and seventeen healthy women were randomly assigned to one of four groups: group 1 – low frequency electrical stimulation and exercise; group 2 – medium frequency electrical stimulation and exercise; group 3 – exercise only; and group 4 – control. Low frequency electrical stimulation included the following parameters: amplitude 0–100 mA; voltage 45 V; frequency 35 Hz; duration 300 µs; interpulse width 25 µs; and waveform biphasic symmetrical balanced rectangular pulse. Medium frequency electrical stimulation included: amplitude 25 mA; voltage 0–105 V; frequency 300 Hz; duration 400–600 µs; and waveform monophasic modified spike wave. Both forms of electrical stimulation were found to significantly influence back muscle endurance compared to the control group. Low frequency electrical stimulation and exercises were shown to significantly increase isokinetic back muscle strength compared to the control and medium frequency groups (Kahanovitz et al 1987).

Electrical stimulation parameters for NMES include pulsed DC or burst-modulated AC current with a pulse duration of 200–1000 µs, and a frequency of 30–75 pulses or bursts per second (Nalty 2001). Isometric contractions are typically generated for 10–15 s followed by 50–120 s of rest to minimize fatigue (Selkowitz 1989) for a total of 10 contractions. The stimulus intensity is gradually increased to the therapeutic level over several seconds to help patient tolerance, however, the ramp time should be added to the total contraction time to ensure appropriate duration of the contraction at an appropriate level. Electrodes are typically placed over the motor point of the muscle and the intensity of stimulation is increased until the force reaches at least 50% of the force generated

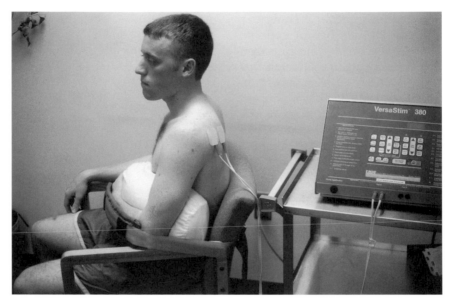

Figure 13.5 Electrode placement for neuromuscular electrical stimulation for strengthening the rotator cuff muscles.

volitionally. Patients should receive the NMES treatment at least three times per week to maximize strength gains (Robinson & Snyder-Mackler 1995). Patient positioning depends on the muscle group to be treated. For example, once precautions following surgery have been removed, NMES can be used to restore rotator cuff strength by stabilizing the arm against the side of the body using a belt or sheet. In the case of stimulating the supraspinatus, placing the electrodes near the spine of the scapula helps minimize upper trapezius recruitment (Fig. 13.5). Amplitude is increased to maximum tolerance until a strong contraction is elicited.

When strengthening lumbar paraspinal muscles with NMES, the pelvis must be stabilized to the table and the spine placed in slight flexion to avoid lumbar hyperextension when the stimulation is applied. (Fig.13.6).

The success of NMES treatments depends on correct preparation of the patient by the clinician. It is essential to help patients tolerate very high force contractions in order to produce strength gains because the intensity of the NMES elicited contractions correlates positively with strength gains (Snyder-Mackler et al 1994). Patients rarely refuse the treatment due to discomfort if they realize its benefits. Strategies to improve patient tolerance include increasing the rest time between contractions, reducing the frequency of stimulation, increasing the ramp-up time and, if available, changing the shape of the waveform. Delitto & Rose (1986) found that although

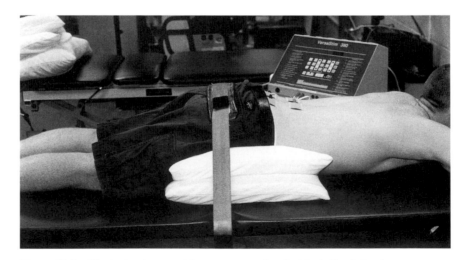

Figure 13.6 Electrode placement for neuromuscular electrical stimulation for strengthening the lumbar paraspinal muscles.

no consistent differences in level of comfort were found between NMES with triangular, sine, or square wave pulses, individual preferences did exist. Clinicians may use this information as evidence to the patient that use of a different waveform may make the NMES treatment more tolerable.

REDUCED TISSUE EXTENSIBILITY

Another aspect of sport and exercise injury that affects the progress in rehabilitation is that of reduced tissue extensibility that may impair joint range of motion. Superficial heat and the thermal effects of continuous US are commonly thought to affect tissue extensibility and improve range of motion.

Although superficial heat is used prior to range of motion activities, research has shown no effect in improving range of motion when used in an athletic population. Henricson et al (1984) studied the use of an electric heating pad for 20 min at 43°C on the posterior-lateral thigh. The use of heat and stretch did not significantly increase hip flexion, abduction, or external rotation. Similarly, Taylor et al (1995) looked at the effect of heat on hamstring length. A 77°C hot pack surrounded by seven dry terry cloth towels for 20 min was used. No significant increase in hamstring flexibility was noted. These studies provide evidence that disputes the use of superficial heat prior to stretching as a way to increase range of motion in an athletic population (Henricson et al 1984, Taylor et al 1995).

In contrast, continuous US, with its thermal effect, is used to improve collagen extensibility by affecting the viscoelastic properties of collagen tissue (Enwemeka 1989, Jackson et al 1991). The 'heat and stretch' technique is often used to improve muscular flexibility (Reed et al 2000). Muscle tissue typically needs to be heated to between 39 and 47°C to increase extensibility (Gersten 1955). Several investigations have demonstrated increased tissue extensibility of the human calf after application of continuous US (Draper & Ricard 1995, Wessling et al 1987). Draper & Ricard (1995) suggested that the stretch must be applied within 3 min of the application of US to achieve the maximum benefits.

TREATMENT OF TISSUE DAMAGE

ELECTRICAL STIMULATION FOR FRACTURE REPAIR

Bone has piezoelectric properties in which tension creates positive charge and compression creates negative charge.

Therefore, electrical stimulation can be beneficial in promoting fracture repair (Uhl 1989, Evans et al 2001).

Direct current (DC) and pulsed electromagnetic fields (PEMF) have been used in promoting fracture repair. Three types of electrical stimulation applications are used for bone healing: invasive, percutaneous (semi-invasive), and non-invasive (Evans et al 2001). Each has advantages and disadvantages and are chosen based on fracture location, complication factors, and patient compliance (Evans et al 2001).

Both DC (Kahanovitz & Arnoczky 1990, Meril 1994) and PEMF (deHass et al 1980, Marks 2000) have been shown to assist bony healing. Application of PEMF is non-invasive and involves a coil worn over the fracture site for at least 10 h a day for maximum benefit. The restriction on daily activities affects compliance with the treatment and may be an important factor in choosing this modality (Patterson 2000, Uhl 1989). PEMF can be effective when displacement is less than 1 mm, no signs of synovial pseudoarthrosis are evident, and no signs of intracarpal collapse in the case of scaphoid non-union are present (Uhl 1989).

The semi-invasive electrical stimulation units are used to deliver DC. The cathode is anchored to the bone and a self-adherent anode electrode is secured to the skin, which also houses the power source. The anodal electrode is replaced daily and a non-weightbearing cast is applied to prevent motion at the fracture site as well as to reduce tension on the electrode cables. This system requires monitoring of the power source, wire connections, and for the possibility of chemical effects associated with DC on the skin under the anode (Evans et al 2001).

Fully invasive units have been utilized in conjunction with spinal fusions to enhance bone formation (Kahanovitz & Arnoczky 1990, Marks 2000, Meril 1994) or when compliance is a concern (Uhl 1989). The electrodes are implanted at the fracture/fusion site and a battery pack is located subcutaneously. Once fusion is achieved, the battery pack may be removed under local anesthesia. The electrodes can remain in the healed fracture site (Uhl 1989).

LASER

Laser is electromagnetic energy found in the visible or infrared spectrums and is used to promote tissue healing. Three properties differentiate laser from other light sources: monochromaticity, coherence and collimated beam. Monochromatic laser contains a single wavelength. Coherent means single wavelengths oscillate in phase. Collimated beams indicate a minimal scattering of photons. Lasers that are used clinically have a frequency of less than 60 milliwatts so the effects are non-thermal. Rather, the effects of laser are due to its ability to alter cellular mechanisms, such as increased phagocytosis or facilitation of collagen synthesis (Basford 1995). Two typical lasers that are used are the helium-neon (HeNe) and the galium-arsenide (GaAs). Wavelengths typically range from 820 to 904 nm and the dose of the treatment is usually between 1–4 J/cm^2 (Basford 1995).

There are two uses of laser in sports medicine; promotion of tissue healing and pain management. However, much of the literature published on laser treatments is anecdotal. There have been few randomized clinical controlled studies on laser (Basford 1995), therefore, the use of laser in sports medicine has not gained acceptance and the Federal Drug Administration has not approved its use in the USA (Basford 1995).

Possible benefits of laser on wound healing may be due to the lasers' effect on stimulation of capillary growth and the formation of granulation tissue (Basford 1995). Mester et al (1985) cited multiple studies of the use of laser in the healing of ulcers and non-healing wounds, but the limitations of the research involve poor randomization, lack of measurements by blinded observers, and lack of control groups. Studies in which blinded researchers were used, found no significant difference in the healing of venous stasis ulcers in response to treatment with HeNe lasers (Lundeberg & Malm 1991, Santoianni et al 1984).

The use of laser in the athletic population has focused predominantly on pain relief. Basford et al (1998) attempted to determine the effectiveness of low-intensity laser therapy on the treatment of pain control for plantar fasciitis. They used a 30 milliwatt continuous wave 0.83 μm GaAlAs diode laser three times a week for 4 weeks and found no statistical difference in pain level and duration of painful walking upon awakening, a common symptom with plantar fasciitis (Basford et al 1998). Similarly, Vecchio et al (1993) investigated the effect of 3-Joule laser treatments using a 30 milliwatt 830 nm GaAlAs diode twice a week for 8 weeks on rotator cuff tendinitis. No significant differences in pain, range of motion or strength were found between the group treated with laser and that treated with the sham laser. Vasseljen et al (1992) showed improvement of pain and strength of lateral epicondylitis with eight treatments of 3.5 J/cm^2 laser using an 18 milliwatt pulsed 904 nm diode. However, the authors state that the benefits of laser alone would not be as great without other forms of therapy (Vasseljen et al 1992). Lowe et al (1997) investigated the effects of low-level laser on ischemic pain at Erb's point, the junction of the midclavicle and sternocleidomastoid muscle. This area is easily irradiated because nerve trunks from the brachial plexus are most superficial at this point. They found no significant decrease in pain using a GaAlAs 830 nm diode for either 5 or 30 s (Lowe et al 1997).

Some possible precautions to the use of laser are pregnancy, cancer, acute hemorrhages, placement over growth plates, and photosensitive skin. Other risks of laser center on the ability of laser to destroy tissue (Basford 1995).

All lasers used in laser therapy are not the same. The possible benefits of one type of diode laser may not yield the same benefits of another diode (Basford 1995). Having many types of lasers available makes comparisons of the study's results difficult. Depth of target tissue can affect the results. The use of laser currently needs more research to support its use in sports medicine when compared to other widely used modalities in sports medicine.

HYPERBARIC OXYGEN

Hyperbaric oxygen (HBO) involves the application of 100% oxygenated air at high pressures (2–3 times atmospheric pressure) to patients who are enclosed in special tanks. The principle behind HBO is that by delivering oxygen under high pressure, alveolar oxygen pressure is increased, thus producing a rise in plasma oxygen content, which results in enhanced tissue oxygen delivery. Studies have shown that when pressures are twice that of atmospheric pressure, blood oxygen content can increase by 2.5% and the oxygenation of local tissue can increase ten-fold (Bassett & Bennett 1977, Jain 1995).

HBO has been useful in decreasing edema, which should facilitate healing by improving oxygenation to the damaged tissues. HBO has been shown to promote granulation tissue formation, revascularization, and epithelialization (Jain 1995, Lavan & Hunt 1990). However, a recent study by Fabian et al (2000) on full-thickness wound healing in rabbits found that HBO therapy did not significantly improve the rate of healing. Only recently has the research focused on the use of HBO in sports medicine (Best et al 1998, Borromeo et al 1997, Staples et al 1999). The use of HBO early after injury (i.e. in the first 4–6 h) has shown the best results for improving the effects of tissue injury (Hunt & Pai 1972, Jain 1995).

Borromeo et al (1997) looked at the effect of HBO on the time to recovery, and ankle range of motion, after acute ankle sprains. HBO had no effect on decreasing the recovery time or increasing the range of motion of the ankle. The time taken to administer HBO may limit its use in sports medicine because typical treatment duration is approximately 90 min. HBO treatment is contraindicated in patients who have a fever, upper respiratory infection, or predisposition to a tension pneumothorax (Staples & Clement 1996). The continued use of HBO needs further prospective randomized trials to demonstrate and elucidate its positive effects on the sports population.

SUMMARY

Tissue damage is associated with most athletic injury. The damage can range from localized cellular damage to ruptured tendon or fracture. The use of electrophysical agents may help to facilitate healing of damaged tissues by addressing inflammation, edema, pain, and loss of muscle strength and function due to disuse or immobilization. This chapter presents the principles of electrophysical agents that are common in sports medicine. The benefits and uses of each electrophysical agent must be carefully evaluated when deciding appropriate intervention strategies.

REFERENCES

Alon G, 1991 Principles of electrical stimulation. In: Nelson R L, Currier D P (eds) Clinical electrotherapy. Appleton and Lange, Norwalk, p 35–101

Bare A C, McAnaw M B, Pritchard A E et al 1996 Phonophoretic delivery of 10% hydrocortisone through the epidermis of humans as determined by serum cortisol concentrations. Physical Therapy 76:738–745

Basford B R 1995 Low intensity laser: still not an established clinical tool. Lasers in Surgery and Medicine 16:331–342

Basford B R, Malanga G A, Krause D A, Harmsen W S 1998 A randomized controlled evaluation of low-intensity laser therapy: plantar fasciitis. Archives of Physical Medicine 79:249–253

Bassett B E, Bennett P B 1977 Introduction to the physical and physiological bases of hyperbaric therapy. In: Davis J C, Hunt T K (eds) Hyperbaric oxygen therapy. Undersea Medical Society, Bethesda, p 11–24

Bassett F H 3rd, Kirkpatrick J S, Engelhardt D L et al 1992 Cryotherapy-induced nerve injury. American Journal of Sports Medicine 20:516–518

Benson H A, McElnay J C, Harland R 1989 Use of ultrasound to enhance percutaneous absorption of benzydamine. Physical Therapy 69:113–118

Bertolucci L E 1982 Introduction of antiinflammatory drugs by iontophoresis. Double blind study. Journal of Orthopaedic and Sports Physical Therapy 4:103–108

Bertoti D B 2000 Electrical stimulation: a reflection on current clinical practices. Assistive Technology 12(1):21–32

Best T M, Loitz-Ramage B, Corr D T et al 1998 Hyperbaric oxygen in the treatment of acute muscle stretch injuries. American Journal of Sports Medicine 26:367–371

Borromeo C N, Ryan J L, Marchetto P A et al 1997 Hyperbaric oxygen therapy for acute ankle sprains. American Journal of Sports Medicine 25:619–624

Braun B L 1987 Treatment of acute anterior disk displacement in the temporomandibular joint: a case study. Physical Therapy 67(8):1234–1236

Byl N 1995 The use of ultrasound as an enhancer for transcutaneous drug delivery: phonophoresis. Physical Therapy 75(6):539–553

Cameron M H, Monroe L G 1992 Relative transmission of ultrasound by media customarily used for phonophoresis. Physical Therapy 72:142–148

Christie A D, Willoughby G L 1990 The effect of interferential therapy on swelling following open reduction and internal fixation of ankle fractures. Physiotherapy Theory and Practice 6:3–7

Ciccone C D, Leggin B G, Callamaro J J 1991 Effects of ultrasound and trolamine salicylate phonophoresis on delayed-onset muscle soreness. Physical Therapy 71:666–678

Crago P E, Peckham P H, Thrope G B 1980 Modulation of muscle force by recruitment during intramuscular stimulation. IEEE Transactions on Biomedical Engineering 27:679–684

Cramp A F, Gilsen C, Lowe A S, Walsh D M 2000 The effect of high- and low-frequency transcutaneous electrical nerve stimulation upon cutaneous blood flow and skin temperature in healthy subjects. Clinical Physiology 20:150–157

deHass W G, Watson J, Morrison D M 1980 Non-invasive treatment of ununited fractures of the tibia using electrical stimulation. Journal of Bone and Joint Surgery (Br) 62–B:465–470

Delacerda F G 1982 A comparative study of three methods of treatment for shoulder girdle myofascial syndrome. Journal of Orthopaedic and Sports Medicine 4:51–54

Delitto A, Rose S J 1986 Comparative comfort of three waveforms used in electrically elicited quadriceps femoris contractions. Physical Therapy 66:1704–1707

Delitto A, Rose S J, McKowen J M, Lehman R C 1988 Electrical stimulation versus voluntary exercise in strengthening thigh musculature after anterior cruciate ligament surgery. Physical Therapy 68:660–663

Draper D O, Ricard M D 1995 Muscle following 3 MHz Ultrasound: the stretching window revealed. Journal of Athletic Training 30:304–307

Enwemeka C S 1989 The effects of therapeutic ultrasound on tendon healing. A biomechanical study. American Journal of Physical Medicine and Rehabilitation 68:283–287

Eston R, Peters D 1999 Effects of cold water immersion on the symptoms of exercise induced muscle damage. Journal of Sports Sciences 17:231–238

Evans T A, Ingersoll C, Knight K et al 1995 Agility following the application of cold therapy. Journal of Athletic Training 30:231–234

Evans R, Foltz D, Foltz K 2001 Electrical stimulation with bone and wound healing. Clinics in Podiatric Medicine and Surgery 18:79–95

Fabian T S, Kauffman H J, Lett E D et al 2000 The evaluation of subatmospheric pressure and hyperbaric oxygen in ischemic full-thickness wound healing. The American Surgeon 66:1136–1143

Gersten J 1955 Effect of ultrasound on tendon extensibility. American Journal of Physical Medicine 34:362–369

Green T, Refshauge K, Crosbie J et al 2001 A randomized controlled trial of a passive accessory joint mobilization on acute ankle inversion sprains. Physical Therapy 81:984–994

Greenberg R S 1972 The effects of hot packs and exercise on local blood flow. Physical Therapy 52:273–278

Griffin J W, Newsome L S, Stralka S W et al 1990 Reduction of chronic posttraumatic hand edema: a comparison of high voltage pulsed current, intermittent pneumatic compression, and placebo treatments. Physical Therapy 70:279–86

Harris P R 1982 Iontophoresis: clinical research in musculoskeletal inflammatory conditions. Journal of Orthopaedics and Sports Physical Therapy 4:109–112

Henricson A S, Fredrikson K, Persson I et al 1984 The effect of heat and stretching on the range of hip motion. Journal of Orthopaedic and Sports Physical Therapy 6:110–115

Hillebrandt F A, Houtz S J 1956 Mechanisms of muscle training in man: experimental demonstration of the overload principle. Physical Therapy Review 38:319–322

Hunt T K, Pai M P 1972 The effect of varying ambient oxygen tensions on wound metabolism and collagen synthesis. Surgery Gynecology Obstetrics 135:561–567

Ingerdand H J, Morgan B J 1995 Effect of interference current on forearm vascular resistance in asymptomatic humans. Physical Therapy 75:306–312

Ingersoll C D, Knight K L, Merrick M A 1992 Sensory perception of the foot and ankle following therapeutic applications of heat and cold. Journal of Athletic Training 27:231–234

Jackson B A, Schwane J A, Starcher B C 1991 Effect of ultrasound therapy on the repair of Achilles tendon injuries in rats. Medicine and Science in Sports and Exercise 23:171–176

Jain K K 1995 Textbook of hyperbaric medicine , 2nd edn. Toronto. Hogrefe and Huber, Toronto

Japour C, Vohra R, Vohra P et al 1999 Management of heel pain syndrome with acetic acid iontophoresis. Journal of the American Podiatric Medical Association 89:251–257

Jensen J E, Conn R R, Hazelrigg G et al 1985 The use of transcutaneous neural stimulation and isokinetic testing in arthroscopic knee surgery. American Journal of Sports Medicine 13:27–33

Kahanovitz N, Arnoczky S P 1990 The efficacy of direct current electrical stimulation to enhance canine spinal fusions. Clinical Orthopaedics and Related Research 251:295–299

Kahanovitz N, Nordin M, Verderame R et al 1987 Normal trunk muscle strength and endurance in women and the effect of exercises and electrical stimulation. Part 2: comparative analysis of electrical stimulation and exercises to increase trunk muscle strength and endurance. Spine 12:112–118

Kandel E R, Schwartz J H, Jessell T M 1995 Essentials of neural science and behavior. Appleton and Lange, Stamford, CT

Karunakara R G, Lephart S M, Pincivero D M 1999 Changes in forearm blood flow during single and intermittent cold application. Journal of Orthopaedic and Sports Physical Therapy 29:177–180

Klaiman M D, Shrader J A, Danoff J V et al 1998 Phonophoresis versus ultrasound in the treatment of common musculoskeletal conditions. Medicine and Science in Sports and Exercise 30:1349–1355

Knight K L 1995 Cryotherapy in sports injury management. Human Kinetics, Champaign, IL

Kots Y M, Babkin D, Timtsenko N 1977 Canadian-Soviet exchange symposium on electrostimulation of skeletal muscles. Concordia University, Montreal, Quebec, Canada, December, p 6–15

Lark M R, Gangarosa L P 1990 Iontophoresis: an effective modality for the treatment of inflammatory disorders of the temporomandibular joint and myofascial pain. Cranio 8:108–119

Lavan F B, Hunt T K 1990 Oxygen and wound healing. Clinical Plastic Surgery 17(3):463–472

Lehman J D, Delateur B J 1990 Therapeutic heat. In: Lehman J F (ed) Therapeutic heat and cold. Williams and Wilkins, Baltimore

Lehman J D, Brunner G D, Stow R W 1958 Pain threshold measurements after therapeutic application of ultrasound, microwaves, and infrared. Archives of Physical Medicine 39:560–565

Levy A S, Lintner S 1997 Penetration of cryotherapy in treatment after shoulder arthroscopy. Arthroscopy 13:461–464

Lowe A S, McDowell B C, Walsh D M et al 1997 Failure to demonstrate any hypoalgesic effect of low intensity laser irradiation (830 nm) of Erb's point upon experimental ischemic pain in humans. Lasers in Surgery and Medicine 20:69–76

Lundeberg T, Malm M 1991 Low-power HeNe laser treatment of venous leg ulcers. Annals of Plastic Surgery 27:537–539

Manal T J, Snyder-Mackler L 1997 Electrotherapy for pain management: high intensity stimulation shows promising results. Rehabilitation Management 65:56–57

Marks R A 2000 Spine fusion for discogenic low back pain: outcomes in patients treated with or without pulsed electromagnetic field stimulation. Advances in Therapy 17(2):57–67

Mendel F, Fish D 1993 New perspectives in edema control via electrical stimulation. Journal of Athletic Training 28:63–74

Meril A J 1994 Direct current stimulation of allograft in anterior and posterior lumbar interbody fusions. Spine 19:2393–2398

Mester E, Mester A F, Mester A 1985 The biomedical effects of laser application. Lasers in Surgery and Medicine 5:31–39

Michlovitz S L 1996 Thermal agents in rehabilitation, 3rd edn. F.A. Davis Company, Philadelphia

Myerson M S, Fisher R T, Burgess A R et al 1986 Fracture dislocations of the tarsometatarsal joints. End results correlated with pathology and treatment. Foot and Ankle 6:225–242

Nalty T 2001 Electrotherapy: clinical procedures manual. McGraw Hill, New York

Nussbaum E, Rush P, Disenhaus L 1990 The effects of interferential therapy on swelling following open reduction internal fixation of ankle fractures. Physiotherapy Canada 76:803–807

Ohkoshi Y, Ohkoshi M, Nagasaki S et al 1999 The effect of cryotherapy on intraarticular temperature and postoperative care after anterior cruciate ligament reconstruction. American Journal of Sports Medicine 27:357–362

Oziomek R S, Perrin D H, Herold D A et al 1991 Effects of phonophoresis on serum salicylate levels. Medicine and Science in Sports and Exercise 23:397–401

Palmer J E, Knight K L 1996 Ankle and thigh skin surface temperature changes with repeated ice pack application. Journal of Athletic Training 31:319–323

Paternostro-Sluga T, Fialka C, Alacamliogliu Y et al 1999 Neuromuscular electrical stimulation after anterior cruciate ligament surgery. Clinical Orthopaedics and Related Research 368:166–175

Patterson M 2000 What's the buzz on external bone growth stimulators? Nursing 30(6):44–45

Picker R I 1988 Current trends: low-volt pulsed microamp stimulation, Part I. Clinical Management in Physical Therapy 9:10–14

Picker R I 1989 Current trends: low-volt pulsed microamp stimulation, Part II. Clinical Management in Physical Therapy 9:28–33

Reed B, Ashikaga T, Fleming B et al 2000 Effects of ultrasound and stretch on knee ligament extensibility. Journal of Sports and Orthopaedic Physical Therapy 30:341–347

Rivenburgh D W 1992 Physical modalities in the treatment of tendon injuries. Clinics in Sports Medicine 11:645–659

Robinson A J, Snyder-Mackler L (eds) 1995 Clinical electrophysiology: electrotherapy and electrophysiologic testing, 2nd edn. Williams and Wilkins, Baltimore

Santoianni P, Monfrecola G, Martellotta D et al 1984 Inadequate effect of helium-neon laser on venous leg ulcers. Photodermatology 1:245–249

Schmidt W 1993 Iontophoresis. Is it drug delivery or electrotherapy? Rehabilitation and Therapy Products Review Sept/Oct:15–20

Selkowitz D 1989 High frequency electrical stimulation in muscle strengthening. American Journal of Sports Medicine 17:103–111

Shin S M, Choi J K 1997 Effect of indomethacin phonophoresis on the relief of temporomandibular joint pain. The Journal of Craniomandibular Practice 15:345–348

Snyder-Mackler L, Ladin Z, Schepsis A et al 1991 Electrical stimulation of the thigh muscles after reconstruction of the anterior cruciate ligament. Effects of electrically elicited contractions of the quadriceps femoris and hamstring muscles on gait and strength of the thigh muscles. Journal of Bone and Joint Surgery (Am) 73-A:1025–1036

Snyder-Mackler L, Delitto A, Stralka S et al 1994 Use of electrical stimulation to enhance recovery of quadriceps femoris muscle force production in patients following anterior cruciate ligament reconstruction. Physical Therapy 74:901–907

Snyder-Mackler L, Delitto A, Bailey S et al 1995 Strength of the quadriceps femoris muscle and functional recovery after reconstruction of the anterior cruciate ligament. Journal of Bone and Joint Surgery (Am) 77-A:1166–1173

Staples J R, Clement D B 1996 Hyperbaric oxygen chambers and the treatment of sports injuries. Sports Medicine 22:219–227

Staples J R, Clement D B, Taunton J E et al 1999 Effects of hyperbaric oxygen on a human model of injury. American Journal of Sports Medicine 27:600–605

Starring D 1991 The use of electrical stimulation and exercise for strengthening lumbar musculature: a case study. Journal of Orthopaedic and Sports Physical Therapy 14(2):61–64

Surbey G D, Andrew G M, Cervenko F W et al 1984 Effects of naloxone on exercise performance. Journal of Applied Physiology 57:674–679

Taylor B F, Warning C A, Brashear T A 1995 The effects of therapeutic application of heat or cold followed by static stretch on hamstring muscle length. Journal of Orthopaedic and Sports Physical Therapy 21:283–286

Taylor K, Newton R A, Personius W J et al 1987 Effects of interferential current stimulation for treatment of subjects with recurrent jaw pain. Physical Therapy 67:346–350

Taylor K, Fish D, Mendel F et al 1992 Effect of electrically induced muscle contractions on posttraumatic edema formation in frog hind limbs. Physical Therapy 72:127–132

Taylor K, Mendel F, Fish D et al 1997 Effect of high-voltage pulsed current and alternating current on macromolecular leakage in hamster cheek pouch microcirculation. Physical Therapy 77:1729–1740

Thornton R, Mendel F, Fish D 1998 Effects of electrical stimulation on edema formation in different strains of rats. Physical Therapy 78:386–394

Thorsson O, Lilja B, Ahlgren L et al 1985 The effect of local cold application on intramuscular blood flow at rest and after running. Medicine and Science in Sports and Exercise 17:710–713

Uhl R 1989 The use of electricity in bone healing. Orthopaedic Review 18:1045–1050

Vasseljen O, Hoeg N, Kjeldstad B et al 1992 Low level laser versus placebo in the treatment of tennis elbow. Scandanavian Journal of Rehabilitation Medicine 24:37–42

Vecchio P, Cave M, King V et al 1993 Doubleblind study of the effectiveness of low level laser treatment of rotator cuff tendonitis. British Journal of Rheumatology 32:740–742

Washington L L, Gibson S J, Helme R D 2000 Age-related differences in the endogenous analgesic response to repeated cold water immersion in human volunteers. Pain 89:89–96

Wessling K C, DeVane D A, Hylton C R 1987 Effects of static stretch versus static stretch and ultrasound combined on triceps surae muscle extensibility in healthy women. Physical Therapy 67:674–679

Zemke J E, Anderson J C, Guion W K et al 1998 Intramuscular temperature responses in the human leg to two forms of cryotherapy: ice massage and ice bag. Journal of Orthopaedic and Sports Physical Therapy 27:301–307

Regional sport and exercise injury management

14

Spine

Henry Wajswelner

INTRODUCTION

The spine is one of the most challenging and problematic regions of sports injury. Serious traumatic injuries to the spine, especially catastrophic fractures or dislocations of the cervical spine, are rare, but are the most feared of all sports injuries. Most injuries to the spine in sports, however, are due to repetitive trauma to soft tissues and are not serious. The spine can be conditioned over time with regular exercise and sport but it is not very adaptable in the short term, and does not cope well with rapidly applied extremes of motion and force. Often the combination of a sedentary job or study and athletic pursuits, without adequate stretching and warm-up in transition from work or study to sport, is a source of problems. Specific sports or exercise-induced injuries to the spine present in recognizable patterns (e.g. defects in the pars interarticularis in the younger athlete, disk rupture in the adult, and degenerative spondylosis in the older athlete).

While back and neck pain is common in the general population and regular exercise is promoted as preventative for back pain, athletes are not immune to the type of spinal pain and injury that happens generally. However, there are very specific spinal injuries in sports, caused by faulty technique, poor motor control or poor biomechanics that require much more detailed thought and rehabilitation. These overuse injuries are much more difficult to resolve, and it is not uncommon to find chronic back pain causing prolonged disability in the athlete or a premature end to a sporting career.

While athletes usually respond well to manual physical therapy such as massage, stretching, mobilization, manipulation and strengthening exercises for acute spinal injuries, motor control of the trunk and spinal segments is a vital aspect to management of chronic spinal conditions in sport. Evidence reviewed by Hodges (2000) suggests that when spinal pain is present, the strategies used by the central nervous system (CNS) to control trunk muscles may be altered. The expertise of the sports physical therapist in optimization of motor control of stability is a crucial part of a sports medicine team approach to an athlete's spinal problem.

SPORT-SPECIFIC APPLIED ANATOMY

The anatomical structures subject to sports and exercise-related injury in the spine include the bone, supporting ligaments, and articular, neural, muscular and fascial tissues. There are patterns of injury to certain structures within each region in certain sports that will be revealed by detailed subjective and physical examination.

BONY ANATOMY

The spinal column is made up of 7 cervical, 12 thoracic, 5 lumbar, and 5 sacral vertebrae. The skull is supported by the atlas (C1), and the 5 sacral vertebrae (which are usually fused as one) are anchored to the pelvis. All of these structures provide stability and mobility of motions, while protecting the spinal cord. A typical vertebra has a vertebral body; a ring which surrounds the spinal cord, created by pedicles, transverse processes, and lamina bilaterally, and a spinous process posteriorly.

The disks between the vertebrae are composed of an outer annulus fibrosis and an inner nucleus pulposus. The annulus is the outer section of each disk, composed of a sheet arrangement of lamellae, arranged concentrically for additional support. The annulus contains type I collagen to resist the tensile forces that the spinal motions create. The inner portion of the disks is the nucleus pulposis, which consists of 70% water, although this varies with age. The nucleus exerts a preload on the annulus, allowing the disk to be ready to accept forces, motions, and it deforms in all directions as the spine moves. The nucleus contains type II collagen to resist the compressive forces of spinal motion.

At the thoracic vertebrae, 12 pairs of ribs protect the visceral organs. The ribs also limit the mobility of this region of the spine.

LIGAMENTOUS ANATOMY

The anterior longitudinal ligament (ALL) attaches to the anterolateral surface of the annulus and disks, extending from C2 into the sacrum. From the occiput to C2, it is named the anterior atlantoaxial ligament. The posterior longitudinal ligament (PLL) attaches to the posterior surface of the annulus and disks, extending from C2 to the sacrum. From the occiput to C2, it is named the

tectoral membrane. The ligamentum flavum (LF) extends from C2 to the sacrum, and fibers connect the posterior surface of the vertebral canal and the lamina of the vertebrae above. The ALL, PLL, and the lumbar portion of LF, are made up of superficial fibers, are long, and bridge several vertebrae, while the deep fibers of the ligament run only from one vertebra to the adjacent vertebrae. The ALL and PLL both attach to the disk at the annulus, and can be affected by disk problems.

The interspinous ligament is segmental, extending from the spinous process of a vertebra to the spinous process of the adjacent vertebrae, and is strongest in the lumbar region. The supraspinous ligament extends from the tip of a spinous process to the tip of a spinous process of an adjacent vertebra, and extends from approximately C7 to L3–4. Above C7, the supraspinous ligament becomes the thick, highly elastic ligamentum nuchae. The intertransverse ligament is also segmental, extending from the transverse process of one vertebra to the adjacent vertebrae; it is most prominent in the lumbar spine.

NERVOUS ANATOMY

Two adjacent vertebrae create an intervertebral foramen, through which spinal nerves exit the canal to innervate muscles and cutaneous sensation. A compression, an osteophyte, or a spondylolysis can compress this opening, interfering with function, and causing the athlete pain.

MUSCULAR ANATOMY

The muscles of the back and spine, commonly referred to as the paraspinals, extend segmentally, the entire length of the spinal column. The muscles of the cervical region, the suboccipitals, stabilize and hold the skull upright. The muscles of the thoracic region add stability to the ribs, and assist with respiration. The muscles of the lumbar region assist with trunk motions, holding the body upright, and organ protection. Injury to these muscles causes pain and may cause loss of function or mobility.

SUBJECTIVE EXAMINATION OF THE SPINE IN THE ATHLETE

The Maitland method of spinal assessment (Maitland et al 2001), which is one approach in guiding the subjective interview with the patient, is suitable for a thorough and meaningful examination of athletes and is a method which lends itself to the systematic recording of findings and treatment outcomes (Table 14.1). Athletes should be

Table 14.1   Subjective examination of the spine in athletes (Modified from Maitland et al 2001)

Question	Purpose	Implications
Sport and level of participation	Likely level of fitness, extent of training and competition intensity, and likelihood of repetitive microtrauma injury	High level athletes – more likely to sustain overuse injuries Lower level athletes – poor conditioning a factor
Main problem and its severity now	To determine the type of symptoms, severity and nature (e.g. pain, weakness, stiffness, spasm, neurological symptoms, lack of function)	Type of symptoms may implicate type of tissue involved (e.g. paresthesia or painless weakness indicate nerve involvement)
Area of problem	To assess the extent and show the pattern of symptoms Obtain reassessment signs	Small area suggests localized injury Large or multiple areas; referred symptoms or poorly localized injury
Other areas	To clear regions above and below symptomatic area of involvement	If all other areas are clear of symptoms, tends to indicate a localized problem
Relationships	To determine if areas of symptoms are related or independent (i.e. one source or multiple sources)	If all symptoms related, indicates one source of symptoms likely
Aggravating factors	Determines which movements or activities bring on the symptoms Reassessment signs	Will indicate which tests are likely to reproduce symptoms
Easing factors	Determines which physical measures, stretches or exercises may ease symptoms	Gives clues to likely beneficial treatment techniques
Irritability	Severity, latency and nature of symptoms when they are provoked	Determines the extent and aggression of the physical examination
24 h behavior of symptoms	Night, am or pm pattern of symptoms reveals mechanical versus inflammatory problem	Determines whether problem is more likely to respond to physical or other modalities
Special questions	General health, weight loss, recent illnesses or surgery, medication and effects, investigations and results	Gives clues to possibility of non-mechanical, systemic or sinister pathology
Current and past history of injury	Mechanism of current injury, presence of any predisposing factors and progression of injury	Indicates likely tissue affected, pathology, stage of recovery and severity
Previous treatments and effects	Which treatments, if any, have been tried and which have been beneficial or not	Improvement without treatments is a good prognostic sign. Successful previous treatments should be used

asked first to clarify their main problem: whether it is pain, restriction of motion, lack of function, or performance. Athletes are often more concerned with lack of strength or limitation of function than with pain (e.g. a feeling of weakness in the lumbar spine on heavy squats).

The area of symptoms should be mapped out by the therapist as indicated by the athlete and recorded on a body chart. The affected areas and those regions immediately above and below and on the contralateral side should be 'cleared' of neurological or other symptoms. If there is more than one symptom or region affected, the relationships between the symptoms or areas should be established.

Aggravating factors of the cervical spine should be explored. These include: turning the head or looking up or down suddenly or constantly during performance of the sport, the application of load to the neck as in wrestling or rugby scrums, repeated movements as in swimming, or sustained postures as in cycling (Brukner & Khan 2001). In the lumbar spine, the most common aggravating factors involve either repeated or prolonged flexion as in rowing, or hyperextension and rotation as in cricket fast bowling (Brukner & Khan 2002). The worst aggravating factor that can be reproduced easily in examination should also be tested for severity, irritability, nature of symptoms provoked, and latency. Can the posture or movement be sustained or repeated or does the athlete actually have to stop doing the activity? How severe are the symptoms? Are they of an extremely serious nature (e.g. paralyzing pain or total numbness or weakness)? Once the athlete has stopped the activity, how long does it take for the symptoms to start to abate? Irritability, severity and latency are warning signs for the physical therapist to take care with the extent of assessment and with the choice of treatment and dosage at the first treatment session. When symptoms are severe or chronic but not irritable, the sports physical therapist can be more aggressive in examination and treatment.

Twenty-four hour behavior of the symptoms helps establish whether the problem is mechanical or inflammatory in nature. Symptoms that are much worse after rest, or at night, early morning on rising, or at the start of activity or movement, indicate inflammatory rather than mechanical conditions. Severe, constant night symptoms that disturb or prevent sleep or that necessitate the use of strong analgesics are a warning sign to the sports physical therapist to refer the athlete to a physician to be cleared of systemic disease, infection or malignancy. Symptoms that are worse at the end of the day, that worsen as the sports activity continues or that abate with rest tend to indicate a more mechanical condition. Mechanical conditions are more amenable to physical treatment such as manual therapy and exercise than conditions with a high inflammatory component (Maitland et al 2001).

The current history of injury must cover the time and mechanism of injury and whether this was obviously traumatic, insidious or repetitive in onset. With non-traumatic spinal injury, there is rarely a clear mechanism, so the questioning must be aimed at detailing the level of activity and any new activity around the time of onset of the problem.

If the sports physical therapist was at the field of play, he or she may already know some of these details better than the athlete. If there was trauma, a description is needed as well as an account of what happened immediately after the injury, and whether there was any severe impact, loss of bodily function or loss of memory, indicating spinal shock or head injury that will necessitate further referral and investigation.

The level of disability following the trauma needs to be established. Was the athlete able to continue playing or training? If so, it is possible that the current symptoms are due to secondary trauma or to continued activity since then, and not just to the initial incident itself. What has been the course of the problem since onset? Have the symptoms improved, changed, worsened or stabilized? What treatment has the athlete already received or self-administered and what has been the effect of treatment?

The past history should focus on any previous trauma to the head and neck or spine, and what previous diagnoses have been given, treatment supplied and the effects of such treatment. These answers will give a clue to what measures are likely to be successful or not if the condition is similar. If any exercises were prescribed for this or a similar condition previously, the athlete should be asked whether these are being continued regularly or not. Chronic spine conditions often reoccur because athletes have stopped their regular exercise routine as the symptoms abated.

Athletes should be asked if they are using medication for their conditions, for example, nonsteroidal anti-inflammatory drugs (NSAIDs) or analgesics, and about the dosage, current usage rate and effect of the medications. They should be asked about X-rays or scans or other medical tests they have had, how long ago they were done, and what the results of these tests were, if known.

The other special questions for the spine are intended to screen for serious pathology such as systemic disease, inflammatory or arthritic conditions, malignancy, spinal cord or cauda equina compression, or vertebro-basilar insufficiency (VBI). These questions should cover: general health, history of serious illness or surgery, any unexplained weight loss, chronic medical conditions, long-term medication including corticosteroids or anabolic steroids, dizziness or other signs of VBI, ataxia, pins and needles in both hands or both feet or problems with balance for the cervical spine, and saddle paresthesia or loss of bowel or bladder function for the lumbar spine.

Finally, athletes with spinal injuries should be asked about their expectations and commitment to treatment in the context of what they already know or think about their injury, their current level of sporting activity and what demands are made on them in terms of upcoming competition, training or selection commitments. Their attitude to their treatment program and course of rehabilitation will be a crucial factor in their recovery.

By the end of the subjective interview, there should be a plan of which areas to examine fully and how extensively to examine, and which areas to clear of involvement. The therapist should also obtain baseline measures of function, pain or disability, using validated and reliable outcome measures, such as the modified McGill Pain Scale (Melzack 1987), the Oswestry Low Back Disability Questionnaire (Fairbank et al 1980), the Roland Morris Disability Questionnaire (Roland & Morris 1983) and the Neck Disability Index (Vernon & Mior 1991) or the Patient Specific Functional Scale (Stratford et al 1995), which is particularly useful for more specific, sports-related disability. The physical examination can then proceed along standard lines described in full detail by Maitland et al (2001) (Table 14.2).

At the end of the physical examination, the sports physical therapist should carry out two or three physical reassessment tests, ideally including one each of function, movement and strength, to assess outcomes of physical treatments in the short and long term.

CERVICAL SPINE INJURIES IN ATHLETES

Sports injuries of the cervical spine are generally of soft tissue origin and fractures are uncommon. Serious injuries to the cervical spine are the domain of medical specialists but the sports physical therapist must have an awareness of the mechanisms of these injuries, particularly in attending the injured athlete at the field of play.

Table 14.2   Physical examination of the spine in athletes (Modified from Maitland et al 2001)

Observe and record	Purpose	Starting position	Tests and method	Implicates
Posture and symmetry (e.g. pelvic levels, leg lengths)	To assess symmetry, muscle balance and effect of posture on symptoms	Cervical and thoracic: sitting. Lumbar: standing Observe from front, side and back	Head, shoulder girdle, chin and spinal posture Record what is observed, instruct change to see if symptoms change	Habitual posture at work, study or sport. Muscle tightness or imbalance
AROM	To assess flexibility. To reproduce and show the pattern of symptoms. To obtain reassessment signs	Sitting or standing, observe from back and front, see how the athlete compensates or tricks to obtain ROM	Flexion, extension, lateral flexions, rotations, flexion rotation, extension rotation, quadrants. Instruct to move to first onset of pain and beyond as appropriate	Muscles especially multijoint muscles such as hamstrings, trapezius, facet joints, intervertebral joints
PROM	To find the restricted segment limiting motion and PROM, to find where to apply Rx	Supine, side lying. Cradle the region and feel the spine as it is moved through ROM	Take through flexion, extension, lateral flexions, and rotations, feeling spinal intersegmental motions	Muscles, facet joints, soft tissues of intervertebral joint segments
Special tests (e.g. VBI, slump, ULTT, neurological)	To test for signs of VBI or neural involvement in symptoms or in preparation for mobilization, manipulation	Sitting, supine and standing as appropriate. Instruct athlete first on what to expect and what to report	Take gently to extremes of RANGE, check premanipulative position, quick rotation and vestibular testing as needed. Gauge effect of change of neural tension on symptoms	Vertebral arteries or vestibular apparatus/middle ear. Nerve roots, nerve trunks, neuromeningeal structures
Palpation	Finding the source of symptoms and a location to trial mobilize first	Prone, with palpating thumbs testing centrally and unilaterally over facet joints, CV joints etc	Press in gently to first onset of pain and resistance, feel for stiffness and spasm, reproduction of symptoms	Muscles, facet joints, CV joints, intervertebral joints, ligaments, other soft tissues
Muscle function and balance, core stability	Find the strength coordination or control-related contributing factors	Functional positions and activities, sports-specific skills that are symptomatic	Activate the core stability muscles (e.g. TA) and challenge the stability with movement demands	Motor control problem, uncontrolled hypermobility problem

AROM: active range of movement; CV: costovertebral; PROM: passive range of movement; ROM: range of movement; Rx: treatment; TA: transversus abdominis; ULTT: upper limb tension test; VBI: vertebro-basilar insufficiency

Traumatic fractures or dislocations of the cervical spine in sport are most frequently seen in the football codes and occur in hyperflexion (e.g. rugby scrum collapse), hyperextension (e.g. head-high tackles) and axial compression (e.g. spear tackles, landing on head) (Torg et al 1990). Axial loading was implicated by Torg et al (1990) as being primarily responsible for severe cervical spine injury in American football. Forceful contraction of the trapezius or rhomboid muscles in power lifting has also been reported to cause a 'clay-shoveler's fracture', which is an avulsion of the spinous process in the lower cervical spine or at T1 (Anderson et al 1998). The sports physical therapist must assume there has been serious injury sustained in all cases of cervical spine trauma where there has been a mechanism involving axial compression, hyperflexion or hyperextension, neurological symptoms or loss of consciousness. The athlete must be removed appro-priately from the field of play and medical assistance obtained, including a full series of cervical spine X-rays.

COMMON SPORTS INJURY SYNDROMES OF THE CERVICAL SPINE

Most cervical injuries in the athlete are not serious and are similar to those encountered in the general population in that they are self-limiting and generally resolve quickly. Some injuries are more recalcitrant and this is due to the fact that they are mostly soft tissue in origin, and are chronic posture-related joint and muscle strains due to repeated positions or movements performed in the sport. Cyclists and triathletes commonly report chronic neck stiffness and headache due to the adoption of a posture of upper cervical extension on the bike. Swimmers or distance runners who report chronic or recurrent neck pain have a postural component to their problem.

Acute wry neck

Acute wry neck syndrome in athletes usually occurs without a specific incident and presents with unilateral stiffness and pain, with or without radiation to the shoulder. The mechanism of injury is generally non-specific, but it may follow the morning after a particularly heavy weight-training session of the upper body, where the shoulder girdle muscles have been used heavily and this has caused strain to their attachments to the cervical spine. The athlete may have simply woken one morning with a stiff neck or just moved the neck suddenly or awkwardly, feeling a sensation in the neck which gradually becomes stiffer and more painful. The athlete will complain of restriction of movement towards the painful side, particularly rotation and lateral flexion towards the painful side. If the problem is in the upper cervical spine, extension is usually more affected than flexion, and vice versa for a problem in the lower cervical spine. There is usually no radiation of pain beyond the point of the shoulder or neurological symptoms, which tend to suggest that the source of symptoms is mechanical impingement of soft tissue, most probably within the zygoapophyseal joints, triggering local muscle spasm. It may coexist with chronic shoulder or upper thoracic and cervical posture syndromes in the athlete. While wry neck is usually self-limiting and of short duration, the contributing factors may be very long-standing and should be addressed within the treatment setting to prevent the possibility of recurrence and more serious pathology in the long term.

Treatment of the acute condition involves careful assessment of the extent and nature of symptoms, checking which movements are most restricted or 'locked' to determine a side and level to treat, and ensuring there are no contraindications to mobilization or manipulation. If the athlete complains of a feeling of constant pain at rest, being unable to support the weight of the head, that it feels as though the head might fall off; or if there is extreme sharp pain and spasm with minor movement precluding passive mobilization; the therapist should be wary of passive mobilization and manipulation in the first instance and stick to heat, massage and the use of a soft collar for support, sending the athlete home or to their physician with advice to seek medical assessment and medication, such as muscle relaxants, analgesics and NSAIDs.

When the constant pain or other acute symptoms have abated, usually in the first 24–48 h, and stiffness replaces pain as the main problem, with pain on movement only, the athlete may be treated more actively. The athlete lies prone with the forehead supported on the palms, but if there is a severe restriction of cervical extension and the prone position is too painful, the athlete can be positioned in a supported, sitting, leaning, slightly forward position with the arms resting on a plinth and head supported on pillows.

Segmental palpation will confirm the level most affected: usually one or two of the facet joints in the mid-cervical spine region on the affected side, though the levels above and below and on the other side are also stiff and can be treated as well. Heat and massage can be used first to lessen coexisting muscle tightness or spasm, then unilateral passive mobilization can be tried. If there is still excessive tenderness or spasm precluding direct palpatory techniques, indirect techniques, such as passive rotary mobilization away from the direction of restriction or manipulation should be attempted. An approach of working above and below the site of injury can give a good measure of relief even when the site of injury is too painful to treat. Therefore, manipulation can be used on day one in the upper thoracic spine or upper cervical spine to treat a midcervical problem.

Facet joint syndrome

Facet joint syndrome in the cervical spine in sports is really the chronic version of acute wry neck syndrome, the difference being that the onset may be much more gradual or associated with recurrent bouts of acute, unilateral stiffness and pain. The primary complaint is stiffness and it is associated with varying degrees of radicular pain referred to the suprascapular region, trigger points found in the upper trapezius, rhomboids and levator scapulae, and referred pain or other neurological symptoms to the upper limb. While the motion restriction in wry neck is temporary and follows a closing pattern, changes such as shortening or thickening in the articular structures in facet joint syndrome lead to more permanent restriction of motion, with symptoms presenting more on stretching the joint, (i.e. rotation and lateral flexion away from the affected side). Chronic neck pain that has not responded to a trial of physical therapy should be investigated fully with X-rays, especially if there is a hard end feel to the restricted motions. If no pathological or degenerative changes in the joints are revealed, a course of passive mobilization, intermittent mechanical traction, manipulation and stretching should be undertaken followed by a specific regular exercise regimen to regain and maintain range of motion.

Cervical spondylosis/nerve root impingement

Cervical spondylosis or nerve root impingement may be the cause of chronic, global neck stiffness in an older athlete, or unilateral cervical symptoms associated with poorly localized shoulder, arm or other upper quarter symptoms, or where there are neurological symptoms. More common in athletes who are over 40 years, degenerative changes in the intervertebral disks, uncovertebral and zygapophyseal joints are the late result of chronic facet joint syndrome which often precedes the onset of cervical spondylosis. Joint degeneration may lead to bony osteophythic encroachment into the lateral recesses and intervertebral foraminae, pressing on the nerve roots and giving radicular pain. These bony changes may be revealed on plain X-rays, computed tomography (CT) or magnetic resonance imaging (MRI) scans and will confirm the clinical impression, and give an idea of the prognosis. The problem may present initially as constant dull ache in the base of the neck or suprascapular region, with or without referred pain or neurological symptoms in the upper limbs. The onset may be insidious or sudden as with wry neck, but while the acute neck pain eases, the referred symptoms do not respond initially to treatment. The course then is usually very long term (3–6 months). Management will involve modification of aggravating activities and sports techniques may have to be altered; a long-term course of anti-inflammatory or anti-arthritic medication may be used. Physical therapy will include all heat, massage and mobilization measures. Although manipulation is contraindicated at the severely affected level, it can be used above and below to add functionality and movement. The main physical modality is traction and if the radicular pain is reduced by a trial of manual traction, a course of progressively increasing doses of mechanical traction may be instituted.

Recurrent headache

Recurrent headache is a repetitive strain condition commonly due to pressure on the pain-sensitive structures of the upper cervical spine. It may be caused by having the upper cervical spine continually extended as in cycling and triathlon sport, due to the neck and head posture adopted on the bike in the aerodynamic position. Contributing factors include pre-existing stiffness of the lower cervical or thoracic spine due to previous injury or pathological/degenerative changes such as previous fractures, congenital conditions or cervical spondylosis. If these areas are limited in extension, there is more demand on upper cervical extension to maintain the desired posture for the sport. In the absence of irreversible pathology, where there is no further potential movement available in the upper cervical spine, a course of passive mobilization at the site of restriction to the atlanto-occipital, atlanto-axial and second and third cervical facet joints should be attempted, with follow-up stretching.

Extra functional range and longer-term prevention can then be achieved by mobilizing and stretching the mid and lower cervical and thoracic spines. The athletes' ergonomics should be assessed (e.g. their bike position set-up).

If the athletes' problems are to do with the adoption of an extended upper cervical posture in their sport, this should be addressed with postural awareness training, muscle stretching and strengthening of deep neck flexors and shoulder retractors.

Efficacy of physical therapies for sports injuries in the cervical spine

There is little information available from randomized controlled clinical trials to support the use of physical modalities for mechanical neck pain, and certainly very few trials testing treatment of neck pain in sports. For the general population, Kjellman et al (1999) critically analyzed randomized clinical trials on neck pain and treatment efficacy by reviewing 27 randomized clinical trials published between 1966 and 1995. Positive outcomes were noted for 18 of the investigations, and treatments used in the studies were effective for pain, range of motion, and activities of daily living. A more recent systematic review by Gross et al (2001) found some support for the use of electromagnetic therapy and against the use of laser therapy with respect to pain reduction for mechanical neck pain. However, there have been no trials to examine functional outcomes of neck treatment in an athletic population.

Outcome measures such as the Patient Specific Functional Scale (Stratford et al 1995) or the neck pain disability index can be used to confirm treatment efficacy.

Passive treatments – Immobilization

Hard collars should be used where rigid immobilization is required, as in cervical spine fractures. For all other cervical conditions, a soft collar is usually sufficient. A makeshift soft collar can be fashioned from a towel and secured with safety pins or tape, for overnight use to support the neck. In the case of soft tissue trauma, neck immobilization should be used for short periods only, as there is evidence to show that prolonged immobilization is of no benefit in painful neck conditions (Spitzer et al 1995).

Heat and cold

While there is insufficient evidence to support the use of either heat or cold therapy in neck conditions in athletes, the application of heat or cold is a widely utilized home remedy that can be used regularly between more active treatments. Ice should be used for acute, traumatic injuries. Hydro-collator or microwave hot packs are a very useful adjunct to treatment in all other cases to help relieve pain and spasm and to warm the treatment area before the application of massage, mobilization, manipulation and stretching.

Electrophysical agents

Ultrasound, microwave or short wave diathermy may be used to afford temporary pain relief or for their deeper warming effects as an adjunct to more active treatment. For example, it may be more effective to treat a facet joint first with ultrasound to reduce the point tenderness and to allow deeper grades of palpatory mobilization to be administered. Laser therapy has been shown to be ineffective (Thorsen et al 1992), and there is limited evidence that interferential or transcutaneous electrical nerve stimulation (TENS) may be utilized for its analgesic effects. There is further discussion of electrophysical agents in physical therapy in Chapter 13.

Massage

Though there is insufficient evidence to support its use, massage is widely used in the treatment of neck strains. Every neck injury involves the muscles and other soft tissues, and massage can be used to address this component of the problem, usually after the application of heat and before mobilization or manipulation.

Passive stretching

Controlled and localized passive stretching techniques can be performed for the upper trapezius (Fig. 14.1) and upper cervical spine muscles (Fig. 14.2). Proprioceptive neuromuscular facilitation (PNF) or hold/relax techniques work well, especially after active range has been restored with mobilization or manipulation. Self-administration of passive stretching is best, as the athletes can gauge the discomfort themselves and apply the correct amount of force. At a later stage, active strengthening of the deep cervical flexor muscles can be incorporated (Fig. 14.3).

Traction

Klaber Moffett et al (1990) investigated the effects of cervical traction in a well-designed trial comparing weighted cervical traction (6–15 lbs) applied according to a technique commonly used by physical therapists with placebo traction, where the weights were applied in exactly the same way, but which produced a force of not more than 1 lb on the head. Both groups were given neck-

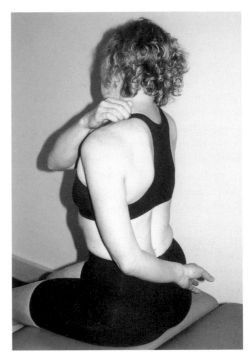

Figure 14.1 Localized upper trapezius stretches.

care education. The weighted group tended to improve slightly more than the placebo group on measures of pain, sleep disturbance, social dysfunction, activities of daily living (ADL) and range of movement at the neck. No significant posttreatment differences were found

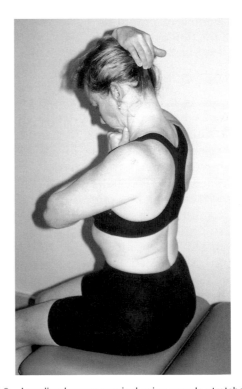

Figure 14.2 Localized upper cervical spine muscle stretches.

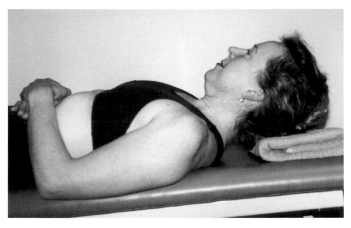

Figure 14.3   Active strengthening of deep cervical flexor muscles.

between the two treatment groups except on flexion and right-side flexion.

In their blinded review of randomized clinical trial methods for the efficacy of traction for back and neck pain, Van der Heijden et al (1995) concluded that the available reports of studies on the efficacy of traction for back and neck pain do not allow clear conclusions because of the methodological flaws in their design and conduct. There were no clear indications, however, that traction was ineffective for neck pain, therefore traction may be a reasonable treatment option for radicular symptoms due to sporting injury or spondylitic neck pain in the older athlete.

Manual or mechanical traction should be used for specific treatment of radicular pain or for general mobilization in cervical spondylosis. A trial of gentle manual traction can be used first to gauge its effect. If there is no immediate or latent exacerbation of symptoms, mechanical traction can be progressed from light doses of intermittent mechanical traction (e.g. 5 kg, on 10 s, off 10 s for 5 min) to higher doses in terms of force, duration, and from intermittent to continuous mode.

Continuous traction is better for nerve root impingement syndromes whereas intermittent traction is better for its mobilization effect on more general conditions (e.g. facet joint syndrome). Traction should be applied with the affected segment in neutral flexion/extension (i.e. the starting position for lower segments should be slightly more flexion).

Passive mobilization

Whilst there is a paucity of specific evidence for the efficacy of passive mobilization in sports injuries of the neck, Maitland et al (2001) describe the full range of mobilization techniques in their book. As most problems are unilateral, unilateral palpatory posteroanterior mobilization can be tried first over the affected facet joints, followed by mobilization in combined or off neutral starting positions. Athletes often present with functional limitation near the limit of range.

When there is a stretch pattern of pain reproduced (i.e. rotation to the left causes pain on the right side of the neck), the mobilization can be performed with the athlete's neck in some left rotation as a starting position. This will mobilize and restore the accessory joint glide at the limit of the physiological range where it is needed. Passive physiological mobilization is usually performed away from the side of pain and is a good choice when more direct techniques are too painful or cause spasm.

High velocity thrust technique (HVTT)/manipulation

The use of cervical HVTT is controversial due to the danger of adverse reactions and complications from this treatment, particularly the risk of damage to the vertebro-basilar arterial system with the concomitant small but real possibility of permanent impairment or death (Maitland et al 2001). Hurwitz et al (1996) conducted a systematic review of the literature and concluded that both cervical spine manipulation and mobilization probably provide at least short-term benefits for some patients with neck pain and headaches. They reported a complication rate for cervical spine manipulation as estimated to be between 5 and 10 per 10 million manipulations. The risk, albeit small, must be weighed against the probable benefit in the sporting context.

To study whether a 3-week series of spinal manipulation had any lasting effect on passive cervical range of motion, Nilsson et al (1996) compared goniometric cervical range of motion between two groups. They found that any changes in the passive range of motion after spinal manipulation were of a temporary nature.

The main benefit of HVTT is the possibility of more rapid return of cervical range of motion than with other modalities. The indications for use of this treatment are: a plateau or lack of improvement with cervical mobilization alone, where there is stiffness greater than pain as the main symptom at the end of range, where there is an acutely locked cervical facet joint, where it has been used successfully before.

Contraindications include any of the signs of vertebro-basilar insufficiency, such as dizziness on head or neck motion, double vision or blurring of vision, ringing in the ears, slurring of speech or difficulty swallowing, and drop attacks or fainting. If manipulation is indicated and no contraindications exist, the patient should be asked for their informed consent before proceeding with vertebral artery testing, and then with the manipulative treatment using the full premanipulative testing and treatment guidelines (Maitland et al 2001).

Neck manipulation can be carried out in sitting or supine positions, and is most often used in combination with other modalities such as massage, mobilization, stretching and exercise. In examining the cervical spine, passive intersegmental motion and palpation should be performed to ascertain the stiffness level. Manipulation should be carried out in a direction away from that which causes pain (i.e. if left rotation is stiff and painful, the neck should be manipulated to the right first). Most HVTT techniques involve sudden and forceful stretching that opens the facet joint surfaces. This is achieved by taking the joint to the limit of the physiological range and applying a quick, forceful but localized and controlled thrust in the desired direction. There are various methods, the most common being the use of the radial side of the therapist's first metacarpophalangeal joint to localize the force for the thrust to the stiff facet joint.

Successful manipulation will provide extra range of cervical motion and should be followed up with more mobilization, stretching and exercises to maintain the improvement. While manipulation often provides dramatic pain relief and improved motion, the effect is commonly temporary and should always be followed up with posture and technique evaluation, stretches and strengthening exercises to address the cause of the problem.

Active treatments: postural correction and postural awareness training

Athletes are accustomed to making changes in their posture and movement patterns as part of their physical training. The typical postural imbalances that may lead to mechanical neck pain include a poking chin (upper cervical extension), shortening of posterior upper cervical muscles and protracted shoulders, which may be a manifestation of poor thoracic mobility or kyphosis. Proprioceptive education, using retraction taping of the shoulders and taping the thoracic spine in extension, and exercises to strengthen the deep neck flexors may be of benefit in chronic neck conditions. It has been suggested that the deep neck flexors have a reduced ability to hold the neck in the neutral position against gravity in subjects with chronic neck conditions (Jull 1997). Sterling et al (2001) showed that manipulative physical therapy may facilitate specific low load exercises to strengthen the deep neck flexors, reducing symptoms associated with cervicogenic headache with long-term beneficial effects. Taimela et al (2000) found that active treatment of chronic neck pain, including proprioceptive exercises, relaxation, and behavioral support, was more effective than active home exercises alone and that active treatment was clearly more effective than just advising on neck care.

Correction of muscle tightness and weakness may commence with localized muscle stretching for the tight upper trapezius (Fig. 14.1), upper cervical extensors (Fig. 14.2), levator scapulae, scalenes, sternomastoids, and pectoralis major and minor. Strengthening of the deep upper cervical muscles may commence in the supine position (Fig. 14.3), focussing on improved holding time, and progressing to more sport-specific functional tasks.

THORACIC SPINE INJURIES IN ATHLETES

In athletes, thoracic spine symptoms are often related to underlying, structural spinal stiffness as occurs as a late sequelae of Scheuermann's disease or due to habitual poor posture. An increased thoracic kyphosis is seen commonly in elite swimmers, and this can be either structural, as with Scheuermann's disease or functional and correctible, as with muscle imbalance or poor core/scapular stability. The structures at risk of becoming injured or symptomatic include: the intervertebral disks, giving central symptoms and referred pain through to the front of the chest; the facet or costovertebral joints, usually giving unilateral pain radiating around the chest wall when severe; and the intercostal nerve roots, giving radicular pain along the rib (Maitland et al 2001).

Stiffness of the intervertebral, paravertebral and costal joints in the thoracic spine is manifested as restriction of range, particularly in rotation and extension, and in some cases, may affect depth of inspiration. Respiratory symptoms, such as catching pain on breathing in deeply or inability to take a full deep breath, can be due to costovertebral/costotransverse joint stiffness or subluxation, and respond well to manual therapy. In rowing, canoeing, kayaking, and golf, rib stress fractures are a common source of thoracic, chest or ribcage pain. Rib stress fractures in these sports are found most frequently between the 4th and 9th ribs, either anterolaterally or posterolaterally, but occasionally they occur posteriorly in the neck of the rib where they can be a source of severe thoracic back pain and mimic thoracic disk injury or facet/costovertebral joint syndromes.

SCHEUERMANN'S DISEASE IN ATHLETES

Scheuermann's disease is a self-limiting form of osteochondrosis in the thoracic or upper lumbar vertebrae, causing degenerative changes in the intervertebral disk and cartilage endplates. It is seen commonly in X-rays of the active adolescent's spine and is thought to be a growth disorder involving an irregular or absent osteocartilaginous growth zone and thinned endplates, allowing herniation of disk material into the vertebral body (Schmorl's nodes) (Corrigan & Maitland 1998). It is

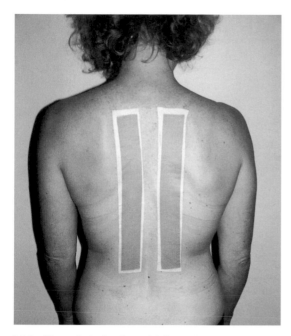

Figure 14.4   Thoracic taping to maintain posture.

more common in males and affects up to 6% of the juvenile population (Corrigan & Maitland 1998). The most common levels affected are around T9. Atypical Scheuermann's disease may also affect the upper lumbar spine leading to apophyseal ring fracture, Schmorl's nodes and associated disk pathology in the younger athlete (d'Hemecourt et al 2000).

The affected thoracic vertebrae may become wedged anteriorly, leading to, or as a result of, dorsal kyphosis and a stooped posture with rounded shoulder girdles and a flexed lower cervical spine. Presence of the typical features in an X-ray of the athlete's spine is of no concern in itself, and the condition is often asymptomatic. If symptoms do arise, they consist of mild to moderate pain in the thoracic spine with a loss of range of movement. This may be treated symptomatically in the short term with rest from aggravating activities (especially weight-lifting), postural correction with a brace or taping, a firmer bed, active exercises to stretch tight muscles such as the hamstrings, and postural correction exercises such as thoracic extension and rotation stretching to prevent progression of existing deformity.

Taping the shoulders back or taping the thoracic spine in a corrected position may offer the young athlete useful feedback on their posture (Fig. 14.4). Manual therapy techniques are generally contraindicated (Corrigan & Maitland 1998).

THORACIC DISK INJURY IN ATHLETES

The lower thoracic spine may be subject to disk degeneration in athletes whose sport involves repeated thoracic rotation, such as golfers, cricketers, discus throwers or sweep rowers (Corrigan & Maitland 1998). The pain and stiffness is usually central but may radiate along the line of the ribs with paresthesia if nerve roots are involved. Pain on movement and night pain is a feature because it is aggravated by extension as in lying down, and rotation as in turning over in bed. The condition can be very irritable so management consists of carefully graded mobilization and pain relief modalities, followed by home exercises involving thoracic strengthening and stretching of thoracic extension and rotation.

COSTOVERTEBRAL AND COSTOTRANSVERSE JOINT SPRAINS

These sprains or hypomobility syndromes may occur in sports involving thoracic flexion and rotation as in sweep rowing, which is often associated with rib stress fractures, or in ribcage compression such as in weightlifting. The pain is sharp and unilateral and the athlete will complain of difficulty in taking a deep breath, rotation, lateral flexion and extension of the thoracic spine. Central and unilateral spinal palpation will reveal a hypomobile segment and corresponding stiff rib. Unless rib stress fracture is suspected (Wajswelner 1996, Wajswelner et al 2000), treatment is oriented to pain relief in the acute stage, and mobilization, manipulation and stretching and strengthening exercises as the symptoms abate.

LUMBAR SPINE INJURIES IN ATHLETES

Despite the fact that low back pain in sport is so common, the source of symptoms is often never detected. In most cases there will be no objective or radiological signs of pathology and the diagnosis will be one of non-specific low back pain (NSLBP) of soft tissue origin. Specific bony injuries such as acute traumatic fractures through vertebral bodies or transverse processes, stress fractures through the pars interarticularis, and congenital defects such as spina bifida occulta and spondylolysis can be detected, and every attempt should be made to reach a diagnosis where possible. However, we do not as yet have the tools to differentiate objectively between causes of most cases of low back pain (LBP), so most cases will be lumped together and given the generic label of NSLBP.

Commonly recognized syndromes such as chronic facet joint sprains, 'bulging' disks, and ligament sprains or muscle strains will not show any signs on objective tests such as X-rays or scans. However, a common causative thread has been suggested: dynamic muscular dysfunction or poor motor control of the deep muscular stabilizing system of the spine (Richardson et al 1999).

While poor motor control may be a common factor in cases of LBP in athletes, acute macrotrauma and repetitive microtrauma related to particular sporting activities can set up specific patterns of symptoms that are recognizable. These are extension syndromes (pars defects, facet joint impingement), flexion syndromes (disk herniation and sciatica) and hypermobility/instability syndromes in the younger athlete; with hypomobility syndromes (lumbar spondylosis and degenerative disk disease) more commonly seen in the older athlete.

SPONDYLOLYSIS/SPONDYLOLISTHESIS

The etiology of spondylolysis/spondylolisthesis in sports is a stress fracture due to repeated stresses leading to mechanical overload in the pars interarticularis (Mandelbaum & Gross 1991). Spondylolisthesis usually occurs later when there is a bilateral defect and slip progression as mechanical loads are imposed on the soft tissues, such as those occurring in sports. Although spondylolysis may be unilateral or bilateral, in sports it is more commonly unilateral, usually occurring on the side opposite to the most active (Corrigan & Maitland 1998).

A structural defect in the pars interarticularis allows this forward slippage of a vertebra, usually L4 or L5, onto the vertebra below. In spondylolysis, there is a defect but no slippage, and it is also possible to have a slippage with no defect by elongation of the pars (Flemming 1990). Spondylolysis and spondylolisthesis in athletes, has an incidence higher than the 5% seen in the general population. It is estimated that 25% of adolescents who present with back pain show radiographic evidence of pars defects and this association is much higher in athletes in some sports (Flemming 1990). Table 14.3 shows that incidence rates in different sports can be as high as 63%.

Sports and sporting activities that involve hyperextension and rotation of the lumbar spine, such as diving, gymnastics, wrestling, and butterfly swimming are often associated with these conditions. The bony defects are thought to be stress reactions within the pars interarticularis caused by repetitive microtrauma that can be manifested as either an acute stress fracture, fibrous

---

Box 14.1 Classification of spondylolysis and spondylolisthesis. (Modified from Mandelbaum & Gross 1991.)

Dysplastic
Congenital deficiency of the facet joints, allowing gradual forward slip of one vertebra onto another

Isthmic
Spondylolysis defect in the pars interarticularis allowing forward slip of one vertebra onto another
    Lytic fracture of the pars interarticularis
    Elongated or attenuated, but intact, pars interarticularis
    Acute fracture of the pars interarticularis

Degenerative
Degeneration of the L5–S1 disk and facet joints, allowing forward displacement

Traumatic
Acute fracture in areas other than the pars interarticularis, such as the pedicle, lamina or facet joint, that allows forward displacement

Pathological
Attenuation of the posterior neural arch secondary to structural weakness in the bone, such as in metabolic bone disease

---

non-union or healing of the pars in an elongated state (Flemming 1990).

Wiltse et al (1976) developed a system of classification based on five modes of pathogenesis, which are dysplastic, isthmic, degenerative, traumatic, and pathological (Box 14.1). Of these, the lesion commonly found in young athletes is isthmic spondylolisthesis (Mandelbaum & Gross 1991).

It is not clear whether it is flexion or extension or a combination of both, producing alternating tension and compression stresses, that causes the lesion in the pars. Mandelbaum & Gross (1991) suggested the latter, as this is the way most flexible structures fail. It is not known whether vigorous participation in sports at a very young age when the spine is immature compounds the cumulative stresses to the pars caused during repetitive hyperflexion, hyperextension and rotation.

Hyperflexion is commonly seen in rowing and forward walkovers in gymnastics (Mandelbaum & Gross 1991). Hyperextension of the lumbar spine occurs in many sports but particularly with backward walkovers in gymnastics, tennis serving, blocking, tackling and the defensive lineman's stance in American football. Ciullo & Jackson (1985) showed that the same high forces that cause a fracture in the pars in the laboratory are reproduced several times during a gymnastics training session (Fig. 14.5). Elliot et al (1995) demonstrated that the counter-rotation of the shoulders and lumbar spine produced by a combination of fully front on and fully side on bowling action in cricket increases the likelihood of spondylolysis in young fast bowlers.

Table 14.3 Incidence of spondylolysis/spondylolisthesis in selected sports. (Modified from Rossi 1988 and Hardcastle et al 1992.)

Sport	Incidence rate (%)
Diving	63.3
Cricket fast bowling	55.0
Weightlifting	36.2
Wrestling	33.0
Gymnastics	32.0
Athletics	22.5
General population	5.0

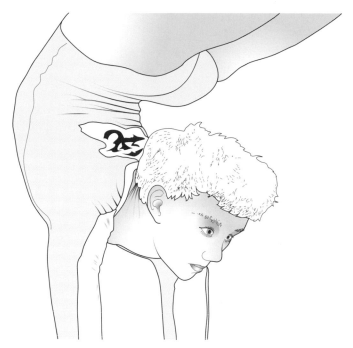

Figure 14.5 Lumbar hyperextension in a gymnastics skill showing 'hinging' spine.

Assessment and diagnosis of pars defects in athletes

The athlete with a pars defect will usually present with unilateral back pain after sport or exercise, which may radiate to the buttock or hamstring and be associated with very tight hamstrings. Local tenderness, the extension/rotation or quadrant test (Corrigan & Maitland 1998), and the one-legged extension test are indicative of possible posterior element pathology that must be diagnosed. The basic points in diagnosis of the athlete with suspected spondylolysis or spondylolisthesis are to determine whether there is a crack or a slip, whether it is new or old, bilateral or unilateral, whether the slip is stable or unstable (progressive) and whether the symptoms are due to the pars defect itself or other pathology (e.g. disk or facet joint problem coming from the levels above or below the slip). For example, if there is a concurrent L5 disk injury, posteroanterior palpatory glide will be painful, whereas with an L5–S1 spondylolisthesis that is symptomatic, the same glide may relieve pain.

The athlete with a suspected pars defect should be referred to a sports physician for the appropriate investigations and definitive management. This will involve plain anteroposterior and lateral X-rays and preferably a single photon emission computed tomography (SPECT) bone scan to localize the lesion and determine if it is new or old. Oblique X-ray views are commonly ordered to reveal the defect which appears as a collar on the 'Scotty

Dog' formed by the 20° cephalad oblique image (Corrigan & Maitland 1998). Congeni et al (1997) reported an 85% incidence of fractures found on CT imaging in patients with negative oblique views and positive bone scans. If focal uptake is seen on the bone scan, a limited CT may be performed at the isolated level to classify the fracture as early, progressive or terminal depending on the extent of sclerosis (d'Hemecourt et al 2000).

Management of spondylolysis/spondylolisthesis in athletes

There are two types of pars defect injuries in athletes, the first being acute pars stress fracture and the second being aggravation of a pre-existing, possibly non-symptomatic pars defect. All symptomatic cases should be treated initially with rest (from the aggravating activities), semirigid immobilization with an antilordotic lumbar brace until healing has occurred, and physical therapy. With a history of recent onset, scans may confirm an acute stress fracture or early lesion. This should be managed with a short period (3–4 weeks) of very rigid immobilization to encourage early primary healing. Morita et al (1995) showed that none of the terminal lesions and 73% of early lesions healed, although Fellander-Tsai & Micheli (1998) reported healing of sclerotic lesions with external electrical stimulation and rigid bracing. However, the most effective form of bracing based on fracture classification is yet to be determined. The treating sports physician should be asked to determine the length of primary healing, protected function, and return to sport stages, depending on severity of the injury and stage of healing.

Physical therapy in the acute stage (4–6 weeks) consists of pain relief modalities, such as interferential treatment (IFT) or TENS (see Ch. 13), postural correction, and pelvic tilt and transversus abdominus (TA) retraining (Fig. 14.6). O'Sullivan et al (1997) reported on an exercise program involving the specific training of the deep abdominal muscles, with coactivation of the lumbar multifidus proximal to the pars defects. The program was effective in reducing pain during functional activities in a randomly assigned group of patients with confirmed listhetic displacement and who underwent a 10-week specific exercise treatment program compared to controls. The activation of these muscles was incorporated into previously aggravating static postures and functional tasks.

During the acute period, stretching of tight hamstrings, gluteals and hip flexors should be performed daily, with the patient taught to do them while avoiding back strain. It is beneficial to mobilize joints above and below the injury, without hyperextending the lumbar spine, so as to spread the range of body extension (e.g. shoulders, thoracic spine, sacroiliac and hip joints). Quadratus lumborum and deep hip flexor releases and stretching

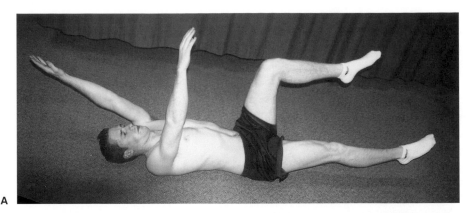

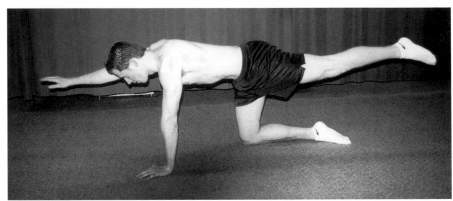

Figure 14.6A & B   Transversus abdominis retraining. **A**: supine. **B**: two-point stance.

have also been found to be beneficial in the short term to improve pain free range of movement by this author (Fig. 14.7).

During the subacute and protected function stage, strengthening may progress to harder abdominal work including deep abdominal, TA, lumbar multifidus (LM), lateral abdominal and stabilized rotatory strengthening

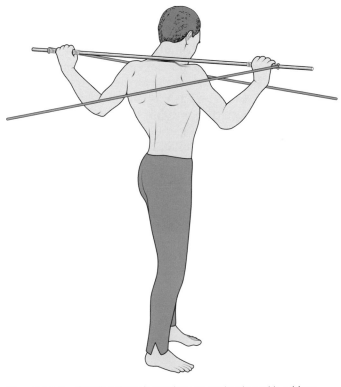

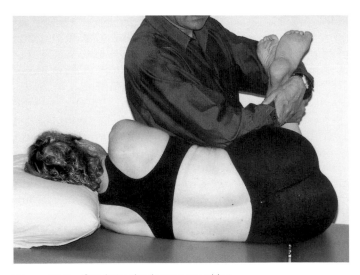

Figure 14.7   Quadratus lumborum stretching.

Figure 14.8   Stabilized trunk rotation strengthening with rubber bands.

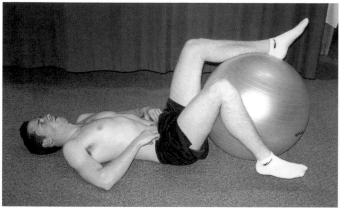

A

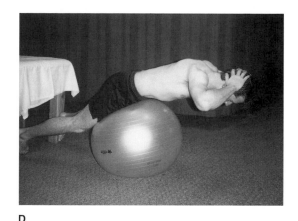

D

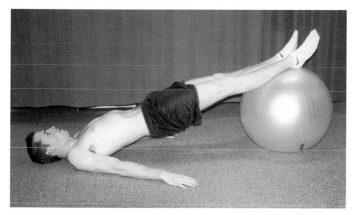

B

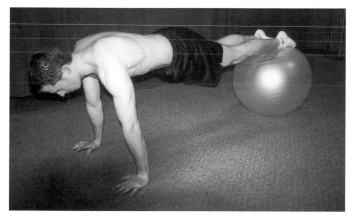

E

Figure 14.9A–E   Progression (from **A–E**) of core stability exercises using Swiss ball.

C

(Figs 14.8 and 14.9). In athletes, strength training exercises are applied to specific sports skills once adequate core stability has been established. If the athlete can perform an isolated TA contraction and keep the spine stabilized under load or postural perturbation, rehabilitation can be progressed from the clinical to more functional tasks. Each movement task may be slowed down and broken down into its components to allow

specific strength work using pulleys, rubber bands or weights to provide stability throughout the whole risk movement (see Fig. 14.8).

Functional taping or bracing can be used to limit hyperextension or rotation on return-to-sports activities to give the athlete further feedback (Fig. 14.10). In the return-to-sport stage (12 weeks or longer), technique modification may also be required.

FACET JOINT SYNDROMES IN ATHLETES

Facet joint syndrome is common in sports with hyperextension and rotation (e.g. tennis, netball) and flexion and rotation (e.g. sweep rowing). It is also common in those who adopt a lordotic posture in running

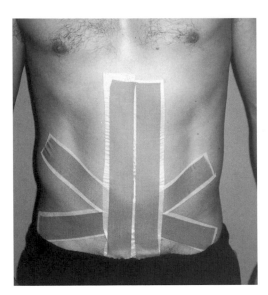

Figure 14.10 Functional taping to limit hyperextension.

(i.e. shorter runners who tend to overstride). The athlete will present with unilateral pain and stiffness that usually does not radiate below the top of the buttock. It can present in two ways, either as a 'closing down' pattern where extension, lateral flexion rotation and the quadrant position on the painful side are worst, or as an 'opening up' pattern where flexion, rotation and lateral flexion away from the painful side are most symptomatic. Palpation in either case will reveal a stiff, painful segment.

Usually the condition responds well to local physical treatment consisting of passive unilateral posteroanterior or rotary mobilization and stretching, particularly of tight thoracolumbar fascia, quadratus lumborum and deep hip flexors. Unless the posture or technique is changed it tends to continue and recur; lower limb biomechanics and orthotics can play an important role here.

STRESS FRACTURES/TRAUMATIC FRACTURES OF THE LUMBAR SPINE

While stress fractures can occur in the pars interarticularis, they also occur in the lateral processes or vertebral bodies in distance runners due to poor lower limb and pelvic biomechanics. These spinal stress fractures will present with a 'bone damage' type pain behavior (i.e. insidious onset, increase in pain with increased use, eased by rest, does not 'warm up' with use, latent aching and night pain). The athlete with this type of presentation must be referred to a physician for definitive diagnosis and management.

Physical therapy will consist of pain relief, functional strengthening and stretching as appropriate with assess-

ment of running biomechanics to help alleviate contributing factors. Athletes with poor biomechanics, manifested as excessive pelvic tilt or rotation in their running gait, are prone to lumbar spine stress fractures. This may be corrected with core stability training, lumbopelvic postural correction in running and correction of foot biomechanics with functional orthoses if needed.

Female athletes may suffer from loss of bone mineral density (leading to stress fracture) and need an intensive sports medicine team approach to their management with input from the sports physician, sports podiatrist, sports nutritionist and sports psychologist (see Ch. 26).

Traumatic fractures are common in contact sports and falls and athletes usually present with swelling, bruising and gross movement restriction. X-rays are required to confirm a fracture, commonly of the transverse or spinous processes and these are generally not serious and can be treated symptomatically. Rehabilitation should commence with alternative training and pain relief, stretching and strengthening the area as symptoms allow. The athlete should wait for the fracture to heal before resuming contact sport, with protective padding used on initial return to play.

LUMBAR DISK INJURIES IN ATHLETES

Lumbar spine disk injuries are seen in athletes in many sports (Brukner & Khan, 2002). Weight-training, especially the clean and squat exercise, done poorly, is one of the major causative factors, but injury can also be due to the combination of a sedentary job or study leading to lumbar stiffness, and playing sport without warming up adequately in between work and sport. Lumbar disk injury is common in weightlifting, rowing, football, court-sports and even in running. The mechanism of injury is usually the same as in the general population (i.e. prolonged flexion or flexion and rotation under load). Acute injuries often follow warning signs that are ignored by the athlete.

There may have been a sudden onset such as with a single heavy weight lift, or a more trivial incident such as bending over to pick up something, or a sneeze; or a more insidious onset such as increasing pain and stiffness with prolonged or repeated flexion and rotation activities.

The athlete with lumbar disk injury will present with a variety of back symptoms depending on the mechanism, severity and stage of the disk injury. There may be central, unilateral or bilateral pain or stiffness, and radiation of pain to the buttock, posterior thigh, knee or calf with neurological symptoms. With acute disk prolapse, there may be more radicular referred pain in the calf or neurological symptoms such as paresthesia than in LBP. Flexion is the main aggravating factor (i.e. prolonged sitting). Increasing stiffness and difficulty on rising from a seated position, with pain on coughing or sneezing, are also indicative of a disk problem.

On physical assessment there is usually pain, restriction, loss of lordosis, deformity and sometimes spasm on active flexion in standing. There may also be positive straight leg raise, neurological and positive slump test findings, and usually hypomobility and pain found on palpation (Maitland et al 2001). In severe or irritable cases, or where disk prolapse is suspected, the slump test is contraindicated. In cases of disk prolapse, the athlete may present with spinal deformity (i.e. a lumbar scoliosis, usually away from the side of pain) (Maitland et al 2001). If these clinical signs are evident, the athlete should be referred for full medical investigation.

Physical therapy for lumbar disk injury in the athlete

Acute lumbar disk injuries can be managed successfully using physical therapy with a systematic and staged approach. The evidence for efficacy of these treatments has been studied in some detail and is outlined below. The acute stage of disk injury may last 2–3 or even 6 weeks in severe cases. It is managed initially with a short period of bed rest (2 days), physical modalities such as TENS, IFT and heat and medication for pain relief, and exercises, passive mobilization or traction. Traction may be the first treatment option if referred leg pain or neurological symptoms are a dominant feature (Maitland et al 2001).

Prevention of further aggravation is important; however, it is equally important to offer options to the athlete even in these early stages, of some alternative form of exercise; for example, gentle walking or swimming may be possible without exacerbation of back or leg pain. Taping or bracing may be used during the day to limit movement, especially flexion, and to add some mechanical support to the lumbar spine during normal activities. The subacute stage (from 3 to 12 weeks) sees the introduction of more mobilizing, stretching and strengthening exercises, however, which exercises are best prescribed, is controversial. McKenzie's extension regimen remains the favored option for regaining range of movement and maintaining lumbar lordosis in lumbar disk injury, except where repeated lumbar extension remains painful.

McKenzie mobilizing exercise programs are adapted easily to athletes as they are basically a self-management regimen in three stages: correction of deformity, prone-lying with passive extension, and finally, more general stretches such as rotation and flexion. These programs are based on the concept that lumbar extension is reshaping the bulging disk back to normal and 'centralizing' the pain over several bouts of exercise performed daily.

Repeated motions that cause back pain to ease and become more proximal are encouraged, while exercises or repeated movements that make the pain radiate more peripherally are avoided. Over several sessions, the regimen is followed in a particular order. First, if there is lateral flexion deformity in standing, this is corrected passively by the therapist and/or actively by the athlete. If there is a list to the right with pain on the left side, the athlete stands with the right shoulder against a wall and shunts the pelvis passively to the right ten times, pushing on the left hip with the left hand, and nudging slightly further into range each time. This maneuvre can often produce severe back pain, leading to dizziness or even passing out. Therefore, it is wise to have a chair nearby just in case.

This is followed by passive extension stretches in standing, using the hands for counterpressure on the iliac crests, and then prone-lying for as long as it takes for the pain to abate. As the pain eases, passive extension exercises are commenced and progressed to a point where the athlete has both elbows fully extended, then downward pressure can be exerted to increase the extension by breathing out and letting the hips sag, or passively by the therapist or with a seat belt. Flexion, especially when sitting, is avoided. Any periods of flexion are countered with extension exercises either while standing or in the prone position to maintain the lordosis and normal disk shape.

Finally, rotation and flexion exercises are gradually introduced using extension in between the exercises to balance the forces on the disk. This process may take just a few days or may continue for several weeks through the whole subacute stage to the 12-week point. At the end of the 12-week period, the condition is, by definition, now chronic. If pain has not resolved, or if there has been a prior history of recurrence with apparently trivial activity, or difficulty getting a comfortable position at night and aggravation from any prolonged posture, instability of a disk segment should be suspected. Instability is basically a clinical diagnosis, and the patient should be referred to a physician. These true instabilities may need bracing as well as the core stability strength exercises, close attention to posture and bedding, modification of sporting activities or even re-evaluation of sporting goals in the long term.

Most cases of long-term disk injuries in athletes are not true disk instabilities but are simply chronic or recurrent LBP. These are cases that persist beyond the 12-week mark and the evidence shows that active treatment in the form of exercise is more effective than passive treatment in these cases. Regaining motor control of spinal segmental stability is vital as there is strong evidence to suggest that a weakened or inhibited TA and LM is associated with recurrent LBP, not only in athletes, but in the general community as well (Richardson et al 1999). Various study findings provide evidence that both conscious and automatic patterns of abdominal muscle activation can be altered by specific exercise interventions (O'Sullivan et al 1998, Richardson et al 1999).

CORE STABILITY TRAINING

Many athletes participate in what is called core stability training (see Chapter 9), emphasizing TA activation. It is important with this approach to correctly activate TA in an isolated fashion to avoid perpetuating poor motor control patterns (Richardson et al 1999). Athletes often demonstrate an overactivation of the external oblique abdominals and this can be very difficult to change. Athletes also often attempt very difficult training exercises, without really stabilizing well enough first (Richardson et al 1999).

Core stability training should begin with the detailed assessment of TA and lumbar multifidus activation and motor control in the lumbopelvic region under no load and then in functional positions such as standing, walking, running, hopping and sport-specific activities. Where there is poor control, it can be observed as excessive lumbopelvic movement during the performance of these activities (e.g. excessive lateral or anterior pelvic tilt). Where instability and poor motor control are confirmed as contributing factors to an athlete's back pain, athletes should be retaught to correctly activate their TA and LM in isolation in the supine, four-point kneeling, sitting, standing, single leg standing, and in walking, etc.

The main problem with athletes in TA training is overactivity of the external oblique abdominals in attempting to achieve an isolated TA contraction, which tend to contract automatically in response to attempts to activate the TA. To this end, real time ultrasound imaging of the TA can be utilized as biofeedback (Richardson et al 1999). Once the athlete can achieve an adequate isolated TA activation, training can progress beyond these static postures to challenge the motor control system more dynamically. Athletes can progress beyond the standard TA and LM activation exercise to include high repetition abdominal, trunk rotation, extension and lateral flexion work. Therapeutic rubber tubing, Pilates training and Swiss balls can be used to challenge the athlete's endurance, strength and stability to make further progress. Swiss Ball rehabilitation (with appropriate progressions) should be commenced when the athlete is comfortable sitting (Fig. 14.9).

With long-term disk problems, there may be postural changes evident that can hamper recovery and contribute to continued back pain. Tightness of hip flexors (psoas), hamstrings and deep gluteal muscles should be addressed with deep massage and stretching. Also, there

may be adverse neural tension signs as described by Butler (1991). Neural stretching, including slump techniques, can be used after the acute stage with care, and can be incorporated in a regular home program of stretching (Fig. 14.11).

Strengthening of the lower back extensors as distinct from that of the LM should only commence with isometrics, back extensions using the Swiss ball and finally the classic hyperextension exercises in a Roman Chair with or without added weights. This must be closely supervised with care taken to ensure that the TA and LM are activated first and that hyperextension is actually avoided during the exercise.

Full rehabilitation of lumbar disk injury in the athlete and prevention of reoccurrence will need a detailed flexibility and strengthening program plus attention to posture and technique, often in consultation with a coach or weight-training coach. The athlete and coach cannot ignore a disk injury, the lumbar spine is now vulnerable, and although the athlete can compensate by continued stretching and strengthening, there will have to be compromises made in the training program to keep the problem manageable. Heavy squats, deadlifts, cleans and bent over rows are the type of strength training exercises that put a weakened disk at high risk, and alternative methods for developing leg and back strength should be used.

NEUROGENIC BACK PAIN IN THE ATHLETE

Primary neuromeningeal pathology is rare, but symptoms of adverse mechanical tension in the nervous system are often the late result of previous severe back injuries (i.e. disk bulges or spondylolisthesis) and may cause chronic back or leg pain (Butler 1991). The slump test can be used to determine whether there is a neuromeningeal component to an athlete's back symptoms (Corrigan & Maitland 1998). The slump test is positive if the athlete's pain is reproduced and if it is altered by changes in tension on the neuromeningeal structures involved. If there is a neuromeningeal component to the problem, neural or dural mobilization may be incorporated, cautiously at first, then more aggressively, in back mobilization techniques (Fig. 14.11A).

It is also important to prescribe neuromeningeal stretches to patients with low back pain, when appropriate, to add to their regular home program. These can commence with simple hamstring, gluteal, and ankle dorsiflexion maneuvres in combination with spinal flexion to mobilize the lumbosacral nerves, or hip extension and knee flexion with spinal flexion for the femoral and upper lumbar nerves (see Fig. 14.11B).

Modifying slump for the gluteals or posterior thigh and femoral slump (Fig. 14.11C) for the groin and

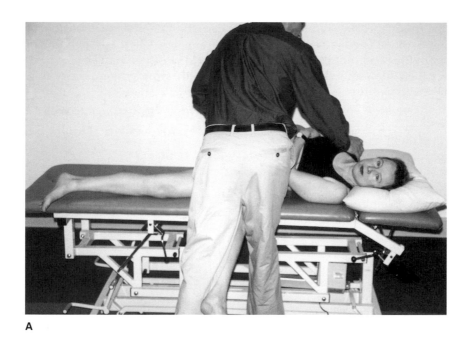

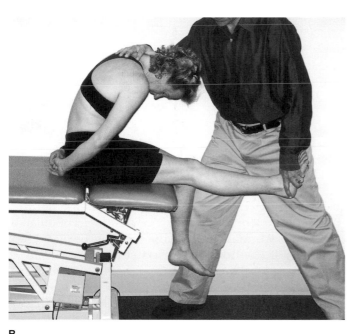

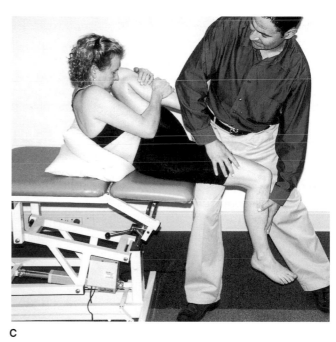

Figure 14.11A–C   **A**: Passive rotation/straight leg raise stretching. **B**: Modified 'slump' stretches to improve neuromeningeal mobility in the gluteals or posterior thigh, knee or leg. **C**: Modified femoral slump stretch to improve neuromeningeal mobility in the anterior thigh, knee or leg.

anterior thigh stretches in various ways is possible to allow the athlete to feel stretch in the symptomatic area. These stretches are best done after all the other exercises, when the back, hamstring and gluteals have warmed up, not first thing in the morning, and are certainly contra-indicated in acute spinal injury or irritable conditions. Instruction should be given to athletes as to when not to do slump stretches, as well as when they should be done.

SACROILIAC JOINT SYNDROMES IN ATHLETES

The sacroiliac joints (see Ch. 18) can be a source of symp-toms in younger athletes or especially those prone to hypermobility. It is common in females postpartum, in ex-dancers, and ex-gymnasts, and in prior participants in callisthenics who were previously very flexible and very well-toned, but who subsequently develop poor abdominal muscle tone and poor pelvic biomechanics. Problems arise when these women begin a new running or exercise program without the benefit of their previous level of fitness to protect their hypermobile joints. It is also common in athletes who require extreme hip or pelvic mobility or those engaging in asymmetric sports activities, such as hurdlers.

One or both of the hypermobile sacroiliac joints may sublux and remain fixated causing pain on the affected side, or on the opposite side, which has more demands placed upon it due to the nature of the closed mechanical system of the pelvis, leading to joint inflammation. There may be a relevant functional or structural leg length discrepancy.

Acute sacroiliitis can be very irritable and refer pain to the buttock, back of the leg and groin but it has a non-dermatomal distribution; it is worse on standing and walking than in sitting. Sacroiliac syndromes respond poorly to mobilization. The use of ultrasound or other forms of heat and gentle exercises first, followed by the dynamic stabilization or muscle energy approach is sometimes used with good success in chosen cases.

ILIAC CREST INJURY IN ATHLETES

An elongated transverse process of L4 or L5 impinging on the iliac crest can cause LBP that is aggravated by ipsilateral lateral flexion in sports, such as tennis, netball or football. It usually has not responded to previous treatment aimed at an apparent soft tissue problem. Traction apophysitis in the adolescent athlete or iliolumbar ligament sprain can also cause acute tenderness of the posterior portion of the iliac crest and can radiate pain into the buttock or lower lumbar spine. Plain X-rays are usually helpful in establishing the cause. Once the diagnosis of soft tissue injury has been confirmed, physical therapy such as electrotherapy, massage, stretching and strengthening programs are beneficial. Local corticosteroid injection may be required where physical therapy has only afforded temporary relief.

TRANSITIONAL VERTEBRAE WITH PSEUDARTHROSES IN THE ATHLETE

X-rays of the lumbar spine in athletes with LBP sometimes reveal an extra lumbar vertebra, sacralization of the fifth lumbar vertebra or lumbarization of the first sacral vertebra, with or without intervening pseudarthroses. These 'false joints' are prone to degenerative conditions that may be the cause of disk degeneration and chronic LBP, especially if one side is fused. Physical therapy will consist of all the available pain relieving modalities, whilst mobilization of the affected level is unlikely to afford relief, mobilizing above the injury and functional

core strengthening may be of benefit, as will be correction of any leg length or pelvic asymmetry. Local corticosteroid injection may be required where physical therapy has only afforded temporary relief.

EFFICACY OF PHYSICAL THERAPIES FOR LUMBAR SPINE INJURIES IN ATHLETES

Bed rest

Hagen et al (2001) concluded that rest compared to advice to stay active will at best have small effects, and at worst might have small harmful effects on acute LBP. Two high quality trials reported no differences in pain intensity between 2 to 3 days of bed rest and 7 days of bed rest.

Massage

Based on studies reviewed by Furlan et al (2001), there is insufficient evidence to recommend massage as a stand-alone treatment for NSLBP. The athletic population was not specifically studied. There is a need for high quality controlled trials to further evaluate the effects of massage for different categories of LBP. However, athletes frequently seek hands-on treatment including back massage and may benefit from massage delivered as an adjunct to evidence-based therapy.

Exercise

The evidence summarized in a systematic review by van Tulder et al (2001b) did not indicate that specific exercises are effective for the treatment of acute LBP. Exercises may be helpful for chronic LBP patients to increase return to normal daily activities and work. The athletic population, however, was not specifically mentioned in the van Tulder et al (2001b) review. Faas et al (1996) concluded that in acute back pain, exercise therapy is ineffective, whereas in subacute back pain, exercises with a graded activity program, and in chronic back pain, intensive exercising, deserve attention. Hilde & Bo (1998) could make no firm conclusions concerning efficacy of exercise in the treatment of chronic LBP drawn from the existing randomized controlled trials (RCTs).

Whilst there is a paucity of evidence to support the use of exercise in acute or chronic LBP in the general population, it is widely believed that specific back and abdominal retraining, and in particular motor relearning for core stability, is a vital part of rehabilitation of athletic back injury (Hodges 2000).

Manipulation

The indications and contraindications for spinal manipulative therapy (SMT) in athletes with LBP are the same as for the general population (Maitland et al 2001). Manipulation is indicated where there has been a poor response or a plateau in improvements from mobilization alone, where there is an acute locked lumbar facet joint, and where stiffness at end of range is greater than pain as the main symptom. In a metaanalysis of clinical trials of spinal manipulation, Anderson et al (1992) concluded that SMT proved to be consistently more effective in the treatment of LBP than were any of the arrays of comparison treatments. The analysis provided some suggestion that manipulation, as such, is more effective than mobilization. For acute LBP, within the first 6 weeks of onset, SMT provides better short-term improvement in pain and activity levels and higher patient satisfaction than other treatments (Waddell 1998). For chronic LBP, the evidence is inconclusive (Koes et al 1996).

Acupuncture

The evidence from a systematic review by van Tulder et al (2001a) did not indicate that acupuncture is effective for the treatment of back pain. The athletic population, however, was not specifically mentioned.

Traction

Lumbar traction is best performed using mechanical or motorized means. Beurskens et al (1997) investigated the efficacy of traction for NSLBP with a randomized clinical trial, and found no statistically significant differences between the groups on all outcome measures. Werners et al (1999) performed a randomized trial comparing interferential therapy with motorized lumbar traction and massage in the management of LBP in a primary care setting, and found a progressive fall in Oswestry Disability Index and pain visual analog scale scores in patients with LBP treated with either interferential therapy or motorized lumbar traction and massage. There was no difference in the improvement between the two groups at the end of treatment. Although there is evidence from several other trials that traction alone is ineffective in the management of LBP, this study could not exclude some effect from the concomitant massage.

BACK PAIN IN THE YOUNG ATHLETE

Back injuries affect between 10–15% of young athletes, including both traumatic and overuse injuries (d'Hemecourt et al 2000). The incidence of back pain increases with higher levels of physical activity, according to a Finnish cohort study in schoolchildren (Kujala et al 1999). While the incidence of traumatic back injuries may be reduced by rule modification for young participants, overuse injuries tend to recur, with a rate of

26% in males and 33% in females reported by Taimela et al (1997). Most back complaints in children and adolescents will be soft tissue in origin and related to growth or to posture. The child that presents with persistent back pain, however, should be fully investigated for the presence of serious pathology. Common back problems encountered in young athletes are juvenile lumbar disk lesions, atypical Scheuermann's disease, and spondylolysis or spondylolisthesis seen in sports involving hyperextension and rotation, such as fast bowling in cricket, defensive line in American football, diving or gymnastics (see Ch. 24).

PREVENTION OF SPINAL INJURIES IN SPORT

For prevention of cervical spine injury, especially in contact sports such as American and Australian football, Rugby League, and Rugby Union, there is no doubt that strict enforcement of rules of play and modification of rules in these sports for young athletes is effective. While there are no RCTs on prevention of spinal injury in sports, review of the current literature on prevention of LBP yields several conclusions. First, there is strong evidence that back schools or other forms of back education are ineffective in prevention of LBP. Also, there is only moderate evidence to show that lumbar supports are ineffective in the prevention of LBP. Finally, there is limited evidence for the positive effect of exercise in the prevention of LBP. Clearly, due to the inconsistent findings of the RCTs reviewed, more studies are needed to clarify the role of exercise in LBP (Maher 2000). Thus, there may be a role for regular exercise in the prevention of LBP, and it is logical that those athletes who have already suffered an episode of spinal injury may benefit from regular maintenance exercise.

While there is insufficient evidence to support the concept at present, preseason or preparticipation spinal screening has been advocated for prevention of sports injury in a wider context, and it would be of benefit to screen young athletes for potential spinal injury in high risk sports such as weightlifting, gymnastics, rowing, the defensive line in American football and fast bowling in cricket (See Ch. 11).

SUMMARY

The spine can be conditioned with regular exercise and sport over time. However in the short term, the spine is not adaptable, and does not cope well with rapidly applied extremes of motion and force. Specific sports or exercise-induced injuries to the spine present in recognizable patterns. As discussed, there are very specific spinal injuries in sports caused by faulty technique, poor motor control or poor biomechanics. Rehabilitation and treatment of spinal injuries in the sport population are not the same as the spinal injuries found in the general population, and awareness of this is required by the physical therapist when developing a rehabilitation program.

REFERENCES

Anderson I F, Read J W, Steinweg J 1998 Atlas of imaging in sports medicine. McGraw Hill, Sydney

Anderson R, Meeker W C, Wirick B E et al 1992 A meta-analysis of clinical trials of spinal manipulation. Journal of Manipulative and Physiological Therapeutics 15:181–194

Beurskens A J, de Vet H C, Koke A J et al 1997 Efficacy of traction for nonspecific low back pain. 12-week and 6-month results of a randomized clinical trial. Spine 22:2756–2762

Brukner P, Khan K 2000 Clinical Sports Medicine, 2nd edn. McGraw Hill, Sydney

Burnett A, Elliot B, Foster O et al 1990 The back breaks before the wicket. The young fast bowler's spine. Sport Health 9(4):11–14

Butler D S 1991 Mobilization of the nervous system. Churchill Livingstone, Edinburgh

Ciullo J V, Jackson D W 1985 Pars interarticularis stress reaction, spondylolysis and spondylolisthesis in gymnasts. Clinics in Sports Medicine 4:95–110

Congeni J, McCulloch J, Swanson K 1997 Lumbar spondylolysis. A study of natural progression in athletes. American Journal of Sports Medicine 25:248–253

Corrigan B, Maitland G D 1998 Vertebral musculoskeletal disorders. Butterworth Heinemann, Oxford

d'Hemecourt P A, Gerbino P G, Micheli L J 2000 Back injuries in the young athlete. Clinics in Sports Medicine 19:663–679

Elliot B, Burnett A, Stockill N et al 1995 The fast bowler in cricket: a sports medicine perspective. Sports, Exercise and Injury 1:201–206

Faas A, Battie M C, Malmivaara A 1996 Exercises: which ones are worth trying, for which patients, and when? Spine 21: 2874–2879

Fairbank J C T, Mbaot J C, Davies J B et al 1980 The Oswestry Low Back Pain Disability Questionnaire. Physiotherapy 66:271–273

Fellander-Tsai L, Micheli L J 1998 Treatment of spondylolysis with external electrical stimulation and bracing in adolescent athletes: a report of two cases. Clinical Journal of Sports Medicine: 8:232–234

Flemming J E 1990 Spondylolysis and spondylolisthesis. In: Hochshuler S H (ed) The spine in sports. Hanley and Belfus, Philadelphia, PA

Furlan A D, Brosseau L, Welch V et al 2001 Massage for low back pain. Cochrane Review. In: The Cochrane Library, 2, 2001. Update Software, Oxford

Gross A R, Aker P D, Goldsmith C H et al 2001 Physical medicine modalities for mechanical neck disorders. Cochrane Review. In: The Cochrane Library, 2, 2001. Update Software, Oxford

Hagen K B, Hilde G, Jamtvedt G et al 2001 Bed rest for acute low back pain and sciatica. Cochrane Review. In: The Cochrane Library, 2, 2001. Update Software, Oxford

Hardcastle P, Annear P, Foster D H et al 1992 Spinal abnormalities in young fast bowlers. Journal of Bone and Joint Surgery (Br) 74B: 421–425

Hilde G, Bo K 1998 Effect of exercise in the treatment of chronic low back pain: a systematic review, emphasising type and dose of exercise. Physical Therapy Reviews 3:107–117

Hodges P W 2000 The role of the motor system in spinal pain: implications for rehabilitation of the athlete following lower back pain. Journal of Science and Medicine in Sport 3:243–253

Hurwitz E L, Aker P D, Adams A H et al 1996 Manipulation and mobilization of the cervical spine: a systematic review of the literature. Spine 21:1746–1760

Jull G 1997 Management of cervical headache. Manual Therapy 2:182–190

Kjellman G V, Skargren E I, Oberg B E 1999 A critical analysis of randomised clinical trials on neck pain and treatment efficacy. A review of the literature. Scandinavian Journal of Rehabilitation Medicine 31:139–145

Klaber Moffett J A, Hughes G I, Griffiths P 1990 An investigation of the effects of cervical traction. Part 1: Clinical effectiveness. Clinical Rehabilitation 4:205–211

Koes B W, Assendelft W J J, Van der Heijden G J M G et al 1996 Spinal manipulation for low back pain: an updated systematic review of randomised clinical trials. Spine 21:2860–2873

Kujala U M, Taimela S, Viljanen T 1999 Leisure physical activity and various pain symptoms among adolescents. British Journal of Sports Medicine 5:325–328

Maher C G 2000 A systematic review of workplace interventions to prevent low back pain. Australian Journal of Physiotherapy 46: 259–269

Maitland G, Hengeveld E, Banks K et al 2001 Vertebral manipulation, 6th edn. Butterworth Heinemann, Oxford

Mandelbaum B R, Gross M L 1991 Spondylolysis and spondylolisthesis. In: Reider B (ed) Sports medicine: the school-age athlete. WB Saunders, Philadelphia, PA

Melzack R 1987 The short-form McGill Pain questionnaire. Pain 30:191–197

Morita T, Ikata T, Katoh S, Miyake R 1995 Lumbar spondylolysis in children and adolescents. Journal of Bone and Joint Surgery Br 77(4): 620–625

Nilsson N, Christensen H W, Hartvigsen J 1996 Lasting changes in passive range motion after spinal manipulation: a randomized, blind, controlled trial. Journal of Manipulative and Physiological Therapeutics 19:165–168

O'Sullivan PB 2000 Lumbar segmental 'instability': clinical presentation and specific stabilizing exercise management. Manual Therapy 5:2–12

O'Sullivan P B, Phyty G D, Twomey LT et al 1997 Evaluation of specific stabilizing exercise in the treatment of chronic low back pain with radiologic diagnosis of spondylolysis or spondylolisthesis. Spine 22:2959–2967

O'Sullivan P B, Twomey L, Allison G T 1998 Altered abdominal muscle recruitment in patients with chronic back pain following a specific exercise intervention. Journal of Orthopaedic and Sports Physical Therapy 27:114–124

Richardson C, Jull G, Hodges P et al 1999 Therapeutic exercise for spinal segmental stabilization in low back pain. Scientific basis and clinical approach. Churchill Livingstone, Edinburgh

Roland M, Morris R 1983 A study of the natural history of back pain. Part 1: Development of a reliable and sensitive measure of disability in low back pain. Spine 8:141–144

Rossi F 1988 Spondyolysis, spondylolisthesis in sports. Journal of Sports Medicine and Physical Fitness 18:317–340

Spitzer W O, Skovron M L, Salmi L R et al 1995 Scientific monograph of the Quebec Task Force on whiplash-associated disorders: redefining 'whiplash' and its management. Spine 20(suppl):1S–73S

Sterling M, Jull G, Wright A 2001 Cervical mobilization: concurrent effects on pain, sympathetic nervous system activity and motor activity. Manual Therapy 6:72–81

Stratford P, Gill C, Westaway M et al 1995 Assessing disability and change on individual patients: a report of a patient specific measure. Physiotherapy Canada 47:258–263

Taimela S, Kujala U M, Salminen J J et al 1997 The prevalence of low back pain among children and adolescents. A nationwide, cohort-based questionnaire survey in Finland. Spine 22:1132–1136

Taimela S, Takala E P, Asklof T et al 2000 Active treatment of chronic neck pain: a prospective randomized intervention. Spine 25:1021–1027

Thorsen H, Gam A N, Svensson B H et al 1992 Low level laser therapy for myofascial pain in the neck and shoulder girdle. A double-blind, cross-over study. Scandinavian Journal of Rheumatology 2:139–141

Torg J S, Vesgo J J, O'Neill M J et al 1990 The epidemiological, pathologic, biomechanical, and cinematographic analysis of football-induced cervical spine trauma. American Journal of Sports Medicine 18:50–57

Van der Heijden G J M G, Beurskens A J H M, Koes B W et al 1995 The efficacy of traction for back and neck pain: a systematic, blinded review of randomized clinical trial methods. Physical Therapy 75:93–104

van Tulder M W, Cherkin D C, Berman et al 2001a Acupuncture for low back pain. Cochrane Review. In: The Cochrane Library, 2, 2001. Update Software, Oxford

van Tulder M W, Malmivaara A, Esmail R et al 2001b Exercise therapy for low back pain. Cochrane Review. In: The Cochrane Library, 2, 2001. Update Software, Oxford

Vernon H, Mior S 1991 The Neck Disability Index: a study of reliability and validity. Journal of Manipulative and Physiological Therapeutics 14:409–415

Waddell G 1998 The back pain revolution. Churchill Livingstone, Edinburgh

Wajswelner H 1996 Management of rowers with rib stress fractures. Australian Journal of Physiotherapy 42:157–161

Wajswelner H, Bennell K, Story I et al 2000 Muscle action and stress on the ribs in rowing. Physical Therapy in Sport 1:75–84

Werners R, Pynsent P B, Bulstrode C J K 1999 Randomized trial comparing interferential therapy with motorized lumbar traction and massage in the management of low back pain in a primary care setting. Spine 24:1579–1580

Wiltse L L, Newman P H, Macnab I 1976 Classification of spondylolysis and spondylolisthesis. Clinical Orthopedics 117:23

15

Shoulder

Mary E Magarey   Mark Jones

INTRODUCTION

The shoulder complex is required to withstand extreme forces with overhead and contact sports and yet has what appears to be relatively few anatomical constraints to generate and support such forces. In reality, the glenohumeral joint consists of an intricate network of interlinked support mechanisms especially designed to withstand large forces, provide extraordinary mobility and yet maintain the stability and control necessary to enable precise function of the upper limb.

The primary focus of this chapter is the glenohumeral joint and its supporting mechanisms, and on those conditions associated with overhead sports, as this is the patient group that presents the most challenge to the sports physical therapist.

SPORT-SPECIFIC APPLIED ANATOMY AND BIOMECHANICS

Descriptions of anatomy can be found in most shoulder texts including Ciullo (1996), Dugas et al (1999), Jobe (1998), O'Brien et al (1998a), Peat & Culham (1994), and Warner & Boardman (1999).

THE CAPSULOLABRAL COMPLEX

The glenoid labrum forms a ring around the periphery of the glenoid and provides anchorage for the capsulo-ligamentous structures (Warner & Boardman 1999) (Fig. 15.1). The labrum contributes to stability by increasing the surface area of the glenoid and acting in a load-bearing capacity for the humeral head (Bowen et al 1992, Rames & Karzel 1993, Soslowsky et al 1991, 1992a,b), as well as increasing the depth and concavity of the glenoid (Fukuda et al 1988, Hata et al 1992, Howell &

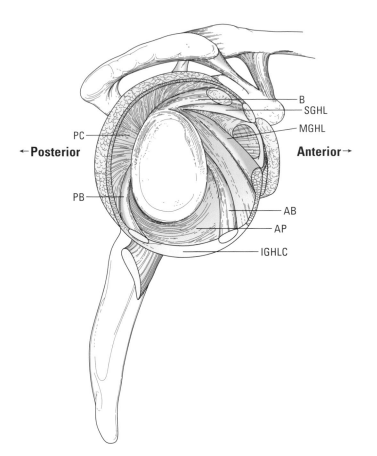

Figure 15.1 Anatomical configuration of the soft tissue structures about the glenohumeral joint. A = anterior, P = posterior, SGHL = superior glenohumeral ligament, MGHL = middle glenohumeral ligament, IGHLC = inferior glenohumeral ligament complex, consisting of an anterior band (AB), a posterior band (PB), and the axillary pouch (AP), PC = posterior capsule, B = tendon of biceps, demonstrating its close association with the SGHL. The configuration of the ligaments shown in this diagram matches that described as most common by Ferrari (1990) with the opening of the subscapularis bursa between the SGHL and MGHL. More superficially (not named in this diagram) surrounding and joint is the rotator cuff, with supraspinatus superiorly, infraspinatus posteriorly, teres minor posteroinferiorly and subscapularis anteriorly. (Reproduced from O'Brien et al 1990, with the permission of The American Orthopaedic Society for Sports Medicine.)

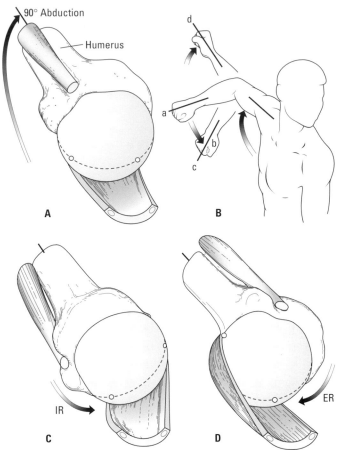

Figure 15.2 The IGHLC and its function during abduction and rotation. **A**: The whole IGHLC is tightened during abduction. **B**: Different parts of the ligament are further tightened during medial or lateral rotation in abduction. **C**: With medial rotation, the posterior band fans out to support the head and the anterior band becomes cord-like. **D**: With lateral rotation, the anterior band fans out to support the head and the posterior band becomes cord-like. (Adapted from O'Brien et al 1998a.)

Galinat 1987, Lippitt et al 1993, Lippitt & Matsen 1993, Pagnani & Warren 1994). The labrum provides the concave space necessary to maintain negative pressure (Habermeyer & Schüller 1990, Habermeyer et al 1992), preventing distraction of the joint surfaces and decreasing available translation. Damage to the labrum breaks the seal and decreases the compression, allowing an increase in the range of translation, independent of capsular venting.

The inferior glenohumeral ligament complex (IGHLC) is the primary passive restraint to movement in all positions other than adduction (Bigliani et al 1992, Branch et al 1995, O'Brien et al 1990, 1995, O'Connell et al 1990, Pagnani & Warren 1994, Pollock et al 2000, Schwartz et al 1987) (Fig. 15.2). With the arm in adduction, the rotator

interval takes on the primary stabilizing role (Field et al 1995, Harryman et al 1992, Helmig et al 1990, Neer et al 1992, Nobuhara & Ikeda 1987, Ozaki 1989, Warner & Boardman 1999, Warner et al 1990, 1992, 1993b, Warren et al 1984).

The capsule and ligaments function predominantly to check and guide movement of the joint, with little direct midrange effect (Matsen et al 1998b). They are responsible for the 'obligate' conjoint rotations and translations that occur towards end range, altering the convex/concave kinematics that function within range (Harryman et al 1990, 1992, Terry et al 1991). The significance of the conjoint movement lies in recognition of normal, as a tightened capsule exaggerates these translations while a lax capsule leads to a reduction in translation or even a reversal, such as seen with anterior laxity in the overhead athlete (Harryman et al 1990, 1992).

A complex interaction exists between the various regions of the shoulder capsule and their labral attachments. The role of any specific component varies with the position of the arm and direction of applied force. The site and nature of damage associated with trauma depends on the age of the subject, the direction and amount of force applied, and the rate and frequency of application of that force. The force required to rupture a glenohumeral capsule and rotator cuff decreases with age (Hertz 1984, Kaltsas 1983, Reeves 1968) such that older subjects tend to rupture through these structures, whereas younger subjects fail at the labralosseous junction or within the labrum itself. Rupture of the rotator cuff concurrent with dislocation of the shoulder is common in subjects over 40 years of age (Craig 1984, Gonzalez & Lopez 1991, Neviaser et al 1988).

DYNAMIC RESTRAINTS OF THE GLENOHUMERAL JOINT

Rotator cuff

The rotator cuff is the primary dynamic restraint of the glenohumeral joint (Ciullo 1996, David et al 2000, Kibler 1998a, Lippitt & Matsen 1993, Lippitt et al 1993, Matsen et al 1998a, 1998b, Schenkman & Rugo de Cartaya 1987, 1994, Souza 1994). It forms a sheath of tissue composed of the tendinous portions of supraspinatus, infraspinatus, teres minor and subscapularis, which surrounds the glenohumeral joint, forming a nearly continuous sleeve (Clark et al 1990, Clark & Harryman 1992, Dugas et al 1999, Harryman & Clark 1996) (Fig. 15.3).

Supraspinatus arises from the supraspinatus fossa, and infraspinatus from the infraspinatus fossa, overlying fascia and the scapular spine (Jobe 1998). Teres minor arises from the middle part of the lateral border of the scapula and the infraspinatus fascia (Jobe 1998). In addition to its tendinous insertion, muscular fibers attach directly to the posterior surgical neck of the humerus and extend inferiorly for up to 2 cm below the greater tuberosity (Harryman & Clark 1996).

Subscapularis arises from the subscapularis fossa. It has two compartments, with the upper 60% forming a collagen-rich tendon, considered to have a significant passive stabilizing role against anterior translation (Ovesen & Neilsen 1985, Symeonides 1972, Terry et al 1991, Turkel et al 1981), while the lower 40% has a fleshy insertion into the humerus inferior to the lesser tuberosity (Jobe 1998). The middle glenohumeral ligament (MGHL) blends with the deep surface of the upper portion of the tendon, while the anterior band of the IGHLC lies deep to the midportion (Clark et al 1990).

The long head of biceps (LHB) is a component of the rotator cuff. It arises from the superior labrum and

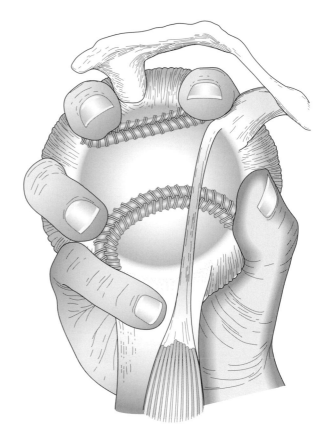

Figure 15.3 The four rotator cuff muscles, arising from different aspects of the scapula, surround and control the position of the head of humerus like the fingers of a baseball pitcher on the ball. By means of synergistic cocontraction of the musculotendinous units, the rotator cuff maintains balanced stability of the glenohumeral joint and therefore controls the position of the entire upper limb. (Reproduced from Harryman D T, Clark J M 1996 Anatomy of the rotator cuff. In: Burkhead W Z (ed) Rotator cuff disorders. Williams and Wilkins, Baltimore, with the permission of Lippincott Williams and Wilkins.)

supraglenoid tubercle (Andrews et al 1985, Blachut & Day 1989, Detrisac & Johnson 1986, Getelman & Snyder 1999, Izaki et al 1994a, 1994b, Refior & Sowa 1995), although variations are reported (Ciullo 1996, Grauer et al 1992, Habermeyer et al 1987, Habermeyer & Walch 1996) (Fig. 15.4). The tendon is intra-articular but extrasynovial, passing over the humeral head and leaving the glenohumeral joint via the intertubercular (bicipital) groove, between the tendons of supraspinatus and subscapularis.

As a result of its attachments to the superior labrum and its intimate association with the coracohumeral ligament (CHL), superior glenohumeral ligament (SGHL) and MGHL, the LHB is an important dynamic stabilizer of the glenohumeral joint to both superior migration and anteroposterior translation (Burkhead 1990, Flatow et al 1997, Habermeyer et al 1987, Habermeyer & Walch 1996, Itoi et al 1993, 1994, Kumar et al 1989, Matsen et al 1998a, 1998b, Warner & McMahon 1994). The tendon of the LHB functions as a 'monorail', guiding humeral rotation, while depressing the humeral head through the rotator

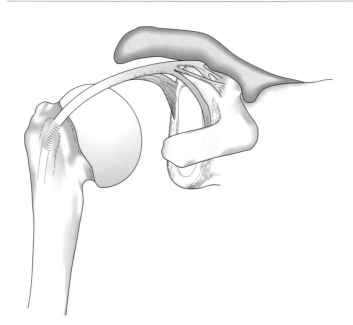

Figure 15.4 Diagrammatic representation of the origin of the LHB tendon, demonstrating its attachment to the anterior and posterior labrum in addition to the supraglenoid tubercle and base of the coracoid process.

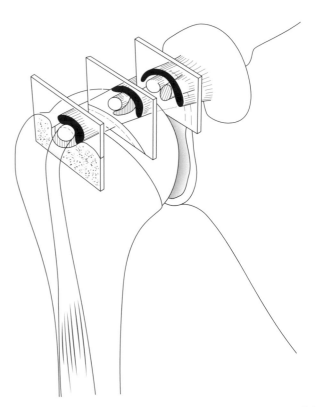

Figure 15.5 Schematic diagram showing the inter-relationship of the coracohumeral and superior glenohumeral ligaments and the LHB tendon in the rotator interval. The coracohumeral ligament (black) forms a crescent shaped root over the LHB tendon (white), while the SGHL (hatched) forms a U-shaped trough underneath the tendon. (Reproduced from Habermeyer P, Walch G 1996 The biceps tendon and rotator cuff disease. In: Burkhead W Z (ed) Rotator cuff disorders. Williams and Wilkins, Baltimore, with the permission of Lippincott Williams and Wilkins.)

interval suspensory system (Fig. 15.5). Any pathology that disrupts the rotator interval can lead to instability of the LHB tendon (Habermeyer & Walch 1996). Lateral rotation tightens the tendon in the floor of its groove, where its efficiency is enhanced and it is able to function more effectively as a stabilizer (Kessell 1982). Both the LHB and the short head of biceps (SHB) contribute to anterior stability in lateral rotation, reducing the load on the inferior stabilizing structures (Itoi et al 1993, Rodosky et al 1994). In extreme ranges of lateral rotation, however, the stabilizing effect becomes significant only when the inferior stabilizing mechanisms are disrupted (Itoi et al 1993). Further information can be found in Ciullo (1996).

The tendons of all rotator cuff tendons intermingle across the bicipital groove in their deeper layers: supraspinatus overlying the LHB tendon and subscapularis lining the bicipital groove, with fibers also blended with those of the rotator interval and the CHL, forming the rotator interval sling (Clark et al 1990, Clark & Harryman 1992, Harryman & Clark 1996). The tendon of infraspinatus interdigitates with the posterior border of the supraspinatus tendon while the inferior fibers of infraspinatus blend with those of teres minor in a similar way. The subscapularis tendon has a different layering pattern, with the terminal fibers angulating and splaying to distribute their insertion over a larger area of fibrocartilage (Benjamin et al 1986).

There is now convincing evidence that most tendon disorders do not relate to inflammation (Astrom & Rausing 1995, Khan et al 1999, Kannus & Josza 1991,

Uhthoff & Sano 1997). Inflammatory changes appear to be present only in the torn tendon (Astrom et al 1995, Josza & Kannus 1997, Khan et al 1998, 1999). Chronic tendon pain as a result of overuse leads to degeneration of tendon tissue, lowering the tensile strength of the tendon and predisposing it to rupture. This is the most likely mechanism associated with partial tendon ruptures in the rotator cuff.

The structural link between the rotator cuff and the capsule influences stability, as contraction tightens the capsular structures and provides compression, thus limiting humeral head translation (Harryman & Clark 1996, Lippitt & Matsen 1993, Lippitt et al 1993, Matsen et al 1998a, 1998b, Warner et al 1993a). Rotator cuff tears lead to significant glenohumeral instability, as a result of disruption to the links with the passive restraints (Hsu et al 1997). When lengthened, the tendons provide a barrier against translation, often opposite to the direction of restraint provided by active contraction. For example, medial rotation lengthens and therefore tightens the posterior capsule and infraspinatus, thus restricting posterior translation, while active contraction of infraspinatus prevents anterior translation of the humeral head (Harryman & Clark 1996). Interestingly, the coracoacromial ligament (CAL) also has a stabilizing role, with its disruption leading to significant increases in anterior and inferior translation, particularly at lower ranges of abduction (Lee et al 2001).

All rotator cuff muscles have their own torque producing role. Infraspinatus is considered to be the primary lateral rotator of the glenohumeral joint (Harryman & Clark 1996). However, teres minor contributes more with the arm in abduction, with infraspinatus more active with the arm adducted, supporting the need to consider their separate functional roles (Jobe & Pink 1994). Two types of motor activation organization patterns have been identified: a 'length-dependent pattern' operating locally around a joint by cocontraction and responsible for stabilization, and a 'force-dependent' pattern acting at several linked joints and responsible for force generation (Kibler 1998a, Nichols 1994). Burkhart's (1991, 1992, 1993, 1994, 1996, Burkhart et al 1993) biomechanical modeling indicates that the lower elements of the rotator cuff (infraspinatus/teres minor and subscapularis) fulfill the characteristics of a length-dependent pattern and, coupled with evidence of activation of the rotator cuff prior to that of the superficial muscles and cocontraction throughout isokinetic rotations in the normal shoulder (David et al 2000), would appear to further support this function for the rotator cuff. The muscular extensions to the insertions of subscapularis and teres minor provide additional depressive/compressive leverage to these muscles, thus facilitating this function. Preliminary work on unstable shoulders indicates substantial disruption to the normal firing pattern, similar to that seen in the lumbar spine and knee (Cowan et al 2001, David et al 1997, Hodges & Richardson 1996, Magarey & Jones, in press a). In addition to the individual and combined functions of the muscles outlined above, the action of all muscles of the shoulder complex varies, depending on the position of the arm and therefore the axis of rotation (Matsen et al 1998b).

The subacromial space

The subacromial space is bounded superiorly by the coracoacromial arch, consisting of the anterior under-surface of the acromion and the coracoacromial ligament (CAL), and inferiorly by the rotator cuff, primarily supraspinatus, on the superior surface of the humeral head. It provides a strong ceiling for the glenohumeral joint, against which the rotator cuff tendons glide during shoulder movements (Matsen et al 1998a). Facilitating movement between the cuff and the arch is the subacromial bursa, which normally consists of two synovially lined surfaces in contact with each other

(Hulstyn & Fadale 1995, Matsen et al 1998a). The normal 'suprahumeral gliding mechanism' of the subacromial space (Kernwein et al 1961, Matsen et al 1998a) is an important contributor to shoulder function, as superior stability is dependent on an intact coracoacromial arch (Burns & Whipple 1993, Flatow et al 1997).

Compressive loading is normal for the rotator cuff between the concentric rings of the coracoacromial arch and the humeral head. The bursal surface of the cuff is adapted for compression and the articular surface for tensile forces (Benjamin et al 1986, Clark & Harryman 1992, Cooper et al 1993, Flatow et al 1997, Fukuda et al 1990a, 1990b, Gohlke et al 1994, Harryman & Clark 1996, Nakajima et al 1994, Woo et al 1988). Problems arise when the coracoacromial and humeral rings are no longer concentric or the cuff or bursal structure is disrupted, highlighting the intricate balance required for routine function between a normal degree of capsular laxity, a normal thickness of rotator cuff and an intact coracoacromial arch (Matsen et al 1998a).

Scapular stabilizers

The angle of inclination of the scapula has a significant effect on inferior stability of the glenohumeral joint, particularly with the arm adducted (Basmajian & Bazant 1959, Itoi et al 1992). An increase in scapular inclination tightens the superior capsule, with the increased upward slope of the glenoid fossa acting as a bony cam, further

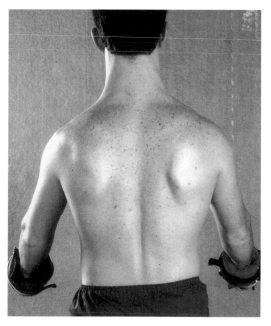

Figure 15.6 A patient demonstrating inferior drooping of the lateral scapula with apparent lengthening of the upper trapezius and possible tightness/overactivity of levator scapulae. Isometric activity to maintain slight abduction against the load of the cuff weight emphasizes inferior angle winging.

tightening the rotator interval structures (Itoi et al 1992, 1993). Inferior drooping of the lateral scapula (Fig. 15.6), from disruption of normal scapular muscle balance, leads to relaxation of the rotator interval stabilizing mechanisms, such that the humeral head is 'dumped' out of the glenoid fossa (Matsen et al 1998b).

Serratus anterior and trapezius are the primary muscles involved in scapular elevation, although their specific contribution changes as the axis of rotation moves from the root of the scapular spine to the acromioclavicular joint (Abelew 2001, Bagg & Forrest 1988, Basmajian 1963, Culham & Laprade 2001, Dvir & Berme 1978, Inman et al 1944, Poppen & Walker 1978, Schenkman & Rugo de Cartaya 1987, 1994). Alterations in function found in painful shoulders of athletes (as described below) indicate that serratus anterior and probably lower trapezius are the primary stabilizers of the scapulothoracic region.

CLINICAL EXAMINATION

Clinical examination of the shoulder is presented in many reference books, for example, the relevant chapters in Andrews & Wilk (1994a), Brukner & Khan (2001), Ciullo (1996), Rockwood & Matsen (1998), and Warren et al (1999). Physical therapy examination is presented by Allingham (1996), Johanson & Gonzalez-King (1997), and Norris (1993), while Anderson & Hall (1995) present an athletic trainer's viewpoint. An impairment based approach is presented in Tovin & Greenfield (2001), rather than the traditional medical model, with the chapter by Jones & Magarey (2001) presenting the clinical reasoning associated with shoulder examination. Knowledge of a basic shoulder examination is assumed or can be obtained from the references provided.

The diagnostic process associated with the shoulder takes time, with the need for repeated visits (Shankwiler & Burkhead 1996). The examination consists of a subjective examination or interview and a physical examination (Scarpinato et al 1991). The physical therapist must screen for activities typically associated with shoulder disorders, such as overhead sport, and the characteristic features of conditions likely to be responsible for symptoms and for those less likely. In particular, with the athletic shoulder, specific details of the sport, the level of commitment and future aspirations, amount of training and competition undertaken must be sought, as well as details of specific aggravating and easing features. If the disorder is associated with trauma, details of the mechanism of injury are important to determinie the structures involved.

Knowledge of the biomechanical and physiological demands of the relevant sports is valuable in assessment of the overhead athlete. Good summaries of the biomechanics of throwing, swimming and tennis, as the most common sports in which overuse shoulder injuries occur, can be found in Andrews & Wilk (1994b) and Ciullo (1996) and the series of papers from the Centinela Hospital Medical Centre (CHMC) Biomechanics Laboratory group (e.g. DiGiovine et al 1992, Glousman et al 1988, Gowan et al 1987, Jobe et al 1983, 1984).

An important component of the subjective examination is the generation of hypotheses from categories such as:

- The patient's disabilities and impairments (WHO 1980), both physical and psychosocial
- Contributing factors, including biomedical, physical, environmental and technique or equipment related
- Precautions and contraindications to examination and treatment; prognosis and management (Gifford 1997, Jones 1995, Jones et al 2000).

Discussion in this chapter is restricted to the physical considerations of a patient's presentation, although recognition that the patient's cognitive/affective psychosocial status influences all pain states (acute to chronic and nociceptive dominant to centrally dominant) is essential to obtaining a complete picture of the disorder and its effect on the patient's life (Gifford 1998, 2000, Jones et al 2002).

Physical examination of the shoulder complex must include detailed evaluation of the acromioclavicular joint (ACJ) and sternoclavicular joint (SCJ) in addition to the scapulothoracic articulation, the subacromial space and the glenohumeral joint. However, here the focus is on the latter three. Within the glenohumeral joint, in addition to routine examination such as active and passive physiological movements, accessory movements, palpation and neural provocation tests, the key features most relevant in the athletic shoulder are:

- Posture and relative muscle contour
- Quality, control and awareness of movement patterns
- Involvement of the rotator cuff tendons in any pain provocative state and evaluation for different types of impingement
- Integrity of the passive stabilizing structures
- Integrity of the glenoid labrum
- Dynamic control of the glenohumeral and scapulothoracic joints (STJ) and the remainder of the kinetic chain.

POSTURE AND RELATIVE MUSCLE CONTOUR

Observation of whole body posture in the context of the patient's functional demands is an integral component of postural assessment of the upper quarter. Lower quarter muscle development and spinal posture can indicate whether whole body integrated movement patterns are adequate for normal upper quarter muscle function. Cervicothoracic posture influences scapular position and mobility and, therefore, also glenohumeral mobility (Crawford & Jull 1991, Culham & Peat 1993, Solem-Bertoff et al 1993).

Specific analysis of scapular and arm position will then provide initial clues to the comparative load carried by the glenohumeral and scapulothoracic joints. Measurement of the amount of the humeral head palpable anterior to the acromion (normally approximately one-third) provides a good reassessment tool. Kibler's (1991, 1998a, 1998b) 'lateral scapular slide test' and the modified lateral scapular slide test (Davies & Dickoff-Hoffman 1993), while addressing scapular position in one plane only, also provide objective measurements that can be reviewed during reassessment. Finally, specific analysis of contour and tone of all relevant muscle groups should be made.

QUALITY, CONTROL AND AWARENESS OF MOVEMENT PATTERNS

Trunk and pelvic stability are important to upper quarter function, particularly at speed or under load (Kibler 1998a, 1998b). Awareness of movement patterns and the ability to dissociate movement of one body segment from another are essential for good motor control, so careful evaluation for substitution strategies should be included, as should control of concentric and eccentric movement at speeds and under loads relevant to the patient's sport.

If abnormal humeral head placement or poor scapular rotation are identified during movement, their impact on pain provocation or quality of movement should be assessed. For example, manual stabilization of the humeral head in the glenoid similar to a mobilization with movement (MWM) technique (Mulligan 1999), preventing anterior translation during active lateral rotation, may reduce the pain of internal impingement, while manually assisted upward scapular rotation during elevation may improve quality of movement and reduce pain. If such maneuvers alter symptoms, they provide a good indication that a motor control pattern to facilitate such dynamic control is indicated.

ROTATOR CUFF AND SUBACROMIAL SPACE AS A SOURCE OF PAIN

Resisted isometric tests of abduction and rotations load the rotator cuff. Pain and weakness associated with a single resisted movement are likely to implicate an isolated component of the cuff. However, as a result of anatomical and functional integration of the individual elements of the cuff (Burkhart 1996, Clark & Harryman 1992), the discriminatory value of these tests becomes limited when multiple resisted movements are positive, although marked weakness on both resisted abduction and lateral rotation is a strong predictor of a full thickness rotator cuff tear (Matsen et al 1998a).

When isometric testing provokes pain, differentiating tests can be used to determine the relative contribution of impingement of the tendons to the pain response (Magarey & Jones 1991, Maitland 1991, Pfund et al 1998a, 1998b). Repetition of the resistive test with a distracting force separating the acromion from the humeral head has no effect on the tendons but eliminates any subacromial impingement during resisted abduction or lateral rotation. Similarly, repeating resisted medial rotation in a degree of lateral rotation eliminates subcoracoid impingement. As with all clinical tests, however, care is needed with interpretations that have not been validated, although informal analysis supports these interpretations (Magarey 1993).

A number of additional tests for the contractile structures may refine our ability to detect pathology. These include:

- The supraspinatus or 'empty can test' described by Jobe & Moynes (1982) as the position in which electromyographic (EMG) activity is maximal in supraspinatus may be useful to identify specific involvement of this muscle.
- The 'reverse empty can test' loads the shoulder elevation component of LHB function. This test is predicated on the biceps' contribution to glenohumeral abduction and flexion irrespective of elbow activity (Burkhead 1990).
- Shoulder flexion added to the isometric test of elbow flexion/supination selectively loads LHB (Itoi et al 1994).
- Resisted LHB function through full range tests involvement of the tendon sheath. Tenderness, soft tissue changes and crepitus may be felt in the groove during the movement.
- The lift off test: an inability to maintain the hand off the back in the hand behind back position indicates a tear of supscapularis (Gerber & Krushell 1991, Gerber et al 1996, Warner et al 2001).

The positions adopted in the traditional orthopedic impingement tests – the Neer (Neer & Welsh 1977) and Hawkins (Hawkins & Kennedy 1980) tests – are not structure specific. They rely for their diagnostic value on elimination of pain with injection of local anesthetic into specific structures – a feature not available to physical therapists. Therefore, their value to the physical therapist is limited. A number of alternative tests are reported in the orthopedic literature, most named after the first person to report them. Descriptions of these tests can be found in the papers cited above.

INTEGRITY OF PASSIVE STABILIZING STRUCTURES

There is a plethora of passive stability tests cited in the shoulder literature, although unfortunately, with little validation of their results (Ellenbecker et al 2000, Jerosch et al 1993). Those tests the authors have found of most clinical benefit were originally described by Gerber & Ganz (1984).

The anterior drawer test measures the range of 'allowed' anterior translation in different ranges of scapular plane abduction, with the arm in neutral rotation. Hence, it fails to test any alteration of obligate translation associated with end range (Harryman et al 1990, 1992). However, addition of lateral rotation to abduction, which would allow evaluation of normal coupled translation, approximates the apprehension position (Glousman & Jobe 1996, Mohtadi 1991) with potential for muscle guarding to limit the value of the test.

The posterior drawer test more closely evaluates the primary passive restraints to posterior translation, as the test involves horizontal flexion and slight medial rotation combined with a posterior translation force and is, therefore, more likely to provide a picture of integrity of these structures. An alternative posterior drawer test can be undertaken in sitting, with the arm in neutral (Allingham 1996), particularly if relaxation is difficult in the supine position.

The inferior glide or sulcus test (Gerber & Ganz 1984) is best performed in the supine position. Subtle instabilities associated with overhead athletes often do not demonstrate a sulcus but increased translation can be detected with palpation of the gap between the bony surfaces. Translation should be applied to the arm in a variety of positions around what would be considered neutral until one is found in which the maximum movement is available, usually in slight abduction or flexion, as the upwardly rotated glenoid will restrict inferior translation in adduction.

An anteroinferior test provides an assessment of translation in the direction in which instability is most common (Dalton & Snyder 1989, Glousman & Jobe 1996, Jobe & Jobe 1983, Matsen et al 1991, 1998b, Mohtadi 1991, Moran & Saunders 1991, Tullos & Bennett 1984, Warner & Caborn 1992, Wirth & Rockwood 1993). This test appears less prone to provocation of apprehension or muscle guarding, allowing a more consistent evaluation of range of movement and end feel (Fig. 15.7).

Traditional assessment of instability includes evaluation of anterior apprehension and relocation (Mohtadi

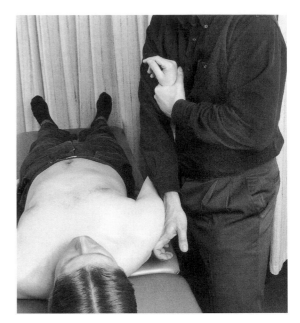

Figure 15.7 Anteroinferior translation test.

1991), although differentiation between pain and apprehension may sometimes be difficult (Altcheck et al 1990). Subjects with atraumatic instability associated with athletic overuse, may not demonstrate the same apprehensive response as following dislocation (Glousman & Jobe 1996). Pain provocation on the apprehension test rather than apprehension, with its elimination on relocation is considered diagnostic of internal impingement (Davidson et al 1995, Jobe et al 1996). Contact between posterior glenoid and rotator cuff may not occur until higher ranges of abduction, highlighting the need to vary abduction angles during testing (Hamner et al 2000).

ASSESSMENT FOR LABRAL INJURY

Overuse shoulder injuries associated with overhead athletes commonly involve disruption to the superior labrum and superior suspensory system (Abrams 1991, Andrews et al 1991, Berg & Ciullo 1998, Ciullo 1996, Gartsman & Hammerman 2000, Glasgow et al 1992, Gross et al 1990, Iannotti & Wang 1992, Jobe et al 1996, Magarey et al 1996, Schmidt & Ciullo 1998, Yoneda et al 1991). Clinical diagnosis of superior labral lesions is difficult, as there are few identifiable clinical features (Ciullo 1996, Magarey et al 1996, Schmitz & Ciullo 1998, Snyder et al 1995). Loading of LHB in different positions, particularly emphasizing the shoulder flexion component, may indirectly load the superior labrum (Andrews et al 1985, Ciullo 1996, Detrisac & Johnson 1986, Grauer et al 1992), thereby provoking pain in the presence of labral damage.

Recently, a number of tests have been reported to evaluate superior labral or superior labral anterior posterior (SLAP) lesions (Ciullo 1996, Liu et al 1996, Mimori et al 1999, O'Brien et al 1998b, Schmitz & Ciullo 1998, Zaslav 2001).

- The SLAP prehension test involves sudden medial rotation of the shoulder in 90° of forward flexion and 30° adduction. Clicking in the shoulder and/or pain radiating down the biceps tendon or in the posterior joint constitutes a positive test (Berg & Ciullo 1998, Ciullo 1996, Schmitz & Ciullo 1998). No research verification of this test was provided.
- The crank test consists of medial and lateral rotation performed in maximal forward flexion with axial compression down the humeral shaft. Reproduction of a click and/or pain is considered positive (Liu et al 1996).
- O'Brien's active compression test is performed in the standing position, with the patient's arm flexed to 90°, then placed into 10–15° of horizontal adduction with medial rotation and full elbow extension. With the forearm pronated, so that the thumb points downwards, the examiner, standing behind the patient, applies a downward resistance to the arm, such that the patient just meets the resistance. Pain response is assessed. The maneuvre is then repeated with the forearm in supination, so that the tension via the biceps tendon on the biceps anchor is altered without altering any other load on the shoulder. The test may be positive for ACJ or labral disorders, with the positive result related to pain provoked or worsened with the arm medially rotated and relieved or lessened in lateral rotation. ACJ pathology leads to local ACJ pain, while labral pathology leads to pain and/or clicking deep in the glenohumeral joint (O'Brien et al 1998b).
- The pain provocation test of Mimori et al (1999) is performed in the sitting position, with the arm in 90–100° of abduction and passive lateral rotation. The test consists of resisted biceps contraction with the arm either maximally pronated or supinated. Subjective reports of compared severity of symptoms in the two positions are used as the basis of diagnosis, with a test positive for labral pathology when pain is worse with forearm pronation. The authors emphasized that this test was useful for SLAP lesions involving the biceps anchor, not those involving superficial fraying of the labrum.
- The internal rotation resistance strength test (IRRST) consists of resisted medial and lateral rotation in a position of 90° abduction in the coronal plane and approximately 80° of lateral rotation. Weakness with or without increased pain on medial rotation, compared with lateral rotation, is positive for intraarticular pathology with the reverse being the case for subacromial pathology (Zaslav 2001).

The latter four procedures have been tested for their clinical usefulness, but given the limitations with the research design in each case, coupled with the danger of overdiagnosis of type II SLAP lesions as a result of failure to recognize normal anatomical variations (Huber & Putz 1997), the results reported should be interpreted cautiously.

Variations of a 'clunk' test may be useful in detecting frank labral pathology (Cordasco et al 1993, Field & Savoie 1993, Glasgow et al 1992, Grauer et al 1992, Payne & Jokl 1993, Rames & Karzel 1993, Resch et al 1993, Snyder et al 1990, 1995), although these tests may not detect labral fraying and minor lesions.

DYNAMIC CONTROL OF THE GLENOHUMERAL JOINT AND SCAPULOTHORACIC JOINT

Dynamic control is essential for high performance during sport and as such, assessment of glenohumeral, scapular and trunk stability should be routine. Evaluation of gross muscle strength is often delayed until stabilizing motor control is reestablished.

The authors use two tests to determine the glenohumeral dynamic stability. The dynamic rotary stability test (DRST) (Magarey & Jones in press a,b) is used to evaluate the ability of the rotator cuff to maintain normal centering of the humeral head when loaded through rotation (Howell & Galinat 1987, Howell et al 1988, Matsen et al 1998b) (Fig. 15.8). In a clearly unstable shoulder, the humeral head can be felt to translate when the rotator cuff is loaded. In more subtle situations, provocation of symptoms, alteration in the quality of contraction, clicking/clunking and compensation by other muscle groups are often noted, without the sensation of humeral head translation. Frequently, the patient's perception of loss of control (i.e. 'it feels less solid') is quite sensitive and therefore also worth attention. Load is applied manually first isometrically, then isotonically, to both rotations in different parts of the range, varying the speed and load to match the patient's functional demands. The aim is to find the position(s) in range where the patient has control of the humeral head as close as possible to the position in which control is lost. With athletes, quick reversals of rotation while holding a weighted ball may facilitate detection of humeral head movement more readily than manual resistance.

The dynamic relocation test (DRT) (Jones & Magarey 2001, Magarey & Jones in press a,b) is a test of the ability of the transverse force couple of the rotator cuff to stabilize the head of humerus in the glenoid against a destabilizing load by means of cocontraction prior to activation of more superficial muscles (David et al 1997, 2000) (Fig. 15.9). Cocontraction stiffens a joint and is an important feature of early stages of skill acquisition (Shumway-Cook & Woollacott 2001). Once the ability to

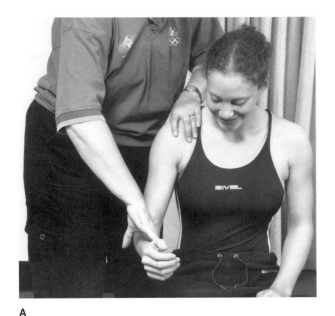

A

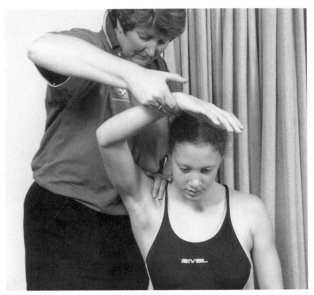

B

Figure 15.8A & B   The Dynamic Rotary Stability Test.

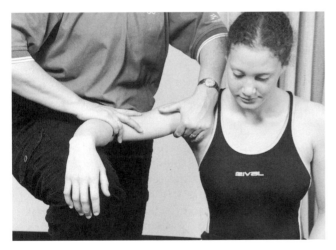

Figure 15.9   The Dynamic Relocation Test.

isolate the cocontraction has been determined in the optimal position of approximately 60–80° of scapular plane abduction, maintenance of this isolated contraction can be evaluated in different positions and during different tasks. The specific techniques for these tests are outlined elsewhere (Magarey & Jones in press a,b).

Scapular stabilizing and movement function can be evaluated in two ways, using weightbearing assessment of scapular control and modified proprioceptive neuromuscular facilitation (PNF) diagonal patterns in isolation from and in conjunction with arm movements.

Weightbearing assessment allows evaluation of scapular control for dissociation of spinal from scapular movement and dissociation of lumbar or cervical from thoracic movement. The standard starting position for

weightbearing assessment is four point kneeling, although evaluation should be undertaken in multiple different positions including leaning against a wall or table, prone on elbows and frontal and scapular plane weightbearing.

In four point kneeling, the patient's ability to protract and retract the scapulae without concurrent spinal movement is assessed. If this can be achieved, the scapula's holding ability in neutral protraction is then evaluated through different stages and types of loading. If loading in this position fails to demonstrate any impairment, the assessment can be progressed to more challenging positions or demands.

One method in which to assess functional muscle performance is through the use of the PNF D1 and D2 arm patterns (Engle 1994, Knott & Voss 1968, Voss et al 1953). During these movements, the scapula moves from retraction/depression/downward rotation to protraction/elevation/upward rotation and from protraction/depression/downward rotation to retraction/elevation/upward rotation respectively. Having first determined that the relevant range is available passively, an initial assessment of the patient's ability to undertake these scapular patterns is undertaken. The rotation component of the scapular movement is minimal when the arm is not involved, but the resultant diagonal movements are regularly dysfunctional with a painful shoulder. Stimulation with passive, active assisted and resisted movement through the patterns is used to determine whether the dysfunction is a result of lack of familiarity. If so, repeated assessment of unassisted active scapular diagonal movement is significantly improved, whereas

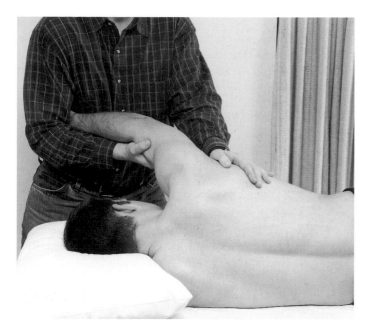

Figure 15.10   Assessment and facilitation of scapula upward rotation.

in the impaired shoulder, such improvement is not immediately evident.

Frequently with overhead athletes, delayed or restricted upward scapular rotation is apparent, so the scapula's ability to rotate upwardly during arm elevation is routinely evaluated, using similar principles to those described for the scapular patterns. The emphasis is on retraction/downward rotation to protraction/upward rotation with less emphasis on depression/elevation (Fig. 15.10).

COMMON SPORTS-RELATED INJURIES

The shoulder is commonly injured during participation in overhead sports. Most of the injuries reported relate to overuse rather than trauma. An understanding of the mechanics of the individual sports is assumed and the references cited above provide good summaries.

SWIMMING

Shoulder pain is the most common musculoskeletal complaint in swimming (Allegrucci et al 1994, Bak 1996, Bak & Faunø 1997, Ciullo & Stevens 1989) with reports of incidence of disabling shoulder pain in competitive swimmers ranging from 27% to 87% (Beach et al 1992, Bak 1996, Bak & Faunø 1997, Ciullo & Guise 1983, McMaster & Troup 1993, McMaster et al 1998, Richardson et al 1980, Stocker et al 1995). In earlier reports, subacromial impingement was the most common injury cited, however, the prevalence of hyperlaxity or instabi-

lity as a component of the problem has been identified more recently (Allegrucci et al 1994, Bak 1996, Bak & Faunø 1997, Bak & Magnusson 1997, Ciullo 1996, Ciullo & Stevens 1989, McMaster 1986, McMaster et al 1998, Murphy 1994, Pink & Jobe 1994, Zemek & Magee 1996).

The extensive EMG and cinematographic work undertaken by Centinela Hospital Medical Center (CHMC) Biomechanics Laboratory on normal swimmers and swimmers with pain during all strokes has enhanced understanding of the muscular contribution to swimming and its alteration with pain (Nuber et al 1986, Perry et al 1992, Pink et al 1991, Pink et al 1992, Pink et al 1993a, 1993b, Ruwe et al 1994, Scovazzo et al 1991). These studies have demonstrated, across all strokes, decreased activity in serratus anterior in the painful shoulder, leading to a floating scapula (Kibler 1998b). The CHMC studies, however, did not collect data from lower trapezius. Wadsworth & Bullock-Saxton (1997) reported a significant delay in timing of onset in serratus anterior and lower trapezius in swimmers with painful shoulders during active abduction, with little variation in activity in upper trapezius and rhomboids. These findings provide an indication that omission of lower trapezius from their data potentially weakens the conclusions of the CHMC studies, an opinion reinforced by Kibler's (1998a, 1998b) observation that serratus anterior and lower trapezius appear to be consistently dysfunctional in painful shoulders.

Altered patterns of muscle contraction of the rotator cuff and deltopectoral group were found in asymptomatic swimmers compared with non-swimmers during isokinetic rotations (Carr et al 1998, Schwabel 1998). The swimmers demonstrated equivalent peak torque readings to the non-swimmers, but with a lower contribution of stabilizing cocontraction by the antagonist rotator cuff/biceps group and earlier activation of the superficial muscle group during concentric lateral rotation. While the sample was small (n = 8), these findings may demonstrate swim-specific muscle function and the potential for such altered function to predispose the swimmer to reduced dynamic control of the glenohumeral joint.

Pathology is considered to occur primarily as a result of fatigue in those muscles which fire almost continuously throughout the swim stroke at 20% maximum voluntary contraction (MVC) or above (Pink et al 1991, Scovazzo et al 1991). The high level of repetitions and long training sessions, with freestyle frequently being the stroke in which most training occurs, are considered the most provocative factors. Stretching, use of training aids such as hand paddles and kickboards, and/or dry land training techniques, including weights and surgical tubing exercises, that overemphasize strengthening of muscle groups involved in the propulsive phase of the stroke, have also been identified as common features

(Ciullo 1986, Ciullo & Stevens 1989, McMaster & Troup 1993, Murphy 1994, Richardson et al 1980).

Faulty technique is usually identified as a key component of the problem, either as a primary cause or a result of antalgic modification. A cross-over hand entry and crossing the mid-line in the mid pull-through phases of the freestyle stroke predispose to impingement while a low elbow during the recovery and early pull-through phases is an important indicator of fatigue (Allegrucci et al 1994, Murphy 1994). A lack of adequate body roll forces the recovering arm into a greater range of horizontal extension and medial rotation in order to clear the hand from the water, while too much encourages arm cross-over at mid pull-through. Optimal body roll allows the arm to stay close to the plane of the scapula, thus reducing the stress of soft tissue structures in the anterior shoulder region (Murphy 1994).

Optimal body roll also allows greater lengthening of the oblique abdominal muscles, shoulder adductors/ medial rotators and scapular retractors, so that at the limit of the reach, immediately prior to initiation of the powerful catch and pull-through, these muscles are on relative stretch. One difference from throwing that is frequently cited, is the lack of eccentric muscle contraction during swimming (McLeod & Andrews 1986). However, at this point in the stroke cycle, the stretch-shortening mechanism will come into play. Some coaches are recognizing the benefit of exploiting this phenomenon, encouraging initiation of the pull-through by the pelvis to incorporate more contribution of the powerful abdominals to the action, thus decreasing the load required of the shoulder rotators.

Clinical findings in swimmers with painful shoulders have been extensively reported (e.g. Allegrucci et al 1994, Bak 1996, Bak & Faunø 1997, Ciullo 1986, Ciullo & Stevens 1989, McMaster 1986, McMaster & Troup 1993, McMaster et al 1998, Murphy 1994, Stocker et al 1995). Box 15.1 provides a summary of reported findings.

Stocker et al (1995) and Pink & Jobe (1994) reported the incidence and management of injuries in a survey of 532 masters and 395 collegiate level swimmers in the USA. The primary emphases in conservative rehabilitation suggested consistently in all reports include:

- temporary reduction in training distance and frequency
- altered training patterns to provide relative rest to the injured shoulder while allowing continued swim-specific training of non-injured structures
- avoidance of provocative training techniques, such as use of hand paddles, kickboards, surgical tubing and weight-training
- strengthening of the specific muscles identified as susceptible to fatigue

---

Box 15.1 Summary of reported clinical findings in swimmers with painful shoulders

Subjective features	Physical features

• Pain usually anterior or anterolateral, radiating to the insertion of deltoid
 • Incidence of bilateral involvement high, associated with longer duration of symptoms
 • Butterfly stroke universally identified as most provocative stroke
 • Sensation of snapping during recovery and/or mid pull-through (trapping of irritated supraspinatus tendon by the CAL or interposition of labral fragment between joint surfaces)
 • Pain and clicking during hand entry may implicate superior labrum
 • Shoulder 'slipping out' or sense of looseness
 • Less commonly, sensation of the 'shoulder being out of its socket' or frank instability
 • May complain of shoulder going 'dead'
 • Neer & Welsh's (1977) four stages of 'swimmer's shoulder':
    I pain only after heavy workouts
    II pain (not disabling) during and after workouts
    III disabling pain during & after workouts that interferes with performance
    IV pain that prevents competitive swimming, pain at rest and sleep disturbance
 • History is not mentioned specifically, but implied usually as a gradual onset
	Vary depending on proposed pathology
	
	 Subcromial impingement
	 • Point tenderness over the coracoacromial ligament
	 • Positive Neer and/or Hawkins tests
	 • Crepitus on circumduction
	 • Pain and weakness on resisted functional abduction at 90°, empty can test
	
	 Labral lesion
	 • Pain and clicking with medial rotation (MR) in 90° abduction
	 • Sliding sensation of humeral head shifting into lateral rotation (LR) as bucket handle tear relocates
	
	 Anteroinferior instability
	 • Positive anterior apprehension test
	 • MR from abduction/LR causes pop anteriorly, related to interposition of damaged labrum
	 • Increased range on translation tests
	
	 Common features reported
	 • Scapulothoracic instability
	 • Relative increase in range of LR and decrease in MR
	 • Generalized hyperlaxity
	 • Altered muscle function of various types reported on isokinetic testing

- stretching of tight structures around the shoulder, particularly any restriction of medial rotation
- technique modification to eliminate inappropriate stresses to the tissues, with this factor emphasized strongly in all programs (Allegrucci et al 1994, Bak 1996, Bak & Faunø 1997, Ciullo & Stevens 1989, Murphy 1994).

There appears to be a strong correlation between maintenance of a central position of the humeral head in the glenoid and altered muscle function, as all pathologies reported relate to abnormal humeral translation leading to disruption of adjacent structures. Traditional weight and resistance strength training programs primarily target the superficial propelling muscles (e.g. pectoralis major, deltoid and latissimus dorsi), but rehabilitation and prevention programs should include specific exercises for the rotator cuff and scapular stabilizers (Bak & Magnusson 1997). An informal analysis using the same protocol as that of Carr et al (1998) indicated a marked delay in onset and activity at peak torque in the rotator cuff of unstable shoulders and would support the need for such a focus (David et al 1997, Magarey & Jones in press a,b).

One key feature of working with swimmers is their reluctance to leave the water (Murphy 1994). There is no suitable substitute dry land equivalent, so modification of training schedules and techniques that allow continued work in the water are important components for the physical therapist in establishing or maintaining credibility with the swimmer (Allegrucci et al 1994, Murphy 1994). This can be quite challenging and, in some instances, impossible, so that a short dry-land period may be required. If this is so, it is important that the swimmer understands the reason for the lay-off and that it be kept as short as possible, even if return to the water means a compromise to the rehabilitation process. It is better to have a compromised program that the athlete will follow than an ideal one that is ignored.

THROWING

The literature associated with throwing and throwing injuries is extensive, and what is presented here represents only a sample of more recent reports. Throwing is an activity frequently associated with shoulder injuries (Andrews & Wilk 1994a, Arroyo et al 1997, Beynnon et al 1993, Cavallo & Speer 1998, Ciullo 1996, [p15], Copeland 1993, Fleisig et al 1994, 1995, 1996, Glousman 1993, Jobe & Pink 1993, Jobe et al 1998, Kvitne et al 1995, Meister 2000, Meister & Andrews 1993, Ruwe et al 1994, Ticker et al 1995). Recognition of the phase of the throw at which pain occurs is important in identifying which mechanism is likely to be primarily responsible. The high forces

---

Box 15.2 Classification of shoulder injury in overhead athletes as proposed by researchers from the Centinela Hospital Medical Center

Group 1
Older athletes
Pure impingement
No instability
Pathology within subacromial space

Group 2
Primary instability because of chronic labral and capsular microtrauma from repetitive overuse
Secondary impingement
- subacromial (Group 2A)
- intraarticular (Group 2B)
  - *apprehension sign positive for pain, pain eliminated with relocation*

Group 3
Primary instability because of generalized ligamentous hyperelasticity
  - *marked mutidirectional increase in translation*
Secondary impingement
- subacromial (Group 3A)
- internal (Group 3B)
  - *apprehension sign positive for pain, pain eliminated with relocation*

Group 4
Pure instability (traumatic)
  - *apprehension positive, relieved by relocation*
No impingement

---

applied at the extremes of range, coupled with the levels of repetition place the structures of the shoulder complex under considerable stress.

Over the past 10 years, understanding of the mechanisms of shoulder injuries in throwing athletes has advanced, with recognition of intraarticular pathology as a significant component. The CHMC research group has developed a classification system of injury common to overhead athletes, and relatively uniformly adopted by others (e.g. Glousman 1993, Jobe & Bradley 1988, Jobe & Pink 1993, Kvitne & Jobe 1993, Kvitne et al 1995) (Box 15.2). These authors also proposed an instability continuum, emphasizing that each of the pathologies does not occur in isolation (Fig. 15.11).

While this classification system appears succinct, it unfortunately does not cover all possibilities, with other authors identifying tensile overload leading to intrasubstance or articular surface tendon failure as a result of extreme eccentric loads during late cocking and deceleration (Andrews & Angelo 1988, Copeland 1993, Fleisig et al 1994, 1995, 1996, Meister & Andrews 1993,). McLeod & Andrews (1986) also described a 'shoulder grinding factor', resulting from humeral head translation during arm acceleration and deceleration, often in a shoulder with normal mobility. Subcoracoid impingement,

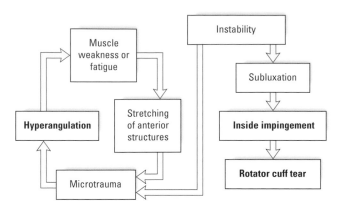

Figure 15.11   The Instability Continuum. (Adapted from Jobe et al 1996, p168.)

whether intra- or extra-articular, associated with posterior instability, may occur during follow-through (Gerber et al 1987, Gerber & Sebesta 2000).

Different mechanisms have been proposed for development of impingement, an understanding of which is fundamental to that of pathology related to the athletic shoulder (Burkhart et al 2000, Davidson et al 1995, Jobe 1995, Jobe et al 1992, 1996, Kvitne et al 1995, Walch 1996, Walch et al 1992a, 1992b). Briefly, the mechanism of intra-articular impingement, that is primarily associated with throwers, and proposed by the CHMC group, relates to underlying anterior laxity resulting in excessive lateral rotation and anterior wedging, allowing abutment of the undersurface of the rotator cuff against the postero-superior glenoid and labrum during the late cocking phase of the throw.

However, Burkhart (Burkart 2000, Burkhart et al 2000) argued strongly that the primary lesion is a type 2 SLAP lesion, which allows repetitive posterosuperior subluxa-tion of the humeral head and twisting of the tendon fibers during late cocking and early acceleration, resulting in fiber fatigue and failure of the cuff in the area of instability. This lesion is proposed to occur as a result of loss of medial rotation in throwers. Associated tight-ness in the posterior capsule causes a posterosuperior shift of the axis of humeral rotation, such that the humerus laterally rotates about a new axis, causing increased con-tact between the rotator cuff and labrum and increased forces at the posterosuperior biceps–labral attachment (Burkhart et al 2000). In their series of 64 athletes, all had greater than 25° restriction of medial rotation compared with the non-throwing shoulder and 94% demonstrated scapular dysfunction at rest and during movement. In the majority of the sample, altered function was also identified at other points in the kinetic chain, empha-sizing the importance of evaluation beyond the shoulder.

A deceleration mechanism has been proposed for biceps anchor tears, associated with the large forces transmitted via the biceps tendon to the superior labrum

as the muscle contracts eccentrically to decelerate the elbow (Andrews et al 1985, Andrews et al 1991, McLeod & Andrews 1986). Certainly, pain initiated and provoked on follow-through is a common clinical finding. However, Kuhn et al (1999) demonstrated that it took 20% less force to produce a posterior SLAP lesion when loading in the late cocking position on cadaver specimens than in the deceleration scenario.

Although Burkhart (Burkhart 2000, Burkhart et al 2000) is adamant that the primary lesion is loss of medial rotation and that evidence of anteroinferior laxity is 'pseudolaxity' associated with disruption of the superior labrum rather than capsular laxity, it seems feasible that each mechanism may occur in different patients.

A less common but associated presentation is that of a Bennett's lesion or symptomatic thrower's exostosis (Ferrari et al 1994, Meister 2000, Meister et al 1999), an osteophyte on the posteroinferior glenoid in the region of the posterior band of the IGHLC. It has been identified in throwing athletes, causing posterior shoulder pain during the late cocking, early acceleration and/or deceleration phases. Its presence is highly predictive of undersurface tearing of the rotator cuff and posterior labral damage, with its formation apparently related to repetitive traction to the capsular insertion during follow-through, increasing posterior humeral impingement.

The biceps muscle and tendon, biceps anchor, and its associated superior stability mechanisms, are extremely important in the mechanics of throwing. In addition to the features identified above, Fleisig et al (1994, 1995, 1996) and Meister (2000) highlighted that normal throwing mechanics should lead to maximal elbow flexion torque occurring prior to maximum shoulder compressive force, the relevance of which relates to the degree of load on the biceps. If, as a result of poor technique, these two occur together, the load on the biceps is increased markedly, increasing the vulnerability to injury of the tendon and its attachments. Similarly, Meister (2000) highlighted the importance of biceps in limiting torsional forces at the shoulder in the abducted externally rotated position, where this muscle fulfills a compressive (stabilizing) function. Anterior and posterosuperior labral strain is greatest in this position, whereas biceps tendon strain is greatest in adduction – a useful differentiating feature during examination. In addition, loss of the biceps anchor reduces torsional rigidity in the late arm cocking position, creating markedly increased strain on the IGHLC, with the potential for late failure of the antero-inferior glenohumeral stabilizing structures. Increased activity in the biceps reported in unstable shoulders (Glousman 1993) is hypothesized to be an attempt to compensate for the loss of passive restraints.

As with swimming, key features identified by most authors include poor technique and overuse, in terms of intensity of the throw, number of throws in a session and number of sessions in a week (Garth et al 1987, Jobe & Kvitne 1989, Jobe et al 1998). Fatigue related alteration of technique is highlighted (Andrews & Bisson 1999). In addition, all mechanisms reported have an element of altered humeral head translation and associated poor dynamic control of both the humeral head in the glenoid and the scapula on the chest wall.

Increased range of lateral rotation coupled with excessively decreased range of medial rotation is also an important factor in both swimmers and throwers (Burkhart et al 2000, Meister 2000), usually interpreted as a result of posterior capsular tightness associated with microtrauma from the high braking forces in these tissues during follow-through. However, increased humeral retroversion has been reported in the dominant arm of throwers (Pieper 1988) similar to that in unstable shoulders (Kronberg & Brostrom 1990) and not reflected in the general population (Edelson 1999, Kronberg et al 1990), such that their total range became biased towards lateral rotation. Interestingly, Peiper (1988) reported this phenomenon in athletes who had thrown during their growing years but not in those who had only starting throwing as adults, also indicating a preponderance of shoulder pain in the latter group.

Clinical features of the conditions highlighted above are similar. Symptoms are often vague and clinical signs subtle (Kvitne et al 1995, Magarey et al 1996). Arroyo et al (1997) and Magarey et al (1996) described non-specific shoulder pain, with athletes frequently denying the presence of symptoms, even to themselves, until the injury affected performance, for example, when there was loss of power or accuracy of throw. The thrower with internal impingement may complain of loss of control associated with early ball release secondary to painful loss of lateral rotation (Meister 2000). Burkhart et al (2000) reported a clear distinction between anterior and posterior SLAP lesions by corresponding site of pain, while the CHMC group reports (Davidson et al 1995, Jobe et al 1992, 1996, Jobe 1995, Kvitne et al 1995, Ruwe et al 1994, Walch 1996, Walch et al 1992a, 1992b) identified posterior pain associated with internal impingement. Episodes of clicking or clunking may be reported related to labral pathology (Andrews et al 1991) and a sensation of 'looseness' associated with instability (Allen & Warner 1995). A 'dead arm' syndrome (recurrent transient anterior subluxation) is not uncommon in association with throwing injuries (Rowe 1987, Rowe and Zarins 1981), although definitions of the condition vary. Burkhart et al (2000, p. 126) redefined the 'dead arm' as a 'pathologic shoulder condition in which the thrower is unable to throw with his preinjury velocity and control because of a combination of pain and subjective unease in the shoulder'. Throwers often have difficulty describing

the sensations of unease although most ascribe it to the late cocking and early acceleration phases. Transient neurological symptoms may also be a component of the problem (Allen & Warner 1995, Rowe & Zarins 1981).

Distinguishing physical features reported by different authors in painful throwing shoulders include:

- Increased range of lateral rotation and decreased medial rotation in the throwing shoulder compared with the non-throwing shoulder – a total rotation range of less than 180° in 90° abduction represents a shoulder at risk (Burkhart et al 2000).
- In the relocation position, application of a posteriorly directed force will cause no change to the pain in the patient with primary impingement, but a reduction in pain with primary anterior instability and secondary impingement (type 2B), as the posterior glide removes the humeral head from the internal impingement position (Kvitne et al 1995).
- A posterior impingement sign – deep posterior shoulder pain with the arm in 90° abduction and maximum lateral rotation, which is considered diagnostic of internal impingement (Meister 2000). The same pain is elicited by deep palpation of the posterior rotator cuff and capsule with the arm in horizontal adduction.
- Speed's test and O'Brien's cross-body test reported by Burkhart et al (2000) as positive for anterior SLAP lesions, reproducing anterior bicipital groove pain, and the relocation test, provoking posterior pain, as positive for posterior SLAP lesions. Tenderness on deep palpation of the bicipital groove appears sensitive in anterior but not posterior SLAP lesions.
- A posterior stress test (posterior and axial pressure through the flexed and medially rotated arm) is likely to distinguish symptomatic posterior instability, seen associated with deceleration and follow-through, often in patients with an element of multidirectional instability (Allen & Warner 1995, Tibone & Bradley 1993). Palpable subluxation over the posterior glenoid rim that reproduces the patient's pain is considered positive.

Diagnostic imaging and arthroscopic findings are well reported in the literature but their description is beyond the scope of this chapter. The relevant chapters in Andrews & Wilk (1994a), Rockwood & Matsen (1998), Warren et al (1999) provide a good starting point.

Treatment reported in the literature for the throwing shoulder extends from conservative to surgical, with arthroscopic debridement and stabilization common recommendations (e.g., Allen & Warner 1995, Andrews et al 1991, Burns & Turba 1992, Ciullo 1996, Copeland 1993, Jobe & Pink 1993, Jobe et al 1998, Kvitne & Jobe 1993, Meister & Andrews 1993, Montgomery & Jobe 1994,

Rubinstein et al 1992, Scarpinato et al 1991), particularly for the elite athlete, in whom a moderate result or delayed outcome is not acceptable. However, Gartsman & Hammerman (2000) highlighted the danger of mistaking normal anatomical variations in superior labral attachment for pathology. Conservative management centers around reduction of pain, reduced training load, stretching of tight posterior capsular and scapulo-thoracic structures and strengthening of the rotator cuff, scapular stabilizers and other power producing muscles. Attention to the whole kinetic chain is also stressed (Burkhart et al 2000, Davies & Dickoff-Hoffman 1993, Kibler 1998a,b). In his numerous publications, Wilk has stressed the value of isokinetic testing and treatment as a component of rehabilitation, arguing that it provides objective evidence of muscle function and therefore can make rehabilitation more specifically directed (Wilk 1994, 1999, Wilk & Arrigo 1994, Wilk et al 1995, 1997). His thorough reports provide a good starting point for further reading. However, isokinetic testing and training devices are not always available, in which case, the therapist must rely on critical reassessment of key clinical impairments found during physical examination. Further discussion on rehabilitation will be covered in the management section.

While there is a wealth of literature related to management of the painful throwing shoulder, no reports of randomized controlled trials of management were found. Most reports consisted of retrospective reviews of clinical findings and surgical procedures, so the evidence base for the proposed management is poor. In most cases, management is based on an understanding of the underlying biomedical features of the condition or on the presenting impairments. Our own approach to management falls into the same category as it is yet to be subjected to the rigors of controlled trial.

TENNIS AND OTHER RACKET SPORTS

The biomechanics of tennis are similar to those of throwing. Excellent descriptions are provided by Ellenbecker (1994, 1995), Kibler (1995), Lee (1995), and Ryu et al (1988) where many of the same principles for throwing apply also to assessment and management in tennis. One key difference highlighted is the influence of the racket, which provides a mechanical advantage in power delivery to the ball, but which may increase the stress on the shoulder because of its weight and lever arm effect (Ryu et al 1988). Lee (1995) provided an excellent exposition on the importance of the stretch-shortening cycle to optimize generation of power throughout the kinetic chain, for example, early arm cocking is characterized by upper extremity concentric contractions and lower extremity eccentric contractions, while in late

cocking, the reverse occurs. The contribution and importance of the scapula and remainder of the kinetic chain was emphasized in most papers reviewed (Burkhart et al 2000, Chandler et al 1990, 1992, Ellenbecker 1994, 1995, Kibler 1995, 1998a, 1998b, Lee 1995, Lehman 1988, McCann & Bigliani 1994, Priest 1988, Ryu et al 1988). The requirements for strokes other than the serve and overhead volley complicate the picture in tennis, although most injuries are reported as related to these more explosive strokes (Ellenbecker 1994, 1995, Kibler 1995, Lee 1995, McCann & Bigliani 1994, Priest 1988).

High injury rates are reported in all levels of tennis, ranging from 10–30% in elite juniors to 74% of world class players (Ellenbecker 1995). The characteristic 'tennis shoulder' is associated with a postural change of shoulder girdle depression associated with an apparent scoliosis (Priest 1988). The etiology appears related either to the service action causing stretching of the shoulder elevating muscles, or to hypertrophy of the playing arm. Anterior pain was reported most frequently, provoked by the serve or forehand smash. Thoracic outlet syndrome may also be related to the downwardly rotated scapular position. Other injury reports indicate that the tennis player is likely to suffer the same problems as the thrower as a result of the comparable mechanics of the sports (Kibler 1995, Lee 1995, Ryu et al 1988). However, Chandler et al (1992) reported relative isokinetic weakness of the lateral rotators in the serving arm compared to the medial rotators, which demonstrated increased strength compared to the non-dominant shoulder. Little difference in lateral rotation strength was reported between the dominant and non-dominant arms, however, Chandler et al (1992) considered the relative imbalance likely to predispose to injury, suggesting that specific strengthening of the lateral rotators to maintain a more even strength balance may reduce the chance of overload injury. These findings contrast with those related to throwing, where Wilk (1994) reported no significant difference between sides. Other racket sports, such as squash and badminton, have similar mechanics, although with some differences unique to each sport. The rackets in both are lighter, possibly creating less influence on the shoulder structures, but the technique of the overhead smash is comparable.

OTHER SPORTS

Gymnastics involves extraordinary ranges of movement and loads about the shoulder, particularly for male gymnasts, with heavy training schedules and little time off. Many gymnasts train for over 20 hours/week for 50 weeks/year. The high bar and rings involve the greatest load on the shoulder, requiring a 'delicate and masterful management of forces through the upper extremities'

(Hemsley 1994, p. 425). Female gymnasts have their own special problems, related to the fact that they must peak while pre-pubescent, as the onset of puberty is frequently career ending. Training intensity for all elite gymnasts predisposes them to overuse injuries, related to impingement or labral damage. Gymnastics is a highly specialized area, with athletes who do not seek treatment until the pain makes them incapable of continuing training. The loads and forces required of the shoulder, the hypermobility, extensive training schedules and the psyche of the gymnast make their management a challenge.

Isolated suprascapular neuropathy appears frequently associated with volleyball (Eggert & Holzgraefe 1993, Ferretti 1994, Ferretti et al 1987, 1998, Hama et al 1992, Holzgraefe et al 1994, Hughes 2001, Montagna & Colonna 1993, Sandow & Ilic 1998). Twelve of 96 athletes at the 1985 European Championships were observed with this disorder (Ferretti 1994), while its presence in six members of the Australian men's volleyball team has been identified since 1990 (Hughes 2001). There are a number of proposed mechanisms (Ferretti 1994, Rengachary et al 1979, Sandow & Ilic 1998, Tengan et al 1993). The clinical presentation consists of vague posterior shoulder pain, significant infraspinatus wasting, most evident when viewed from above, and weakness of lateral rotation, with normal supraspinatus (Sandow & Ilic 1998). Patients with this disorder are often unaware of the wasting, presenting only when the muscle imbalance leads to other complaints. Hughes (2001) reported that it is frequently benign with minimal disability.

The suprascapular nerve may be tensioned in scapular depression, protraction and horizontal flexion with either glenohumeral lateral rotation (Mayfield & True 1973, Narakas 1989, Pratt 1986, Seddon 1943, Solheim & Roaas 1978, Sunderland 1978) or resisted lateral rotation and passive medial rotation (Skurja & Monlux 1985), with any of these positions potentially provoking symptoms.

Weightlifting can understandably lead to shoulder damage, particularly when using heavy weights with techniques forcing the arm into extension and lateral rotation (Gross et al 1993). These authors reported on 23 shoulders in 20 patients with recurrent instability related to weightlifting, in whom the cause of the instability was anteroinferior labral and capsular damage rather than the superior labral injuries associated with throwing and swimming. From a conservative management perspective, modification of use of the equipment such that the shoulder is not placed under load in extreme ranges of movement is a good starting point, while reduction in load is essential until symptoms have settled and motor control of the shoulder and scapula is reestablished. Neviaser (1991) reported that regular use of anabolic steroids gives the athlete a quicker recovery time between sessions and a systemic euphoria, leading to a false sense of security. A decrease in stiffness and pain following training was reported, potentially masking significant injury. Osteolysis of the distal clavicle has also been reported in weightlifters (Cahill 1982, Matthews et al 1993), possibly as a result of excessive stress on the acromioclavicular joint, leading to subchondral stress microfractures.

All sports may lead to shoulder problems but others in which overuse injuries are more common include golf, handball, field events such as shotput, discus, javelin and hammer throw, water polo and wheelchair sports (e.g. Burnham et al 1993, Greenan et al 1993, Kao et al 1995, McMaster et al 1991).

OTHER CAUSES OF SHOULDER PAIN IN ATHLETES

Traumatic injuries of the shoulder include fractures, dislocations and subluxations of the glenohumeral, acromioclavicular and sternoclavicular joints and the associated bony structures, ruptures of ligamentous supports and muscle or tendon rupture. Branch et al (1992) reported 12 cases of spontaneous fracture of the humerus during pitching. Early postinjury management of traumatic disorders is dependent on the preference of the physician or surgeon, while physical therapy management should follow the principles outlined below. Details of traumatic injuries can be found in most texts on the shoulder (e.g. Rockwood & Matsen 1998) and will not be further discussed here.

Schulte & Warner (1995) have provided an excellent summary of uncommon causes of shoulder pain in the athlete, including: a number of neurovascular disorders, thoracic outlet syndrome, effort thrombosis, ruptures of muscles and/or tendons other than the rotator cuff, the 'snapping scapula' syndrome, stress fractures, osteochondritis dissecans and tumors. These conditions should be considered as part of a differential diagnosis of shoulder pain in the athlete.

Gerber & Sebesta (2000) described a new site of impingement – of the deep surface of subscapularis tendon and the reflection pulley (or rotator interval sling) on the anterosuperior glenoid rim. The impingement of subscapularis occurs in a position of approximately 90° of flexion and medial rotation, as in early pull-through in freestyle, while that of the biceps occurs in higher ranges of flexion, such as holding the pole over the head in pole vaulting, during the follow-through of a tennis serve, or in the non-dominant shoulder of a golfer during the backswing.

Posterior instability in athletes may occur as a result of direct trauma or, more commonly, as a recurrent subluxation (Tibone & Bradley 1993). Activities that predispose to posterior instability include follow-through in throwing and volleyball, backstroke in swimming, backhand in tennis. Common to all activities is the position of forward flexion combined with active adduction and medial rotation. These patients complain of pain rather than instability, with pain located posteriorly or in typical impingement positions. Apprehension is uncommon. The athlete may remember a specific minor incident that resolves, with symptoms becoming evident some time later. Alternatively, overuse may lead to an insidious onset. Examination reveals posterior joint line tenderness and posterior joint crepitus, pain on forward flexion combined with medial rotation and increased posterior translation (Tibone & Bradley 1993). Athletes with minor posterior instability also often present with anterior pain associated with subcoracoid impingement during follow-through. In these patients, the posterior instability is not usually symptomatic and can be readily detected with a posterior translation test.

Multidirectional instability (MDI) is not uncommon in the shoulder of athletes (Beasley et al 2000). The sports commonly associated with MDI are gymnastics, the butterfly stroke in swimming and the follow-through of a throw or tennis serve (Beasley et al 2000, Cordasco & Bigliani 1998). Kuroda et al (1997) found a correlation between the age of onset of sport and onset of symptoms. The principal symptoms are pain and weakness, initially following exertion, but with progression, becoming more constant and affecting athletic performance. Fatigue and a sense of instability are also common (Cooper & Brems 1992). Less commonly, patients describe paresthesia (Cooper & Brems 1992, Neer & Foster 1980, Yamaguchi & Flatow 1995). The most significant directions of instability are demonstrated by the athlete's identification of provoking movements or activities (Yamaguchi & Flatow 1995). For example, a dominance of posterior instability causes pain with the follow-through of a throw, whereas an athlete with predominantly anterior instability has more difficulty with late arm cocking. Inferior instability is manifested in activities such as carrying a heavy object and often includes neurological symptoms (Beasley et al 2000, Neer & Foster 1980, Yamaguchi & Flatow 1995). Frequently, the shoulder may be lax in all directions, but only symptomatically unstable in one (Mallon & Speer 1995).

Typically, physical examination reveals inferior subluxation with a positive sulcus sign (Altcheck et al 1991, Foster 1983, Lebar & Alexander 1992, Mallon & Speer 1995, Neer & Foster 1980) with most authors also describing increased range of translation in all directions. Abnormal scapulothoracic mechanics frequently coexist with MDI, in particular, with a downwardly rotated scapula, leading to loss of the bony cam provided by the inferior lip of the glenoid (Beasley et al 2000, Itoi et al 1992).

MANAGEMENT OF SHOULDER DISORDERS

Management of shoulder disorders in the overhead athlete with a predominance of nociceptive involvement is multidimensional. Selection of treatment is based on interpretations of and the priority placed on findings from both the subjective and physical examination, combined with knowledge of the requirements of the athlete's sport and the level and stage of competition (e.g. in season or between seasons). Clearly such considerations are different for the elite, professional athlete than the casual recreational participant.

The authors support the approach advocated by Maitland (1991) of impairment-based management, tempered by our growing knowledge of pathomechanics and pathophysiology of the structures within the shoulder complex (Jones & Magarey, 2001) and influences of psychosocial factors on all pain states (Gifford 1997, 1998, 2000, Jones et al 2000). Knowledge of an accurate tissue-specific diagnosis, assuming a peripherally-based nociceptive source, influences management more in terms of prognosis than specific direction of treatment. It certainly helps to understand the underlying causes of the impairments with which the athlete presents, and directs management towards correction of specific contributing factors. It also allows the physical therapist to provide a detailed explanation to the patient of the likely pathology, its implications for the sport and the most appropriate approach to management. As primary contact practitioners, physical therapists must be aware of their limitations. For example, extended conservative management of an elite throwing athlete with shoulder pain may be inappropriate, given that the pathology is likely to include disrupted integrity of the superior articular structures, which will not heal with conservative measures. If alteration of contributing factors does not alter symptoms relatively quickly, such an athlete should be counseled to seek an orthopedic opinion promptly as to the benefit of arthroscopic investigation and/or management.

The physical therapist's role, therefore, is to identify the specific impairments present in each case and to address them within the context of the likely pathology. If the presentation includes pain, the findings on examination will determine whether the most appropriate approach to decreasing that pain is direct treatment of the apparent source or alteration of provocative contributing factors. Selection of passive treatment techniques is covered elsewhere (Austin et al 1996, Jones et al 1994, Magarey 1986, Maitland 1991), while choice of passive movement, soft tissue techniques or electrotherapy appears dependent on personal preference and skill, as there is no research evidence to support one approach over another. Whichever approach is chosen, it should be based on detailed assessment of the athlete's impairments, both physical and psychosocial, with the outcome critically reassessed, in terms of specific impairments and functional activities, and with progression based on sound reflective reasoning (Jones & Magarey 2001).

Our experience has shown that passive movement can be useful in the treatment of the overhead athlete. Specific limitations of movement – in particular, the relative loss of medial rotation – may be addressed with localized stretches to the glenohumeral joint, combined with judicious use of home stretching, ensuring the stretch is to the glenohumeral joint and not to the already lengthened scapulothoracic structures. Soft tissue mobilization to stretch tight posterior capsular and muscular structures may also be effective in reducing the imbalance of rotation range, such that the adaptive loss of medial rotation is not too great (Burkhart et al 2000). Gentle passive mobilization techniques are frequently effective in reducing pain associated with an acute injury, allowing quicker and more effective inclusion of dynamic control strategies. Evidence of the neurophysiological basis for effective pain relief with passive movement is building slowly (Vicenzino et al 2000, Wright 1995). Specific, useful techniques are presented in Jones & Magarey, 2001.

Most rehabilitation programs reported in the literature are based on strengthening the rotator cuff and scapular stabilizers, in conjunction with attention to the remainder of the kinetic chain. David et al (2000) demonstrated that the rotator cuff performs a dynamic stabilizing role based on cocontraction, even during a rotational task where the torque-producing characteristics of the muscle would predominate. There is also preliminary evidence of delayed activation of the rotator cuff in the presence of glenohumeral instability (David et al 1997), similar to that reported in transversus abdominis in the presence of low back pain and vastus medialis oblique with patellofemoral pain (Cowan et al 2001, Hodges & Richardson 1996, O'Sullivan et al 1997). Altered function of serratus anterior and lower trapezius in painful shoulders has also been demonstrated (Kibler 1998a, 1998b, Wadsworth & Bullock-Saxton 1997).

General strengthening exercise without training of the specific stabilizers has been shown to be less effective in controlling back pain than specific dynamic stabilizing programs (O'Sullivan et al 1997). Equally, strengthening torque-producing functions of the rotator cuff may have limited effect on its stabilizing function, leaving the joint without the normal cocontraction necessary for adequate concavity-compression (Lippitt & Matsen 1993, Lippitt et al 1993).

Since stabilizing muscle function involves only small levels of activity, facilitation of normal neural control to ensure preparatory activation of the stabilizers prior to, and low-level cocontraction during, movement would seem a more appropriate initial step in rehabilitation than individual muscle strengthening. Therefore, if examination of dynamic control of the glenohumeral and scapulothoracic regions demonstrates impairment, our management includes a motor control rehabilitation program, on which more advanced and sport-specific retraining can be based. Our clinical experience has shown that most athletes with shoulder pain present with an inability to cocontract the rotator cuff in isolation from the superficial muscles, associated with a failure to maintain the humeral head centered in the glenoid during rotational tasks, and coupled with altered patterning of scapular rotation, irrespective of their sport or the specific pathology in the shoulder. Reestablishment of these functions becomes our primary goal of management.

Just as a coach breaks a skilled task within a sport down to its component parts during training for mastery, so a motor control rehabilitation program uses the concept of breaking down function into interim steps (Schmidt 1991, Winstein 1991). Goals of the program include facilitation and training of deep stabilizer activation of the region prior to that of the more superficial torque-producing muscles, with maintenance of that activation combined with reestablishment of optimal movement patterns during functional tasks. This can be achieved either through strategies of isolation or controlled posture and movement facilitated by imagery (Magarey & Jones in press a).

A key component to the success of any motor control rehabilitation program is cooperation with the patient, who must understand the purpose of the program to ensure compliance. This is particularly so for the athlete used to vigorous training and the concept that exercise must be hard work to be effective. It is a challenge to persuade the injured athlete that the hard work required in the early stages is cognitive not physical, and that the cognitive component is essential to mastery of the skill and progression to the more physical aspects of the rehabilitation. The analogy to learning a sport-based skill and the use of mental imagery to facilitate isolated cocontraction of deep stabilizing muscles are useful strategies in achieving success.

We encourage frequent practice of the facilitatory technique throughout the day, as this improves awareness and activation far more than an isolated exercise session once a day (Catalano & Kleiner 1984, Shumway-Cook & Woollacott 2001). It is also not necessary to wait for pain to settle before starting a motor control program. Positions can always be found in which pain-free activation is possible. Initially, each region is trained in isolation (i.e. the rotator cuff is worked with the scapula in an unchallenged position and vice versa) in cocontraction in their relevant force couples, with the contractions initially isometric and isotonic with low load, developing a gradual build-up and release.

Training should always occur in those positions in which the patient has control, to avoid use of substitution strategies to achieve the task, but as close as possible to the position where that control is lost in order to make use of overflow principles. Isometric and isotonic training can be undertaken concurrently, as long as the patient is aware of the different sensations associated with control and loss of control. Teaching this difference in feel may be time-consuming initially, but is essential to the success of the program, as training in a position in which control is lacking may reinforce poor movement patterns.

Once mastery is achieved, progression depends on the functional needs of the athlete. Kibler (1998a) stated that muscle activation around the shoulder is a closed chain activity, with emphasis on cocontraction muscle forces at both the glenohumeral and scapulothoracic joints. Closed chain activity also simulates normal proprioceptive pathways during the throwing motion and, by decreasing deltoid activation, decreases the tendency for superior humeral migration, thus making it easier to achieve dynamic relocation. Therefore, closed kinetic chain activities are a logical progression from basic cognitive challenges in the neutral position, as described by Magarey & Jones (in press a).

In various degrees of weightbearing, depending on level of control (with the hand against the wall, a table or a moving surface such as a ball, or on all fours) movement in all directions can be added to the dynamic relocation and scapular setting, with progressive increase in the cognitive challenge and physical load of the exercise. Such exercises can be done with the focus on movement of the scapula on a stable glenohumeral joint or vice versa. Kibler (1998a) considered that closed chain rehabilitation was a major improvement in their rehabilitation protocol as it allowed smoother and more rapid transition from below to above shoulder height activities.

While attending to pain relief and establishment of localized dynamic control of the glenohumeral and scapulothoracic regions, the remainder of the kinetic chain should be addressed (Burkhart et al 2000, Kibler 1995, 1998a, 1998b, Lee 1995, McCann & Bigliani 1994, Priest 1988, Ryu et al 1988), making use of the principles of specificity of muscle function and the importance of functional relevance for transfer of training (Kibler 1998a, Kibler & Chandler 1994, Shumway-Cook & Woollacott 2001). Emphasis is placed initially on core trunk and pelvic control, moving quickly into drills where some of the components are sport-specific. For example, abdominal muscle function is emphasized, as it is an important component of the action of all overhead sports. In particular, oblique abdominal work into outer range,

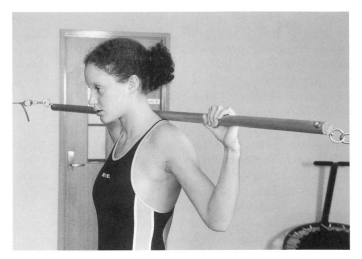

Figure 15.12 Working with a 'twisties' bar. Rubber tubing is attached to the ends of a bar and attached to the wall at right angles to each other. The patient sets the hips and pelvis and twists the trunk against the resistance of the tubing. Once the technique has been mastered, movement can be initiated from the pelvis, followed by trunk rotation, mimicking initiation of body-roll or a throw. The technique can be further progressed by increasing the strength of the rubber tubing or performing the exercise while standing on one leg, with the other supported on a stool or exercise ball. The exercise can also be performed with the twisties bar on a diagonal, so that the twist is from extension/right rotation to flexion/left rotation (e.g. with the potential to incorporate some plyometric component at the limits of the movement).

with plyometric reversals, once trunk control is sufficient, are incorporated to simulate the action required of these muscles in the changeover from late arm cocking to acceleration and hand entry to early catch. Achievement of outer range control is facilitated by working over a Swiss ball, which has the added advantage of incorporating the need for total trunk stabilization during the exercise. Plyometric abdominal work is also encouraged through partner exercises, throwing and catching a weighted ball while seated on the Swiss ball and by use of a 'twisties' bar (Fig. 15.12). Gluteals, hamstring, quadriceps and calves are all included, with each activity incorporating some aspect that is relevant to the athlete's sport. We integrate the Swiss ball in many exercises because of the advantages provided by the unstable surface coupled with the simple fun of working on the ball – it encourages compliance. An example of the program of kinetic chain exercises for an elite swimmer can be found in Magarey (in press).

For many non-athletic patients, addressing the motor control issues and teaching the patient appropriate strategies to continue monitoring and stimulating the control are sufficient for a return to normal function. However, the overhead athlete must also address other issues, including:

• Retraining the physiological needs of specific muscles required in the particular sport, e.g. strength, power or endurance. At this point, many programs reported in the literature, in particular those from the CHMC group (Abrams 1991, Carson 1989, Dines & Levinson 1995, Ellenbecker 1995, Jobe & Pink 1993, Kamkar et al 1993, Kelly 1995, Litchfield et al 1993, Pink & Jobe 1991, Townsend et al 1991) encourage strengthening directed at isolated muscles, with suggestions for specific exercises that emphasize individual muscles. Wilk (Wilk 1994, 1999, Wilk & Arrigo 1994, Wilk et al 1995, 1997) also encourages the use of isokinetics for retraining. Our experience is that we achieve better results if we address the functional requirements of the sport, ensuring correct technique, in developing the physiological needs of the muscles. Therefore, the emphasis is on functional muscle group activity rather than isolated individual muscle strengthening. For example, we would use PNF based elastic tubing or pulley exercises in the directions relevant for throwing, so that the muscles are working in the patterns relevant for the sport, increasing the load and speed as appropriate to the athlete's level of performance and stabilizing control, emphasizing eccentric control in addition to concentric strengthening.

• As early as possible, the inclusion of mini-plyometric drills, with progression to more challenging functional plyometric exercises (Wilk & Voight 1994), focussing on both the glenohumeral and scapulothoracic areas, which enhances functional recovery, as stretch-shortening activities are fundamental to optimize generation of power throughout the kinetic chain in all overhead sports (Lee 1995).

• The correction of faulty technique which is essential to all athletes with a painful shoulder. It seems surprising that athletes can achieve elite levels of participation with poor technique, but it is our experience that this is often the case. Evaluation of technique by video and working closely with an experienced coach, preferably familiar with the athlete, can facilitate technique correction, which should always be superimposed on deliberate stabilizing activation during retraining, so that the activation becomes integrated in the developing feed-forward mechanism.

Fundamental alteration to technique may be required to reduce the overall number of injuries associated with a sport. The need for extraordinary ranges of lateral rotation to develop speed during baseball pitching is emphasized in many reviewed papers (e.g. Fleisig et al 1994, 1995), such that acceleration is encouraged with the body already front on to the plate. Sufficient throwing speed appears possible by field players without the need for this range of lateral rotation. Some throwing coaches associated with cricket, baseball and softball within Australia encourage an arm cocking position that does not go beyond the median frontal plane, with the elbow

extended slightly beyond 90° and the wrist pronated and slightly flexed. From this position, forward momentum of the body during acceleration will still take the arm behind the median frontal plane, but not to the exaggerated ranges encouraged in pitching, thereby reducing the stress on the anterior shoulder structures. In addition, throwing athletes are encouraged to initiate acceleration with a forward thrust from their ipsilateral leg and powerful plyometric contraction of the oblique abdominal muscles, rather than the glenohumeral medial rotators alone, as these muscles are better designed to cope with the forces generated by the stretch-shortening contraction. Forceful cross-body adduction of the abducted glove hand during acceleration also increases the power generated. An exaggerated follow-through facilitates dissipation of forces associated with deceleration of the arm, reducing stress on the posterior structures. There is no formal evidence to demonstrate that this change in throwing technique relates to a reduction in injury rate, but anecdotal evidence from coaches and players supports its benefits.

Similarly, strengthening of oblique abdominals, particularly with outer range drills and use of fin belts in training encourages initiation of body roll from the pelvis and therefore facilitates the plyometric abdominal contribution to the catch in swimming, while strengthening hip flexors and gluteals to encourage an increased emphasis on the kick may decrease the load through the shoulder.

• Alteration of training routines if they are detrimental to recovery or likely to lead to an exacerbation. Adequate, preferably dynamic, warm-up relevant to the specific sport is essential, as is progressive increase in intensity of activity. Throwing drills, for example, should always start short and progress to long and hard only when the athlete is suitably warmed up. Inclusion of rest periods during training and rest days between training sessions to allow recovery is appropriate – a particularly difficult concept to sell to a swimmer or gymnast! Preventative recovery practices, such as icing the shoulder after training, can also be helpful, though again, there is no research evidence to support this practice.

• We have found that deliberate preactivation of the dynamic stabilizers, included as a component of the warm-up before training or competition facilitates return to sport and prevention of recurrence. For the swimmer, elastic tubing can be used to replicate water resistance during movement from simulated hand entry to catch and early pull-through, following deliberate presetting of the scapular stabilizers and rotator cuff, immediately before entry to the pool (Fig. 15.13). A thrower can preset the scapular and glenohumeral stabilizers and work the shoulder through rotations with a small weighted ball in the hand, progressively increasing the speed of rotation

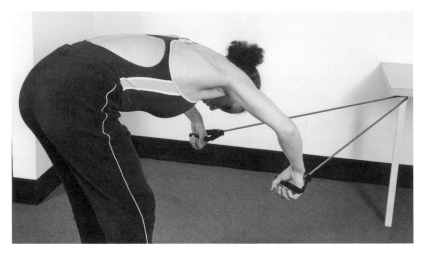

Figure 15.13 Elastic tubing can be used to replicate water resistance during movement from simulated hand entry to catch and early pull-through, following deliberate presetting of the scapular stabilizers and rotator cuff, and as part of the athlete's warm-up immediately before entry to the pool.

and the position in which it is performed, with the last set in the late cocking/acceleration position of the shoulder. In each case, care should be taken that the humeral head remains centered in the glenoid and the scapula stabilized on the chest wall during the exercise, as failure indicates poor control by the dynamic stabilizers and therefore, incorrect muscle activation.

Throughout the period of injury, as with any sporting injury, the athlete should maintain general cardio-respiratory fitness through running, cycling, modified activity in the water, making this activity as relevant to the sport as possible. Prior to return to sport, the athlete must work through sports-specific drills at training, concentrating on gradual return to full activity. For example, throwing should start over short distance, with gradual increase in speed, distance and number of throws, and swimming should begin on alternate days over shorter distances with no speed work. Focus on correct technique should be an integral part of the regimen. Return to competition should also occur gradually, playing part of a game, if possible, with full return occurring ideally when the shoulder is pain-free with good intrinsic dynamic control, good integration of kinetic chain function and appropriate strength and endurance of the shoulder and scapulothoracic muscles. The coach should be satisfied with the technique and the athlete should pass a sport-specific fitness test with no discomfort the next morning. Facilitatory taping may be appropriate for additional proprioceptive input during the early stages of rehabilitation and may be continued as added protection once full activity is resumed, until the athlete is fully match-hardened. In most instances, elastic tape rather than restrictive sports tape is adequate to achieve the facilitation of rotator cuff function, applied over a non-allergenic undertape.

Alternative forms of management, such as hydrotherapy, can be important components to the rehabilitation program, with cocontraction combined with movement through water. However, further discussion is beyond the scope of this chapter (Speer et al 1993, Tovin 2001). If surgery is appropriate, postoperative physical therapy management should follow similar principles, under guidance from the surgeon, ensuring that healing structures are not compromised.

SUMMARY

There is a wide range of sport-related conditions of the shoulder. If management of the sporting shoulder is approached from a sound knowledge base of the structure and biomechanics of the region and of the sport involved, a good understanding of relevant clinical patterns, and thorough clinical examination that explores impairment in addition to seeking structural diagnosis, success with this challenging region can be enhanced.

REFERENCES

Abelew T 2001 Kinesiology of the shoulder. In: Tovin B J, Greenfield B H (eds) Evaluation and treatment of the shoulder: an integration of the guide to physical therapist practice. F A Davis Co, Philadelphia, ch 2, p 25

Abrams J S 1991 Special shoulder problems in the throwing athlete: pathology, diagnosis, and nonoperative management. Clinics in Sports Medicine 10(4):839–861

Allegrucci M, Whitney S L, Irrgang J J 1994 Clinical implications of secondary impingement of the shoulder in freestyle swimmers. Journal of Orthopaedic and Sports Physical Therapy 20(6):307–318

Allen A A, Warner J J P 1995 Shoulder instability in the athlete. Orthopedic Clinics of North America 26(3):487–504

Allingham C 1996 The shoulder complex. In: Zuluaga M, Briggs C, Carlisle J et al (eds) Sports physiotherapy: applied science and practice. Churchill Livingstone, Melbourne, ch 23, p 357–406

Altcheck D W, Warren R F, Skyhar M J 1990 Shoulder arthroscopy. In Rockwood C A, Matsen F A (eds) The shoulder. W B Saunders, Philadelphia, ch 8, p 258–277

Altcheck D W, Warren R F, Skyhar M J et al 1991 T-plasty modification of the Bankart procedure for multidirectional instability of the anterior and inferior types. Journal of Bone and Joint Surgery (Am) 73A(1):105–112

Anderson M K, Hall S J 1995 Sports injury management. Williams and Wilkins, Baltimore, ch 10, p 363–418

Andrews J R, Angelo R L 1988 Shoulder arthroscopy for the throwing athlete. Techniques of Orthopaedics 3:75–81

Andrews J R, Wilk K E 1994a The athlete's shoulder. Churchill Livingstone, New York

Andrews J R, Wilk K E 1994b Shoulder injuries in baseball. In: Andrews J R, Wilk K E (eds) The athlete's shoulder. Churchill Livingstone, New York, ch 32, p 369–390

Andrews J R, Bisson L J 1999 Instability mechanisms in the throwing athlete. In: Warren R F, Craig E V, Altcheck D W (eds) The unstable shoulder. Lippincott-Raven, Philadelphia, ch 4, p 77–92

Andrews J R, Carson W G, McLeod W D 1985 Glenoid labrum tears related to the long head of biceps. American Journal of Sports Medicine 13(5):337–341

Andrews J R, Kupferman S P, Dillman C J 1991 Labral tears in throwing and racquet sports. Clinics in Sports Medicine 10(4):901–911

Arroyo J S, Hershon S J, Bigliani L U 1997 Special considerations in the athletic throwing shoulder. Orthopedic Clinics of North America 28(1):69–78

Astrom M, Rausing A 1995 Chronic achilles tendinopathy. A survey of surgical and histological findings. Clinical Orthopaedics and Related Research 316:151–164

Austin L, Maitland G D, Magarey M 1996 Manual therapy: when and why? In: Zuluaga M, Briggs C, Carlisle J et al (eds) Sports physiotherapy: applied science and practice. Churchill Livingstone, Melbourne, ch 12, p 181–206

Bagg S D, Forrest W J 1988 A biomechanical analysis of scapular rotation during arm abduction in the scapular plane. American Journal of Physical Medicine and Rehabilitation 67(6):238–245

Bak K 1996 Nontraumatic glenohumeral instability and coracoacromial impingement in swimmers. Scandinavian Journal of Medicine and Science in Sports 6:132–144

Bak K, Fauno P 1997 Clinical findings in competitive swimmers with shoulder pain. American Journal of Sports Medicine 25(2):254–260

Bak K, Magnusson S P 1997 Shoulder strength and range of motion in symptomatic and pain-free elite swimmers. American Journal of Sports Medicine 25(4):454–460

Basmajian J V 1963 The surgical anatomy and function of the arm-trunk mechanism. Surgical Clinics of North America 43:1471

Basmajian J V, Bazant F J 1959 Factors preventing downward dislocation of the adducted shoulder joint: an electromyographic and morphological study. Journal of Bone and Joint Surgery (Am) 41A:1182–1186

Beach M L, Whitney S L, Dickoff-Hoffman S A 1992 Relationship of shoulder flexibility, strength and endurance to shoulder pain in competitive swimmers. Journal of Orthopaedic and Sports Physical Therapy 16(6):262–268

Beasley L, Faryniarz D A, Hannafin J A 2000 Multidirectional instability of the shoulder in the female athlete. Clinics in Sports Medicine 19(2):331–349

Benjamin M, Evans E J, Copp L 1986 The histology of tendon attachments to bone in man. Journal of Anatomy 149:89–100

Berg E E, Ciullo J V 1998 A clinical test for superior glenoid labral or 'SLAP' lesions. Clinical Journal of Sports Medicine 8(2):121–123

Beynnon B D, Nichols C E, Pope M H 1993 The kinematics of throws and strokes. In: Matsen F A, Fu F H, Hawkings R J (eds) The shoulder: a balance of mobility and stability. American Academy of Orthopaedic Surgeons, Rosemont, ch 11, p 193–204

Bigliani L U, Pollock R G, Soslowsky L J et al 1992 Tensile properties of the inferior glenohumeral ligament. Journal of Orthopaedic Research 10(2):187–197

Blachut P A, Day B 1989 Arthroscopic anatomy of the shoulder. Journal of Arthroscopic and Related Surgery 5(1):1–10

Bowen M K, Deng X H, Warner J J P et al 1992 The effect of joint compression on stability of the glenohumeral joint. Transactions of the Orthopaedic Research Society 17:289

Branch T, Partin C, Chamberland P et al 1992 Spontaneous fractures of the humerus during pitching. A series of 12 cases. American Journal of Sports Medicine 20(4):468–470

Branch T P, Lawton R L, Iobst C A et al 1995 The role of the glenohumeral capsular ligaments in internal and external rotation of the humerus. American Journal of Sports Medicine 23(5):632–637

Brukner P, Khan K 2001 Clinical Sports Medicine, 2nd edn. McGraw-Hill, Roseville, ch 14, p 229–273

Burkhart S S 1991 Arthroscopic treatment of massive rotator cuff tears: clinical results and biomechanical rationale. Clinical Orthopaedics and Related Research 267:45–56

Burkhart S S 1992 Fluoroscopic comparison of kinematic patterns in massive rotator cuff tears: a suspension bridge model. Clinical Orthopaedics and Related Research 254:29–34

Burkhart S S 1993 Arthroscopic debridement and decompression for selected rotator cuff tears: clinical results, pathomechanics and patient selection based on biomechanical parameters. Orthopedic Clinics of North America 24:111–123

Burkhart S S 1994 Reconciling the paradox of rotator cuff repair versus debridement: a unified biomechanical rationale for the treatment of rotator cuff tears. Journal of Arthroscopic and Related Surgery 10(1):4–19

Burkhart S S 1996 A unified biomechanical rationale for the treatment of rotator cuff tears: debridement versus repair. In: Burkhead W Z (ed) Rotator cuff disorders. Williams & Wilkins, Baltimore, ch 21, p 293–312

Burkhart S S 2000 Burkhart's internal impingement/SLAP presentation in slide format. Online. Available: http://www.shoulder.com/ppt/BurkhartSLAP_Internalimpingement/ index/htm/ 10 Sept 2001

Burkhart S S, Esch J C, Jolson R C 1993 The rotator crescent and rotator cable: an anatomic description of the shoulder's 'suspension bridge'. Journal of Arthroscopic and Related Surgery 9(6):611–616

Burkhart S S, Morgan C D, Kibler W B 2000 Shoulder injuries in overhead athletes. The 'dead arm' revisited. Clinics in Sports Medicine 19(1):125–158

Burkhead W Z 1990 The biceps tendon. In Rockwood C A, Matsen F A (eds) The Shoulder. W B Saunders, Philadelphia, ch 20, p 791–836

Burnham R S, May L, Nelson E et al 1993 Shoulder pain in wheelchair athletes. The role of muscle imbalance. American Journal of Sports Medicine 21(2):238–242

Burns T P, Turba J E 1992 Arthroscopic treatment of shoulder impingement in athletes. American Journal of Sports Medicine 20(1):13–16

Burns W C, Whipple T L 1993 Anatomical relationships in the shoulder impingement syndrome. Clinical Orthopaedics and Related Research 294:96–102

Cahill B R 1982 Osteolysis of the distal part of the clavicle in male athletes. Journal of Bone and Joint Surgery (Am) 64A:1053–1057

Carr A, David G, Magarey M et al 1998 Rotator cuff muscle performances during glenohumeral joint rotations: an isokinetic and electromyographic study of freestyle swimmers. In: Proceedings: Australian Conference of Science and Medicine in Sport, Adelaide, p 84

Carson W B 1989 Rehabilitation of the throwing shoulder. Clinics in Sports Medicine 8(4):657–689

Catalano J F, Kleiner B M 1984 Distant transfer and practice variability. Perceptual and Motor Skills 58:851–856

Cavallo R J, Speer K P 1998 Shoulder instability and impingement in throwing athletes. Medicine and Science in Sports and Exercise 30(4, suppl):S18–S25

Chandler T J, Kibler W B, Uhl T L et al 1990 Flexibility comparisons of junior elite tennis players to other athletes. American Journal of Sports Medicine 18(2):134–136

Chandler J, Kibler B, Stracener E C et al 1992 Shoulder strength, power and endurance in college tennis players. American Journal of Sports Medicine 20(4):455–458

Ciullo J V 1986 Swimmer's shoulder. Clinics in Sports Medicine 5(1):115–137

Ciullo J V 1996 Shoulder injuries in sport. Human Kinetics, Champaign, IL

Ciullo J V, Guise E R 1983 Adolescent swimmer's shoulder. Orthopedic Transactions 7(1):171

Ciullo J V, Stevens G G 1989 The prevention and treatment of injuries to the shoulder in swimming. Sports Medicine 7:182–204

Clark J C, Harryman D T 1992 Tendons, ligaments and capsule of the rotator cuff. Journal of Bone and Joint Surgery (Am) 74A:5713–5725

Clark J, Sidles J A, Matsen F A 1990 The relationship of the glenohumeral joint capsule to the rotator cuff. Clinical Orthopaedics and Related Research 254:29–34

Cooper R A, Brems J J 1992 The inferior capsular-shift procedure for multidirectional instability of the shoulder. Journal of Bone and Joint Surgery (Am) 74A(10):1516–1521

Cooper D E, O'Brien S J, Warren R F 1993 Supporting layers of the glenohumeral joint. An anatomic study. Clinical Orthopaedics and Related Research 289:144–155

Copeland S 1993 Throwing injuries of the shoulder. British Journal of Sports Medicine 27(4):221–227

Cordasco F A, Bigliani L U 1998 Multidirectional shoulder instability. In: Warren R F, Craig E V, Altcheck D W (eds) The unstable shoulder. Lippincott-Raven, Philadelphia, ch 16, p 249–261

Cordasco F A, Steinmann S, Flatow E L et al 1993 Arthroscopic treatment of glenoid labral tears. American Journal of Sports Medicine 21(3):425–431

Cowan S M, Bennell K L, Hodges P W et al 2001 Delayed onset of electromyographic activity of vastus medialis obliquus relative to vastus lateralis in subjects with patellofemoral pain syndrome. Archives of Physical Medicine and Rehabilitation 82:183–189

Craig 1984 The posterior mechanism of acute anterior shoulder dislocations. Clinical Orthopaedics and Related Research 190:212–216

Crawford H J, Jull G A 1991 The influence of thoracic form and movement on range of shoulder flexion. Physiotherapy, Theory and Practice 9:143–148

Culham E, Peat M 1993 Functional anatomy of the shoulder complex. Journal of Orthopaedic and Sports Physical Therapy 18(1):342–350

Culham E, Laprade J 2001 Biomechanics of the shoulder complex. In: Dvir Z (ed) Clinical biomechanics. Churchill Livingstone, Philadelphia, ch 6, p 141–164

Dalton S E, Snyder S J 1989 Glenohumeral instability. Bailliere's Clinical Rheumatology 3(3):511–534

David G, Jones M A, Magarey M E et al 1997 Rotator cuff muscle performance during glenohumeral joint rotations: an isokinetic, electromyographic and ultrasonographic study. Tenth Biennial Conference, Manipulative Physiotherapists Association of Australia, Melbourne

David G, Magarey M, Jones M et al 2000 EMG and strength correlates of selected shoulder muscles during rotations of the glenohumeral joint. Journal of Clinical Biomechanics 15(2):95–102

Davidson P A, El Attrache N S, Jobe C M et al 1995 Rotator cuff and posterior-superior glenoid labrum injury associated with increased glenohumeral motion: a new site of impingement. Journal of Shoulder and Elbow Surgery 4(5):384–390

Davies G J, Dickoff-Hoffman S 1993 Neuromuscular testing and rehabilitation of the shoulder complex. Journal of Orthopaedic and Sports Physical Therapy 18(2):449–458

Detrisac D A, Johnson L L 1986 Arthroscopic shoulder anatomy. Pathologic and surgical implications. Slack, New Jersey

DiGiovine N M, Jobe F W , Pink M et al 1992 An eletromyographic analysis of the upper extremity in pitching. Journal of Shoulder and Elbow Surgery 1(2):15–25

Dines D M, Levinson M 1995 The conservative management of the unstable shoulder including rehabilitation. Clinics in Sports Medicine 14(4):797–816

Dugas J R, Cooper D E, O'Brien S J 1999 Gross and microscopic anatomy of the shoulder. In: Warren R F, Craig E V, Altcheck D W (eds) The unstable shoulder. Lippincott-Raven, Philadelphia, ch 2, p 27–50

Dvir Z, Berme N 1978 The shoulder complex in elevation of the arm: a mechanism approach. Journal of Biomechanics 11:219

Edelson G 1999 Variations in the retroversion of the humeral head. Journal of Shoulder and Elbow Surgery 8(2):142–145

Eggert von S, Holzgraefe M 1993 Compression neuropathy in volleyball players. Sportverl Sportschad 7:136–142

Ellenbecker T S 1994 Shoulder injuries in tennis. In: Andrews J R, Wilk K E (eds) The athlete's shoulder. Churchill Livingstone, New York, ch 34, p 399–409

Ellenbecker T S 1995 Rehabilitation of shoulder and elbow injuries in tennis players. Clinics in Sports Medicine 14:107–108

Ellenbecker T S, Mattalin A J, Elam E et al 2000 Quantification of anterior translation of the humeral head in the throwing shoulder. American Journal of Sports Medicine 28(2):161–167

Engle R P 1994 Proprioceptive neuromuscular facilitation for the shoulder. In: Andrews J R and Wilk K E (eds) The athlete's shoulder. Churchill Livingstone, New York, ch 38, p 451

Ferrari D A 1990 Capsular ligaments of the shoulder. Anatomical and functional study of the anterior superior capsule. The American Journal of Sports Medicine 18(1):20–24

Ferrari J D, Ferrari D A, Coumas J et al 1994 Posterior ossification of the shoulder: the Bennett lesion. Etiology, diagnosis and treatment. American Journal of Sports Medicine 22(2):171–176

Ferretti A, De Carli A, Papandrea P 1994 Volleyball injuries: a colour atlas of volleyball traumatology. Fédération Internationale de Volleyball, Lausanne, p 105–113

Ferretti A, Cerullo G, Russo G 1987 Suprascapular neuropathy in volleyball players. Journal of Bone and Joint Surgery (Am) 69A:260–263

Ferretti A, DeCarli A, Fontana M 1998 Injury of the suprascapular nerve at the spinoglenoid notch. The natural history of infraspinatus atrophy in volleyball players. American Journal of Sports Mecidine 26:759–763

Field L D, Savoie F H 1993 Arthroscopic suture repair of superior labral detachment lesions of the shoulder. American Journal of Sports Medicine 21(6):783–790

Field L D, Warren R F, O'Brien S J et al 1995 Isolated closure of rotator interval defects for shoulder instability. American Journal of Sports Medicine 23(6):557–564

Flatow E L, Raimondo, Kelkar R et al 1997 Active and passive restraints against superior humeral translation: the biceps tendon and the coracoacromial arch. Journal of Shoulder and Elbow Surgery 6(2):172

Fleisig G S, Dillman C J, Andrews J R 1994 Biomechanics of the shoulder during throwing. In: Andrews J R, Wilk K E (eds) The athlete's shoulder. Churchill Livingstone, New York, ch 31, p 355–368

Fleisig G S, Andrews J R, Dillman C J et al 1995 Kinetics of baseball pitching with implications about injury mechanisms. American Journal of Sports Medicine 23(2):233–239

Fleisig G S, Barrentine S W, Escamilla R F et al 1996 Biomehanics of overhand throwing with implications for injuries. Sports Medicine 21(6):421–437

Foster C R 1983 Multidirectional instability of the shoulder in the athlete. Clinics in Sports Medicine 2(2):355–368

Fukuda K, Chen C M, Cofield R H et al 1988 Biomechanical analysis of stability and fixation strength of total shoulder prostheses. Orthopaedics 11:141

Fukuda H, Hamada K, Yamanaka K 1990a Pathology and pathogenesis of bursal-side rotator cuff tears viewed from en bloc histologic sections. Clinical Orthopaedics and Related Research 254:75–80

Fukuda H, Hamada K, Nakajima T et al 1990b Pathology and pathogenesis of joint-side rotator cuff tears (rim rents) viewed from en bloc histologic sections. Read at Meeting of American Shoulder and Elbow Surgeons, Chicago, Illinois

Garth W P, Allman F L, Armstrong W S 1987 Occult anterior subluxations of the shoulder in noncontact sports. American Journal of Sports Medicine 15(6):579–585

Gartsman G M, Hammerman S M 2000 Superior labrum, anterior and posterior lesions. When and how to treat them? Clinics in Sports Medicine 19(1):115–124

Gerber C, Ganz R 1984 Clinical assessment of instability of the shoulder, with special reference to anterior and posterior drawer tests. Journal of Bone and Joint Surgery (Br) 66B(4):551–556

Gerber C, Krushell R J 1991 Isolated rupture of the tendon of the subscapularis muscle: clinical features in 16 cases. Journal of Bone and Joint Surgery (Br) 73B:389–394

Gerber C, Sebesta A 2000 Impingement of the deep surface of the subscapularis tendon and the reflection pulley on the anterosuperior glenoid rim: a preliminary report. Journal of Shoulder and Elbow Surgery 9(6):483–490

Gerber C, Terrier F, Zehnder R et al 1987 The subcoracoid space: an anatomic study. Clinical Orthopaedics and Related Research 215:132–138

Gerber C, Hersche O, Farron A 1996 Isolated rupture of subscapularis tendon. Journal of Bone and Joint Surgery (Am) 78A:1015–1023

Getelman M H, Snyder S J 1999 SLAP lesions and lesions of the long head of the biceps tendon. Treatment considerations. In: Warren R F, Craig E V, Altcheck D W (eds) The unstable shoulder. Lippincott-Raven, Philadelphia, ch 23, p 347–366

Gifford, L S 1997 Pain. In: Pitt-Brooke J (ed): Rehabilitation of movement: theoretical bases of clinical practice. WB Saunders, London, p 196

Gifford L S (ed) 1998 Topical issues in pain 1. Whiplash – science and management. Fear avoidance beliefs and behaviour. CNS Press, Falmouth

Gifford L S 2000 Topical issues in pain 2. Biopsychosocial assessment. Relationships and pain. CNS Press, Falmouth

Glasgow S G, Bruce R A, Yacobucci G N et al 1992 Arthroscopic resection of glenoid labrum tears in the athlete: a report of 29 cases. Journal of Arthroscopic and Related Surgery 8(1):48–54

Glousman R E 1993 Instability versus impingement syndrome in the throwing athlete. Orthopedic Clinics of North America 24(1):89–99

Glousman R, Jobe F W 1996 Anterior shoulder instability, impingement and rotator cuff tear. In: Jobe F W (ed) Operative techniques in upper extremity sports injuries. St Louis, Mosby, Ch 7, Section C: Anterior and multidirectional glenohumeral instability, p 191–210

Glousman R, Jobe F, Tibone J et al 1988 Dynamic electromyographic analysis of the throwing shoulder with glenohumeral instability. Journal of Bone and Joint Surgery (Am) 70A(2):220–226

Gohlke F, Essigkrug B, Schmitz F 1994 The pattern of the collagen fiber bundles of the capsule of the glenohumeral joint. Journal of Shoulder and Elbow Surgery 3:111–128

Gonzalez D, Lopez R A 1991 Concurrent rotator-cuff tear and brachial plexus palsy associated with anterior dislocation of the shoulder. Journal of Bone and Joint Surgery (Am) 73A(4):620–621

Gowan I D, Jobe F W, Tibone J E et al 1987 A comparative eletromyographic analysis of the shoulder during pitching. Professional versus amateur pitchers. American Journal of Sports Medicine 15(6):586–590

Grauer J D, Paulos L E, Smutz W P 1992 Biceps tendon and superior labral injuries. Arthroscopy 8(4):488–497

Greenan T J, Zlatkin M B, Dalinka M K et al 1993 Posttraumatic changes in the posterior glenoid and labrum in a handball player. American Journal of Sports Medicine 21(1):153–156

Gross M L, Seeger L L, Smith J B et al 1990 Magnetic resonance imaging of the glenoid labrum. American Journal of Sports Medicine 18(3):229–234

Gross M L, Brenner S L, Esformes I et al 1993 Anterior shoulder instability in weight lifters. American Journal of Sports Medicine 21(4):599–603

Habermeyer P, Schüller U 1990 Die bedeutung des labrum glenoidale für die stabilität des glenohumeralgelenkes. Eine experimentelle studio. Unfallchirurgie 93:19–26

Habermeyer P, Walch G 1996 The biceps tendon and rotator cuff disease. In: Burkhead W Z (ed) Rotator cuff disorders. Williams and Wilkins, Baltimore, ch 10, p 142–159

Habermeyer P, Kaiser E, Knappe M et al 1987 Functional anatomy and biomechanics of the long biceps tendon. Unfallchirurgie 90(7):319–329

Habermeyer P, Schüller U, Wiedemann E 1992 The intra-articular pressure of the shoulder: an experimental study on the role of the glenoid labrum stabilizing the joint. Arthroscopy 8(2):166–172

Hama H, Ueba Y, Norinaga T et al 1992 A new strategy for treatment of suprascapular nerve entrapment. Journal of Shoulder and Elbow Surgery 1:253–260

Hamner D L, Pink M M, Jobe F W 2000 A modification of the relocation test: arthroscopic findings associated with a positive test. Journal of Shoulder and Elbow Surgery 9(4):263–267

Harryman D T, Clark J M 1996 Anatomy of the rotator cuff. In: Burkhead W Z (ed) Rotator cuff disorders. Williams and Wilkins, Baltimore, ch 2, p 23–35

Harryman D T, Sidles J A, Matsen F A 1990 The humeral head translates on the glenoid with passive motion. In: Post M, Morrey B F, Hawkins R J (eds) Surgery of the shoulder. Mosby Year Book, St Louis, ch 43, p186

Harryman D T, Sidles J A, Harris S L et al 1992 The role of the rotator interval capsule in passive motion and stability of the shoulder. Journal of Bone and Joint Surgery (Am) 74A(1):53–66

Hata Y, Nakatsuchk Y, Saitoh S et al 1992 Anatomic study of the glenoid labrum. Journal of Shoulder and Elbow Surgery 1(4):207–214

Hawkins R J, Kennedy J C 1980 Impingement syndrome in athletes. American Journal of Sports Medicine 8(3):151–158

Helmig P, Søjbjerg J O, Kærsgaard-Andersen P et al 1990 Distal humeral migration as a component of multidirectional shoulder instability. Clinical Orthopaedics and Related Research 252:139–143

Hemsley K P 1994 Shoulder injuries in gymnastics. In: Andrews J R, Wilk K E (eds) The athlete's shoulder. Churchill Livingstone, New York, ch 36, p 425–433

Hertz H 1984 Die bedeutung des limbus glenoidalis fur die stabilitat des schultergelenks. Wien Klin Wochenschr Suppl 152:1–23

Hodges P W, Richardson C A 1996 Inefficient muscular stabilisation of the lumbar spine associated with low back pain: a motor control evaluation of transversus abdominis. Spine 21:2640–2650

Holzgraefe M, Kukowski B, Eggert S 1994 Prevalence of latent and manifest suprascapular neuropathy in high-performance volleyball players. British Journal of Sports Medicine 28:177–179

Howell S M, Galinat B J 1987 The containment mechanism: the primary stabilizer of the glenohumeral joint. Paper read at Annual Meeting of American Academy of Orthopaedic Surgeons, San Francisco, 23 January 1987

Howell S M, Galinat B J, Renzi A J et al 1988 Normal and abnormal mechanics of the glenohumeral joint in the horizontal plane. Journal of Bone and Joint Surgery (Am) 70A(2):227–232

Hsu H-C, Luo Z-P, Cofield R H et al 1997 Influence of rotator cuff tearing on glenohumeral stability. Journal of Shoulder and Elbow Surgery 6(5):413–422

Huber W P, Putz R V 1997 Periarticular fiber system of the shoulder joint. Journal of Arthroscopy and Related Research 13(6):680–691

Hughes A 2001 Volleyballer's shoulder. Sportslink (Sports Physiotherapy Australia) 4–5 September

Hulstyn M J, Fadale P D 1995 Arthroscopic anatomy of the shoulder. Orthopedic Clinics of North America 26(4):597–612

Iannotti J P, Wang E D 1992 Avulsion fracture of the supraglenoid tubercle: a variation of the SLAP lesion. Journal of Shoulder and Elbow Surgery 1(1):26–30

Inman V T, Saunders J B de C M, Abbott L C 1944 Observations on the function of the shoulder joint. Journal of Bone and Joint Surgery (Am) 26A:1–30

Itoi E, Motzkin N E, Morrey B F et al 1992 Scapular inclination and inferior stability of the shoulder. Journal of Shoulder and Elbow Surgery 1(3):131–139

Itoi E, Motzkin N E, Morrey B F et al 1993 Bulk effect of rotator cuff on inferior glenohumeral stability as function of scapular inclination angle: a cadaver study. Tohoku Journal of Experimental Medicine 171(4):267–276

Itoi E, Motzkin N E, Morrey B F et al 1994 Stabilizing function of the long head of the biceps in the hanging position. Journal of Shoulder and Elbow Surgery 3(3):135–142

Izaki T, Midorikawa K, Shibata Y et al 1994a Biceps labrum complex (BLC) lesions. Paper read to the Third Scandinavian – Japanese Congress on Shoulder Surgery, Aarhus, Denmark, 7–9 June 1993, Journal of Shoulder and Elbow Surgery 3:1 (Part 2), S41

Izaki T, Midorikawa K, Shibata Y et al 1994b The histological study of biceps labrum complex and its attachment to the glenoid. Paper read to the Twentieth Annual Meeting of the Japan Shoulder Society, Nagasaki, 1–2 October 1993, Journal of Shoulder and Elbow Surgery 3(1) (Part 2):S47

Jerosch J, Castro W H M, Drescher H 1993 Does the glenohumerral joint capsule have proprioceptive capability? Knee Surgery, Sports Traumatology, Arthroscopy 1:80–84

Jobe C M 1995 Posterior superior glenoid impingement: expanded clinical spectrum. Arthroscopy 11:530–536

Jobe C M 1998 Gross anatomy of the shoulder. In: Rockwood C A, Matsen F A (eds) The shoulder, 2nd edn. WB Saunders, Philadelphia, ch 2, p 34–98

Jobe F W, Moynes D R 1982 Delineation of diagnostic criteria and a rehabilitation program for rotator cuff injuries. American Journal of Sports Medicine 10(6):336–339

Jobe F W, Jobe C M 1983 Painful athletic injuries of the shoulder. Clinical Orthopaedics and Related Research 173:117–124

Jobe F W, Bradley J P 1988 Rotator cuff injuries in baseball: prevention and rehabilitation. Sports Medicine 6:378–387

Jobe F W, Kvitne R S 1989 Shoulder pain in the overhand or throwing athlete. The relationship of anterior instability and rotator cuff impingement. Orthopaedic Review 18(9):963–975

Jobe F W, Pink M 1993 Classification and treatment of shoulder dysfunction in the overhead athlete. Journal of Orthopaedic and Sports Physical Therapy 18(2):427–432

Jobe F W, Pink M 1994 The athlete's shoulder. Journal of Hand Therapy April-June:107–110

Jobe F W, Tibone J E, Perry J et al 1983 An EMG analysis of the shoulder in throwing and pitching. A preliminary report. American Journal of Sports Medicine 11(1):3–5

Jobe F W, Moynes D R, Tibone J E et al 1984 An EMG analysis of the shoulder in pitching. A second report. American Journal of Sports Medicine 12(3):218–220

Jobe C M, Walch G, Sidles J 1992 Evidence for a superior glenoid impingement upon the rotator cuff: anatomic, kinesiologic, MRI and arthroscopic findings. Orthopaedic Transactions, American Shoulder and Elbow Surgeons, p 763

Jobe C M, Pink M, Jobe F W et al 1996 Anterior shoulder instability, impingement and rotator cuff tear. In: Jobe F W (ed) Operative techniques in upper extremity sports injuries, ch 7, section A: theories and concepts. Mosby, St Louis, p 164–176

Jobe F W, Tibone J E, Pink M M, et al 1998 The shoulder in sports. In: Rockwood C A, Matsen F A (eds) The shoulder, 2nd edn. WB Saunders, Philadelphia, ch 25, p 1214–1238

Johanson M A, Gonzalez-King B Z 1997 Differential soft tissue diagnosis. In: Donatelli R A (ed) Physical therapy of the shoulder. 3rd edn. ch 3, p 57–94

Jones M A 1995 Clinical reasoning and pain. Manual Therapy 1:17–24

Jones M A, Magarey M E 2001 Clinical reasoning in the use of manual therapy techniques for the shoulder girdle. In: Tovin B, Greenfield B H (eds) Evaluation and treatment of the shoulder. An integration of the guide to physical therapist practice. FA Davis, Philadelphia, ch 13, p 317–346

Jones H M, Jones M A, Maitland G D 1994 Evaluation and treatment by passive movement. In: Grant R (ed) Physical therapy of the cervical and thoracic spine. Churchill Livingstone, New York, ch 12 p 245

Jones, M A, Jensen, G, Edwards, I 2000 Clinical reasoning in physiotherapy. In: Higgs, J, Jones, M A (eds): Clinical reasoning in the health professions, 2nd Edn. Butterworth Heinemann, Oxford, ch 12, p 117–127

Jones M A, Edwards I, Gifford L 2002 Conceptual models for implementing biopsychosocial theory in clinical practice. Manual Therapy 7(1):2–9

Josza L, Kannus P 1997 Human tendons. Human Kinetics, Champaign

Kaltsas D S 1983 Comparative study of the properties of the shoulder joint capsule with those of other joint capsules. Clinical Orthopaedics and Related Research 173:20–26

Kamkar A, Irrgang J J, Whitney S L 1993 Nonoperative management of secondary shoulder impingement syndrome. Journal of Orthopaedic and Sports Physical Therapy 17(5):212–224

Kannus P, Josza L 1991 Histopathological changes preceding spontaneous rupture of a tendon. A controlled study of 891 patients. Journal of Bone and Joint Surgery 73:1507–1525

Kao J T, Pink M, Jobe F W et al 1995 Electromyographic analysis of the scapular muscles during a golf swing. American Journal of Sports Medicine 23(1):19–23

Kelly M J 1995 Anatomic and biomechanical rationale for rehabilitation of the athlete's shoulder. Journal of Sport Rehabilitation 4:122–154

Kernwein G H, Rosenburg B, Sneed W R 1961 Aids in the differential diagnosis of the painful shoulder syndrome. Clinical Orthopaedics and Related Research 20:11–20

Kessell L 1982 Clinical disorders of the shoulder. Churchill Livingstone, Edinburgh

Khan K M, Maffulli N, Coleman B D et al 1998 Patellar tendinopathy: some aspects of basic science and clinical management. British Journal of Sports Medicine 32:346–355

Khan K M, Cook J L, Bonar F et al 1999 Histopathology of common tendinopathies: update and implications for clinical management. Sports Medicine 27:393–408

Kibler W B 1991 Role of the scapula in the overhead throwing motion. Contemporary Orthopedics 22(5):525–533

Kibler W B 1995 Biomechanical analysis of the shoulder during tennis activities. Clinics in Sports Medicine 14(1):79–85

Kibler W B 1998a Shoulder rehabilitation: principles and practice. Medicine and Science in Sports and Exercise 30 (4, suppl):S40–50

Kibler B 1998b The role of the scapula in athletic shoulder function. American Journal of Sports Medicine 26 (2):325–339

Kibler W B, Chandler T J 1994 Sports-specific conditioning. American Journal of Sports Medicine 22(3):424–432

Knott M, Voss D 1968 Proprioceptive neuromuscular facilitation. Harper and Row, New York

Kronberg M, Brostrom L-A 1990 Humeral head retroversion in patients with unstable humeroscapular joints. Clinical Orthopaedics and Related Research 260:207–211

Kronberg M, Brostrom L-A, Soderlund V 1990 Retroversion of the humeral head in the normal shoulder and its relationship to the normal range of motion. Clinical Orthopaedics and Related Research 253:113–117

Kuhn J E, Lindblom S R, Huston L J et al 1999 Failure of the biceps-superior labral complex in the throwing athlete: a cadaveric biomechanical investigation comparing the positions of late cocking and early deceleration. Presented at the Arthroscopy Association of North America Specialty Day, AAOS Annual Meeting, Anaheim, CA, 7 February 1999

Kumar V P, Satku K, Balasubramaniam P 1989 The role of the long head of biceps brachii in the stabilization of the head of the humerus. Clinical Orthopaedics and Related Research 244:172–175

Kuroda S, Sumiyoshi T, Moriishi J et al 1997 Onset and spontaneous recovery of multidirectional instability (MDI) of the shoulder. Journal of Shoulder and Elbow Surgery 6(2):242–243

Kvitne R S, Jobe F W 1993 The diagnosis and treatment of anterior instability in the throwing athlete. Clinical Orthopaedics and Related Research 291:107–123

Kvitne R S, Jobe F W, Jobe C M 1995 Shoulder instability in the overhead or throwing athlete. Clinics in Sports Medicine 14(4):917–935

Lebar R D, Alexander A H 1992 Multidirectional shoulder instability. Clinical results of inferior capsular shift in an active-duty population. American Journal of Sports Medicine 20(2):193–198

Lee H W M 1995 Mechanisms of neck and shoulder injuries in tennis players. Journal of Orthopaedics and Sports Physical Therapy 21(1):28–37

Lee T Q, Blac, A D, Tibone J E et al 2001 Release of the coracoacromial ligament can lead to glenohumeral laxity: a biomechanical study. Journal of Shoulder and Elbow Surgery 10(10):68–72

Lehman R C 1988 Shoulder pain in the competitive tennis player. Clinics in Sports Medicine 7(2):309–327

Lippitt S, Matsen F 1993 Mechanisms of glenohumeral joint stability. Clinical Orthopaedics and Related Research 291:20–28

Lippitt S B, Vanderhooft E, Harris S L et al 1993 Glenohumeral stability from concavity-compression: a quantitative analysis. Journal of Shoulder and Elbow Surgery 2(1):27–35

Litchfield R, Hawkins R, Dillman C J et al 1993 Rehabilitation for the overhead athlete. Journal of Orthopaedic and Sports Physical Therapy 18(2):433–441

Liu S H, Henry M H, Nuccion S et al 1996 Diagnosis of glenoid labral tears: a comparison between magnetic resonance imaging and clinical examinations. American Journal of Sports Medicine 24(2):149–154

McCann P D, Bigliani L U 1994 Shoulder pain in tennis players. Sports Medicine 17(1):53–64

McLeod W D, Andrews J R 1986 Mechanisms of shoulder injuries. Physical Therapy 66(12):1901

McMaster W C 1986 Anterior glenoid labrum damage: a painful lesion in swimmers. American Journal of Sports Medicine 14(5):383–387

McMaster W C, Troup J 1993 A survey of interfering shoulder pain in United States competitive swimmers. American Journal of Sports Medicine 21(1):67–70

McMaster W C, Long S C, Caiozzo V J 1991 Isokinetic torque imbalances in the rotator cuff of the elite water polo player. American Journal of Sports Medicine 19(1):72–75

McMaster W C, Roberts A, Stoddard T 1998 A correlation between shoulder laxity and interfering pain in competitive swimmers. American Journal of Sports Medicine 26(1):83–87

Magarey M E 1986 The first treatment session. In: Greive G P (ed) Modern manual therapy of the vertebral column. Churchill Livingstone, Edinburgh, ch 61, p 661

Magarey M E 1993 The shoulder complex: how useful are our differentiating procedures? In: Singer K (ed) Proceedings, Eighth Biennial Conference, Manipulative Physiotherapists Association of Australia, p 43

Magarey M E in press Case study: patient with shoulder pain. In: Jones M A, Rivett D, Clinical Reasoning for Clinicians, Butterworth-Heinemann

Magarey M E, Jones M A 1991 Clinical examination and management for minor instability of the shoulder complex. Australian Journal of Physiotherapy 38:260–280

Magarey M E, Jones M A in press a Dynamic evaluation and early management of altered motor control around the shoulder complex. Submitted to Manual Therapy, June 2001

Magarey M E, Jones M A in press b Specific evaluation of the function of force couples relevant for stabilisation of glenohumeral joint. Submitted to Manual Therapy, June 2001

Magarey M E, Jones M A, Grant E R 1996 Biomedical considerations and clinical patterns related to disorders of the glenoid labrum in the predominantly stable glenohumeral joint. Manual Therapy 1(5):242–249

Maitland G D 1991 Peripheral manipulation, Butterworth Heinemann, London

Mallon J W, Speer K P 1995 Multi-directional instability. Journal of Shoulder and Elbow Surgery 4(1):54–64

Matsen F A, Harryman D T, Sidles J A 1991 Mechanics of glenohumeral stability. Clinics in Sports Medicine 10(4):783–788

Matsen F A, Arntz C T, Lippitt S B 1998a Rotator cuff. In: Rockwood C A, Matsen F A (eds) The shoulder. 2nd edn. WB Saunders Co, Philadelphia, ch 15, p 755–839

Matsen F A, Thomas S C, Rockwood C A et al 1998b Glenohumeral instability. In: Rockwood C A, Matsen F A (eds) The shoulder, 2nd edn. WB Saunders Co, Philadelphia, Vol 2, ch 14, p 611–754

Matthews L S, Simonson B G, Wolock B S 1993 Osteolysis of the distal clavicle in a female body builder. A case report. American Journal of Sports Medicine 21(1):150–152

Mayfield F H, True C W 1973 Chronic injuries to peripheral nerves by entrapment. In: Youmans J (ed) Neurological Surgery, WB Saunders, Philadelphia, p 1158–1159

Meister K 2000 Injuries to the shoulder in the throwing athlete. Part One: Biomechanics/pathophysiology/classification of injury. American Journal of Sports Medicine 28(2):265–274

Meister K, Andrews J R 1993 Classification and treatment of rotator cuff injuries in the overhand athlete. Journal of Orthopaedic and Sports Physical Therapy 18(2):415–421

Meister K, Andrews J R, Batts J et al 1999 Symptomatic thrower's exostosis. American Journal of Sports Medicine 27(2):133–142

Mimori K, Muneta T, Nakagawa T et al 1999 A new pain provocation test for superior labral tears of the shoulder. American Journal of Sports Medicine 27(2):137–146

Mohtadi N G H 1991 Advances in the understanding of anterior instability of the shoulder. Clinics in Sports Medicine 10(4):863–870

Montagna P, Colonna S 1993 Suprascapular neuropathy restricted to the infraspinatus muscle in volleyball players. Acta Neurologica Scandinavica 87:248–250

Montgomery W H, Jobe F W 1994 Functional outcoes in athletes after modified anterior capsulolabral reconstruction. American Journal of Sports Medicine 22(3):352–358

Moran C A, Saunders S R 1991 Evaluation of the shoulder: a sequential approach. In Donatelli R (ed) Physical therapy of the shoulder, 2nd edn. Churchill Livingstone, New York, ch 2, p 19–62

Mulligan B R 1999 Manual Therapy 'Nags', 'Snags', 'MWMs' etc, 4th edn. Hutcheson Bowman and Stewart, Wellington

Murphy T C 1994 Shoulder injuries in swimming. In: Andrews J R, Wilk K E (eds) The athlete's shoulder. Churchill Livingstone, New York, ch 35, p 411–424

Nakajima T, Rokuuma N, Hamada K et al 1994 Histologic and biomechanical characteristics of the supraspinatus tendon : reference to rotator cuff tearing. Journal of Shoulder and Elbow Surgery 3(2):79–87

Narakas A 1989 Compression syndromes about the shoulder including brachial plexus. In: Szabo R M (ed) Nerve compression syndromes. Diagnosis and treatment. Slack, Thorofare, ch 15, p 227

Neer C S, Welsh P 1977 The shoulder in sports. Orthopedic Clinics of North America 8:583–590

Neer C S, Foster C R 1980 Inferior capsular shift for involuntary inferior and multidirectional instability of the shoulder; a preliminary report. Journal of Bone and Joint Surgery (Am) 62A(6):897–908

Neer C S, Satterlee C C, Dalsey R M et al 1992 The anatomy and potential effects of contracture of the coracohumeral ligament. Clinical Orthopaedics and Related Research 280:182–185

Neviaser T J 1991 Weight lifting. Risks and injuries to the shoulder. Clinics in Sports Medicine 10(3):615–621

Neviaser R J, Neviaser T J, Neviaser J S 1988 Concurrent rupture of the rotator cuff and anterior dislocation of the shoulder in the older patient. Journal of Bone and Joint Surgery (Am) 70A(9):1308–1311

Nichols R T 1994 A biomechanical perspective on spinal mechanisms of coordinated muscular action. Acta Anatomica 15:1–13

Nobuhara K, Ikeda H 1987 Rotator interval lesion. Clinical Orthopaedics and Related Research 223:44–50

Norris C M 1993 Sports injuries: diagnosis and management for physiotherapists. Butterworth Heinemann, Oxford, ch 20, p280–292

Nuber G W, Jobe F W, Perry J et al 1986 Fine wire electromyography analysis of muscles of the shoulder during swimming. American Journal of Sports Medicine 14(1):7–11

O'Brien S J, Neves M C, Arnoczky S P et al 1990 The anatomy and histology of the inferior glenohumeral ligament complex of the shoulder. American Journal of Sports Medicine 18(5):449–456

O'Brien S J, Schwartz R S, Warren R F et al 1995 Capsular restraints to anterior-posterior motion of the abducted shoulder: a biomechanical study. Journal of Shoulder and Elbow Surgery 4:298–308

O'Brien S J, Allen A A, Fealy S et al 1998a Developmental anatomy of the shoulder and anatomy of the glenohumeral joint. In: Rockwood C A, Matsen F A (eds) The shoulder, 2nd edn. WB Saunders Co, Philadelphia, ch 1, p 1–27

O'Brien S J, Pagnani M J, Fealy S et al 1998b The active compression test: a new and effective test for diagnosing labral tears and acromioclavicular joint abnormality. American Journal of Sports Medicine 26(5):610–614

O'Connell P W, Nuber G W, Mileski R A et al 1990 The contribution of the glenohumeral ligaments to anterior stability of the shoulder joint. American Journal of Sports Medicine 18(6):579–584

O'Sullivan P B, Twomey L T, Allison G T 1997 Evaluation of specific stabilizing exercise in the treatment of chronic low back pain with radiologic diagnosis of spondylolysis or spondylolisthesis. Spine 22:295–296

Ovesen J, Neilsen 1985 Stability of the shoulder joint. Cadaver study of the stabilising structures. Acta Orthopaedica Scandinavica 56:149–151

Ozaki J 1989 Glenohumeral movement of the involutary inferior and multidirectional instability. Clinical Orthopaedics and Related Research 238:107–111

Pagnani M J, Warren R F 1994 Stabilisers of the glenohumeral joint. Journal of Shoulder and Elbow Surgery 3(3):173–190

Payne L Z, Jokl P 1993 The results of arthroscopic debridement of glenoid labral tears based on tear location. Arthroscopy 9(5):560–565

Peat M, Culham E 1994 Functional anatomy of the shoulder complex. In: Andrews J R, Wilk K E (eds) The athletes shoulder, Churchill Livingstone, New York, ch 1, p 1–15

Perry J, Pink M, Jobe F W et al 1992 The painful shoulder during the backstroke: an EMG and cinematographic analysis of 12 muscles. Clinical Journal of Sports Medicine 2:13–20

Pfund R, Jones M A, Magarey M E et al 1998a Manueller Test zur differenzierung von strukturen im subakromialen raum, Teil II. Manuelle Therapie 1:164–174

Pfund R, Jones M A, Magarey M E et al 1998b Manueller Test zur differenzierung von strukturen im subakromialen raum, Teil I. Manuelle Therapie 2:114–119

Pieper H G 1988 Humeral torsion in the throwing arm of handball players. American Journal of Sports Medicine 26(2):247–253

Pink M, Jobe F W 1991 Shoulder injuries in athletes. Orthopedics 11(6):39–47

Pink M M, Jobe F W 1994 Biomechanics of swimming. In: Athletic injuries and rehabilitation, ch 16, p 317–331

Pink M, Perry J, Browne A et al 1991 The normal shoulder during freestyle swimming. An eletromyographic and cinematographic analysis of twelve muscles. American Journal of Sports Medicine 19(6):569–576

Pink M, Jobe F W, Perry J et al 1992 The normal shoulder during the backstroke: an EMG and cinematographic analysis of 12 muscles. Clinical Journal of Sports Medicine 2:6–12

Pink M, Jobe F W, Perry J et al 1993a The painful shoulder during the butterfly stroke: an electromyographic and cinematographic analysis of twelve muscles. Clinical Orthopaedics and Related Research 288:60–72

Pink M, Jobe F W, Perry J et al 1993b The normal shoulder during the butterfly swim stroke: an electromyographic and cinematographic analysis of twelve muscles. Clinical Orthopaedics and Related Research 288:48–59

Pollock R G, Wang V M, Bucchieri J S et al 2000 Effects of repetitive subfailure strains on the mechanical behaviour of the inferior glenohumeral ligament. Journal of Shoulder and Elbow Surgery 9(5):427–435

Poppen N K, Walker P S 1978 Forces at the glenohumeral joint in abduction. Clinical Orthopaedics and Related Research 135:165–170

Pratt N E 1986 Neurovascular entrapment in the regions of the shoulder and posterior triangle of the neck. Physical Therapy 66(12):1894–1900

Priest J D 1988 the shoulder of the tennis player. Clinics in Sports Medicine 7(2):387–402

Rames R D, Karzel R P 1993 Injuries to the glenoid labrum, including SLAP lesions. Orthopedic Clinics of North America 24(1):45–53

Reeves B 1968 Experiments on the tensile strength of the anterior capsular structures of the shoulder in man. Journal of Bone and Joint Surgery (Br) 50B(4):858–865

Refior H J, Sowa D 1995 Long tendon of the biceps brachii: sites of predilection for degenerative lesions. Journal of Shoulder and Elbow Surgery 4(6):436–440

Rengachary S S, Burr D, Lucas S et al 1979 Suprascapular entrament neuropathy: a clinical, anatomical and comparative study. Part 2: anatomical study. Journal of Neurosurgery 5:447–451

Resch H, Golser K, Thoeni H et al 1993 Arthroscopic repair of superior glenoid labral detachment (the SLAP lesion). Journal of Shoulder and Elbow Surgery 2(3):147–155

Richardson A B, Jobe F W, Collins H R 1980 The shoulder in competitive swimming. American Journal of Sports Medicine 8(3):159–163

Rockwood C A, Matsen F A (eds) 1998 The Shoulder, 2nd edn. WB Saunders Co, Philadelphia

Rodosky M W, Harner C D, Fu F H 1994 The role of the long head of the biceps muscle and superior glenoid labrum in anterior stability of the shoulder. American Journal of Sports Medicine 22(1):121–130

Rowe C R 1987 Recurrent transient anterior subluxation of the shoulder. The 'dead arm' syndrome. Clinical Orthopaedics and Related Research 223:11–19

Rowe C R, Zarins B 1981 Recurrent transient subluxation of the shoulder. Journal of Bone and Joint Surgery (Am) 63A:863–872

Rubinstein D S, Jobe F W, Glousman R E et al 1992 Anterior capsulolabral reconstruction of the shoulder in athletes. Journal of Shoulder and Elbow Surgery 1(5):229–237

Ruwe P A, Pink M, Jobe F W et al 1994 The normal and the painful shoulders during the breaststroke. Electromyographic and cinematographic analysis of twelve muscles. American Journal of Sports Medicine 22(6):789–796

Ryu R K N, McCormick J, Jobe F W et al 1988 An electromyographic analysis of shoulder function in tennis players. American Journal of Sports Medicine 16(5):481–485

Sandow M J, Ilic J 1998 Suprascapular nerve rotator cuff compression syndrome in volleyball players. Journal of Shoulder and Elbow Surgery 7(5):516–521

Scarpinato D R, Bramhall J P, Andrews J R 1991 Arthroscopic management of the throwing athlete's shoulder: indications, techniques and results. Clinics in Sports Medicine 10(4):913–927

Schenkman M, Rugo de Cartaya V 1987 Kinesiology of the shoulder complex. Journal of Orthopaedic and Sports Physical Therapy 8:438

Schenkman M, Rugo de Cartaya V 1994 Kinesiology of the shoulder complex. In: Andrews J R, Wilk K E (eds) The athlete's shoulder. Churchill Livingstone, New York, ch 2, p 15

Schmidt R A 1991 Motor learning principles for physical therapy. Contemporary management of motor control problems. Proceedings of the II Step Conference, Alexandria, VA: APTA

Schmitz M A, Ciullo J 1998 The recognition and treatment of superior labral anterior-posterior (SLAP) lesions in the shoulder. Medscape Orthopaedics and Sports Medicine 2(6)Available online: http://orthopaedics.medscape.com/medscape/orthosportsmed/journal/public/archive/1998/TOC-0206.html

Schulte K R, Warner J J P 1995 Uncommon causes of shoulder pain in the athlete. Orthopedic Clinics of North America 26(3):505–528

Schwabel A 1998 Timing of onset of rotator cuff and delto-pectoral activity during isokinetic glenohumeral joint rotations in asymptomatic swimmers. Unpublished Master of Applied Science (Sports Physiotherapy) thesis, University of South Australia

Schwartz E, O'Brien S J, Torzilli P A et al 1987 Capsular restraints to anterior-posterior motion of the shoulder. Transactions of the Orthopaedic Research Society 12:78

Scovazzo M L, Browne A, Pink M et al 1991 The painful shoulder during freestyle swimming. American Journal of Sports Medicine 19(6):577–582

Seddon H J 1943 Three types of nerve injury. Brain 66:237

Shankwiler J A, Burkhead W Z 1996 Evaluation of painful shoulders: entities that may be confused with rotator cuff disease. In: Burkhead W Z (ed) Rotator cuff disorders. Williams and Wilkins, Baltimore, ch 5, p 59–72

Shumway-Cook A, Woollacott M J 2001 Motor control: theory and practical applications. Lippincott Williams and Wilkins, Philadelphia

Skurja M, Monlux J H 1985 Case studies: the suprascapular nerve and shoulder dysfunction. Journal of Orthopaedic and Sports Physical Therapy 6(4):254–258

Snyder S J, Karzel R P, Del Pizzo W et at 1990 SLAP lesions of the shoulder. Journal of Arthroscopic and Related Research 6(4):274–279

Snyder S J, Banas M P, Karzel R P 1995 An analysis of 140 injuries to the superior glenoid labrum. Journal of Shoulder and Elbow Surgery 4(4):243–248

Solem-Bertoff E, Thuomas K-A, Westerberg C-E 1993 The influence of scapular retraction and protraction on the width of the subacromial space. An MRI study. Clinical Orthopaedics and Related Research 296:99–103

Solheim L F, Roaas A 1978 Compression of the suprascapular nerve after fracture of the scapular notch. Acta Orthopaedica Scandinavica 49:338

Soslowsky L J, Pawluk R J, Ark J W et al 1991 In situ articular contact at the glenohumeral and subacromial joints. Transactions of the Orthopaedic Research Society, p 569

Soslowsky L J, Flatow E L, Bigliani L U et al 1992a Articular geometry of the glenohumeral joint. Clinical Orthopaedics and Related Research 285:181–190

Soslowsky L J, Flatow E L, Bigliani L U et al 1992b Quantitation of in situ contact areas at the glenohumeral joint: a biomechanical study. Journal of Orthopaedic Research 10(4):524–534

Souza T A 1994 General biomechanics. In: Souza T A (ed) Sports injuries of the shoulder. Churchill Livingstone, New York, ch 2, p 37

Speer K P, Cavanaugh J T, Warren R F et al 1993 A role for hydrotherapy in shoulder rehabilitation. American Journal of Sports Medicine 21:850

Stocker D, Pink M, Jobe F W 1995 Comparison of shoulder injury in collegiate- and master's-level swimmers. Clinical Journal of Sport Medicine 5:4–8

Sunderland S 1978 Nerves and nerve injuries, 2nd edn. Churchill Livingstone, Edinburgh

Symeonides P P 1972 The significance of the subscapularis muscle in pathogenesis of recurrent anterior dislocation of the shoulder. Journal of Bone and Joint Surgery (Br) 54B:476–483

Tengan C H, Oiviero A S B, Kiymoto B H et al 1993 Isolated and painless infraspinatus atrophy in top-level volleyball players: report of two cases and review of the literature. Arq Neuropsiqiatri 51:125–129

Terry G C, Hammon D, France P et al 1991 The stabilizing function of passive shoulder restraints. American Journal of Sports Medicine 19(1):26–34

Tibone J E, Bradley J P 1993 The treatment of posterior subluxation in athletes. Clinical Orthopaedics and Related Research 291:124–137

Ticker J B, Fealy S, Fu F H 1995 Instability and impingement in the athlete's shoulder. Sports Medicine 19(6):418–426

Tovin B J, Greenfield B H 2001 Evaluation and treatment of the shoulder. An integration of the guide to physical therapist practice. FA Davis, Philadelphia

Townsend H, Jobe F W, Pink M, Perry J 1991 Electromyographic analysis of the glenohumeral muscles during a baseball rehabilitation program. American Journal of Sports Medicine 19(3):264–272

Tullos H S, Bennett J B 1984 The shoulder in sports. In Scott W N, Nisconson B, Nicholas J A (eds) Principles of sports medicine. Williams and Wilkins, Baltimore

Turkel S J, Panio M W, Marshall J L et al 1981 Stabilizing mechanisms preventing anterior dislocation of the glenohumeral joint. Journal of Bone and Joint Surgery (Am) 63A:1208–1217

Uhthoff H K, Sano H 1997 Pathology of failure of the rotator cuff tendon. Orthopedic Clinics of North America 28:31–41

Vicenzino B, Buratowski S, Wright A 2000 A preliminary study of the initial hypoalgesic effect of a mobilisation with movement treatment for lateral epicondylalgia. In: Singer K (ed) Proceedings, 7th Scientific Conference of the International Federation of Orthopaedic Manipulative Therapists, Perth, p 460–464

Voss D E, Knott M, Kabat M 1953 Application of neuromuscular facilitation in the treatment of shoulder disabilities. Physical Therapy Review 33:536

Wadsworth D J S, Bullock-Saxton J E 1997 Recruitment patterns of the scapular rotator muscles in freestyle swimmers with subacromial impingement. International Journal of Sports Medicine 18:618–624

Walch G 1996 Posterosuperior glenoid impingement. In: Burkhead W Z (ed) Rotator cuff disorders. Baltimore, Williams and Wilkins, ch 14, p 193–198

Walch G, Liotard J P, Noel E 1992a Postero-superior impingement: another shoulder impingement. Journal of Orthopaedic Surgery 6:78–81

Walch G, Boileau P, Noel E et al 1992b Impingement of the deep surface of the supraspinatus tendon on the posterosuperior glenoid rim: an arthroscopic study. Journal of Shoulder and Elbow Surgery 1:238–245

Warner J J P, Caborn D N 1992 Overview of shoulder instability. Critical Reviews in Physical and Rehabilitation Medicine 4(3,4):145–198

Warner J J P, McMahon P J 1994 Abnormal shoulder kinematics following isolated rupture of the long head of biceps brachii muscle. Paper read to the Seventh Congress of the European Society for Surgery of the Shoulder and Elbow, Aarhus, Denmark, 10–12 June, 1993, Journal of Shoulder and Elbow Surgery 3:1 (Part 2) S31

Warner J J P, Boardman N D 1999 Anatomy, biomechanics and pathophysiology of glenohumeral instability. In: Warren R F, Craig E V, Altcheck D W (eds) The unstable shoulder. Lippincott-Raven, Philadelphia, ch 2, p 51–76

Warner J J P, Micheli L J, Arslanian L E et al 1990 Patterns of flexibility, laxity, and strength in normal shoulders and shoulder with instability and impingement. American Journal of Sports Medicine 18:366–375

Warner J J P, Deng X H, Warren R F et al 1992 Static capsuloligamentous restraints to superior-inferior translation of the glenohumeral joint. American Journal of Sports Medicine 20:675–685

Warner J J P, Caborn D N M, Berger R et al 1993a Dynamic capsuloligamentous anatomy of the glenohumeral joint. Journal of Shoulder and Elbow Surgery 2(3):115–133

Warner J J P, Deng Z, Warren R F et al 1993b Superoinferior translation in the intact and vented glenohumeral joint. Journal of Shoulder and Elbow Surgery 2(2):99–105

Warner J J P, Higgins L, Parsons I M et al 2001 Diagnosis and treatment of anterosuperior rotator cuff tears. Journal of Shoulder and Elbow Surgery 10:37–46

Warren R F, Kornblatt I B, Marchard R 1984 Static factors affecting posterior shoulder stability. Orthopaedic Transactions 8:89

Warren R F, Craig E V, Altcheck D W (eds) 1999 The unstable shoulder. Lippincott-Raven, Philadelphia

Wilk K E 1994 Current concepts in the rehabilitation of athletic shoulder injuries. In: Andrews J R, Wilk K E (eds) The athlete's shoulder. Churchill Livingstone, New York, ch 30, p 335–354

Wilk K E 1999 Rehabilitation after shoulder stabilisation surgery. In: Warren R F, Craig E V, Altcheck D W (eds) The unstable shoulder. Lippincott-Raven, Philadelphia, ch. 24, p 367–402

Wilk K E, Arrigo C A 1994 Isokinetic exercise and testing for the shoulder. In: Andrews J R, Wilk K E (eds) The athlete's shoulder. Churchill Livingstone, New York, ch 44, p 543–566

Wilk K E, Voight M L 1994 Plyometrics for the shoulder complex. In: Andrews J R, Wilk K E (eds) The athlete's shoulder. Churchill Livingstone, New York, ch 44, p 543–566

Wilk K E, Andrews J R, Arrigo C A 1995 The abductor and adductor strength characteristics of professional baseball pitchers. American Journal of Sports Medicine 23(3):307–311

Wilk K E, Arrigo C A, Andrews J R 1997 Current concepts: the stabilizing structures of the glenohumeral joint. Journal of Orthopaedic and Sports Physical Therapy 25(6):355–376

Winstein C J 1991 Designing practice for motor learning: clinical implications. Contemporary management of motor control problems. Proceedings of the II Step Conference, Alexandria, VA: APTA

Wirth M A, Rockwood C A 1993 Traumatic glenohumeral instability: pathology and pathogenesis. In Matsen F A, Fu F H, Hawkins R J (eds) The shoulder: a balance of mobility and stability. American

Academy of Orthopaedic Surgeons, Rosemont, Illinois, ch 17, p 279–304

Woo S, Maynard J, Butler D et al 1988 Ligaments, tendon and joint capsule insertions to bone. In Woo S L Y and Buckwalter J A (eds) Injury and repair of the musculoskeletal soft tissues. American Academy of Orthopaedic Surgeons, Park Ridge, Illinois, p 133–166

World Health Organization (WHO) 1980 International classification of impairments, disabilities and handicaps. Geneva, Switzerland

Wright A 1995 Hypoalgesia post-manipulative therapy: a review of a ptoential neurophysiological mechanism. Manual Therapy 1(1):11–16

Yamaguchi K, Flatow E L 1995 Management of multidirectional instability. Clinics in Sports Medicine 14(4):885–902

Yoneda M, Hirooka A, Saito S et al 1991 Arthroscopic stapling for detached superior glenoid labrum. Journal of Bone and Joint Surgery (Br) 73B(5):746–750

Zaslav K R 2001 Internal rotation resistance strength test: a new diagnostic test to differentiate intra-articular pathology from outlet (Neer) impingement syndrome in the shoulder. Journal of Shoulder and Elbow Surgery 10(1):23–27

Zemek M J, Magee D J 1996 Comparison of glenohumeal joint laxity in elite and recreational swimmers. Clinical Journal of Sports Medicine 6:40–47

16

Elbow

Michael M Reinold   Kevin E Wilk

INTRODUCTION

Injuries to the elbow joint complex occur frequently in the athletic population. Rehabilitation following these injuries is often challenging to the clinician due to the significant amount of stress applied to the unique anatomy of the elbow joint during sport-specific movements. Mechanisms of injuries include repetitive microtraumatic forces from overuse, as well as macrotraumatic overload of excessive forces (Wilk et al 1993a, Wilk & Levinson 2001). Athletes experience sport-specific injury patterns based on the unique demands involved with each particular sport. Overhead athletes such as throwers and tennis players typically present with injuries caused by chronic stress overload or repetitive traumatic stress (Fleisig & Barrentine 1995). Conversely, athletes participating in contact sports such as football, ice hockey, wrestling, gymnastics and soccer are more susceptible to traumatic injuries including fractures and dislocations due to the aggressive nature of each sport.

Rehabilitation of the elbow joint requires a thorough knowledge of the anatomical, biomechanical, and pathomechanical factors associated with athletic participation. The purpose of this chapter is to overview the anatomy and biomechanics of the elbow joint during sports, followed by a detailed description of common clinical examination techniques for the injured athlete. Several non-operative and postoperative rehabilitation programs will be discussed for specific sport injuries utilizing a multiphased, progressive rehabilitation approach based on current scientific research and clinical experience. The ultimate goal of rehabilitation is to gradually restore function and return the athlete to competition as quickly and safely as possible.

ANATOMY

Sport-specific applied anatomy of the elbow joint complex can be broken down into osseous, capsulo-ligamentous, musculotendinous, and neurological structures.

OSSEOUS STRUCTURES

The elbow joint complex includes the humerus, radius, and ulna, articulating to form the humeroulnar, humeroradial, proximal radioulnar, and distal radioulnar joints.

The humeroulnar joint is generally considered a uniaxial, diarthrodial joint with one degree of freedom allowing flexion and extension in the sagittal plane around a coronal axis. Morrey (1985) described the humeroulnar joint as a modified hinge joint due to the small amounts of internal and external rotation that occur at extreme ranges of flexion and extension. The anterior aspect of the distal humerus contains the convex trochlea, an hourglass shaped surface covered with articular cartilage. The trochlear groove is located centrally within the trochlea and runs obliquely in the anterior–posterior direction. The distal end of the humerus exhibits 30° of anterior rotation with respect to the long axis of the humerus. A corresponding version is seen at the proximal ulna with 30° of posterior rotation in respect to the shaft of the ulnar. This anatomical rotation of the humerus and ulna allow for excessive elbow flexion from 145° to 150° and enhances static stability when the elbow is in full extension (Lehmkuhl & Smith 1983).

The proximal ulna contains a centrally located ridge that runs between two bony prominences, the coronoid process anteriorly and the olecranon posteriorly. Two fossae are located on each side of the corresponding articular surfaces of the humerus. Anteriorly, the coronoid fossa articulates with the coronoid process of the ulna during flexion. Posteriorly, the olecranon fossa receives the olecranon process of the ulna, serving to limit extension. The congruency achieved by these articulations makes the humeroulnar joint one of the most stable joints in the human body (Morrey & An 1983).

Also of significance to the humeroulnar joint is the medial epicondyle of the humerus. Located proximal and medial to the trochlea, the medial epicondyle serves as the attachment site of the flexor-pronator muscle group and the ulnar collateral ligament (UCL). Hoppenfeld (1976) states that the size and prominence of the medial epicondyle provides an important mechanical advantage for the medial stabilizing structures of the elbow joint. The cubital tunnel is located posterior to the medial epicondyle and serves to protect the ulnar nerve as it transverses distally.

The humeroradial joint is similarly a diarthrodial, uniaxial joint allowing elbow flexion and extension with the humeroulnar joint. In addition, the humeroradial joint pivots around a longitudinal axis to allow rotation movements in association with the proximal radioulnar joint, thus making the joint a combination hinge and pivot joint (Norkin & Levangie 1985).

The articular surfaces of the humeroradial joint include the concave radial head and the spherical convex capitulum on the distal aspect of the humerus (Kapandji 1970). The capitulum and trochlea are separated by a groove within the humerus, the capitulotrochlear groove. This groove guides the radial head as the elbow moves in flexion and extension.

Immediately proximal to the capitellum on the anterior aspect of the humerus is the radial fossa. The radial fossa receives the anterior aspect of the radial head in the maximally flexed elbow position. The lateral epicondyle lies laterally to the radial fossa and serves as an attachment site of the wrist extensor muscle group. The radial tuberosity is located on the radius just distally to the radial head. This area serves as the attachment site for the biceps brachii tendon.

The proximal and distal radioulnar joints are intricately related, together allowing for one degree of freedom in the transverse plane around a longitudinal axis. These two joints allow forearm supination and pronation. During supination and pronation, the head of the radius rotates within a ring formed by the annular ligament and radial notch of the ulna. Little motion occurs in the ulna. The radius and ulna lie parallel to each other while in the supinated position. As the forearm rotates into pronation, the radius crosses over the ulna. The radius and ulna are also connected midway between the two bony shafts by an interosseous membrane, which serves as an additional attachment site for the forearm musculature.

The bony articulation of the elbow joint forms the carrying angle of the elbow. This is defined as the angle formed by the long axis of the humerus and the ulna and results in the abducted position of the forearm in relation to the humerus. This angle is measured in the frontal plane with the elbow extended and averages 11–14° in males and 13–16° in women (Atkinson & Elftman 1945, Keats et al 1966). The carrying angle changes linearly as the elbow joint is flexed and extended, diminishing in flexion and increasing with extension (Morrey 1985).

CAPSULOLIGAMENTOUS STRUCTURES

The joint capsule is a relatively thin but significantly strong structure. The anterior capsule is normally a thin transparent structure that allows visualization of the bony prominence when the elbow is fully extended. The anterior capsule inserts proximally above the coronoid and radial fossa. Distally, the capsule attaches to the anterior margin of the coronoid medially and into the annular ligament laterally. Posteriorly, the capsule attaches just above the olecranon fossa and distally along the medial and lateral margins of the trochlea. The capsule exhibits significant strength from the transverse and obliquely directed fibrous bands. The anterior capsule is taut into extension and lax with elbow flexion. The greatest capacity occurs at approximately 80° of flexion (Johansson 1962). The synovial membrane lines the joint capsule and is attached anteriorly above the radial and coronoid fossa to the medial and lateral margins of the articular surface, and posteriorly to the superior margin of the olecranon fossa.

The ligaments of the elbow consist of thickened parts of the medial and lateral capsules. The UCL is located on the medial aspect of the elbow. This ligamentous complex can be divided into three distinct portions, the anterior, posterior and transverse bundles. The anterior bundle originates from the inferior surface of the medial epicondyle and inserts at the medial aspect of the coronoid process. Due to the posterior orientation of the ligament in relation to the center of rotation, the anterior bundle is taut throughout the range of motion. The anterior bundle can be further divided into two bands: the anterior band, which is taut in extension, and the posterior band, which tightens in flexion (Schwab et al 1980, Morrey et al 1985). The anterior bundle of the UCL is the main ligamentous support to valgus strain at the elbow.

The transverse bundle of the UCL originates from the medial olecranon and inserts into the coronoid process. The posterior bundle originates from the medial epicondyle posteroinferiorly and fans out to attach onto the posteromedial aspect of the olecranon. Several authors report that these two bundles provide minimal amounts of medial elbow stability (Morrey & An 1983, Morrey et al 1985, Schwab et al 1980).

Laterally, the ligamentous complex helps stabilize against varus stress and is made up of several components including the radial collateral ligament, the annular ligament, the accessory lateral collateral ligament, and the lateral ulnar collateral ligament (Morrey & An 1983).

The radial collateral ligament (RCL) is not as well defined as the UCL. Originating from the lateral epicondyle, the RCL fans out and inserts into the annular ligament. The RCL origin is in line with the axis of joint rotation, allowing little change in length as the elbow moves through full range of motion.

The annular ligament is a strong fibro-osseous ring that encircles and stabilizes the radial head in the radial notch of the ulna. Its origin and insertion occur along the anterior and posterior radial notch of the ulna. The anterior portion of this ligament becomes taut with

Table 16.1 Contributing forces to displacement of the elbow (modified from Morrey & An 1983)

Elbow position	Stabilizing structure	Distraction (%)	Varus (%)	Valgus (%)
Elbow Extended (0°)	UCL	6	–	31
	LCL	5	14	–
	Capsule	85	32	38
	Articulation	–	55	31
Elbow flexed (90°)	UCL	78	–	54
	LCL	10	9	–
	Capsule	8	13	10
	Articulation	–	75	33

supination while the posterior portion becomes taut with pronation (Spinner & Kaplan 1970).

The accessory lateral collateral ligament (ALCL) originates from the inferior margin of the annular ligament and inserts discretely into the tubercle of the supinator crest of the ulna. The ALCL further assists the annular ligament in varus stabilization (Martin 1958).

The lateral ulnar collateral ligament (LUCL) originates from the lateral epicondyle and inserts into the tubercle of the crest of the supinator. This ligament provides posterolateral stability of the humeroulnar joint (O'Driscoll et al 1991).

The elbow joint is one of the most congruent joints in the human body and is thus one of the most stable (Morrey & An 1983). Stability is provided by the interaction of soft tissue and articular constraints. The static soft tissue stabilizers include the capsular and ligamentous structures. Table 16.1 summarizes the influence of the ligamentous and articular components of the elbow joint (Morrey & An 1983). When the elbow is in full extension, the anterior capsule provides approximately 70% of the restrain to distraction, whereas the UCL provides approximately 78% of the distraction at 90° of elbow flexion. The restraint to valgus displacement varies significantly depending on the elbow flexion angle. When the elbow is in full extension, the capsule provides 38% of the restraint, the UCL provides 31%, and the articulation provides the remaining 31%. Conversely, at 90° of flexion, the primary restraint is the UCL, which provides 54% of the restraint, followed by the osseous articulation, which provides 33%, and the capsule, which provides 13%. Varus stress is controlled in extensions by the joint articulation (54%), RCL (14%), and joint capsule (32%). As the elbow flexes, the RCL and capsule contribute 9% and 13%, respectively, while the joint articulation provides 75% of the stabilizing force (Morrey & An 1983).

MUSCULOTENDINOUS STRUCTURES

The elbow joint musculature can be divided into six groups based on the functions of each muscle. These groups include the elbow flexors, extensors, flexor pronators, extensor supinators, primary pronators and primary supinators.

The three primary flexor muscles of the elbow include the biceps brachii, the brachioradialis, and the brachialis. The biceps brachii typically consists of a long head and a short head. The long head of the biceps brachii originates on the superior glenoid and attaches directly to the glenoid labrum. The long head passes directly through the glenohumeral joint capsule and through the intertubercular groove of the humerus until it joins with the short head of the biceps brachii. The short head of the biceps originates from the coracoid process of the scapula. The two heads of the biceps brachii join to form a common attachment onto the posterior portion of the radial tuberosity and via the bicipital aponeurosis, which attaches to the anterior capsule of the elbow joint. The biceps is responsible for the vast majority of elbow flexion strength when the forearm is supinated and generates its highest torque values when the elbow is flexed between 80–100° (Norkin & Levangie 1985). The biceps also acts secondarily as a supinator of the forearm, principally when the elbow is in a flexed position.

The brachialis muscle originates from the lower half of the anterior surface of the humerus. The brachialis muscle extends distally to cross the anterior aspect of the elbow joint and inserts into the ulnar tuberosity and coronoid process. The brachialis muscle is active in flexing the elbow in all positions of the forearm (Basmajian & DeLuca 1985).

The brachioradialis muscle originates from the proximal two thirds of the lateral supracondylar ridge of the humerus and along the lateral intermuscular septum distal to the spiral groove. The brachioradialis muscles insert into the lateral aspect of the base of the styloid process of the radius. The brachioradialis muscle inserts distant from the joint axis; therefore, exhibiting a significant mechanical advantage as an elbow flexor (Norkin & Levangie 1985).

The triceps brachii and the anconeus muscles serve as the primary extensors of the elbow. The triceps brachii is a large three-headed (long, lateral, and medial) muscle that comprises almost the entire posterior brachium. The long head of the triceps originates from the infraglenoid tubercle, crossing the shoulder joint. The other two heads, the lateral and medial heads, originate from the posterior and lateral aspects of the humerus. At the distal portion of the humerus, the three heads converge to form a common muscle that inserts into the posterior surface of the olecranon.

The small anconeus muscle originates from a broad area on the posterior aspect of the lateral epicondyle and inserts into the olecranon. The anconeus muscle covers the lateral portion of the annular ligament, the radial head, and the posterior surface of the proximal ulna. Electromyographic (EMG) activity of the anconeus muscle during the early phases of elbow extension has been noted, and this muscle appears to have a stabilizing role during pronation and supination movements (Pavly et al 1967).

The flexor pronator muscles include the pronator teres, flexor carpi radialis, palmaris longus, flexor carpi ulnaris, and flexor digitorum superficialis. All these muscles originate completely or in part from the medial epicondyle, and all serve secondary roles as elbow flexors. Their primary roles are associated with the wrist and hand. This muscle group may provide a limited amount of dynamic stability to the medial aspect of the elbow against valgus stress (Jobe et al 1984).

The extensor supinator muscles include the brachioradialis, extensor carpi radialis brevis and longus, supinator, extensor digitorum, extensor carpi ulnaris, and extensor digiti minimi muscles. Each muscle originates near or directly from the lateral epicondyle of the humerus. The primary functions of the extensor supinator muscles involve the wrist and hand and provide dynamic support over the lateral aspect of the elbow. This muscle group, as well as the flexor pronator musculature, is susceptible to various overuse muscle strains.

The pronator quadratus and pronator teres muscles act on the radioulnar joints to produce pronation. The pronator quadratus originates from the anterior surface of the lower ulna. Insertion occurs at the distal and lateral border of the radius. The pronator quadratus acts as a significant pronator in all positions of the elbow and forearm.

The pronator teres, which possesses humeral and ulnar heads, originates from the medial epicondyle and coronoid process of the ulna. The two heads join together and insert along the middle of the lateral surface of the radius. The pronator teres is a strong pronator muscle that generates its highest contractile force during rapid or resisted pronation (Soderberg 1981). However, the pronator teres' contribution to pronation strength diminishes when the elbow is positioned in full extension (Norkin & Levangie 1985). The flexor carpi radialis and brachioradialis also act as secondary pronators.

The biceps brachii and the supinator muscles are the primary supinators of the forearm, while the brachioradialis also acts as an accessory supinator. The supinator muscle originates from three separate locations: the lateral epicondyle, the proximal anterior crest and depression of the ulnar distal to the radial notch, and the radial collateral and annular ligaments. The supinator muscle then winds around the radius to insert into the dorsal and lateral surfaces of the proximal radius. The supinator is the primary supinator of the forearm but appears to be generally weaker than the biceps (Morrey 1985). The supinator acts alone with unresisted slow supination in all elbow and forearm positions and with unresisted fast supination with the elbow extended (Kapandji 1970). The effectiveness of the supinator is not altered by elbow position; however, elbow position does significantly affect the biceps. The supinator originates at the radial collateral and annular ligaments, suggesting that the muscle may also act as a supportive or stabilizing muscle to the lateral aspect of the elbow.

NEUROLOGICAL STRUCTURES

The four nerves that play significant roles in normal elbow function and pathologies are the median, ulnar, radial, and musculocutaneous nerves. Box 16.1 shows the effect of injury to specific peripheral nerves.

The median nerve arises from branches of the lateral and medial cords of the brachial plexus. Nerve root levels include C5 to C8 and T1. This nerve proceeds distally over the anterior brachium, continuing to the medial aspect of the antecubital fossa. From the fossa, the nerve continues its course under the bicipital aponeurosis and passes most often between the two heads of the pronator teres. The median nerve can be compressed between the two heads of the pronator teres or by the bicipital aponeurosis, resulting in either pronator syndrome or anterior interosseous syndrome. Although relatively uncommon, highly repetitive and strenuous pronation movements of the forearm can also lead to entrapment of the median nerve (Magee 1987).

The ulnar nerve emanates from the C8 and T1 levels and descends into the proximal aspect of the upper extremity from the medial cord of the brachial plexus. The ulnar nerve passes from the anterior to posterior compartments of the brachium through the arcade of Struthers. This arcade represents a fascial bridging between the medial head of the triceps and medial intermuscular septum. The nerve continues distally, passing behind the medial epicondyle and through the cubital tunnel. At the cubital tunnel, bony anatomy provides little protection for the nerve. Ulnar nerve injury, which can occur by compression or stretching, takes place most frequently in the cubital tunnel. The cubital tunnel retinaculum flattens with elbow flexion, thus decreasing the capacity of the cubital tunnel. This can be noted clinically as stimulating nerve symptoms when osteophytes are present on the ulna or medial epicondyle (St John & Palmaz 1986). Injury to the medial capsular ligaments can result in increased traction forces against the medial elbow, resulting in a change in length of the ulnar nerve. This change in length may result in neuropathy or ulnar nerve subluxation. The nerve enters the forearm by passing between the two heads of the

flexor carpi ulnaris and continues distally between the flexor digitorum profundus and the flexor carpi ulnaris.

The radial nerve originates from the posterior cord of the brachial plexus and derives its nerve supply from the C6, C7, and C8 levels with variable contributions from

---

Box 16.1   The effects of injury to specific peripheral nerves

Musculocutaneous nerve (C5, C6, C6)
Sensory supply
Lateral half of the anterior surface of the forearm from the elbow to the thenar eminence

Effect of injury
- Severe weakness of elbow flexion
- Weakness of supination
- Loss of biceps deep tendon reflex
- Loss of sensation, cutaneous distribution

Radial nerve (C5, C6, C7, C8, T1)
Sensory supply
Back of arm, forearm, wrist, radial half of the dorsum of the hand, back of thumb, index finger, and part of the middle finger

Effect of injury
- Loss of triceps deep tendon reflex
- Weakness of elbow flexion
- Loss of supination (when elbow is extended)
- Loss of wrist extension
- Weakness of ulnar and radial deviation
- Loss of extension at the MCP joints
- Loss of extension and abduction of the thumb

Median nerve (C5, C6, C7, C8, T1)
Sensory supply
Radial half of the palm, palmar surface of the thumb, index, middle, and radial half of the ring finger, and dorsal surface of the same fingers

Effect of injury
- Loss of complete pronation (brachioradialis can bring the forearm to midpronation but not beyond)
- Weakness with flexion and radial deviation (ulnar deviation with wrist flexion)
- Loss of flexion at MCP joints
- Loss of thumb opposition or abduction, loss of flexion at IP and MCP joints

Ulnar nerve (C7, C8, T1)
Sensory supply
Dorsal and palmar surfaces of the ulnar side of the hand, including the little finger, and ulnar half of the ring finger

Effect of injury
- Weakness of wrist flexion and ulnar deviation (radial deviation with wrist flexion)
- Loss of flexion of DIP joints of ring and little fingers
- Inability to abduct or adduct fingers
- Inability to adduct thumb
- Loss of flexion of fingers, especially ring and little fingers at the MCP joints
- Loss of extension of fingers, especially ring and little fingers at the IP joint

IP – interphalangeal; MCP – metacarpophalangeal; DIP – distal interphalangeal

the C5 and T1 levels. At the midpoint of the brachium, the radial nerve descends laterally through the radial groove of the humerus and continues in a path lateral and distal. The nerve descends anteriorly behind the brachioradialis and brachialis muscles, and at the level of the joint, the nerve divides into the posterior interosseous and superficial radial branches.

The musculocutaneous nerve originates from the lateral cord of the brachial plexus at nerve root levels C5 to C7. The nerve passes between the biceps and brachialis muscles to pierce the brachial fascia lateral to the biceps tendon. The nerve continues distally and terminates as the lateral antebrachial cutaneous nerve, which provides sensation over the anterolateral aspect of the forearm. Compression between the biceps tendon and the brachialis fascia can cause entrapment of the musculocutaneous nerve.

Sensory nerves innervate the elbow cutaneously and are derived from specific nerve root levels. The lateral arm is innervated by branches of the axillary nerve of the C5 root level while the lateral forearm is innervated by the musculocutaneous nerve of the C6 root level (Andrews et al 1993). The medial arm is innervated by the brachial cutaneous nerve from the T1 nerve root level. The medial forearm is innervated by branches of the antebrachial cutaneous nerve from the C8 root level (Andrews et al 1993). The T2 dermatome extends from the axilla to the posteromedial elbow (Magee 1987). Variability exists regarding the extent of each nerve root innervation; overlap between dermatome distribution occurs.

ELBOW BIOMECHANICS IN SPORT

Injuries to the elbow may occur in many different sports. The repetitive motions required for competition in many athletic events result in several common elbow injuries. These injuries are most often related to the tremendous amounts of force applied to the elbow joint during these sport-specific motions. The following section discusses the biomechanics and pathomechanics of the elbow during three sports that commonly produce elbow injuries: baseball pitching, tennis, and golf.

BIOMECHANICS OF BASEBALL PITCHING

The biomechanics of the elbow during overhead baseball pitching can be broken down into six phases: windup, stride, arm cocking, arm acceleration, arm deceleration, and follow through.

During the windup and stride, minimal elbow kinetics and muscle activity are present. As the foot contacts the ground, the elbow is flexed to approximately 85° (Werner et al 1993).

The arm cocking phase begins as the foot comes into contact with the ground and continues until the point of maximum shoulder external rotation. As the arm moves into external rotation, a varus torque is produced at the elbow to prevent valgus stress (Werner et al 1993). Shortly before maximum external rotation, the elbow is flexed to 95° and a varus torque of approximately 64 Nm is produced (Fleisig & Barrentine 1995). At this critical instant, excessive valgus strain may cause injury to the medial stabilizing structures of the elbow, particularly the UCL. As previously discussed, Morrey & An (1983) report that at this moment, the UCL is contributing approximately 54% of the valgus strain. Assuming that the UCL produces 54% of the 64 Nm of valgus strain observed during the arm cocking phase, 35 Nm would be applied to the UCL approaching the maximum capacity of load before failure in the UCL (Fleisig et al 1995, Fleisig & Barrentine 1995).

Also, as the elbow joint sustains a valgus strain, lateral compression is applied, possibly leading to compressive injuries of the lateral compartment of the elbow as the radial head and humeral capitellum are approximated. This compression may lead to avascular necrosis, osteochondritis dissecans, or osteochondral chip fractures.

As the arm accelerates from maximal external rotation to ball release, the elbow extends at approximately 2500°/s (Fleisig & Barrentine 1995). As the elbow extends and resists valgus strain simultaneously, the olecranon can impinge against the medial aspect of the trochlear groove and olecranon fossa (Fleisig & Barrentine 1995). This impingement may lead to posteromedial osteophyte formation and loose body formations. This has been described by Wilson et al (1983) as valgus extension overload.

As the arm decelerates and continues into the follow-through phase, eccentric contraction of the elbow flexors must control the distractive forces at the elbow joint. Moderate activity of the biceps brachii and brachioradialis has been reported (Werner et al 1993). Muscular activity of the elbow flexors may assist in the prevention of olecranon impingement as the elbow is rapidly extended. The elbow remains in a flexed position of approximately 20° as the arm continues into follow through. Minimal kinetic and muscular activity is present during this final phase.

BIOMECHANICS OF THE ELBOW DURING TENNIS

The kinematic and kinetic data during tennis varies dependent on the type of stroke, and the biomechanics of the serve and groundstrokes will be discussed separately.

The overhead serve has been compared to the mechanics of overhead throwing (Fleisig & Barrentine 1995). The elbow has been reported to extend at 982°/s and pronate at 347°/s during acceleration and deceleration phases of the tennis serve (Kibler 1994). Morris et al (1989) report high activity of the triceps and pronator teres during the tennis serve in order to produce significant racket velocity. Because of this excessive angular velocity, the eccentric contraction of the elbow flexors and supinators is critical for the prevention of injuries to the elbow.

During groundstrokes, in both the forehand and the backhand, the wrist extensors are predominantly active as the athlete prepares the racket for impact (Morris et al 1989). The extensor carpi radialis longus, brevis, and extensor communis musculature are active during both strokes, with the forehand showing additional muscle activity of the biceps brachii and brachioradialis (Kelley et al 1994, Morris et al 1989, Rhu et al 1988). As the racket comes into contact with the ball and begins the follow through, continued activity of the extensor carpi radialis brevis is noted, while the backhand produces additional activity of the biceps brachii as the elbow decelerates into extension (Kelley et al 1994, Morris et al 1989, Rhu et al 1988).

Kelley et al (1994) compared the muscular activity of the elbow during the backhand stroke in subjects with and without lateral epicondylitis. Results indicated that the group of subjects exhibiting lateral epicondylitis showed a significant increase in EMG activity of the extensor carpi radialis longus and brevis, pronator teres, and flexor carpi radialis. These retrospective findings may have an impact in explaining the etiology of lateral epicondylitis.

BIOMECHANICS OF THE GOLF SWING

The biomechanics of the golf swing pertaining to elbow and wrist injuries can be broken down into five phases: the backswing, transition, downswing, impact, and follow through. As the athlete swings the club, the lead arm and back arm are susceptible to injuries at various moments of the swing.

The backswing phase produces few injuries to the elbow. As the backswing progresses, the lead wrist pronates, flexes, and radially deviates. The back arm flexes at the elbow and the wrist supinates, extends, and radially deviates. The wrist flexors exhibit minimal EMG activity, whereas the wrist extensors exhibit 33% of a maximum voluntary isometric contraction (MVIC) (Glazebrook et al 1994). As the clubhead approaches the top of the backswing, the musculature of the elbow must eccentrically contract to control the clubhead and transition from the backswing to the downswing. This motion places a great deal of stress on the stretched flexor pronator mass of the back arm (Stanish et al 1994).

As the downswing progresses, the wrists must uncoil to produce clubhead speed. The wrist and elbow uncoil to return to the neutral position initially observed at setup to prepare for impact. The downswing is characterized by increased muscle activity of both the wrist extensors, which exhibit 45% MVIC, and the wrist flexors, which exhibit 35% MVIC. During impact, the wrist and hands decelerate due to the force of impact (Glazebrook et al 1994). McCarroll & Gioe (1982) report that more than twice as many injuries occur during the downswing compared to the backswing, as the elbow and wrist move approximately three times as fast during this phase. This deceleration of force places a great deal of strain on the forearm musculature as it attempts to maintain control of the club (Stanish et al 1994). The majority of elbow injuries take place during impact as the lateral epicondyle of the lead arm and the medial epicondyle of the backarm are placed under significant strain. The lead elbow extensor mass has been reported to be under even greater stress at impact due to the compressive force from ball impact and divots (McCarroll 1985) At ball contact, the wrist flexor activity significantly increases to 91% MVIC. Additionally, the wrist extensors exhibit EMG activity of approximately 58% MVIC (Glazebrook et al 1994).

Following impact, the arm continues into the follow through. Minimal injuries occur during this phase. The wrist and hands follow the pattern of the backswing in reverse; the lead arm flexes at the elbow, supinates, extends and radially deviates while the back arm pronates, flexes, and radially deviates at the wrist. During the follow through, the wrist extensors EMG activity is approximately 60 to 70% MVIC. The repetitive nature of elbow and wrist motion observed may be responsible for overuse injuries to the forearm musculature.

When comparing the muscular activity patterns of golfers with medial epicondylitis and golfers without injuries, the golfers with medial epicondylitis exhibit significantly greater wrist flexor muscle activity during the backswing, transition, and downswing (Glazebrook et al 1994).

CLINICAL EXAMINATION

The clinical examination of the athletic elbow relies on a complete and thorough history, extensive knowledge of the anatomy and biomechanics of the joint, and a well organized physical examination. The goal of the examination is to identify the areas of dysfunction and determine an appropriate course of rehabilitation.

HISTORY

Before the examination begins, a complete and thorough history is imperative. The location, intensity, and duration of pain should be clearly identified. The date and mechanism of injury should be explained thoroughly, as this will assist in determining involved structures. Other subjective reports such as aggravating factors, previous injuries, and primary complaints should be recorded to assist in the assessment and development of patient specific treatment and goals.

OBSERVATION

For a thorough inspection, the patient should completely expose the trunk and arms to provide a full view of the neck, shoulder, and elbow. The skin should be evaluated for areas of contusion, ecchymosis, swelling, burns, surgical scars, redness, blanching, petechiae, and venous congestion. The carrying angle should also be assessed during this portion of the examination.

PALPATION

The palpation of the elbow begins with the identification of specific bony landmarks. The clinician should palpate each to determine if tenderness or deformity exists.

The medial epicondyle may exhibit tenderness for various reasons including epicondylitis, muscle strains and UCL injury. The medial supracondylar ridge should be examined for osteophytes, which may be entrapping the median nerve. The olecranon is easily palpated and is covered by the insertion of the triceps and the olecranon bursa, both of which may be tender if pathological. Osseous changes on the posteromedial olecranon may be associated with valgus extension overload in overhead athletes. The ulnar border should also be palpated for stress fractures, which are sometimes present in the throwing population. The lateral epicondyle is often irritable when palpated in the presence of epicondylitis. Lastly, the radial nerve lies approximately 2 cm distally from the lateral epicondyle and should be palpated during passive supination and pronation.

When palpating the soft tissues of the elbow, it is helpful to divide the elbow into four distinct regions: the medial, posterior, lateral, and anterior aspects. The major structures of the medial aspect of the elbow include the ulnar nerve, flexor pronator muscle group, the UCL, and the supracondylar lymph nodes. The clinician should determine if the ulnar nerve is capable of dislocating from the bony sulcus. This is done by abduction, externally rotating the shoulder with the patient supine, while the elbow is flexed to 20–70° (Andrews et al 1993). The medial epicondyle is palpated to determine tenderness to the flexor pronator muscle mass or the UCL.

The posterior elbow contains the olecranon, which should be palpated for inflammation of a swollen bursa. The triceps insertion points should also be palpated for tenderness.

Laterally, the wrist extensor group is palpated. The brachioradialis is made prominent by having the patient close their fist, place the forearm in a neutral position, and resist elbow flexion. Resisted wrist flexion allows for easy palpation of the extensor carpi radialis longus and brevis.

The anterior structures of the elbow pass through the cubital fossa. These structures from medial to lateral are the median nerve, brachial artery, and the biceps tendon. The biceps can be made prominent by resistance in elbow flexion.

RANGE OF MOTION

The normal range of motion (ROM) of the elbow is 0° of extension, 140–150° of flexion, 80° of pronation, and 80° of supination (Norkin & White 1995). Passive ROM is assessed in each direction and compared to the contralateral elbow.

In addition, the end feel of movement should be assessed. Normal end feels of the elbow are different for each movement; elbow extension exhibits a bony end feel, flexion a soft tissue approximation, and forearm pronation and supination a capsular end feel (Cyriax 1982).

MUSCLE TESTING

Muscle testing of the elbow musculature begins with the patient seated (Kendall & McCreary 1983). The brachialis is tested with the elbow flexed and forearm pronated. The biceps is tested with the forearm supinated and shoulder flexed to 45–50°. The brachioradialis is tested with the elbow flexed with neutral wrist rotation. Triceps extension is performed with the shoulder flexed to 90° and elbow flexed 45–90°. Pronation and supination of the elbow is performed with the arm by the side and elbow flexed to 90° and neutral wrist rotation. Resistance is applied at the distal forearm as the patient attempts to rotate in either direction. Wrist extension and flexion are performed with the elbow flexed to 30° and with the elbow fully extended. Isokinetic testing may also be applied to determine specific objective data of muscular strength.

SPECIAL TESTS

Special tests for the elbow joint are used to elicit specific signs or symptoms of pathologies. Laxity assessment is used to evaluate the integrity of the medial and lateral stabilizing structures. Varus and valgus testing may be performed by stabilizing the arm with one hand and applying a fulcrum at the elbow joint with the other. The examiner imparts a varus or valgus stress and notes the amount of gapping and the end-feel motion. The tests are compared bilaterally and may be performed at 0° of extension and at 30° of flexion. Pain, excessive gapping, or a soft end feel may all indicate pathology to the stabilizing structures.

The clinical test for valgus extension overload involves the examiner grasping the elbow in a flexed position. As the examiner forces the elbow into extension, a valgus stress is simultaneously applied to the elbow. The examiner palpates the posteromedial joint for tenderness and/or crepitation. Pain over the posteromedial olecranon process signifies a positive test (Wilson et al 1983).

A lateral pivot shift test is used to assess posterolateral rotatory instability (O'Driscoll et al 1991). Patients that have sustained an elbow dislocation often report a posterolateral rotatory mechanism of injury that is replicated during this test. The patient is supine and the examiner holds the arm over the head with 90° of shoulder flexion and maximal external rotation. The examiner applies a valgus and supination moment while flexing the elbow, resulting in the semilunar notch of the ulna displacing from the trochlea of the humerus; maximal displacement occurs at approximately 40° (O'Driscoll et al 1991). This test is often not tolerated by the patient without general anesthesia, however, signs of apprehension during testing indicate a positive clinical test in the awake patient (Kelly & Weiland 2001).

NEUROLOGICAL TESTING

The deep tendon reflexes that are significant in examination of the elbow are the biceps reflex, brachioradialis reflex, and the triceps reflex, which are controlled by spinal levels C5, C6, and C7 respectively. A slight response is normal whereas an increased response could signify an upper motor neuron lesion, and a decreased response may indicate the presence of a lower motor neuron lesion.

The biceps tendon reflex can be elicited with the elbow relaxed and in a flexed position; the examiner places their thumb over the biceps tendon in the cubital fossa and gently taps the thumb with a reflex hammer. The brachioradialis reflex is elicited by tapping the tendon at the lateral distal end of the radius with the flat edge of a reflex hammer. The triceps tendon reflex is elicited by tapping over the triceps tendon with a reflex hammer.

Sensory perception is assessed by using a pinprick or light touch to the skin and noting the patient's response.

The contralateral extremity is used for comparison. The lateral arm is innervated by the axillary nerve (C5) and the lateral forearm is innervated by branches of the musculocutaneous (C6). The medial arm is innervated by the brachial cutaneous (C8) and the medial forearm is innervated by the antebrachial cutaneous (T1) nerve.

DIAGNOSTIC IMAGES

Plane view radiographs, computed tomography (CT) arthrogram, and magnetic resonance imaging (MRI) may be useful adjuncts to the clinical examination. Radiographs will allow the clinician to identify the presence of fractures, loose bodies, and posterior olecranon osteophytes.

A diagnostic CT arthrogram is extremely useful when a UCL tear is suspected. Contrast dye is injected into the elbow, and X-rays are taken to determine if the dye has escaped the capsule through a tear. Complete UCL tears will provide a positive arthrogram. A CT scan, performed immediately following the arthrogram, can enhance visualization of a capsuloligamentous injury.

MRI of the elbow is also helpful in diagnosing complete UCL tears, particularly when the elbow is injected with saline prior to testing. A UCL tear is indicated by a leakage of dye along the medial side of the elbow proximally and distally along the medial olecranon. Timmerman & Andrews (1994) referred to this as a 'T-sign'.

OVERVIEW OF ELBOW REHABILITATION

Rehabilitation following elbow injury or elbow surgery follows a sequential and progressive multiphased approach. The ultimate goal of elbow rehabilitation is to return the athlete to their previous functional level as quickly and safely as possible. Several key principles must be addressed when rehabilitating the athlete's elbow: (1) the effects of immobilization must be minimized, (2) healing tissue must not be overstressed, (3) the patient must fulfill certain criteria throughout the phases of rehabilitation, (4) the program must be based on current scientific and clinical research, (5) the process must be adaptable to each patient and their specific goals, and (6) the rehabilitation program must be a team effort between the physician, physical therapist, athletic trainer, and patient. Communication between each team member is essential to successful outcomes. The following section will provide an overview of the rehabilitation process following elbow injury (Box 16.2) and surgery (Box 16.3); rehabilitation protocols for specific pathologies will follow.

Box 16.2 Non-operative rehabilitation program for elbow injuries

PHASE I. **ACUTE (WEEK 1)**
Goals
• Improve motion
• Diminish pain and inflammation
• Retard muscle atrophy

Exercises
1. Stretching for wrist and elbow joint, stretches for shoulder joint
2. Strengthening exercises, isometrics for wrist, elbow, and shoulder musculature
3. Pain and inflammation control cryotherapy, high voltage stimulation, ultrasound, and whirlpool

PHASE II. **SUBACUTE (WEEKS 2–4)**
Goals
• Normalize motion
• Improve muscular strength, power, and endurance

WEEK 2
1. Initiate isotonic strengthening for wrist and elbow muscles
2. Initiate exercise, tubing exercises for shoulder
3. Continue use of cryotherapy, etc

WEEK 3
1. Initiate rhythmic stabilization drills for elbow and shoulder joint
2. Progress isotonic strengthening for entire upper extremity
3. Initiate isokinetic strengthening exercises for elbow flexion/extension

WEEK 4
1. Initiate Thrower's Ten program
2. Emphasize eccentric biceps work, concentric triceps and wrist flexor work
3. Program endurance training

4. Initiate light plyometric drills
5. Initiate swinging drills

PHASE III. **ADVANCED STRENGTHENING (WEEKS 4–8)**
Goals
• Preparation of athlete for return to functional activities

Criteria to progress to advanced phase:
1. Full non-painful range of motion
2. No pain or tenderness
3. Satisfactory isokinetic test
4. Satisfactory clinical examination

WEEKS 4–5
1. Continue strengthening exercises, endurance drills, and flexibility exercises daily
2. Thrower's Ten program
3. Progress plyometric drills
4. Emphasize maintenance program based on pathology
5. Progress swinging drills (i.e. hitting)

WEEKS 6–8
1. Initiate interval sport program once determined by physician Phase I program

PHASE IV. **RETURN TO ACTIVITY (WEEKS 6–9)**
Weeks 6 through 9
When you return to play depends on your condition and progress, your physician will determine when it is safe

1. Continue strengthening program, Thrower's Ten program
2. Continue flexibility program
3. Progress functional drills to unrestricted play

PHASE I – IMMEDIATE MOTION PHASE

The first phase of elbow rehabilitation is the immediate motion phase. The goals of this phase are to minimize the effects of immobilization, reestablish non-painful range of motion, decrease pain and inflammation, and to retard muscular atrophy. The rehabilitation specialist must not overstress healing tissues during this phase.

Early range of motion activities are performed to nourish the articular cartilage and assist in the synthesis, alignment, and organization of collagen tissue (Coutts et al 1981, Dehne & Tory 1971, Haggmark & Eriksson 1979, Noyes et al 1987, Perkins 1954, Salter et al 1980, 1984, Tipton et al 1978, Wilk et al 1993a). Range of motion (ROM) activities are performed for all planes of elbow and wrist motions to prevent the formation of scar tissue and adhesions. Reestablishing full elbow extension is the primary goal of early ROM activities to minimize the occurrence of elbow flexion contractures (Akeson et al 1980, Green & McCoy 1979, Nirschl & Morrey 1985). The elbow is predisposed to flexion contractures due to the intimate congruency of the joint articulations, the tightness of the joint capsule, and the tendency of the anterior capsule to develop adhesions following injury. The brachialis muscle also attaches to the capsule and crosses the elbow joint before becoming a tendinous

structure. Injury to the elbow may cause excessive scar tissue formation of the brachialis muscle as well as functional splinting of the elbow.

Grade I and II joint mobilizations may be performed during this early phase of rehabilitation as tolerated (Maitland 1977). Posterior glides with oscillations are performed in the midrange of motion to assist in regaining full elbow extension. Aggressive mobilization techniques are not utilized until later stages of rehabilitation when pain has subsided. Grade I and II mobilization techniques are also utilized to neuromodulate pain by stimulating type I and type II articular receptors (Maitland 1977, Wyke 1966).

If the patient continues to have difficulty achieving full extension using ROM and mobilization techniques, a low load, long duration (LLLD) stretch may be performed to produce a creep of the collagen tissue, which will result in tissue elongation (Kottke et al 1966, Sapega et al 1976, Warren et al 1971, 1976). We have found this exercise to be extremely beneficial for regaining full elbow extension (Wilk et al 1993a, Wilk & Levinson 2001). The patient lies supine with a towel roll placed under the brachium to act as a cushion and fulcrum. Light resistance exercise tubing is applied to the wrist of the patient and secured to the table or a dumbbell on the ground

Box 16.3 Postoperative rehabilitation protocol for elbow arthroscopy

PHASE I. **INITIAL (WEEK 1)**
Goal
Full wrist and elbow range of motion, decrease swelling, decrease pain, retardation of muscle atrophy

A. Day of surgery
Begin gently moving elbow in bulky dressing

B. Post-op day 1 and 2
1. Remove bulky dressing and replace with elastic bandages
2. Immediate post-op hand, wrist, and elbow exercise
   a. Putty/grip strengthening
   b. Wrist flexor stretching
   c. Wrist extensor stretching
   d. Wrist curls
   e. Reverse wrist curls
   f. Neutral wrist curls
   g. Pronation/supination
   h. Active/active-assisted range of motion elbow ext/flex

C. Post-op day 3 through 7
1. Passive range of motion elbow ext/flex (motion to tolerance)
2. Begin progressive resistance exercises with 1 lb weight
   a. Wrist curls
   b. Reverse wrist curls
   c. Neutral wrist curls
   d. Pronation/supination
   e. Broomstick roll-up

PHASE II. **INTERMEDIATE (WEEKS 2–4)**
Goal
Improve muscular strength and endurance; normalize joint arthrokinematics

A. Week 2 ROM exercises (overpressure into extension)
1. Addition of biceps curl and triceps extension
2. Continue to progress progressive resistance exercise weight and repetitions as tolerable

B. Week 3
1. Initiate biceps and triceps eccentric exercise program
2. Initiate rotator cuff exercises program
   a. External rotators
   b. Internal rotators
   c. Deltoid
   d. Supraspinatus
   e. Scapulothoracic strengthening

PHASE III. **ADVANCED (WEEKS 4–8)**
Goals
Preparation of athlete for return to functional activities

Criteria to progress to advanced phase:
1. Full non-painful range of motion
2. No pain or tenderness
3. Isokinetic test that fulfills criteria to throw
4. Satisfactory clinical exam

A. 3 through 6 weeks
1. Continue maintenance program, emphasizing muscular strength, endurance, and flexibility
2. Initiate interval throwing program phase I

(Fig. 16.1). The patient is instructed to relax as much as possible for 10–12 min. The amount of resistance applied should be of low magnitude to enable the patient to perform the stretch for the entire duration without pain or muscle spasm.

The aggressiveness of stretching and mobilization techniques is dictated based on healing constraints of involved tissues as well as the amount of motion and end feel. If the patient presents with a decrease in motion and hard end feel without pain, aggressive stretching

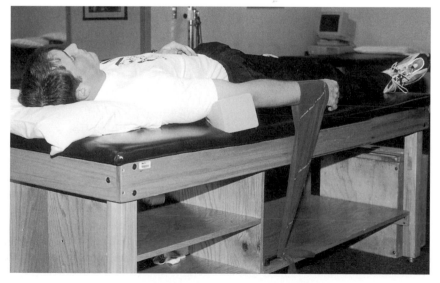

Figure 16.1 Low load, long duration stretch into elbow extension.

and mobilization technique may be used. Conversely, a patient exhibiting pain before resistance and/or empty end feel will be progressed slowly with gentle stretching.

Cryotherapy and high voltage stimulation may be performed as required to assist in reducing pain and inflammation. Once the acute inflammatory phase has passed, moist heat, warm whirlpool, and ultrasound may be used at the onset of treatment to prepare the tissue for stretching and to improve the extensibility of the capsule and musculotendinous structures.

The early phases of rehabilitation must also focus on retarding muscular atrophy. Subpainful and submaximal isometrics are performed initially for the elbow flexor and extensor, as well as the wrist flexor, extensor, pronator, and supinator muscle groups. Isometrics should be performed at multiple angles for 2–3 sets of 10 repetitions, holding each contraction for 6–8 s. Shoulder isometrics may also be performed during this phase with caution against internal and external rotation exercises if painful. Alternating rhythmic stabilization drills for shoulder flexion/extension/horizontal abduction/ adduction and shoulder internal/external rotation are performed to begin reestablishing proprioception and neuromuscular control of the upper extremity.

PHASE II – INTERMEDIATE PHASE

Phase II, the intermediate phase, is initiated when the patient exhibits full ROM, minimal pain and tenderness, and a good (4/5) manual muscle test of the elbow flexor and extensor musculature. The emphasis of this phase includes enhancing elbow and upper extremity mobility, improving muscular strength and endurance, and reestablishing neuromuscular control of the elbow complex.

Stretching exercises are continued to maintain full elbow flexion and extension. Mobilization techniques may be progressed to more aggressive grade III techniques, as needed, to apply a stretch to the capsular tissue and end range. Flexibility is progressed during this phase to focus on wrist flexion, extension, pronation, and supination. Shoulder flexibility is also maintained in athletes with emphasis on flexion, external and internal rotation, and horizontal adduction.

Strengthening exercises are progressed during this phase to include isotonic contractions. Emphasis is placed on elbow flexion and extension, wrist flexion and extension, and forearm pronation and supination. The weight of the arm is initially used before progressing to a 1lb dumbbell. Resistance is then progressed by 1lb per week to gradually stress the involved tissues. The shoulder and scapular muscles are also placed on a progressive resistance program during the later stages of

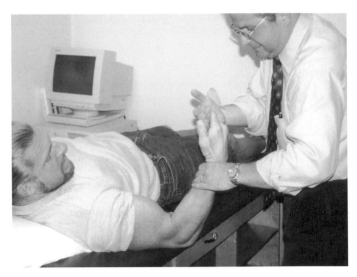

Figure 16.2 Manual resisted elbow and wrist flexion using both concentric and eccentric contractions of the elbow flexors.

this phase. Emphasis is placed on strengthening the shoulder external rotators and scapular muscles, and training eccentric control of the elbow flexors. Shoulder internal and external rotation are performed with exercise tubing at 0° of abduction; standing scaption with external rotation (full can), standing abduction, prone horizontal abduction, and prone rowing are all included in this phase.

Muscular endurance activities are also performed during this phase. High repetition, low resistance dumbbell exercises, as previously described, and the upper body ergometer may be used.

Neuromuscular control exercises are initiated in this phase to enhance the muscles' ability to control the elbow joint during athletic activities. These exercises include proprioceptive neuromuscular facilitation exercises with rhythmic stabilizations (Wilk et al 2001b) and slow reversal manual resistance elbow/wrist flexion drills (Fig. 16.2).

PHASE III – ADVANCED STRENGTHENING PHASE

The third phase involves a progression of activities to prepare the athlete for sport participation. The goals of this phase are to gradually increase strength, power, endurance, and neuromuscular control, to prepare for a gradual return to sport. Specific criteria that must be met before entering this phase include full non-painful ROM, no pain or tenderness, and strength that is 70% of the contralateral extremity.

Advanced strengthening activities during this phase include aggressive strengthening exercises emphasizing high speed and eccentric contraction and plyometric activities. Strengthening exercises are progressed to

The Thrower's Ten Program is designed to exercise the major muscles necessary for throwing. The Program's goal is to be an organized and concise exercise program. In addition, all exercises included are specific to the thrower and are designed to improve strength, power and endurance of the shoulder complex musculature.

1A Diagonal Pattern D2 Extension:
Involved hand will grip tubing handle overhead and out to the side. Pull tubing down and across your body to the opposite side of leg. During the motion, lead with your thumb.
Perform _____ sets of _____ repetitions _____ times daily.

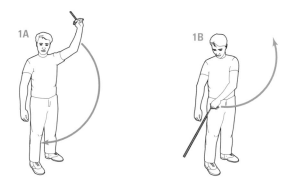

1B Diagonal Pattern D2 Flexion:
Gripping tubing handle in hand of involved arm, begin with arm out from side 45° and palm facing backward. After turning palm forward, proceed to flex elbow and bring arm up and over involved shoulder. Turn palm down and reverse to take arm to starting position.
Perform _____ sets of _____ repetitions _____ times daily.

2A External Rotation at 0° Abduction:
Stand with involved elbow fixed at side, elbow at 90° and involved arm across front of body. Grip tubing handle while the other end of tubing is fixed. Pull out arm, keeping elbow at side. Return tubing slowly and controlled.
Perform _____ sets of _____ repetitions _____ times daily.

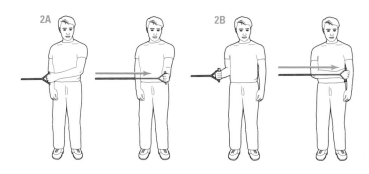

2B Internal Rotation at 0° Abduction:
Standing with elbow at side fixed at 90° and shoulder rotated out. Grip tubing handle while other end of tubing is fixed. Pull arm across body keeping elbow at side. Return tubing slowly and controlled.
Perform _____ sets of _____ repetitions _____ times daily.

2C (Optional) External Rotation at 90° Abduction:
Stand with shoulder abducted 90°. Grip tubing handle while the other end is fixed straight ahead, slightly lower than the shoulder. Keeping shoulder abducted, rotate shoulder back keeping elbow at 90°. Return tubing and hand to start position.
I Slow Speed Sets: (slow and controlled)
Perform _____ sets of _____ repetitions _____ times daily.
II Fast Speed Sets:
Perform _____ sets of _____ repetitions _____ times daily.

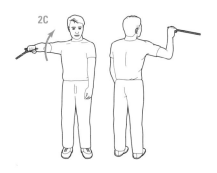

2D (Optional) Internal Rotation at 90° Abduction:
Stand with shoulder abducted to 90°, externally rotated 90° and elbow bent to 90°. Keeping shoulder abducted, rotate shoulder forward, keeping elbow bent at 90°. Return tubing and hand to start position.
I Slow Speed Sets: (slow and controlled)
Perform _____ sets of _____ repetitions _____ times daily.
II Fast Speed Sets:
Perform _____ sets of _____ repetitions _____ times daily.

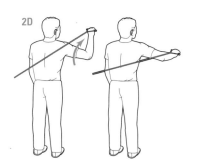

Figure 16.3   The Thrower's Ten program.

3 Shoulder Abduction to 90°:
Stand with arm at side, elbow straight, and palm against side. Raise arm to the side, palm down, until arm reaches 90° (shoulder level).
Perform _____ sets of _____ repetitions _____ times daily.

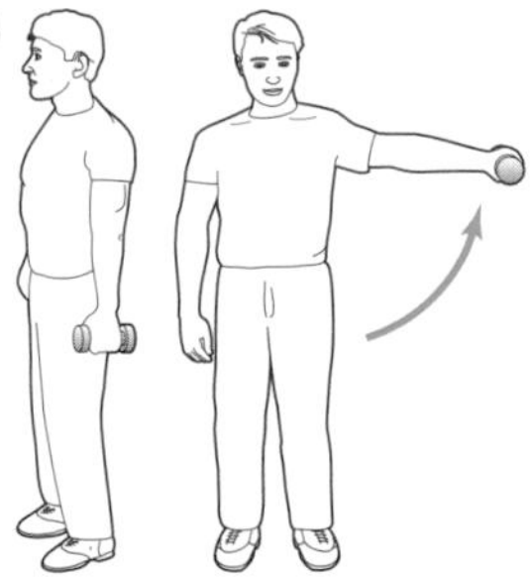

4 Scaption, External Rotation:
Stand with elbow straight and thumb up. Raise arm to shoulder level at 30° angle in front of body. Do not go above shoulder height. Hold 2 seconds and lower slowly.
Perform _____ sets of _____ repetitions _____ times daily.

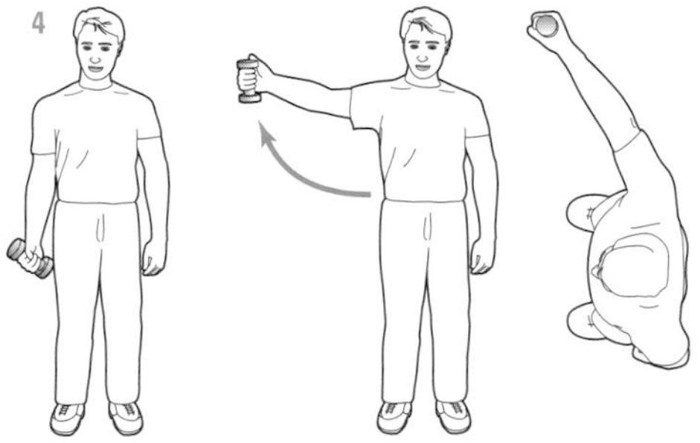

5 Sidelying External Rotation:
Lie on uninvolved side, with involved arm at side of body and elbow bent to 90°. Keeping the elbow of involved arm fixed to side, raise arm. Hold 2 seconds and lower slowly.
Perform _____ sets of _____ repetitions _____ times daily.

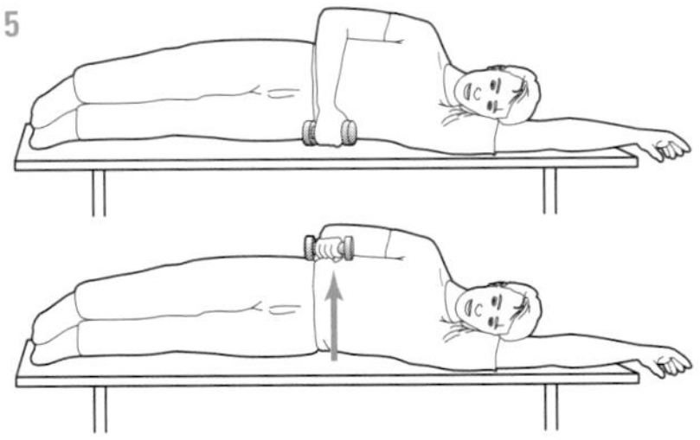

6A Prone Horizontal Abduction (Neutral):
Lie on table, face down, with involved arm hanging straight to the floor, and palm facing down. Raise arm out to the side, parallel to the floor. Hold 2 seconds and lower slowly.
Perform _____ sets of _____ repetitions _____ times daily.

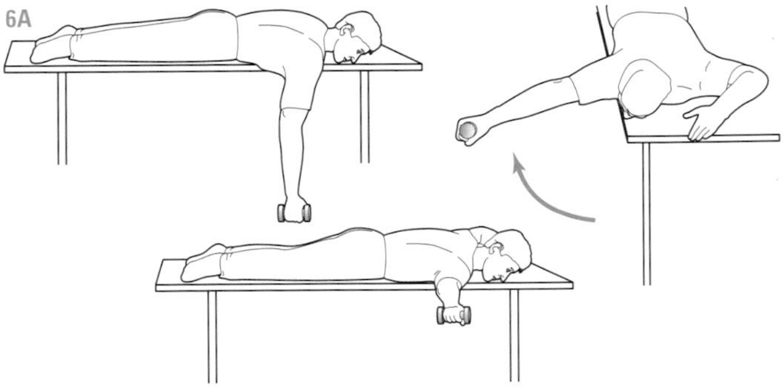

6B Prone Horizontal Abduction (Full ER, 100° ABD):
Lie on table face down, with involved arm hanging straight to the floor and thumb rotated up (hitchhiker). Raise arm out to the side with arm slightly in front of shoulder, parallel to the floor. Hold 2 seconds and lower slowly.
Perform _____ sets of _____ repetitions _____ times daily.

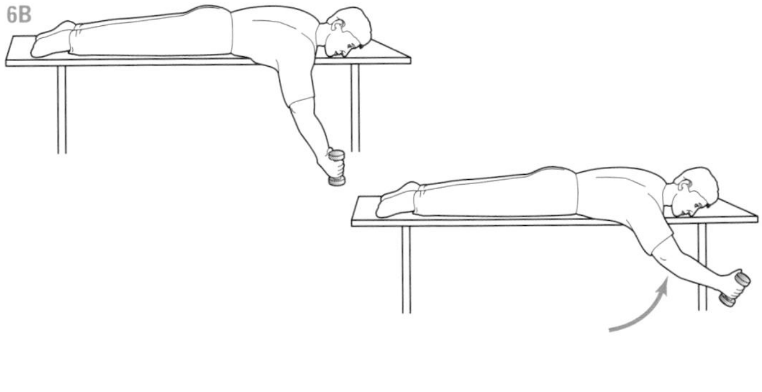

Figure 16.3 (*Cont'd*)

6C Prone Rowing:
Lying on your stomach with your involved arm hanging over the side of the table, dumbbell in hand and elbow straight. Slowly raise arm, bending elbow, and bring dumbbell as high as possible. Hold at the top for 2 seconds, then slowly lower.
Perform _____ sets of _____ repetitions _____ times daily.

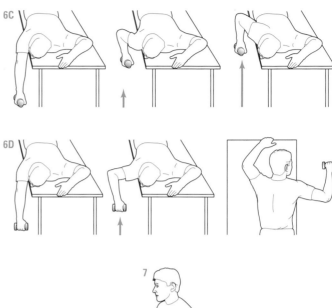

6D Prone Rowing into External Rotation:
Lying on your stomach with your involved arm hanging over the side of the table, dumbbell in hand and elbow straight. Slowly raise arm, bending elbow, up to the level of the table. Pause 1 second. Then rotate shoulder upward until dumbbell is even with the table, keeping elbow at 90°. Hold at the top for 2 seconds, then slowly lower taking 2–3 seconds.
Perform _____ sets of _____ repetitions _____ times daily.

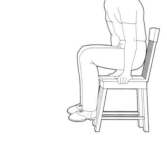

7 Press-ups:
Seated on a chair or table, place both hands firmly on the sides of the chair or table, palm down and fingers pointed outward. Hands should be placed equal with shoulders. Slowly push downward through the hands to elevate your body. Hold the elevated position for 2 seconds and lower body slowly.
Perform _____ sets of _____ repetitions _____ times daily.

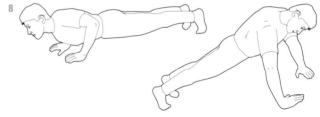

8 Push-ups:
Start in the down position with the arms in a comfortable position. Place hands no more than shoulder width apart. Push up as high as possible, rolling shoulders forward after elbows are straight. Start with a push-up into wall. Gradually progress to table top and eventually to floor as tolerable.
Perform _____ sets of _____ repetitions _____ times daily.

9A Elbow Flexion:
Standing with arm against side and palm facing inward, bend elbow upward turning palm up as you progress. Hold 2 seconds and lower slowly.
Perform _____ sets of _____ repetitions _____ times daily.

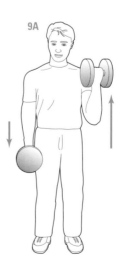

Figure 16.3 *(Cont'd)*

9B Elbow Extension (Abduction):
Raise involved arm overhead. Provide support at elbow from uninvolved hand. Straighten arm overhead. Hold 2 seconds and lower slowly.
Perform _____ sets of _____ repetitions _____ times daily.

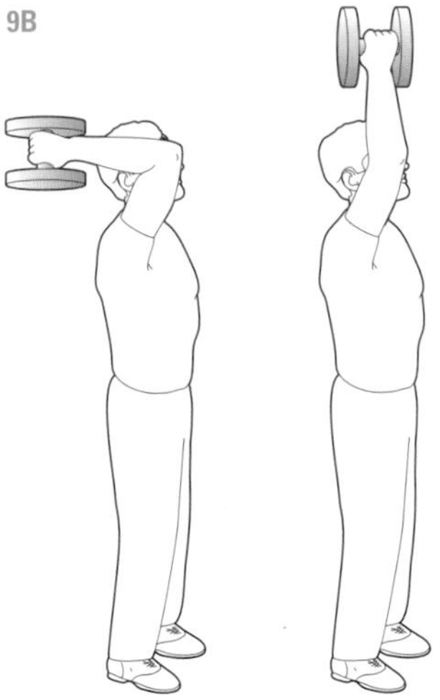

10A Wrist Extension:
Supporting the forearm and with palm facing downward, raise weight in hand as far as possible. Hold 2 seconds and lower slowly.
Perform _____ sets of _____ repetitions _____ times daily.

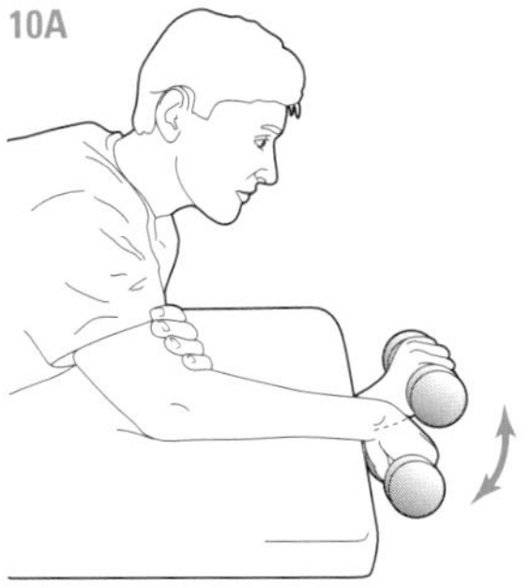

10B Wrist Flexion:
Supporting the forearm and with palm facing upward, lower a weight in hand as far as possible and then curl it up as high as possible. Hold for 2 seconds and lower slowly.
Perform _____ sets of _____ repetitions _____ times daily.

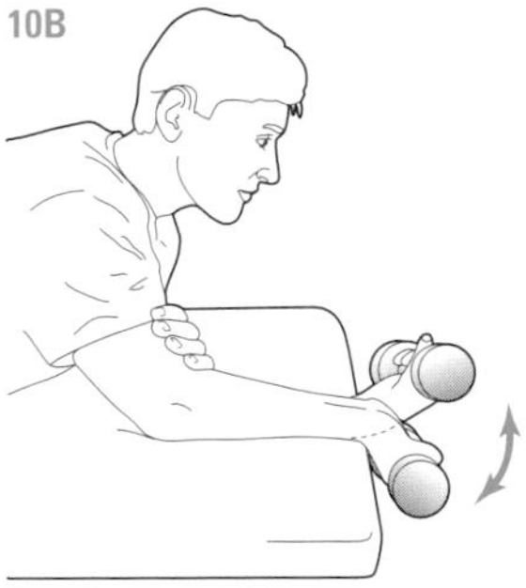

10C Supination:
Forearm supported on table with wrist in neutral position. Using a weight or hammer, roll wrist taking palm up. Hold 2 seconds and return to starting position.
Perform _____ sets of _____ repetitions _____ times daily.

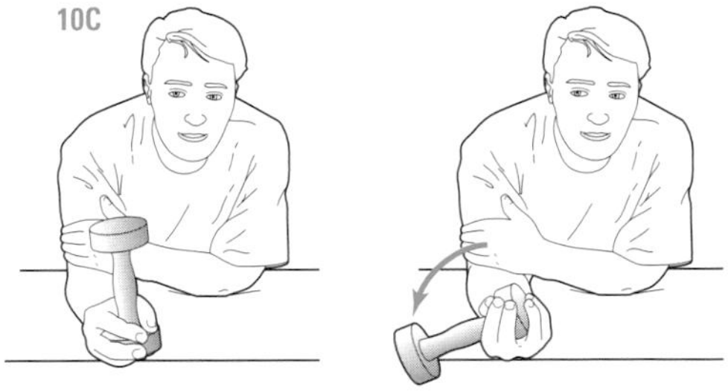

10D Pronation:
Forearm should be supported on a table with wrist in neutral position. Using a weight or hammer, roll wrist taking palm down. Hold 2 seconds and return to starting position.
Perform _____ sets of _____ repetitions _____ times daily.

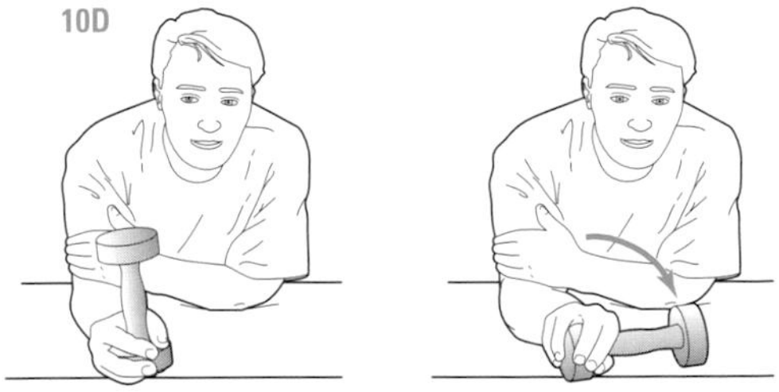

Figure 16.3 (Cont'd)

include the Thrower's Ten program (Fig. 16.3). The design of these exercises is based on numerous EMG studies (Blackburn et al 1990, Fleisig & Escamilla 1996, Moseley et al 1992, Townsend et al 1991) and they are designed to strengthen all of the shoulder, scapular, elbow, and wrist muscles that are utilized during upper extremity athletic activities. Internal and external rotation exercises with exercise tubing are progressed to a function position of 90° abduction with 90° elbow flexion. Exercises may be performed at slow and fast speeds. Scapulothoracic exercises are progressed to include prone horizontal abduction at 100° and full external rotation as well as prone rows into external rotation.

Elbow flexion exercises are progressed to emphasize eccentric control. The biceps muscle is an important stabilizer during the follow-through phase of overhead throwing to eccentrically control the deceleration of the elbow, preventing pathological abutting of the olecranon within the fossa (Andrews & Frank 1985, Fleisig & Escamilla 1996). Elbow flexion can be performed with elastic tubing to emphasize slow and fast speed concentric and eccentric contractions.

Aggressive strengthening exercises with weight machines are also incorporated during this phase. These most commonly begin with bench press, seated rowing, and front latissimus dorsi pull-downs.

Neuromuscular control exercises are progressed to include side-lying external rotation with manual resistance. Concentric and eccentric external rotation is

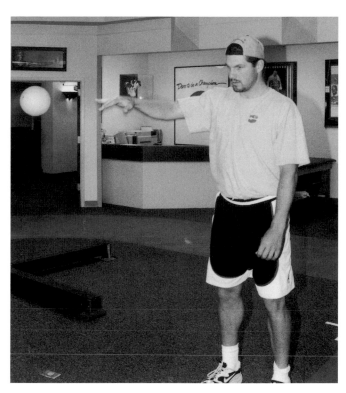

Figure 16.5 One-handed plyometric throws at 90° of shoulder abduction and 90° of elbow flexion using a 2 lb weighted ball.

performed against the clinician's resistance with the addition of rhythmic stabilizations (Wilk et al 2001b). This manual resistance exercise may be progressed to standing external rotation with exercise tubing at 0° and finally at 90° (Fig. 16.4).

Plyometric drills are an extremely beneficial form of exercise for training the upper extremity musculature (Wilk et al 1993b). The physiological principles of plyometric exercise utilize an eccentric prestretch of the muscle tissue, thereby stimulating the muscle spindle to produce a more forceful concentric contraction. Plyometric exercises are performed using a weighted medicine ball during the later stages of this phase to train the upper extremity musculature to develop and withstand high levels of stress. Plyometric exercises are initially performed with two hands performing a chest pass, side-to-side throw, and overhead soccer throw. These may be progressed to include one hand activities such as 90/90 throws (Fig. 16.5), external and internal rotation throws at 0° of abduction and wall dribbles (Wilk et al 1993b, 2001b). Specific plyometric drills for the forearm musculature include wrist flexion flips (Fig. 16.6) and extension grips.

PHASE IV – RETURN-TO-ACTIVITY PHASE

The final phase of elbow rehabilitation, the return-to-activity phase, allows the athlete to return progressively

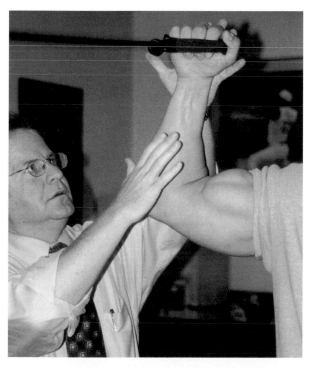

Figure 16.4 External rotation at 90° of shoulder abduction with tubing and manual resistance.

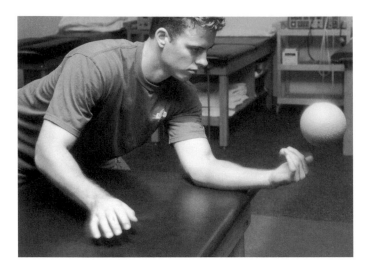

Figure 16.6　Plyometric wrist flips.

Table 16.2　Satisfactory isokinetic test results

	Bilateral comparisons			
Velocity °/s	Elbow Flex	Elbow Ext		
180	110–120%	105–115%		
300	105–115%	100–110%		
Velocity °/s	Shoulder ER	Shoulder IR	Shoulder Abd	Shoulder Add
180	98–105%	110–120%	98–105%	110–128%
300	85–95%	105–115%	96–102%	111–129%
	Unilateral muscle ratios			
Velocity °/s	Elbow Flex/Ext	Shoulder ER/IR	Shoulder Abd/Add	Shoulder ER/Abd
180	70–80%	66–76%	78–84%	67–75%
300	63–69%	61–71%	88–94%	60–70%
	Peak torque to body weight ratios			
Velocity °/s	Shoulder ER	Shoulder IR	Shoulder Abd	Shoulder Add
180	18–23%	28–33%	26–33%	32–38%
300	12–20%	25–30%	20–25%	28–34%

Abd – abducation; Add – adduction; ER – external rotation; Ext – extension; Flex – flexion; IR – internal rotation

to full competition using an interval return to sport program (Wilk et al 2001a). Sport-specific functional drills are performed to prepare the athlete for the stresses involved with each particular sport.

Before an athlete is allowed to begin the return-to-activity phase of rehabilitation, the athlete must exhibit full ROM, no pain or tenderness, a satisfactory isokinetic test, and a satisfactory clinical examination. Isokinetic testing is commonly utilized to determine the readiness of the athlete to begin an interval sport program. Athletes are routinely tested at 180°/s and 300°/s. Successful results of isokinetic testing are listed in Table 16.2.

Upon achieving the previously mentioned criteria to return to sport, we begin a formal interval sport program. For the overhead thrower, we initiate a long-toss interval

---

Box 16.4　Interval throwing program for baseball players – phase I

The interval throwing program (ITP) is designed to gradually return motion, strength and confidence in the throwing arm after injury or surgery by slowly progressing through graduated throwing distances. The ITP is initiated upon clearance by the athlete's physician to resume throwing, and performed under the supervision of the rehabilitation team (physician, physical therapist and athletic trainer).

The program is set up to minimize the chance of reinjury and emphasize prethrowing warm-up and stretching. In the development of the ITP, the following factors are considered most important:

1. The act of throwing the baseball involves the transfer of energy from the feet through the legs, pelvis, trunk, and out of the shoulder through the elbow and hand. Therefore, any return to throwing after injury must include attention to the entire body.
2. The chance for reinjury is lessened by a graduated progression of interval throwing.
3. Proper warm-up is essential.
4. Most injuries occur as the result of fatigue.
5. Proper throwing mechanics lessen the incidence of reinjury.
6. Baseline requirements for throwing include:
   - Pain-free range of motion
   - Adequate muscle power
   - Adequate muscle resistance to fatigue.

Because there is an individual variability in all throwing athletes, there is no set timetable for completion of the program. Most athletes, by nature, are highly competitive individuals and wish to return to competition at the earliest possible moment. While this is a necessary quality of all athletes, the proper channeling of the athlete's energies into a rigidly controlled throwing program is essential to lessen the chance of reinjury during the rehabilitation period. The athlete may have the tendency to want to increase the intensity of the throwing program. This will increase the incidence of reinjury and may greatly retard the rehabilitation process. It is recommended to follow the program rigidly as this will be the safest route for return to competition.

During the recovery process the athlete will probably experience soreness and a dull, diffuse aching sensation in the muscles and tendons. If the athlete experiences sharp pain, particularly in the joint, stop all throwing activity until this pain ceases. If pain continues, the physician should be contacted.

Weight-training. The athlete should supplement the ITP with a high repetition, low weight exercise program. Strengthening should address a good balance between anterior and posterior musculature so that the shoulder will not be predisposed to injury. Special emphasis must be given to posterior rotator cuff musculature for any strengthening program. Weight-training will not increase throwing velocity, but will increase the resistance of the

Box 16.4 (Cont'd)

arm to fatigue and injury. Weight-training should be done the same day as the athlete throws; however, it should be after throwing is completed, using the day in between for flexibility exercises and a recovery period. It should be stressed at this point that a weight-training pattern or routine is a 'maintenance program.' This pattern can and should accompany the athlete into and throughout the season as a deterrent to further injury. It must be stressed that weight-training is of no benefit unless accompanied by a sound flexibility program.

Individual variability. The ITP is designed so that each level is achieved without pain or complications before the next level is started. This sets up a progression that a goal is achieved prior to advancement instead of advancing to a specific timeframe. Because of this design, the ITP may be used for different levels of skills and abilities, from those in high school to professional levels. The reasons for being in the ITP will vary from person to person. Example: one athlete may wish to use alternate days throwing with or without using weights in between; another athlete may have to throw every third or fourth day due to pain or swelling. 'Listen to your body – it will tell you when to slow down'. Again, completion of the steps of the ITP will vary from person to person. There is no set timetable in terms of days to completion.

Warm-up. Jogging increases blood flow to the muscles and joints, thus increasing their flexibility and decreasing the chance of reinjury. Since the amount of warm-up will vary from person to person, the athlete should jog until developing a light sweat, then progress to the stretching phase.

Stretching. Since throwing involves all muscles in the body, all muscle groups should be stretched prior to throwing. This should be done in a systematic fashion beginning with the legs and including the trunk, back, neck and arms. Continue with capsular stretches and L-bar range of motion exercises.

Throwing Mechanics. A critical aspect of the ITP is maintenance of proper throwing mechanics throughout the advancement. The use of the crow-hop method simulates the throwing act, allowing emphasis of the proper body mechanics. This throwing method should be adopted from the set in the ITP. Throwing when flat-footed encourages improper body mechanics, placing increased stress on the throwing arm and, therefore, predisposing the arm to reinjury. The pitching coach and sports biomechanist (if available) may be valuable allies to the rehabilitation team with their knowledge of throwing mechanics.

Components of the crow-hop method are first a hop, then a skip, followed by the throw. The velocity of the throw is determined by

the distance, whereas the ball should have only enough momentum to travel each designed distance. Again, emphasis should be placed upon proper throwing mechanics when the athlete begins phase two: 'throwing off the mound' or from the athlete's respective position, to decrease the chance of reinjury.

Throwing. Using the crow-hop method, the athlete should begin warm-up throws at a comfortable distance (approximately 30–45 ft.) and then progress to the distance indicated for that phase. The program consists of throwing at each step, 2 to 3 times without pain or symptoms, before progressing to the next step. The object of each phase is for the athlete to be able to throw the ball the specified number of feet without pain (45, 60, 90, 120, 150, 180 ft), 75 times at each distance. After being able to throw at the prescribed distance without pain the athlete will be ready for throwing from flat ground 60 ft 6 in. in the normal pitching mechanics or return to the athlete's respective position (step 14). At this point, full strength and confidence should be restored in the athlete's arm. It is important to stress the crow-hop method and proper mechanics with each throw. Just as the advancement to this point has been gradual and progressive, the return to unrestricted throwing must follow the same principles. A pitcher should first throw only fast balls at 50%, progressing to 75% and 100%. At this time, the pitcher may start more stressful pitches such as breaking balls. The position player should simulate a game situation, again progressing at 50–75 to 100%. Once again, if an athlete has increased pain, particularly at the joint, the throwing program should be backed off and re-advanced as tolerated, under the direction of the rehabilitation team.

Batting. Depending on the type of injury that the athlete has, the time of return to batting should be determined by the physician. It should be noted that stress placed upon the arm in the batting motion is very different from the throwing motion. Return to unrestricted use of the bat should also follow the same progression guidelines as seen in the training program. Begin with dry swings progressing to hitting off the tee, then soft toss and finally live pitching.

Summary. In using the ITP in conjunction with a structured rehabilitation program, the athlete should be able to return to full competition status, minimizing any chance of reinjury. The program and its progression should be modified to meet the specific needs of each individual athlete. A comprehensive program consisting of a maintenance strength and flexibility program, appropriate warm-up and cool-down procedures, proper pitching mechanics, and progressive throwing and batting will assist the baseball player in returning safely to competition.

	45 ft Phase		**60 ft Phase**		**90 ft Phase**		**120 ft Phase**
Step 1:	A. Warm-up throwing B. 45 ft (25 throws) C. Rest 5–10 min D Warm-up throwing E. 45 ft (25 throws)	Step 3:	A. Warm-up throwing B. 60 ft (25 throws) C. Rest 5–10 min D. Warm-up throwing E. 60 ft (25 throws)	Step 5:	A. Warm-up throwing B. 90 ft (25 throws) C. Rest 5–10 min D. Warm-up throwing E. 90 ft (25 throws)	Step 7:	A. Warm-up throwing B. 120 ft (25 throws) C. Rest 5–10 min D. Warm-up throwing E. 120 ft (25 throws)
Step 2:	A. Warm-up throwing B. 45 ft (25 throws) C. Rest 5–10 min D. Warm-up throwing E. 45 ft (25 throws) F. Rest 5–10 min G. Warm-up throwing H. 45 ft (25 throws)	Step 4:	A. Warm-up throwing B. 60 ft (25 throws) C. Rest 5–10 min D. Warm-up throwing E. 60 ft (25 throws) F. Rest 5–10 min G. Warm-up throwing H. 60 ft (25 throws)	Step 6:	A. Warm-up throwing B. 90 ft (25 throws) C. Rest 5–10 min D. Warm-up throwing E. 90 ft (25 throws) F Rest 5–10 min G. Warm-up throwing H. 90 ft (25 throws)	Step 8:	A. Warm-up throwing B. 120 ft (25 throws) C. Rest 5–10 min D. Warm-up throwing E. 120 ft (25 throws) F. Rest 5–10 min G. Warm-up throwing H. 120 ft (25 throws)

Box 16.4 *(Cont'd)*

150 ft Phase

Step 9:
- A. Warm-up throwing
- B. 150 ft (25 throws)
- C. Rest 5–10 min
- D. Warm-up throwing
- E. 150 ft (25 throws)

Step 10:
- A. Warm-up throwing
- B. 150 ft (25 throws)
- C. Rest 5–10 min
- D. Warm-up throwing
- E. 150 ft (25 throws)
- F. Rest 5–10 min
- G. Warm-up throwing
- H. 150 ft (25 throws)

Step 11:
- A. Warm-up throwing
- B. 180 ft (25 throws)
- C. Rest 5–10 min
- D. Warm-up throwing
- E. 180 ft (25 throws)

Step 12:
- A. Warm-up throwing
- B. 180 ft (25 throws)
- C. Rest 5–10 min
- D. Warm-up throwing
- E. 180 ft (25 throws)
- F. Rest 5–10 min
- G. Warm-up throwing
- H. 180 ft (25 throws)

180 ft Phase

Step 13:
- A. Warm-up throwing
- B. 180 ft (25 throws)
- C. Rest 5–10 min
- D. Warm-up throwing
- E. 180 ft (25 throws)

Step 14: Begin throwing off the mound or return to respective position

The throwing program should be performed every other day, unless otherwise specified by the physician or rehabilitation specialist.

Perform each step ___ times before progressing to next step

Flat ground throwing
- A. Warm-up throwing
- B. Throw 60 ft (10–15 throws)
- C. Throw 90 ft (10 throws)
- D. Throw 120 ft (10 throws)
- E. Throw 60 ft (flat ground) using pitching mechanics (20–30 throws)

Flat throwing
- A. Warm-up throwing
- B. Throw 60 ft (10–15 throws)
- C. Throw 90 ft (10 throws)
- D. Throw 120 ft (10 throws)
- E. Throw 60 ft (flat ground) using pitching mechanics (20–30 throws)
- F. Throw 60–90 ft (10–15 throws)
- G. Throw 60 ft (flat ground) using pitching mechanics (20 throws)

throwing program (Box 16.4). The athlete throws three times per week with a day off from throwing in between each session. Each step is performed at least twice on separate days before we allow the athlete to progress to the next step. Throwing should be performed without pain or significant increase in symptoms. If the athlete experiences symptoms at a particular step within the program, the athlete is instructed to regress to the prior step until symptoms subside. We believe it is important for the overhead athlete to perform stretching and an abbreviated strengthening program prior to and after performing the interval sport program. Typically, our overhead throwers warm-up, stretch, and perform one set of their exercise program before throwing, followed by two additional sets of exercises after throwing. This provides an adequate warm-up but also ensures maintenance of necessary range of motion and flexibility of the shoulder joint.

Following the completion of a long-toss program, pitchers will progress to phase II of the throwing program – throwing off a mound (Box 16.5). In phase II, the number of throws, intensity, and type of pitch are progressed to gradually increase stress on the shoulder joint.

Interval sport programs for tennis and golf follow the same guidelines as the baseball program. A specific interval program for tennis is outlined in Box 16.6. As the athlete progresses, the number of forehand and backhand shots are gradually increased. Overhead serving is typically initiated during the third week of the program and games are allowed during the fourth week if symptoms have not exacerbated.

Box 16.7 outlines an interval golf program. The program begins with simple putting and chipping and progresses to include short iron swings by the end of week 1, medium irons by week 2, and long irons by week 3. Medium and long iron shots are hit using a tee, to minimize the forces at the elbow observed while taking a divot. Woods are initiated at the end of week 3 and progressed to include drives by the fourth week. The athlete can play 9 holes during the end of the fourth week if asymptomatic.

The following sections will briefly overview the clinical presentations, findings, and rehabilitation programs of numerous elbow joint disorders commonly seen in athletes, followed by several non-common sport related pathologies. Non-operative injuries will be presented first, followed by postoperative procedures.

COMMON SPORT-RELATED INJURIES

MEDIAL AND LATERAL EPICONDYLITIS

Medial and lateral epicondylitis may result from numerous factors, many of which have been previously

---

Box 16.5 Interval throwing program for baseball players – throwing off the mound – phase II

After the completion of phase I of the interval throwing program (ITP) and when able to throw to the prescribed distance without pain, the athlete will be ready for throwing off the mound or to return to the athlete's respective position. At this point, full strength and confidence should be restored in the athlete's arm. Just as the advancement to this point has been gradual and progressive, the return to unrestricted throwing must follow the same principles. A pitcher should first throw only fast balls at 50%, progressing to 75% and 100%. At this time, the athlete may start more stressful pitches such as breaking balls. The position player should simulate a game situation, again progressing at 50–75–100%. Once again, if an athlete has increased pain, particularly at the joint, the throwing

program should be backed off and re-advanced as tolerated, under the direction of the rehabilitation team.

Summary. In using the ITP in conjunction with a structured rehabilitation program, the athlete should be able to return to full competition status, minimizing any chance of reinjury. The program and its progression should be modified to meet the specific needs of each individual athlete. A comprehensive program consisting of a maintenance strength and flexibility program, appropriate warm-up and cool-down procedures, proper pitching mechanics, and progressive throwing and batting will assist the baseball player in returning safely to competition.

STAGE ONE: FASTBALLS ONLY

Step 1: Interval throwing
15 throws off mound 50%

Step 2: Interval throwing
30 throws off mound 50%

Step 3: Interval throwing
45 throws off mound 50%

Step 4: Interval throwing
60 throws off mound 50%

Step 5: Interval throwing
70 throws off mound 50%

Step 6: 45 throws off mound 50%
30 throws off mound 75%

Step 7: 30 throws off mound 50%
45 throws off mound 75%

Step 8: 65 throws off mound 75%
10 throws off mound 50%

STAGE TWO: FASTBALLS ONLY

Step 9: 60 throws off mound 75%
15 throws in batting practice

Step 10: 50–60 throws off mound 75%
30 throws in batting practice

Step 11: 45–50 throws off mound 75%
45 throws in batting practice

STAGE THREE

Step 12: 30 throws off mound 75% warm-up
15 throws off mound 50% BREAKING BALLS
45–60 throws in batting practice (fastball only)

Step 13: 30 throws off mound 75%
30 breaking balls 75%
30 throws in batting practice

Step 14: 30 throws off mound 75%
60–90 throws in batting practice (gradually increase breaking balls)

Step 15: SIMULATED GAME: PROGRESSING BY 15 THROWS PER WORKOUT (pitch count)
(Use interval throwing to 120 ft Phase as warm-up)

ALL THROWING OFF THE MOUND SHOULD BE DONE IN THE PRESENCE OF THE PITCHING COACH TO STRESS PROPER THROWING MECHANICS

(Use speed gun to aid in effort control)

---

discussed. The majority of causes are related to repetitive microtrauma and poor biomechanics, which are sport specific. Medially, overhead throwers most often exhibit pronator tendonitis, and golfers present with wrist flexor tendonitis, whereas lateral epicondylitis is most often seen in tennis players. Patients most often present with tenderness near the epicondyle and along the flexor pronator and extensor supinator muscle masses, which may be exacerbated by contraction or stretching of the musculature.

Clinical examination should attempt to distinguish the structures involved. For medial epicondylitis, manual resistance of wrist flexion should be performed as well as pronation to determine if a pronation strain has occurred. For lateral epicondylitis, testing the extensor carpi radialis longus is performed with the elbow flexed to 30° and resistance given to the second metacarpal bone (Kendall & McCreary 1983). The extensor carpi radialis brevis is tested with the elbow fully flexed and resistance given

to the third metacarpal bone (Kendall & McCreary 1983). In addition, the extensor carpi ulnaris can be differentiated by resisting ulnar deviation (Kendall & McCreary 1983).

The non-operative approach for treatment of epicondylitis (Box 16.8) focuses on diminishing pain and gradually improving muscular strength. The primary goals of rehabilitation are to control the applied loads and create an environment for healing. The initial treatment consists of warm whirlpool, phonophoresis, transverse friction massage, stretching exercises, and light strengthening exercises to stimulate a healing response. High voltage stimulation and cryotherapy are used following treatment to decrease pain and post-exercise inflammation. The athlete should be cautioned against excessive gripping activities. Once the patient's symptoms have subsided, an aggressive stretching and strengthening program with emphasis on eccentric contractions is initiated. Wrist flexion and extension

Box 16.6 Interval tennis program

The same principles should be followed with the interval tennis program as for the interval baseball program. Proper warm-ups, stretching, and strengthening should still be implemented throughout the entire interval tennis rehabilitation program. As you start your program, remember that mechanics play an important role in your recovery. If you have any further questions, please contact your physician or therapist.
OH – overhead shots
FH – forehand shots
BH – backhand shots

	MONDAY	WEDNESDAY	FRIDAY
1st week	12 FH	15 FH	15 FH
	8 BH	8 BH	10 BH
	10 min rest	10 min rest	10 min rest
	13 FH	15 FH	15 FH
	7 BH	7 BH	10 BH
2nd week	25 FH	30 FH	30 FH
	15 BH	20 BH	25 BH
	10 min rest	10 min rest	10 min rest
	25 FH	30 FH	30 FH
	15 BH	20 BH	15 BH
			10 BH
3rd week	30 FH	30 FH	30 FH
	25 BH	25 BH	30 BH
	10 OH	15 OH	15 OH
	10 min rest	10 min rest	10 min rest
	30 FH	30 FH	30 FH
	25 BH	25 BH	15 OH
	10 OH	15 OH	10 min rest
			30 FH
			30 BH
			15 OH
4th week	30 FH	30 FH	30 FH
	30 BH	30 BH	30 BH
	10 OH	10 OH	10 OH
	10 min rest	10 min rest	10 min rest
	Play 3 games	Play set	Play 1½ sets
	10 FH	10 FH	10 FH
	10 BH	10 BH	10 BH
	5 OH	5 OH	3 OH

Ice after each day of play

Box 16.7 Interval golf program

The same principles should be followed with the interval golf program as for the interval baseball program. Proper warm-up, stretching, and strengthening should still be implemented throughout the entire interval golf rehabilitation program. As you start your program, remember that mechanics play an important role in your recovery. If you have any further questions, please contact your physician or rehabilitation specialist.

	MONDAY	WEDNESDAY	FRIDAY
1st week	10 putts	15 putts	20 putts
	10 chips	15 chips	20 chips
	5 min rest	5 min rest	5 min rest
	15 chips	25 chips	20 putts
			20 chips
			5 min rest
			10 chips
			10 short irons
2nd week	20 chips	20 chips	15 short irons
	10 short irons	15 short irons	20 medium irons
	5 min rest	10 min rest	(5 iron/tee)
	10 short irons	15 short irons	10 min rest
	15 medium irons	15 chips	20 short irons
	(5 iron off tee)	Putting	
		15 medium irons	
		(5 iron/tee)	
3rd week	15 short irons	15 short irons	15 short irons
	20 medium irons	15 medium irons	15 medium irons
	10 min rest	10 long irons	10 long irons
	5 long irons	10 min rest	10 min rest
	15 short irons	10 short irons	10 short irons
	15 medium irons	10 medium irons	10 medium irons
	10 min rest	5 long irons	10 long irons
	20 chips	5 wood	10 wood
4th Week	15 short irons		
	15 medium irons		
	10 long irons	Play 9 holes	Play 9 holes
	10 drives		
	15 min rest		
	Repeat		
5th week	9 holes	9 holes	18 holes

Key to golf programs
Flexibility exercises before hitting
Use ice after hitting
Chips – pitching wedge; short irons – W, 9, 8; medium irons – 7, 6, 5; long irons – 4, 3, 2; woods – 3, 5; drives – driver

activities should be performed initially with the elbow flexed 30–45°. Once the athlete can perform these isotonic exercises with a 3 lb weight, they can be performed with the elbow fully extended. A gradual progression through plyometric and throwing activities precedes the initiation of the interval sport program. Because poor mechanics are often a cause of this condition, an analysis of sport mechanics and proper supervision through the interval sport program are critical.

ULNAR NEUROPATHY

There are several theories regarding the cause of ulnar neuropathy of the elbow in athletes (Glousman 1990).

Ulnar nerve changes can result from tensile forces, compressive forces, or nerve instability. Any one or a combination of these mechanisms may be responsible for ulnar nerve symptoms (Glousman 1990).

A leading mechanism for tensile force on the ulnar nerve is valgus stress. This may be coupled with an external rotation-supination stress overload mechanism. The traction forces are further magnified when underlying valgus instability from UCL injuries is present (Andrews & Whiteside 1993). Ulnar neuropathy is often a secondary pathology of UCL insufficiency.

Box 16.8 Epicondylitis rehabilitation protocol

PHASE I. ACUTE
Goals
- Decrease inflammation
- Promote tissue healing
- Retard muscular atrophy

Cryotherapy
Whirlpool
Stretching to increase flexibility
    wrist extension/flexion
    elbow extension/flexion
    forearm supination/pronation
Isometrics
    wrist extension/flexion
    elbow extension/flexion
    forearm supination/pronation
High voltage stimulation
Phonophoresis
Friction massage
Iontophoresis (with anti-inflammatory, e.g. dexamethasone)
Avoid painful movements (e.g. gripping, etc)

PHASE II. SUBACUTE
Goals
- Improve flexibility
- Increase muscular strength/endurance
- Increase functional activities/return to function

Exercises
Emphasize concentric/eccentric strengthening
Concentration on involved muscle group
Wrist extension/flexion
Forearm pronation/supination
Elbow flexion/extension
Initiate shoulder strengthening (if deficiencies are noted)
Continue flexibility exercises
May use counterforce brace
Continue use of cryotherapy after exercise/function
Gradual return to stressful activities
Gradually re-initiate once painful movements

PHASE III. CHRONIC
Goals
- Improve muscular strength and endurance
- Maintain/enhance flexibility
- Gradual return to sport/high level activities

Exercises
Continue strengthening exercises (emphasize eccentric/concentric)
Continue to emphasize deficiencies in shoulder and elbow strength
Continue flexibility exercises
Gradually decrease use of counterforce brace
Use of cryotherapy as needed
Gradual return-to-sport activity
Equipment modification (grip size, string tension, playing surface)
Emphasize maintenance program

Compression of the ulnar nerve is often due to hypertrophy of the surrounding soft tissues or the presence of scar tissue. The nerve may also be trapped between the two heads of the flexor carpi ulnaris (Glousman 1990).

Repetitive flexion and extension of the elbow with an unstable nerve can irritate or inflame the nerve. The nerve may sublux or rest on the medial epicondyle, rendering it vulnerable to direct trauma. Complete dislocation of the nerve may occur anteriorly leading to friction neuritis.

There are three stages of ulnar neuropathy (Alley & Pappas 1995). The first stage includes an acute onset of radicular symptoms. The second stage is manifested by a recurrence of symptoms as the athlete attempts to return to competition. The third stage is associated with persistent motor weakness and sensory changes. Once the athlete presents in the third stage of injury, conservative management may not be effective.

Clinical examination often reveals tenderness along the cubital tunnel. Additionally, the examiner may perform a Tinel test by tapping on the cubital tunnel (Magee 1987). A positive Tinel test results in paresthesia or tingling over the ulnar nerve distribution.

The non-operative treatment of ulnar neuropathy focuses on diminishing ulnar nerve irritation, enhancing dynamic medial joint stability, and gradually returning the athlete to competition.

Following the diagnosis of ulnar neuropathy, throwing athletes are instructed to discontinue throwing activities for at least 4 weeks. The athlete progresses through the immediate motion and intermediate phases over the course of 4 to 6 weeks with emphasis placed on eccentric and dynamic stabilization drills. Plyometric exercises are utilized to facilitate dynamic stabilization of the medial elbow. The athlete is allowed to begin an interval throwing program when the following criteria are fulfilled: (1) full pain-free ROM, (2) a satisfactory clinical examination, (3) no neurological symptoms, (4) adequate medial stability, and (5) satisfactory muscular performance. The athlete may gradually return to play if progression through the interval sport program does not reveal neurological symptoms.

ULNAR NERVE TRANSPOSITION

Surgical transpositioning of the ulnar nerve involves stabilizing the nerve with fascial slings. Caution is taken so that the soft tissue structures involved in the relocation of the nerve are not overstressed. The rehabilitation following an ulnar nerve transposition is outlined in Box 16.9. A posterior splint at 90° of elbow flexion is used for the first 2 weeks postoperatively to prevent excessive ROM and tension on the nerve. The splint is discharged at week 2 and light ROM activities are initiated. Full ROM is usually restored by weeks 3–4. Gentle isotonic

---

Box 16.9 Postoperative rehabilitation following ulnar nerve transposition

PHASE I. IMMEDIATE POSTOPERATIVE (WEEK 0–2)
Goals
- Allow soft tissue healing of relocated nerve
- Decrease pain and inflammation
- Retard muscular atrophy

A. Week 1
1. Posterior splint at 90° elbow flexion with wrist free for motion (sling for comfort)
2. Compression dressing
3. Exercises such as gripping exercises, wrist range of motion, shoulder isometrics

B. Week 2
1. Remove posterior splint for exercise and bathing
2. Progress elbow range of motion (passive range of motion 15° to 120°)
3. Initiate elbow and wrist isometrics
4. Continue shoulder isometrics

PHASE II. INTERMEDIATE (WEEKS 3–7)
Goals
- Restore full pain-free range of motion
- Improve strength, power, and endurance of upper extremity musculature
- Gradually increase functional demands

A. Week 3
1. Discontinue posterior splint
2. Progress elbow range of motion, emphasize full extension

3. Initiate flexibility exercise for wrist extension/flexion, forearm supination/pronation, and elbow extension/flexion
4. Initiate strengthening exercises for wrist extension/flexion, forearm supination/pronation, elbow extensors/flexors, and a shoulder program

B. Week 6
1. Continue all exercises listed above
2. Initiate light sport activities

PHASE III. ADVANCED STRENGTHENING (WEEKS 8–12)
Goals
- Increase strength, power, endurance
- Gradually initiate sporting activities

A. Week 8
1. Initiate eccentric exercise program
2. Initiate plyometric exercise drills
3. Continue shoulder and elbow strengthening and flexibility exercises
4. Initiate interval throwing program

PHASE IV. RETURN TO ACTIVITY (WEEKS 12–16)
Goals
- Gradually return to sporting activities

A. Week 12
1. Return to competitive throwing
2. Continue Thrower's Ten Exercise Program

---

strengthening is begun during week 4 and progressed to the full Thrower's Ten program by 6 weeks following surgery. Aggressive strengthening including eccentric and plyometric training is incorporated by weeks 7 to 8 and an interval sport program at weeks 8 to 9, if all previously outlined criteria are met. A return to competition usually occurs between weeks 12 and 16 postoperatively.

VALGUS EXTENSION OVERLOAD

Valgus extension overload occurs in repetitive sport activities such as throwing, tennis serving, and swimming. Injury usually occurs during the acceleration or deceleration phase as the olecranon wedges up against the medial olecranon fossa during elbow extension (Wilson et al 1983). This mechanism may result in osteophyte formation and potentially loose bodies. Repetitive extension stress from the triceps may further contribute to this injury. There is often a certain degree of underlying valgus instability in these athletes, further facilitating osteophyte formation through compression of the radiocapitellar joint and the posteromedial elbow (Anderson 2001).

Athletes typically present with pain in the posteromedial aspect of the elbow that is exacerbated with forced extension and valgus stress. The clinical test for valgus extension overload involves the examiner grasping the elbow in a flexed position. As the examiner forces the

elbow into extension, a valgus stress is simultaneously applied to the elbow (Fig. 16.7). The examiner palpates the posteromedial joint for tenderness and/or crepitation. Pain over the posteromedial olecranon process signifies a positive test (Wilson et al 1983).

A conservative treatment approach is often attempted before considering surgical intervention. Initial treatment involves relieving the posterior elbow of pain and inflam-

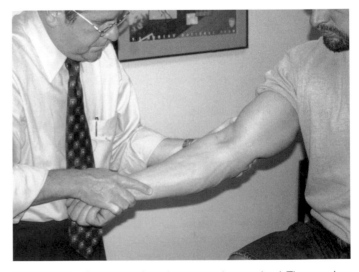

Figure 16.7 Clinical test for valgus extension overload. The examiner forcefully extends the elbow while applying a valgus stress.

mation. As symptoms subside and ROM normalizes, strengthening exercises are initiated. Emphasis is placed on improving eccentric strength of the elbow flexors in an attempt to control the rapid extension that occurs at the elbow during athletics. Manual resistance exercises of concentric and eccentric elbow flexion are performed, as well as elbow flexion with exercise tubing.

POSTERIOR OLECRANON OSTEOPHYTE EXCISION

Surgical excision of posterior olecranon osteophytes is performed using an osteotome or motorized burr. Approximately 5–10 mm of the olecranon tip is removed concomitantly and a motorized burr is used to contour the coronoid, olecranon tip and fossa to prevent further impingement with extreme flexion and extension (Martin & Baumgarten 1996).

The rehabilitation program following arthroscopic posterior olecranon osteophyte excision is slightly more conservative in restoring full elbow extension secondary to postsurgical pain. ROM is progressed within the patient's tolerance; by 10 days postoperatively, the patient should exhibit at least 15–100° of ROM, and 10–110° by day 14. Full ROM is typically restored by day 20 to 25 postsurgery. The rate of ROM progression is most often limited by osseous structure pain and synovial joint inflammation.

The strengthening program is similar to the previously discussed progression. Isometrics are performed for the first 10 to 14 days and isotonic strengthening from weeks 2 to 6. The full Thrower's Ten program is initiated by week 6. An interval sport program is included by weeks 10 to 12. The rehabilitation focus is similar to the non-operative treatment of valgus extension overload. Emphasis is placed on eccentric control of the elbow flexors and dynamic stabilization of the medial elbow.

Andrews & Timmerman (1995) reported on the outcome of elbow surgery in 72 professional baseball players. 65% of these athletes exhibited a posterior olecranon osteophyte and 25% of the athletes who underwent an isolated olecranon excision, later required an ulnar collateral ligament reconstruction (Andrews & Timmerman 1995). This may suggest that subtle medial instability may accelerate osteophyte formation.

Conversely, there is a certain amount of concern related to the effects of excising the posterior olecranon on medial elbow stability; by altering the static stability of the humeroulnar articulation, medial elbow stability may be compromised. Andrews et al (2001) examined the amount of stress applied to the anterior bundle of the UCL with varying amounts of posterior olecranon excisions. UCL strain was measured with intact olecranons and with 2 mm incremental resections of the medial

olecranon up to 8 mm. A further resection of 13 mm was also performed. The UCL was then strained to failure during an applied valgus stress at varying degrees of elbow flexion from 50° to 100°. Results indicate no significant differences in strain on the UCL with change in level of osteotomy for a given applied load and angle of flexion. Thus, it appears that UCL strain is not significantly increased with posterior olecranon resection.

ULNAR COLLATERAL LIGAMENT INJURY

Injuries to the UCL are becoming increasingly more common in overhead throwing athletes, although the higher incidence of injury may be due to our increased ability to diagnose these injuries. As described briefly in the biomechanics section, the elbow experiences a tremendous amount of valgus stress during overhead throwing. These stresses approach the ultimate failure load of the ligament with each throw. The repetitive nature of overhead sport activities such as baseball pitching, football passing, tennis serving, and javelin throwing, further increase susceptibility to UCL injury by exposing the ligament to repetitive microtraumatic forces.

The athlete with an injury to the UCL usually presents with pain and tenderness to the medial elbow. Generalized joint effusion may also be present. The patient's subjective history typically reveals either recurring medial elbow symptoms or a single traumatic incident of medial elbow pain while throwing, etc. The patient recalls a sudden, sharp, medial elbow pain, often with a popping sensation.

There are several clinical tests that are used to test the integrity of the UCL. We will describe the two most common techniques that we utilize in our clinic. The patient is positioned supine while the examiner holds the elbow and externally rotates the shoulder, blocking the upper extremity from further rotating (Fig. 16.8). The UCL is easily palpated in this position. The elbow is tested at 5° and 25–30° of flexion. A valgus stress is imparted upon the elbow to determine the integrity of the ligament. The amount of opening, or gapping, is assessed as well as the end feel of motion. Excessive gapping, a soft end feel, or localized medial pain, may all be indicative of UCL injury (Andrews et al 1993).

Next, the patient moves to the prone position with the involved arm hanging over the edge of the table. The examiner internally rotates the shoulder and stabilizes the elbow before placing a valgus stress on the elbow at 5° and 25–30° of flexion (Fig. 16.9). Again the amount of opening and end feel are assessed.

Furthermore, an MRI enhanced with intra-articular dye injection may be useful in the athlete with a suspected UCL injury. A UCL tear is indicated by a T-sign as previously discussed (Timmerman & Andrews 1994).

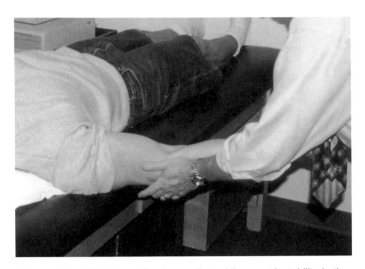

Figure 16.8 Clinical test for ulnar collateral ligament instability in the supine position.

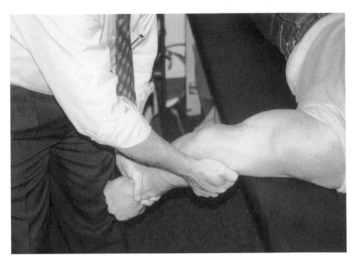

Figure 16.9 Clinical test for ulnar collateral ligament instability in the prone position.

Box 16.10 Conservative treatment following ulnar collateral sprains of the elbow

PHASE I. IMMEDIATE MOTION (WEEKS 0 THROUGH 2)
Goals
- Increase range of motion
- Promote healing of ulnar collateral ligament
- Retard muscular atrophy
- Decrease pain and inflammation

1. *ROM*
   Brace (optional) nonpainful ROM (20–90°)
   AAROM, PROM elbow and wrist (non-painful range)

2. *Exercises*
   Isometrics – wrist and elbow musculature
   Shoulder strengthening (no ext. rotation strengthening)

3. *Ice and compression*

PHASE II. INTERMEDIATE (WEEKS 3 THROUGH 6)
Goals
- Increase range of motion
- Improve strength/endurance
- Decrease pain and inflammation
- Promote stability

1. *ROM*
   Gradually increase motion 0° to 135° (increase 10° per week)

2. *Exercises*
   Initiate isotonic exercises:
       wrist curls
       wrist extensions
       pronation/supination
       biceps/triceps
       dumbbells: external rotation, deltoid, supraspinatus,
           rhomboids, internal rotation

3. *Ice and compression*

PHASE III. ADVANCED (WEEKS 6 AND 7 THROUGH 12 AND 14)
Criteria to progress:
1. Full range of motion
2. No pain or tenderness
3. No increase in laxity
4. Strength 4/5 of elbow flexor/extensor

Goals
- Increase strength, power and endurance
- Improve neuromuscular control
- Initiate high speed exercise drills

Exercises
Initiate exercise tubing, shoulder program:
   Thrower's Ten program
   Biceps/triceps program
   Supination/pronation
   Wrist extension/flexion
   Plyometrics throwing drills

PHASE IV. RETURN TO ACTIVITY (WEEK 12 THROUGH 14)
Criteria to progress to return to throwing:
1. Full non-painful ROM
2. No increase in laxity
3. Isokinetic test fulfills criteria
4. Satisfactory clinical examination

Exercises
Initiate interval throwing
Continue Thrower's Ten program
Continue plyometrics

AAROM – active-assisted range of motion; PROM – passive range of motion; ROM – range of motion

Box 16.11 Postoperative rehabilitation following chronic ulnar collateral ligament reconstruction using autogenous graft

PHASE I. IMMEDIATE POSTOPERATIVE (0–3 WEEKS)
Goals
• Protect healing tissue
• Decrease pain/inflammation
• Retard muscular atrophy

A. Postoperative week 1
1. Posterior splint at 90° elbow flexion
2. Wrist AROM extension/flexion
3. Elbow compression dressing (2–3 days)
4. Exercises such as gripping exercises, wrist ROM, shoulder isometrics (except shoulder ER), biceps isometrics
5. Cryotherapy

B. Postoperative week 2
1. Application of functional brace 30° to 100°
2. Initiate wrist isometrics
3. Initiate elbow flex/ext isometrics
4. Continue all exercises listed above

C. Postoperative week 3
Advance brace 15–110° (gradually increase ROM; 5° extension/10° flexion per week)

PHASE II. INTERMEDIATE (WEEKS 4–8)
Goals
• Gradual increase in range of motion
• Promote healing of repaired tissue
• Regain and improve muscular strength

A. Week 4
1. Functional brace set (10–120°)
2. Begin light resistance exercises for arm (1 lb) wrist curls, extensions pronation/supination elbow ext/flexion
3. Progress shoulder program, emphasize rotator cuff strengthening (avoid ER until 6th week)

B. Week 6
1. Functional brace set 0–130°); AROM 0–145° (without brace)
2. Progress elbow strengthening exercises
3. Initiate shoulder external rotation strengthening
4. Progress shoulder program

PHASE III. ADVANCED STRENGTHENING (WEEKS 9–13)
Goals
• Increase strength, power, endurance
• Maintain full elbow ROM
• Gradually initiate sporting activities

A. Week 9
1. Initiate eccentric elbow flexion/extension
2. Continue isotonic program; forearm and wrist
3. Continue shoulder program – Thrower's Ten program
4. Manual resistance diagonal patterns
5. Initiate plyometric exercise program

B. Week 11
1. Continue all exercises listed above
2. May begin light sport activities (i.e. golf, swimming)

PHASE IV. RETURN TO ACTIVITY (WEEKS 14 THROUGH 26)
Goals
• Continue to increase strength, power, and endurance of upper extremity musculature
• Gradual return-to-sport activities

A. Week 14
1. Initiate interval throwing program (phase 1)
2. Continue strengthening program
3. Emphasis on elbow and wrist strengthening and flexibility exercises

B. Weeks 22 through 26
Return to competitive throwing

Various opinions exist regarding the efficacy of non-operative treatment for UCL strains or partial tears for the throwing athlete. If an injury to the UCL is suspected, the rehabilitation program outlined in Box 16.10 is initiated. Range of motion is initially permitted in a non-painful arc of motion, usually 10–100°, to allow for a decrease in inflammation and the alignment of collagen tissue. A brace may be used to restrict motion as well as prevent valgus strain. Isometric exercises are performed for the shoulder, elbow, and wrist to prevent muscular atrophy. Ice and anti-inflammatory medications are prescribed to control pain and inflammation.

Range of motion of both flexion and extension is gradually increased during the second phase of treatment as tolerated. Full ROM should be achieved by at least 3–4 weeks. Rhythmic stabilization exercises are initiated to develop dynamic stabilization and neuromuscular control of the upper extremity. As dynamic stability is advanced, isotonic exercises are incorporated for the entire upper extremity.

The advanced strengthening phase is usually initiated at 6 to 7 weeks postinjury. During this phase, the athlete is progressed to the Thrower's Ten isotonic strengthening program and plyometric exercises. An interval return to sport program is initiated once the athlete regains full motion, adequate strength, and dynamic stability of the elbow. The athlete is allowed to return to competition following the asymptomatic completion of the interval sport program. If symptoms continue to persist, the athlete is reassessed and possible surgical intervention is considered.

ULNAR COLLATERAL LIGAMENT RECONSTRUCTION

Surgical reconstruction of the UCL attempts to restore the stabilizing functions of the anterior bundle of the UCL (Andrews et al 1996). The palmaris longus or alternate graft source, is taken and passed in a figure-8 pattern through drill holes in the sublime tubercle of the ulna and the medial epicondyle (Andrews et al 1996). An ulnar nerve transposition is often performed at the time of reconstruction (Andrews et al 1996).

The rehabilitation program following UCL reconstruction varies based on the surgical technique, method of transpositioning of the ulnar nerve, and the overall extent of injury to the elbow. The rehabilitation program we currently use following UCL reconstruction is outlined in Box 16.11. The athlete is placed in a posterior splint with the elbow immobilized at 90° of flexion for the first 7 days postoperatively. This allows adequate healing of the UCL graft and soft tissue slings involved in the nerve transposition. The patient is allowed to perform wrist ROM, and gripping and submaximal isometrics, for the wrist and elbow. The patient is progressed from the posterior splint to an elbow ROM brace, which is adjusted to allow ROM from 30–100° of flexion. Motion is increased by 5° of extension and 10° of flexion thereafter to restore full ROM by the end of week 6 (0–145°). The brace is discontinued by weeks 5 to 6.

Isometric exercises are progressed to include light resistance isotonic exercises at week 4 and the full Thrower's Ten program by week 6. Sport-specific exercises are incorporated at weeks 8 to 9. Focus is again placed on developing dynamic stabilization of the medial elbow. Due to the anatomical orientation of the flexor carpi ulnaris and flexor digitorum superficialis overlaying the UCL, isotonic and stabilization activities for these muscles may assist the UCL in stabilizing valgus stress at the medial elbow.

Aggressive exercises involving eccentric and plyometric contractions are included in the advanced phase, usually weeks 9 through 14. An interval sport program is allowed at week 16 postoperatively. In most cases, throwing from a mound is progressed within 4 to 6 weeks following the initiation of an interval throwing program and a return to competitive throwing at approximately 6 to 7 months following surgery.

LESS COMMON SPORT-RELATED INJURIES

OSTEOCHONDRITIS DISSECANS

Osteochondritis dissecans of the elbow may develop due to the valgus strain on the elbow joint, which produces not only medial tension but also a lateral compressive force. This is observed as the capitulum of the humerus compresses with the radial head. Patients often complain of lateral elbow pain upon palpation and valgus stress. Morrey (1994) described a three-stage classification of pathological progression. Stage one describes patients without evidence of subchondral displacement or fracture, whereas stage two referred to lesions showing evidence of subchondral detachment or articular cartilage fracture. Stage three lesions involve detached osteochondral fragments, resulting in intra-articular loose bodies. Non-surgical treatment is attempted for

stage one patients only and consists of relative rest and immobilization until elbow symptoms have resolved.

Non-operative treatment includes 3 to 6 weeks of immobilization at 90° of elbow flexion. ROM activities for the shoulder, elbow, and wrist are performed 3–4 times a day. As symptoms resolve a strengthening program is initiated with isometric exercises. Isotonic exercises are included after approximately 1 week of isometric exercise. Aggressive high speed, eccentric, and plyometric exercises are progressively included to prepare the athlete for the start of an interval sport program.

If non-operative treatment fails, or evidence of loose bodies exists, surgical intervention including arthroscopic abrading and drilling of the lesion with fixation or removal of the loose body is indicated (Roberts & Hughes 1950). Long-term follow-up studies regarding the outcome of patients undergoing surgery to drill or reattach the lesions have not produced favorable results, suggesting that prevention and early detection of symptoms may be the best form of treatment (Baur et al 1992, Woodward & Bianco 1975).

DEGENERATIVE JOINT DISEASE

Degenerative joint disease (DJD) of the elbow may occur prematurely in certain athletes who participate in sport activities that repetitively load the articular surfaces of the elbow joint. Acceleration of joint degeneration and osteophyte formation may occur. Pain and joint effusion may be observed during examination, as well as tenderness to palpation over the joint lines. Although this particular pathology may not restrict normal function and activities of daily living, the pain and motion loss associated with DJD may restrict further participation in sports.

Conservative treatment is thus focused on first diminishing pain and inflammation and secondly, improving ROM and soft tissue flexibility. Warm whirlpool prior to stretching and gentle joint mobilization techniques may be beneficial to enhance soft tissue extensibility. As pain and ROM normalize, an overall enhancement of upper extremity strength and endurance is emphasized. In the event that conservative treatment does not produce favorable results, an open or arthroscopic debridement may be indicated to alleviate symptoms.

SYNOVITIS

Generalized joint synovitis may occur from the repetitive nature of throwing and other overhead sports. Patients often complain of a diffuse joint pain not specific to one area and a flexion contracture is revealed upon examination. Initial treatment includes anti-inflammatory medications and activity modification to allow for a period of rest and recovery.

The rehabilitation program is focused on restoring elbow extension. ROM, stretching and mobilization exercises are performed as necessary to restore and maintain full ROM. The clinician must be cautioned against overaggressive stretching and mobilization during the acute phases of recovery to avoid contributing to the inflammatory synovial reaction. Tepid to warm whirlpool treatment may be used prior to ROM exercises. Contrast treatment (cold to warm) may also be beneficial. Submaximal isometric exercises are performed until the inflammatory response has diminished, followed by the initiation of an isotonic strengthening program. A return to sport-specific drills and an interval sport program are instituted once the patient has achieved proper strength and a satisfactory clinical examination.

DISLOCATIONS

Dislocations of the elbow joint most commonly occur in contact sports such as football and wrestling or in non-contact sports as the athlete lands onto an outstretched hand. A hyperextension injury occurs as the olecranon is forced into the olecranon fossa and the trochlea translates posteriorly or posterolaterally over the coronoid process (Andrews & Whiteside 1993). Disruption of the UCL and possibly the RCL may occur. Fractures of the radial head or capitulum may also be seen concomitantly (Andrews & Whiteside 1993).

A lateral pivot shift test may be used to assess posterolateral stability of the elbow (O'Driscoll et al 1991). Initial reduction of the injury may be performed by applying traction to the forearm and humerus with the elbow in 30° of flexion (Andrews & Whiteside 1993). Neurovascular integrity should be assessed immediately and surgical intervention may be necessary to repair concomitant ligament instability and osseous fractures.

Treatment depends greatly on the severity of injury and the associated injuries that are present. An initial period of rest and immobilization may be warranted to allow for soft tissue healing and a decrease in pain and inflammation. Early motion should be initiated within the first week following injury to minimize the chances of motion loss, which is one of the primary complications following elbow dislocation (Richardson & Iglarsh 1994). Progression through rehabilitation follows a progressive sequence similar to the previously described program to regain motion and strength of the elbow and forearm.

FRACTURES

Various fractures of the elbow may occur in the athletic population, including extra- and intra-articular distal humerus fractures, radial head fractures, and olecranon fractures (Richardson & Iglarsh 1994). Stress fractures of the olecranon have been reported in overhead throwers and can occur in any part of the olecranon, especially in the midarticular area (Bennett 1941). The most likely cause of injury involves repetitive stresses applied to the olecranon as the elbow extends from triceps contraction during the acceleration, deceleration, and follow-through phases of throwing. Patients often subjectively report an insidious onset of pain in the posterolateral elbow while throwing. Symptoms appear similar to triceps tendonitis; however, tenderness over the involved site of the olecranon is often detected upon palpation. Plane radiographs are typically taken and diagnosis may be further enhanced with the aid of a bone scan and/or an MRI.

Aggressive stretching and strengthening exercises are restricted for the first 6 to 8 weeks to allow adequate healing of the fracture site. The athlete should maintain motion with light ROM exercises. Heavy lifting, plyometrics, and sport-specific drills are not allowed until bony healing is seen on radiographic evaluation, typically by 8 to 12 weeks. Once adequate healing has been documented, an interval sport program may be allowed. Complete recovery occurs in approximately 3 to 6 months following injury. An open reduction internal fixation may be indicated if conservative management fails.

ARTHROLYSIS

Many of the previous pathologies that have been discussed have involved motion loss as a primary complication. The elbow joint is one of the most frequent joints to develop motion loss (Timmerman & Andrews 1994, Green & McCoy 1979). Following injury, the elbow flexes in response to pain and hemarthrosis. The periarticular soft tissue and joint capsule become shortened, fibrotic, and loss of motion develops. An arthroscopic arthrolysis may be necessary in patients that do not respond to conservative treatment.

During the first postoperative week, the patient is instructed to perform elbow and wrist range of motion exercises hourly. Treatment to regain ROM at this time is cautiously aggressive (Wilk 1994). Full motion should be obtained quickly; however, a pace that does not cause additional inflammation of the joint capsule is necessary to avoid further pain and reflexive splinting. LLLD stretching has been an extremely beneficial treatment technique for us clinically. Full passive ROM is usually restored by day 10 to 14.

Isometric strengthening is begun during week 2 and progressed to isotonic dumbbell exercises during the third to fourth week. Strengthening exercises are progressed as tolerated by the patient. Emphasis during the later phases of rehabilitation continues to be placed on maintaining motion. Patients are educated to continue a motion maintenance program several times per day and before and after sport activities for at least 2 to 3 months following surgery.

SUMMARY

The elbow joint is a common site of injury in the athletic population. Injuries vary widely from repetitive microtraumatic injuries to gross macrotraumatic dislocations. A thorough understanding of the sport-specific anatomy and biomechanics of the joint are necessary for a successful clinical examination, assessment, and rehabilitation prescription. Rehabilitation of the elbow, whether post-injury or postsurgical, must follow a progressive and sequential order to ensure that healing tissues are not overstressed. A rehabilitation program that limits immobilization, achieves full ROM early, progressively restores strength and neuromuscular control, and gradually incorporates sport-specific activities is essential to successfully return athletes to their previous level of competition as quickly and safely as possible.

REFERENCES

Akeson W H, Amiel D, Woo S L Y 1980 Immobilization effects on synovial joints. The pathomechanics of joint contracture. Biorheology 17:95–107

Alley R M, Pappas A M 1995 Acute and performance-related injuries of the elbow. In: Pappas A M (ed) Upper extremity injuries in the athlete. Churchill Livingstone, New York, p 339–364

Anderson K 2001 Elbow arthritis and removal of loose bodies and spurs, and techniques for restoration of motion. In: Altchek D W, Andrews J R (eds) The athlete's elbow. Lippincott Williams and Wilkins, Philadelphia, p 219–230

Andrews J R, Frank W 1985 Valgus extension overload in the pitching elbow. In: Andrews J R, Zarins B, Carson W B (eds) Injuries to the throwing arm. WB Saunders, Philadelphia, p 250–257

Andrews J R, Whiteside J A 1993 Common elbow problems in the athlete. Journal of Orthopaedic and Sports Physical Therapy 17(6):289–295

Andrews J R, Timmerman L 1995 Outcome of elbow surgery in professional baseball players. American Journal of Sports Medicine 23:245–250

Andrews J R, Wilk K E, Satterwhite Y E et al 1993 Physical examination of the thrower's elbow. Journal of Orthopaedic and Sports Physical Therapy 17(6):296–304

Andrews J R, Jelsma R D, Joyse M E et al 1996 Open surgical procedures for injuries to the elbow in throwers. Operative Techniques in Sports Medicine 4(2):109–113

Andrews J R, Heggland E J H, Fleisig G S et al 2001 Relationship of ulnar collateral ligament strain to amount of medial olecranon osteotomy. American Journal of Sports Medicine 29(6):716–721

Atkinson W B, Elftman H 1945 The carrying angle of the human arm as a secondary sex character. The Anatomical Record 91:49–54

Basmajian J V, DeLuca C J 1985 Muscles alive: their function revealed by electromyography. Williams and Wilkins, Baltimore, p 279–280

Baur M, Jonsson K, Josefson P O et al 1992 Osteochondritis dissecans of the elbow: a long-term follow-up study. Clinical Orthopaedics and Related Research 284:156–160

Bennett G E 1941 Shoulder and elbow lesions of the professional baseball player. Journal of the American Medical Association 117:510–514

Blackburn T A, McCleod W D, White B 1990 EMG analysis of posterior rotator cuff exercises. Journal of Athletic Training 25:40–45

Coutts R, Rothe C, Kaita J 1981 The role of continuous passive motion in the rehabilitation of the total knee patient. Clinical Orthopaedics and Related Research 159:126–132

Cyriax J 1982 Textbook of Orthopedic Medicine (vol 1), Diagnosis of soft tissue lesions, 8th edn. Baillière Tindall, London, p 52–54

Dehne E, Tory R 1971 Treatment of joint injuries by immediate mobilization based upon the spiral adaptation concept. Clinical Orthopaedics and Related Research 77:218–232

Fleisig G S, Barrentine S W 1995 Biomechanical aspects of the elbow in sports. Sports Medicine and Arthroscopy Review 3:149–159

Fleisig G S, Escamilla R F 1996 Biomechanics of the elbow in the throwing athlete. Operative Techniques in Sports Medicine 4(2):62–68

Fleisig G S, Andrews J R, Dillman C J et al 1995 Kinetics of baseball pitching with implications about injury mechanisms. American Journal of Sports Medicine 23:233–239

Glazebrook M A, Curwin S, Islam M N et al 1994 Medial epicondylitis. an electromyographic analysis and an investigation of intervention strategies. American Journal of Sports Medicine 22:674–679

Glousman R E 1990 Ulnar nerve problems in the athlete's elbow. Clinics in Sports Medicine 9:365–377

Green D P, McCoy H 1979 Turnbuckle orthotic correction of elbow flexion contractures. Journal of Bone and Joint Surgery (Am) 61(A):1092

Haggmark T, Eriksson E 1979 Cylinder or mobile cast brace after knee ligament surgery: a clinical analysis and morphologic and enzymatic studies of changes of the quadriceps muscle. American Journal of Sports Medicine 7:48–56

Hoppenfeld S 1976 Physical examination of the spine and extremities. Appleton-Century-Crofts, New York, p 35–55

Jobe F W, Moynes D R, Tibone J E et al 1984 An EMG analysis of the shoulder in pitching. American Journal of Sports Medicine 12:218–220

Johansson O 1962 Capsular and ligament injuries of the elbow joint. Acta Chirurgica Scandinavica (suppl):287

Kapandji I A 1970 The physiology of the joints (vol 1). E & S Livingston, London, p 82–83, 112–117

Keats T E, Teeslink R, Diamond A E et al 1966 Normal axial relationships of the major joints. Radiology 87:904

Kelley B T, Weiland A J 2001 Posterolateral rotatory instability of the elbow. In: Altchek D W, Andrews J R (eds) The athlete's elbow. Lippincott Williams and Wilkins, Philadelphia, p 175–189

Kelley J D, Lombardo S J, Pink M et al 1994 EMG and cinematographic analysis of elbow function in tennis players with lateral epicondylitis. American Journal of Sports Medicine 22:359–363

Kendall F P, McCreary E K 1983 Muscles, testing, and function 3rd edn. Williams and Wilkins, Baltimore, p 86–87

Kibler W B 1994 Clinical biomechanics of the elbow in tennis: implications for evaluation and diagnosis. Medicine and Science in Sports and Exercise 26:1203–1206

Kottke F J, Pauley D L, Ptak R A 1966 The rationale for prolonged stretching for connective tissue. Archives of Physical Medicine and Rehabilitation 47:345–352

Lehmkuhl D L, Smith L R 1983 Brunnstrom's clinical kinesiology. FA Davis, Philadelphia, p 149–170

McCarroll J R 1985 Golf. In: Schneider R C et al (eds) Sports injuries: mechanisms, prevention, and treatment. Williams and Wilkins, Baltimore, p 290–294

McCarroll J R Gioe T J 1982 Professional golfers and the price they pay. Physician and Sports Medicine 10(7):64–70

Magee D J 1987 Orthopaedic physical assessment. WB Saunders, Philadelphia

Maitland G D 1977 Peripheral manipulation. Butterworth, Boston

Martin B F 1958 The annular ligament of the superior radioulnar joint. Journal of Anatomy 52:473

Martin S D, Baumgarten T E 1996 Elbow injuries in the throwing athlete: diagnosis and arthroscopic treatment. Operative Techniques in Sports Medicine 4(2):100–108

Morrey B F 1985 Anatomy of the elbow. In: Morrey B F (ed) The elbow and its disorders. Saunders, Philadelphia, p 7–40

Morrey B F 1994 Osteochondritis dissecans. In: DeLee J C, Drez D (eds) Orthopedic sports medicine. Saunders, Philadelphia, p 908–912

Morrey B F, An K N 1983 Articular and ligamentous contributions to the static stability of the elbow joint. American Journal of Sports Medicine 11:315–319

Morrey B F, An K N, Dobyns J 1985 Functional anatomy of the elbow ligaments. Clinical Orthopaedics and Related Research 201:84

Morris M, Jobe F W, Perry J et al 1989 EMG analysis of elbow function in tennis players. American Journal of Sports Medicine 17:241–247

Moseley V B, Jobe F W, Pink M 1992 EMG analysis of the scapular muscles during a shoulder rehabilitation program. American Journal of Sports Medicine 20(3):128–134

Nirschl R P, Morrey B F 1985 Rehabilitation. In: Morrey B F (ed) The elbow and its disorders. WB Saunders, Philadelphia, p 147–152

Norkin C, Levangie P 1985 Joint structure and function: a comprehensive analysis. FA Davis, Philadelphia, p 191–210

Norkin C C, White D J 1995 Measurement of joint motion: a guide to goniometry, 2nd edn. FA Davis, Philadelphia

Noyes F R, Mangine R E, Barber S E 1987 Early knee motion after open and arthroscopic anterior cruciate ligament reconstruction. American Journal of Sports Medicine 15:149–160

O'Driscoll S W, Bell D F, Morrey B F 1991 Posterolateral rotatory instability of the elbow. Journal of Bone and Joint Surgery (Am) 73A:440–446

Pavly J E, Rushing J L, Scheving L E 1967 Electromyographic study of some muscles crossing the elbow joint. Journal of Anatomy 159:47–53

Perkins G 1954 Rest and motion. Journal of Bone and Joint Surgery (Br) 35(B):521–539

Rhu K N, McCormick J, Jobe F W et al 1988 An electromyographic analysis of shoulder function in tennis players. American Journal of Sports Medicine 16:481

Richardson J K, Iglarsh Z A 1994 Clinical orthopaedic physical therapy. WB Saunders, Philadelphia, p 227–230

Roberts W, Hughes R 1950 Osteochondritis dissecans of the elbow joint: a clinical study. Journal of Bone and Joint Surgery (Br) 32(B):348–360

St John J N, Palmaz J C 1986 The cubital tunnel in ulnar entrapment neuropathy. Musculoskeletal Radiology 158:119

Salter R B, Simmonds D F, Malcolm B W et al 1980 The effects of continuous passive motion on healing of full thickness defects in articular cartilage. Journal of Bone and Joint Surgery (Am) 62A:1232–1251

Salter R B, Hamilton H W, Wedge J H 1984 Clinical application of basic research on continuous passive motion for disorders and injuries of synovial joints. A preliminary report of a feasibility study. Journal of Orthopedic Research 1:325–342

Sapega A A, Quedenfeld T C, Moyer R A et al 1976 Biophysical factors in range of motion exercise. Archives of Physical Medicine and Rehabilitation 57:122–126

Schwab G H, Bennett J B, Woods G W et al 1980 The biomechanics of elbow stability: the role of the medial collateral ligament. Clinical Orthopaedics and Related Research 146:42

Soderberg G L 1981 Kinesiology application to pathological motion. Williams and Wilkins, Baltimore, p 131–136

Spinner M, Kaplan E B 1970 The quadrate ligament of the elbow – its relationship to the stability of the proximal radioulnar joint. Acta Orthopaedica Scandinavica 41:632

Stanish W D, Loebenberg M I, Kozey J W 1994 The elbow. In: Stover C N, McCarroll J R, Mallon W J (eds) Feeling up to par: medicine from tee to green. FA Davis, Philadelphia, p 143–149

Timmerman L A, Andrews J R 1994 Undersurface tears of the ulnar collateral ligament in baseball players. A newly recognized lesion. American Journal of Sports Medicine 22:33–36

Tipton C M, Mathies R D, Martin R F 1978 Influence of age and sex on strength of bone-ligament junctions in knee joints in rats. Journal of Bone and Joint Surgery (Am) 60(A):230–236

Townsend H, Jobe F W, Pink M et al 1991 Electromyographic analysis of the glenohumeral muscles during a baseball rehabilitation program. American Journal of Sports Medicine 19(3):264–272

Warren C G, Lehmann J F, Koblanski J N 1971 Elongation of rat tail tendon: effect of load and temperature. Archives of Physical Medicine and Rehabilitation 52:465–474

Warren C G, Lehmann J F, Koblanski J N 1976 Heat and stretch procedures: an evaluation using rat tail tendon. Archives of Physical Medicine and Rehabilitation 57:122–126

Werner S, Fleisig G S, Dillman C J et al 1993 Biomechanics of the elbow during baseball pitching. Journal of Orthopaedic and Sports Physical Therapy 17:274–278

Wilk K E 1994 Rehabilitation of the elbow following arthroscopic surgery. In: Andrews J R, Soffer S R (eds) Elbow arthroscopy. Mosby, St. Louis, p 109–116

Wilk K E, Levinson M 2001 Rehabilitation of the athlete's elbow. In: Altchek D W, Andrews J R (eds) The athlete's elbow. Lippincott Williams and Wilkins, Philadelphia, p 249–273

Wilk K E, Arrigo C, Andrews J R 1993a Rehabilitation of the elbow in the throwing athlete. Journal of Orthopaedic and Sports Physical Therapy 17(6):305–317

Wilk K E, Voight M, Keirns M D et al 1993b Plyometrics for the upper extremities: theory and clinical application. Journal of Orthopaedic and Sports Physical Therapy 17:225–239

Wilk K E, Andrews J R, Arrigo C A et al 2001a Preventive and rehabilitative exercises for the shoulder and elbow, 6th edn. American Sports Medicine Institute, Birmingham

Wilk K E, Reinold M M, Andrews J R 2001b Postoperative treatment principles in the throwing athlete. Sports Medicine and Arthroscopy Review 9:69–95

Wilson F D, Andrews J R, Blackburn T A et al 1983 Valgus extension overload in the pitching elbow. American Journal of Sports Medicine 11(2):83–88

Woodward A H, Bianco A J Jr 1975 Osteochondritis dissecans of the elbow. Clinical Orthopaedics and Related Research 110:35–41

Wyke B D 1966 The neurology of joints. Annals of the Royal College of Surgeons (London) 41:25–29

17

Wrist and hand

Paul LaStayo   Susan Michlovitz

INTRODUCTION

The incidence of all sport-related injuries occurring to the wrist and hand is 3–9% (Arendt 1999). These injuries are more common in the adolescent athlete than in the adult. Wrist injuries typically occur during contact sports or with frequent weightbearing activities through the upper extremity (e.g. gymnastics). Athletic finger injuries such as sprains, fractures, dislocations, and tendon ruptures occur more often in ball-handling sports (e.g. basketball, baseball, and volleyball) (Arendt 1999). This chapter will focus on wrist and hand sport-related injuries, including the examination and management of these injuries.

SPORT-SPECIFIC APPLIED ANATOMY

THE WRIST COMPLEX

The distal radius, distal ulna and two rows of carpal bones make up the wrist complex. The distal articular surface of the radius angles palmarly 10–15° and inclines ulnarly 15–25° (Palmer 1993). Restoration of these angles and the bony relationships is imperative after injury (Kaukonen et al 1988, Laseter & Carter 1996, McQueen 1988) because badly united fractures, especially dorsal angulation and shortening of the radius (relative to the ulna), can lead to limited range of motion (ROM) (Kazuki et al 1993), mid-carpal instability (Taliesnik & Watson 1984), ulnar wrist pain (due to alterations in the transmission of axial forces) (Short et al 1987) and reduced grip strength (Villar & Marsh 1987).

Both the radiocarpal and mid-carpal joints contribute to wrist motion. Normally the wrist flexion/extension arc is 160–180° and the radial/ulnar deviation arc is 60°. Functional ROM, however, is 40° for both flexion and extension and a 40° arc of deviation (Ryu et al 1991). The

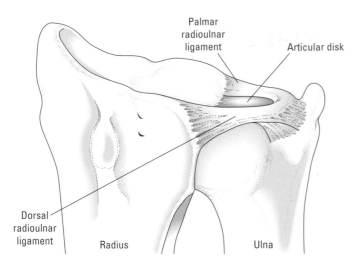

Figure 17.1 Triangular fibrocartilage complex (TFCC) ligaments and articular disk. The ligaments of the TFCC that provide stability to the distal radioulnar joint (DRUJ) are the dorsal and palmar radioulnar ligaments. The centrally located articular disk is the fibrocartilaginous component of the TFCC which does not provide stability to the DRUJ.

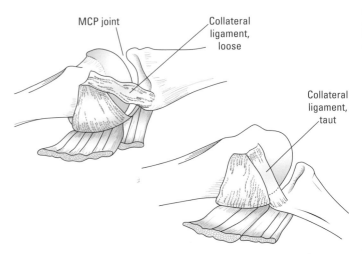

Figure 17.2 The metacarpophalangeal (MCP) joint collateral ligament is loose in joint extension and taut in joint flexion. If immobilized in extension, the collateral ligaments structurally shorten, thereby preventing MCP flexion.

distal radioulnar joint (DRUJ), in concert with the proximal radioulnar joint, is responsible for the 170° arc of forearm rotation (Chidgey 1995). Within the proximal carpal row, two of the most important intrinsic stabilizing ligaments are the scapholunate (SL) and lunotriquetral (LT) while at the DRUJ, the critical soft tissues are encompassed in the triangular fibrocartilage complex (TFCC) (Berger & Garcia-Elias 1991, Horii et al 1991, Ruby et al 1987). The radioulnar ligamentous components of the TFCC and the interosseous membrane are the primary stabilizers of the DRUJ. The articular disk (triangular fibrocartilage) of the TFCC, however, does not contribute to joint stability (Chidgey 1995, Kihara et al 1995) (Fig. 17.1).

THE FINGER JOINTS

The finger joints include the metacarpophalangeal (MCP), proximal interphalangeal (PIP) and distal interphalangeal (DIP) joints. A disruption of the surrounding soft tissue structures can cause a characteristic deformity or motion loss. PIP joint dislocations, extensor and flexor tendon ruptures and collateral ligament sprains or tears will be discussed later in this chapter.

The MCP joints of the digits are formed by the cam-shaped distal end of the metacarpal and the biconcave proximal end of the proximal phalanx. This osseous arrangement provides little bony stability. Flexion/extension and radial/ulnar deviation, with a small amount of supination and pronation, occurs at the MCP joints. In extension, the true or band fibers of the MCP collateral ligaments are in their slack position, and in a fully flexed position, these ligaments are lengthened to a taut position (Fig. 17.2). For this reason, there is minimal radial and ulnar deviation at the MCP joint when it is fully flexed. Injury to the true collateral ligament will cause excessive deviation (radial/ulnar) on passive motion when the joint is fully flexed. On the volar joint surface, the main supporting structure is the volar or palmar plate. The volar plate at the MCP joint is less constraining than at the PIP and DIP, thus allowing significant hyperextension (30–45°) at that joint. This motion, coupled with ulnar deviation, is important for activities requiring palmar push off or ball handling. MCP flexion values greater than 90° occur at the 5th digit for a strong and tight fist (Werner 1996).

The PIP and DIP joints have more inherent bony stability and a stiffer, less compliant volar plate than the

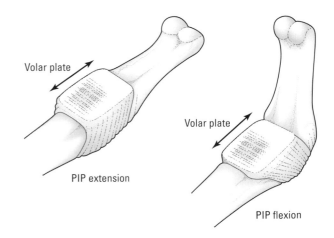

Figure 17.3 The proximal interphalangeal joint (PIP) volar plate is relatively non-compliant and does not change length with joint motion, hence it is a primary stabilizer to the PIP joint. To allow PIP joint movement the volar plate glides proximally and distally. If the excursion of the volar plate is restricted, particularly the distal excursion, loss of PIP extension occurs.

MCP joint. Unlike the MCP joint, the true collateral ligaments are taut throughout the range of motion. The injured PIP joint has a propensity for flexion deformity, initially due to joint effusion and ultimately due to limited gliding of the volar plate (Fig. 17.3). Normal flexion ROM at the PIP is 100–110° and at the DIP it can be up to 90° (Freeland & Sennett 1996).

CARPOMETACARPAL JOINTS (INCLUDING THE THUMB)

The carpometacarpal (CMC) joints act as a link between the wrist and the digits. The first CMC joint, termed the basal joint of the thumb, has 3° of freedom, permitting flexion/extension, abduction/adduction and opposition/reposition. There is 40° abduction, 50° flexion and 80° opposition (Cooney et al 1981). During pinch, the forces at this joint are 12 times that at the tips of the fingers (Cooney et al 1981). The primary stabilizing structure preventing posterior translation of the metacarpal on the trapezium during pinch is the volar oblique (beak) ligament (Pellegrini 1991). Attenuation of this ligament has been implicated in the commonly occurring instability/osteoarthritis of the basal joint. This arthritis has its highest prevalence in postmenopausal women. The 2nd and 3rd CMC joints are relatively immobile and act to transmit weightbearing loads from the metacarpals through the capitate and trapezoid. A degenerative osteophyte, termed a carpal boss, can occur about these joints. The 4th and 5th CMCs have 20–25° of flexion, motion that is necessary for 'cupping' of the hand around spherical and conical objects as well as making a full fist.

The two distal joints of the thumb, the MCP and interphalangeal (IP), work in concert with the CMC to position the thumb. The thumb is rotated 90° from the plane of the fingers and has the added motion of opposition to position the thumb against the fingers for prehension and precision activities. Because of the position of the thumb, it is vulnerable to lateral stresses, such as that which occur with the so-called 'ski pole' injury (injury to the ulnar collateral ligament of the MCP joint). In addition to the stability provided by the collateral ligaments, stability against lateral stress is provided by the aponeurosis of the adductor pollicis muscle, which inserts on the base of the proximal phalanx and has an intimate relationship with the ulnar collateral ligament (UCL).

MUSCLE/TENDON STRUCTURES OF THE WRIST AND HAND

Extensor tendons and compartments of the wrist

The three primary wrist extensors are: the extensor carpi radialis longus (ECRL) and brevis (ECRB) in the second compartment, and the extensor carpi ulnaris (ECU) in the sixth compartment. The ECRL is most effective as a wrist extensor when the elbow is extended and when radial deviation is balanced by the primary ulnar deviator (the ECU) (Brand & Hollister 1993). The ECRB is a more effective wrist extensor due to its insertion on the base of the third metacarpal, its larger moment arm for wrist extension, and the fact it is not influenced by elbow position (Brand & Hollister 1993).

The first dorsal compartment contains the abductor pollicis longus (APL) and the extensor pollicis brevis (EPB) tendons. The APL and EPB tendons may be separated by septations (fibrous or osseofibrous divisions), which create separate compartments and potential sites of compression (Kirkpatrick 1990). Septations are commonly found in patients with De Quervain's disease, also known as stenosing tenovaginitis (Kirkpatrick 1990).

Ruptures of tendons that cross the wrist are more commonly seen at the third compartment where the extensor pollicis longus (EPL) tendon turns radially at Lister's tubercle. This is most common in patients with rheumatoid arthritis and/or fractures of the distal radius (Rosenthal 1990). Blending with the dorsal wrist capsule are the floor of the fourth and fifth compartments, which contain the extensor digitorum communis (EDC), extensor indicis proprius and the extensor digiti quinti. They become primary wrist extensors when extension of the wrist follows digital extension in an obligate fashion. This is, however, an unnatural functional sequence as it limits the spatial positioning of the hand and grasping power and is often limited during rehabilitation following wrist fractures (Rosenthal 1990).

Finger extensors and extensor mechanism of the fingers

EDC tendons are maintained in position over the dorsum of MCP joints by sagittal bands, which are components of the dorsal hood. Injury to sagittal bands results in painful subluxation of these tendons during digital flexion and extension. The EDC tendons are also maintained in position through their juncturae tendinae on the dorsum of the hand. The conjoint lateral bands of the lumbricals and interossei travel dorsally to the axis of motion of the PIP and DIP. Injury to the extensor tendon, the central slip component, over the PIP joint and/or the triangular membrane over the middle phalanx can cause volar migration of the lateral bands and a subsequent boutonnière deformity (PIP flexion + DIP hyperextension). Dorsal displacement of the lateral bands can cause a swan neck deformity (PIP hyperextension + DIP flexion). Distally, the terminal tendon inserts onto the distal phalanx for DIP extension. Direct impact to the tip of the finger can tear or avulse the terminal tendon and result in an extension deficit called mallet finger. The mallet finger can also precipitate a swan neck deformity.

Finger flexors of the digits

The tendons which flex the digits stem from the muscle bellies of the flexor digitorum superficialis (FDS) and the flexor digitorum profundus (FDP). Both tendons travel through a synovial sheath in the fingers. Nutrition to the tendons occurs via perfusion extrinsically via vincula, and diffusion intrinsically as the tendons move through synovial fluid within the tendon sheath. The confined structure of the tenosynovial sheath, with its two tendons within, is an area for adhesion formation after phalangeal fractures, crush injuries and flexor tendon injuries and repair. The tendons are reinforced within their tendon sheaths, to maintain their moment arms and mechanical advantage, via fibrous annular (A) pulleys. The A1 pulley is the location where a tendon stenosis can occur resulting in a trigger finger. The A2 and A4 pulleys are the most important as they maintain optimal moment arms and facilitate optimal tendon excursion. All tendons travel in a synovial sheath through the carpal tunnel with the median nerve. In addition to carpal tunnel syndrome, flexor tenosynovitis can occur at the wrist. The flexor pollicus longus (FPL) tendon also travels through the carpal tunnel with the long finger flexors (FDS and FDP) and has a continuous tendon sheath to its insertion on the distal phalanx of the thumb.

NEUROLOGICAL AND VASCULAR STRUCTURES OF THE WRIST AND HAND

The median nerve, originating from the nerve roots of C5–7, provides cutaneous innervation to the radial side of the palm, volar thumb, index, middle and radial half of the ring finger, and the dorsum of these digits over the distal phalanx (Pratt 1996). The palmar cutaneous branch of the median nerve branches off proximal to the wrist joint and primarily innervates the skin of the thenar eminence. The remainder of the median nerve has cutaneous and motor branches and travels under the transverse carpal ligament, through the carpal tunnel. The common and proper digital nerves provide cutaneous innervation to the aforementioned digits, with the recurrent branch innervating the muscles of the thenar eminence. Carpal tunnel syndrome involves the median nerve distal to the palmar cutaneous branch.

The radial nerve, originating from the nerve roots of C6–8, only has a cutaneous branch at the level of the hand, supplying the skin to the dorsum of the thumb and hand including digits 2 and 3 and the radial half of the

ring finger to the level of the distal phalanx. This superficial branch originates near the elbow, deep to the brachioradialis as the radial nerve splits to the superficial and deep (posterior) interosseous branches. This nerve can become irritated due to a blow to the radial side of the wrist or with surgery (particularly external fixation of distal radius fractures) on that side of the wrist, often producing dysesthesia and hyperesthesia, both of which are difficult to treat.

The ulnar nerve, originating from the nerve roots of C8–T1, splits into two branches before entering the wrist and hand. One branch travels dorsally (dorsal cutaneous branch of the ulnar nerve) to provide sensation to the ulnar dorsum of the hand and the dorsum of the ulnar half of the ring finger and to the little finger. On the volar surface, the other branch of the ulnar nerve travels between the pisiform and hamate to innervate the hypothenar muscles, interossei, 4th and 5th lumbricales, adductor pollicus and 50% of the flexor pollicus brevis. The ulnar nerve also provides sensation to the volar surfaces of the little and ulnar half of the ring fingers.

The blood supply to the hand is via the ulnar and radial arteries, with two major 'arches' formed. The superficial palmar arterial arch is supplied by the ulnar artery, and the superficial palmar branch of the radial artery. This superficial arch forms the digital arteries to all but the thumb and radial aspect of the index finger. These lateral digits are perfused by the radial artery. The deep palmar arterial arch is formed by the radial artery and deep branch of the ulnar artery (Pratt, 1996). With arterial occlusion, there will be a spontaneous onset of digital pain. Inadequate blood flow results in pain, cold sensitivity, weakness and may lead to ulceration and tissue necrosis (Coleman & Anson 1961).

EXAMINATION – GENERAL CONCEPTS RELATED TO THE WRIST AND HAND

Taking a thorough history, performing a meticulous physical examination and corroborating these findings with additional studies (e.g. imaging and electro-physiology) is the hallmark of the assessment of wrist/hand pain and impairment (Beckenbaugh 1984, Cyriax 1982). The tenets of the examination are:

- The patient should describe and perform the task or maneuver that precipitates their symptoms, starting at the least symptomatic region and concluding with the most symptomatic region.
- The exam progression, as suggested by Cyriax (1982), is: active range of motion→ passive range of motion→ isomeric resistive tests→ provocative maneuvers → palpation.

- Provocative maneuvers (predicted to be painful) should be the last maneuver performed.
- Assessing the status of cutaneous nerves with sensory testing if a nerve injury is suspected, e.g. reduced or abnormal sensations.
- Grip strength testing is an index of muscle performance and of a joint's ability to withstand a load.
- Electromyography (EMG) and nerve conduction velocity (NCV) can help locate an area of nerve injury/entrapment and can determine the nerve and muscle's status.
- Radiographic images (see Ch. 29) directly reveal the integrity, relationships and contours of the wrist/hand osseous structures and indirectly, the ligamentous status.
- A generic and/or condition-specific outcome measure can assess a patient's perception of disability and should be coupled with physical measures (see Ch. 12).

COMMON SPORT-RELATED INJURIES

MANAGEMENT OF WRIST AND HAND PAIN AND IMPAIRMENT

In this section, the following will be presented: (1) an algorithmic approach toward managing radial (Fig. 17.4), central (Fig. 17.5) and ulnar-based (Fig. 17.6) wrist pain and impairment, (2) management principles for sport-specific hand and finger injuries and, (3) treatment concepts, options and caveats (Table 17.1) for major diagnostic categories that affect the hand and wrist.

RADIAL WRIST PAIN AND IMPAIRMENT

Fractures

Scaphoid fractures encompass 70% of all carpal fractures, which are more often noted in young males participating in athletic events (Botte & Gelberman 1987, Zemel & Stark 1986). Unfortunately, scaphoid non-unions are not uncommon due to the scaphoid's dependence on a single interosseous blood supply that is often disrupted after fracture (Gelberman et al 1983, Prosser & Herbert 1996). Hyperextension and carpal supination forces, due to a fall on an outstretched hand (FOOSH), are the typical mechanisms of action in distal radius and scaphoid fractures (and/or ligamentous instability) (Mayfield 1981, Weber & Chao 1978). The distal radius osteoporotic fracture in the elderly is common (Laseter & Carter 1996). The higher velocity distal radius fracture, the most common snowboarding injury, tends to have greater soft tissue damage than the typical osteoporotic-type elderly

fracture, hence, problems with swelling and return of ROM are more pronounced in the former than the latter. Following the immobilization and fracture healing of either the scaphoid or distal radius, there is often a limitation of wrist extension (additionally forearm supination in the latter) and pain at the extremes of motion (Weber 1980). Grip strength is also reduced by more than 50% (Laseter & Carter 1996, Prosser & Herbert 1996). Overcoming wrist stiffness and a return to functional wrist motion is a priority. Treatment options and approaches are presented in Figure 17.7 and Table 17.1.

After addressing the passive range of motion (PROM) limitations, one must not underestimate the importance of reconstituting active wrist extension via the ECRL and ECRB, rather than the digital extensors prior to strengthening activities. Treatment guidelines for radius and scaphoid fractures are outlined in Table 17.2. In the pediatric wrist patient, especially gymnasts, epiphyseal plate injuries are not uncommon. Radiographic findings are often negative, but the clinical signs of pain (with palpation) and swelling over the physis are indicative of this injury (Sotereanos et al 1994).

Tenderness in the anatomical snuff box following a FOOSH is thought to be pathopneumonic for a scaphoid fracture in younger individuals. This region, however, needs to be explored proximally in the older athlete, at the distal radius where the radial styloid process is located, as symptomatic degenerative changes in the posttraumatic and aged patient are not uncommon. Tenderness and edema in this region may be present (and accentuated with radial deviation) especially when the radial styloid is fractured and/or a scaphoid irritation is occurring on the radial styloid (radial styloid impingement). If the latter is noted on radiograph and coupled with pain on forced radial deviation, as with decelerating a golf club at the peak of a backswing, rest and protection with a long opponens splint (Fig. 17.8) coupled with an alteration of the task are required. (Watson & Ryu 1986, Whipple 1992). Instability of the scaphoid (via non-union or a ligamentous disruption) can be associated with the scapholunate advanced collapse (SLAC) wrist condition. SLAC wrist pathology is a pattern of degenerative changes that are based on and caused by articular alignment problems between the scaphoid, lunate, capitate and the radius. Pain and impairments are pronounced and are exacerbated by axial loading (gripping) and radial deviation (Watson & Ballet 1984).

Instability

In addition to fractures, a FOOSH can result in isolated ligamentous damage, with injury to the scapholunate (SL) ligament being the most common (Wright &

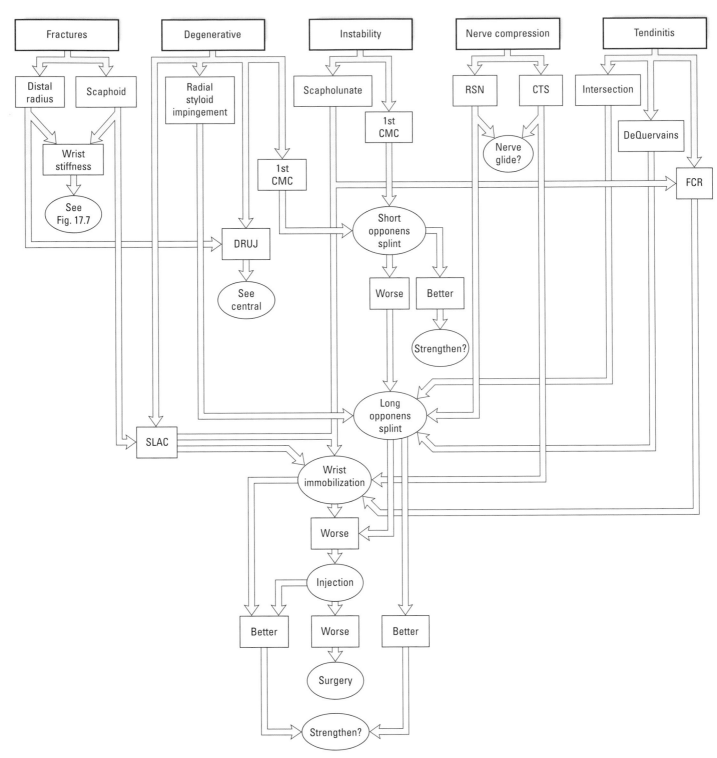

Figure 17.4 An algorithm to guide the differential diagnosis and treatment concepts of radial wrist pain and impairment. SLAC = scapholunate advanced collapse, DRUJ = distal radioulnar joint, CMC = carpometacarpal joint, RSN = radial sensory neuritis, CTS = carpal tunnel syndrome, FCR = flexor carpi radialis.

Michlovitz 1996). Ligament injuries in association with fractures occur frequently (>50%) (Richards et al 1997). In SL dissociations (e.g. rotary subluxation of the scaphoid), there is a characteristic dorsal/radial swelling of the wrist, lack of ROM, pain with gripping, a positive scaphoid shift test (Watson's Test) (Watson et al 1988, 1993) (Table 17.3), and a radiographic carpal instability pattern will sometimes be noted (Weber 1984). An intact

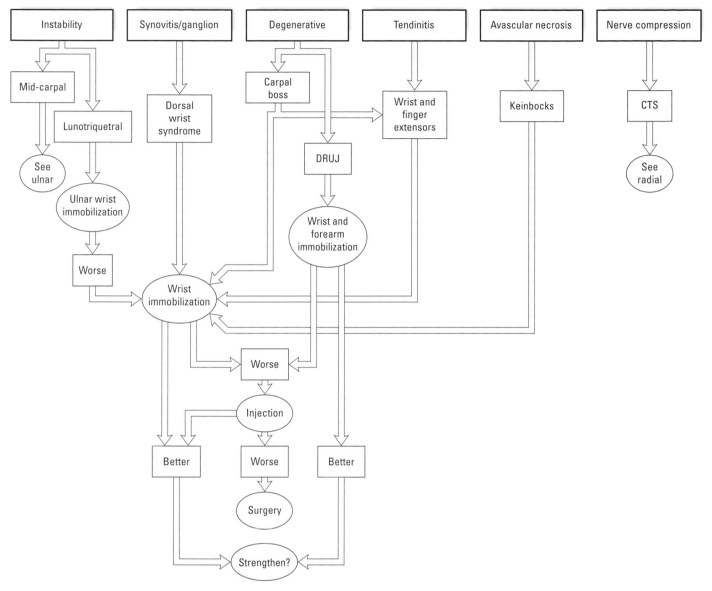

Figure 17.5 An algorithm to guide the differential diagnosis and treatment concepts of central wrist pain and impairment. DRUJ = distal radioulnar joint.

SL ligament forces the lunate to move with the scaphoid into palmar flexion with radial deviation. With a disrupted SL ligament, however, the lunate is free to assume its natural (and triquetrum-influenced) dorsi-flexed position, while the scaphoid continues to palmar-flex (hence the rotary subluxation of the scaphoid). This instability pattern, a dorsiflexion intercalated segment instability (DISI), is in reference to the lunate's position (Wright & Michlovitz 1996). In many instances a dynamic instability is present, especially in those with a diagnosis of a 'wrist sprain', whereby an axial load (gripping) must be employed to create the DISI and pain (Wright & Michlovitz 1996). Often a carpal instability radiographic series with the patient making a fist (axially loaded film)

is required to pick up dynamic instabilities (Gilula & Yin 1996). The flexor carpi radialis (FCR) can often become inflamed with overuse in racket sports and with throwing. This tendon's intimate relationship to the scaphoid warrants close assessment of an underlying scaphoid instability.

Vigorous ROM activities are contraindicated in the presence of wrist instabilities. Stability can sometimes be restored with wrist splinting, either a long opponens (Fig. 17.8) or a wrist control (Fig. 17.9) and avoidance of axial loading (resistive fisting), but surgical stabilization is often required. To ensure no fisting activity, a distal block of finger flexion may need to be incorporated into the splint. Treatment options and caveats are outlined in

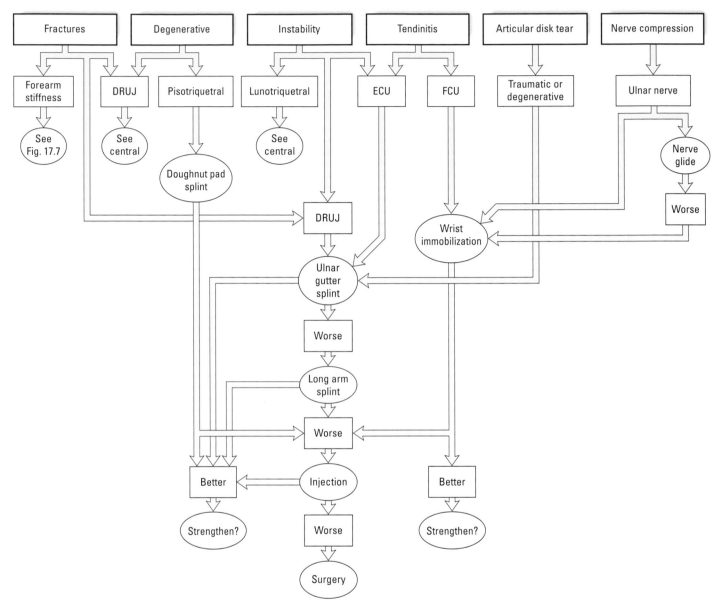

Figure 17.6   An algorithm to guide the differential diagnosis and treatment concepts of ulnar wrist pain and impairment. ECU = extensor carpi ulnaris, DRUJ = distal radioulnar joint, FCR = flexor carpi radialis.

Table 17.1, while Table 17.2 describes management during the phases of recovery from a wrist instability.

Degenerative disorders

The 1st CMC joint of the thumb has the greatest amount of ROM in the wrist and hand and experiences relatively high loads (4–5 times the applied external load) with pinching and grasping (Cooney & Chao 1977). Therefore, the impairments related to osteoarthritis of the basal joint of the thumb include a spectrum of disorders ranging from instability (in the young) and degenerative joint disease (DJD)/deformities (in older individuals).

Problems with pinching and grasping in tasks such as writing or swinging a racket or club are usually coupled with pain and swelling. The axial compression-adduction 'grind test' (Table 17.3) (Eaton & Littler 1969) is used to identify CMC joint arthrosis and to assess the stability of the CMC joint.

Splinting (Figs 17.8 and 17.10) or taping (Fig. 17.11) that will allow both protection and rest of the unstable 1st CMC joint can be fashioned in many ways, however, the principle of providing stability at the joint while pinching is essential. Several splint designs can provide the needed support, however, the short opponens is typically preferred (Fig. 17.10) (Weiss et al 2000).

Table 17.1 Treatment of wrist and hand pain and impairment: concepts, applications, adjuncts, and caveats

	Concept	Treatment Application	Caveats	Treatment Adjunct(s)
Protection/Rest (Shultz-Johnson 1996)	Rigid immobilization	Casting	Too long duration = stiffness Too short duration = non/delayed union, instability	Anti-inflammatories by mouth and/or transdermally (e.g. iontophoresis, phonophoresis Ch. 13) Electrophysiological agents (Ch. 13)
	Semi-rigid immobilization	Pre-fabricated or custom splinting		
	Incomplete immobilization and/or athletic participation	Athletic taping, silicone rubber, neoprene, foam rubber		
Strengthening (See Ch. 9)	To overload or not with wrist/hand patients?	Resistance exercises (see Ch. 9).	The potential risks (overstressing structures before they are biologically prepared for such stressors, promoting inflammation and pain) versus benefits (increasing muscle mass, function, and overall performance) must be considered before implementing a strengthening program	Consider eccentric muscle loading for high muscle tensions
Joint Stiffness (Flowers & LaStayo 1994, Threlkeld 1992)	HLBS (Threlkeld 1992) LLPS (TERT) (Flowers & LaStayo 1994)	Joint mobilization Dynamic splinting, prolonged positioning	Pain, inflammation, increased stiffness See algorithm (Fig. 17.7) (McClure et al 1994)	Manipulation under anesthesia, or surgical joint release
Instability (Wright & Michlovitz 1996)	Protect and rest (complete or partial) 4–8 weeks No pain prior to strengthening/ROM	See protection and rest as above	Transient joint stiffness may not be detrimental Joint pain indicates inadequate protection and/or excessive joint loading	Anti-inflammatories and modalities as above Surgical stabilization
Degenerative joint disease (Eaton & Littler 1969, Jaffe et al 1996, Michlovitz & Kozin 2000)	Avoid provocative activities Protect/rest as above	Behavioral modification See protection and rest as above	Strengthening not always a good option if it aggravates degenerative region	Anti-inflammatories and modalities as above Injections (e.g. anesthetic, corticosteroid)
Tendonitis/synovitis (Mennell 1964, Cyriax 1982)	Avoid provocative activities Protect/rest as above	Behavioral modification See protection and rest as above	Gentle stretching and resistance exercises can be helpful if the dosages are minimal to moderate	Anti-inflammatories and modalities as above Injections (e.g. anesthetic, corticosteroid)
Nerve (Mackinnon & Novak 1997, Sweeney & Harms 1996)	Protection/rest or nerve mobilization	See protection and rest as above Avoid traction to nerve Nerve gliding	If protection increases symptoms add motion If traction/gliding increases symptoms stop nerve mobilization	Anti-inflammatories and modalities as above Surgical decompression

HLBS = high load brief stress, LLPS = low load prolonged stress, ROM = range of motion

Tendonitis

De Quervain's tenosynovitis of the EPB and APL in the first dorsal compartment of the wrist is common with repetitive sporting activities or tasks requiring ulnar deviation and thumb movement (Keon-Cohen 1951). Palpation of the first extensor compartment proximal to the anatomical snuff box may reveal tenderness, swelling and tendinous nodules (Berger & Dobyns 1996). More proximally, intersection syndrome (see table for provocative test), where the APL and EPB muscles lie across the radial wrist extensors (~3cm proximal to the radial styloid), is a disorder that mimics de Quervain's and frequently causes crepitus and swelling along the radial forearm in weightlifters and rowers (Wood & Dobyns 1986). A Finkelstein's test (Table 17.3) is the classic evaluative provocative maneuver for de Quervain's and is positive if intense pain is experienced along the styloid process of the radius in the region of the 1st dorsal compartment (Finkelstein 1930). In addition, however, the Finkelstein testing position may irritate thumb CMC

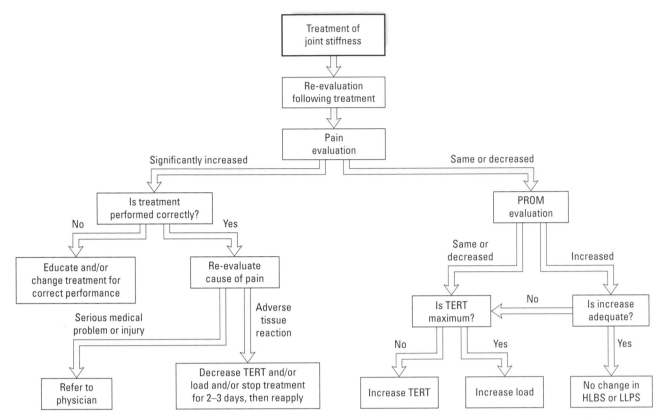

Figure 17.7 An algorithm to guide the use of treatments for joint stiffness secondary to structural changes to periarticular soft tissues. HLBS = high load brief stress, LLPS = low load prolonged stress, TERT = total end range time (duration × frequency of treatment per treatment session), Load = the amount of force applied during treatment session. Adverse tissue reaction = swelling, heat, pain (Adapted from McClure P W, Blackburn L G, Dusold C 1994 The use of splints in the treatment of joint stiffness: biologic rationale and an algorithm for making clinical decisions. Physical Therapy: 74: 1101–1107, with permission of the American Physical Therapy Association.)

DJD and/or provoke an established radial sensory neuritis or intersection syndrome.

The primary goal of treatment is to reduce pain and inflammation with splinting (Fig. 17.8) and modalities such as iontophoresis (Table 17.1). Education as to postures and sport-related techniques that both irritate (thumb adduction and wrist radial deviation) and relieve de Quervain's tensosynovitis is essential. Taping (Fig. 17.11) during sport can provide temporary relief. Strengthening of the small thumb tendons should be progressed slowly or omitted. If pain is elicited with strengthening activities, these exercises should be stopped. Factors that affect tendonitis and synovitis (Table 17.1), and specifically the recovery of de Quervain's, are outlined in Table 17.4.

Nerve compression and traction

The radial sensory nerve (RSN) along the radial aspect of the wrist is susceptible to compression and traction injuries. Symptoms can vary from paresthesias to pain or numbness. The RSN can get irritated 7–9 cm proximal to the radial styloid, where the nerve becomes superficial from under the distal aspect of the brachioradialis, that is, with forearm pronation and wrist flexion as with racket sport strokes (Dellon & Mackinnon 1986). The nerve is further strained when ulnar deviation accompanies these motions (Table 17.3); hence avoiding these composite postures with educational training and/or a long arm splint (Fig. 17.12), which must cross proximal to the elbow for controlling forearm rotation, is essential for the nerve to recover. Tinel's percussion testing over the nerve can help localize the lesion (Tinel 1915). Light touch perception may be altered over the first dorsal web space distribution of the nerve. In many instances, gentle nerve gliding (using the progressive positioning noted in the RSN traction test (Table 17.3) may be helpful, especially following a nerve release. Other effective interventions may simply involve removing the irritant (watch band, strap, tight jewelry) and changing the hand and wrist posture during activity.

Table 17.2   Treatment guidelines for wrist fractures (radius and scaphoid) and carpal instabilities

	Protective phase (immobilization)	Motion phase (following immobilization)	Strength and function phase
Time frame	6–12 wks (longer duration typically required for scaphoid fractures) – duration of immobilization will be less with some internal fixation techniques	Starting immediately after immobilization	PROM >>AROM PROM >25% normal Wrist joint is not painful
Goals	Protect fracture and/or stabilized segment Control swelling, avoid pin site (if present) infections Full finger ROM, no grip strengthening	Active wrist extension, flexion, and forearm supination PROM 1 week later if needed	Increase wrist extension, forearm supination and grip strength
Techniques	Cast, splint, surgical fixation/ stabilization, external fixator Elevation, retrograde massage, compressive wraps, daily pin site cleaning Active and passive gentle fisting	AROM: wrist extension with finger flexion PROM: manual, gravity assisted, weight assisted, dynamic splinting	Isometric progressing to isotonic exercises Putty grip exercises
Comments and precautions	Finger ROM should be attained during this phase Nerve symptoms, 'pins and needles', and any CRPS must be monitored closely	Pain, swelling secondary too vigorous ROM exercise Avoid excessive ROM following instability Wrist flexion is a priority following stabilization to the dorsal wrist Any stabilization procedure that fuses one of the carpal rows should result in ~50% return of wrist ROM	Excessive overload, irritated tissues (i.e. tendonitis, joint instability) Any stabilization procedure that fuses one of the carpal rows should result in ~75% return of grip strength

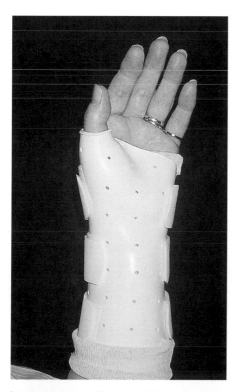

Figure 17.8   Long opponens splint is used for many of the problems that plague the radial side of the wrist/hand.

CENTRAL WRIST PAIN AND IMPAIRMENT

Degenerative

The DRUJ lies in the center of this region. Degenerative changes to the articular surfaces of the DRUJ are not uncommon, especially after distal radius fractures with or without ulnar variance discrepancies. If the normally smooth motion of the sigmoid notch of the radius rotating around the ulnar head, with concomitant ulnar translation, is disrupted, then pain, swelling, crepitus and limitation of forearm rotation are often present. A simple provocative grind and rotate maneuver (Table 17.3) is often helpful in identifying these patients. As with the conservative management of other forms of DJD in the upper extremity, the primary course of treatment is rest with a long arm splint (Fig. 17.12) to prevent forearm rotation, anti-inflammatory medication and patient education (Table 17.1).

In this central region, pain can be due to a carpal boss, which is an osteoarthritic spur that develops at the base of the second and/or third carpometacarpal joints. A carpal boss is often confused with a dorsal wrist ganglion (Watson 1979). A wrist splint, limiting wrist extension (Fig. 17.9), can control symptoms, but often an injection, aspiration or surgical excision is required (Angelides 1999).

Table 17.3 Provocative tests for radial, central, and ulnar lesions that cause pain and impairment

Radial tests	Technique	Central tests	Technique	Ulnar tests	Technique
Scaphoid shift for scaphoid instability (LaStayo & Howell, 1995, Watson et al 1988)	Stabilize wrist. Thumb pressure on palmar scaphoid. Passive wrist movement into ulnar deviation/extension, then radial deviation and flexion. Remove thumb pressure. Positive test = Relocating 'thunk', reproduction of pain	DRUJ Grind & Rotate for DJD of DRUJ (Schernberg 1990)	Manual compression of ulnar head into sigmoid notch while rotating forearm. Positive test = reproduction of pain	AD shear for AD tears (LaStayo & Howell 1995)	Dorsal glide of the piso-triquetral complex coupled with a volar glide of ulnar head, thereby shearing the AD. Positive test = reproduction of painful symptoms and/or excessive laxity in TFCC region.
1st CMC grind for DJD (Eaton & Littler 1969)	Axial compression and adduction of metacarpal on trapezium. Palpate for instability or crepitus. Positive test = painful crepitus and/or instability	Ballottement for lunotriquetral joint instability (Reagan et al 1984, LaStayo & Howell 1995)	Stabilize lunate and glide piso-triquetral complex volarly and dorsally. Positive test = laxity and/or a reproduction pain	GRIT for ulnar impaction syndrome (LaStayo & Weiss 2001)	Grip strength in 3 forearm positions: first in neutral, then in full supination and finally in pronation. Calculate a ratio (supination:pronation) grip strength. Positive test = GRIT ratio on involved side > 1.0 while on the uninvolved side the GRIT ratio is no different than 1.0
Finkelstein for De Quervain's (Finkelstein 1930)	Thumb actively adducted and held tightly in the palm with the other fingers. Wrist actively in ulnar deviation. Positive test = sharp lancinating pain at the first dorsal compartment	Volar/dorsal translation for DRUJ instability (Chidgey 1995)	Volar/dorsal glide of ulna on radius in various positions of forearm rotation (initially in neutral forearm rotation then in extreme positions of supination and pronation). Positive test = ulnar translation at extremes of rotation equals that of the neutral translation	Catch up clunk for CIND instability (Lichtman et al 1981)	Active wrist radial and ulnar deviation. Positive test = clunk or thud and pain at a point just beyond neutral as the wrist moves into ulnar deviation
Traction for radial sensory neuritis (Kenneally et al 1988)	Radial nerve tensioning. Positioning: (1) elbow extension, (2) forearm pronation, (3) wrist flexion, (4) wrist ulnar deviation (5) digital flexion (6) sidebending of cervical spine to contralateral side. Positive test = reproduction of pain	Middle finger extension for dorsal wrist syndrome (Watson & Weinzweig 1997)	Resisted middle finger extension (over the PIPJ) with wrist flexed. Positive test = pain in the scapholunate/dorsal wrist region	Piso-triquetral grind for piso-triquetral DJD (Schernberg 1990)	Compress and translate the pisiform against the triquetrum. Positive test = reproduction of pain
Intersection for intersection syndrome	Active wrist extension with concomitant active thumb circumduction. Positive test = pain, crepitus +/- squeaking sound from intersection region			ECU subluxation for instability (Burkhart et al 1982)	Passive supination followed by wrist ulnar deviation +/- resistance to ulnar deviation. Positive test = visible and palpable painful subluxation

AD = articular disk, CMC = carpometacarpal joint, CIND = carpal instability non-dissociative, DJD = degenerative joint disease, DRUJ = distal radioulnar joint, ECU = extensor carpi ulnaris, PIPJ = proximal interphalangeal joint, TFCC = triangular fibrocartilage complex

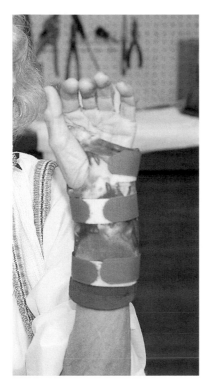

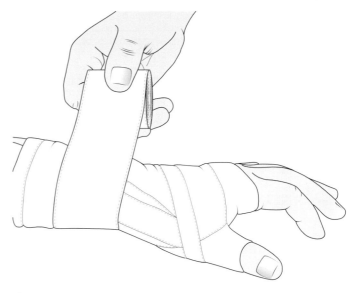

Figure 17.11 An example of protection and rest with incomplete immobilization using athletic taping. Taping can provide protection and rest of the wrist and thumb as depicted here. Also, taping can be used at the hand and with the fingers.

Figure 17.9 Wrist control splint. The splint most often used to limit wrist motion.

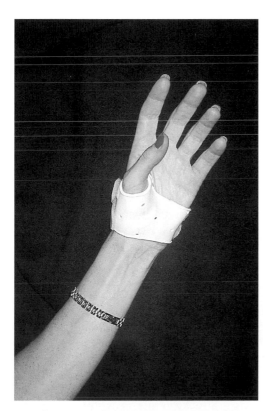

Figure 17.10 Short opponens splint protects the thumb carpometacarpal joint. The distal margin of the thumb component can be extended distally to also incorporate the metacarpophalangeal joint.

Instability

Injury to the LT joint can precipitate central wrist pain, but like DRUJ instability, is often described as a source of ulnar wrist pain. Signs and symptoms of LT injury include: diminished motion, weakness of grip, a sensation of instability or giving way, ulnar nerve paresthesias and a positive ballottement test (Table 17.3) (Bishop & Reagan 1998). Typically, a simple wrist control resting splint (Fig. 17.9) will suffice in LT strains but conservative and postoperative management principles described in Table 17.1 and 17.2 should be followed. As with any carpal instability, care must be taken when applying axial loads (e.g. fisting and/or FOOSH) to the wrist so as not to compromise the healing of ligamentous/capsular tissue.

Synovitis and ganglion

Dorsal wrist pain postactivity and/or with forced wrist extension, especially in sporting activities that require weightbearing through the wrist, can be the result of a dorsal wrist syndrome. Watson describes dorsal wrist syndrome as localized SL synovitis secondary to overstress to ligaments in this area, or it may represent an occult ganglia (Watson et al 1997, Watson & Weinzweig 1997). Dorsal wrist ganglia, which comprise 60–70% of all hand and wrist ganglia, can be either palpable or occult and may indicate a dorsal wrist syndrome. Clicks and palpable subluxation from this region should also increase the examiner's suspicion that underlying SL

Table 17.4   Factors that affect recovery from de Quervain's stenosing tenovaginitis

	Protective phase (immobilization)	Motion phase (following immobilization)	Strength and function phase
Time frame	Surgical repair: 6–8 weeks Debridement: 1–3 weeks Longer (6 weeks) if ulnar shortening osteotomy with plate fixation is performed	Surgical repair: Starting immediately after immobilization Debridement: Typically protected intermittent ROM during immobilization phase Followed by unrestricted ROM in motion phase	Surgical repair/debridement: PROM >>AROM PROM >25% normal Wrist complex is not painful
Goals	Surgical repair: Protect stabilized DRUJ, no forearm rotation Control swelling, full finger ROM Debridement: Avoid painful forearm rotation positions Control swelling, full finger ROM No forceful gripping	Surgical repair/debridement: Active forearm rotation PROM 1 week later if needed	Surgical repair/debridement: Increase forearm rotation, wrist and grip strength
Techniques	Surgical repair: Cast, splint, surgical fixation/stabilization Elevation, retrograde massage, compressive wraps, active gentle fisting Debridement: Cast, splint Elevation, retrograde massage, compressive wraps, active gentle fisting	Surgical repair/debridement: AROM forearm rotation PROM manual, gravity assisted, weight assisted, dynamic splinting	Surgical repair/debridement: Isometric progressing to isotonic exercises Putty grip exercises
Comments and precautions	Surgical repair: must be rigorously protected Debridement alone needs little protection, debridement with ulnar osteotomy/plate fixation requires bone healing Surgical repair/debridement: Finger ROM should be attained during this phase Nerve symptoms, 'pins and needles', and any CRPS must be monitored closely	Surgical repair/debridement: Pain, swelling secondary to vigorous ROM exercise Functional forearm rotation is 50° supination and 50° pronation. Many sport activities, however, require more ROM	Surgical repair/debridement: Excessive overload, irritated tissues (i.e. tendonitis, joint instability)

pathology is present (Watson et al 1988, Watson et al 1997). Tenderness in the SL region, coupled with a positive middle finger extension test (Table 17.3), are indicators of a dorsal wrist syndrome (Watson et al 1997). A wrist splint, limiting wrist extension (Fig. 17.9), can control symptoms, but often an injection, aspiration or surgical excision is required.

Avascular necrosis

The lunate, located ulnar to the scaphoid along the proximal margin of the mid-carpal joint, may also cause central wrist pain and impairment. Tenderness over the lunate is suggestive of a fracture and/or Kienbock's disease (idiopathic osteonecrosis) (Skirvin 1996, Watson et al 1997). The latter is often associated with an ulnar negative variance. Ulnar variance is a measure (obtained radiographically) of the distance that the ulnar head extends below (negative) or above (positive) the articular surface of the radius. In all carpal bone or joint lesions causing central wrist pain and impairment, a rigid or semi-rigid block of wrist extension (Fig. 17.9) and diminished axial loading (fisting) is required.

Tendonitis

It is important to differentiate tenderness in this central region as either coming from the lunate or the tendons of the fourth extensor compartment where tenosynovitis can occur. If tendonitis is present at the insertion of the ECRL and ECRB at the base of the 2nd and 3rd metacarpal, one must identify if a carpal boss is the irritant. Also, any systemic cause of inflamed tendons, e.g., rheumatoid arthritis, needs to be ruled out. Using the selective tensioning of tissue approach advocated by Cyriax (Cyriax 1982) is helpful in diagnosing tendonitis.

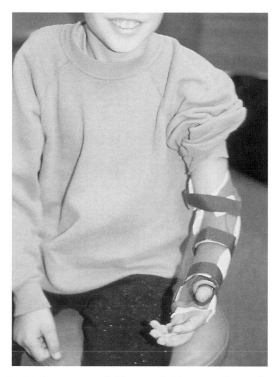

Figure 17.12 Long arm splint is essential for protecting and restricting the wrist and hand from forearm rotation. The proximal margin must have components that sit medially and laterally over the epicondyles of the elbow, but the volar proximal portion should be flared distally to allow some elbow flexion and extension.

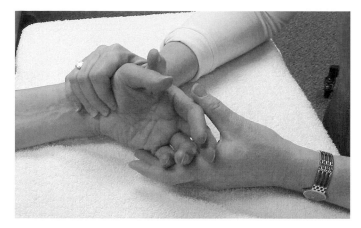

Figure 17.13 Median nerve compression coupled with wrist flexion is a provocative position used to identify carpal tunnel syndrome as the external compression and flexed position increase pressures on the median nerve.

AROM may be painful, while PROM is generally painless; PROM tends to selectively tension inert, non-contractile tissues. Tendonitis should be suspected when pain is elicited with isometric resistance. Wrist motion should be avoided with a protective device (Fig. 17.9) or taping (Fig. 17.11). Modalities should be used as needed and an emphasis on education should be employed in all cases. If strengthening is required after a resolution of pain, an eccentric component to the strengthening exercise is suggested. Guidelines for treatment are described in Table 17.1.

Nerve compression

Carpal tunnel syndrome, the most common entrapment neuropathy, is due to compression/traction injury to the median nerve within the carpal tunnel. Various etiologies including anatomical anomalies, repetitive activity, hormonal changes that occur in pregnancy and systemic diseases such as diabetes mellitus have been implicated in contributing to the occurrence of this disorder. The signs and symptoms of carpal tunnel syndrome are paresthesias with or without pain in the volar thumb, index, middle and radial half of the ring fingers (paresthesia may only occur in portions of median distribution); paresthesias awaken the individual at night

and worsen with repetitive activity. There is a feeling of clumsiness in handling small objects and a weakness of grip and pinch. Provocative maneuvers for carpal tunnel include a positive reproduction of symptoms and a median nerve compression/wrist flexion test (Fig. 17.13) (Tetro et al 1998, Massey-Westropp et al 2000). A sensory evaluation (Breger 1987, Gellman et al 1986), the differential Tinel's percussion test over the nerve, can help isolate the compression site (Tinel 1915). Quantifying symptoms using the symptoms severity scale (Levine et al 1993) is also suggested. The judicious use of nerve and muscle electrodiagnostic studies that can clarify the location and extent of the injury are often helpful. Surgical decompression of the nerve is reserved for cases resistant to conservative care or in instances when nerve compression has led to muscle atrophy.

Conservative treatment (Table 17.1) involves techniques to reduce compression of the median nerve within the carpal tunnel. These interventions include splinting the wrist in neutral (Fig. 17.9) (Burke et al 1994, Kuo et al 2001, Walker et al 2000, Weiss et al 1995) and avoiding sustained pressure on the palm (Cobb 1995) and/or sustained grip activities (Seradge et al 1995). Nerve and tendon gliding exercises (Fig. 17.14) have also been suggested (Rozmaryn et al 1998). If conservative treatment fails or if there is atrophy of the thenar intrinsic muscles, then surgical release of the transverse carpal ligament is indicated.

Following surgery, grip and pinch strengths will be diminished, sometimes for up to 6 months. There will often be pillar (Ludlow et al 1997) and/or scar tenderness limiting the ability to bear weight on the palm for a number of weeks. Postoperative therapy may assist the individual to return to activity sooner than without therapy (Provinciali et al 2000). General guidelines for

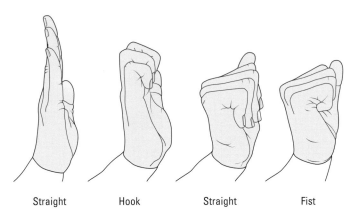

Straight   Hook   Straight   Fist

Figure 17.14 Tendon gliding exercises: different fist positions accentuating active differential tendon gliding of the extrinsic flexors and active/passive gliding of the extrinsic extensors.

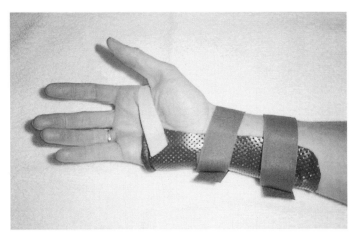

Figure 17.15 Ulnar gutter splint for blocking wrist ulnar deviation and partially limiting wrist flexion and extension.

postoperative care include: tendon and nerve gliding exercises (Wehbe & Hunter 1985), and strengthening of grip and pinch beginning at about 4 weeks (Maser et al 2001).

ULNAR WRIST PAIN AND IMPAIRMENT

Fractures

Any fracture of the distal radius or ulna can compromise the DRUJ, limit ROM and/or produce instability in the distal forearm joint, especially if it is intra-articular in nature and/or has resulted in a malunion. Even what appears to be a benign ulnar styloid fracture can cause instability or wrist/forearm stiffness. An uncommon, yet debilitating sport-related fracture is to the hook of the hamate. Typically, ulnar wrist pain localized to the hook of the hamate after a forceful swing, either with a bat or golf club, is the mechanism of injury.

If stiffness is the primary problem then the clinician must be ensured that a bony abnormality is not blocking motion. This can be done using imaging studies as a primary resource and supplementing that clinically with the type of end feel that is present at the joints end range; which is either soft or hard indicating the absence of presence of an osseous limitation respectively. If soft tissue structural changes are causing stiffness then appropriate treatments for joint stiffness should be used as described in Figure 17.7 and Table 17.1. A bevy of splints and end-range positioning devices are now available to help restore forearm rotation (Schultz-Johnson 1996, Jaffe et al 1996).

Distal, radioulnar joint instability

If DRUJ/TFCC instability and pain are the main concerns, due either to a lack of bony support from the DRUJ, (an ulnar styloid non-union with or without a torn

TFCC), or an isolated TFCC (dorsal radial ulnar ligament or palmar ulnar ligament specifically) tear, a supportive splint or cast is necessary. DRUJ/TFCC instability can cause central (+/– ulnar) pain. To test the stability of the DRUJ, and concomitantly the supportive function of the TFCC, one can use a simple volar/dorsal translation provocative maneuver (Table 17.3).

The DRUJ/TFCC stabilizing options can include circumferential taping around the wrist/DRUJ, a simple ulnar gutter (Fig. 17.15) or a long arm splint (Fig. 17.12) (Jaffe et al 1996). The taping and ulnar gutter splint does not prevent forearm rotation, but often provides enough support for palliative relief. If the ulnar gutter is not therapeutic then seguing to a long arm splint is necessary (Jaffe et al 1996). For restricting forearm rotation a long arm splint, which crosses the wrist as well as the elbow joint, can be fashioned to allow flexion and extension of the elbow while preventing supination and pronation. Adequate protection (limited forearm rotation) for 6–8 weeks is necessary. If stability of the DRUJ is not restored with conservative treatment then surgical repair of the torn structures is necessary. Table 17.5 describes the postoperative management.

Degenerative disorders

An ulnar-based site of DJD is between the sesamoid pisiform bone and the triquetrum at the base of the hypothenar eminence. Although most commonly seen in the elderly, any individual can have volar ulnar pain if there is a history of direct injury to the pisiform. Typically, there is a complaint of pain when pressure is exerted on the pisiform, as in resting the hand on a table when writing, or gripping a racket, bat or club handle. A grinding type of provocative maneuver (Table 17.3) is typically positive when this DJD is present.

Table 17.5 Postoperative management guidelines after TFCC surgery (repair and debridement)

Factors affecting recovery: de Quervain's	
Acute versus chronic	*Acute:* typically resolved with complete rest, avoidance of thumb adduction and wrist ulnar deviation, and judicious use of NSAIDs *Chronic:* often complete rest is not a panacea Gentle (non-painful) wrist ROM, modalities, intermittent splinting/taping, and biomechanical/ergonomic education is required
Concomitant lesions	Irritation to the radial sensory nerve, 1st CMC joint, or the intersection-region delay recovery. Fortunately, the avoidance of thumb adduction and ulnar deviation will facilitate healing of all of these lesions
Conservative versus operative	The prognosis for conservative treatment is good if symptoms resolve within 1–2 weeks. The surgical prognosis is good if all septations are released, the tendons are painlessly mobilized postoperatively, and there are no concomitant lesions.

NSAID = non-steroidal anti-inflammatory drug

The splinting options here should include a pad interface between an ulnar gutter splint (Fig. 17.15) and the pisiform. This pad is shaped like a doughnut, so as to prevent compressive forces across the joint when laying the hands on a hard surface.

Articular disk of the triangular fibrocartilage tear

Isolated tears in the articular disk will not typically result in instability of the DRUJ or the ulnar carpal structures of the TFCC. They do, however, often cause clicking, and ulnar-sided wrist pain, which is worsened with gripping and forearm pronation. The articular disk shear test and gripping rotatory impaction test (GRIT) can help identify articular disk lesions (Table 17.3). Ulnar impaction syndrome, secondary to a positive ulnar variance, can precipitate articular disk tears. The pain increases with ulnar deviation, being most profound with gripping and during forearm pronation (due to maximal potential for a positive ulnar variance).

During axial loading (gripping), the radiocarpal joint transmits 80% of the force through the radial aspect of the wrist and forearm while the ulna, through its articulation with the ulnar carpus and the TFCC, carries 20% of the load (Palmer 1993). With malunited distal radius fractures and DRUJ incongruity, loads through the radius

and ulna shift, and can exceed physiological limits (Palmer & Werner 1984). Ulnar variance can also affect this force distribution markedly. Ulnar positive variance increases ulnar-sided forces and conversely, ulnar negative variance increases radial-sided forces (hence it also decreases forces transmitted through the ulnar side) (Palmer & Werner 1984). Ulnar variance changes in a positive direction with forearm pronation and gripping (Epner et al 1982, Palmer et al 1982, LaStayo & Weiss 2001). Gripping and pronating can adversely impact ulnar-sided structures such as the TFCC, lunate and LT ligament, and may be a source of pain during such maneuvers as a tennis serve, swinging a bat or any sports requiring gripping in a pronated position.

Traumatic or degenerative tears within the centrally located avascular articular disk region cause pain which is often recalcitrant, having very minimal to no potential for healing. Radially-based tears, however, have some vascularity and are surgically repairable (Cooney 1998). Table 17.5 outlines the postoperative care following debridement or repair of articular disk tears.

Non-surgical management options include taping (Fig. 17.11) for sport activities, an ulnar gutter splint (Fig. 17.15) and education which emphasizes avoiding functional activities that require forearm pronation and gripping. This education is most effectively imprinted when you get patients to reproduce their pain by having them grip with simultaneous movement into forearm pronation. If the patient is having problems modifying this painful behavior, and/or the pain is not improving with the static ulnar gutter splint, then forearm pronation must be limited with a long arm splint (Fig. 17.12). If the clinician feels that strengthening is appropriate, i.e. grip strength, then care must be taken to progress the resistive gripping program from a supinated position, to a neutral forearm position and then finally into pronation if there is no pain.

Instability

Mid-carpal row instability is a non-dissociative type of carpal instability, classified as carpal instability non-dissociative (CIND) and is typically difficult to diagnose, as static imaging studies are often unremarkable. The typical patient has a ligamentous laxity at the wrist and other joints. Typically, this instability is noticed first on clinical examination and then confirmed with cineradiography. If excessive laxity is noted, the tests for dissociative conditions within the proximal row (i.e. the scaphoid shift and ballotement tests for SL and LT tears respectively) may produce false positives. Perhaps the most notable clinical characteristic of mid-carpal instability is the abrupt carpal shift that occurs with ulnar deviation during the catch-up clunk test (Table 17.3)

(Lichtman et al 1981). Since gripping and deviation of the wrist are common in sport activities, taping (Fig. 17.11) is essential during training or competition. A special pad addition to the wrist splint, along the pisiform for boosting it dorsally, is helpful in reducing the painful clunk.

The ECU tendon can also be the source of ulnar sided pain as it is apt to move about in its groove in the ulna if the 6th dorsal extensor compartment of the wrist can no longer stabilize it. The ECU subluxation test (Table 17.3) amplifies this instability. Visible or palpable subluxation of the ECU with this maneuver indicates instability. Attempts have been made with wrist cuffs and/or wrist circumferential taping to stabilize the ECU in a conservative manner, but often the tendon still exhibits excessive motion with ulnar deviation. Consequently, preventing ulnar deviation with an ulnar gutter splint (Fig. 17.15) is often effective. If this is unsuccessful then, a surgical procedure for stabilization of the ECU tendon is performed.

Tendonitis

Irritation or inflammation (tendonitis) of the flexor carpi ulnaris (FCU) and ECU tendons is thought to contribute to ulnar wrist pain. This diagnosis should be based on findings of swelling and crepitus over the tendons and pain with manual isometric resistance of wrist flexion/ulnar deviation (for FCU) and wrist extension/ulnar deviation for (ECU). The selective tensioning of musculo-tendinous tissue via isometric resistance should be accompanied by active and passive ROM testing in the assessment format put forth by Cyriax (1982). These lesions, however, may present themselves only as a result of some other primary lesion. A classic example is an ECU tendonitis resulting from a subtle ECU instability. Unfortunately, if the primary lesion is not addressed, often the secondary tendonitis remains recalcitrant. Splinting or taping (Fig. 17.11), in the form of an ulnar gutter (Fig. 17.15), for the FCU and ECU problems can often be helpful in both classic tendonitis and/or tendon instability. Modalities that address inflammation when present are often helpful, but heat also can be comforting when tenosynovitis is the culprit. Additionally, taping/splinting to rest the tendon and, ultimately, eccentric exercise after the tendon has healed, are appropriate (Table 17.1).

Nerve compression

Compression of the ulnar nerve can cause an aching pain and paresthesias on the ulnar side of the hand, however, it more often occurs when the lesion is at the level of the wrist than the elbow. It is important then to rule out compression of the ulnar nerve in the cubital tunnel at the elbow, which is a commonly occurring entrapment neuropathy. Ulnar nerve compression at the wrist can occur with prolonged weightbearing activities, such as bicycling without adequate palmar padding or when the straps to the bike gloves are fastened too tightly during a long ride. When ulnar nerve compression at the wrist is causing the ulnar wrist pain then the use of a wrist control splint (Fig. 17.9) with a protective pad over the hypothenar eminence is the first option in the conservative care. If the clinician is interested in using any nerve mobilization to treat this lesion, care must be taken to avoid straining the nerve. Unfortunately, compression of the nerve in Guyon's canal may not be detected until there is intrinsic muscle atrophy. The option for intervention then is surgical, with the postoperative course including nerve gliding exercise and avoidance of pressure over the thenar eminence.

MANAGEMENT OF FINGER AND THUMB JOINT AND SKELETAL INJURIES

Joint injuries and fractures of the hand are commonly seen as a result of sports activities. Some supposed 'simple' injuries of the hand, such as PIP joint sprains, may not be taken seriously by the initial treating practitioner, and consequently are not treated accurately or aggressively. This can lead to stiffness, deformity and disability. The care of a fracture of the hand includes fracture reduction, immobilization so the fracture fragment(s) can heal, and subsequent mobilization and strengthening to regain function. The clinician must know when it is safe to mobilize the hand and how to protect the hand, when necessary, during sports activities.

ULNAR COLLATERAL LIGAMENT INJURIES – THUMB METACARPOPHALANGEAL JOINT

During pinch activities, stability of the MCP joint of the thumb is critical. The UCL, dorsal joint capsule and volar plate, in conjunction with the adductor pollicus aponeurosis, stabilize the ulnar side of that joint (Minami et al 1985). When the thumb is torqued into an abducted or valgus position, such as can occur when falling forward with the hand gripping a 'planted' ski pole, damage can occur to the UCL of the thumb MCP joint. The magnitude of the force will determine the extent of the injury.

A mild valgus force can cause a grade I sprain and a severe force can tear the ligament completely, resulting in a grade III sprain. A grade II is intermediary (Wright & Rettig 1995). When the UCL is completely torn, the proximal ligament stump may get 'stuck' under the adductor pollicus muscle's aponeurosis, creating the so-called Stener's lesion (Stener 1962). In this case, surgical intervention is required to remove the aponeurosis from between the two ends of the UCL.

Grade I and II thumb MCP UCL injuries

The MCP joint is frequently swollen, tender, and painful to valgus stress. The initial treatment consists of rest, ice, compression, and elevation. Grade I or mild sprains can be treated with early mobilization and a thermoplastic splint (Figs 17.8 and 17.10) for pain control. When a partial tear of the ligament is suspected (grade II) a thumb spica cast, with the interphalangeal joint left free, is worn for 4–5 weeks (Wright & Rettig 1995). Some physicians will manage this injury with a forearm or hand based cast or thermoplastic removable splint (Fig. 17.10), rather than a thumb spica cast that crosses the wrist.

After cast immobilization is concluded, a removable splint is fabricated (Figs 17.8 and 17.10) and gradual mobilization is started. Progression of exercise is from active MCP flexion and extension to active abduction/adduction and opposition. Pain can be used as a guideline for progressing exercise. High-load brief stressors (HLBS) via joint mobilization, using high-grade (III or IV) volar glide of the proximal phalanx on the metacarpal, followed by passive flexion via a manual stretch, can be used to restore flexion of the MCP joint. With resistant flexion limitations, a low-load prolonged stress (LLPS) program with a progressive static flexion splint may be necessary (Table 17.1). A volar glide mobilization of the distal phalanx on the proximal phalanx can be performed for gaining IP flexion. The goal for flexion is to match the uninjured side. Side-to-side comparison is essential due to the wide variability in thumb MP range of motion, from about 25° to 70° (Bostock & Morrie 1993).

Strengthening activities, such as grip and lateral pinch, are instituted at approximately 4 weeks for grade I injuries and 6 weeks for grade II injuries. Activities that stress the thumb in an abducted and opposed position, for example, tip pinch, should be avoided for up to 8 weeks after injury (Brody 1999). Specialized foam or rubber playing casts are also options that can be explored (Wright & Rettig 1995).

Grade III or complete UCL tears

Complete tears require surgery to repair or reconstruct the ligament and adductor aponeurosis. With a grade III injury, a Stener's lesion may exist (Stener 1962). Following surgery, the MCP joint is immobilized for 4 weeks in a thumb spica cast (Zeiman et al 1998). The principles for management during this phase are the same as with the non-operative case. Because surgery has been performed, there may be more swelling of the hand and more of a necessity for patient education than in the non-operative case. A general schema for management guidelines during recovery after a repair or reconstruction of the UCL is outlined in Table 17.6. Losses of

Table 17.6 General schema of rehabilitation after repair or reconstruction of the thumb metacarpophalangeal (MCP) ulnar collateral ligament (UCL)

	Protective phase	Motion phase	Strength and function phase
Timeframe	Weeks 0–3	Weeks 3–6	Weeks 6–10
Goals	Prevent loss of motion of fingers and thumb IP Control digital swelling	Restore thumb MCP flexion	By discharge should have use of thumb for pinch and torque activities (e.g. using tools, opening jars)
Techniques	Instruction in elevation AROM of thumb IP and all joints of four fingers Prevent adherent and sensitive scar	AROM and PROM of MCP and IP P–A[a] and A–P[b] glides to restore MCP flexion and extension. If regaining flexion is difficult, splinting can be used. Scar massage. Silicone mold over scar. Desensitization techniques if scar hypersensitive	Pinch and grip strengthening activities
Precautions	If a thermoplastic splint is used, education of patient about risks of removing splint Must protect repair/reconstruction	Avoid radially directed torque to the MCP joint (resisted adduction, forced abduction, or resisted opposition)	

[a] posterior to anterior (P–A) glide (joint mobilization)
[b] anterior to posterior (A–P) glide (joint mobilization)

ROM of the MCP after surgery can be about 20% (Mitsionis et al 2000) to 30% (Downey et al 1995). Grip and pinch strengths usually are between 90–100% of the uninjured side (Downey et al 1995, Melone et al 2000).

PROXIMAL INTERPHALANGEAL JOINT SPRAIN AND DISLOCATION

Common consequences of 'jamming' or hyperextending the finger during activities like volleyball and basketball include proximal interphalangeal joint dislocations and sprains, or disruption of the digital extensor tendon (the central slip and/or the terminal tendon), leading to a boutonnière or mallet finger deformity respectively. Good emergent care and regular follow-up of these injuries is necessary to prevent flexion contractures, in the case of the proximal interphalangeal (PIP) injury, and loss of active terminal finger extension in the case of an extensor tendon injury. With these injuries, regaining joint extension is more challenging than regaining flexion. Injuries of the PIP joint always result in edema and stiffness of that joint. Therapy is implemented to minimize these problems, maximize motion and protect the healing structures about the joint. Overzealous treatment can contribute to prolonged swelling, a flexion deformity and disability. Edema control should be emphasized and implemented by string wrapping and retrograde massage (Flowers 1988) with compression wraps of the digit used between therapy sessions.

The management of PIP joint injuries varies with the diagnosis and the stability of the joint. Dorsal dislocations or subluxations are most common and require anatomical reduction. Most PIP joint dislocations are stable and will not redislocate during active motion.

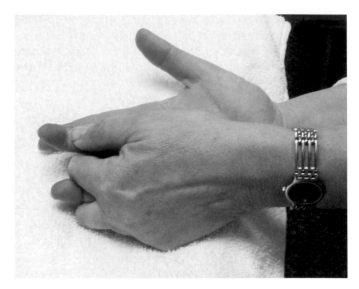

Figure 17.16 Isolated distal interphalangeal joint flexion and extension with blocking of PIP motion.

These injuries can be treated by a brief period of splinting (3–5 days) and early motion. In contrast, injuries that are not aligned, and that are unstable after closed reduction, require physical blocks to full PIP extension and longer protection (2–3 weeks).

If the PIP joint is stable (i.e. without evidence of dorsal subluxation or medial or lateral deformity) it may be protected by buddy strapping the injured finger to the adjacent finger, or by immobilization for 3 to 5 days in full extension. The goals of therapy are to maintain gliding of the tendons that cross the PIP joint and prevent a PIP flexion contracture. If the injured finger is 'buddy' strapped to the adjacent finger, active range of motion exercises of the PIP and DIP joints should be imple-

Table 17.7 General schema of rehabilitation after PIP joint injury

	Protective phase	Motion phase	Strength and function phase
Time frame	0 to 2–3 weeks	3 to 6 weeks	6 to 10 weeks
Goals	Control digit edema Promote flexor and extensor tendons excursions	Restore active and passive PIP flexion and extension Prevent or reduce a PIP flexion contracture	Restore functional grip strength
Techniques	Compression wraps Buddy strap injured finger to uninjured Splint PIP joint in full extension at night	AROM, PROM PIP joint PIP flexion contracture should be aggressively managed using a low load prolonged stress (serial cast)	Putty exercise Graded hand held grippers
Precautions	Monitor for extension lag	Increased PIP joint swelling indicates that the vigor of exercise may be excessive; adjust exercise accordingly	

Note: In the case of an unstable injury where surgery is required, the protective phase is extended and limits on motion are more stringent.

mented to reduce the likelihood of adhering tendons, collateral ligaments and the proximal portion of the volar plate. In addition, exercises should include DIP flexion and extension with the PIP joint blocked in extension (Fig. 17.16). This is done to promote volar and distal glide of the lateral bands and to prevent adherence of the oblique retinacular ligament. If the PIP joint is immobilized in a splint, the DIP joint is left free for range of motion exercises. Full DIP motion should be encouraged to maximize tendon gliding of the FDP and lateral bands of the extensor mechanism. It may be necessary to splint the PIP joint in full available extension at night to reduce the likelihood of a flexion deformity secondary to joint effusion. A general schema of rehabilitation after a PIP joint injury is outlined in Table 17.7.

If the PIP joint has been immobilized, it is likely to be stiff. Therapy should emphasize regaining flexion while preventing a flexion contracture. PIP flexion contractures which are not fixed (i.e. not resistant to stress) may respond to a period of LLPS. LLPS techniques utilizing progressive static splinting, such as serial casting, can be effective in reducing flexion contractures (Table 17.1) (Flowers & LaStayo 1994). An additional advantage of serial casting is the circumferential pressure to control and reduce edema. If this treatment is successful, gains of 5° to 10° per week can be expected. When the flexion contracture is less than 20°, dynamic splinting via spring-wire splints can be used intermittently during the day to promote extension. At that point the patient can also work on regaining PIP flexion through passive flexion strapping and light resisted grip exercises. The balance between regaining full flexion and extension can be challenging. Even though full motion would be ideal, the goal should be at least 90° to 95° of flexion at the PIP joint. An extension deficit of 10° to 15° is an acceptable outcome for most functional activities. Surgical release of a chronic unremitting flexion contracture may be needed to optimize function (Abbiati et al 1995).

Strengthening exercises can begin 4–6 weeks after injury, when swelling and pain are controlled. An additional increase in flexion may occur with grip strengthening exercises due to high forces transmitted through the flexor tendons by the extrinsic flexor muscles, which have a relatively greater cross-sectional area than the extensors. The therapy program during this phase should include sport-specific grip activities to prepare for return to maximum function, e.g. impact activities like hammering nails into wood. If vibration, such as in batting or racket sports is an issue, a support wrap around the digit and buddy strapping can be used during activity until the joint can tolerate vibration and impact. While swelling may persist for months after this injury, return to full function can be expected within 8 to 10 weeks.

With severe disruption of the PIP joint, the joint may be unstable, and emergency care should emphasize restoration of joint stability. If an unstable fracture/dorsal dislocation has adequate joint contact, the goal is to maintain the reduction while allowing a safe ROM. Extension block (approximately 30°) splinting is used in these circumstances (Hamer & Quinton 1992). This technique maintains joint reduction within a safe range by limiting extension. The same principle can be applied to managing volar plate injuries. Immediate active motion (both flexion and extension) to encourage healing of periarticular structures and promote good collagen alignment is permitted within the confines of the dorsal blocking splint.

When reduction cannot be maintained with extension block splinting, then a volar plate arthroplasty (Durham-Smith & McCarten 1992) may be indicated to restore the stability of the PIP joint by constructing a volar 'check-rein' to subluxation of the middle phalanx. The repair is protected using a short arm dorsal extension-blocking splint. Flexor tendon gliding exercises (Fig. 17.14) are important as there may be adhesions within the flexor tendon sheath after manipulation of the tendons in surgery. The exercises, performed within the confines of the extension block splint, can include flexion of the PIP with the MCP blocked in extension (Fig. 17.17) and flexion of the DIP with the PIP stabilized in extension (Fig. 17.16). This procedure is continued for 4 weeks, after which the extension block is removed. Therapeutic measures (Table 17.1) (Fig. 17.7) for joint stiffness can then be instituted to regain extension. A PIP flexion or extension contracture is inevitable, but an anatomical reduction must be the goal.

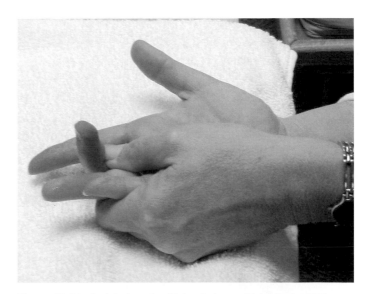

Figure 17.17 Isolated proximal interphalangeal joint flexion and extension with blocking of MCP motion.

METACARPAL FRACTURES

The tendons of the flexors and extensors as well as the intrinsics (interossei and lumbrical) muscles are aligned by the position of the metacarpal bones. This close proximity and dependent relationship between the metacarpals and surrounding musculotendinous structures can produce deforming forces across the fracture site and adversely influence function.

Metacarpal fractures can be caused by a direct blow to the metacarpal or an indirect twisting force through the finger. As with other hand fractures, the soft tissue injury that occurred with the fracture will influence outcome and is often underestimated because the initial focus is often on the fracture. The treatment of the metacarpal fractures must provide a stable bony construct to allow early motion (Kozin et al 2000). Undisplaced and stable fractures are allowed to heal in a hand- or forearm-based splint. After the cast or brace is removed, gradual mobilization and exercise is encouraged. Specific hand motions include: a full fist, a claw fist into the intrinsic minus position (Fig. 17.18), and a table-top posture into the intrinsic plus position (Fig. 17.19); these are used to regain movement.

Irreducible fractures, open fractures, multiple fractures, fractures with bone loss, and fractures associated with tendon laceration usually require surgery to restore stability to the metacarpal(s) and hand. Stable fixation, which is usually obtained with screw, or plate and screw,

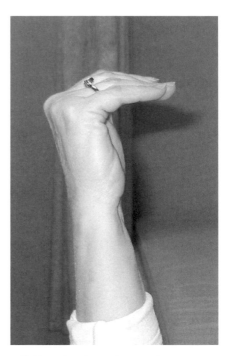

Figure 17.19   'Table-top' intrinsic plus position.

fixation can be treated by early active range of motion as soon as the acute pain from surgery subsides. This is important to prevent contracture, disuse osteopenia and muscle atrophy. A dorsal surgical approach can limit extensor tendon gliding. Active and active assisted motion of the fingers and wrist promotes tendon gliding, primarily of the extensor tendons, and limits adhesion formation. An extension assist splint may be useful in providing resistance during flexion to promote tendon gliding. Selective gliding of the extensor digitorum tendons can be done by actively extending the MCP joints while the PIP and DIP joints are held in flexion: the hook fist. Scar management techniques can include a silicone mold worn over the scar, and vibration, scar massage and gentle suction over the scar.

Passive motion should be limited until bony union is apparent, as aggressive movement can disrupt the fracture fixation. A splint is used between exercise sessions and is necessary to rest the hand, protect the healing fracture, and prevent contracture. The therapy goals are to maintain MCP flexion while minimizing PIP flexion contractures. The splint should be made to position the MCP joint in flexion and the interphalangeal joints in extension (Fig. 17.19). When more vigorous attempts to regain flexion are permitted (and this is guided by evidence of fracture consolidation), buddy strapping of the injured digit to the adjacent digit can be used. The uninjured digit, which presumably has more flexion will drag the other finger along with it into flexion.

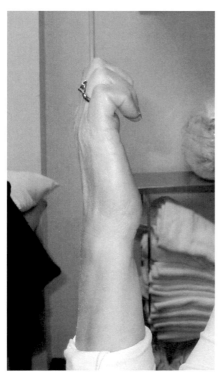

Figure 17.18   'Claw fist' intrinsic minus position.

PHALANGEAL FRACTURES

Extra-articular distal phalangeal fractures (i.e. tuft fractures) are usually the result of a crush injury and have a concomitant nail bed laceration. These fractures are treated with splint immobilization until fracture union. Pain and limited function following this injury are seldom from the fracture and more likely to be from the nail bed injury. Therapy is warranted if the magnitude of sensitivity causes the patient to guard the use of the hand. In this case, therapy is done using progressive exercises for functional use of the hand for prehension and precision activities. In contrast, proximal and middle phalangeal fractures are more problematic and can result in hand impairment due to the likelihood of PIP flexion contractures and limited tendon gliding (see Fig. 17.14 for tendon gliding exercises) due to scar.

Stable phalangeal fractures are either not displaced or stable after closed reduction. A non-displaced fracture can be treated by immobilization for a few days until the swelling subsides and then with protected motion (using buddy taping) until union. The hand is immobilized in the 'safe position' with MCP flexion and IP extension (Fig. 17.19) to prevent contracture. Since the interossei muscles traverse volar to the MCP joint, this position also relaxes the interossei, which can act as deforming forces in phalangeal fractures. Protected motion, where the fractured digit is buddy taped to the adjacent digit, should be used continuously for 4–6 weeks until union occurs, to promote tendon gliding. Clinical fracture union is indicated by lack of tenderness at the fracture site and will precede radiographic union (bony bridging across fracture site). This can create confusion as an X-ray report may still indicate a visible fracture line despite clinical union. At this point, strengthening and resistive exercises can be initiated as the strength across the fracture site can withstand these forces.

Unstable, displaced fractures are managed surgically by closed reduction and percutaneous pinning or open reduction and internal fixation using compression screws, interosseous wiring, screws or mini-plate and screws (Oulette & Freeland 1996). There is a greater propensity for adhesions and loss of tendon gliding in phalangeal fractures in comparison to metacarpal fractures due to the intimate proximity of the dorsal extensor hood. Therefore, a fixation that allows early motion is preferred, to diminish the consequences of immobilization.

To plan an exercise program, the therapist must know the status of the fixed fracture. Stable rigid fixation can be treated by early range of motion to encourage tendon gliding and to prevent contracture and atrophy (Oulette & Freeland 1996). Non-rigid fixation, however, must be protected. Static splinting is necessary between exercise sessions to rest the injured digit(s) and to prevent surrounding joint contracture. This early motion regimen, in rigidly fixed fractures, is usually instituted 3–7 days after surgery and requires careful supervision.

Active and active assisted motion exercises are utilized until union. MCP, PIP (Fig. 17.17) and DIP (Fig. 17.16) blocking exercises with appropriate support are used. Passive motion can be started after fracture union, usually at about 4–6 weeks. This should be verified with the patient's physician who performed the fracture reduction. HLBS joint mobilization (Table 17.1) to restore both flexion and extension are then cautiously instituted. LLPS-like activities (Table 17.1) (Fig. 17.7) such as strapping of the fractured digit into flexion or the use of a progressive static splint may be needed to regain flexion. Potential complications following hand fractures include: scarring of the soft tissues in the skin, around tendons, or in joint capsules leading to stiffness; mal-union which is typically characterized by malrotation, angulation or shortening (Page & Stern 1998). Nerve or artery injuries can result from the initial trauma or be iatrogenic (from surgery). Sensory nerves along the dorsum of the hand are particularly prone to neuroma formation. Complex regional pain syndrome type I or II (reflex sympathetic dystrophy) may also occur. The general schema of rehabilitation after unstable digit or metacarpal fractures is described in Table 17.8.

MANAGEMENT OF FINGER TENDON INJURIES

Flexor tendons

Active finger flexion is necessary to perform many tasks including manipulation of small objects and grasping around objects. The long flexors of the digits are integral in performing these tasks. Following a laceration of a flexor tendon, the desirable outcome after intervention is to flex the finger to touch the palm. Surgical repair and subsequent postoperative management are designed to restore anatomy as closely as possible and to facilitate healing and maximum gliding of the tendon within its tendon sheath. There must be a balance of sufficient scar at the repair site to maximize tensile strength, yet avoidance of excessive scar within the tendon sheath, to maximize tendon gliding.

Unlike some other areas of rehabilitation, much valuable information on rehabilitation following flexor tendon repair exists (Evans 1989). The quantity of basic science and clinical research addressing flexor tendon management parallels or exceeds that of injuries to the ACL of the knee. Studies have addressed healing in animal models, tensile strengths with various suturing techniques, techniques of protection (i.e. splinting after tendon repair) and methods of exercise, which are

Table 17.8   General schema of rehabilitation after unstable hand fractures treated by surgical intervention

	Protective phase	Motion phase	Strength and function phase
Timeframe	A few days for fractures with rigid fixation Up to a few weeks for fracture less rigid fixation (e.g. k-wire) Consult with physician regarding timing of motion	3–5 days to 6 weeks following rigid fixation 3 (or more) to 6 weeks for less rigid fixation	6 weeks and onward May be delayed if complications such as delayed union of fracture
Goals	Edema control Motion of uninvolved joints	Promote maximum joint motion Prevent flexion contractures Promote tendon gliding.	Promote maximum grip and pinch strength Sports-specific functional training
Techniques	Elevation String wrap and retrograde massage Compressive wraps Protective padding and/or splinting if physician allows sports participation	Active and active assisted ROM Tendon gliding exercises Joint mobilization if fracture consolidated May need protective padding	Putty and hand held grippers Closed chain grip and torque activities Upper body strengthening and conditioning Functional activities to match sports-specific requirements
Precautions	Avoid undue stresses across fracture site Reduce motion exercises if edema increases or if pain increases and persists for more than 2 h following exercise	Avoid undue passive joint motion or joint loading if articular surfaces are damaged; motion goals will be reduced Monitor for complications	Delay introduction of activities if pain increases

outlined in Table 17.9 (Chow et al 1988, Duran & Houser 1975, Kleinert et al 1973, May et al 1992).

Flexor tendon injuries usually occur by a laceration that directly cuts the tendon(s). The treatment of the lacerated flexor tendon(s) is by direct repair. The ultimate goal of the suture method is to allow earlier active motion which will often decrease adhesion formation and optimize functional outcome. Closed rupture of the flexor tendons is less common than open lacerations. The FDP can rupture distally with an extension force against a flexed DIP joint. This occurs often in football as the flexed digit (most commonly in the ring finger) is holding onto the jersey and is quickly extended during an attempted tackle. This injury has been termed the rugger or football jersey injury. The jersey injury involves rupture or avulsion of the FDP tendon from its bony insertion and occurs most commonly in the ring finger (Stamos & Leddy 2000). Often a fragment of the distal phalanx will avulse. A recovery period of 12 weeks is necessary for maximizing the strength of the repair (in the case of ruptured tendon) or good bony consolidation (in the case of avulsion with bony fragment).

Closed ruptures are treated by early repair of the avulsed FDP tendon to its insertion at the base of the distal phalanx. In order to protect the repaired tendon from rupture or attenuation (gapping) at the repair site, the hand and wrist are immobilized in flexion in the operating room. Within 2–5 days after surgery, the surgical dressings and posterior cast shell are removed and replaced by a thermoplastic molded splint. Postoperative splint application and immobilization depends upon the rehabilitation method selected, strength of the suture technique and magnitude of associated injuries.

The general schema of rehabilitation is outlined in Table 17.10. During the first few days after surgery, intervention is directed toward pain and edema control, fabrication and application of a thermoplastic splint and initiating motion. Early postoperative management during the protective phase varies from complete immobilization for 3 weeks to early active motion in flexion and progressing to more vigorous blocked tendon exercises (Fig. 17.16 and Fig. 17.17) and tendon gliding exercises (Fig. 17.14). The greatest variations in treatment techniques occur during the first 3 weeks following repair.

Extensor tendons

In sports, closed injuries to extensor tendons can commonly occur. A direct blow to the tip of the finger can often cause a tearing/avulsion of the terminal extensor tendon or the central slip. The respective mallet finger (DIP) or bouttonnieère deformity (PIP) is treated with static extension splinting, with the uninjured IP joint free, for 6 weeks. This is followed by motion (active motion initially) exercises to restore finger flexion. A night splint to hold the respective IP joint fully extended is worn for 6 more weeks (Newport 1997). Problems in recovery include an extension lag of the joint. If a lag occurs,

Table 17.9 Techniques used during protective phase after flexor tendon repair

		Immobilization	Passive flexion/passive extension[a]	Passive flexion/active extension[b]	Early active (or short arc) motion[c]
Candidates		Children Unreliable adult	Reliable adult	Reliable adult	Minimum: 4-strand epitenon
Splint	Wrist	30–40° flexion	same	same	same
	Digit(s)	MCP 50–60° flexion IPs extended	MCP: same Rubber band traction to flex IPs or straps over IPs removed for exercise	MCP: same Rubber band traction to flex IPs	MCP: same Rubber band traction to flex MCPs
Exercises		Maintain motion of non-immobilized joints	Passively flex finger joints Passively extend finger joints within confines of splint		

[a] Duran & Houser (1975)
[b] Kleinert et al (1973)
[c] Silverskold & May (1994)

Table 17.10 General schema of rehabilitation following flexor tendon repair in the digits

	Protective phase	Motion phase	Strength and function phase
Timeframe	0 to 3 (or 4) weeks	3 weeks (or longer) to 8 weeks	8 weeks through 12 weeks
Goals	Prevent tendon rupture Restore full passive digital flexion Prevent PIP flexion contracture Control edema	Restore active flexion Reduce flexion contractures if present Protect against tendon rupture	Promote tendon glide if active insufficiency of digit flexion is occuring
Techniques	Splint wrist/hand to protect repair Splint PIP in extension at night Digit compression wrap/elevation Protected motion	Use a wristlet with rubber band traction for digits to protect from grabbing and lifting objects	Putty Free weights Progress to functional activities
Precautions	No simultaneous wrist and digit extension	If tendon gliding is freely occurring, protect longer If tendon is adhered, motion attempts can be more vigorous	No more than 5 lb grip force until about 10 weeks

further extension splinting, coupled with resistance extensor tendon gliding exercises are indicated.

Overall, extensor tendon injuries in the hand are easier to surgically repair than their synovially bathed flexor antagonists. Hence, longer periods of protection and immobilization are needed which can often result in tendon adherence and some residual active extension deficit (Newport 1997).

LESS COMMON SPORT-RELATED INJURIES OF THE WRIST AND HAND

OSTEOCHONDROSIS – KIENBOCK'S

The progressive collapse of the lunate, secondary to avascular necrosis can cause significant wrist impairment and disability. Although no single factor can be attributed to Kienbock's, it is likely that in the athletic population, repetitive compressive forces can cause cancellous fractures. This is especially relevant in those with an ulnar minus variant, as axial forces are shifted predominately across the lunate and scaphoid, and those with an osseous vascular compromise (Gelberman et al 1975, 1983). Immobilization in the early stages can rectify the impairment and disability, but later stages require surgical redistribution of forces across the radiocarpal joint with either an ulnar lengthening or radial shortening. A limited carpal fusion or salvage procedure like a proximal row carpectomy are also utilized if collapse of the carpus is advanced (McCue & Bruce 1994). Postoperatively, the emphasis is on return of ROM and strength.

VASCULAR THROMBOSIS

Thrombosis of the ulnar artery in Guyon's canal (also in a persistent median artery in the carpal tunnel) can occur following blunt and/or repetitive trauma to the palm (Costigan et al 1959). Generally, the thrombosis can precipitate an acute neuropathy and a tender mass in the hypothenar area. Allen's test will be abnormal with poor filling through the ulnar artery. Doppler ultrasound and/or an arteriogram can help confirm the diagnosis. Although splinting of the wrist is helpful, the most widely accepted treatment is surgical resection. Vigorous activity is restricted for 6 weeks and the wrist is protected in sport for 3 months after surgery (McCue & Bruce 1994).

MALLET THUMB

Disruption of the EPL insertion into the base of the distal phalynx, most often secondary to contact with a ball, can result in flexion deformity similar to that seen in the fingers. Splinting dorsally across the interphalangeal joint only in slight hyperextension for 6 weeks is often helpful, however, operative repair of the extensor tendon is more predictably effective if the tendon is lacerated or avulsed (Miura et al 1986).

SUMMARY

Although injuries to the wrist and hand are not the most common injury type in sport and exercise, some sporting activities place participants at greater risk. Given the large number of structures in the wrist and hand, injuries can involve several joints and soft tissue structures. The examination of wrist and hand injuries is complex and involves many different joints. Fractures, instability, degenerative disorders, tendonitis, and nerve injuries are the most common injuries found in this region.

REFERENCES

Abbiati G, Delaria G, Saporiti E et al 1995 The treatment of chronic flexion contractures of the proximal interphalangeal joint. Journal of Hand Surgery (Br) 3B:385–389

Angelides A C 1999 Ganglions of the hand and wrist. In: Green D P, Hotchkiss R N, Pederson W C (eds) Operative hand surgery (4th edn). Churchill Livingstone, New York

Arendt E A 1999 Orthopaedic knowledge update: sports medicine 2. American Academy of Othopaedic Surgeons, Rosemont, IL

Beckenbaugh R D 1984 Accurate evaluation and management of the painful wrist following injury. Orthopedic Clinics of North America 15:289–306

Berger R A, Garcia-Elias M 1991 General anatomy of the wrist. In: An K N, Berger R A, Cooney W P (eds). Biomechanics of the wrist joint. Springer-Verlag, New York

Berger R A, Dobyns J H 1996 Physical examination and provocative maneuvers of the wrist. In: Gilula L A, Yin Y (eds). Imaging of the wrist and hand. WB Saunders, Philadelphia

Bishop A T, Reagan D S 1998 Lunotriquetral sprains. In: Cooney W P, Linscheid R L, Dobyns J H (eds) The wrist: diagnosis and operative treatment. Mosby, St Louis, MO

Bostock S, Morrie M A 1993 The range of motion of the MP joint of the thumb following operative repair of the ulnar collateral ligament. Journal of Hand Surgery (Br) 18B:710–711

Botte M J, Gelberman R H 1987 Fractures of the carpus, excluding the scaphoid. Hand Clinics 3:149–61

Brand P W, Hollister A 1993 Clinical mechanics of the hand. Mosby Year Book, St Louis, MO

Breger D 1987 Correlating Semmes-Weinstein monofilament mappings with sensory nerve conduction parameters in Hansen's disease patients: an update. Journal of Hand Therapy 1:33–37

Brody L T 1999 The elbow, forearm wrist and hand. In: Hall C M, Brody L T. Therapeutic exercise: moving toward function. Lippincott Williams and Wilkins. Philadelphia

Burke D T, McHale-Burke M, Stewart G W 1994 Splinting for carpal tunnel syndrome: in search of the optimal angle. Archives of Physical Medicine and Rehabilitation 75:1241–1244

Burkhart S S, Wood M B, Linscheid R L 1982 Post-traumatic recurrent subluxation of the extensor carpi ulnaris tendon. Journal of Hand Surgery (Br) 7B:1–3.

Chidgey L K 1995 The distal radioulnar joint: problems and solutions. Journal of the American Academy of Orthopaedic Surgeons 3:105–109

Chow J A, Thomes L J, Dovell S 1988 Controlled motion rehabilitation after flexor tendon repair and grafting: a multi-centre study. Journal of Bone and Joint Surgery (Br) 70B:591–595

Cobb T K, An K-N, Cooney W P 1995 Externally applied forces to the palm increase carpal tunnel pressure. Journal of Hand Surgery 20A:181–185

Coleman S S, Anson B J 1961 Arterial patterns in the hand based upon a study of 650 specimens. Surgery, Gynecology and Obstretrics 113:409–424

Cooney W P 1998 Tears of the triangular fibrocartilage of the wrist. In: Cooney W P, Linscheid R L, Dobyns J H (eds) The wrist: diagnosis and operative treatment. Mosby, St Louis, MO.

Cooney W P, Chao E Y S 1977 Biomechanical analysis of static forces in the thumb during hand function. Journal of Bone and Joint Surgery (Am) 59A:27

Cooney W, Lucca M, Chao E et al 1981 The kinesiology of the thumb trapeziometacarpal joint. Journal of Bone and Joint Surgery (Am) 63A:1371

Costigan D G, Riley J M, Coy F E 1959 Thrombofibrosis of the ulnar artery in the palm. Journal of Bone and Joint Surgery (Am) 41A:702–704

Cyriax J 1982 Textbook of orthopaedic medicine, vol I. The diagnosis of soft tissue lesions, 8th edn. Ballière-Tindall, London

Dellon A L, Mackinnon S E 1986 Radial sensory nerve entrapment. Archives of Neurology 43:833–837

Downey D J, Monheim M S, Omer G E 1995 Acute gamekeepers thumb. Quantitative outcome of surgical repair. American Journal of Sports Medicine 23:222–226

Duran R J, Houser R G 1975 Controlled passive motion following flexor tendon repair in Zones II and III. In: American Academy of Orthopaedic Surgeons Symposium on Tendon Surgery of the Hand. CV Mosby, St Louis, MO

Durham-Smith G, McCarten G M 1992 Volar plate arthroplasty for closed proximal interphalangeal joint injuries. Journal of Hand Surgery (Br) 14B:422–428.

Eaton R G, Littler J W 1969 A study of the basal joint of the thumb. Treatment of its disabilities by fusion. Journal of Bone and Joint Surgery (Am) 51A:661–668

Epner R A, Bowers W H, Guilford W B 1982 Ulna variance: the effect of wrist positioning and roentgen filming technique. Journal of Hand Surgery (Br) 7B:298–305

Evans R 1989 Management of the healing tendon: what must we question? Journal of Hand Therapy 2:61–65

Finkelstein H 1930 Stenosing tenovaginitis at the radial styloid process. Journal of Bone and Joint Surgery 12:509–540

Flowers K R 1988 String wrapping versus massage for reducing digital volume. Physical Therapy 68:57–59

Flowers K R, LaStayo P C 1994 Effect of total end range time on improving passive range of motion. Journal of Hand Therapy 7:150–157

Freeland A E, Sennett B J 1996 Phalangeal fractures. In: Peimer C A (ed) Surgery of the hand and upper extremity, vol 1. McGraw Hill, New York

Gelberman R H, Salamon P B, Jurist J M 1975 Ulnar variance in Kienbock's disease. Journal of Bone and Joint Surgery (Am) 57A:674–676

Gelberman R H, Panagis J S, Taleisnik J et al 1983 The arterial anatomy of the human carpus. Journal of Hand Surgery (Am) 8A:367–375

Gellman H, Gelberman R H, Tan A M et al 1986 Carpal tunnel syndrome: an evaluation of the provocative diagnostic tests. Journal of Bone and Joint Surgery 68:735–737

Gilula L A, Yin Y 1996 Imaging of the wrist and hand. WB Saunders, Philadelphia

Gunther S F 1985 Dorsal wrist pain and the occult scapholunate ganglion. Journal of Hand Surgery (Am) 10A:697–703

Hamer D W, Quinton D N 1992 Dorsal fracture subluxation of the distal interphalangeal joint of the finger and the interphalangeal joint of the thumb treated by extension blockage splint. Journal of Hand Surgery 17:591–594

Horii E, Garcia-Elias M, An K N et al 1991 A kinematic study of lunotriquetral dissociations. Journal of Hand Surgery (Am) 16A:355–362

Jaffe R, Chidgey L K, LaStayo P C 1996 The distal radioulnar joint: anatomy and management of disorders. Journal of Hand Therapy 9:129–138

Kaukonen J P, Karaharju E O, Porras M et al 1988 Functional recovery after fractures of the distal forearm. Analysis of radiographic and other factors affecting the outcome. Annales Chirurgiae et Gynaecologiae 77:27–31

Kazuki K, Kusunoki M, Yamada J et al 1993 Cineradiographic study of wrist motion after fracture of the distal radius. Journal of Hand Surgery (Am) 18A:41–46

Kenneally M, Rubenach H, Elvey R 1988 The upper limb tension test: the SLR test of the arm. In: Grant R (ed) Physical therapy of the cervical and thoracic spine. Churchill Livingstone, New York

Keon-Cohen B 1951 De Quervain's disease. Journal of Bone and Joint Surgery (Br) 33B:96–99

Kihara H, Short W H, Werner F W et al 1995 The stabilizing mechanisms of the distal radioulnar joint during supination and pronation. Journal of Hand Surgery (Am) 20A:930–936

Kirkpatrick W H 1990 De Quervain's disease. In: Hunter J M, Schneider L H, Mackin E J et al (eds) Rehabilitation of the hand: surgery and therapy. CV Mosby, St Louis, MO

Kleinert H E, Kutz J E, Atasoy E et al 1973 Primary repair of flexor tendons. Orthopedic Clinics of North America 4:865–876

Kozin S H, Thoder J T, Lieberman G 2000 Operative treatment of metacarpal and phalangeal shaft fractures. Journal of the American Academy of Orthopaedic Surgeons 8:111–121

Kuo M-H, Leong C-P, Cheng Y-F et al 2001 Static wrist position associated with least median nerve compression. American Journal of Physical Medicine and Rehabilitation 80:256–260

Laseter G F, Carter P R 1996 Management of distal radius fractures. Journal of Hand Therapy 9:114–128

LaStayo P C, Howell J 1995 Clinical provocative tests used in evaluating wrist pain: a descriptive study. Journal of Hand Therapy 8:10–17

LaStayo P C, Weiss S 2001 The GRIT: a quantitative measure of ulnar impaction syndrome. Journal of Hand Therapy 14:173–179

Levine D W, Simmons B P, Koris M J et al 1993 A self-administered questionnaire for the assessment of severity of symptoms and functional status in carpal tunnel syndrome. Journal of Bone and Joint Surgery (Am) 75A:1585–1592

Lichtman D M, Schneider J R, Swafford A R et al 1981 Ulnar midcarpal instability of the wrist: clinical and laboratory analysis. Journal of Hand Surgery 6:515–523

Ludlow K S, Merla J L, Cox J A et al 1997 Pillar pain as a postoperative complication of carpal tunnel release: a review of the literature. Journal of Hand Therapy 10:277–282

McClure P W, Blackburn L G, Dusold C 1994 The use of splints in the treatment of joint stiffness: biologic rationale and an algorithm for making clinical decisions. Physical Therapy 74:1101–1107

McCue F C, Bruce J F 1994 Hand and Wrist. In: DeLee J C, Drez D (eds) Orthopaedic sport medicine: principles and practice. WB Saunders, Philadelphia

Mackinnon S E, Novak C B 1997 Repetitive strain in the workplace. Journal of Hand Surgery (Am) 22A:2–18

McQueen M 1988 Colles fracture: does the anatomical result affect the final function? Journal of Bone and Joint Surgery (Br) 70B:649–651

Maser B M, Clark C M, Girard D 2001 Carpal tunnel syndrome: postoperative management. In: Maxey L, Magnusson J (eds) Rehabilitation for the postsurgical orthopedic patient. Mosby, St Louis, MO

Massey-Westropp N, Grimmer K I, Bain G 2000 A systematic review of the clinical diagnostic tests for carpal tunnel syndrome. Journal of Hand Surgery (Am) 25A:120–127

May E J, Silfverskiold K L, Sollerman C J 1992 Controlled mobilization after flexor tendon repair in zone II: a prospective comparison of three methods. Journal of Hand Surgery (Am) 17A:942–952

Mayfield J K 1981 Mechanisms of carpal injuries. Clinical Orthopaedics and Related Research 149:45–54

Melone C P, Beldner S, Basuk R S 2000 Thumb collateral ligament injuries: an anatomic basis for treatment. Hand Clinics 16:345–357

Mennell J 1964 Joint Pain. Little Brown and Company, Boston

Michlovitz S L, Kozin S H 2000 Osteoarthritis and traumatic arthritis of the upper quadrant. Journal of Hand Therapy 13(2):77–78

Minami A, An K-N, Cooney W P et al 1985 Ligament stability of the metacarpophalangeal joint: a biomechanical study. Journal of Hand Surger (Am) 10A:255–260

Mitsionis G I, Varitimidis S E, Sotereanos G G 2000 Treatment of chronic injuries of the ulnar collateral ligament of the thumb using a free tendon graft and bone suture anchors. Journal of Hand Surgery (Br) 25B:208–211

Miura T, Nakamura R, Torii S 1986 Conservative treatment for a ruptured extensor tendon on the dorsum of the proximal phalanges of the thumb (mallet thumb). Journal of Hand Surgery (Am) 11A:229–233

Newport M L 1997 Extensor tendon injuries in the hand. Journal of the American Academy of Orthopaedic Surgeons 5:59–66.

Oulette E A, Freeland A E 1996 Use of the minicondylar plate in metacarpal and phalangeal fractures. Clinical Orthopaedics and Related Research 327:38–46

Page S M, Stern P J 1998 Complications and range of motion following plate fixation of metacarpal and phalangeal fractures. Journal of Hand Surgery (Am) 23A:827–832.

Palmer A K 1993 Fractures of the distal radius. In: Green D P (ed) Operative hand surgery. Churchill Livingstone, New York

Palmer A K, Werner F W 1984 Biomechanics of the distal radioulnar joint. Clinical Orthopaedics and Related Research 187:26–35

Palmer A K, Glisson R R, Werner F W 1982 Ulnar variance determination. Journal of Hand Surgery 7:376–379

Pellegrini V D Jr 1991 Osteoarthritis of the thumb trapeziometacarpal joint: a study of the pathophysiology of articular cartilage degeneration. Part I: anatomy and pathology of the aging joint. Journal of Hand Surgery (Am) 16A:967–974

Pratt N E 1996 Clinical musculoskeletal anatomy. JB Lippincott, Philadelphia

Prosser R, Herbert T 1996 The management of carpal fractures and dislocations. Journal of Hand Therapy 9:139–147

Provinciali L, Giattini A, Splendiani G et al 2000 Usefulness of hand rehabilitation after carpal tunnel surgery. Muscle and Nerve 23:211–216

Reagan D S, Linscheid R L, Dobyns J H 1984 Lunotriquetral sprains. Journal of Hand Surgery (Am) 9A:502–514

Richards R S, Bennett J D, Roth J H et al 1997 Arthroscopic diagnosis of intra-articular soft tissue injuries associated with distal radius fractures. Journal of Hand Surgery (Am) 22A:772

Rosenthal E A 1990 The extensor tendons. In: Hunter J M, Schneider L H, Mackin E J et al (eds) Rehabilitation of the hand: surgery and therapy. CV Mosby, St Louis, MO

Rozmaryn L M, Douvelle S, Rothman E R 1998 Nerve and tendon gliding exercises and the conservative management of carpal tunnel syndrome. Journal of Hand Therapy 11:171–179

Ruby L K, An K N, Linscheid R L et al 1987 the effects of scapholunate ligament section on scapholunate motion. Journal of Hand Surgery (Am) 12A:767–771

Ryu J Y, Cooney W P 3rd, Askew L J et al 1991 Functional ranges of motion of the wrist joint. Journal of Hand Surgery (Am) 16A:409–419

Schernberg F 1990 Roentgenographic examination of the wrist: a systematic study of the normal, lax and injured wrist. Journal of Hand Surgery (Br) 15B:210–228

Schultz-Johnson K 1996 Splinting the wrist: mobilization and protection. Journal of Hand Therapy 9:165–178

Seradge H, Jia Y-C, Owens W 1995 In vivo measurement of carpal tunnel pressure in the functioning hand. Journal of Hand Surgery (Am) 20A:855–859

Short W H, Palmer A K, Werner F W et al 1987 A biomechanical study of distal radial fractures. Journal of Hand Surgery (Am) 12A:523–534

Silverskold K L, May E J 1994 Flexor tendon repair in Zone II with a new suture technique and an early mobilization program combining passive and active flexion. Journal of Hand Surgery (Am) 19A:53–60

Skirvin T 1996 Clinical examination of the wrist. Journal of Hand Therapy 9:96–107

Sotereanos D G, Levy J A, Herndon J H 1994 Hand and wrist injuries. In: Fu F H, Stone D A (eds) Sports injuries: mechanisms, prevention and treatment. Williams and Wilkins, Baltimore

Stamos B D, Leddy J P 2000 Closed flexor tendon disruption in athletes. Hand Clinics 16:359–365

Stener B 1962 Displacement of the ruptured ulnar collateral ligament of the metacarpophalangeal joint of the thumb: a clinical and anatomical study. Journal of Bone and Joint Surgery (Br) 44B:869–879

Sweeney J, Harms A 1996 Persistent mechanical allodynia following injury of the hand: treatment through mobilization of the nervous system. Journal of Hand Therapy 9:328–338

Taliesnik J, Watson H K 1984 Midcarpal instability caused by mal-united fractures of the distal radius. Journal of Hand Surgery (Am) 9A:350–357

Tetro A M, Evanoff B A, Hollstien S B et al 1998 A new provocative test for carpal tunnel syndrome. Journal of Bone and Joint Surgery (Br) 80B:493–498

Threlkeld A J 1992 The effects of manual therapy on connective tissue. Physical Therapy 72:893–902

Tinel J 1915 Le Signe du 'Fourmillement' dans les lesions des Nerfs Peripheriques. Press Med 47:388–389

Villar R N, Marsh D 1987 Three years after Colle's fracture: a prospective review. Journal of Bone and Joint Surgery (Br) 69B:635–638

Walker W C, Melzler M, Cifu D X et al 2000 Neutral wrist splinting in carpal tunnel syndrome: a comparison of night-only versus full-time wear instructions. Archives of Physical Medicine and Rehabilitation 81:424–429

Watson H K 1979 The carpal boss: surgical treatment and etiological considerations. Plastic and Reconstructive Surgery 63:88–93

Watson H K, Ballet F L 1984 The SLAC wrist: scapholunate advanced collapse pattern of degenerative arthritis. Journal of Hand Surgery (Am) 9A:358–365

Watson H K, Ryu J 1986 Evolution of arthritis of the wrist. Clinical Orthopaedics and Related Research 202:57–67

Watson H K, Weinzweig J 1997 Physical examination of the wrist. Hand Clinics 13:17–34

Watson H K, Ashmead D, Makhlouf M V 1988 Examination of the scaphoid. Journal of Hand Surgery (Br) 13B:657–660

Watson H K, Ottoni L, Pitts E C et al 1993 Rotary subluxation of the scaphoid: a spectrum of instability. Journal of Hand Surgery (Br) 18B:62–64

Watson H K, Weinzweig J, Zeppieri J 1997 The natural progression of scaphoid instability. Hand Clinics 13:39–49

Weber E R 1980 Biomechanical implications of scaphoid wrist fractures. Clinical Orthopaedics and Related Research 149:83–90

Weber E R 1984 Concepts governing the rotational shift of the intercalated segment of the carpus. Orthopaedic Clinics of North America 15:193–207

Weber E R, Chao E Y 1978 An experimental approach to the mechanism of scaphoid wrist fractures. Journal of Hand Surgery (Am) 3A:142–148

Wehbe M A, Hunter J M 1985 Flexor tendon gliding in the hand. Part II. Differential gliding. Journal of Hand Surgery (Am) 10A:626–632

Weiss N D, Gordon L, Bloom T et al 1995 Position of the wrist associated with the lowest carpal-tunnel pressure: implications for splint design. Journal of Bone and Joint Surgery (Am) 77A:1695–1699

Weiss S, LaStayo P C, Mills A et al 2000 Prospective analysis of splinting the first carpometacarpal joint: an objective, subjective and radiographic assessment. Journal of Hand Therapy 13:218–226

Werner F W 1996 Principles of musculoskeletal biomechanics-hand. In: Peimer C A (ed) Surgery of the hand and upper extremity, vol 1. McGraw-Hill, New York

Whipple T L 1992 Preoperative evaluation and imaging. In: Whipple T L Arthroscopic surgery: the wrist. JG Lippincott, Philadelphia

Wood M, Dobyns J 1986 Sports related extra-articular wrist syndromes. Clinical Orthopaedics and Related Research 202:93–102

Wright H H, Rettig A C 1995 Management of common sports injuries. In: Hunter J M, Mackin D J, Callahan A D (eds) Rehabilitation of the hand: surgery and therapy, 4th edn. CV Mosby, St Louis, MO

Wright T W, Michlovitz S L 1996 Management of carpal instabilities. Journal of Hand Therapy, 9:148–156

Zeiman C, Hunter R E, Freeman J R et al 1998 Acute skier's thumb repaired with a proximal phalanx suture anchor. American Journal of Sports Medicine 26:644–649

Zemel N, Stark H 1986 Fractures and dislocations of the carpal bones. Clinics in Sports Medicine 5:709–772

18

Pelvis, hip and groin

Michael T Cibulka

INTRODUCTION

The pelvis, hip, and groin share one common anatomical component, the innominate bone. The innominate bone comprises three bones, the ilium, pubis, and the ischium, which are fused together as one. All three bones fuse together at the acetabulum, with each contributing a third to the make up of the acetabulum. The pelvis consists of the paired left and right innominate bones along with the sacrum. The hip joint consists of the acetabulum along with the head of the femur bone. The groin or adductor triangle consists of the hip flexor muscles, the adductor muscles, and the femoral nerve, artery, and vein. While the pelvis and hip have some of the strongest and thickest ligaments, muscles, and bones in the body (Solonen 1957), it is no wonder that it is often the joints in this area that are the frequent sites of problems; for example, many runners, especially in middle and long distance, develop anterior hip joint pain. Unilateral low back pain, from the sacroiliac joint, is common in many athletes. The pelvis is a vital structure; it is where our center of gravity is located and it evenly distributes the weight of our upper extremities and trunk to the lower extremities.

SPORT-SPECIFIC APPLIED ANATOMY

KINESIOLOGY OF THE SACROILIAC AND SYMPHYSIS PUBIS JOINTS

Anatomy and arthrology

The sacroiliac joints are two paired joints formed by the connection of the left and right iliac bones to the sacrum. The sacrum consists of five fused vertebrae. The joint capsule differentiates into two structures, an external fibrous capsule and an inner synovial layer (Bernard &

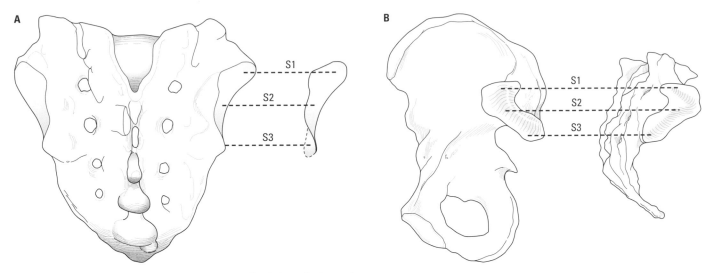

Figure 18.1 **A**: Sacrum. **B**: Iliac bone and sacroiliac joint articular surfaces.

Cassidy 1991, Schunke 1938). On the sacral side, the cartilage is hyaline (3–4 mm thick); the iliac side is also hyaline but less thick (1–2 mm) (Kampen & Tillman 1998, Sasabili et al 1995, Sashin 1930, Schunke 1938). By the third decade after birth, the iliac surface develops a convex ridge that runs centrally along the entire length of the joint surface. Motion is then limited to anterior/posterior tilting (rotation) (Brunner et al 1991, Wilder et al 1980).

The sacroiliac joints are diarthrodial (synovial) joints with the characteristic features of synovial joints including a joint capsule, synovial fluid, hyaline cartilage, surrounding ligaments, and movement between the joint surfaces (Alderink 1991, Bernard & Cassidy 1991, Portefield & DeRosa 1990, 1991, Sashin 1930, Schunke 1938, Solonen 1957). The joint is formed through the connection of the ilium to the sacrum. The joint articular surface has been described as 'C','L', or 'kidney bean' shaped (Fig. 18.1) with its convexity located anteriorly (Alderink 1991, Beal 1982, Bernard & Cassidy 1991, Portefield & DeRosa 1990,1991, Sashin 1930, Schunke 1938, Solonen 1957). The sacroiliac joint (SIJ) follows the ventral portion of the bodies of the sacral segments of the S1, S2, and S3 fused vertebrae. The sacrum's articular surfaces are predominantly concave, while the two ilial articular surfaces of the SIJs are convex (Weisl, 1955a).

JOINT MOVEMENTS OF THE BICONDYLAR SACROILIAC JOINTS

Movements at the sacroiliac joints (SIJs) are restricted to motion along their curved articular surfaces. Movement of the SIJ has been described as an oblique sagittal plane motion with movement primarily developing in an anterior or posterior direction. Some minor motion also occurs in both the frontal and horizontal planes (Smidt et al 1995, Sturreson et al 1989, 2000, Weisl 1955b, Wilder et al 1980). Smidt et al (1997) confirmed this in a recent cadaveric study where he showed that the innominate bones move in all three planes, however, with most of the motion developing in the sagittal plane. The sellar SIJs are also identified as bicondylar joints (Lavignolle et al 1983, Weisl 1955a). Bicondylar joints, so called because they articulate with two distinct articular condyles, have only two degrees of freedom (MacConaill & Basmajian 1977). The two degrees of freedom consequently limit joint motion around just two axes of motion, each lying perpendicular to each other (MacConaill & Basmajian 1977). As with all bicondylar joints, a movement of one joint must be accompanied by a correlative movement at the other (MacConaill & Basmajian 1977).

A characteristic feature of synovial joints is that the shape and orientation of the articular surfaces determine to some extent the type of movement that can occur (MacConnaill & Basmajian 1977). It therefore follows that the SIJ, being a synovial joint, follows the curvature of its articular surfaces during movement. The characteristic movement of the SIJ is a simultaneous anterior or posterior oblique movement of the left and right innominate bones on the sacrum. This motion develops during symmetrical trunk movements or symmetrical hip motion, for example, trunk forward bending, performing a pelvic tilt, or when moving from sitting to standing (Egund et al 1978, Sturesson et al 1989). The second and only other movement possible at the SIJs must therefore be an equal yet opposite (antagonistic) movement where one innominate bone moves anteriorly while the other side moves posteriorly. This occurs in accordance with the rules that govern movement of bicondylar joints where movement of one side must be accompanied by a correlative movement of the other side (MacConaill & Basmajian 1977). Sturesson et al (1989) suggest that the two innominate bones rotate as a unit around the sacrum. Presumably innominate bone motion could thus develop as either agonistic (in the same direction) or antagonistic (in opposite directions) motion. Although agonistic motion has been accepted for years, only recently has evidence for antagonistic motion of the innominate bones been demonstrated. During asymmetrical hip motions, where one hip flexes and the other extends, for example in walking, running, or kicking a ball, antagonistic innominate motion has been demonstrated (Barakatt et al 1996, Sturesson et al 2000). However, the first reported description of antagonistic movement of the innominate bones was by Pitkin & Pheasant (1936) who proposed that an unpaired unilateral motion of one innominate bone would rupture the symphysis pubis. Using asymmetrical standing positions and an inclinometer to measure innominate bone tilt, they showed that the left and right innominate bones tilt in opposite (antagonistic) directions. Later, Lavignolle et al (1983) showed antagonistic (dissymmetrical) innominate motion after orthogonally measuring the pelvis while flexing one hip and extending the other. Cibulka et al (1988), observed antagonistic innominate movement after applying a manipulative technique directed at the SIJ in patients who had low back pain with signs of SIJ dysfunction. Cummings et al (1993) repeated Pitkin & Pheasant's (1936) work, using a different type of inclinometer, but still found the same antagonistic motion between the innominate bones when an imposed leg length discrepancy was artificially created. Finally, Barakatt et al (1996), using a Metrecom, showed that with asymmetrical hip positions (one hip maximally flexed and the other maximally extended), the left and right innominate bones move in an equal and opposite direction (antagonistic motion) from each other. So far, no evidence (other than anecdotal evidence) has shown that innominate bone motion can occur independently, except in disruption of the pelvic ring. Conversely, considerable evidence does exists to show antagonistic motion (Barakatt et al 1996, Smidt et al 1997, Sturesson et al 2000), thus supporting the concept that the SIJs are bicondylar joints.

Thus, research studies have shown that the SIJ's rotatory motion ranges from 1° to 19° (Barakatt et al 1996, Colachis et al 1963, Egund et al 1978, Frigerio et al 1974, Lavignolle et al 1983, Smidt et al 1995, 1997, Sturesson et al 1989, 2000). Although all reports agree that motion primarily develops in the sagittal (x) plane, motion also develops in both the frontal and transverse planes (y, z) during different movements. Regardless of how much motion actually takes place at the SIJ, which is probably somewhere in between these ranges, perhaps the most important point is that all studies do agree that both agonistic and antagonistic movements of the innominate bones take place at the SIJ.

JOINT MOVEMENT OF THE AMPHIARTHRODIAL SYMPHYSIS PUBIS

For the SIJs to function as bicondylar joints, motion must be absent or severely limited at the symphysis pubis joint. The symphysis pubis is an amphiarthrodial joint (a fibrous joint with little or no motion available) (Walheim et al 1984). The reported amount of movement measured at the symphysis pubis is no more than 2 mm in females (less than ⅛ of an inch) and 0.5 mm in males (Chamberlain 1930, Walheim & Selvik 1984, Walheim et al 1984). Sturesson et al (1989) reports that the symphysis pubis allows the two innominate bones to rotate only as a unit around the sacrum, therefore allowing both paired innominate motion and antagonistic innominate motion on the sacrum. Pregnancy, of course, can significantly increase the symphysis pubis mobility (Borrel & Fernestrom 1957, Death et al 1982). In pregnancy, the amount of movement possible at the pubis increases (Borrel & Fernestrom 1957). Therefore, except for pregnancy, the symphysis pubis should probably be regarded functionally as a 'fused' joint.

LIGAMENTS AND THEIR ROLE IN LIMITING SACROILIAC JOINT MOVEMENT

The ligaments of the pelvis are among the strongest in the body. In the SIJ, most of the ligaments are short and thick (Walker 1992). Anteriorly, the SIJ ligament is loose and thin, while posteriorly, the dorsal sacroiliac and interosseous ligaments are very thick and strong. The dorsal SIJ ligaments run in two directions, one along the length of the articular surface and the second in a ventral to dorsal direction (Weisl 1954). The primary purpose of the dorsal SIJ ligaments is to prevent the sacrum from falling into the pelvic brim or outlet (Weisl 1954). Since the sacrum is tapered dorsally, the sacrum is limited in moving dorsally by its wedge shape. The majority of the ligaments of the SIJ are short (25 mm in length) (Weisl 1954), perhaps explaining why no study has described ligament strain as the cause of SIJ dysfunction.

The sacrotuberous and sacrospinous ligaments are the only long ligaments of the SIJ, and they limit ventral sacral motion (Weisl 1954). The sacrotuberous ligament is continuous with the origin of the hamstring muscles and is thought to play some unexplained role in function. No study has yet shown that either of these two ligaments is a common cause of pain or is commonly strained.

MUSCLES AND THEIR EFFECT ON SACROILIAC JOINT MOVEMENT

Any muscle that is attached to the pelvis, theoretically has the potential to have a an effect on movement of the SIJ. However, not all muscles attached to the pelvis are aligned in such a way that they may produce SIJ motion. For example, since the SIJ moves primarily in the sagittal plane and the abductor and adductor muscles lie in the frontal plane, their line of pull could not theoretically create sagittal plane movement. Thus, the primary muscles that theoretically can create movement of the pelvis are muscles in the sagittal plane, which include the trunk muscles (specifically, the erector spinae and the abdominal muscles), and the hip muscles, which include the hip flexors, extensors, medial and lateral rotators.

NEUROLOGY OF THE SACROILIAC JOINT

Solonen (1957) describes the innervation of the SIJ ventrally from the spinal nerves of L3 to S2 and the superior gluteal nerve, and dorsally from the first and second spinal sacral nerves (S1–S2). Therefore, the widespread innervation suggests that pain from the SIJ may radiate anywhere in the lower extremity if irritated enough.

CLINICAL CONSIDERATIONS WHEN CONSIDERING PROBLEMS WITH THE PELVIS

The evidenced-based pactice (EBP) approach described by Sackett et al (1985) allows for an unbiased choice when selecting the best tests and intervention for a problem or condition (Sackett et al 1998). Many clinicians currently use the method of differential diagnosis in selecting tests and not EBP. When using the differential diagnosis method, the first step is to develop a list of possible causes that may explain the signs and symptoms. Different strategies often help to refine the examiner's thought processes when making the diagnosis, for example, when using the anatomical method, each specific tissue (e.g. ligament) is tested or stressed to determine its response (Friedland et al 1998). The major problem when using this approach is that tests and interventions may be selected in a biased fashion. Conversely, when using EBP (Sackett et al 1998), evidence is assembled in an unbiased fashion using the best available evidence to select and interpret the best diagnostic tests and for guidance in the assessment of potentially useful interventions.

The most common pelvic problem seen by physical therapists is low back pain related to impairment of the

SIJs (Broadhurst 1989, DonTigny 1979, 1985, Erhard & Bowling 1977, Goldthwaite & Osgood 1905, Schwarzer et al 1995, Shaw 1992). Symphysis pubis problems are much less common. Muscle pulls of one joint hip flexor, and the extensor muscles, external and internal rotators, and abductor muscles are extremely rare. Muscle strains or 'pulls' of two joint hip/thigh muscles, for example, the hamstring and adductor or groin muscles, are much more frequent, especially in sports. Hamstring muscle pulls will be covered in another chapter, while groin muscle pulls will be covered later in this chapter.

HISTORY

When using EBP, the prevalence of the disorder is established before any diagnostic tests are selected (Freidland et al 1998, Sackett et al 1998). It is important to determine the prevalence because if the likelihood of a disorder is low (i.e. it has low prevalence), most diagnostic tests will have limited diagnostic importance (Diamond & Forrester 1979). Moreover, as prevalence of the disorder decreases, the predictive value of a positive test decreases and thus the possibility of finding a false positive test result increases (Diamond & Forrester 1979, Sackett et al 1985). Consequently, it is important to determine the prevalence of the disorder before any specific diagnostic tests are performed (Diamond & Forrester 1979).

If prevalence is not known, which is common, the EBP method to increase prediction of the prevalence of a disorder is to estimate its pretest probability, (Sackett et al 1985,1998). Pretest probability, defined, is the prior assessment of diagnostic possibilities before any tests are performed (Sackett et al 1985). Pretest probabilities most often come from the patient's history or presentation (Sackett et al 1998); using clinical experience, an estimate of the probability of the presence of the disorder can be made. Pretest probabilities may also come from published literature or data and can be expressed in rank order as high, medium, and low or be given a percentage to reflect relative probability (Sackett et al 1985,1998).

Pretest probability data on SIJ dysfunction is sparse. Most of the data describing SIJ dysfunction has been obtained from textbooks as few published studies exist. Calvillo et al (2000) suggest that adjacent spinal structures may cause pain to be referred to the SIJ; precise diagnosis can be difficult. However, studies have shown that pain near the posterior superior iliac spine (PSIS) is suggestive of SIJ dysfunction. In one recent study, Fortin et al (1994) injected the SIJ with an irritant and found unilateral pain around the PSIS. Fortin et al (1994) also showed that pain can refer down the leg in the dermatomal region from L3 to S2. Although often described, no specific or single mechanism of SIJ dysfunction has been

Box 18.1 Pretest probability for sacroiliac joint dysfunction in an outpatient physical therapy clinic

1. Unilateral pain in or around the posterior superior iliac spine
2. No mechanism of injury
3. No neurological signs or symptoms
4. Full painless trunk range of motion
5. Minimal to moderate pain (2–4 on a 0–10 pain scale)

For all five 75%: pretest probability
For four 50%: pretest probability
For three or less 40%: pretest probability

Box 18.2 Pretest probability for no sacroiliac joint dysfunction in an outpatient physical therapy clinic

1. Central low back pain or pain radiating below the knee
2. Specific mechanism of injury
3. Neurological signs and symptoms
4. Painful limited trunk range of motion
5. Constant pain
6. Moderate severe or severe low back pain (above 5 on a 0–10 pain scale)

shown to create SIJ pain (Dreyfuss et al 1996). SIJ dysfunction usually develops without provocation or incident. Other features of SIJ dysfunction included moderate pain (e.g. Modified Oswestry score around 38%) (Fritz & George 2000). A list of the pretest probabilities that was developed from my own experience is in Box 18.1. Also, a list of pretest probabilities not associated with SIJ dysfunction, and which can help rule out SIJ dysfunction, is listed in Box 18.2.

EXAMINATION OF THE PELVIS

Confirmation of SIJ dysfunction has been a continued source of controversy. No doubt this is exacerbated by the fact that so far, no 'gold standard' of diagnosis has been established for the presence of SIJ dysfunction. Reasons include its deep location, small motion, irregular shape and orientation of articular surfaces, all of which make direct examination, visual appraisal of motion, and injection difficult (Bernard & Cassidy 1991). Therefore, it is easy to understand that most individual tests used to detect SIJ dysfunction have been shown to be unreliable (Delitto et al 1992, Potter & Rothstein 1985). Clinicians, however, rarely use just one test to detect SIJ dysfunction (Beal 1982, Cibulka & Koldehoff 1999, Delitto et al 1992). Recent research shows that when SIJ tests are combined, reliability as well as diagnostic specificity improves (Cibulka & Koldehoff 1999, Diamond & Forrester 1979). Cibulka & Koldehoff (1999) and Dreyfuss et al (1996) found high specificity in identifying patients with SIJ

dysfunction when combining SIJ tests. Recently, Levangie (1999) also found high test specificity when using the Gillet test and sitting flexion test (93%) to detect pelvic asymmetry, an often described feature of SIJ dysfunction. Laslett & Williams(1994) also found good reliability, when using SIJ provocation tests. Freburger & Riddle (2001) recently evaluated the use of pelvic calipers in the clinic and found unacceptable reliability; however, few therapists routinely use pelvic calipers in the clinic to assess pelvic landmarks on patients.

Most SIJ tests can be divided into three different groups. The first group includes tests that attempt to detect limited or abnormal motion of the SIJ, the second group tests for signs of pelvic obliquity, and the last group uses tests that provoke the joint to determine irritability. Tests used to detect abnormal SIJ motion usually try to compare motion on one side with the other side. A major problem with using tests to detect abnormal or limited motion is that since bicondylar joint motion is relative, (i.e. both sides move together), it is highly unlikely that abnormal or limited motion can be palpated. Also, the few studies that have been performed on patients with SIJ dysfunction have shown no difference in motion between healthy subjects and those identified with SIJ dysfunction (Sturesson et al 1989, 2000). However, admittedly, in these studies, the sample size was small, no control group was used, and the roentgen stereo-phonogrammetric analysis (RSA) setup that was used to make these studies was difficult to interpret. However, currently, we do not have any other convincing evidence that motion at the SIJ is increased, decreased, or altered in patients with SIJ dysfunction. Nevertheless, since no study has yet to show that movement is altered in SIJ dysfunction, I do not suggest using specific tests to detect movement, at this time, for the SIJ.

The second most common method of testing for SIJ dysfunction is to use four tests for pelvic obliquity (Cibulka & Koldehoff 1988). Pelvic obliquity has long been considered a common element of SIJ dysfunction (Bourdillon & Day 1987, Cibulka et al 1988, Erhard & Bowling 1977, Mennell 1960, Mitchell et al 1979). Detecting the presence of pelvic obliquity, especially when sitting, suggests SIJ dysfunction (Cibulka et al 1986, Mitchell et al 1979). The sitting position eliminates the possible chance that any difference in leg lengths could create pelvic asymmetry. When sitting, the landmarks of the pelvis should normally be level. Uneven pelvic landmarks (e.g. the PSIS) when sitting, suggest innominate bone asymmetry (Fig. 18.2). Innominate bone asymmetry, which is not the result of leg length disparity, can only be produced by an antagonistic innominate bone tilt, where one innominate bone is tilted anteriorly and the other posteriorly. Normally, the innominate bones should remain symmetrical while sitting. It is not

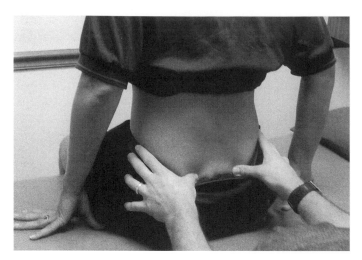

Figure 18.2 Observation of pelvic landmarks in sitting. The position of the physical therapist's thumbs on the posterior superior iliac spine suggests innominate asymmetry.

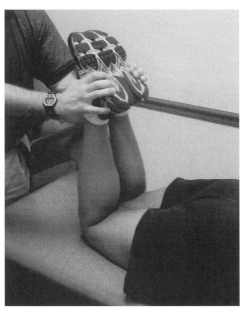

Figure 18.4 Prone knee flexion test for sacroiliac joint dysfunction.

known how the innominate bones assume this asymmetrical position however, some have suggested hip muscle imbalance, although there is presently no evidence available to confirm this (Cibulka 1992, Porterfield & DeRosa 1990,1991). A major caveat in detecting pelvic bone landmarks is that palpation often depends on working with a patient in whom it is possible to reliably and accurately detect uneven pelvic landmarks. Janos (1992) found poor reliability when palpating pelvic landmarks. However, when using a cluster of similar tests (Cibulka & Koldehoff 1999, Delitto et al 1992), the reliability of detecting SIJ dysfunction was found to have improved considerably. The four tests used by Cibulka &

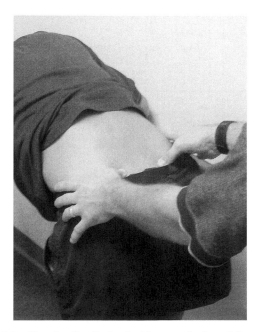

Figure 18.3 The standing flexion test for examination of the pelvis.

Koldehoff (1999) are different methods used to detect pelvic obliquity and include the standing flexion test (Fig. 18.3), the prone knee flexion test (Fig. 18.4), the supine long sitting test, and uneven PSIS heights when sitting (Fig. 18.2). It is important when interpreting the results of a cluster of tests that all of the results converge, that is, that they should all suggest the same direction of innominate bone tilt and not contradict each other. Therefore, SIJ dysfunction is defined by the presence of antagonistic innominate bone asymmetry that is present when, normally, the innominate bones should be symmetrical. Thus the two normal antagonistic movements possible, the first where the left innominate bone tilts posteriorly and the right anteriorly, and the second where the right innominate bone tilts posteriorly and the left anteriorly, define the two types of SIJ dysfunctions that can develop. Knowledge of the direction of the innominate bone's tilt is extremely important when planning treatment of SIJ dysfunction.

Provocation tests are used to try and recreate a similar painful response by provoking the SIJ through compression or gapping of the SIJs. Laslett & Williams (1994) have shown the reliability of some provocation tests and have suggested their use in identifying SIJ dysfunction. Potter & Rothstein (1985) also found good reliability with provocation tests. Other studies, however, have shown poor test specificity with individual provocation tests (Dreyfuss et al 1994, Maigne et al 1996). Recently, Broadhurst & Bond (1998) showed that when provocation tests are combined, they have a high predictive value for detecting SIJ dysfunction. A major problem is that although provocation tests may indeed be useful in identifying the presence of SIJ dysfunction, they have limited clinical usefulness because they have not shown any ability to either guide prognosis or treatment. Also, positive provocation tests have been found in asymptomatic patients (Dreyfuss et al 1994), which can lead to false positive findings. Therefore, provocation tests have limited clinical usefulness.

Using the EBP approach, where pretest probabilities are combined with one or more tests that have good measurement properties (e.g. high likelihood ratios, or high specificity or sensitivity), is the best method of making the diagnosis of SIJ dysfunction. Box 18.1 lists pretest probabilities that are used in my clinic to help increase prediction of the prevalence of SIJ dysfunction. A next step is to go online and via the sites PUBMED (www.ncbi.nlm.nih.gov/pubmed/) and Grateful Med (www.igm.nlm.nih.gov/gratefulmed/), to search for those tests that have shown high sensitivity, specificity, or likelihood ratios and that are used to determine the post-test probability, and therefore rule in the diagnosis of SIJ dysfunction. The tests used include the four tests for pelvic obliquity mentioned earlier (Cibulka & Koldehoff 1999). Positive results in at least three out of four tests suggest SIJ dysfunction (Cibulka & Koldehoff 1999). Also, all of the SIJ tests must converge or agree suggesting that the exact same problem exists in all of them (e.g. a left posterior innominate bone). The problem with using a cluster of tests is that a gold standard currently does not exist, however using a cluster as a clinical standard has already shown its usefulness in helping physical therapists guide successful intervention, which is the primary purpose of any examination.

A diagnosis of SIJ dysfunction is made by finding a high post-test probability from the results of the pretest probability for the disorder, and the likelihood ratio generated from the positive test results. For example, one could predict a pretest probability of 75% if the patient had unilateral PSIS pain primarily, had no trauma, had full trunk range of motion, and indicated a pain score of around 4/10 on a 1–10 analog pain scale. Then, on examination, if all four SIJ tests were found to be positive (all suggesting a left posterior innominate SIJ dysfunction), the positive likelihood ratio of finding at least three out of four tests positive for SIJ dysfunction is 6.83. Thus, as a result of doing the mathematics, the pretest probability of 0.75 and the likelihood ratio of 6.83 would give a post-test probability of 96%. A post-test probability of 96% strongly suggests that it is likely that the patient has SIJ dysfunction.

PROGNOSIS IN SACROILIAC JOINT DYSFUNCTION

No published data exists on the prognosis of SIJ dysfunction. Numerous reports describe SIJ dysfunction

as a recurring problem. The ubiquitous use of SIJ fixation belts is one example of the clinician's quest to reduce the incidence of this problem. Although unilateral low back pain is the most common symptom of SIJ dysfunction, hip pain and hamstring muscle strain have also been shown to be related to SIJ dysfunction (Cibulka & Delitto 1993, Cibulka et al 1992).

INTERVENTION STRATEGIES

Much has been written on the treatment of the SIJ; unfortunately most is anecdotal and no randomized clinical trials have been performed so far, therefore, little published evidence is available to guide clinicians. In the only randomized clinical trial (Erhard et al 1994) on SIJ intervention, treatment involved both the SIJ and the lumbar spine, thus making inferences difficult. In another study (Cibulka et al 1988), manipulation, presumably directed at the SIJ, was shown to restore innominate bone symmetry in patients with previous innominate bone asymmetry and with signs and symptoms of SIJ dysfunction; unfortunately no data was collected on symptomatic improvement. Most of the non-peer-reviewed literature on the treatment of the SIJ is extremely confusing. Some treatments aim to restore mobility while others seek to restrict mobility. However, without a reliable or valid measure of motion, these treatments currently appear speculative at best. Since, so far, no data has shown that SIJ mobility is altered in patients with SIJ dysfunction, I believe it may be better to abandon the idea of treating the joint with too much or too little motion until we have some convincing evidence.

Mobilization, although used widely, has not been performed in any randomized control trial so far, therefore, we are left with primarily anecdotal descriptions of mobilizations that were successful in patients with SIJ dysfunction. When using mobilization, unlike manipulation, the direction that the innominate bones tilt must be known for this technique to be effective (Freburger & Riddle 2001). Many textbooks describe these techniques, which primarily include the movement of one or both innominate bones in a direction that would restore innominate bone symmetry (Bourdillon & Day 1987, Lee 1989, Stoddard 1959, Wells 1986, Woerman 1989).

As already mentioned, manipulation has been shown to restore pelvic symmetry in patients with SIJ dysfunction who previously had innominate bone asymmetry (Cibulka et al 1988). Tullberg et al (1998), however, recently questioned the effect manipulation has on the SIJ. Using an RSA technique, where markers were placed only on the dorsal surface of the pelvis of the 'dysfunctional side', Tullberg et al (1998) found no change in position between the side of the dysfunctional ilium and the sacrum, before and after a manipulative treatment aimed at the SIJ. The technical setup of this RSA study is questionable primarily because of Tullberg's marker placement. As previously discussed, inadequate marker placement limits the interpretation of movement between the innominate bones and sacrum. The data acquired from the frontal plane markers cannot possibly describe sagittal plane motion between the sacrum and innominate bones. The study by Cibulka et al (1988), in which pelvic calipers were used, showed that in patients who had a cluster of SIJ signs, a manipulative technique aimed at the SIJ restored innominate bone symmetry in all 10 patients who previously had measurable innominate bone asymmetry. A weakness of this study was that reliability of the pelvic calipers was not determined before the study. However, despite this, and with the examiner also being blinded to who was being treated, a significant difference in pelvic tilt was noted in all 10 patients in the experimental group. Also, the cluster of tests not only agreed with the innominate bone measurement of tilt, as to the direction of innominate bone tilt, but also was able to predict that no movement developed in 9 of the 10 patients in the control group. Therefore, in this study, a manipulative technique aimed at the SIJ convincingly restored innominate bone symmetry.

How does a unilateral manipulative technique restore bilateral innominate bone symmetry? I am not sure, however, since the two SIJs are considered to be one bicondylar joint, manipulating one side must also move the opposite side. More research is needed on this interesting subject.

PREVENTION OF SACROILIAC JOINT DYSFUNCTION RECURRENCE

Recurrence is considered a problem in patients with low back pain from the SIJ. A significant part of the problem, I believe, is ignorance. Many clinicians believe that the SIJ moves with three degrees of freedom, describing these motions as unilateral innominate bone movement, sacral flexions, rotations, and upslips (Mitchell et al 1979, Oldrieve 1996, 1998). All of these movements are impossible at this bicondylar joint. Furthermore, no data exists to prove that any of these motions exist. Puzzlingly, many of these motions often describe the exact same phenomena. I believe that what is important in the prevention of recurrence is to define the diagnosis of SIJ dysfunction and determine the possible reason for innominate bone symmetry. The movements of the SIJs are related to the motion of the hip and lumbar spinal joints; evaluation of these two areas are mandatory in recalcitrant SIJ problems. Interestingly, a number of studies have shown the importance of the hip in SIJ mechanics; for example, patients with hip joint

impairments, including patients with amputations of the thigh (Matanovic & Granic-Husic 1991), osteoarthritis of the hip and total hip replacements (Aalam & Hoffman 1975, Hebling 1978, Pap et al 1987), have all demonstrated significant changes in their SIJ. Furthermore, studies have reported that unilateral limited hip rotation is related to low back and SIJ dysfunction (Barbee et al 1990, Cibulka et al 1998, LaBan et al 1978). I recommend that with any recurrent SIJ problem, the hip and lumbar spine should be assessed.

HIP JOINT

JOINT MOVEMENTS OF THE HIP

The hip joint is the connection between the head of the femur bone and the acetabulum of the innominate bone. The hip joint is an ovoid, or ball and socket joint, and is the largest synovial joint in the body. The joint is very stable and strong because of its ligamentous attachments and its congruent fit. The hip joint's major function is to allow movement for walking and running, however, hip joint motion is important in movement of the trunk.

The two identical synovial joints of the left and right hip are considered to be unmodified ovoid joints with three degrees of freedom of movement, flexion/extension, abduction/adduction, and medial/lateral rotation. The head of the femur forms about two-thirds of a sphere with a diameter of 4–5 cm (Kapandji 1970). The head is supported by the femoral neck which runs obliquely from the femoral shaft at an angle of about 125° (within a range of 90–135°). The femoral neck enhances hip motion by placing the femoral shaft away from the pelvis laterally. The concave acetabulum faces in an oblique, anterior, lateral, and inferior direction.

The close-pack position of the hip, where the capsule and majority of the ligaments are taut and the joint articular surfaces are congruent, is where the hip is extended, internally rotated and abducted (MacConaill & Basmajian 1977). The loose-pack position, where the capsule and most of the hip ligaments are slackened and the joint articular surfaces are incongruent, is where the hip is flexed, externally rotated, and adducted (MacConaill & Basmajian 1977). Walmsley (1928) reports that the hip is in full congruence only when the hip transmits weight and is incongruent in all other positions. The hip joint moves from a loose-pack position at heel-strike to a close-pack position at heel-off and then back again. The loose-pack position at heel-strike is necessary so that the eccentrically contracting muscles of the hip and thigh can absorb the force of ground impact over time; while at heel-off, the hip must be in the close-pack position in order to push off a rigid lever to propel the body forward as the hip and thigh muscles contract primarily concentrically.

The hip joint has three degrees of freedom allowing motion in the frontal, sagittal and transverse planes. The hip moves primarily in the sagittal plane with 10–15° of extension and 135° of flexion. Movement in the frontal and transverse planes is more varied with measures of: abduction 30–45°, adduction 20–30°, internal rotation 30–75°, and external rotation 25–75°. The frontal and transverse plane hip movements have a wider variation of motion. Although the range is quite wide, very little difference is found when comparing left and right sides of the same motion (e.g. left and right medial rotation) in the asymptomatic and young.

LIGAMENTS AND THEIR ROLE IN HIP JOINT MOTION

The hip joint is surrounded by a strong and dense articular capsule that has a cylindrical shape and that runs from the iliac bone to the upper end of the femur. The hip joint capsule consists of two sets of fibers, one circular and the other longitudinal. The circular fibers are deeper and form a collar around the neck of the femur, while most of the longitudinal fibers are in the anterior aspect of the joint capsule. The capsule is partially blended with the posterior and anterior ligaments.

The hip joint has three very strong ligaments that strengthen the hip anteriorly and posteriorly: the ischiofemoral, pubofemoral, and iliofemoral ligaments (Grubel Lee 1983). The ischiofemoral ligament is the only posterior ligament. The pubofemoral ligament runs from the pubis to the trochanteric fossa, while the iliofemoral ligament runs from the lower part of the anterior inferior iliac spine to the trochanter line. All of the three hip ligaments become taut in extension and are relaxed during flexion. During medial hip rotation, the anterior ligaments are relaxed while the posterior ligament (the ischiofemoral ligament) remains taut, and during external rotation, the anterior ligaments (the iliofemoral and pubofemoral) become taut while the ischiofemoral becomes relaxed (Kapandji 1970). During adduction, the ischiofemoral and pubofemoral ligaments relax, while during abduction, they tighten (Kapandji 1970). The iliofemoral ligament, however, becomes taut during adduction.

The ligamentum teres is a minor supporting ligament with adduction being the only movement where it becomes taut; however, the role of the ligamentum teres in the development of osteophytes is interesting.

Functionally, the transverse ligament of the acetabulum is a portion of the acetabular labrum, however, it is not cartilagenous. It consists of strong fibers which cross the acetabular notch, forming a foramen. The acetabular labrum is a fibrocartilagenous rim attached to the margin of the acetabulum, thereby deepening the hip joint socket.

MUSCLE AND ITS ROLE IN HIP JOINT MOVEMENT

The hip joint is an ovoid joint with three degrees of freedom, and as described above, movement occurs in the sagittal plane (flexion and extension), the frontal plane, (abduction and adduction), and the transverse plane (internal and external rotation). Many of the muscles surrounding the hip have hybrid functions: they may be prime movers in one direction and assist in one or more other motions. The muscles that allow flexion of the hip include the iliopsoas, pectineus, sartorious, tensor fascia latae, and rectus femoris. The hip extensor muscles include the gluteus maximus and the hamstring muscle group. The hip abductor muscles include the gluteus medius, the gluteus minimus, and the tensor fascia latae. The hip adductor muscles include the gracilis, and the three adductor muscles – the longus, magnus, and brevis. The hip internal rotator muscles include the gluteus minimus, the anterior fibers of the gluteus medius, and the tensor fascia latae. The hip external rotator muscles include the piriformis, quadratus femoris, gemelli superior and inferior, and obturator internus and externus. Muscles of the hip may change their role according to the position the hip joint is in, for example, with the hip in 90° of hip flexion, the angle of pull of hip external rotators allows hip abduction instead of hip external rotation.

NEUROLOGY OF THE HIP JOINT

The hip joint is densely supplied with nerves formed from articular nerves that also innervate the surrounding muscles of the hip. The hip joint innervation is supplied primarily by the obturator nerve (Warwick & Williams 1973). Three articular nerves supply the hip joint and they include the posterior branch, the medial articular branch, and the nerve to the ligamentum capitus femoris. The posterior articular nerve has the greatest nerve supply to the hip; it supplies the posterior and inferior aspects of the hip joint capsule (Dee 1969). The medial articular nerve arises from the anterior division of the obturator nerve (from the ventral rami of the second, third, and fourth lumbar nerves) and divides into two branches (Dee 1969); the medial branch of this nerve supplies the anteromedial and inferior aspects of the joint capsule. The nerve to the ligamentum capitis femoris arises from the muscular branch of the posterior division of the obturator nerve (Warwick & Williams 1973) and it primarily supplies the ligamentum teres. The hip joint may also be supplied by a small number of nerves, coming from accessory articular nerves, which are from surrounding muscle supplied by the femoral nerve (from the dorsal branches of the ventral rami of the second, third, and fourth lumbar nerves) (Dee 1969).

BLOOD SUPPLY

The hip joint receives its blood supply from the obturator, gluteal, and femoral arteries. These arteries supply the acetabulum, and the femoral head and neck (Warwick & Williams 1973). The blood supply is clinically important in a number of hip disorders. The acetabulum branch of the obturator artery supplies blood to the medial aspect of the acetabulum. A small branch of this artery also supplies the ligamentum teres and therefore a limited portion of the superior aspect of the femoral head (Warwick & Williams 1973). The superior and inferior gluteal artery supplies part of the acetabulum. The femoral artery gives rise to the medial and lateral circumflex arteries (ascending branches) that supply the proximal end of the femur, from the femoral neck to the subcapital sulcus, and give rise to the retinacular arteries which supply the head of the femur (Warwick & Williams 1973). The retinacular arteries that supply the femoral head do not have any anastomoses, thus preventing the femoral head from having access to an alternative blood supply in case of injury.

HIP PROBLEMS IN THE ATHLETE

The two most common athletic problems that trouble the hip include hip joint pain from incongruence which creates capsular or labral problems, and hip pointers. Other conditions such as rheumatoid arthritis, ankylosing spondylitis, as well as childhood diseases and conditions, such as septic arthritis, Legg–Calvé–Perthes disease, slipped capital femoral epiphysis, and congenital hip dislocation, can and do affect the hip, however, these diseases and conditions are rare in the athlete. Hip dislocation, although rare, can occur during contact sports such as American football.

HISTORY

In most non-traumatic hip pain, the history of the pain is often unremarkable. Those who have had a childhood disease, such as Legg–Calvé–Perthes disease or slipped capital femoral epiphysis, are often more likely to develop hip pain later in life. The primary complaint is one of either anterior groin pain or lateral greater trochanter region pain (Roberts & Williams 1998). Pain posteriorly, in the buttock region, is more suggestive of a

lumbar problem than hip pain (Roberts & Williams 1988). Published data on hip pain (Khan & Woolson 1998) show that hip pain is usually referred to the groin and occasionally to the knee. Acute hip pain in a child of 3–10 years with weightbearing, spasm, and fever is suggestive of septic synovitis that should be referred on immediately (Hart 1996). If there is anterior hip pain in the prepubescent child, Legg–Calvé–Perthes disease should be suspected (Adkins & Figler 2000), while in adolescents, slipped capital femoral epiphysis should not be overlooked (Adkins & Figler 2000, O'Kane 1999). Stress fracture of the femoral neck should be suspected if there is a history of anterior hip pain in distance runners (Adkins & Figler 2000, Sterling et al 1993). Pain along the iliac crest is more suggestive of a hip pointer, often with a history of a direct blow, pain on palpation, occasional ecchymosis, and frequently pain with a valsalva maneuver (e.g. coughing or sneezing), or abdominal muscle contraction. Hip dislocation during sport is always traumatic and very painful.

PHYSICAL EXAMINATION OF THE HIP

Only a few studies give any kind of measurement properties (e.g. sensitivity, specificity, predictive value) for clinical hip tests. Birrel et al (2001), showed that restricted hip internal rotation was the most predictive of radiographic osteoarthritis (OA) of the hip. They found that restricted hip internal rotation had a sensitivity of 86% for moderate OA and 100% severe OA, while specificity was 54% and 42% respectively. Restriction in all three planes had greater discrimination with a sensitivity for moderate and severe OA with 33% and 54% respectively, while specificity was 93% and 88% respectively (Birrel et al 2001). Altman (1987) proposed that OA of the hip may be suggested by a combination of clinical criteria including: age greater than 40 years, weightbearing pain, pain relieved by sitting, antalgic gait, and decreased painful range of motion. No data on sensitivity or specificity was given. Later, Altman et al (1991) proposed new criteria that classified a patient as having OA of the hip if pain was present in combination with: hip internal rotation less than or equal to 15°, pain present on hip internal rotation, morning stiffness of the hip for less than or equal to 1h, age greater than 50 years, hip flexion less than or equal to 115°. The sensitivity and specificity for this criteria was 86% and 75% respectively.

As there is little in the way of publications on diagnostic ruling tests at present, ruling out diagnoses, such as septic arthritis or Legg–Calvé–Perthes disease in the evaluation of a hip joint often helps to crystalize the diagnostic process. The history and age, as described above, are important in helping to guide the clinician's thought process.

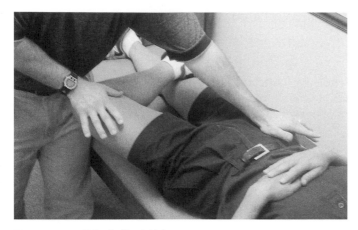

Figure 18.5 Faber's (Patrick's) test.

The examination of the hip starts first with active hip motion during functional movements. Functional movements depend on age and agility, and such activities can include squatting, going from sitting to standing, trunk forward bending, one legged standing, walking and running. Passive hip range of motion is assessed next, especially hip rotation, since internal rotation is often the first motion lost in OA (Altman et al 1991, Birrel 2001). Muscle length (Thomas and Ober tests) and strength are also assessed. Guidance for the examination of these tissues can be found in many textbooks. An examination of the pelvis, including leg lengths, is also performed on all patients with hip pain, since any alteration in innominate bone tilt can result in unequal concentration of pressure on the hip joints. Other tests for the hip include FABER's (Patrick's) test (Fig. 18.5) to determine hip joint irritability, tests for leg length to detect pelvic obliquity, and the Trendelenburg test to test the hip abductor muscles functionally for strength. Altman et al (1991) also proposes a test where passive internal rotation of the hip is used to determine hip joint irritability.

In the adult hip, where trauma is not involved, few mechanical disorders develop. The most common hip problem is pain that comes from the hip joint itself. This is usually just called hip pain (Grubel Lee 1983, Reynolds & Freeman 1989). Other diagnoses, like bursitis and tendinitis, around the hip are rare. Ligament strain of the hip joint has not been described in the literature. Muscle injury to the one-joint muscles surrounding the hip is very uncommon, although the two-joint rectus femoris, adductor, and hamstring muscles are frequently strained during athletic activity. The most common problem within the hip is joint inflammation that is usually the result of capsular shortening, which leads to incongruence leading to abnormal joint contact pressures and eventually arthritic changes (Loyd-Roberts 1953, Pauwels 1976, Reynolds & Freeman 1989, Walmsley 1928).

Abnormal stress imposed on the hip has also been related to tears of the acetabular labrum (Dorrell & Catterall 1986) which may also create anterior hip pain. In traumatic conditions, such as hip dislocation, motion is very painful, weightbearing is impossible, and deformity of the hip, such as shortening and angulation is visually obvious.

The problem of congruence between the head of the femur and acetabulum and the development of abnormal hip joint pressure is important in understanding the development of hip OA (Bullough et al 1973, Pauwels 1976, Walmsley 1928). The reduction or realignment of stress on the hip joint is of major importance in treating hip joint pain (Pauwels 1976). Many potential risk factors can influence joint congruence within the hip joint including joint range of motion, hip joint muscle force (including both muscle length and strength), pelvic obliquity, and a history of childhood hip disease. Many of these factors may alter hip joint motion, which in turn can either increase or decrease hip joint pressure by not allowing the hip joint to attain a full close-pack or loose-pack position during gait (Grubel Lee 1983). Articular cartilage is dependant on the repetitive loading and unloading of the hip for nutrition and lubrication, therefore reducing hip joint mobility through either capsular shortening or muscle weakness can diminish the health of the hip joint (Grubel Lee 1983, Loyd-Roberts 1953, Reynolds & Freeman 1989).

During heel-strike, the joints of the hip are primarily in their loose-pack position, allowing the eccentrically contracting muscles of the hip, and not the hip joint, to withstand the impact of ground force. However, if the hip joint cannot attain a full position of loose-pack (flexion, adduction, and external rotation) at the time of heel-strike, excessive compressive forces may develop within the hip. At heel-off, just the opposite problem may develop. At heel-off, the majority of the hip muscles are contracting concentrically to push the limb from the ground,

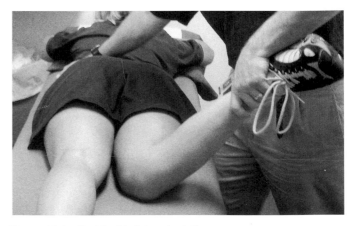

Figure 18.6 Test for hip internal rotation.

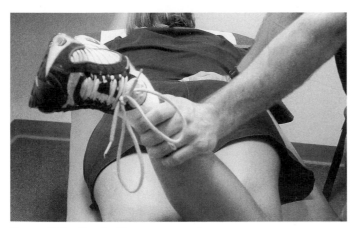

Figure 18.7   Test for hip external rotation.

therefore the hip joint must attain a close-pack position to allow the muscle enough momentum to push off. However, if the hip joint cannot attain full close-pack position (the combined movement of internal rotation, extension, and abduction), force cannot be equally disseminated across the hip joint and thus excessive pressures can develop leading to hip pain and eventually arthritis.

The presence of anterior or groin pain, pain with weightbearing relieved by rest, limited hip internal rotation (Fig. 18.6) (when comparing the left and right sides), excessive hip external rotation (Fig. 18.7), signs of pelvic obliquity, short hip flexor muscles with the Thomas test, and hip muscle weakness also suggest hip joint pain. Birrell et al (2001) or Altman (1987, 1991) criteria and data can be used for those who are unsure in the diagnosis of OA of the hip. Radiographic measurements, however, especially in more advanced cases, are more accurate as well as specific in making the diagnosis of hip OA (Birrel et al 2001).

PROGNOSIS FOR HIP PROBLEMS

The prognosis for almost all non-surgical hip problems in the athlete is very good. Usually hip pain in the young is self-limiting and eventually goes away with or without intervention, especially if activity is restricted. Persistent hip pain in the adult that is related to capsular shortening, diminished range of motion, and incongruence, may lead to OA (Grubel Lee 1983, Reynolds & Freeman 1989). Also, those with persistent anteversion of the hip may also be at higher risk for development of hip OA (Halpern et al 1979, Terjesen et al 1982). In non-traumatic conditions, the athlete who develops a femoral head stress fracture is of particular concern. Stress fracture of the femoral head is uncommon but has been described in distance runners who ignore their hip pain (Adkins & Figler 2000, Sterling et al 1993).

INTERVENTION STRATEGIES

Strategies for dealing with problems attaining the close-pack position

Problems with the close-pack position include those where the hip cannot achieve the full close-pack position, or congruence, especially during the heel-off portion of the gait when muscles are contracting concentrically. Three major reasons exists for this. First, the joint does not have full range of motion in abduction, extension, or medial rotation (in any or all of these movements). Lack of motion can be due to muscular or capsular problems, or both. The Thomas test can determine if the hip flexor muscles are shortened. Second, muscle strength may not be sufficient to achieve full close-pack, that is, any or all of the hip abductors, hip extensors, and hip medial rotator muscles may be weak. Third, the hip may not be able to attain full close-pack range of motion because the pelvis is oblique. Two types of pelvic obliquity can develop, one from a leg length disparity and the second, from SIJ dysfunction, as described previously. In all types of pelvic obliquity, the change in acetabular orientation creates a frontal plane shift in the hip joint, on the long leg side, where the hip is adducted; while on the short leg side, the hip is abducted (Gofton 1971, Morscher 1977). In SIJ dysfunction, the hip joint adducts on the posterior tilted side and abducts on the anterior tilted side. Treatment strategies include restoring joint mobility, muscular strength, and eliminating the reason for pelvic obliquity (by leveling leg lengths or treating the SIJ).

Strategies for dealing with problems attaining the loose-pack position

Strategies for achieving a loose-pack position of the hip are just the opposite of those for a close-pack position problem. Problems with loose-pack position include those where the hip cannot achieve the full loose-pack position. The loose-pack position is needed during heel-strike and during the swing phase of the gait. Three major reasons can prevent the hip from gaining the loose-pack position. First, the hip joint has lost some of its range of motion in the direction of adduction, flexion, or lateral rotation movements. Lack of motion can be due to muscular or capsular problems, or both. Second, hip muscle strength may not be sufficient to achieve full loose-pack, that is, any or all of the hip abductors, hip flexors, and hip lateral rotator muscles may be weak, thus not allowing full loose-pack. Third, the hip may not be able to attain full loose-pack range of motion because the pelvis is oblique. Pelvic obliquity creates hip adduction on the long leg side, while on the short leg side, the hip is abducted (Gofton 1971). In SIJ dysfunction, the hip is adducted on the posterior tilted side and abducted on the

anterior tilted side. Treatment strategies are aimed at restoring hip joint mobility, muscular strength, and eliminating any pelvic obliquity.

PREVENTION OF RECURRENT HIP PAIN

The lack of research and data on the recurrence of hip pain helps to explain why the prevention of recurrent hip pain is not very well understood. Some suggest that the persistence of pelvic obliquity is one possible reason for recurrent hip pain (Bjerkreim 1974, Cibulka & Delitto 1993, Halpern et al 1979, Jorring 1980) while Terjesen et al (1982) suggest that increased femoral anteversion is also a predisposing factor in OA of the hip. This factor is similar to unilateral hip rotation asymmetry, which has been shown to be related to anterior and posterior hip pain (Cibulka & Delitto 1993, Cibulka et al 1998). Presumably, anything that does not allow the hip to gain its full close-pack or full loose-pack position may be considered a potential risk factor in the development of recurrent hip pain. Therapists should determine the best course of intervention to insure attainment of full hip range of motion.

GROIN INJURIES IN ATHLETES

The groin region, which may also be termed the inguinal area or femoral triangle region, is a common site for athletic injuries. The most common athletic problems in this region include adductor muscle strains (also including gracilis muscle strain), osteitis pubis, and less commonly, hernia. Therapists must be aware of the specific signs and symptoms of each in order to determine a quick referral or an effective treatment for each problem. The groin region consists of: the symphysis pubis, described previously, an amphiarthrodial or cartilagenous joint, which has very little movement (2 mm or less normally); the adductor muscles, including the brevis, longus, magnus; the gracilis muscle; and the medial hip flexor muscles, primarily the pectineus, and iliopsoas muscles. The neurology of the groin region is slightly more complex than other regions, owing to the vast amount of different nerves supplying the genitals, as well as the skin, muscles, and surrounding joints. The lumbar plexus (L2, L3, L4) gives rise to the iliohypogastric nerve (L1) which supplies a branch (the anterior cutaneous branch) to the skin of the abdomen above the pubis (Warwick & Williams 1973). The ilioinguinal nerve, which also arises from the first lumbar nerve, supplies the skin of the genitals and the skin of the superiomedial area of the thigh (Warwick & Williams 1973), the most common area of groin pain. The genitofemoral nerve supplies the genitals and the area of skin over the upper part of the femoral triangle, just lateral to the groin region.

HISTORY

Most of the injuries in and around the groin are traumatic injuries. Muscle strains always have a mechanism of injury. Muscle does not develop fatigue failure like bone, therefore there has to be another reason for the muscle strain. Most commonly, lateral running, skating, jumping, or any other quick motion in the frontal plane that requires a forceful contraction of the involved muscle, often while the muscle is also elongating, is the mechanism of muscle injury. As muscle ruptures, it bleeds which results in ecchymosis and later, the appearance of integumentary contusion. Blood will often migrate distally with the amount of ecchymosis dependent on the degree of muscle injury. Pain from muscle strain is never referred beyond the boundary of the injured muscle; for example, pain from an adductor muscle strain stays within the adductor muscle.

Osteitis pubis is usually characterized by a forceful contraction of the adductor or rectus abdominus muscles (Briggs et al 1992). Adductor muscle strains and osteitis pubis are usually caused by the same adduction motion. The mechanism of injury of osteitis pubis, like adductor muscle strain, includes sudden changes in direction or sprinting (Batt et al 1995) Osteitis pubis is often aggravated by exercise, specifically movements such as running, kicking, or pivoting on one leg and is usually relieved by rest (Andrews & Carek 1998). Pain distribution for osteitis pubis can be in several areas including the pubic, groin, lower abdominal, perineal, testicular, suprapubic, and inguinal regions (Andrews & Carek 1998). Climbing stairs, coughing or sneezing can create groin symptoms (Andrews & Carek 1998).

PHYSICAL EXAMINATION OF THE GROIN REGION

Examination of the groin includes: examining hip active and passive range of motion, to rule out referred pain from the hip; sacroiliac examination, since Major & Helms (1997) demonstrated that SIJ problems are associated with osteitis pubis; muscle testing (both muscle length and strength) to rule out adductor muscle and abdominal muscle strain; and if no physical impairments are found, examination for possible hernia. Adductor muscle strain (including the gracilis muscle), is tested by examining muscle length and strength. Muscle strains are characterized by reproduction of pain on elongating muscle and on resisted contraction. Thus passive abduction of the hip usually aggravates most adductor muscle

---

Box 18.3 Diagnosis of groin muscle strain

1. Described mechanism of muscle injury
2. Pain localized only to the muscle itself, no radiation of pain
3. Pain on palpation of the injured muscle
4. Pain on elongation of the injured muscle
5. Pain on contraction of the injured muscle

---

strains. Also, resisted muscle contraction of adduction for the adductor muscles, and resisted adduction and knee flexion for the gracilis usually reproduces pain. Lastly palpation is useful as a strained muscle is usually painful when palpated, especially over the anatomical location of the strain (Box 18.3).

Osteitis pubis is characterized by pubic tenderness and pain with active hip abduction. Osteitis pubis is the most common inflammatory condition affecting the symphysis pubis (Andrews & Carek 1998). Adductor muscle strain must be ruled out when osteitis pubis is considered. Williams suggests that radiographic examination (using a flamingo view) that shows more than 2 mm vertical displacement would indicate pubic symphysis instability (Williams et al 2000).

TREATMENT

Treatment of adductor muscle strains includes restoring adductor muscle length and strength. Initially, like all acute injuries, the area is treated with ice, elevation, and compression and avoidance of activities that aggravate the pain. Once symptoms subside, gentle stretching exercises to the involved muscle can begin. As the muscle regains approximately 75% of its length, muscle strengthening exercises follow. The goal in the rehabilitation of injured muscle is to restore the full length and strength of the injured muscle. Additional physical modalities can be used to hasten the rehabilitation process. Later, once muscle length and strength is restored, sport-specific training can begin.

Treatment of osteitis pubis is usually in the form of symptomatic relief, with physical modalities, rest, and anti-inflammatory medications; surgery is rarely indicated and reserved only for those whose symptoms are not relieved by conservative therapy (Vincent 1993).

SUMMARY

This chapter demonstrates the complexity of the anatomy around the pelvis, hip, and groin area. A thorough knowledge of the anatomical structures and their relationship to each other is necessary to accurately diagnose pain and injuries in this region. When considering treatment options for such injuries, the nature of the sport or exercise activity that the athlete is involved in should be considered, and appropriate biomechanical analysis of movements carried out. In managing injuries in this region both manual and exercise treatment should be combined with biomechanical correction of movement patterns.

REFERENCES

Aalam M, Hoffman P 1975 Deterioration of the ilio-sacral joints through serious unilateral hip joint disease. Archiv fur Orthopadische und Unfall-Chirurgie 82:257–262
Adkins S B 3rd, Figler R A 2000 Hip pain in athletes. American Family Physician 61(7):2109–2118
Alderink G J 1991 The sacroiliac joint: review of anatomy, mechanics, and function. Journal of Orthopaedic and Sports Physical Therapy 13:71–84
Altman R D 1987 Criteria for the classification of osteoarthritis of the knee and hip. Scandinavian Journal of Rheumatology 65(suppl):31–39
Altman R D, Alarcon G, Appelrouth D et al 1991 The American College of Rheumatology criteria for the classification and reporting of osteoarthritis of the hip. Arthritis and Rheumatism 34(5):505–514
Andrews S K, Carek P J 1998 Osteitis pubis: a diagnosis for the family physician. Journal of the American Board of Family Practice 11:291–295
Barakatt E, Smidt G L, Dawson J D et al 1996 Interinnominate motion and symmetry: comparison between gymnast and nongymnast. Journal of Orthopaedic and Sports Physical Therapy 23:309–319
Batt M E, McShane J M, Dillingham M F 1995 Osteitis pubis in collegiate football players. Medicine and Science in Sports and Exercise 27:629–633

Beal M C 1982 The sacroiliac problem: review of anatomy, mechanics, and diagnosis. Journal of the American Osteopathic Association 81:667–679
Bernard T N, Cassidy J 1991 The sacroiliac joint syndrome: pathophysiology, diagnosis, and management. In: Frymoyer J W (ed) The adult spine: principle and practice. Raven Press, New York
Birrell F, Croft P, Cooper C et al 2001 Predicting radiographic hip osteoarthritis from range of movement. Rheumatology 40(5):506–512
Bjerkreim I 1974 Secondary dysplasia and osteoarthrosis of the hip in functional and fixed obliquity of the pelvis. Acta Orthopaedica Scandinavica 45:873–882
Blankevoort L 1988 The envelope of passive knee joint motion. Journal of Biomechanics 21:705–720
Bourdillon J F, Day E A 1987 Spinal manipulation. William Heinemann Medical, London
Borrel U, Fernestrom I 1957 The movements of the sacro-iliac joints and their importance to changes on pelvic dimensions during parturition. Acta Obstetrica Gynecologica Scandinavica 36:42–57
Briggs R C, Kolbjornsen P H, Southall R C 1992 Osteitis pubis, Tc-99m MDP, and professional hockey players. Clinical Nuclear Medicine 17:861–863
Broadhurst N A 1989 Sacroiliac joint dysfunction as a cause of low back pain. Australian Family Physician 18(6):626–627
Broadhurst N A, Bond M J 1998 Pain provocation tests for the

assessment of sacroiliac joint dysfunction. Journal of Spinal Disorders 11:341–345

Brunner C, Kissling R, Jacob H 1991 The effects of morphology and histopathology. Spine 16:1111–1117

Bullough P, Goodfellow J, O'Conner J 1973 The relationship between degenerative changes and load bearing in the human hip. Journal of Bone and Joint Surgery (Br) 55B:746–758

Calvillo O, Skaribas I, Turnispeed J 2000 Anatomy and pathophysiology of the sacroiliac joint. Current Reviews in Pain 4(5):356–361

Chamberlain W E 1930 The symphysis pubis in the roentgen examination of the sacroiliac joint. American Journal of Roentgenology 24:621–624

Cibulka M T 1992 The treatment of the sacroiliac joint component to low back pain: a case report. Physical Therapy 72:917–922

Cibulka M T, Delitto A 1993 A comparison of two different methods to treat hip pain in runners. Journal of Orthopaedic and Sports Physical Therapy 17:172–176

Cibulka M T, Koldehoff R M 1999 Clinical usefulness of a cluster of sacroiliac joint tests in patients with and without low back pain. Journal of Orthopaedic and Sports Physical Therapy 29:83–92

Cibulka M T, Rose S J, Delitto A et al 1986 Hamstring muscle strain treated by mobilizing the sacroiliac joint. Physical Therapy 66(8):1220–1223

Cibulka M T, Delitto A, Koldehoff R M 1988 Changes in innominate tilt after manipulation of the sacroiliac joint in patients with low back pain: an experimental study. Physical Therapy 68:1359–1363

Cibulka M T, Erhard R E, Delitto A 1992 Pain patterns in patients with and without sacroiliac joint dysfunction. In: Vleeming A, Mooney V, Snijders C et al (eds) Proceedings of the First Interdisciplinary World Congress on Low Back Pain and its Relation to the Sacroiliac Joint. San Diego, CA

Cibulka M T, Sinacore D R, Cromer G S et al 1998 Unilateral hip rotation range of motion asymmetry in patients with sacroiliac joint regional pain. Spine 23:1009–1015

Colachis S C, Warden R E, Bechtol C O et al 1963 Movement of the sacroiliac joint in the adult male: a preliminary report. Archives of Physical Medicine and Rehabilitation 44:490–498

Cummings G, Scholz J P, Barnes K 1993 The effect of imposed leg length difference on pelvic bone symmetry. Spine 18:368–373

Death A B, Kirby R I, MacMillan C L 1982 Pelvic ring mobility: assessment by stress radiography. Archives of Physical Medicine and Rehabilitation 63:129–135

Dee R 1969 Structure and function of hip joint innervation. Annals of the College of Surgeons England 45:357–374

Delitto A, Shulman A D, Rose S J 1992 Reliability of a clinical examination to classify patients with low back syndrome. Physical Therapy Practice 1:1–9

Diamond G A, Forrester J S 1979 Analysis of probability as an aid in the clinical diagnosis of coronary artery disease. New England Journal of Medicine 300:1350–1358

DonTigny R L 1979 Dysfunction of the sacroiliac joint and its treatment. Journal of Orthopaedic and Sports Physical Therapy 1:23–35

DonTigny R L 1985 Function and pathomechanics of the sacroiliac joint, a review. Physical Therapy 65:35–44

Dorrell J H, Catterall A 1986 The torn acetabular labrum. Journal of Bone and Joint Surgery (Br) 68B(3):400–403

Dreyfuss P, Dreyer S, Griffin J 1994 Positive sacroiliac screening tests in the asymptomatic adults. Spine 19:1138–1143

Dreyfuss P, Michaaelsen D C, Pauza K et al 1996 The value of medical history and physical examination in diagnosing sacroiliac joint pain. Spine 21:2594–2602

Egund N, Olsson T H, Schmid H et al 1978 Movements in the sacroiliac joints demonstrated with roentgen stereophotogrammetry. Acta Radiologica Diagnostica 19:833–846

Ellison J V, Rose S J, Sahrmann S A 1990 Patterns of hip rotation range of motion: a comparison between healthy subjects and patients with low back pain. Physical Therapy 70:537–541

Erhard R, Bowling R 1977 The recognition and management of the pelvic component of low back pain and sciatica pain. Bulletin of the Orthopaedic Section, American Physical Therapy Association 2:4–15

Erhard R E, Delitto A, Cibulka M T 1994 Relative effectiveness of an extension program and a combined program of manipulation and flexion and extension exercises in patients with acute low back syndrome. Physical Therapy 74:1093–1100

Fortin J, Aprill C N, Ponthieux R T et al 1994 Sacroiliac joint: pain referral maps upon applying a new injection/arthrography technique. Part II: clinical evaluation. Spine 19:1483–1489

Freburger J K, Riddle D L 2001 Using published evidence to guide the examination of the sacroiliac joint region. Physical Therapy 81:1135–1143

Friedland D J, Go S A, Davoren J B et al 1998 Evidence-base medicine. A framework for clinical practice. Appleton and Lange, Stamford, CT

Frigerio N A, Stowe R R, Howe J W 1974 Movement of the sacroiliac joint. Clinical Orthopaedics and Related Research 100:370–377

Fritz J M, George S 2000 The use of a classification approach to identify subgroups of patients with acute low back pain. Spine 25:106–114

Gofton J P 1971 Studies in osteoarthrosis of the hip: Part II. Osteoarthrosis of the hip and leg length disparity. Canadian Medical Association Journal 104:791–799

Goldthwaite J E, Osgood R B 1905 A consideration of the pelvic articulation from an anatomical, pathological and clinical standpoint. Boston Medical and Surgical Journal 152:593–601

Grubel Lee D M 1983 Disorders of the hip. JB Lippincott, Philadelphia, PA

Halpern A A, Tanner J, Rinsky L 1979 Does persistent fetal femoral anteversion contribute to osteoarthritis. Clinical Orthopaedics and Related Research 145:213–215

Hart J J 1996 Transient synovitis of the hip in children. American Family Physician 54(5):1587–1591

Hebling R 1978 The sacroiliac joint after hip arthrodesis. Zeitschrift fur Orthopadie 116:113–23

Janos S C 1992 Palpation of selected bony landmarks in the lumbopelvic region. In: Proceedings of the International Federation of Orthopaedic Manipulative Therapists, Fifth International Conference, Vail, CO

Jorring K 1980 Osteoarthritis of the hip, epidemiology and clinical role. Acta Orthopaedica Scandinavica 51:523–530

Kampen W U, Tillmann B 1998 Age-related changes in the articular cartilage of human sacroiliac joints. Anatomy and Embryology (Berlin)198:505–513

Kapandji I A 1970 Physiology of the Joints, vol 2, 2nd edn. Churchill Livingstone, London

Khan N Q, Woolson S T 1998 Referral patterns of hip pain in patients undergoing total hip replacement. Orthopedics 21(2):123–126

LaBan M M, Meerschaert J R, Taylor R S et al 1978 Symphyseal and sacroiliac joint pain associated with pubic symphysis instability. Archives of Physical Medicine and Rehabilitation 59:470–472

Laslett M, Williams M 1994 The reliability of selected pain provocation tests for sacroiliac joint pathology. Spine 19:1243–1249

Lavignolle B, Vital J M, Senegas J et al 1983 An approach to the functional anatomy of the sacroiliac joints in vivo. Anatomica Clinica 5:169–176

Lee D 1989 The pelvic girdle. Churchill Livingstone, Edinburgh

Levangie P K 1999 Four clinical tests of sacroiliac joint dysfunction: the association of test results with innominate torsion among patients with and without low back pain. Physical Therapy 79:1043–1057

Loyd-Roberts G C 1953 The role of the capsular changes in osteoarthritis of the hip joint. Journal of Bone and Joint Surgery (Br) 35B:627–642

MacConaill M A, Basmajian J V 1977 Muscles and movements. Robert E. Krieger Publishing, Huntington, NY

Maigne J, Aivaliklis A, Pfefer F 1996 Results of sacroiliac joint double block and value of sacroiliac joint pain provocation tests in 54 patients with low back pain. Spine 15:1889–1892

Major N M, Helms C A 1997 Pelvis stress injuries: the relationship between osteitis pubis (symphysis pubis stress injury) and sacroiliac joint abnormalities in athletes. Skeletal Radiology 26:711–717

Matanovic B, Granic-Husic M 1991 Degenerative changes in the sacroiliac joint in persons with amputations of the thigh and biomechanical disorders of gait. Reumatizam 38:9–13

Mennell J M 1960 Back pain: diagnosis and treatment using manipulative techniques. Little, Brown and Company, Boston, MA

Mitchell F L, Moran P S, Pruzzo N A 1979 An evaluation and treatment manual of osteopathic muscle energy technique procedures. Mitchell, Moran and Pruzzo, Valley Park, MO

Morscher E 1977 Progress in orthopaedic surgery 1. In: Hungerford DS (ed) Leg length discrepancy – the injured knee. Springer-Verlag, Berlin

O'Kane J W 1999 Anterior hip pain. American Family Physician 60(6):1687–1696

Oldrieve W L 1996 A critical review of the literature on the anatomy and biomechanics of the sacroiliac joint. Journal of Manual and Manipulative Therapy 4:157–165

Oldrieve W L 1998 A classification of, and a critical review of the literature on, syndromes of the sacroiliac joint. Journal of Manual and Manipulative Therapy 6:24–30

Pap A, Maager M, Kolarz G 1987 Functional impairment of the sacroiliac joint after total hip replacement. International Rehabilitation Medicine 8:145–147

Pauwels F 1976 Biomechanics of the normal and diseased hip. Springer-Verlag, Berlin

Pitkin H C, Pheasant, H C 1936 Sacrarthrotgenic telagia. Journal of Bone and Joint Surgery (Am) 18A:111–133

Porterfield J A, DeRosa C 1990 The sacroiliac joint. In: Gould J A (ed) Orthopaedic and sports physical therapy. CV Mosby, St Louis, MO

Porterfield J A, DeRosa C P 1991 Mechanical low back pain: perspectives in functional anatomy. WB Saunders, Philadelphia, PA

Potter N A, Rothstein J M 1985 Intertester reliability for selected clinical tests of the sacroiliac joint. Physical Therapy 65:1671–1675

Reynolds D, Freeman M 1989 Osteoarthritis of the young adult hip. Churchill Livingstone, Edinburgh

Roberts W N, Williams R B 1988 Hip Pain. Primary Care 15(4):783–793

Sackett D L, Haynes R B, Tugwell P 1985 Clinical epidemiology. A basic science for clinical medicine. Little Brown, Boston, MA

Sackett D L, Richardson W S, Rosenberg W et al 1998 Evidence-based medicine. How to practice and teach EBM. Churchill Livingstone, Edinburgh

Sasabili N, Valojerdy M R, Hogg D A 1995 Variation in thickness of articular cartilage in the human sacroiliac joint. Clinical Anatomy 8:388–390

Sashin D 1930 A critical analysis of the anatomy and the pathological changes of the sacroiliac joint. Journal of Bone and Joint Surgery (Am) 12A:891–910

Schunke G 1938 The anatomy and development of the sacroiliac joint in man. The Anatomical Record 72:313–331

Schwarzer A C, Aprill C N, Bogduk M 1995 The sacroiliac joint in chronic low back pain. Spine 20:31–37

Shaw J L 1992 The role of the sacroiliac joint as a cause of low back pain and dysfunction. In: Vleeming A, Mooney V, Snijders C et al (eds) Proceedings of the First Interdisciplinary World Congress On Low Back Pain and its Relation to the Sacroiliac Joint, San Diego, CA

Smidt G L, McQuade K, Wei S H et al 1995 Sacroiliac kinematics for reciprocal straddle positions. Spine 20:1047–1054

Smidt G L, Wei S H, McQuade K et al 1997 Sacroiliac motion for extreme hip positions. A fresh cadaver study. Spine 22:2073–2082

Solonen K A 1957 The sacro-iliac joint in the light of anatomical, roentgenological and clinical studies. Acta Orthopaedica Scandinavica (suppl)27:1–27

Sterling J C, Webb R F, Meyers M C et al 1993 False negative bone scan in a female runner. Medicine and Science in Sports and Exercise 25(2):179–185

Stoddard A 1959 Manual of osteopathic technique. Hutchinson, London

Sturesson B, Selvik G, Uden A 1989 Movements of the sacroiliac joint. A roentgen stereophotogrammetric analysis. Spine 14:162–165

Sturesson B, Uden A, Vleeming A 2000 A radiostereometric analysis of the movement of sacroiliac joints in the reciprocal straddle position. Spine 25:214–217

Terjesen T, Benum P, Anda S et al 1982 Increased femoral anteversion and osteoarthritis of the hip joint. Acta Orthopaedica Scandinavica 53:571–575

Tullberg T, Blomberg S, Branth B et al 1998 Manipulation does not alter the position of the sacroiliac joint. A roentgen stereophotogrammetric analysis. Spine 23:1124–1128

Vincent C 1993 Osteitis pubis. Journal of the American Board of Family Practice 6:492–496

Walheim G G, Selvik F 1984 Mobility of the pubis symphysis. In vivo measurements with an electromechanic method and a roentgen stereophotogrammetric method. Clinical Orthopaedics and Related Research 191:129–135

Walheim G G, Olerud S, Ribbe T 1984 Mobility of the pubis symphysis. Measurements by an electromechanical method. Acta Orthopaedica Scandinavica 55:203–208

Walker J M 1992 The sacroiliac joint. A critical review. Physical Therapy 72:903–916

Walmsley T 1928 The articular mechanism of the diarthrosis. Journal of Bone and Joint Surgery (Am) 10A:40–45

Warwick R, Williams P 1973 Gray's Anatomy, 35th British edn. WB Saunders, Philadelphia, PA

Weisl H 1954 The ligaments of the sacro-iliac joint examined with particular reference to function. Acta Anatomica 20:201–213

Weisl H 1955a The articular surfaces of the sacro-iliac joint and their relation to the movement of the sacrum. Acta Anatomica 23:80–91

Weisl H 1955b The movement of the sacro-iliac joint. Acta Anatomica 23:80–91

Wells P E 1986 The examination of the pelvic joints. In: Grieve G P (ed) Modern manual therapy of the vertebral column. Churchill Livingstone Edinburgh

Wilder D G, Pope M H, Frymoyer J W 1980 The functional topography of the sacroiliac joint. Spine 5:575–579

Williams P R, Thomas D P, Downes E M 2000 Osteitis pubis and instability of the pubic symphysis. When nonoperative measures fail. American Journal of Sports Medicine 28:350–355

Woerman A L 1989 Evaluation and treatment of dysfunction in the lumbar-pelvic-hip complex In: Donatelli R, Wooden M J (eds) Orthopedic physical therapy. Churchill Livingstone, Edinburgh

19

Thigh

Suzanne Werner

INTRODUCTION

Injuries to the thigh are relatively common in athletes, with soft tissue and muscle injuries predominating (Peterson & Renström 2001). Typically, thigh injuries are incurred in sport and exercise activities that involve contact (e.g. football), or in those that involve rapid stopping and starting of running (e.g. basketball) and change of running direction.

SPORT-SPECIFIC APPLIED ANATOMY

BONE

The femur is the largest and strongest bone in the human body. The shaft of femur is a long bone with a tubular shape and a predominantly thick cortical rim. There is also an anterolateral bow in the proximal and middle third of the bone, which helps to absorb stresses that are placed on the femur (e.g. during standing, walking, running, and jumping). The femur is subjected to a large amount of stress; for example, the running cycle applies a stress on the femur that is approximately three times body weight (Sherman et al 1981). Due to the bowed configuration of the femoral shaft, the medial side will be under compression, while the lateral side will be under tension during weightbearing. Great forces are generated through muscle attachments to the femur, and in particular, at the junction of the proximal and middle third of the femur.

MUSCLES
Anterior thigh muscles

Knee extension is performed by the quadriceps femoris on the anterior aspect of the thigh. This is the biggest muscle group of the body (with a weight of approximately 1.5 kg) and consists of four components: the rectus femoris, vastus medialis, vastus lateralis, and vastus intermedius, which converge through a conjoined tendon at the basis of the patella and insert at the tuberositas tibiae. The vastus medialis and vastus lateralis are the most prominent of the four muscles with the medialis extending slightly more inferiorly. The vastus medialis can be functionally classified into two distinct portions: the vastus medialis longus, having more vertically oriented fibers, and the vastus medialis obliquus with an oblique fiber orientation of 40° to 60° medially from the longitudinal femoral axis (Lieb & Perry 1968). The quadriceps muscle group is innervated by the femoral nerve, L2, L3, and L4. The rectus femoris is a biarticular muscle originating from the spina iliaca anterior inferior and sometimes there is also a thin tendon from the os ilium just above the acetabulum, with both inserting at the basis of the patella. Since the rectus femoris crosses the hip joint, its function is not only knee extension but also hip flexion.

The sartorius is the longest muscle in the body. It originates from the anterior superior iliac spine, crosses the anterior aspect of the thigh medially in an oblique vertical direction, and continues along the medial side of the thigh and knee joint in order to insert at the anterior, upper part of the medial side of the tibia, in the so-called pes anserinus. It can be visualized by a combined flexion–abduction–external rotation of the hip joint and flexion of the knee joint. The sartorius is most easy to palpate at the proximal anteromedial aspect of the thigh, just distal to its origin. The function of the sartorius is to flex, externally rotate, and abduct the hip joint and to flex and assist in internal rotation of the knee joint. It is innervated by the femoral nerve, L2 and L3.

Posterior thigh muscles

The hamstring muscle group on the posterior aspect of the thigh consists of the biceps femoris (long and short heads) on the lateral side, and the semitendinosus and semimembranosus on the medial side. The biceps femoris inserts at the lateral side of the head of the fibula, at the lateral condyle of the tibia and at the deep fascia on the lateral side of the leg. The semitendinosus inserts at the proximal part of the medial surface of the tibia, at the deep fascia on the medial side of the leg, and also at the so-called pes anserinus. The semimembranosus inserts at the posteromedial aspect of the medial condyle of the tibia. The long head of the biceps femoris, semitendinosus, and semimembranosus originate from the ischial tuberosity and are innervated by the tibial branch of the sciatic nerve, L5, S1, and S2. The short head of the biceps femoris originates from the linea aspera and posterior

femur and is innervated by the peroneal branch of the sciatic nerve, L5, S1, and S2. Subsequently, all hamstring muscles, except for the short head of the biceps femoris, cross both the hip and knee joints and are thereby functioning as both hip extensors and knee flexors.

The gracilis, on the posterior thigh, acts together with the medial hamstrings as a knee flexor. The gracilis, semitendinosus and sartorius insert together to form the pes anserinus on the posteromedial aspect of the knee; it is attached to the inferior portion of the medial tibial plateau, approximately 6 cm below the medial joint line.

BIOMECHANICS OF THIGH MUSCLES CROSSING TWO JOINTS

The hamstring muscles and the rectus femoris are believed to be prone to injury because they span two joints (Sash 1981, Wilson 1972). The short head of the biceps femoris is the most frequently strained hamstring muscle. It has two motor points, one innervated by the tibial part of the sciatic nerve and the other by the peroneal part of the same nerve. The dual innervation may cause problems as the short head may contract at the same time as the quadriceps, resulting in a hamstring strain (Burkett 1976).

MUSCLE INJURIES

Muscle strain

The definition of a muscle strain is a partial or complete tear of the musculotendinous junction (Burkett 1970). Muscle strains may be graded into mild (grade I), moderate (grade II) and severe, complete tears (grade III). A grade I strain means that the athlete might experience slight discomfort with pain and tenderness and minimal swelling but with full range of motion. A grade II strain means that palpation is painful and reveals a small to moderate defect in the area of torn fibers; which, combined with swelling and decreased range of motion might lead to impaired gait. A grade III strain means that a moderate to extensive defect can be palpated in the site of injury and it is characterized by a higher degree of swelling, less range of motion and more intense pain in comparison with grade I and II injuries (Kirkendall et al 2001).

The vast majority of strains involve muscles that pass over two joints or more, and muscles with complex architecture. In the anterior thigh, the rectus femoris is most vulnerable to strains, while in the posterior thigh, the hamstring group, especially the short head of the biceps femoris is usually the one where strains occur. However, muscle strains can occur in each one of the different thigh muscles, as well as anteriorly and posteriorly (Brewer 1962, Craig 1973).

Muscle strains are due to dynamic overload, often occurring during an eccentric muscle action (Glick 1980, Zarins & Ciullo 1983). The typical cause is a violent muscle contraction simultaneous with an excessively forced stretch (Arner & Lindholm 1958, Fuller 1984, Garrett 1983, Garrett et al 1984, Zarins & Ciullo 1983), and usually happening at the musculotendinous junction (Garrett et al 1987, 1988, Norfray et al 1980, Safran et al 1988).

Muscle strains are common in explosive sports involving the movements of sprinting and jumping. A sudden acceleration for extra speed during running or a sudden deceleration might result in a muscle strain. Furthermore, muscle strains are common in other sports such as soccer due to the kicking action (Burkett 1970, Glick 1980, Peterson & Renström 2001). Grade I strain is a minor injury, where the fibers either have been stretched or torn. This injury is characterized by pain and tenderness on resisted active contraction as well as on passive stretching. An area of local spasm is palpable at the site of pain.

Generally, there is full, or close to full, range of motion. The athlete might not be aware of the moment of injury and will notice it when cooling down after physical exercise or even on the next day. Conservative treatment is to be recommended (Table 19.1) (Kirkendall et al 2001).

Grade II strain is a moderate injury with torn muscle/tendon fibers. The athlete complains of significant pain on passive stretching and on opposed active contraction. Usually this injury will result in a moderate area of inflammation and a limitation of range of motion due to swelling. The athlete generally ceases the physical activity at the moment of being injured. Conservative treatment is to be recommended (Table 19.1) (Kirkendall et al 2001).

Grade III strain is a major injury with complete rupture of the muscle belly, muscle tendon junction or tendon insertion. The athlete experiences an intense pain and there is a palpable muscle fiber defect recognized when the muscle is contracted. This injury will cause tenderness over a large area, a 50% or more loss of range of

Table 19.1 Treatment protocol for mild, moderate, and severe muscle strains

	Mild muscle strain	Moderate muscle strain	Severe muscle strain
Days 1–3	Compression Ice Elevation Active range of motion Isometric training Electrical muscle stimulation	Compression Ice Elevation Pain-free active range of motion Electrical muscle stimulation Crutch walking	Compression Ice Elevation Crutch walking
From day 4	Pool training Pain-free stretching Isotonic training (progress from light to heavier weights and from concentric to eccentric actions) Bicycle training Functional exercises	Pain-free isometric training	Electrical muscle stimulation
From day 7	Isokinetic training (progress from fast to slow angular velocities and from concentric to eccentric actions) Plyometric training Sport-specific exercises	Pool training Pain-free stretching Isotonic training (progress from fast to slow angular velocities and from concentric to eccentric actions) Bicycle training Functional exercises	Pain-free active range of motion Pain-free isometric training
From week 2		Isokinetic training (progress from fast to slow angular velocities and from concentric to eccentric actions) Plyometric training Sport-specific exercises	Pool training Pain-free stretching Isotonic training (progress from fast to slow angular velocities and from concentric to eccentric actions) Bicycle training Functional exercises
From week 3			Isokinetic training (progress from fast to slow angular velocities and from concentric to eccentric actions) Plyometric training Sport-specific exercises

motion and functional loss of muscle strength leading to difficulties with full weightbearing. In the long term, however, most athletes with grade III strains will resolve with physical therapy (Table 19.1) (Kirkendall et al 2001).

Muscle contusion

A muscle contusion is likely to be the result of a direct impact to the muscle. On this direct impact, the contracted muscle is compressed against the underlying bone, often causing a deep rupture and bleeding. Muscle tissue injury and hemorrhage occur, directly followed by an inflammatory response; then granulation tissue develops and matures into dense collagenous scar tissue. Muscle contusions mainly occur deep in the muscle, adjacent to the bone (Peterson & Renström 2001, Ryan 1969, Walton & Rothwell 1983) but can also be superficial (Peterson & Renström 2001) and may occur anywhere within the muscle. Contusions may be graded in severity by restriction in range of motion of the subtended joints. A mild contusion causes a loss of less than one-third of the normal range of motion, whereas severe contusions cause limitations of greater than one-third of normal excursion (Peterson & Renström 2001).

Intramuscular hematoma

A rupture or an impact to the muscle may result in intramuscular bleeding. This will lead to an increase in intramuscular pressure counteracting further bleeding by compressing the blood vessels (Peterson & Renström 2001). Swelling occurs and persists beyond the first 48 h and is accompanied by tenderness, pain, and reduced mobility (Peterson & Renström 2001). Due to osmosis, the bleeding draws fluid from the surrounding tissue, which may lead to a risk of further swelling, thereby leading to completely impaired muscle function (Peterson & Renström 2001).

Intermuscular hematoma

When a muscle fascia and its adjacent blood vessels are damaged, bleeding may occur between muscles. Due to the effect of gravity, bruising and swelling will appear distal to the damaged area 24–48 h after the injury. No increase in pressure and temporary swelling will result in a fast return of muscle function (Peterson & Renström 2001).

Acute muscle injury

The acute management of muscle injuries is important in order to limit the hematoma and thereby promote the return to sport. The repair mechanism following a muscle injury is unstable during the first 24–36 h (Peterson & Renström 2001). This means that further bleeding may

occur as a result of another impact, violent muscle contraction or unprotected weightbearing concerning moderate and severe injuries. A precise diagnosis can be difficult in the acute phase and, therefore, a muscle injury should be considered as potentially serious for the first 2 to 3 days (Peterson & Renström 2001). There is a need for early and repeated examinations of the injured area in order to distinguish between intramuscular and intermuscular bleeding. An early ultrasound (US) examination can be used to distinguish between the two types of hematomas (Peterson & Renström 2001).

The basic concepts of acute management of muscle injuries are:

- Encouraging rest (temporary cessation of sports activity)
- Immediate compression (as firm as possible) for approximately 15 min in order to limit the amount of bleeding, and continuing with compression, bandaged half as hard for further 1 to 3 days
- Keeping the injured extremity immobile during the first minutes
- Cooling the affected area in order to limit pain; however, do not apply the cold pack (or ice) directly onto the skin
- Keeping the injured extremity elevated as much as is practical for 1 to 3 days
- Relieving the load, especially if the injury is moderate or severe; crutches can be used if a leg is affected until a definite diagnosis has been made.

One should pay attention to the following questions 48–72 h after a muscle injury: (a) has the swelling resolved?, (b) has the bleeding spread and caused bruising at some distance from the injured area?, and (c) has the ability of muscle contraction returned or improved? If the answers to these questions are 'no', an intramuscular bleeding is most probably present. Furthermore, it is important to define the severity of the injury in order to give the athlete the correct and adequate treatment (Peterson & Renström 2001).

An accurate diagnosis is of paramount importance due to the fact that a premature physical loading of a muscle affected by intramuscular bleeding, or a complete rupture, might result in further bleeding, and increase scar tissue formation. This can lead to a delayed healing process and sometimes even permanent disability (Peterson & Renström 2001).

EXAMINATION

It is important to obtain an accurate and thorough subjective history from the athlete. Paying attention to history combined with clinical examination, establishes a diagnosis that will greatly aid the clinician in making an accurate assessment of the athlete's condition, and based on that, in designing an appropriate rehabilitation program.

CLINICAL EXAMINATION

The site of pain and the injury mechanism are the most important factors in thigh injuries. The aim of the clinical examination is to reveal the exact site of pain and to assess range of motion and muscle strength. Furthermore, sports-related functional tests should be used in order to evaluate the athlete from the physical point of view of a sport. The clinical examination of athletes with thigh injuries should include sites that might refer pain to the thigh, usually in posterior thigh injuries (e.g. the lumbar spine, the sacroiliac and hip joints and the gluteal muscle) (Brukner & Khan 2001).

Clinical examination protocol of athletes with anterior or posterior thigh injuries

Clinical examination of anterior or posterior thigh injuries should include the following:

- *Inspection* should be performed in standing, walking, supine (anterior thigh injuries) and prone (posterior thigh injuries) positions.
- *Palpation* of the quadriceps and hamstring muscles should be performed in supine and prone positions. Special attention should be paid to possible tenderness and swelling. A focal muscle defect might appear during muscle contraction (Brukner & Khan 2001). When dealing with posterior thigh injuries, where trigger points may refer pain to the hamstrings, palpation of the ischial tuberosity as well as of the gluteal muscles is advisable (Brukner & Khan 2001).
- *Active range of motion* should be controlled with regards to flexion and extension of the knee and hip joints. The mobility of the lumbar spine and the sacroiliac joints should also be controlled.
- *Muscle flexibility/tightness* should be controlled concerning the quadriceps muscle group, the rectus femoris in particular (anterior thigh injuries), and the hamstring muscles (posterior thigh injuries).
- *Muscle action*, both concentric and eccentric, should be controlled with regards to extension and flexion of both the knee and hip joints.
- *Activities of daily living* limitations can be checked by the single leg squat test, the single leg chair test (raise–sit down), the single leg step test (up–down) and the stair climbing test (up–down). These tests involve both concentric and eccentric muscle contractions. Special attention should be paid to the possibility of reproducing pain, which can be evaluated (see

Ch. 8) using either the Borg's pain scale (Borg et al 1981) or the visual analog scale (VAS) (Price et al 1983).
- *Sports activities* can be checked by jumping, kicking, and different running exercises involving both acceleration and deceleration movements.

SPECIAL TESTS

Tests – anterior thigh

Ely's test (Gross et al 1996) is a flexibility test of the rectus femoris. It is performed with the athlete lying supine, with the knee of the symptomatic leg hanging over the edge of the bench. The hip and knee joints of the asymptomatic leg are maximally flexed and the leg is held by the hands toward the chest. Extension of the symptomatic knee joint is a sign of rectus femoris tightness.

Test of action of the quadriceps muscle group. The function of the quadriceps is usually tested by having the subject sitting with the legs hanging over the edge of the bench. With one hand, the examiner stabilizes the thigh by holding it firmly down on the bench. A test of concentric muscle action is performed when the subject is instructed to extend the knee, while the examiner applies a pressure in the direction of flexion with the other hand above the ankle. A test of eccentric muscle action is performed when the subject is instructed to try to maintain the knee in a chosen knee flexion angle, while the examiner applies a pressure and moves the leg in the direction of flexion with the other hand above the ankle. When comparing the symptomatic leg with the asymptomatic one this test may give the examiner a rough measure of whether there is a side-to-side difference in quadriceps strength. However, it should be pointed out that a more appropriate way of evaluating quadriceps strength is by performing an isokinetic measurement.

When performing this test of quadriceps strength, we must also be aware that painful resisted knee extension, in particular eccentrically, might be due to patellofemoral pain and/or patellar tendinosis, so-called jumper's knee (see Ch. 21). Subsequently, due to pain inhibition, these patients can not produce a proper test of muscle strength, meaning that this test might give an answer of pain instead of muscle strength. In order to control whether there is any pain inhibition or not, one can use the isokinetic method with twitch interpolation technique by adding electrical muscle stimulation (McKenzie et al 1992). However, to some extent, the Borg's pain scale (Borg et al 1981) or the visual analog scale (VAS) (Price et al 1983) can also be used.

Tests – posterior thigh

The Wallace test is an appropriate test for flexibility of the hamstring muscle group specifically. The patient lies supine with extended hips and knees. The patient then flexes the hip and knee to be tested to 90° while stabilizing the thigh in that position with the hands, and from this position tries to fully extend the knee with the hip maintained in 90° of flexion. Decreased hamstring flexibility is demonstrated by the number of degrees that are lacking from a complete knee extension (Wallace 1979).

A tightness of the hamstrings will appear either when there is a restriction of knee extension when the hip is flexed, or when there is a restriction of hip flexion when the knee is extended. This is due to the muscles that cross the knee joint as well as the hip joint.

The straight leg raising test for hamstring length is a combination of hip flexion and flexion of the lumbar spine. The patient lies supine on the bench, and with one hand, the examiner passively raises the 'test-leg', with the knee maintained in extension, to an angle of 80–90° of hip flexion in normal cases. The contralateral leg is held down with the other hand to stabilize the pelvis and prevent excessive flexion of the lumbar spine. To find out whether the patient's symptom is caused by tight hamstrings or is of a neurogenic origin, the examiner can raise the leg up to the subject's pain threshold. When slightly lowering the leg the pain should decrease or disappear. A passive ankle dorsiflexion that causes pain in this slightly lowered leg position reveals a neurogenic pain, while no pain means tight hamstring muscles.

The slump test, which is a neural tension test (see Ch. 14), can be used to differentiate between hamstring injuries and referred pain to the hamstring from the lumbar spine. The patient sits on the edge of the bench, with the thighs fully supported and the hands behind the back. The patient slumps forward making a kyphosis of the lumbar and thoracic spine and a maximal flexion of the cervical spine ('chin to chest'), while maintaining the sacrum vertical. In this position, the patient extends one knee and dorsiflexes the ankle of the same leg, and then slowly releases the flexion of the cervical spine. The test is positive when the patient's hamstring pain is reproduced and relieved with reduction of the neural tension by releasing the flexion of the cervical spine.

Test of action of the lateral hamstrings (biceps femoris). The patient lies prone on the bench with the 'test-leg' in somewhat less than 90° of knee flexion and the hip externally rotated. The examiner holds the thigh down firmly on the bench with one hand, and with the other hand, presses against the leg proximal to the ankle in the direction of knee extension.

Test of action of the medial hamstrings (semitendinosus and semimembranosus). The patient lies prone on the bench with the 'test-leg' in somewhat less than 90° of knee flexion and the hip internally rotated. The examiner holds the thigh down firmly on the bench with one hand and pressures with the other hand against the leg proximal to the ankle in the direction of knee extension.

Test of action of the medial hamstrings and gracilis. The gracilis is activated during knee flexion and assists in internal rotation of the knee. It will be activated by the same test position and pressure as used for the medial hamstrings (explained above). The difference in knee flexion action between the medial hamstrings and the gracilis is due to the fact that the medial hamstrings originate from the ischium, while the gracilis originates from the pubis.

INVESTIGATIONS

A plain radiographic examination is not helpful in diagnosing or determining the extent of muscle strains (see Ch. 29). Here, X-rays are only useful to identify a possible avulsion fracture of the ischial tuberosity. If a quadriceps contusion does not respond to treatment, a plain radiographic examination approximately 3 weeks after the injury can reveal the presence of myositis ossificans (Brukner & Khan 2001). A plain radiographic examination of the hip joint may be indicated if the patient presents with impaired range of motion of the hip or complains of painful hip movements (Brukner & Khan 2001).

US examination can be used to confirm muscle strains and the presence of a hematoma in the early stage. Furthermore, it may be helpful in differentiating between a mild muscle strain and muscle contusion (Brukner & Khan 2001).

Magnetic resonance imaging (MRI) rapidly reveals muscle strains, but is not thought to be cost effective and generally does not influence or change the treatment (Brunet & Hontas 1994). It should also be remembered that MRI cannot visualize a hematoma until the hemoglobin has changed into methemoglobin after 3–4 days.

An isotopic bone scan can immediately reveal a stress fracture (e.g. of the shaft of femur) and is therefore to be recommended when a stress fracture is suspected (Blatz 1981, Blickenstaff 1966, Norfray et al 1980, Rosen et al 1982, Rupani et al 1985, Thorstensson & Karlsson 1976, Wilcox et al 1977, Wilson 1969).

COMMON SPORT-RELATED INJURIES

QUADRICEPS STRAIN

Strains within the quadriceps muscle group usually involve the rectus femoris at the level of the middle third of the thigh. Quadriceps muscle fibers are predominantly type II, and therefore best suited to rapid, forceful activity. Typically, the athlete feels the injury as a sudden pain in the anterior thigh when the quadriceps muscle requires a vigorous explosive contraction (e.g. during sprinting, jumping, or kicking).

Strain of the rectus femoris can be confirmed by eliciting pain when the hip joint is extended and the knee joint is flexed. Because the muscle is subcutaneous and overlies the remainder of the quadriceps, a localized swelling or a defect is readily apparent. This can be confirmed with the athlete lying supine and flexing the hip with the knee held in approximately 45° of flexion. If present, a localized swelling or defect will be apparent in this position.

QUADRICEPS CONTUSION

Quadriceps contusion is the most frequent form of muscle contusion (Kirkendall et al 2001) and is therefore the example of contusions to be presented in this chapter. The Jackson & Feagin (1973) classification in assessing prognosis and rate of recovery is useful (Table 19.2).

The treatment recommended for the management of mild, moderate, and severe quadriceps contusions is outlined in Table 19.3.

Strain versus contusion of the quadriceps muscle

An athlete suffering from a muscle strain should progress more slowly through the rehabilitation program (see later section) than an athlete with a muscle contusion. The athlete with a thigh muscle strain should avoid rapid acceleration and deceleration movements during the early phase of rehabilitation (Brukner & Khan 2001).

MYOSITIS OSSIFICANS OF THE QUADRICEPS

Occasionally, after a thigh contusion with intramuscular bleeding, the hematoma calcifies developing myositis ossificans (Brukner & Khan 2001). The onset of myositis ossificans has been related to the severity of contusion.

Table 19.2 Classification of quadriceps contusions based on the classification suggested by Jackson & Feagin (1973)

Severity	Symptoms	Range of movement	Functional ability
Mild	Local tenderness	> 90°	Normal gait Normal knee bend
Moderate	Tender muscle mass Swelling	< 90°	Antalgic gait Pain on climbing stairs Pain on rising from chair
Severe	Marked tenderness Marked swelling	< 45°	Severe limp (crutches needed) Ispilateral knee pain

Myositis ossificans developed in 72% of athletes with moderate or severe contusions, whereas there was none in those with a mild contusion (Jackson & Feagin 1973).

Development of myositis ossificans is a possible complication of deep muscle contusions, especially to the anterior thigh and the quadriceps muscles (Walton & Rothwell 1983). The exact mechanism of onset still remains unknown. It may start with a muscle trauma leading to an inflammation, cellular proliferation, concentration of growth factors, induction of bone forming cells, and ossification.

Pain, a palpable mass, and flexion contracture following a muscle injury strongly suggest the possibility of myositis ossificans (Cushner & Morwessel 1992). Clinically, there might be local tenderness and localized warmth. Intramuscular calcification is generally delayed and can be visualized with X-ray, 6–8 weeks after onset (Cushner & Morwessel 1992, Estwanik & McAlister 1990). To the athlete, myositis ossificans can be a source of a long-term and considerable disability due to inflammatory pain and contracture (Estwanik & McAlister 1990, Garrett 1990).

In patients with myositis ossificans, the pain and size of the mass decrease as the lesion matures but they increase as time progresses in patients with osteosarcoma (Cushner & Morwessel 1992). Young patients engaging in sports can develop malignant tumors. When these cause pain, patients often go to their sports medicine doctor or sports physical therapist (Maffulli et al 1990). Osteosarcoma is the most important differential diagnosis and should be ruled out in every young athlete that presents with a soft tissue mass (Dudkiewicz et al 2001).

There is very little that can be done to accelerate the resorptive process of myositis ossificans. Electrical stimulation in order to reduce muscle spasm, gentle pain-free range of motion exercises, and ice therapy might lead to improvement. Non-steroidal anti-inflammatory drugs are known to decrease calcification, and irradiation has also been suggested for prevention of calcification. It should also be pointed out that a proper treatment of a muscle contusion usually prevents myositis ossificans. However, some cases still have pain in spite of conservative treatment. One year after the original injury, surgical removal of the mass may be helpful in these cases (Kirkendall et al 2001).

HAMSTRING STRAIN

Hamstring strains and ruptures are the most common muscle injuries in the thigh (Kulund 1982) and rank second in all injuries in sports. The biceps femoris is the most commonly injured muscle of the hamstring group (Burkett 1976, Heiser et al 1984, Kulund 1982).

The etiology of hamstring strains in athletes is complex

Table 19.3 Treatment protocol for mild, moderate, and severe muscle contusions

	Mild muscle contusion	Moderate muscle contusion	Severe muscle contusion
Day 1	Compression Ice Gentle stretching	Compression Ice Electrical muscle stimulation Crutch walking	
Day 1–3			Compression Ice Rest Electrical muscle stimulation Crutch walking
Days 2 or 3	Strengthening exercises progressing from isometric through to isotonic training (light to heavy weights), and then to isokinetic training (fast to slow angular velocities, concentric to eccentric actions)	Pain-free isometric training Pain-free active range of motion	
Days 5–7		Pool training Isotonic training (progress from light to heavy weights and from concentric to eccentric actions) Bicycle training	Pain-free isometric training Pain-free active range of motion
Days 7–10		Isokinetic training (progress from fast to slow angular velocities and from concentric to eccentric actions)	
Day 10		Stretching exercises	Pool training Isotonic training (progress from light to heavy weights and from concentric to eccentric actions) Bicycle training
Day 14			Isokinetic training (progress from fast to slow angular velocities and from concentric to eccentric actions) Stretching exercises

and many factors have been reported as being responsible for this injury. These include inadequate warm-up, inadequate stretching, poor hamstring strength, muscle fatigue, poor hamstring flexibility, poor technique, poor posture, and previous incomplete injury (Agre 1985, Burkett 1970, Casperson 1982, Dornan 1971, Garrett 1983, Heiser et al 1984, Kulund 1982, Liemohn 1978, Oakes 1984, O'Neill 1976, Stafford & Grana 1984).

Hamstring strains result from overstretching or a rapid contraction causing different degrees of tearing within the musculotendinous unit. The hamstring muscles are shown to have a relatively high proportion of 'fast twitch' fibers (Garrett et al 1984). The hamstring group crosses

two joints, leading to greater changes in length when compared to muscles that cross only one joint. Therefore, the high levels of intrinsic tensions, produced by the 'fast twitch' fibers, combined with the extrinsic stretch, involved with length changes over two joints, might make the hamstrings prone to injury during high intensity sprinting and jumping activities.

The athlete usually experiences a sudden onset of pain in the posterior thigh during rapid activity. Occasionally, there might be an audible 'pop', identifying a grade II or III strain. The muscle area involved and a local tenderness can be identified by palpation, while the athlete lies prone with the knee slightly flexed against resistance.

Hamstring flexibility and muscle strength, as well as hamstring-to-hamstring and hamstring-to-quadriceps imbalances, appear to be the variables most often considered when dealing with hamstring strains. Subsequently, tests that attempt to stimulate conditions in which hamstring strains occur appear to be the most valid indicators of predisposition to hamstring injury.

HAMSTRING SYNDROME

Compression of the sciatic nerve by tendinous structures within the hamstring muscles can be the cause of the hamstring syndrome. It has been predominantly found in sprinters and hurdlers but athletes in other explosive sports may also suffer from this syndrome. The symptomatic athlete characteristically complains of pain in the sitting position with local tenderness around the ischial tuberosity. Resistance against hamstring contraction will cause pain in the buttock, which might, in some cases, radiate down the leg and which increases with physical activity (Peterson & Renström 2001).

The treatment is usually conservative with sufficient rest and adequate physical therapy similar to that for hamstring strain. Occasionally, surgical excision of damaged tissue and freeing the nerve may be indicated (Peterson & Renström 2001).

GENERAL REHABILITATION PRINCIPLES FOR ANTERIOR AND POSTERIOR THIGH MUSCLE INJURIES

Rehabilitation for anterior and posterior thigh muscle injuries usually involves a combination of the following activities: electrical stimulation of the quadriceps muscle (Fig. 19.1), stretching of the rectus femoris (Fig. 19.2), stretching of the hamstrings (Fig. 19.3), strengthening of the quadriceps without weight applied in a limited range of motion (Fig. 19.4), strengthening of the quadriceps with weight applied in full range of motion (Fig. 19.5), leg presses for quadriceps strengthening (Fig. 19.6), leg curls for hamstring strengthening (Fig. 19.7), functional step-up exercises (Fig. 19.8), functional step-down exercises (Fig. 19.9), StairMaster exercises as a functional form of training (Fig. 19.10), isokinetic training of the quadriceps and hamstrings (Fig. 19.11), and jumping exercises (Fig. 19.12). In addition, sport-specific functional activities are used to gradually retrain the lower limb to the demands of the sporting activity that the patient will be returning to.

RETURN TO SPORT

The goal of rehabilitation is to return the athlete to sport participation in the least amount of time. Sports activity puts heavy demands on physical fitness and conditioning, which is especially important to pay attention to when a recently injured athlete is returning to sport. Therefore, the rehabilitation should lead to a normal function before the athlete can return to sporting activities. The following criteria are suggested to be fulfilled before allowing the athlete with a muscle injury of the anterior or posterior thigh to return to sport participation:

- Full range of motion of both the knee and hip joints
- Good muscle flexibility of quadriceps and hamstrings
- Good muscle strength of quadriceps and hamstrings, < 10% side-to-side differences
- Good muscle balance, hamstring/quadriceps ratio ≥ 55%
- Sport-related functional tests, such as running tests with acceleration and deceleration, sprint and hop tests, performed at full speed without residual of symptoms.

Prevention of muscle injuries

Different preventive strategies for developing muscle injuries have been suggested. Several authors recommend that athletes routinely practice stretching (Beaulieu 1981, Wiktorsson-Möller et al 1983). However, the recommendation of stretching exercises is mainly empirical, because it is believed to prevent muscle injuries. A careful warm-up program is also cited as a way of preventing muscle injuries (Wiktorsson-Möller et al 1983) and an appropriate level of muscle strength can protect a musculotendinous unit from injury (Garrett et al 1987, Safran et al 1988). Furthermore, muscle imbalance has been reported as a cause of hamstring strain and the data from these studies might be of importance in identifying muscle imbalance for preventive purposes (Burkett 1970, Casperson 1982, Kulund 1982, Rankin & Thompson 1983).

LESS COMMON SPORT-RELATED INJURIES

COMPARTMENT SYNDROME

A severe thigh contusion with rapid bleeding may result in development of an acute compartment syndrome and require urgent surgical fasciotomy. Long-distance runners, cross-country skiers and ice-hockey players, who activate their thigh muscles intensively might experience pain in the thigh, weakness and fatigue, which are associated with their sports activity (Peterson & Renström 2001). The pain that can appear suddenly is not associated with any trauma. It can be present in different portions or in

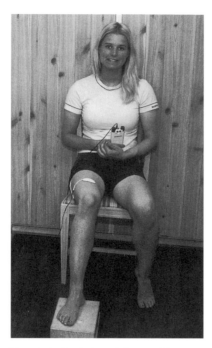

Figure 19.1   Electrical stimulation of the quadriceps muscle.

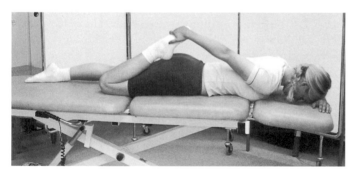

Figure 19.2   Stretching of the rectus femoris.

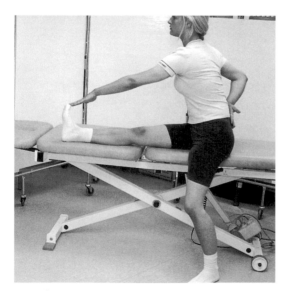

Figure 19.3   Stretching of the hamstrings.

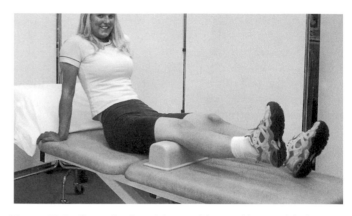

Figure 19.4   Strengthening of the quadriceps without weight in a limited range of motion.

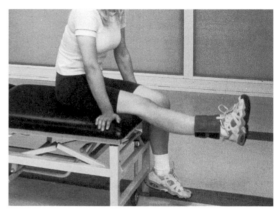

Figure 19.5   Strengthening of the quadriceps with weight applied in full range of motion.

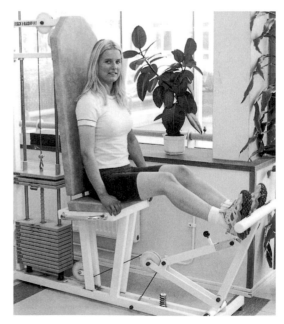

Figure 19.6   Leg press for quadriceps strengthening.

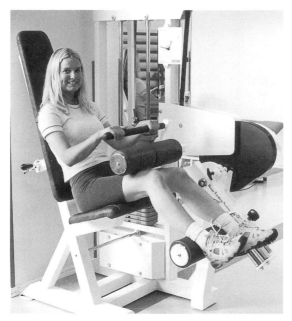

Figure 19.7   Leg curls for hamstring strengthening.

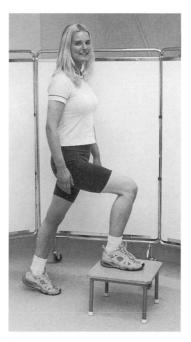

Figure 19.8   Functional step-up exercises.

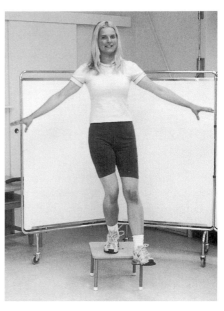

Figure 19.9   Functional step-down exercises.

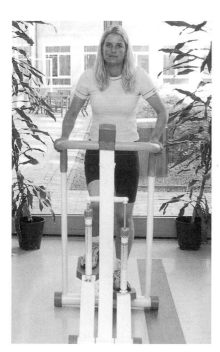

Figure 19.10   StairMaster exercise as a functional form of training.

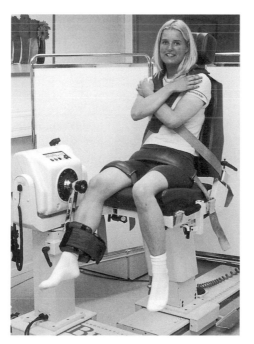

Figure 19.11   Isokinetic training of the quadriceps and hamstrings.

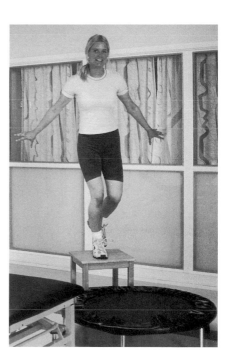

Figure 19.12   Jumping exercises.

the entire thigh. Usually there are either neurological symptoms or abnormal intramuscular pressure measurements. The diagnosis is mainly confirmed by exclusion criteria. When no improvement has been made with physical therapy, fasciotomy should be considered (Peterson & Renström 2001).

STRESS FRACTURE OF THE SHAFT OF FEMUR

Stress fracture of the femoral shaft is uncommon. However, due to the increase in running and jogging among the population a higher number of stress fractures of the femoral shaft has been seen. Distance running is also the most common activity associated with stress fracture of the shaft of femur (Brukner & Khan 2001).

A stress fracture is a microfracture in the bone that results from repetitive physical loading below the single cycle failure threshold. This can happen either through the redistribution of impact forces, resulting in increased stress at focal points in bone or the action of muscle pull across bone. The muscle insertion site at the junction of the proximal and middle third of the femur is often involved. The typical causative factors are a sudden increase in training mileage, intensity, frequency of training, a change in the running surface, improper or inappropriate sport shoes, or a combination of these factors (Fitch 1984).

Usually patients complain of pain either localized in the groin or in the thigh. This onset of pain is commonly insidious and becomes worse with physical activity or sport and is relieved with rest. Sometimes, however, the pain has a sudden onset with severe symptoms. If the patient continues with sporting activities, despite symptoms, the pain will progress to include activities of daily living and pain at night as well (Peterson & Renström 2001).

One must consider osteopenia as a possible underlying cause of femoral stress fractures (see Ch. 5), particularly in female athletes. The strength of bone is relative to the square of its density and a 10% reduction of bone density leads to a strength decrease of that particular bone by a factor of 100 (Carter & Hayes 1976). Amenorrheic female athletes have a lower bone-mineral density meaning that this population has a higher risk for developing femoral stress fractures (Cook et al 1987, Linnell et al 1984).

Clinical findings are sparse making the diagnosis a challenge for the examiner. However, palpation may reveal local tenderness at the site of the fracture. External rotation of the hip joint greater than 65° has been found to be a risk factor for sustaining femoral stress fracture (Giladi et al 1987) and bilateral femoral stress fractures have been reported in runners. Therefore, the clinical

examination should pay extra attention to these parameters.

Plain radiographic findings are typically delayed from 2 to 6 weeks after the onset of pain, when the stress fracture is in its reparative phase (Blickenstaff 1966, Rosen et al 1982, Savoca 1971, Wilcox et al 1977, Wilson 1969). Therefore, plain radiographs are solely of use for late confirmation of the diagnosis (Bargren et al 1971, Daffner et al 1982, Fitch 1984, Provost & Morris 1969, Torg et al 1981, Weber 1988). Scintigraphy (bone scan) has become the gold standard for early confirmation of stress fractures (Blatz 1981, Blickenstaff 1966, Norfray et al 1980, Rosen et al 1982, Rupani et al 1985, Thorstensson & Karlsson 1976, Wilcox et al 1977, Wilson 1969). An early diagnosis of a femoral stress fracture in athletes is important, since this gives the possibility to an appropriate treatment by preventing a possible fracture displacement. MRI can also confirm the diagnosis, while computed tomography (CT) scan may be used, but its role as it relates to stress fractures has not yet been defined.

The rehabilitation of femoral stress fractures can be divided into the following three phases: phase I (weeks 1–4), phase II (weeks 5–7), and phase III (week 8 onwards).

Phase I (weeks 1–4)

The initial treatment of patients with femoral stress fractures usually includes a period of protected weight-bearing by using crutches (Black 1974, Fitch 1984, Hallel et al 1976, Lombardo & Benson 1982, Provost & Morris 1969, Weber 1988). Progress to full weightbearing is allowed when the patient can ambulate without any pain. Cardiovascular fitness, such as stationary armcycle training and upper extremity exercises are encouraged.

Phase II (weeks 5–7)

This phase begins when the patient does not use crutches anymore and daily living activities are pain-free. Exercises of the lower extremity, such as swimming and stationary bicycle training, are started and continue with a gradual increase of intensity based on the patient's symptoms.

Phase III (from week 8)

The third phase can begin when cycling for at least 30 min can be carried out without pain. Exercises such as walking, jogging and later running on a soft surface can be allowed and gradually increased in both mileage and on different types of surfaces, as long as the patient is pain-free. After approximately 10 weeks from the onset of pain, the patient can start a walking–jogging–running protocol, which means that week 10 allows walking, week 11 jogging and week 12 running, for 5–8 km. Return to sport can start with a gradual approach in intensity and duration (mileage) when the athlete has performed the walking–jogging–running protocol without any pain. The entire treatment program can be followed as long as the physical exercises can be performed pain-free. However, if symptoms reoccur, the athlete is dropped back to the previous phase for some 2–3 weeks.

SUMMARY

This chapter provides an outline of a range of injuries related to the thigh. Muscle strains, contusions, and hematomas are the most common injury to the thigh and the rehabilitation management usually involves a range of modalities from rest to active functional strengthening. The less common injuries to this region include compartment syndrome and femoral shaft stress fractures.

REFERENCES

Agre J C 1985 Hamstring injuries: proposed aetiological factors, prevention and treatment. Sports Medicine 2:21–33

Arner O, Lindholm A 1958 What is tennis leg? Acta Orthopaedica Scandinavica 116:73–77

Bargren J H, Tilson D H, Bridgeford O E 1971 Prevention of displaced fatigue fractures of the femur. Journal of Bone and Joint Surgery (Am) 53A:1115–1117

Beaulieu J E 1981 Developing a stretching program. Physician and Sportsmedicine 9:59–65

Black J 1974 Failure of implants for internal hip fixation. Orthopedic Clinics of North America 5:833–844

Blatz D J 1981 Bilateral femoral and tibial shaft stress fractures in a runner. American Journal of Sports Medicine 9:322–325

Blickenstaff L 1966 Fatigue fracture of the femoral neck. Journal of Bone and Joint Surgery (Am) 48A:1031–1047

Borg G, Holmgren A, Lindblad I 1981 Quantitative evaluation of chest pain. Acta Medica Scandinavica 644 (suppl):43–45

Brewer B J 1962 Athletic injuries: musculotendinous unit. Clinical Orthopaedics and Related Research 23:30–37

Brukner P, Khan K 2001 Clinical Sports Medicine, 2nd edn., McGraw-Hill, Sydney

Brunet M E, Hontas R B 1994 The thigh. In: DeLee J C, Drez D (eds) Orthopaedic sports medicine. Principles and practice. WB Saunders, Philadelphia, PA

Burkett L N 1970 Causative factors in hamstring strain. Medicine and Science in Sports and Exercise 2:39–42

Burkett L N 1976 Investigation into hamstring strains: the case of the hybrid muscle. Journal of Sports Medicine 3:228–231

Carter D R, Hayes W C 1976 Bone compressive strength: the influences of density and strain rate. Science 10:1174–1175

Casperson P C 1982 Groin and hamstring injuries. Athletic Training 17:43–45

Cook S D, Harding A F, Thomas K A et al 1987 Trabecular bone density in menstrual function in women runners. American Journal of Sports Medicine 15:503–507

Craig T T 1973 American Medical Association Comments in Sports Medicine. American Medical Association, Chicago

Cushner F D, Morwessel R M 1992 Myositis ossificans traumatica. Orthopaedic Review 21:1319–1326

Daffner R H, Martinez S, Gehweiler J A 1982 Stress fractures of the femoral neck. Journal of the American Medical Association 247:1039–1041

Dornan P 1971 A report on 140 hamstring injuries. Australian Journal of Sports Medicine 4:30–36

Dudkiewicz I, Salai M, Chechik A 2001 A young athlete with myositis ossificans of the neck presenting as a soft-tissue tumour. Archives of Orthopaedic and Trauma Surgery 121(4):234–237

Estwanik J J, McAlister J A 1990 Contusions and the formation of myositis ossificans. Physician and Sportsmedicine 18(4):53–64

Fitch K D 1984 Stress fractures of the lower limbs in runners. Australian Family Physician 13:511–515

Fuller P J 1984 Musculotendinous leg injuries. Australian Family Physician 13:495–498

Garrett W E 1983 Strains and sprains in athletes. Postgraduate Medicine 73(3):200–209

Garrett W E 1990 Muscle strain injuries: clinical and basic aspects. Medicine in Science and Sports and Exercise 22:436–443

Garrett W E, Califf J C, Bassett F H 1984 Histochemical correlates of hamstring injuries. American Journal of Sports Medicine 12:98–103

Garrett W E, Safran M R, Seaber A V et al 1987 Biomechanical comparison of stimulated and nonstimulated skeletal muscle pulled to failure. American Journal of Sports Medicine 15:448–454

Garrett W E, Nikolaou P K, Ribbeck B M et al 1988 The effect of muscle architecture on the biomechanical failure properties of skeletal muscle under passive extension. American Journal of Sports Medicine 16:7–12

Giladi M, Milgrom C, Stein M et al 1987 External rotation of the hip: a predictor of risk for stress fractures. Clinical Orthopaedics and Related Research 216:131–134

Glick J M 1980 Muscle strains. Prevention and treatment. Physician and Sportsmedicine 8:72–77

Gross J, Fetto J, Rosen E 1996 Musculoskeletal examination. Blackwell Science, Cambridge, MA

Hallel T, Amit S, Sega F 1976 Fatigue fractures of tibial and femoral shaft in soldiers. Clinical Orthopaedics and Related Research 118:35–43

Heiser T M, Weber J, Sullivan G et al 1984 Prophylaxis and management of hamstring muscle injuries in intercollegiate football players. American Journal of Sports Medicine 12:368–370

Jackson P, Feagin J 1973 Quadriceps contusions in young athletes. Journal of Bone and Joint Surgery (Am) 55A:95–105

Kirkendall D T, Prentice W E, Garrett W E 2001 Rehabilitation of muscle injuries. In: Puddu G, Giombini A, Selvanetti A (eds) Rehabilitation of sports injuries. Springer Verlag, Berlin

Kulund D N 1982 The injured athlete. JB Lippincott, Philadelphia, PA

Lieb F J, Perry J 1968 Quadriceps function: an anatomical and mechanical study using amputated limbs. Journal of Bone and Joint Surgery (Am) 50A:1535–1548

Liemohn W 1978 Factors related to hamstring strains. Journal of Sports Medicine 18:71–76

Linnell S, Stager J, Blue P et al 1984 Bone mineral content and menstrual regularity in female runners. Medicine and Science in Sports and Exercise 16:343–348

Lombardo S J, Benson D W 1982 Stress fractures of the femur in runners. American Journal of Sports Medicine 10:219–227

McKenzie D K, Bigeland-Ritchie B, Gorman R B et al 1992 Central and peripheral fatigue of human diaphragm and limb muscles assessed by twitch interpolation. Journal of Physiology 454:643–656

Maffulli N, Pintore E, Petricciuolo F 1990 Tumours mimicking sports injury in two young athletes. British Journal of Sports Medicine 24:207–208

Norfray J F, Schlachter L, Kernahan W T et al 1980 Early confirmation of stress fractures in joggers. Journal of the American Medical Association 243:1647–1649

Oakes B W 1984 Hamstring muscle injuries. Australian Family Physician 13(8):587–591

O'Neill R 1976 Prevention of hamstring and groin strains. Athletic Training 11:27–31

Peterson L, Renström P 2001 Sports injuries. Their prevention and treatment, 3rd edn. Martin Dunitz, London

Price D D, McGrath P A, Rafii A et al 1983 The validation of visual analog scale measures for chronic and experimental pain. Pain 17:45–56

Provost R A, Morris J M 1969 Fatigue fracture of the femoral shaft. Journal of Bone and Joint Surgery (Am) 51A:487–498

Rankin J M, Thompson C B 1983 Isokinetic evaluation of quadriceps and hamstring function: normative data concerning body weight and sport. Athletic Training 18:110–113

Rosen P R, Micheli L J, Treves S 1982 Early scintigraphic diagnosis of bone stress and fractures in athletic adolescents. Pediatrics 70:11–15

Rupani H D, Holder L E, Espinola D A et al 1985 Three-phase radionuclide bone imaging in sports medicine. Radiology 156:187–196

Ryan A J 1969 Quadriceps strain, rupture and charlie horse. Medicine and Science in Sports 1:106–111

Safran M R, Garrett W E, Seaber A V et al 1988 The role of warm-up in muscular injury prevention. American Journal of Sports Medicine 16:123–129

Sash L 1981 Medical problems in association football. Practitioner 225:1047–1050

Savoca C 1971 Stress fractures: a classification of the earliest radiographic signs. Radiology 100:519–524

Sherman W M, Plyley M J, Vogelgesand D et al 1981 Isokinetic strength during rehabilitation following arthrotomy: specificity of speed. Athletic Training 18:138–141

Stafford M G, Grana W A 1984 Hamstring/quadriceps ratios in college football players: a high velocity evaluation. American Journal of Sports Medicine 12:209–211

Thorstensson A, Karlsson J 1976 Fatiguability and fiber composition of human skeletal muscle. Acta Physiologica Scandinavica 98:312–322

Torg J S, Pavlov H, Morris V B 1981 Salter-Harris type III fracture of the medial femoral condyle occurring in the adolescent athlete. Journal of Bone and Joint Surgery (Am) 63A:586–591

Wallace L 1979 Flexibility measurement. In: Blackburn T A, Milne M, DoHollow J et al (eds) Guidelines for pre-season athletic participation evaluation. Diversified Printing Services, Columbus, GA

Walton M, Rothwell A G 1983 Reactions of thigh tissues of sheep to blunt trauma. Clinical Orthopaedics and Related Research 176:273–281

Weber P C 1988 Salter-Harris type II stress fracture in a young athlete: a case report. Orthopaedics 11:309–311

Wiktorsson-Möller M, Öberg B, Ekstrand J et al 1983 Effects of warming up, massage, and stretching on range of motion and muscle strength in the lower extremity. American Journal of Sports Medicine 11:249–252

Wilcox J R, Moniot A L, Green J P 1977 Bone scanning in the evaluation of exercise-related stress injuries. Nuclear Medicine 123:699–703

Wilson E 1969 Stress fractures. Radiology 92:481–486

Wilson J N 1972 Specific injuries of sport. Physiotherapy 58:194–199

Zarins B, Ciullo J V 1983 Acute muscle and tendon injuries in athletes. Clinics in Sports Medicine 2:167–182

20

Knee

*Terese L Chmielewski   Ryan L Mizner
William Padamonsky II   Lynn Snyder-Mackler*

INTRODUCTION

The knee joint is a common site for sports injuries, particularly ligamentous injuries, because ligaments contribute a great deal to knee joint stability. A solid knowledge of knee anatomy and biomechanics is necessary to properly assess the injury and devise a rehabilitation program that creates the best environment for healing. Criterion-based rehabilitation protocols are used because they outline milestones that must be met for progression, eliminating subjectivity. The rate of progression can differ between athletes and is dependent on the individual rate of healing and the demands of the athlete's activity level. Within each phase of the protocol, clinicians must choose therapeutic exercises that gradually introduce stresses to the healing tissue and that are tailored to preparing the athlete to return to the demands of the sport. Only after completing all phases of rehabilitation and meeting functional testing criteria are athletes allowed to return to sport activities.

ANATOMY AND BIOMECHANICS

BONY STRUCTURE

The tibiofemoral joint is created by the interface of the distal femur and proximal tibia. The distal femur is characterized by two bony prominences, the medial and lateral condyles, which are separated by an intercondylar notch. Both condyles are rounded inferiorly and project posteriorly, but the medial femoral condylar projection is longer. The longer projection of the medial femoral condyle partially dictates the biomechanics of the knee joint. The greater surface area of the medial condyle requires greater accessory motion in the medial half of the knee in comparison to the lateral half. Thus, when the knee is flexed, the tibiofemoral joint undergoes a small

379

but significant amount of internal rotation to sustain congruency between the condyles. When the knee approaches full extension, the tibiofemoral joint undergoes a subsequent external rotation, as the medial aspect of the knee must exhibit greater motion to maintain joint congruency.

When viewed from above, the proximal tibia appears flattened with a raised central region that divides the surface into medial and lateral components. The central region is known as the intercondylar region, or tibial eminence, and serves as a ligamentous attachment site. The tibial eminence protrudes into the corresponding intercondylar notch of the femur. On either side of the tibial eminence lie the medial and lateral tibial plateaus. The tibial plateaus articulate with their respective femoral condyles.

Surrounding the tibiofemoral joint is a joint capsule, which runs along the femoral condyles proximally and attaches distally around the circumference of the tibia. The joint capsule travels more superiorly on the anterior aspect of the femur and much closer to the joint line as it moves posteriorly. The capsule is deficient posteriorly at the lateral femoral condyle to allow passage of the popliteus tendon. The knee joint capsule is lined with a synovial membrane that surrounds, but does not encompass, the cruciate ligaments. The superior projection of the synovial membrane, anteriorly, is called the suprapatellar pouch. On the posterior aspect of the knee, the synovium projection is not as extensive, as it is dictated by the capsular insertion closer to the joint line.

Slightly distal to the lateral aspect of the tibial plateau is the proximal tibiofibular joint, composed of the fibular head and the fibular notch located on the lateral tibia. This articulation is mentioned here due to its proximity to the tibiofemoral joint. The tibiofibular joint has its own joint capsule and is not continuous with the tibiofemoral joint.

LIGAMENTS

Ligaments of the tibiofemoral joint serve to provide structural stability and to guide knee motion. The ligaments can be subclassified as capsular, intracapsular, and extracapsular, based on the relationship of the ligament to the joint capsule. Capsular ligaments are distinct thickenings of the joint capsule, intracapsular ligaments are located within the joint capsule, and extracapsular ligaments are located outside of the joint capsule. The medial collateral ligament (MCL), posterior oblique ligament (POL), and arcuate ligament are all capsular ligaments of the tibiofemoral joint. The lateral collateral ligament (LCL) is a capsular ligament at its superior end; however, distally it is extracapsular. The anterior cruciate ligament (ACL), posterior cruciate

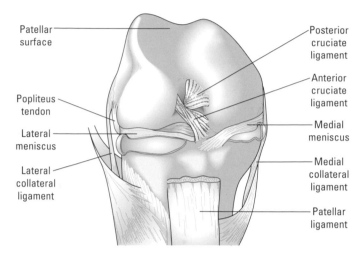

Figure 20.1   Anterior view of the knee with the patella removed.

ligament (PCL), and meniscofemoral ligaments are all intracapsular ligaments.

The MCL is located on the medial aspect of the knee and is composed of both superficial and deep fibers (Fig. 20.1). The superficial fibers of the MCL extend from the medial femoral condyle, anterior to the adductor tubercle, to the anteromedial aspect of the tibial plateau. The deep fibers of the MCL travel from the same origin to insert onto the medial meniscus. On the posteromedial aspect of the knee lies the POL, which originates from the adductor tubercle and inserts onto the posterior aspect of the capsule.

On the lateral side of the knee joint, the LCL courses between the lateral femoral condyle to the fibular head (Fig. 20.1). The arcuate ligament arises from the posterior fibular head and spans the posterolateral aspect of the knee, inserting on the intercondylar region of the tibia and the posterior region of the lateral femoral condyle (Fig. 20.2). The LCL, the arcuate ligament, the popliteus tendon, and the lateral head of the gastrocnemius are collectively considered the arcuate complex.

The ACL originates on the posteromedial aspect of the lateral femoral condyle and inserts on the tibial ridge of the tibial plateau (Fig. 20.1). The ACL is composed of fascicles that can be divided into two bundles: an anteromedial bundle and a posterolateral bundle. The significance of the bundles is that they each are taut in different portions of the range of motion, allowing tension to be produced in the ACL throughout the full range. The posterolateral bundle is taut when the knee is extended, whereas the anteromedial bundle becomes tight as the knee is flexed.

The PCL has a more vertical orientation, originating on the medial aspect of the intercondylar notch and inserting on the tibial ridge of the tibial plateau, just posterior to the ACL (Fig. 20.1). The PCL is comprised of two bundles, an anterolateral bundle and a postero-

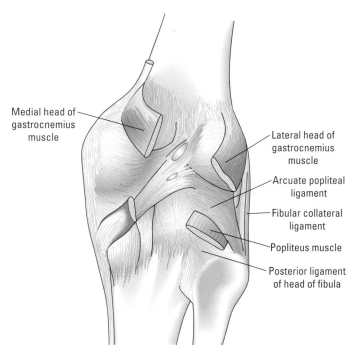

Medial head of gastrocnemius muscle

Lateral head of gastrocnemius muscle

Arcuate popliteal ligament

Fibular collateral ligament

Popliteus muscle

Posterior ligament of head of fibula

Figure 20.2   Posterior view of the knee.

medial bundle. Similar to the ACL, the bundles are tight in reciprocal fashion. The anterolateral bundle becomes tight when the knee is flexed, and the posteromedial bundle is tight with knee extension.

The meniscofemoral ligaments, the ligament of Humphries and the ligament of Wrisberg, are accessory ligaments that surround and augment the PCL (Heller & Langman 1964). These ligaments are variably present; however, at least one ligament has been found in 70–100% of knees (Girgis et al 1975, Heller & Langman 1964). When present, these ligaments are located in the intercondylar notch, forming an attachment between the posterior horn of the lateral meniscus and the lateral border of the medial femoral condyle. The ligament of Humphries is located anterior to PCL, and the ligament of Wrisberg is located posteriorly.

MENISCI

The menisci, located on the surface of the tibial plateaus (Fig. 20.1), are vascularized by the genicular arteries at birth; however, this vascularity recedes with increasing age until only the peripheral 10–30% is vascularized (Arnoczky & Warren 1982, Clark & Ogden 1983). The menisci are slightly concave superiorly, increasing the congruity between the tibia and femur interface, and creating a greater contact area for distribution of load. The menisci further assist in load transmission through their compression.

The amount of movement during knee motion differs between the medial and lateral menisci. Both menisci are secured to the anterior tibial plateau through attachments called coronary ligaments. The medial meniscus, however, has firm attachments through extensions of the joint capsule, whereas the capsular attachments to the lateral meniscus are less firm. Consequently, the medial meniscus translates about 2–5 mm on the tibial plateau during knee motion, and the lateral meniscus about 9–11 mm (Fu & Baratz 1994).

Femoral contact on the menisci changes during knee motion. With increasing knee flexion, there is greater contact on the posterior part, or posterior horn, of the mensici. Conversely, as the knee moves into extension, the femur contacts the anterior aspect, or anterior horn (Fu & Baratz 1994).

KNEE EXAMINATION

GENERAL GUIDELINES

Every knee examination begins with a patient interview during which information is gathered about the mechanism of injury and the location and severity of pain. The patient interview assists the clinician in generating a hypothesis about which structure has been injured. This hypothesis guides the examination, helping the examiner avoid superfluous testing and in the development an examination sequence. Tests that may provoke pain in the structure that is hypothesized to be injured are typically performed near the end of the evaluation, since pain can cause muscle guarding which in turn, can confound the results of subsequent testing procedures.

In most sport injury evaluations, three basic principles can be used to improve the accuracy and validity of the physical examination. First, the patient should be positioned comfortably during the examination. If the patient is not relaxed, muscle contraction may obviate proper technique during testing maneuvers. Second, the knee examination tests should be performed on the contralateral side before testing the injured side. Testing the contralateral side first reveals the amount of normal laxity inherent to the individual, to form a baseline against which the injured side can be compared. Also, patients are more likely to be relaxed when they know what to expect during testing. Finally, examination tests must isolate a structure to conclusively test the integrity of the structure. Structures that contribute the majority of the restraint against a force in a given direction are called primary restraints. Secondary restraints are structures that contribute less to counteracting forces in a specific direction or structures that become a more significant restraint only after the primary restraint is injured. The most sensitive examination procedure is one in which the tested structure is the primary restraint.

Many knee examination tests are designed to assess the integrity of a ligament. A positive ligamentous test is indicated either by pain in the ligament when force is applied, or an increase in laxity compared to the uninjured side. The examiner may also evaluate ligament integrity by the quality of the end feel in comparison to the other side.

Grading scales are often used to allow clinicians to communicate information about the severity of ligament compromise. A scale that assigns a grade based on the amount of laxity during testing is grade 1+ = 0–5 mm, grade 2+ = 5–10 mm, and grade 3+ = 10–15 mm (Hughston & Andrews 1976). The principle consideration concerning grading scales is that clinicians that work together must use a common scale to ensure clear communication.

LIGAMENT TESTING

Medial collateral ligament

The medial collateral ligament (MCL) is best suited to protect the knee against valgus forces because of its location on the medial side of the knee. When the knee is in full extension, the superficial and deep portions of the MCL share the role of primary restraint against valgus stress (Grood et al 1981, Inoue et al 1987). With the knee in 30° of flexion, the superficial portion of the MCL, the portion most commonly injured, is the primary restraint.

To perform a valgus stress test, the patient is positioned supine with the leg to be tested near the edge of the examining table (Fig. 20.3). The examiner faces the patient, supporting the lateral aspect of the distal femur and the medial aspect of the distal tibia, with the knee

joint in approximately 30° of flexion. The distal femur is held in position while a laterally directed force is applied to the distal tibia, producing a valgus force at the knee joint.

Posterior oblique ligament

The posterior oblique ligament (POL) contributes to resisting valgus stress when the knee is extended, and becomes slack when the knee is in 30° of flexion (Grood et al 1981). External rotation of the tibia moves the POL from a posteromedial position to nearly a pure medial arrangement. Once the POL is in this medial position, applying a valgus stress with the knee in extension can test POL integrity.

Lateral collateral ligament

The lateral collateral ligament (LCL) is well suited to resist varus forces at the knee secondary to its lateral location. At full knee extension, the LCL shares the protective role with the arcuate complex (Gollehon et al 1987, Grood et al 1981), however as the knee becomes more flexed, the LCL becomes a primary restraint (Grood et al 1981).

For varus stress testing, the patient is positioned supine, with the test leg close to the edge of the table (McGee 1992). The examiner faces the patient and abducts the leg to allow the examiner to stand between the edge of the table and the test leg (Fig. 20.4). The distal femur is supported medially, and the distal tibia is supported laterally, with the knee flexed to approximately 30°. While firmly stabilizing the femur, the examiner applies a medially directed force to the distal tibia to produce varus force at the knee joint. An alternate way to perform this test, in order to improve femur stabilization, is to hold the distal femur against the edge of the table

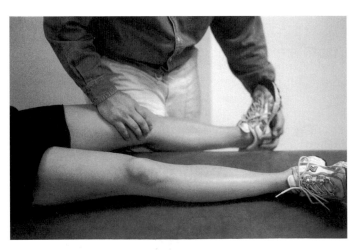

Figure 20.3   Valgus stress test for the knee.

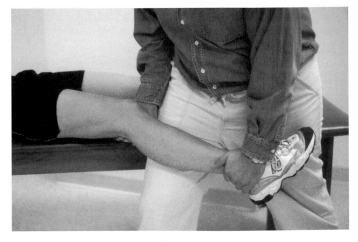

Figure 20.4   Varus stress test for the knee.

while applying the force at the distal tibia, using the edge of the table as a fulcrum to cause a varus stress at the knee joint.

Anterior cruciate ligament

The anterior cruciate ligament (ACL) is the primary restraint against anterior displacement of the tibia on the femur. With the knee flexed to 30°, the ACL provides 87% of the restraint against anterior displacement (Butler et al 1980). In addition, the ACL acts as a secondary restraint for valgus stress at full extension (Inoue et al 1987, Markolf et al 1990).

Many tests have been described to test the integrity of the ACL. The Lachman test has been found to be both sensitive and specific for testing the ACL (Liu et al 1995). To perform a Lachman test, the patient is positioned supine (McGee 1992). The examiner stands facing the patient, supporting the lateral aspect of the distal femur and grasping the medial aspect of the proximal tibia, keeping the knee flexed to approximately 20° (Fig. 20.5). The examiner then pulls the proximal tibia anteriorly, keeping the femur stabilized. If the femur is adequately stabilized, the applied stress will not be localized to the knee. The examiner should also palpate the hamstrings while stabilizing the femur, to ensure that the anterior pull is not being impaired by hamstring contraction.

Another test to assess injury to the ACL is the pivot shift test (Galway et al 1972). This test reproduces the 'giving way' sensation of the knee; therefore patient relaxation is problematic. A greater percentage of positive results in ACL deficient knees are obtained during testing under anesthesia (Donaldson et al 1985). To perform a pivot shift test, the examiner holds the patient's lower leg with one hand and applies a valgus stress at the lateral aspect of the knee joint with the other hand while the

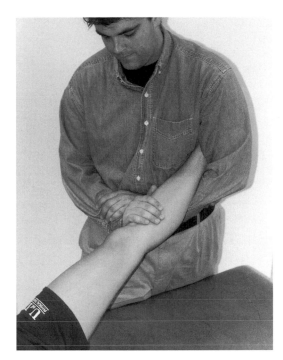

Figure 20.6   Pivot shift test for the anterior cruciate ligament of the knee.

patient's knee is in a fully extended position (Fig. 20.6). In this position, the valgus force produces a rotational subluxation of the lateral tibia. The examiner then moves the knee into approximately 30° of flexion, maintaining the valgus stress at the knee joint. A positive pivot shift test will be perceived as a 'sliding' motion of the tibia as the knee reaches approximately 20–30° of flexion, which is actually a reduction of the tibia. The tibial reduction is caused by the pull of the iliotibial band, which becomes a knee flexor at approximately 20° of flexion.

Posterior cruciate ligament

The posterior cruciate ligament (PCL) is the primary restraint to posterior displacement of the tibia on the femur (Fukubayashi et al 1982, Gollehon et al 1987), thus most examination tests involve the measurement of posterior laxity. The PCL additionally acts as a secondary restraint to varus stress at 0° and 30° knee flexion (Gollehon et al 1987).

Injury to the PCL can be assessed by many tests. One test is called the posterior drawer (Veltri & Warren 1993). To perform the posterior drawer test, the patient is positioned supine with the knee flexed to 90° (Fig. 20.7) The examiner grasps the proximal tibia with both hands, with the thumbs on the anterior aspect of the tibia, and applies a posteriorly directed force. Position of the tibial condyles and the amount of laxity are compared to the uninjured side.

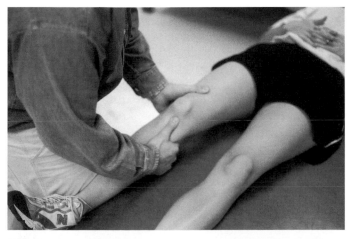

Figure 20.5   Lachman test for the anterior cruciate ligament of the knee.

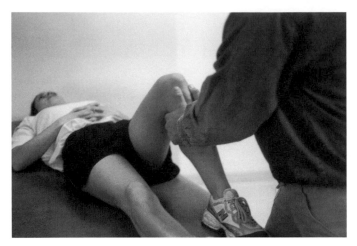

Figure 20.7 Posterior drawer test for the posterior cruciate ligament of the knee.

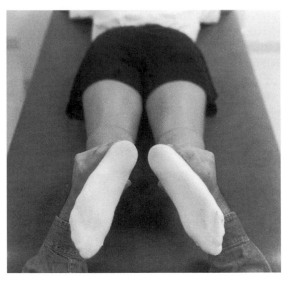

Figure 20.8 Prone external rotation test for the arcuate complex.

Another useful test is the posterior sag test (Veltri & Warren 1993). For this test, the patient is positioned supine while the examiner passively flexes the hips and knees to 90°. To maintain the 90–90 position, the examiner either cradles the distal tibia or places the patient's foot on a chair of appropriate height. If the tibial tubercle on the injured side is less prominent than the tibial tubercle on the uninvolved side, the test is considered positive. The 'sag', or posterior displacement, of the tibia during this test is a consequence of gravitational pull.

The third test commonly used to assess PCL integrity is the quadriceps active test (Veltri & Warren 1993). The patient is positioned supine with the knee flexed to approximately 90°. The examiner stabilizes the patient's foot on the examining table and instructs the patient to try to extend the knee. This will result in an isometric contraction of the quadriceps. If there is PCL compromise, the posteriorly subluxed tibia will be drawn anteriorly by the quadriceps, causing the tibial tubercle to become more prominent.

Arcuate complex

The arcuate complex is the primary restraint to external rotation of the tibia (Gollehon et al 1987). The arcuate complex is tested by the prone external rotation test with the knee at 30° of flexion (Veltri & Warren 1993). The test is performed with the patient prone (Fig. 20.8). Both knees are flexed to 30° by the examiner and the feet are externally rotated, causing tibial external rotation. External rotation of the foot relative to the thigh is compared between the injured and uninjured legs. An increase in the amount of external rotation by 10° or more compared to the uninjured side is considered a positive test (Veltri & Warren 1993).

MENISCAL TESTS

Meniscal tears are difficult to diagnose by physical examination. McMurray's test is commonly used to diagnose meniscal tears and is performed by fully flexing the patient's injured knee, then grasping the foot and rotating the tibia on the femur while the knee remains flexed (Corea et al 1994). Although McMurray's test is commonly used, the sensitivity of the test is only 59% (Corea et al 1994). Clinicians should have a high index of suspicion for a meniscal tear when symptoms of joint line tenderness, clicking in the knee, and knee locking are present (Anderson & Lipscomb 1986, Shakespeare & Rigby 1983).

EFFUSION

Assessing knee effusion allows the clinician to monitor the patient's recovery after injury and the patient's response to treatment progression. Girth measurements do not adequately quantify effusion, particularly if the effusion is small. Instead, the stroke test can give more meaningful information about the presence and amount of effusion (McGee 1992). The stroke test is performed with the patient supine and the knee relaxed in full extension. The test starts with the examiner performing several strokes upward from the medial joint line towards the suprapatellar pouch in an attempt to move effusion from the medial aspect of the knee. The examiner then strokes downward on the lateral side of the knee from the suprapatellar pouch towards the lateral joint line, observing the medial aspect of the knee in an effort to appreciate a fluid wave emanating from the suprapatellar pouch (McGee 1992). At our facility, we use four different grades to describe the amount of effusion. If no wave is produced with the downward stroke, there is no effusion present. If the downward stroke produces a small wave on the medial side of the knee, the effusion is given a 'trace' grade; a larger bulge is given a '1+' grade. If the effusion returns to the medial side of the knee without a downward stroke, the effusion is given a '2+' grade. The inability to move the effusion out of the medial aspect of the knee equates to a '3+' grade.

SPECIAL TOPICS RELATED TO KNEE EVALUATION

Arthrometer testing

Arthrometer testing is most often used to quantify knee joint laxity when ACL injury is suspected. Many different knee arthrometers have been developed, however, results obtained with these different systems are not necessarily generalizable to each other (Anderson et al 1992). The KT 1000 arthrometer (Medmetrics, San Diego, CA, USA) is a commonly used arthometer. Results using KT 1000 with a manual maximum pull have shown a 3 mm difference between sides to be greater than 90% sensitive for an ACL rupture (Liu et al 1995, Rangger et al 1993).

Quadriceps strength testing

Quadriceps weakness is a common sequela after a knee injury, therefore measurement of quadriceps strength is important to ensure full resolution of this impairment prior to return to sport. Biomechanical studies have demonstrated that a quadriceps strength deficit is correlated with altered gait (Snyder-Mackler et al 1995).

A variety of methods can be used to test quadriceps strength. The two most common methods used in the clinical setting are manual muscle testing and isokinetic testing. Manual muscle testing is one of the easiest to employ; however, results are less accurate when a patient is able to generate high force or when the strength difference between limbs is minimal. Isokinetic testing offers the benefit of objective measurement through a force transducer, but there is controversy about which is the most clinically significant testing speed. Faster speeds better approximate speed of joint motion during function; however, they underestimate strength deficits (Gapeyeva et al 2000, Keays et al 2000).

Neither manual muscle testing nor isokinetic testing measure the patient's effort or offer a method for quadriceps inhibition (inability to fully activate the quadriceps voluntarily). Quadriceps can be inhibited after knee injury (Snyder-Mackler et al 1994). The burst-superimposition method of testing quadriceps strength is not used as commonly in the clinical setting as in research studies, but this method offers the ability to measure inhibition (Snyder-Mackler et al 1994). For this type of testing, an electrical stimulus is administered (super-imposed) while the patient produces a maximal voluntary isometric contraction. If the patient has fully activated the quadriceps, there will be no force augmentation when the electrical stimulus is delivered. If the burst-super-imposition method of testing is not available to the clinician, targets should be set and verbal encouragement given during testing to improve quality of effort.

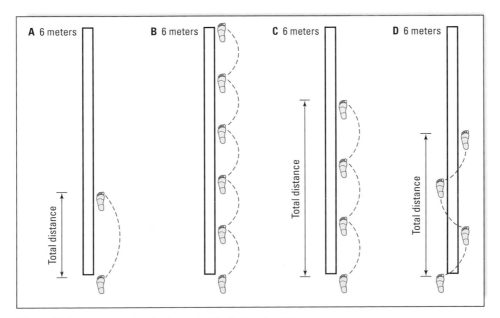

Figure 20.9   Hop tests for the knee. **A**: Single hop for distance.
B: Timed hop. **C**: Triple hop for distance. **D**: Cross-over hop for distance.

Hop testing

Hop testing is a commonly used clinical test of function. Many clinics use one or all of the hop tests described by Noyes et al (1991), which include: the single hop test, triple hop test, cross-over triple hop test and timed hop test (Fig. 20.9). Testing in an uninjured population showed that 92–93% had a symmetry index (side-to-side comparison) of at least 85% for the single hop and timed hop tests (Barber et al 1990); thus a score less than 85% on the hop tests can be indicative of disability. Hop testing has been shown to have good reliability, particularly when patients are given more than one practice trial (Bolgla & Keskula 1997).

Self-report questionnaires

Self-report questionnaires can assist the clinician in measuring disability and monitoring changes in functional status during the course of treatment. The knee-specific (e.g. Lysholm Scale [Lysholm & Gillquist 1982], Cincinnati Knee Rating Scale [Noyes et al 1989]) and general health status questionnaires (e.g. SF-36 [Ware & Shelbourne 1992]), both provide important, but very different information. Knee-specific questionnaires give insight into disability caused by the knee injury, whereas general health status questionnaires reveal mental and emotional states that may impact on rehabilitation. Clinicians should select knee-specific questionnaires that include questions related to high-level activities; otherwise, an athlete may reach the highest score even when some disability remains. Furthermore, clinicians should check the literature to make sure the selected questionnaire has high reliability and is able to measure changes in functional status.

REHABILITATION OF COMMON SPORTS-RELATED INJURIES

GENERAL REHABILITATION GUIDELINES

Rehabilitation guidelines are structured to direct the clinician in returning athletes to preinjury activity levels as quickly and safely as possible. Guidelines should be based upon current scientific evidence and have criteria for progression in rehabilitation. Criterion-based protocols eliminate subjective progression through rehabilitation by dictating the milestones that must be reached in order to progress to the next phase. The rate of progression can differ between athletes and is dependent on the individual rate of healing and the demands of the athlete's activity level. Also, clinicians should prescribe therapeutic interventions within each phase that are tailored to the patient's needs. Prescribing therapeutic interventions in a 'cookbook' fashion for each particular diagnosis is committing a disservice to the patient.

PHASES OF REHABILITATION

Three phases of rehabilitation will be discussed: the acute phase, advanced phase, and return-to-play phase (Box 20.1). It should be noted that many variations on rehabilitation programs for knee injuries are possible and that only some of these approaches are presented in the chapter.

Acute phase

In the acute phase of rehabilitation, strategies are focused on controlling the effects of inflammation (pain, effusion,

---

Box 20.1 Phases of rehabilitation

Acute phase

Goals
Decrease pain
Increase range of movement
Retard muscle atrophy
Unassisted ambulation

Common interventions
Cryotherapy
NMES
Patellar mobilization
Soft tissue mobilization at incision site (if surgical intervention)
Isometric exercise (quadriceps sets)
Range of motion exercises
Gait training
Cardiovascular exercise (stationary bike, swimming)

Advanced phase

Criteria to enter
Full range of motion and effusion controlled (below 2+)

Goal
Increase muscle strength and endurance

Common interventions
Isotonic (both open and closed chain) and isokinetic exercise
NMES
Proprioception exercise
Flexibility exercise
Running program
Cardiovascular exercise (stationary bike, StairMaster, elliptical machine)

Return-to-play phase

Criteria to enter
Quadriceps strength ≥80% of the uninjured side

Goal
Prepare athlete for a return to competition

Common interventions
Isotonic (both open and closed chain) and isokinetic exercise
Agility training
Sport-specific exercise

loss of motion, and muscle atrophy). The goal of the acute phase is to restore full range of motion, reduce effusion, retard muscle atrophy, and ambulate without an assistive device (Box 20.1). Ice, compression, and elevation of the injured limb can assist in counteracting the effects of inflammation. Relative rest is usually indicated to allow for healing to occur without the detrimental effects of strict immobilization, such as arthrofibrosis and deconditioning.

In the acute stage, ambulation with an assistive device is indicated if the athlete is unable to walk without a limp. A knee brace that limits tibiofemoral motion is often used in conjunction with an assistive device to safely allow increased weightbearing. Use of an assistive device is maintained until the athlete can walk without a limp, joint effusion has been controlled, and when the quadriceps have recovered sufficiently to provide protection of healing tissues (typically 60% of the uninvolved side).

Range of motion deficits should also be resolved in this portion of rehabilitation. Most often, regaining knee extension is more difficult, so priority should be placed on achieving extension. The clinician should evaluate the numerous possible sources contributing to a restricted range of motion including: decreased patella mobility, poor quadriceps recruitment, decreased quadriceps strength, decreased accessory motion of the tibiofemoral joint, and muscle guarding and tightness. Interventions should be chosen that address the specific cause of restricted range. A combination of low-load sustained stretching, joint mobilizations of the patella and tibiofemoral joints, and modalities to control pain and resultant muscle spasm are commonly performed following most injuries and surgeries.

Rapid and significant quadriceps femoris weakness is a common concern following injuries to the tibiofemoral joint (Morrissey 1989, Nyland 1999, Snyder-Mackler et al 1994). Efforts to retard atrophy and facilitate volitional quadriceps activation form the basis of early progressive strengthening programs (Snyder-Mackler et al 1991). Successful early quadriceps strengthening will facilitate efforts to gain full knee extension, restore normal patellar mobility, and correct antalgic gait patterns. Reciprocally, early emphasis on obtaining full knee extension during weightbearing will assist in efforts to regain knee extensor strength.

If the athlete is experiencing difficulty producing a strong quadriceps contraction, neuromuscular electrical stimulation (NMES) is indicated (see Ch. 13). Parameters for NMES of athletes include: frequency of 50–75 Hz, wavelength of 200–400 μs, ramp time of 2 s, 10 s of on time, 50 s of off time, and ten contractions during a session, 2–3 sessions a week. The success of NMES depends upon achieving adequate levels of electrical stimulation to provide stimulus to promote strength gains. Patients are counseled to try and relax while the electrically elicited isometric contractions are increased in an effort to achieve 50% of the injured leg's maximal volitional isometric contraction. Intensity levels that are below 50% of maximal voluntary isometric contraction (MVIC) have limited capacity to assist in strength gain beyond volitional exercise alone. Use of this high intensity NMES is maintained until the involved limb achieves strength equal to 80% of the uninvolved side.

Advanced phase

The advanced phase of rehabilitation is initiated when range of motion is full and effusion controlled (below grade 2+) (Box 20.1). The goal of this phase is to increase muscle strength and endurance. Higher intensity resistance training can be initiated and should include exercises for all muscles of lower extremity. If the intensity of therapeutic exercise creates an increase in effusion, intensity levels are reduced to the previous level. Progression to higher activity is dictated by the presence of soreness after exercise (Box 20.2).

Rehabilitation exercises are commonly categorized as open or closed chain exercises. Open chain exercises are those in which the distal end is free to move (e.g. knee extension), and closed chain exercises are those in which the distal end is fixed (e.g. squat). Optimal strengthening requires a combination of both open and closed chain exercises (Fitzgerald 1997, Mikkelson et al 2000, Morrissey et al 2000). When athletes perform closed chain exercises, clinicians should be cognizant of the tendency to compensate for weak muscles in the kinetic chain. Reliance of the ankle plantar flexors and the hip extensors is a common substitution with closed chain exercises following knee injury.

Often, exercises designed to improve dynamic stability are added in this phase. Although there is no literature to support the inclusion of such exercises, there is a theoretical framework for including such exercises based on basic science and applied research. Balance exercises using unstable surfaces and perturbation devices are included.

Box 20.2 Exercise progression guidelines based on soreness

- If no soreness is present from previous exercise, progress exercise by modifying one variable.
- If soreness is present from previous exercise, but recedes with warm-up, stay at same level.
- If soreness is present from previous exercise, but does not recede with warm-up, decrease exercise to the level prior to progression. Consider taking the day off if soreness is still present with the reduced level of exercise. When exercise is resumed, it should be at the reduced level.

Progression of aerobic condition often includes a running program that is usually initiated in this phase of rehabilitation. To start running, the athlete's injured side quadriceps strength must be restored to at least 80% of the uninvolved side, and sufficient healing of the injured structure must have occurred (e.g. ACL reconstruction approximately 8 weeks, grade I MCL injury at 1–2 weeks). Soft tissue healing is usually sufficient at 4–6 weeks. Running progression starts on a treadmill and will move to running on a track. Track workouts are initiated with running the straight-a-ways and walking corners. The intensity is gradually increased until the athlete can run the full length of the track. Road running and finally off-road running represent the least controlled training situations and are instituted as a final stage in running progression. Jogging duration may start with as much as 2 miles and may be progressed on a weekly basis if there is no pain or swelling (Box 20.2). Completing a full running progression can take as long as 2–3 months.

Return-to-play phase

The goal of the return-to-play phase is to prepare the athlete to return to the demands of competition (Box 20.1). The athlete is allowed to enter this phase when intense resistance training and a running program do not increase effusion. Therapeutic exercise interventions should follow the SAID (Specific Adaptations to Imposed Demands) principle. This concept is based in the notion that the body will adapt to accommodate to the stress and strains applied to it. Therefore, exercises should attempt to mimic the demands of activities required for the athlete to successfully return to sport.

The return-to-play phase is characterized by agility training and sport-specific exercise. Less complex agility drills (e.g. shuffle, shuttle run) should be used initially, moving to more complex agility drills (e.g. figure of 8, braiding). The volume of agility activities should be graded by frequency, duration, and intensity. Only one variable should be modified at one time, otherwise it is difficult to determine what was the factor that caused an adverse response (increased pain or effusion) to the treatment. Sport-specific activities are introduced and progressed in the same manner. Practice drills are started, leading to competition level activities.

Athletes are cleared to return to sport when they have progressed through all phases of rehabilitation without symptoms and have met the criteria of return-to-play testing. Return-to-play testing involves quadriceps strength testing, hop testing and self-report questionnaires. Athletes must score 90% on all tests before returning to competition (Manal & Snyder-Mackler 1996).

ANTERIOR CRUCIATE LIGAMENT

Mechanism of injury

The ACL is injured when the tibia translates too far anteriorly relative to the femur. The majority of ACL injuries (around 70%) occur by non-contact mechanisms; the remaining injuries involve contact (Boden et al 2000). Non-contact injuries typically involve a sharp deceleration with the knee close to extension, with or without a change in direction, or landing from a jump (Boden et al 2000). Injury to the ACL can also occur when the knee is hyperextended, or when contact results in valgus collapse of the knee (Boden et al 2000).

Non-operative treatment

Most athletes with an ACL tear experience knee instability during sports that involve cutting or jumping (Shelton et al 1997). Non-operative treatment has primarily been reserved for those willing to reduce their activity level; however, non-operative treatment can be a short-term option for athletes if certain conditions are met. A screening examination has been developed to assess an athlete's potential for dynamically stabilizing the injured knee, to determine if an athlete is a good candidate for non-operative treatment. The screening examination is composed of a variety of clinical tests and is administered when there is no knee effusion present, full knee range of motion has been restored, and the patient experiences no pain with unilateral hopping. In order to qualify for non-operative treatment, the athlete must: (1) have no more than one episode of giving way (i.e. buckling) since the initial injury, (2) score at least 80% on the timed hop test, (3) score at least 80% on the Knee Outcome Survey-Activities of Daily Living Scale (Irrgang et al 1998), and (4) score at least 60% on the Global Rating Scale (Fitzgerald et al 2000a). If the athlete meets the criteria of the screening examination, then non-operative treatment can be offered as a viable option, otherwise surgical intervention is recommended. Non-operative treatment should only be considered when there is no concomitant ligamentous injury greater than grade I, no repairable meniscal tear, and no full-thickness articular cartilage defect.

Athletes who pass the criteria of the screening examination are enrolled in a ten session rehabilitation program that includes lower extremity strengthening exercises, agility training, and perturbation training (Fitzgerald et al 2000b). In a randomized controlled trial, perturbation training augmented rehabilitation was compared to a program consisting of only strengthening exercises and agility training, and was found to result in greater success in returning to sport without episodes of giving way (Fitzgerald et al 2000b). Perturbation training involves the application of controlled forces to the lower extremity through support surface movement. Rockerboard, rollerboard, and rollerboard with a stationary platform are used to apply the perturbations during this type of training (Figs 20.10–20.12). The force, direction and predictability of the perturbations are progressed throughout the ten sessions. Athletes wear a functional brace during agility training and when they return to sport activity. This protocol is given as a short-

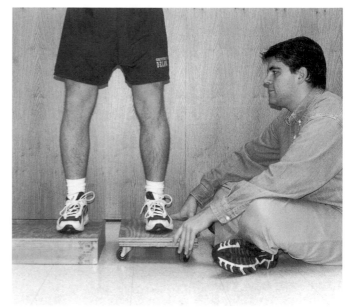

Figure 20.12   Perturbation training for non-operative ACL rehabilitation (rollerboard with stationary platform technique).

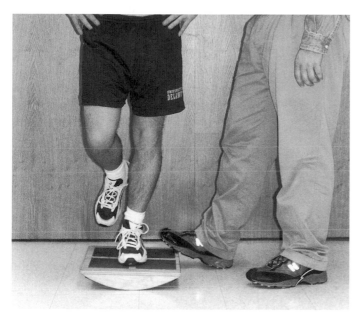

Figure 20.10   Perturbation training for non-operative ACL rehabilitation (rockerboard technique).

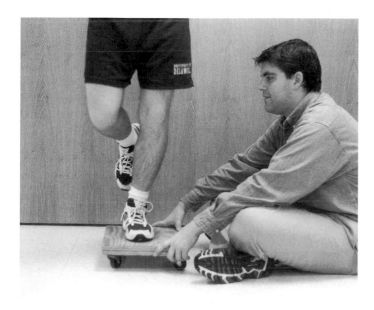

Figure 20.11   Perturbation training for non-operative ACL rehabilitation (rollerboard technique).

term option for athletes who wish to complete their competitive season; operative intervention is recommended when the competitive season is finished.

Operative treatment

Operative treatment should be considered for any athlete who wishes to return to sports that require cutting, jumping, and lateral movement. Athletes may benefit from preoperative rehabilitation to decrease inflammation and improve knee motion. Surgery less than 1 month from injury was found to be one of the factors related to a loss of motion following surgery (Harner et al 1992).

ACL reconstructions are performed with a variety of grafts. Typical autogenous graft choices include the middle third of the patellar tendon or doubled semitendinosis-gracilis tendons. Allograft choices include fresh frozen Achilles or patellar tendon.

Advances in surgical fixation allow for full weight-bearing and the ability to obtain full knee extension in the immediate postoperative phase without concern for graft failure. Considerable research has been conducted to determine which exercises may impose harmful strain to the ACL graft, thus contributing to graft stretching. Some studies suggest that performing knee extension in a range from 0–40° may impose high strain on the ACL; however, other studies show that the amount of strain may be comparable to that during weightbearing (Beynnon et al 1997, Escamilla et al 1998, Lutz et al 1993). Clinicians should, therefore, prescribe knee extension exercises in a terminal range judiciously. It is important to remember that absence of strain can also be detrimental, since strain is essential for graft remodeling. Unfortunately, the optimal strain level has not yet been determined.

Postoperative treatment

Immediately after surgery, patients may experience difficulty producing a quadriceps contraction, particularly if an autogenous patellar tendon graft was used. An inability to produce a quadriceps contraction, coupled with donor site healing, can lead to a restriction of superior patellar mobility. Superior patellar mobilization is therefore essential for these patients. Patients should be positioned at 60° of knee flexion for NMES. By the second week after surgery, 90° of active knee flexion should be achieved, and by 6–8 weeks after surgery, the patient should achieve full active range of motion (Manal & Snyder-Mackler 1996).

In the advanced phase of rehabilitation (6–12 weeks postoperatively), strengthening exercises should be progressed. Approximately 8 weeks after surgery, a running program can be initiated if the patient's involved side quadriceps strength is 80% of the uninvolved side (Manal & Snyder-Mackler 1996).

In the return-to-play phase (12–20 weeks postoperatively), athletes are allowed to gradually increase the complexity and intensity of activities. Athletes are allowed to return to sport approximately 4–6 months after surgery, provided they have met all clinical milestones and progressed through all phases of rehabilitation. The athlete should demonstrate quadriceps strength and hop testing scores that are 90% of the uninjured side before being cleared to return to sport (Manal & Snyder-Mackler 1996). A functional brace is typically prescribed for a return to sport and is worn until the patient feels confident in the stability of the knee.

MEDIAL COLLATERAL LIGAMENT

Mechanism of injury

The majority of isolated MCL injuries involve lateral impact to the lower thigh or upper leg (Indelicato 1995). Injury to the MCL can also occur in combination with an ACL injury, and possibly a POL injury, when the knee is subjected to a large valgus force with external rotation (Indelicato 1995).

Non-operative treatment

Non-operative treatment is recommended for most MCL injuries because the MCL has a rich blood supply and associated high healing potential. Non-operatively managed, incomplete (grade I and II) MCL injuries typically result in an unrestricted return to activity (Derscheid & Garrick 1981, Holden et al 1983). Isolated, complete MCL ruptures can also have good outcomes, although the recovery time will be longer and greater residual laxity will remain (Indelicato et al 1990, Jones et al 1986).

The duration of the acute phase may be as brief as a few days for a grade I MCL sprain and as long as 4 weeks for grade III MCL injuries. In the acute phase of rehabilitation, valgus stress to the knee is avoided to allow initial healing of the MCL. Patients may complain of pain when the knee nears full extension because the MCL is in a lengthened position in extension. For grade II and III MCL sprains, an immobilizer or brace that prohibits knee extension past 30° may be used to reduce pain and to decrease strain of the MCL. Often, an immobilizer is worn initially, then the athlete is progressed to a brace which restricts range of motion. Total duration of motion restriction is 1–4 weeks, dependent on the severity of the sprain (Holden et al 1983, Indelicato 1983). Patients who are limited from full knee extension should be encouraged to perform range of motion exercises in a pain-free range, gradually working on increasing range of motion.

In the advanced phase of rehabilitation, valgus stress to the knee can gradually be introduced. Either side-stepping over cones or hip adduction exercises can be used to introduce valgus stress at the knee. Resistance for hip adduction exercises should initially be placed proximally on the tibia and move distally as the patient is able to tolerate and control a longer lever arm. If the patient was limited from full knee extension in the acute phase, resistance in a terminal range should be progressed gradually.

In the return-to-play phase, agility drills should be initiated in the sagittal plane and progressed to the frontal plane. Agility drills in the frontal plane, such as shuffles, braiding or side jumping, all increase valgus stress across the knee and should be progressed with caution. Functional braces may be worn when the athlete returns to sport, but long-term use is discouraged (Indelicato 1995).

Operative treatment

Operative treatment is usually reserved for complete (grade III) ruptures of the MCL, or complete MCL ruptures in combination with other ligamentous ruptures. The operative procedure is usually primary repair.

Postoperative treatment

Postoperative treatment after MCL repair follows a protocol similar to non-operative treatment of grade III MCL injuries, with the exception that attention must be paid to incision site mobility. An immobilizer is typically worn for 2 weeks, and crutches are used for ambulation. Patient comfort and ability to meet clinical milestones dictate progression to the next phase (Indelicato 1995).

MENISCI

Mechanism of injury

Meniscal tears can occur in isolation or in combination with a ligamentous injury. One mechanism for an isolated meniscal injury is pivoting, in which the femur rotates on the meniscus while the meniscus is compressed. Another mechanism for meniscal injury is rising from a squat. This results because weight is transferred to the posterior horns with increasing knee flexion, then as the athlete begins the ascent phase of the squat, the menisci are pushed forward while the posterior horn remains trapped.

Non-operative treatment

Non-operative treatment may be recommended for an isolated meniscal tear that is stable and non-symptomatic. Rehabilitation is directed at resolving knee impairments, and progression is based on symptoms.

Operative treatment

Repair of the meniscus is always preferred to excision or debridement; however, healing potential dictates what procedure is performed. The meniscal rim is vascularized and has been termed the 'red zone'; whereas the central portion of the meniscus is devoid of vascularity and has been termed the 'white zone' (DeHaven & Arnoczky 1994). A tear in the white zone has poor healing potential and is usually treated with debridement. Tears that occur in the red zone or the transition to the white zone (red–white zone) have greater healing potential and may be treated with a repair, if deemed appropriate by the physician.

Postoperative treatment

Postoperative rehabilitation depends on whether the meniscal tear was debrided or repaired. If the tear was treated with debridement, progression is entirely based on symptoms. There is little tissue morbidity associated with meniscal debridement resulting in a fairly rapid progression in rehabilitation. The clinician should be aware that removal of the meniscus has been associated with increased risk of osteoarthritic changes, therefore, attention should be paid to quadriceps strength deficits, since improving quadriceps strength can provide potential chondroprotective benefits (Slemenda et al 1998).

Protocols reported for postoperative meniscal repair rehabilitation vary in the initiation of weightbearing and motion exercises. Some protocols allow motion from 0° to 90° immediately after surgery (Cooper et al 1991); others recommend keeping the knee in full extension for 2 weeks, then beginning a range of motion progression (DeHaven & Arnoczky 1994). Weightbearing to tolerance after surgery has not been associated with any detrimental effects to the repair (Shelbourne et al 1996); although an immobilizer that keeps the knee in full extension may be used for the first couple of weeks to protect the repair site. Patients are advised to avoid deep squatting for the first 4 weeks to allow healing of the repair site if it is in the posterior part of the meniscus. Patient tolerance and ability to meet clinical milestones dictate progression through the phases of rehabilitation.

REHABILITATION OF LESS COMMON INJURIES

POSTERIOR CRUCIATE LIGAMENT AND POSTEROLATERAL CORNER INJURIES

Mechanism of injury

Compared to the ACL and MCL, the PCL is less commonly injured; however, there is suspicion that many injuries go unreported or are misdiagnosed. PCL injuries during sports usually occur as a result of a posteriorly directed blow to the proximal tibia. Often this occurs when the athlete falls onto a flexed knee with the foot plantar-flexed. This injury is common in ice hockey players or figure skaters who slip and fall on the ice. The PCL can also be compromised in a knee hyperextension injury.

Injuries to the PCL classically create long-term impairments and functional limitations due to secondary pathology of degenerative arthritic changes in the tibiofemoral and patellofemoral joints (Harner & Höher 1998, Keller et al 1993). Some authors have gone so far as to state that degenerative changes in the tibiofemoral joint following PCL injury 'are inevitable' (Cross & Powell 1984). Concomitant quadriceps weakness found after PCL tears often compounds the disability of these conditions.

The posterolateral corner is described as the LCL, the popliteus complex, the arcuate ligament complex, fabellofibular ligament, biceps tendon, and the posterolateral capsular structures (Covey 2001). Injury to these ligamentous and muscular components that surround the posterior aspect of the lateral femoral condyle rarely occurs in isolation; rather, it is usually a concomitant injury with the PCL. The posterolateral corner is typically injured with a posteriorly direct force to the anteromedial tibia with the knee in hyperextension (Baker et al 1985, Covey 2001). Injury to the posterolateral corner can often be missed in an examination of knee ligamentous support, especially with a concomitant PCL injury (Harner & Höher 1998, Noyes & Barber-Westin 1996). Those patients with combined PCL and posterolateral corner injuries have a greater predisposition to degenerative changes than isolated PCL injured patients (Baker et al 1985, Torg et al 1989). Also, the addition of a posterolateral corner to a PCL injury is unlikely to be satisfactorily stabilized with sole reconstruction of the PCL (Harner et al 2000).

Non-operative treatment

Non-operative treatment is usually recommended after a grade I or II injury to the PCL. This corresponds with an isolated PCL injury with posterior translation of less than 10 mm (Veltri & Warren 1993). Multiple directional laxity as a result of concomitant ACL, MCL, or posterolateral corner injury usually undergoes operative reconstruction (Harner & Höher 1998, Harner et al 2000).

Restoring quadriceps strength is the cornerstone of conservative rehabilitation following PCL injury (Torg et al 1989, Wilk 1994). Early efforts to improve quadriceps strength must be tempered by the potentially detrimental posterior stresses that are generated by some types of strengthening exercises. Several studies have investigated the potential posterior translation with open and closed chain knee extension exercises. Open chain knee extension exercises from 0–60° produce anterior shear forces at the tibiofemoral joint while open chain knee extensions beyond 60° can create posterior tibial translations (Jurist & Otis 1985, Kaufman et al 1991, Lutz et al 1993). Studies that have investigated closed chain exercise also report high posterior displacement forces which seem to increase with increased flexion (Lutz et al 1993, Stuart et al 1996). Caution should be taken in using open chain knee flexion exercises in rehabilitation programs following PCL injury, due to the undesired posterior forces associated with these types of strengthening.

During the first 2 weeks following injury, the athlete typically wears a knee brace that limits motion to near full extension. Range of motion exercises from 0–60° are performed 3–4 times a day along with isometric and short arc (0–30°) open chain quadriceps exercises. Use of isometric NMES usually starts at 30° of flexion (Axe et al 2001).

After 2 weeks, biking may be used for range of motion efforts (Wilk 1994). The open chain knee extension exercise range is progressed to 0–60° with progressive resistance. General strengthening of the calf musculature can

be initiated at this time. Range of motion is typically progressed until the patient achieves 0–110° by their fourth week.

At the start of the fourth week, the patient should have restored gait without a limp. Limited range, closed chain strengthening exercises can be initiated if they are purely sagittal plane exercises of no deeper than 45° of flexion (Wilk 1994). The main emphasis of strengthening should continue to be open chain knee extension in limited range. Anterior knee pain is common in this patient population and modifications to open chain exercises to avoid painful strengthening should be employed. Full range of motion should be achieved by 4–6 weeks after injury. By approximately 8 weeks after injury, rehabilitation may progress to the return-to-play phase with close monitoring of patellofemoral joint pain and changes in posterior laxity.

Posterolateral corner instability in combination with PCL injury usually slows the speed of progression in non-operative and operative rehabilitation. There are a number of operative techniques to correct this instability, but currently there is no 'gold standard' for operative measures (Covey 2001). Attempts to improve the dynamic stability of the knee using techniques comparable to non-operative rehabilitation following ACL injury appear to be the best non-operative treatment option to correct for knee instability that lacks a viable surgical correction. A combination of perturbation training and completion of a functional progression represent the non-operative treatment of posterolateral corner injuries.

Operative treatment

Reconstruction as operative management of posterior laxity is typically indicated if the patient has functional instability or pain, early degenerative changes in the tibiofemoral joint, or combined ligamentous injuries (Harner et al 2000). Typical autograft material for reconstruction consists of bone–patellar tendon–bone, semitendinous and gracilis, and quadriceps tendon–bone (Axe et al 2001). Most allografts use Achilles tendon, bone–patellar tendon–bone, or allograft (Bullis & Paulos 1994). A surgical repair may be performed if a bone fragment has avulsed with the PCL. Relatively little is known concerning fixation strength and graft incorporation following PCL operative treatment.

Postoperative treatment

Rehabilitation following surgery is governed by the relatively poor strength of the fixation of the reconstructed ligament. Increased posterior laxity is a more frequent complication than arthrofibrosis and subsequent loss of flexion range of motion. Therefore, early rehabilitative efforts are focused on controlling inflammatory processes, and preventing arthrofibrosis and atrophy without excessively stressing the newly reconstructed graft.

Physical therapy following surgery is very similar to conservative treatment for a grade III PCL tear but involves a longer protective phase to insure that posterior laxity does not develop. Again, open chain knee flexion exercises are avoided as they will likely cause deleterious posterior stress on the newly reconstructed ligament. Patients are usually braced in full extension for at least 2 weeks and as long as 4 weeks. One to two weeks after surgery, preservation of knee extensor musculature is initiated, as this will be crucial for eliminating posterior tibial translation to provide graft protection in later stages of therapy. Knee extension stretches typically are performed in the prone position to minimize possible posterior translation due to gravitational forces on the tibia. Early knee flexion stretches are also performed in the prone position, with careful instructions to the patient to avoid active knee flexion during stretches. A manual anterior displacement of the tibia on the femur should be maintained during passive flexion stretching for the first 4 weeks. A knee range of motion of 0–60° is the milestone for 2 weeks after surgery. Quadriceps control should improve to the point that, at 2 weeks, the patient is able to maintain full knee extension without a lag against gravity.

At 3–4 weeks, the athlete can start to be weaned from the brace and gait training should be initiated if there is demonstration of adequate quadriceps control (Wilk 1994). Open chain knee extensions can be performed from 0–60° of flexion. Closed chain exercises can be incorporated at this point as the patient moves through the advanced rehabilitation stage. Progression into the return-to-play phase will start at approximately 3 months after surgery if the corresponding criteria is met.

Reconstruction for posterior laxity with a combined posterolateral corner injury requires an even greater protection period. Combined posterolateral corner laxity has been identified as a potential cause of graft failure in PCL reconstruction (Harner et al 2000). There are no clear guidelines to perform a reconstruction or repair of this rotational laxity, even when it is recognized (Harner et al 2000). The athlete must be counseled regarding a diminished likelihood of a rapid return to sport with an injury involving combined posterior and posterolateral instability. Clinical milestones should be delayed by 2 weeks compared to isolated PCL injury, and return to cutting and rotational activities will be implemented in a more gradual fashion.

Combined PCL and posterolateral corner reconstructions involve the greatest amount of restrictions following surgery due to the severity of the injury and the reconstruction (Wilk 1994). Crutches are typically discontinued after about 2 weeks but a knee immobilizer is used to lock the knee in full extension for 6 weeks with no motion allowed during this period. At about 6 weeks, strengthening moves beyond isometric quadriceps activities to active and active assisted motions and is progressed as for PCL reconstruction. Typically, full range of motion is achieved at about 8 weeks postoperatively (Wilk 1994). Return to strenuous activities varies from 18 to 21 weeks following surgery.

TIBIAL PLATEAU FRACTURE

Mechanism of injury

A significant varus, valgus or compressive force at the knee can cause a fracture of the tibial plateau. Tibial plateau fractures commonly occur in loaded, twisting injuries or direct blows to the knee causing a direct compressive force through a femoral condyle into the tibial plateau. Due to the natural valgus angulation of the knee, lateral tibial plateau fractures are more common than medial fractures (Kennedy & Bailey 1968). Tibial plateau fractures are categorized as medial, lateral or bicondylar; non-displaced or displaced; and depressed or non-depressed.

Non-operative treatment

If a tibial plateau fracture is treated non-operatively, there is no attempt to restore the anatomical position of the joint surface through surgical reduction. The knee is commonly placed in a cast-brace, with or without traction. Many researchers believe that traction will allow spontaneous reduction via 'ligamentotaxis'; early motion will further contribute to reduction by 'molding' displaced bone fragments (Apley 1979). Allowing at least 2 weeks of immobilization before beginning motion exercises has resulted in greater gains in knee flexion range of motion (Gausewitz & Hohl 1986). Weightbearing can be initiated within the first 7–14 days for all types of tibial plateau fractures, except fractures that are both displaced and depressed, and has positive effects on knee range of motion and avoidance of valgus deformity (Segal et al 1993).

Rehabilitation is dictated first and foremost by the need for physiological healing of the fracture. Weightbearing exercises like squatting are avoided for the first 4–6 weeks in order to allow the fracture sufficient time to heal. Quadriceps strength and knee extension should be a focus of treatment in the acute phase; however, given the fact that tibial plateau fractures are placed in a cast-brace, regaining knee flexion will also become a priority once the cast-brace is removed. Patients are allowed to progress to strenuous weightbearing exercise, such as deep squatting, in the advanced phase, once callus formation is seen on X-ray. Progression in the return-to-play phase is dictated by patient symptoms.

Operative treatment

Operative management of tibial plateau fractures begins with the decision of whether or not the patient needs internal fixation of the fracture. Open reduction with internal fixation (ORIF) is currently the surgical choice, where most tibial plateau fractures are displaced or display more than 4 mm of tibial plateau depression (Lachiewicz & Funcik 1990, Segal et al 1993). Bone grafting into the fracture site or into the depressed tibial plateau is a common adjunct to surgery. Lachiewicz & Funcik (1990) found that the absence of a bone graft with ORIF was associated with less than excellent results postoperatively. Surgical reduction can also help to prevent arthritic changes to the tibiofemoral joint surfaces by restoring joint congruency and correcting for damaging varus/valgus joint instability.

Postoperative treatment

Postoperatively, tibial plateau fractures are treated similarly to non-displaced, non-surgical fractures. Weightbearing, in a cast-brace, is best initiated within 7–14 days for the best range of motion and valgus deformity results (Segal et al 1993). In surgically treated displaced fractures, early motion before 2 weeks postinjury has allowed for the most knee flexion range of motion at 6 month follow-ups (Gausewitz 1986). Like non-operative treatment of tibial plateau fractures, rehabilitation must allow for physiological healing of the reduced joint surface. Weightbearing exercises should be avoided for the first 4–6 weeks. Progression in the advanced and return-to-play phases of rehabilitation is similar to the non-operative treatment protocol.

ARTHRITIS AND THE ATHLETE

More people are remaining active for longer periods of their life. Decisions regarding treatment of an athlete should be based on their desired activity level and not their biological age. The eventual consequence of sports injuries such as meniscal tears, maintaining high body mass index, ligamentous sprains, and articular surface damage, play a substantial role in developing secondary joint disease (Felson et al 2000, Gelber et al 1999, 2000, Kujala et al 1994, Lundberg & Messner 1997, Messner et al 2001). An important factor to remember in treating

athletes with these injuries is that there is no cure for osteoarthritis. Once cartilage damage has occurred, it cannot be perfectly repaired with more hyaline cartilage (Buckwalter 1998). Thus, to slow continued deterioration is a goal of rehabilitative interventions.

Non-operative treatment for osteoarthritis

Counseling is one of the most important aspects in the course of treatment for osteoarthritis. Efforts to reduce weight should be strongly encouraged as obesity is a recognized risk factor in the development of osteoarthritis (Felson et al 1997, Stürmer et al 2000). Loss of body weight can have a pronounced affect on stresses at the knee as the loss of a 1 lb of body weight can correlate to a loss of 3 lb of force at the knee (Schipplein & Andriacchi 1991).

Joint-sparing activities should be used as a mainstay to provide minimal risk to the knee joint while still providing adequate stimulus to maintain strength and conditioning. Non-impact aerobic exercises take the place of running type activities. Examples include, but are not limited to, cross-country skiing, swimming, bicycling, roller-blading, elliptical running simulators, walking, and water aerobics. Avoidance of aerobic exercise should not be counseled, as increased weight associated with inactivity would be likely to have a detrimental affect on the knee. If the athlete insists on the need to continue impact activities, instruction on improved footwear choices, and encouraging exercise on a more forgiving surface, will help to attenuate stresses on the arthritic knee.

Quadriceps strength can play an important role in preserving activity level and potentially decreasing the risk for progressive osteoarthritis (O'Reilly et al 1998, Slemenda et al 1998). Several studies that have investigated strengthening protocols for knee osteoarthritis have reported modest strength gains, but significant reduction in pain and increased function (Fisher et al 1991, Fisher et al 1997, Hurley & Newham 1993, Hurley & Scott 1998). In general, strengthening programs should include an emphasis on open chain exercise to avoid the additional compressive force present during weighted, closed chain strengthening exercise. Efforts should be taken to prescribe exercises that do not cause pain during their execution and do not stimulate an inflammatory response. A process of trial and error is used to prescribe the best exercises for each patient.

In patients that have unicompartmental arthritis, additional mechanical interventions can be attempted to reduce load to the affected compartment. Medial involvement is the most common site of unicompartment joint degeneration. An unloading brace or a lateral heel wedge can potentially decrease the external valgus moment at the knee and decrease pain in patients with this form of the disease (Hewett et al 1998, Keating et al 1993, Pollo 1998, Tohyama et al 1991).

Typically, pain management for osteoarthritis can be achieved through the simple use of analgesics such as acetiminophen (Bradley et al 2001, Brandt 2000). Non-steroidal anti-iflammatory drugs (NSAIDs) can be used as well, but have higher risk for gastrointestinal, renal, or hepatic side-effects from long-term use. For arthritic knees that present with continual effusion, NSAIDs may be more effective in controlling symptoms than analgesics. Joint aspiration and intra-articular corticosteroid injections may also provide pain relief for patients who have effused joints (Creamer 1997, Fadale & Wiggins 1994, Livesley et al 1991). In the knee that is painful without the presence of an effusion, injections of hyaluronic acid have been shown to have pain-reducing properties that are similar to NSAIDs. This relief can last for months after treatment (Altman & Moskowitz 1998, Brandt et al 2001). This treatment usually consists of 3–5 injections given over 15 days and presents a relatively high financial risk for the patient due to the high cost of this form of management.

Recent studies have also supported the use of some 'neutracuticals' in managing symptoms and potentially protecting remaining articular cartilage in knee osteoarthritis. In particular, the oral supplements, chondroitin sulphate and glucosamine, have some efficacy in decreasing symptoms of pain in patients with mild osteoarthritis, with few to no known side-effects (Bourgeois et al 1998, Lippiello et al 2000, Mazieres et al 2001, Muller-Fassbender et al 1994, Reginster et al 2001). These supplements have been hypothesized to provide some chondroprotective effects and can have an impact on pain with osteoarthritis of the knee.

Operative treatment

Several operative treatments are available to reduce the signs and symptoms of an arthritic knee. Procedures as simple as arthroscopic lavage have been proven to provide relief, albeit temporary, from the pain associated with osteoarthritis (Kalunian et al 2000, Livesley et al 1991). Little soft tissue injury is involved in these procedures and the majority of rehabilitation is centered around resolving impairments of pain, loss of range of motion, and weakness.

Chondral lesions, either chronic degenerative injuries or traumatic blows such as involved in an ACL tear, have limited potential for repair or reconstruction. Operative procedures involve evoking a vascular response from the underlying subchondral bone and bone marrow to 'scar' the lesion with fibrocartilage (Buckwalter 1998, Buckwalter & Lohmander 1994). The repaired cartilage has inferior

mechanical properties when compared to hyaline cartilage for joint preservation (Walker 1998). This is achieved through the use of surgical burr (i.e. abrasion chondroplasty, or some form of microfracture where holes are poked through the cartilage defect) (Friedman et al 1984). If a full thickness lesion is present, an OATS (Osteochondral Autograft Transfer System) procedure is performed using a chondral graft to transplant into an area of chondral defect (Bobic 1996, Matsusue et al 1993). Severe chondral lesions can also be addressed with autologous chondrocyte transplantation. Autologous chondrocyte transplantation is where donor chondrocytes are cultured in a laboratory and then reintroduced into the chondral defect under a protective, autologous periosteal flap. This procedure may allow the defect to fill with hyaline-like cartilage (Brittberg et al 1994, Gillogly et al 1998).

Postoperative treatment

Rehabilitation following chondroplasty procedures is focused on limiting early weightbearing to allow for fibrocartilage to mature at the site of microfracture or abrasion. Patients are typically restricted to no greater than touch down weightbearing for 4–6 weeks following these procedures (Irrgang & Pezzullo 1998, Suh et al 1997). Isometric exercises and NMES at joint angles that do not engage the repaired tissue are used to improve muscle function during this period of limited weightbearing (Irrgang & Pezzullo 1998). Stretching efforts are encouraged as immobilization has a detrimental effect on chondrocytes, cartilage thickness, and proteoglycan concentration (Behrens et al 1989, Palmoski & Brandt 1982).

Weightbearing is slowly progressed from this point. Closed chain exercise is used sparingly with a slow progression. Use of an unloading brace and/or heel wedge(s) for 3 months after surgery, with assistive devices during activity, assists in potential unweighting of the repaired chondral defect. Chances for joint effusion are high following these procedures and if patients demonstrate increased effusion, then they step back in activity level. This may mean they go back to the use of crutches to assist in efforts to control inflammation.

Slowly advancing impact to return to play can easily be achieved through the use of aerobics in the pool. Walking in progressively shallow water and instituting aqua-jogging can assist in facilitating conditioning while providing progressive stress to assist in remodeling the healing cartilage surface. Returning to impact activities such as jogging will be instituted as late as 8 months after the repair (Gillogly et al 1998). Most patients who undergo chondroplasty procedures should be counseled in joint-sparing lifestyle changes.

SUMMARY

A thorough knowledge of knee anatomy and biomechanics is needed for proper diagnosis and rehabilitation of the injured athlete. Without this knowledge, healing tissue may be overly stressed, impeding an expedient return to activity. It is also important for clinicians working with athletes to know the demands of the athlete's sport, so that they can properly prepare the athlete for the stresses that will be encountered.

Non-operative rehabilitation and rehabilitation following surgery both follow criterion-based protocols, which outline clinical milestones that must be met in order to progress to the next phase of rehabilitation. Pain and effusion dictate progression within a rehabilitative phase. Athletes must progress through all phases of rehabilitation in order to ensure that they are adequately prepared to return to sport; however, exercises within each phase should be tailored to the athlete's needs and certain exercises may be excluded, based on surgical considerations.

REFERENCES

Altman R D, Moskowitz R 1998 Intraarticular sodium hyaluronate (Hyalgan) in the treatment of patients with osteoarthritis of the knee: a randomized clinical trial. Hyalgan Study Group 25(11):2203–2212

Anderson A F, Lipscomb A B 1986 Clinical diagnosis of meniscal tears. Description of a new manipulative test. American Journal of Sports Medicine 14(4):291–293

Anderson A F, Snyder R B, Federspiel C F et al 1992 Instrumented evaluation of knee laxity: a comparison of five athrometers. American Journal of Sports Medicine 20(2):135–140

Apley A G 1979 Fractures of the tibial plateau. Orthopaedic Clinics of North America 10:61–74

Arnoczky S P, Warren R F 1982 Microvasculature of the human meniscus. American Journal of Sports Medicine 10(2):90–95

Axe M J, Swigart K H, Snyder-Mackler L 2001 Surgical options and procedure-modified rehabilitation for PCL injury. Athletic Therapy Today 6:16–22

Baker C L Jr, Norwood L A, Hughston J C 1985 Acute combined posterior cruciate and posterolateral instability of the knee. American Journal of Sports Medicine 12:204–208

Barber S D, Noyes F R, Mangine R E et al 1990 Quantitative assessment of functional limitations in normal and anterior cruciate ligament-deficient knees. Clinical Orthopaedics and Related Research Jun(255):204–214

Behrens F, Kraft E L, Oegema T R Jr 1989 Biochemical changes in articular cartilage after joint immobilization by casting or external fixation. Journal of Orthopaedic Research 7(3):335–343

Beynnon B D, Johnson R J, Fleming B C et al 1997 The strain behavior of the anterior cruciate ligament during squatting and active flexion-extension. A comparison of an open and a closed kinetic chain exercise. American Journal of Sports Medicine 25(6):823–829

Bobic V 1996 Arthroscopic osteochondral autograft transplantation in anterior cruciate ligament reconstruction: a preliminary clinical study. Knee Surgery, Sports Traumatology, Arthroscopy 3(4):262–264

Boden B P, Dean G S, Feagin J A Jr et al 2000 Mechanisms of anterior cruciate ligament injury. Orthopedics 23(6):573–578

Bolgla L A, Keskula D R 1997 Reliability of lower extremity functional performance tests. Journal of Orthopaedic and Sports Physical Therapy 26(3):138–142

Bourgeois P, Chales G, Dehais J et al 1998 Efficacy and tolerability of chondroitin sulfate 1200 mg/day vs chondroitin sulfate 3 × 400 mg/day vs placebo. Osteoarthritis and Cartilage 6(suppl A):25–30

Bradley J D, Katz B P, Brandt K D 2001 Severity of knee pain does not predict a better response to an anti-inflammatory dose of ibuprofen than to analgesic in patients with osteoarthritis. Journal of Rheumatology 28:1073–1076

Brandt K D 2000 The role of analgesics in the management of osteoarthritis pain. American Journal of Therapeutics 7:75–90

Brandt K D, Block J A, Michalski J P et al 2001 Efficacy and safety of intraarticular sodium hyaluronate in knee osteoarthritis. Clinical Orthopaedics and Related Research 385:130–143

Brittberg M, Lindahl A, Nilsson A et al 1994 Treatment of deep cartilage defects in the knee with autologous chondrocyte transplantation. New England Journal of Medicine 331(14):889–895

Buckwalter J A 1998 Articular cartilage: injuries and potential for healing. Journal of Orthopaedic and Sports Physical Therapy 28(4):192–202

Buckwalter J, Lohmander S 1994 Current concepts review: operative treatment of osteoarthrosis. Journal of Bone and Joint Surgery (Am) 76-A(9):1405–1418

Bullis D W, Paulos L E 1994 Reconstruction of the posterior cruciate ligament with allograft. Clinics in Sports Medicine 13(3):581–597

Butler D L, Noyes F R, Grood E S 1980 Ligamentous restraints to anterior-posterior drawer in the human knee. A biomechanical study. Journal of Bone and Joint Surgery (Am) 62-A(2):259–270

Clark C R, Ogden J A 1983 Development of the menisci of the human knee joint. Morphological changes and their potential role in childhood meniscal injury. Journal of Bone and Joint Surgery (Am) 65-A(4):538–547

Cooper D E, Arnoczky S P, Warren R F 1991 Meniscal repair. Clinics in Sports Medicine 10(3):529–548

Corea J R, Moussa M, Al Othman A 1994 McMurray's test tested. Knee Surgery, Sports Traumatology, Arthroscopy 2:70–72

Covey D C 2001 Current concepts review injuries of the posterolateral corner of the knee. Journal of Bone and Joint Surgery (Am) 83-A(1):106–118

Creamer P 1997 Intra-articular corticosteroid injections in osteoarthritis: do they work and if so, how? Annals of Rheumatic Diseases 56(11):634–636

Cross M J, Powell J F 1984 Long-term followup of posterior cruciate ligament rupture: A study of 116 cases. American Journal of Sports Medicine 12(4):292–297

DeHaven K E, Arnoczky S P 1994 Meniscus repair: basic science, indications for repair and open repair. Instructional Course Lectures 43:65–76

Derscheid G L, Garrick J G 1981 Medial collateral ligament injuries in football: nonoperative management of grade I and grade II sprains. American Journal of Sports Medicine 9:365–368

Donaldson W F, Warren R F, Wickiewicz T 1985 A comparison of acute anterior cruciate ligament examinations. Initial versus examination under anesthesia. American Journal of Sports Medicine 13(1):5–9

Escamilla R F, Fleisig G S, Zheng N et al 1998 Biomechanics of the knee during closed kinetic chain and open kinetic chain exercise. Medicine and Science in Sports and Exercise 30(4):556–569

Fadale P D, Wiggins M E 1994 Corticosteroid Injections: their use and abuse. Journal of the American Academy of Orthopaedic Surgeons 2(3):133–140

Felson D T, Zhang Y, Hannan M T et al 1997 Risk factors for incident radiographic knee osteoarthritis in the elderly. Arthritis and Rheumatism 40(4):728–733

Felson D T, Lawrence R C, Dieppe P A et al 2000 Osteoarthritis: new insights. Part 1: the disease and its risk factors. Annals of Internal Medicine 133(8):635–646

Fisher N D, Pendergast D R, Gresham G E et al 1991 Muscle rehabilitation: its effect on muscular and functional performance of patients with knee osteoarthritis. Archives of Physical Medicine and Rehabilitation 72:367–374

Fisher N M, White S C, Yack H J et al 1997 Muscle function and gait in patients with knee osteoarthritis before and after muscle rehabilitation. Disability and Rehabilitation 19(2):47–55

Fitzgerald G K 1997 Open versus closed kinetic chain exercises: issues in rehabilitation after anterior cruciate ligament reconstructive surgery. Journal of Orthopaedic and Sports Physical Therapy 77(12):1747–1754

Fitzgerald G K, Axe M J, Snyder-Mackler L 2000a A decision-making scheme for returning patients to high-level activity with nonoperative treatment after anterior cruciate ligament rupture. Knee Surgery, Sports Traumatology, Arthroscopy 8(2):76–82

Fitzgerald G K, Axe M J, Snyder-Mackler 2000b The efficacy of perturbation training in nonoperative anterior cruciate ligament rehabilitation programs for physically active individuals. Physical Therapy 80(2):128–140

Friedman M, Berasi C, Fox J et al 1984 Preliminary results with abrasion arthroplasty in the osteoarthritic knee. Clinical Orthopaedics and Related Research 82:200–205

Fu F H, Baratz M 1994 Meniscal injuries. In: DeLee J C, Drez D Orthopaedic sports injuries. WB Saunders, Philadelphia

Fukubayashi T, Torzilli P A, Sherman M F et al 1982 An in vitro biomechanical evaluation of anterior-posterior motion of the knee. Tibial displacement, rotation, and torque. Journal of Bone and Joint Surgery (Am) 64A(2):258–264

Galway H R, Beaupre A, MacIntosh D L 1972 Pivot shift: a clinical sign of symptomatic anterior cruciate deficiency. Journal of Bone and Joint Surgery (Br) 54-B:763–764

Gapeyeva H, Paasuke M, Ereline J et al 2000 Isokinetic torque deficit of the knee extensor muscles after arthroscopic partial meniscectomy. Knee Surgery, Sports Traumatology, Arthroscopy 8(5):301–304

Gausewitz S, Hohl M 1986 The significance of early motion in the treatment of tibial plateau fractures. Clinical Orthopaedics 202:135–138

Gelber A C, Hochberg M C, Mead L A et al 1999 Body mass index in young men and the risk of subsequent knee and hip osteoarthritis. American Journal of Medicine 107:542–548

Gelber A C, Hochberg M C, Mead L A et al 2000 Joint injury in young adults and risk for subsequent knee and hip osteoarthritis. Annals of Internal Medicine 133:321–328

Gillogly S D, Voight M, Blackburn T 1998 Treatment of articular cartilage defects of the knee with autologous chondrocyte implantation. Journal of Orthopaedic and Sports Physical Therapy 28(4):241–251

Girgis F G, Marshall J L, Monajem A R S 1975 The cruciate ligaments of the knee: anatomical, functional and experimental analysis. Clinical Orthopedics 106:216–231

Gollehon D L, Torzilli P A, Warren R F 1987 The role of the posterolateral and cruciate ligaments in the stability of the human knee. A biomechanical study. Journal of Bone and Joint Surgery (Am) 69A(2):233–242

Grood E S, Noyes F R, Butler D L et al 1981 Ligamentous and capsular restraints preventing straight medial and lateral laxity in intact human cadaver knees. Journal of Bone and Joint Surgery (Am) 63A(8):1257–1269

Harner C D, Höher J 1998 Evaluation and treatment of posterior cruciate ligament injuries. American Journal of Sports Medicine 26(3):471–82

Harner C D, Irrgang J J, Paul J et al 1992 Loss of motion after anterior cruciate ligament reconstruction. American Journal of Sports Medicine 20(5):499–506

Harner C D, Vogrin T M, Höher J et al 2000 Biomechanical analysis of a posterior cruciate ligament reconstruction. Deficiency of the posterolateral structures as a cause of graft failure. American Journal of Sports Medicine 28(1):32–39

Heller L, Langman J 1964 The menisco-femoral ligaments of the human knee. Journal of Bone and Joint Surgery (Br) 46-B:307–313

Hewett T E, Noyes F R, Barber-Westin S D et al 1998 Decrease in knee joint pain and increase in function in patients with medial compartment arthrosis: a prospective analysis of valgus bracing. Orthopedics 21(2):131–138

Holden D L, Eggert A W, Butler J E 1983 The nonoperative treatment of Grade I and II medial collateral ligament injuries to the knee. American Journal of Sports Medicine 11(5):340–343

Hughston J C, Andrews J R 1976 Classification of knee ligament instabilities. Part I. The medial compartment and cruciate ligaments. Journal of Bone and Joint Surgery (Am) 58A:159–172

Hurley M V, Newham D J 1993 The influence of arthrogenous muscle inhibition on quadriceps rehabilitation of patients with early, unilateral osteoarthritic knees. British Journal of Rheumatology 32:127–131

Hurley M V, Scott D L 1998 Improvements in quadriceps sensorimotor function and disability of patients with knee osteoarthritis following a clinically practicable exercise regime. British Journal of Rheumatology 37:1181–1187

Indelicato P A 1983 Nonoperative treatment of complete tears of the medial collateral ligament of the knee. Journal of Bone and Joint Surgery (Am) 65A:323–329

Indelicato P A 1995 Isolated medial collateral ligament injuries in the knee. Journal of the American Academy of Orthopaedic Surgeons 3(1):9–14

Indelicato P A, Hermansdorfer J, Huegel M 1990 Nonoperative management of complete tears of the medial collateral ligament of the knee in intercollegiate football players. Clinical Orthopaedics and Related Research Jul (256):174–177

Inoue M, McGurk-Burleson E, Hollis J M et al 1987 Treatment of the medial collateral ligament injury: the importance of anterior cruciate ligament on the valgus-varus knee laxity. American Journal of Sports Medicine 15(1):15–21

Irrgang J J, Pezzullo D P 1998 Rehabilitation following surgical procedures to address articular cartilage lesions in the knee. Journal of Orthopaedic and Sports Physical Therapy 28(4):232–240

Irrgang J J, Snyder-Mackler L, Wainner R S et al 1998 Development of a patient-reported measure of function of the knee. Journal of Bone and Joint Surgery (Am) 80A(8):1132–1145

Jones R E, Henley M B, Francis P 1986 Nonoperative management of isolated Grade III collateral ligament injury tears in high school football players. Clinical Orthopaedics 213:137–140

Jurist K A, Otis J C 1985 Anteroposterior tibiofemoral displacements during isometric extension efforts. The roles of external load and knee flexion angle. American Journal of Sports Medicine. 13(4):254–258

Kalunian K C, Moreland L W, Klashman D J et al 2000 Visually-guided irrigation in patients with early knee osteoarthritis: a multicenter randomized, controlled trial. Osteoarthritis and Cartilage 8:412–418

Kaufman K R, An K N, Litchy W J et al 1991 Dynamic joint forces during knee isokinetic exercise. American Journal of Sports Medicine 19(3):305–316

Keating E M, Faris P M, Ritter M A et al 1993 Use of lateral heel and sole wedges in the treatment of medial osteoarthritis of the knee. Orthopaedic Review 22(8):921–924

Keays S L, Bullock-Saxton J, Keays A C 2000 Strength and function before and after anterior cruciate ligament reconstruction. Clinical Orthopaedics and Related Research Apr (373):174–183

Keller P M, Shelbourne K D, McCarroll J R et al 1993 Nonoperatively treated isolated posterior cruciate ligament injuries. American Journal of Sports Medicine 21(1):132–136

Kennedy J C, Bailey W H 1968 Experimental tibial plateau fractures: studies of mechanism and a classification. Journal of Bone and Joint Surgery (Am) 50A:1522

Kujala U M, Kaprio J, Sarno S 1994 Osteoarthritis of weight bearing joints of lower limbs in former elite male athletes. British Medical Journal 308:231–234

Lachiewicz P F, Funcik T 1990 Factors influencing the results of open reduction and internal fixation of tibial plateau fractures. Clinical Orthopaedics 259:210–215

Lippiello L, Woodward J, Karpman R et al 2000 In vivo chondroprotection and metabolic synergy of glucosamine and chondroitin sulfate. Clinical Orthopaedics and Related Research 381:229–240

Liu S H, Osti L, Henry M et al 1995 The diagnosis of acute complete tears of the anterior cruciate ligament. Comparison of MRI, arthrometry and clinical examination. Journal of Bone and Joint Surgery (Br) 77-B(4):586–588

Livesley P J, Doherty M, Needoff M et al 1991 Arthroscopic lavage of osteoarthritic knees. Journal of Bone Joint Surgery (Br) 73-B(6):922–926

Lundberg M, Messner K 1997 Ten-year prognosis of isolated and combined medial collateral ligament ruptures: a matched comparison in 40 patients using clinical and radiographic evaluations. American Journal of Sports Medicine 25(1):2–6

Lutz G E, Palmitier R A, An K N et al 1993 Comparison of tibiofemoral joint forces during open-kinetic-chain and closed-kinetic-chain exercises. Journal of Bone and Joint Surgery (Am) 75-A(5):732–739

Lysholm J, Gillquist J 1982 Evaluation of knee ligament surgery results with special emphasis on use of a scoring scale. American Journal of Sports Medicine 10(3):150–154

McGee D J 1992 Orthopedic physical assessment, 2nd edn. WB Saunders, Philadelphia

Manal T J, Snyder-Mackler L 1996 Practice guidelines for anterior cruciate ligament rehabilitation: a criterion-based rehabilitation progression. Operative Techniques in Orthopaedics 6(3):190–196

Markolf K L, Gorek J F, Kabo J M et al 1990 Direct measurement of resultant forces in the anterior cruciate ligament. An in vitro study performed with a new experimental technique. Journal of Bone and Joint Surgery (Am) 72-A(4):557–567

Matsusue Y, Yamamuro T, Hama H 1993 Arthroscopic multiple osteochondral transplantation to the chondral defect in the knee associated with anterior cruciate ligament disruption. Arthroscopy 9(3):318–321

Mazieres B, Combe B, Van A P et al 2001 Chondroitin sulphate in osteoarthritis of the knee: a prospective, double blind, placebo controlled multicenter clinical study. Journal of Rheumatology 28:173–181

Messner K, Fahlgren A, Persliden J et al 2001 Radiographic joint space narrowing and histologic changes in a rabbit meniscectomy model of early knee osteoarthrosis. American Journal of Sports Medicine 29(2):151–160

Mikkelsen C, Werner S, Eriksson E 2000 Closed kinetic chain alone compared to combined open and closed kinetic chain exercises for quadriceps strengthening after anterior cruciate ligament reconstruction with respect to return to sports: a prospective matched follow-up study. Knee Surgery, Sports Traumatology, Arthroscopy 8(6):337–342

Morrissey M C 1989 Reflex inhibition of thigh muscles in knee injury. Causes and treatment. Sports Medicine 7(4):263–276

Morrissey M C, Hudson Z L, Drechsler W I et al 2000 Effects of open versus closed kinetic chain training on knee laxity in the early period after anterior cruciate ligament reconstruction. Knee Surgery, Sports Traumatology, Arthroscopy 8(6):343–348

Muller-Fassbender H, Bach G L, Haase W et al 1994 Glucosamine sulfate compared to ibuprofen in osteoarthritis of the knee. Osteoarthritis and Cartilage 2(1):61–69

Noyes F R, Barber S D, Mooar L A 1989 A rationale for assessing sports activity levels and limitations in knee disorders. Clinical Orthopaedics and Related Research Sep(246):238–249

Noyes F R, Barber S D, Mangine R E 1991 Abnormal lower limb symmetry determined by function hop tests after anterior cruciate ligament rupture. American Journal of Sports Medicine 19(5):513–518

Noyes F R, Barber-Westin S D 1996 Surgical restoration to treat chronic deficiency of the posterolateral complex and cruciate ligaments of the knee joint. American Journal of Sports Medicine 24(4):415–426

Nyland J 1999 Rehabilitation complications following knee surgery. Clinics in Sports Medicine 18(4):905–925

O'Reilly S C, Jones A, Muir K R et al 1998 Quadriceps weakness in knee osteoarthritis: the effect on pain and disability. Annals of Rheumatic Diseases 57(10):588–594

Palmoski M, Brandt K 1982 Immobilisation of the knee prevents osteoarthritis after anterior cruciate ligament resection. Arthritis and Rheumatism 25:1201–1208

Pollo F E 1998 Bracing and heel wedging for unicompartmental osteoarthritis of the knee. American Journal of Knee Surgery 11(1):47–50

Rangger C, Daniel D M, Stone M L et al 1993 Diagnosis of an ACL disruption with KT-1000 arthrometer measurements. Knee Surgery, Sports Traumatology, Arthroscopy 1(1):60–66

Reginster J Y, Deroisy R, Rovati L C et al 2001 Long-term effects of glucosamine sulphate on osteoarthritis progression: a randomised, placebo-controlled clinical trial. Lancet 357(9252):247–248

Schipplein O D, Andriacchi T P 1991 Interaction between active and passive knee stabilizers during level walking. Journal of Orthopaedic Research 9(1):113–119

Segal D, Mallik A R, Wetzler M J et al 1993 Early weight bearing of lateral tibial plateau fractures. Clinical Orthopaedics 294:232–237

Shakespeare D T, Rigby H S 1983 The bucket-handle tear of the meniscus. A clinical and arthrographic study. Journal of Bone and Joint Surgery (Br) 65-B:383–387

Shelbourne K D, Patel D V, Adsit W S et al 1996 Rehabilitation after meniscal repair. Clinics in Sports Medicine 15(3):595–612

Shelton W R, Barrett G R, Dukes A 1997 Early season anterior cruciate ligament tears. A treatment dilemma. America Journal of Sports Medicine 25(5):656–658

Slemenda C, Heilman D K, Brandt K D et al 1998 Reduced quadriceps strength relative to body weight. A risk factor for knee osteoarthritis in women? Arthritis and Rheumatism 41(11):1951–1959

Snyder-Mackler L, Ladin Z, Schepsis A A et al 1991 Electrical stimulation of the thigh muscles after reconstruction of the anterior cruciate ligament. Effects of electrically elicited contractions of the quadriceps femoris and hamstring muscles on gait and on strength of the thigh muscles. Journal of Bone and Joint Surgery (Am) 73-A(7):1025–1036

Snyder-Mackler L, De Luca P F, Williams P R et al 1994 Reflex inhibition of the quadriceps femoris muscle after injury or reconstruction of the anterior cruciate ligament. Journal of Bone and Joint Surgery (Am) 76-A(4):555–560

Snyder-Mackler L, Delitto A, Bailey S L et al 1995 Strength of the quadriceps femoris muscle and functional recovery after reconstruction of the anterior cruciate ligament. A prospective, randomized clinical trial of electrical stimulation. Journal of Bone and Joint Surgery (Am) 77-A(8):1166–1173

Stuart M J, Meglan D A, Lutz G E et al 1996 Comparison of intersegmental tibiofemoral joint forces and muscle activity during various closed kinetic chain exercises. American Journal of Sports Medicine 24(6):792–799

Stürmer T, Klaus-Peter G, Brenner H 2000 Obesity, overweight and patterns of osteoarthritis: the Ulm Osteoarthritis Study. Journal of Clinical Epidemiology 53:307–313

Suh J, Åroen A, Muzzonigro T et al 1997 Injury and repair of articular cartilage: related scientific issues. Operative Techniques in Orthopaedics 7(4):270–278

Tohyama H, Yasuda K, Kaneda K 1991 Treatment of osteoarthritis of the knee with heel wedges. International Orthopaedics 15(1):31–33

Torg J S, Barton T M, Pavlov H et al 1989 Natural history of the posterior cruciate deficient knee. Clinical Orthopaedics and Related Research 246:208–216

Veltri D M, Warren R F 1993 Isolated and combined posterior cruciate ligament injuries. Journal of the American Academy of Orthopaedic Surgeons 1(2):67–75

Walker J M 1998 Pathomechanics and classification of cartilage lesions, facilitation of repair. Journal of Orthopaedics and Sports Physical Therapy 28(4):216–231

Ware J E Jr, Shelbourne C D 1992 The MOS 36-item short-form health survey (SF-36). I. Conceptual framework and item selection. Medical Care 30(6):473–483

Wilk K E 1994 Rehabilitation of isolated and combined posterior cruciate ligament injuries. Clinics in Sports Medicine 13(3):649–677

21

Patellofemoral joint

*Kay Crossley   Kim Bennell
Jenny McConnell*

INTRODUCTION

Patellofemoral pain syndrome (PFPS) describes anterior or retropatellar pain in the absence of other knee pathology. It occurs commonly, with prospective cohort studies reporting incidence rates of 7–15% in sporting and general populations (Almeida et al 1998, 1999, Heir & Glomsaker 1996, Jones et al 1993, Kowal 1980, Milgrom et al 1991, Schwellnus et al 1990, Shwayhat et al 1994, Witvrouw et al 2000a). In addition, PFPS is one of the most common conditions presenting to clinicians involved in the management of sports injuries, accounting for 2–30% of all presentations (Baquie & Brukner 1997, Clement et al 1981, DeHaven & Lintner 1986, Devereaux & Lachmann 1984, James et al 1978, Kannus et al 1987, Macintyre et al 1991, Matheson et al 1989, Pagliano & Jackson 1987).

This chapter will examine the relevant anatomy and biomechanics of the patellofemoral joint, outline the signs and symptoms of conditions of patellofemoral origin to assist in differential diagnosis, and provide assessment procedures and intervention strategies for the clinician.

APPLIED ANATOMY

PATELLOFEMORAL JOINT

The patella articulates with the femoral trochlea during knee flexion and extension. The patella is a sesamoid bone located within the patellar ligament. Its posterior surface has five facets, which articulate with the femur: superior, inferior, medial, lateral, and odd. The geometry of the articular facets of the patella varies between individuals and may affect patellar tracking (Ahmed et al 1987, Heegard et al 1994, van Kampen & Huiskes 1990). In normal subjects, a static restraint on the natural tendency of the patella to track laterally (Farahmand et al 1998) is provided by the lateral aspect of the femoral trochlea, which extends further anteriorly than the medial aspect (Grelsamer & Klein 1998). Thus, the bony components of the patellofemoral joint provide inherent stability once the patella is within the confines of the trochlea (from 20–30° knee flexion). Prior to this point, there is no bony support for the patella, and passive stability is provided by the medial and lateral retinaculum and the joint capsule.

SOFT TISSUE STRUCTURES

The lateral side of the knee is made up of various fibrous layers, forming the superficial and deep lateral retinaculum. The anterior portion of the superficial layer of the lateral retinaculum consists of the fibrous expansion of the vastus lateralis, running longitudinally along the lateral border and inserting into the patellar tendon (Reider et al 1981a). Fibers from the iliotibial band interdigitate with fibers from the vastus lateralis and the patellar tendon to form the superficial oblique retinaculum. In particular, lateral support is provided by the two distal components of the iliotibial band, the iliopatellar band and the iliotibial tract (Terry et al 1986, Williams & Warrick 1989). Most of the lateral retinaculum arises from the iliotibial band, thus excessive lateral tracking, lateral patellar tilt and compression may arise if the iliotibial band is tight.

The medial retinaculum is thinner than the lateral retinaculum, and is thought to play a lesser role in influencing patellar position or tracking. Three ligaments, the patellofemoral, patellomeniscal and patellotibial, lie beneath the retinaculum and are described as palpable thickenings in the joint capsule (Fulkerson & Shea 1990, Reider et al 1981a). The medial patellofemoral ligament forms the primary restraint to lateral patellar translation, the medial patellomeniscal ligament is less important (Conlan et al 1993, Desio et al 1998, Hautamaa et al 1998), and the patellotibial ligament and superficial fibers of the medial retinaculum are not functionally useful (Desio et al 1998).

MUSCULAR STRUCTURE

Most of the active stabilization of the patella is provided by the quadriceps muscle, and in particular, the vastus medialis and vastus longus (VL) components. The vastus medialis is commonly divided into the oblique portion, the vastus medialis oblique (VMO), and the more vertical component, the vastus medialis longus (VML) (Bose et al 1980, Lieb & Perry 1968, Lieb & Perry 1971, Raimondo et al 1998, Scharf et al 1985, Thiranagama 1990). While there is often difficulty accurately distinguishing the VMO and

VML as separate entities, most authors agree that they act as two distinct functional units due to their fiber orientation and attachments, and thus angle of force on the patella.

The VMO is more obliquely aligned than the VML or VL, thus providing a mechanical advantage to promote a medial stabilizing force to the patella. This is supported by studies of muscle fiber type, which indicate that vastus medialis functions more as a stabilizer than the VL. The mechanical advantage gained by the fiber orientation is required to counter the relatively larger cross-sectional area and thus force producing capacity of the VL.

The VML acts with the rest of the quadriceps to extend the knee. Although the VMO does not extend the knee, it is active throughout knee extension to keep the patella centered in the trochlea of the femur, thus enhancing VL efficiency during knee extension (Bull et al 1998, Goh et al 1995, Lieb & Perry 1968).

This synergistic relationship between the medial and lateral vastii, which appears to be important in maintaining the alignment of the patella within the femoral trochlea is supported by electromyographic (EMG) studies. Consistently, studies have demonstrated that the EMG activity of VMO and VL in the normal population is relatively balanced in terms of activation magnitude and timing in a wide variety of static, dynamic, weight-bearing and non weightbearing activities (Baecke et al 1982, Brownstein et al 1985, Gryzlo et al 1994, Isear et al 1997, Karst & Willett 1997, Lange et al 1996, Mariani & Caruso 1979, Morrish & Woledge 1997, Powers et al 1996, Reynolds et al 1983, Signorile et al 1995, Smith et al 1995, Wild et al 1982). These results conflict with a common belief that the VMO needs to activate prior to the VL to counter the larger force producing capacity of the VL and maintain patellar alignment (Grabiner et al 1994). It is possible that the mechanical advantage gained by superior fiber alignment of the VMO may be sufficient to balance the greater force and velocity generating capacities of the VL.

PATELLOFEMORAL BIOMECHANICS

Kinematics

A number of studies have used cadaveric models to investigate the three-dimensional motion of the patella relative to the femur (Ahmed et al 1983, Chew et al 1997, Heegard et al 1994, Nagamine et al 1995, Reider et al 1981b, van Kampen & Huiskes 1990). Differences in results may be attributed to the different methodologies, and in particular, the relative fixing of the tibia or femur as a reference point. In general, the pattern of patellar motion during knee flexion is predominantly patellar flexion accompanied by a wavy (from medial to lateral) patellar tilt and a lateral displacement.

Kinetics

The magnitude of the patellofemoral joint (PFJ) reaction force is dependent on the angle of knee flexion, the quadriceps muscle tension and the patellar tendon tension. A greater quadriceps muscle tension is required to resist the flexion moment of body weight as knee flexion increases and the resultant PFJ reaction force increases. Thus, during daily activities, such as stair ascent and descent, the PFJ reaction force can reach 3.3 times body weight (Hungerford & Barry 1979, Reilly & Martens 1972). The increase of PFJ reaction force with flexion offers an explanation for the aggravation of patellofemoral symptoms experienced by individuals during bent knee activities.

PATELLAR TRACKING

Patellar tracking describes the patella articulation with the femur and its motion during knee flexion. The normal function of the patellar tracking system is to enhance quadriceps function in various static and dynamic activities. Patellar motion may be described as the interaction between osseoligamentous structures, muscles and neuromotor control systems (Cowan 2002). These are interdependent components of the patellar tracking system, with one system capable of compensating for deficits in another. Therefore, patellar tracking affects the magnitude and distribution of the forces acting at the PFJ and thus PFJ contact pressures (Grabiner et al 1994).

It is commonly believed that abnormal patellar tracking contributes to the development of patellofemoral pain (Fulkerson & Shea 1990). Altered patellar tracking may lead to an uneven distribution of normal patellofemoral loads, and thus increase the stress or strain on one or more structures around the PFJ.

Sources of pain

There are a number of structures in the PFJ that are susceptible to damage when subjected to loads greater than the load that the structure is able to withstand. There are two important components of patellofemoral load: (1) magnitude of load, which is influenced by the degree of knee flexion during weightbearing and by the quadriceps muscle force and (2) distribution of load, which is related to patellar tracking (structural alignment and muscle balance).

The pathology of PFPS is not clearly understood. Since a variety of pathologies may present with similar signs and symptoms, PFPS is an 'umbrella' term used to encompass all anterior or retropatellar pain in the absence of other pathology. It is likely that the cause of the pain is not the same for all patients. The subjective nature of this condition is a major limitation to determining the exact pathology and hence it may be more appropriate to discuss the potential sources of patellofemoral pain (Dye & Vaupel 1994).

Current evidence indirectly indicates that various intra-articular components of the knee generate neurosensory signals that ultimately result in conscious perception. Dye and coworkers (1998) found that palpation of the anterior synovium and fat pad elicited the strongest sensation of pain, followed by the medial and lateral retinacula, tibial and femoral insertions of the anterior cruciate ligament (ACL) and posterior cruciate ligament (PCL), then the mid regions of the ACL and PCL, the capsular margins of the menisci and the articular cartilage surfaces. This study confirms the findings of Bierdert et al (2000) who described the highest number of afferent nerve fibers in the retinacula and medial/posteromedial capsuloligamentous structures; and of Witonski & Wagrowska-Danielewicz (1999) who found nerve fibers that were immunoreactive for substance-P in the fat pad retinacula and synovium, but not the articular cartilage, in subjects with anterior knee pain. There were more substance-P positive nerve fibers in the medial and lateral retinacula and in the fat pad of patients with PFPS, compared with patients undergoing surgery for ACL reconstruction or with knee joint osteoarthritis (OA).

PATELLOFEMORAL JOINT CARTILAGE

While it is accepted that patellofemoral articular cartilage cannot directly be a source of pain, there are a number of mechanisms for patellofemoral chondropathy to evoke patellofemoral pain. Damage to the articular cartilage may originate in the superficial layer, or deeper within the intermediate or deep layers of the cartilage. Superficial cartilage lesion may lead to chemical or mechanical synovial irritation (see later section) or may progress to subchondral bone erosion (Fulkerson & Hungerford 1997, Insall et al 1976, Moller et al 1989, Ohno et al 1988, Outerbridge 1961). Alternatively, matrix degeneration in the intermediate of deep layers of the cartilage may lead to synovial irritation, altered pressure and thus pain perception in subchondral bone (Goodfellow et al 1976, Ohno et al 1988).

SUBCHONDRAL BONE

A number of studies have revealed that increased intraosseous pressure of the patella can result in pain (Arnoldi 1991, Dye & Vaupel 1994, Schneider et al 2000), possibly secondary to transient venous outflow obstruction (Arnoldi 1991). Osteotomies of the patella provided short-term relief in a number of patients (Arnoldi 1991, Schneider et al 2000). Studies that have investigated the damage to subchondral bone as a source of patello-femoral pain include descriptive human cadaveric studies (Abernathy et al 1978), animal studies that induce mechanical loads (Newberry et al 1997, Radin et al 1973) and in vivo studies using imaging (Dye & Chew 1993, Leppala et al 1998, Lindberg et al 1986, Outerbridge & Dunlop 1975).

LATERAL RETINACULUM

The lateral retinaculum has been implicated as a potent source of patellofemoral pain. A number of quantitative and qualitative histological studies have found evidence of nerve damage in the lateral retinaculum of patients with patellofemoral pain, including nerve fibrosis (Fulkerson & Gosling 1980), neuroma formation (Fulkerson et al 1985, Sanchis-Alfonso et al 1998), increased number of myelinated and unmyelinated nerve fibers with a predominant nociceptive component (Sanchis-Alfonso & Rosello-Sastre 2000, Witonski & Wagrowska-Danielewicz 1999), and increased vascularity (Sanchis-Alfonso & Rosello-Sastre 2000, Sanchis-Alfonso et al 1998, Witonski & Wagrowska-Danielewicz 1999). Based on this information, it was hypothesized that division of the lateral retinaculum could improve pain, independent of its effect on patellar tilt, by effectively denervating an area of chronic nerve injury (Fulkerson et al 1985).

SYNOVIUM

Since large amounts of free nerve endings (IVa) were found in the synovia of fresh cadaver knees (Bierdert et al 1992) peripatellar synovitis must be considered as one of the main causes for patellofemoral pain. This was confirmed by Dye et al (1998) who observed that both knees exhibited severe pain in the anterior synovium during arthroscopic palpation. Therefore it is likely that the synovium is a potential cause of patellofemoral pain. Despite the evidence supporting the synovium as a potential pain source, it appears that the histological changes in the synovium of patients with patellofemoral pain are moderate (Arnoldi 1991, Insall et al 1976, Vaatainen et al 1998). The potential for the synovium to be a source of pain appears to increase with progressive joint disease.

INFRAPATELLAR FAT PAD

The infrapatellar fat pad is a highly potent source of pain, due to its rich innervation, and relationship with the highly innervated synovium. This was confirmed recently by Dye et al (1998) who observed severe pain during arthroscopic palpation of the fat pad. Since the fat pad innervation is linked to that of the entire knee joint structure, it is possible that this structure may be affected by pathology in various knee joint components (Duri et al 1996). Studies have confirmed the infrapatellar fat pad as a source of pain through the positive results of surgical resection (Tsirbas et al 1991). Furthermore, Witonski & Wagrowska-Danielewicz (1999) found nerve fibers that were immunoreactive for substance-P in the fat pad. Therefore the infrapatellar fat pad must be considered as a potent source of patellofemoral pain.

EXAMINATION

CLINICAL EXAMINATION

Subjective examination (history)

In the history, the clinician needs to elicit the area of pain, the type of activity precipitating the pain, the history of pain onset, the behavior of the pain and any associated clicking, giving way or swelling. This gives an indication of the structure involved and the likely diagnosis.

The patient usually complains of a diffuse ache in the anterior knee, which is exacerbated by activities that load the knee (e.g. stair climbing, squats) (Brukner & Khan 2001, Fulkerson & Hungerford 1997, Jacobson & Flandry 1989). The knee may ache during prolonged sitting with the knee flexed. Some may have crepitus, which may be present in 62% of the population (Abernathy et al 1978). Some patients experience 'giving way' or 'locking' of their knee, which must be differentiated from similar symptoms associated with an anterior cruciate deficient knee, loose body or meniscal locking (Brukner & Khan 2001). The reader is referred to Chapter 20 for further information on ACL and meniscal injuries.

Objective examination

Observation

Clinical examination establishes the diagnosis and determines the underlying contributing factors so that the appropriate treatment can be implemented. The patient is initially examined in the standing position for assessment of static lower extremity alignment. The patient can be viewed from the front, back and side (see Table 21.1). Thus, from the patient's static alignment, the clinician can anticipate how the patient will move. Any deviations from the anticipated movement provide information about the muscle control of the activity.

Table 21.1   Observation of static lower limb alignment

Observation	Implication
Front	
Internal femoral rotation	Femoral anteversion or soft tissue adaptation
– 'Squinting patella'	As above
– No 'squinting patellae'	As above with tight lateral patellar structures
VMO muscle bulk	Size, especially asymmetry may indicate weakness
Q angle	
Enlarged or 'puffy' fat pad	Possible fat pad impingement
Tibia varus/valgus/torsion	Knee alignment
Subtalar joint	Excessive or inadequate foot pronation
Arch height	Excessive or inadequate foot pronation
Side	
Anterior/posterior pelvic tilt/sway back	Lumbopelvic mechanics
Knee hyperextension	Presence of enlarged fat pad, possible impingement
Back	
PSIS level	Leg length asymmetry
Gluteal bulk	Size, especially asymmetry may indicate weakness
Resting calcaneal posture	Excessive or inadequate foot pronation

Table 21.2   Assessment of the patellofemoral joint in the lying position

Tests	Purpose
Supine	
Differential diagnostic tests	To exclude other causes of knee pain
Joint line palpation	
Tibiofemoral tests	
Meniscal tests	
Ligament tests	
Hip joint tests	
Muscle length tests	To assess potential contributing factors
Thomas test: psoas, rectus femoris, TFL	
Hamstrings, gastrocnemius	
Neuromeningeal tests	To assess potential contributing factors
Slump	
Femoral nerve tension test (modified Thomas test)	
Patellar orientation tests	To assess position of the patella relative to the femur
Glide	
Mediolateral tilt	
Anteroposterior tilt	
Rotation	
Sidelying	
Tests for tightness of lateral structures	To assess the contribution of the lateral retinaculum
Medial glide	
Medial tilt	
Ober's test	ITB length
Prone	
Lumbar palpation	To confirm lumbar involvement
Foot posture assessment	To assess potential contributing factors
Femoral nerve mobility	To assess potential contributing factors

Dynamic examination

The aim of dynamic examination is to evaluate the effect of muscle action on the static mechanics and to reproduce the patient's symptoms, thus establishing an objective reassessment activity. The least stressful activity of walking is examined first. If the patient's symptoms are not provoked in walking, then evaluation of more stressful activities such as stair climbing, squats and single leg squat may be examined and used as a reassessment activity.

Examination in the lying position

With the patient in a lying position, the clinician begins to confirm the diagnosis. A checklist of the examination procedures is outlined in Table 21.2. Careful palpation will enable the clinician to ascertain areas of tenderness and thus structures under stress. In addition, the clinician can get an appreciation of restrictions to optimal movement of the PFJ and surrounding joints.

Pain in the infrapatellar region is difficult to distinguish between infrapatellar fat pad irritation and patellar tendonopathy. If pain is elicited in the infrapatellar region, the clinician should shorten the fat pad by lifting it towards the patella. If on further palpation, the pain is gone, then the clinician may suspect a fat pad irritation. If the pain remains, patellar tendonopathy is the most likely diagnosis. The symptoms of fat pad irritation can often be reproduced with knee extension overpressure.

The retinacular tissue can be specifically tested for elasticity with the patient in a side-lying position and the knee flexed to 20°. Superficial retinacular fiber tightness will prevent a medial patellar glide. An anteroposterior pressure on the medial border of the patella (medial tilt) assesses deep retinacular fiber tightness.

In the prone position, the flexibility of the anterior hip structures is examined using a figure-of-four position, with the underneath foot at the level of the tibial tubercle (Fig. 21.1). The distance of the anterior superior iliac spine from the plinth is measured. A modification of the test position can be used as a treatment technique.

Assessment of patellar position

An integral component of patellofemoral evaluation in the supine position is assessment of the patellar orientation relative to the femur. An optimal patellar position is one where the patella is parallel to the femur in the frontal and the sagittal planes; and the patella is midway between the two condyles when the knee is flexed to 20°

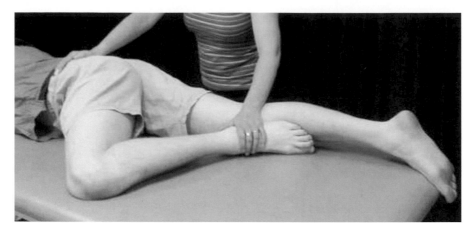

Figure 21.1 Figure-of-four position used to examine the flexibility of the anterior hip structures.

(McConnell 1986). The position of the patella is determined in a static and dynamic manner by examining four discrete components; glide, lateral tilt, antero-posterior tilt and rotation. Table 21.3 outlines the optimal alignment and most common abnormalities seen with static and dynamic assessment of patellar position. In addition, during quadriceps contraction, the VMO and the VL should be activated simultaneously, or even slightly earlier for the VMO (Voight & Weider 1991). In patients with patellofemoral pain, the VMO activity may be delayed (Voight & Weider 1991).

Once the PFJ has been thoroughly examined, and the primary problems have been identified the patient is ready for treatment.

INVESTIGATIONS

Different radiological procedures have been recommended to measure patellofemoral alignment. Wide variability in the radiographic findings of patients with patellofemoral dysfunction, and the difficulty demonstrating radiographic abnormalities consistent with clinical findings, have contributed to the confusion in the diagnosis and classification of patellofemoral pain disorders. Despite this, numerous authors report that in using certain techniques, the radiological evidence of malposition can be accurately and reliably evaluated.

The Merchant's X-ray view quantifies the position of the patella relative to the femoral trochlea in the frontal

Table 21.3 Assessment of patellar position

Optimal static alignment	Abnormal static alignment	Abnormal dynamic alignment	Implication
Glide Midpole of the patella is equidistant (+/− 5mm) to the medial and lateral femoral epicondyles	Midpole of patella sits closer to the lateral femoral epicondyle (lateral glide)	Patella moves lateral, when the quadriceps contracts	Lateral patellar displacement of the patella decreases VMO tension
Mediolateral tilt Medial and lateral patellar borders equal height and the posterior edge of both borders can be palpated	Medial borders higher than lateral (lateral tilt) Posterior edge of the lateral border will be difficult to palpate	Medial patella displacement results in increased lateral tilt	Tight lateral retinacular structures
Anteroposterior tilt Superior and inferior patellar borders are the same height	Inferior pole is displaced posteriorly Often embedded in the fat pad (posterior tilt)	Quadriceps contraction results in increased posterior tilt, particularly with knee hyperextension	Fat pad irritation, often manifests as inferior patella pain – exacerbated by knee extension
Rotation Long axis of the patella should be parallel to the long axis of the femur	Inferior pole sits lateral to the long axis of the femur (external rotation)		Tightness in retinacular structures

Table 21.4 Radiological examination of patellar position

Parameter	Definition	Abnormal values
Patellofemoral congruence angle (PFCA)	PFCA represents lateral patella glide where a positive angle indicates a laterally positioned patella and a negative angle indicates a medially positioned patella	> +5°
Lateral patellofemoral angle (LPFA)	LPFA quantifies the position of the patella in the transverse plane within the sulcus angle and represents lateral patellar tilt where a smaller LPFA angle indicates greater lateral patellar tilting. While some authors refer to the patellar rotation angle as the LPFA, the two angles are not synonymous.	LPFA ≥ 1°
Lateral patellar displacement (LPD)	The LPD quantifies the position of the patella in the frontal plane relative to the medial femoral condyle in mm. A positive LPD indicates a lateral position of the patella, while a negative LPD indicates a medial displacement of the patella	LPD ≥ 1 mm

plane. Using this technique, values for healthy controls and subjects with patellar subluxation or chondromalacia (Aglietti et al 1983, Laurin et al 1978, Merchant et al 1974) have been established (Table 21.4).

Studies using computed tomography (CT) or magnetic resonance imaging (MRI) (Powers 2000b, Powers et al 1998, Sheehan & Drace 1999, Witonski & Goraj 1999) noted that in asymptomatic individuals, the patella was laterally tilted at all angles of knee flexion, starting in approximately 5° of lateral tilt, and then gradually increasing the amount of lateral tilt during the first 50° of knee flexion, especially at 35° knee flexion. Also, the sulcus angle demonstrated increasing values as the knee extended from 45° to 0° (Powers 2000b, Powers et al 1998, Schutzer et al 1986, Witonski & Goraj 1999).

MANAGEMENT

OVERVIEW OF PHYSICAL THERAPY MANAGEMENT

Most patellofemoral conditions may be successfully managed with physical therapy (i.e. non-surgical management). Physical therapy interventions attempt to restore the biomechanics of the patellar tracking system through active (quadriceps or VMO retraining) and/or passive (realignment procedures such as tape, brace, stretching) interventions, thus decreasing the patient's symptoms. The following sections discuss the individual components of taping, VMO retraining, stretching, and orthoses and then discuss the evidence to support or refute the use of physical therapy interventions for PFPS.

PATELLAR TAPING

Theory

Patellar taping aims to create a mechanical realignment of the patella, thus centralizing it within the trochlea groove and improving patellar tracking (McConnell 1986). Theoretically, using tape to provide a sustained stretch of the tight lateral structures makes use of the creep phenomenon, which occurs in viscoelastic material when a constant low load is applied. It has been widely documented that the length of soft tissues can be increased with sustained stretching and the magnitude of increased displacement is dependent on the duration of the applied stretch (Mckay-Lyons 1989, Taylor et al 1990).

In addition, it has been proposed that tape may unload painful structures, provide a mechanical advantage to the quadriceps muscle, improve VMO activation and reduce pain (McConnell 1986, 1996). Consequently, taping facilitates recovery, by enabling the patient to participate without pain in activities, while specifically training the VMO. This pain relief is desirable since knee pain and effusion may inhibit the quadriceps (Spencer et al 1984, Stokes & Young 1984).

Patellar taping is designed to correct patellar malalignments noted on the assessment of patellar position and it has four basic components; medial glide, medial tilt, anterior tilt and rotation. Further taping may be required to unload painful structures (e.g. the infrapatellar fat pad) or inhibit the activation of VL. The choice of taping techniques is partly based on assessment of the patellar position (see the examination section) and partly on the attainment of pain reduction. Appropriate taping combinations should decrease the patients' pain by at least 50% during provocative activities and may require a number of taping components.

Evidence

The evidence to support or refute the effects of patellar taping has been recently reviewed (Crossley et al 2000). Short-term pain reduction is attained with patellar taping (Bockrath et al 1993, Cerny 1995, Conway et al 1992, Handfield & Kramer 2000, Herrington 2001, Herrington & Payton 1997, Kenna 1991, Powers et al 1995, Somes et al 1997, Worrell et al 1994) and research continues to focus on mechanisms to explain this pain relief. Two randomized clinical trials failed to find any benefits of using patellar tape in addition to physical therapy intervention (Clark et al 2000, Kowall et al 1996). Therefore, while it appears as though taping may play a role in short-term pain reduction, thus promoting effective implementation of quadriceps exercises, this requires further confirmation in controlled trials.

A few studies have evaluated the effects of patellar taping on radiographic patellar alignment in PFPS patients with conflicting results. While improvements have been noted in some studies (Roberts 1989, Somes et al 1997, Worrell et al 1994), other studies failed to find radiological evidence of changed patellar position (Bockrath et al 1993, Gigante et al 2001, Worrell et al 1998). A number of factors including different measurement procedures (weightbearing versus non weightbearing), taping techniques, and subject attributes may contribute to the disparate results.

Quadriceps function is decreased in subjects with PFPS (Bennett & Stauber 1986, Powers et al 1997, Thomee et al 1995), possibly resulting from adaptive mechanisms to decrease quadriceps force and thus reducing PFJ load. Patellar tape significantly increases isokinetic quadriceps torque (Conway et al 1992, Handfield & Kramer 2000, Herrington 2001) and knee extensor moments and power during a vertical jump and lateral step up (Ernst et al 1999).

While there is no evidence that patellar tape can change the activation magnitude of the VMO or VL, there is one published study that has investigated the effect of tape on the onset timing of the VMO and/or VL. VMO EMG activity was found to occur earlier in the movement during stair ambulation when the patella was taped (Gilleard et al 1998). Unfortunately, the authors presented the data on the onset of VMO and VL EMG activity in terms of knee angle at muscle onset rather than as a direct measure of EMG timing. Our research group recently investigated the effects of patellar tape on the onset timing of VMO and VL during stair ambulation (Cowan et al 2001a). The study used a randomized, crossover design in which participants with PFPS were required to complete their stair-stepping task under three experimental conditions: no tape, therapeutic tape and control tape. During the stair-stepping task, the application of

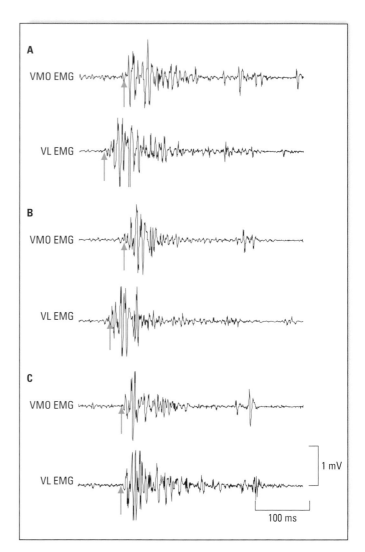

Figure 21.2A–C EMG data of a representative subject from the **A**: PFPS group with no tape, **B**: PFPS with control tape, and **C**: PFPS group therapeutic patellar tape. Note in the no tape and control tape conditions (**A** and **B**) the EMG onset of VL precedes that of VMO, while in the patellar tape condition (**C**) the onsets of VMO and VL are simultaneous.

therapeutic tape was found to alter the temporal characteristics of VMO and VL activation, whereas control tape had no effect (Fig. 21.2). This data supports the use of patellar taping as an adjunct to treatment in individuals with PFPS.

In addition to taping the patella, taping of the lateral thigh has been proposed as a technique that can alter the balance of VL and VMO activity. This tape is applied very firmly in a horizontal direction across the VL muscle belly and the mid thigh level, and is proposed to inhibit the activity of VL (Fig. 21.3). A recent within-subject, placebo controlled trial found that this inhibitory tape significantly reduced the EMG activity of VL compared with no tape or placebo tape in a stair descent task (Tobin

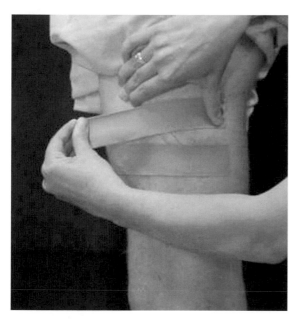

Figure 21.3 Taping of the lateral thigh to alter the balance of VL and VMO activity. The tape is applied very firmly in a horizontal direction across the VL muscle belly and the mid thigh level to inhibit the activity of VL.

& Robinson 2000). The effects of this inhibitory tape on VMO were inconclusive.

Practice

Patellar taping is unique to each patient. The components corrected, the order of correction, and the tension of the tape is tailored for each individual, based on the assessment of patellar position. The worst component is always corrected first and the effect of each piece of tape on the patient's symptoms should be evaluated by reassessing the painful activity. It may be necessary to correct more than one component. The tape should always improve a patient's symptoms immediately. If not, then the order in which the tape was applied or the components corrected should be re-examined. In most cases, hypoallergenic tape is placed underneath the rigid sports tape to provide a protective layer for the skin. If skin problems persist, a plastic coating (applied as either a spray, roll-on or plastic film) may be applied to the skin prior to the tape. The patient must be taught how to apply the tape with the leg fully extended and the quadriceps relaxed.

If a posterior tilt problem has been ascertained on assessment, it must be corrected first, as taping over the inferior pole of the patella will aggravate the fat pad and exacerbate the patient's pain. The posterior component is corrected together with glide or lateral tilt but the tape is placed on the superior aspect of the patella to lift the inferior pole out of the fat pad (Fig. 21.4A).

If there is no posterior tilt problem, glide may be corrected by placing a piece of non-stretch tape from the lateral patellar border, and firmly pulling it, to just past the medial femoral condyle (Fig. 21.4B). At the same time, the soft tissue on the medial aspect of the knee is lifted towards the patella to create a tuck or fold in the skin superomedially. This provides a more effective correction of the glide component and also minimizes the friction rub (friction between the tape and the skin), which can occur when patients have extremely tight lateral structures.

The mediolateral tilt component is corrected by placing a piece of tape firmly from the middle of the patella to the medial femoral condyle (Fig. 21.4C). The object is to lift the lateral border anteriorly so that the patella becomes parallel with the femur in the frontal plane. Again the soft tissue on the medial aspect of the knee is lifted towards the patella.

External rotation is the most common rotation problem and to correct this, the tape is positioned at the inferior pole and pulled upwards and medially towards the opposite shoulder while the superior pole is rotated laterally. Care must be taken so that the inferior pole is not displaced into the fat pad (Fig. 21.4D). Internal rotation, on the other hand, is corrected by taping from the superior pole downwards and medially.

The principle of unloading is based on the premise that inflamed soft tissue does not respond well to stretch. For example, if a patient presents with a sprained medial collateral ligament, applying a valgus stress to the knee will aggravate the condition, whereas a varus stress will decrease the symptoms. To unload the fat pad, the tape commences at the tibial tubercle and comes out in a wide 'V' to the medial and lateral joint lines. As the tape is being pulled towards the joint line, the skin is lifted towards the patella, thus shortening the fat pad (Fig. 21.4E).

The tape is kept on all day, every day, until patients have learnt how to activate their VMO. The tape is removed with care in the evening, allowing the skin time to recover. The tape can cause a breakdown in the skin either through a friction rub or as a consequence of an allergic reaction. Table 21.5 summarizes the problems and the solutions to the problems of skin irritation due to taping.

If the patient experiences a return of the pain, then the patient should readjust the tape. If the activity is still painful, the patient should cease the activity immediately. The tape will loosen quickly if the lateral structures are extremely tight or the patient's job or sport requires extreme amounts of knee flexion. The patient needs to wear the tape until the muscles have adequate endurance, which may take a considerable time for some. Box 21.1 includes a suggested test sequence that the therapist can give the patient to determine if the patient is ready to be without the tape for daily activities.

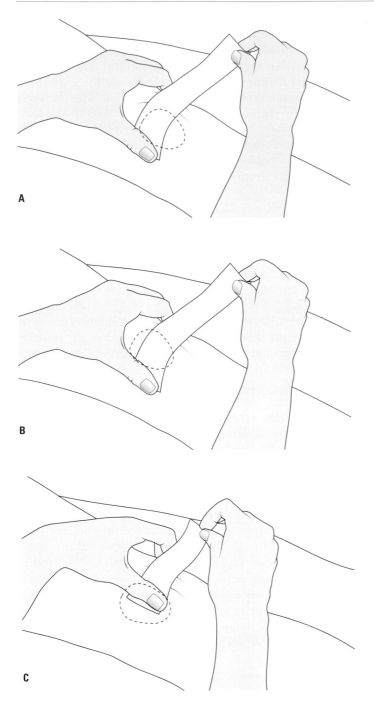

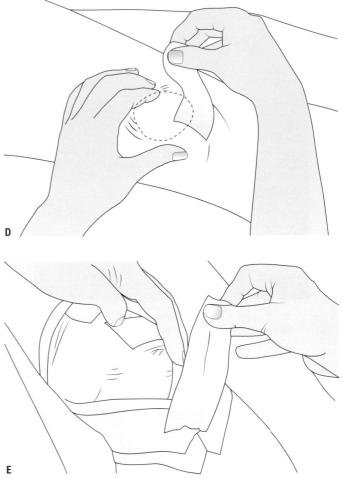

Figure 21.4A–E **A**: Anterior tilt. Correction of an anteroposterior tilt component involves placing tape on the superior aspect of the patella prior to correcting a glide component. **B**: Medial glide. Place tape on the lateral border, lift the skin on the medial side towards the patella and pull tape medially, just short of the hamstring tendons. **C**: Medial tilt. Place tape in the middle of the patella, lift the skin on the medial side towards the patella, and pull the tape medially just short of the hamstring tendons. This tilts the lateral patellar border away from the femur. **D**: Internal rotation. Place tape on the inferior patellar pole, rotate the superior patellar border outward, and use the tape to rotate the inferior pole inward. **E**: Unloading fat pad with tape. Commence tape at the tibial tubercle and lift the soft tissue towards the patella, while firmly pulling the tape to the medial and lateral joint lines.

VASTUS MEDIALIS OBLIQUE RETRAINING

Theory

Under normal circumstances, the synergistic relationship between the VMO and VL maintains the alignment of the patella within the femoral trochlea, especially in the first 30° of knee flexion, when stability of the PFJ cannot be provided by its bony configuration.

It has been proposed that this balanced activation of the VMO and VL is disrupted in patients with PFPS.

Dysfunction of the VMO may result in lateral patellar shift (Sakai et al 2000) or increased lateral patellar pressures (Neptune et al 2000). Individuals with PFPS produce less quadricep torque than those without knee pain (Powers et al 1997, Thomee et al 1995), but the evidence to support imbalance in vastii activation (either decreased activation of VMO or enhanced activation of VL) is contentious (Boucher et al 1992, Mariani & Caruso 1979, Miller et al 1997, Morrish & Woledge 1997, Petschnig et al 1991, Powers 2000a, Powers et al 1996,

Table 21.5 Skin problems associated with taping, and solutions

Problem	Solution
Friction rub	
On the medial aspect of the knee due to friction between tape and skin	Lift the skin on the medial aspect of the knee during taping
Occurs within 1 week; becomes less of a problem as skin toughens	Remove tape carefully, peel back slowly and use the other hand to decrease the pull on the skin
Common (up to 80% of patients)	Use a tape remover
	Rub hand cream into medial aspect of the knee after tape removal
	Use skin preparation (spray, roll-on or plastic film) to provide a barrier
Allergic reaction	
Raised itchy rash where the tape has been	Leave tape off. Apply ice to relieve the itch
Occurs within 1 day if there is previous exposure; may take 10 days if no previous exposure	If severe, may need to seek medical advice
	If possible, identify high risk individuals (previous allergies to tape or adhesive plasters)
Rare (5%)	Use hypoallergenic tape only
	Tape for very short periods

Box 21.1 Example of progression of weaning from tape use

The patient should be able to perform the following exercises pain-free to determine if they are ready to discontinue taping for daily activities:

5 sets of 10 steps performed slowly and controlled with a 10 s rest between each set
1 min quarter squat against the wall
1 min half squat against the wall
A further 5 sets of 10 continuous steps

If the tape is ready to come off, then the patient wears the tape alternate days for 1 week
If the knee has survived 1 week with no recurrence of symptoms, the patient may take the tape off for daily activities, but keep it on for sport
If the patient has been pain-free for a month and is not taped for daily activities, the tape may be removed for sport, provided the patient is able to do the test described above, being untaped and pain-free during the test

---

Sheehy et al 1998, Souza & Gross 1991). Differences in methodology (particularly with respect to the use of EMG) and the inherent heterogeneity in the PFPS population may account for some of the inconsistencies in study results.

While there is inconclusive evidence to support or refute an imbalance in the magnitude of vastii activation in patients with PFPS, disrupted activation of the vastii may take the form of delayed activation of the VMO relative to the VL. It has been hypothesized that the VMO, which has a smaller cross-sectional area than the VL, must receive a feedforward enhancement of its

excitation level in order to track the patellar optimally (Grabiner et al 1994, Wickiewicz et al 1983). Many studies that have examined individuals with PFPS have supported this hypothesis, by demonstrating that the EMG activity and reflex onset time of the VMO relative to the VL is delayed, when compared with asymptomatic individuals (Cowan et al 2001b, Cowan et al 2000, Mariani & Caruso 1979, Perez et al 1995, Voight & Weider 1991, Witvrouw et al 1997). However, there is some conflict regarding the onset of VMO and VL in symptomatic individuals, with a number of authors describing no differences in EMG onsets (Grabiner et al 1992, Karst & Willet 1995, Morrish & Woledge 1997, Powers et al 1996, Sheehy et al 1998). Our research group has attempted to clarify these results by investigating the onset of EMG activity of the VMO and VL in patients with PFPS and asymptomatic controls (Cowan et al 2000, Cowan et al 2001b, 2001c). We observed that in the PFPS population, the EMG onset of VL occurred before that of VMO, while the EMG onsets of VMO and VL occurred simultaneously in the control subjects (Fig. 21.5).

The perceived imbalance between VMO and VL has led to a strong clinical focus on retraining of the VMO in the treatment of PFPS. The goal of this treatment is to restore dynamic patellar stability to correct altered patellar tracking through the appropriate timing and intensity of VMO activation, relative to VL activation.

Physical therapy interventions for PFPS have mostly focussed on strengthening the VMO without increasing the load on the PFJ. Traditionally, standard quadriceps

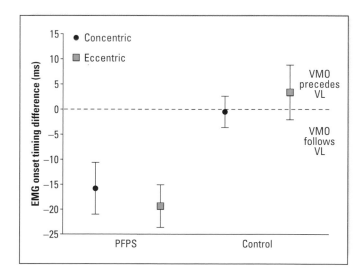

Figure 21.5 Mean differences in EMG onsets of the VMO and VL for the PFPS and control groups in the concentric and eccentric phases of the stair-stepping task. The midpoint of each line indicates the mean EMG onset timing difference. The standard error of the mean is also indicated. Note in the control subjects the average EMG onset of VMO and VL occur almost at the same time, whilst the EMG onset of the VMO occurs after the VL in both the eccentric and concentric phases of the stair-stepping task in the subjects with PFPS.

strengthening consisted of isometric contraction, inner range (non-weightbearing open kinetic chain) contractions and straight leg raises. Often these were progressed through incremental increases in resistance. By exercising the quadriceps in the inner range (30–0°), load on the PFJ is minimized, thus avoiding aggravation of pain. More recently, McConnell (1986) proposed that the VMO should be retrained using motor learning principles (see Ch. 7). This entails utilizing a weightbearing position (closed kinetic chain), thus enabling motor retraining in activities that are more functional and specific.

Although isolated strengthening of the VMO appears to be desirable from a biomechanical standpoint, there is little evidence to suggest that this is possible. The evidence to support or refute the ability to retrain the VMO is presented in the following sections.

Evidence

The effectiveness of VMO retraining may be assessed by studies that investigate whether quadriceps exercises can target VMO activation. It is not possible to measure the strength of the VMO or VL in isolation, therefore EMG has been used to measure the relative activation of these muscles.

There are three main open kinetic chain exercises that are used to strengthen the quadriceps: (1) isometric knee extension, (2) inner range knee extension (terminal or short arc knee extension), and (3) straight leg raises. All three utilize knee flexion less than 30° in order to minimize PFJ contact stress. The available evidence suggests that the VMO is not preferentially activated compared with VL during isometric knee extension (Cerny 1995, Cuddeford et al 1996, Gryzlo et al 1994, Karst & Jewett 1993, Souza & Gross 1991, Zakaria et al 1997), inner range quadriceps (Boucher et al 1992, Cerny 1995, Cuddeford et al 1996, Gryzlo et al 1994, Mirzabeigi et al 1999, Ng & Man 1996) or straight leg raises, regardless of the hip rotation bias (Cuddeford et al 1996, Gryzlo et al 1994, Karst & Jewett 1993, Soderberg & Cook 1983, Wild et al 1982). In fact, all studies evaluating both the straight leg raise and isometric quadriceps setting have shown less EMG activity in the single joint extensors (VL, VML and VMO) during a straight leg raise (even when resistance is applied) than during the isometric quadriceps setting exercise (Wild et al 1982). The addition of hip rotation (internal or external) does not appear to have a beneficial effect on the activation of VMO (Cerny 1995, Mirzabeigi et al 1999, Ng & Man 1996). There are mixed results regarding the addition of hip adduction on the relative activation of VMO and VL, with some authors finding that hip adduction enhances the VMO/VL ratio (Hanten & Schulthies 1990, Hodges & Richardson 1993), while others found no benefits (Cerny

1995, Karst & Jewett 1993, Laprade et al 1998, Zakaria et al 1997).

Closed kinetic chain exercises (step-up, step-down, squats and lunges) are more likely to produce a VMO/VL ratio greater than 1.0 (i.e. VMO activity greater than VL). This has been demonstrated for a squat (Cuddeford et al 1996, Gryzlo et al 1994, Hung & Gross 1999, Souza & Gross 1991), although not by Cerny 1995, Mirzabeigi et al 1999 for step-up (Cuddeford et al 1996, Miller et al 1997, Sheehy et al 1998, Souza & Gross 1991, Willett et al 1998), step-down (Cerny 1995, Miller et al 1997, Sheehy et al 1998, Souza & Gross 1991), and a lunge (Cerny 1995, Miller et al 1997).

Conflicting results from these studies may be partly accounted for by differences in experimental technique (surface electrode vs. fine wire electrodes), methods of quantifying the EMG data (normalized vs. non-normalized), specific conditions of the exercises (e.g. hip flexion or extension) and the inherent variability of EMG measurements.

The available evidence cannot support the premise that VMO functions independent of the VL, and controversy remains over whether the VMO can be selectively recruited relative to the VL. This indicates that isolated recruitment of the VMO does not occur with exercises that are commonly prescribed for the treatment of PFPS. Emphasis on selective strengthening of the VMO most likely results in a balanced activation of the VMO and VL and may translate into a general quadriceps strengthening effect.

Practice

Weightbearing activities should be commenced early in the retraining program, as long as the therapist can ensure that the activities are pain-free with patellar taping. Since the patient will be performing weightbearing activities during activities of daily living, it is desirable to do some carefully monitored practice of a functional activity in a pain-free range.

The essential aspect of training in early stages of rehabilitation is that emphasis should be given to the timing and intensity of the VMO contraction relative to the VL. While surface EMG biofeedback devices provide non-normalized data, in clinical practice they appear to be extremely useful (particularly the dual channel device) in facilitating VMO activation because they give patients immediate feedback and reinforcement when the correct pattern is achieved (LeVeau & Rogers 1980, Wild et al 1982).

A useful starting exercise is small range knee flexion and extension movements (the first 30°) in the standing position, with the feet positioned pelvis-width apart, facing forward and with the weight distributed either equally on both feet, or partially through the symptomatic limb. The patient is instructed to maintain the pelvis, hips, knees and feet in a forward-facing alignment while the knees are slowly flexed to 30° and then returned to full extension without locking the knees back. If the patient's pain returns, then the tape should be readjusted so the patient can proceed with the training. Muscle stimulation may be used to facilitate a VMO contraction.

VMO retraining could progress to small range flexion and extension movements in the walk stance position, with the VMO constantly active. This position not only simulates the motion of the knee during the stance phase of walking, but it is also the position where VMO recruitment is poor and the seating of the patella in the trochlea is critical. Again, emphasis should be given to the timing and intensity of the contraction of VMO relative to VL.

Many patients experience pain during stair ascent and descent, therefore one of the aims of treatment is to improve the patient's ability to negotiate stairs without reproducing symptoms. The patients need to practice stepping up and down, initially using a small step. This should be performed slowly, in front of a mirror, so that changes in limb alignment can be observed and deviations can be observed and corrected (Fig. 21.6). Some patients may be able to do only a small number of repetitions with correct lower limb alignment. Since inappropriate practice can be detrimental to learning, using a small number of exercises with correct alignment is sufficient until the patient can perform larger numbers, pain-free and with correct lower limb alignment. Initially, small numbers of exercises should be performed frequently throughout the day and the number of repetitions should be increased as the skill level improves.

For further progression, the patients can move to a larger step, initially decreasing the number of contractions and then slowly increasing them again. As the control improves, patients can alter the speed of their stepping activity and may vary the place on descent where they stop going down. Weights may be introduced in the hands or in a backpack on the back. Initially, the number of repetitions and the speed of the movement should be decreased, then built back up again.

The aim of retraining is to make the transition from functional exercises to functional activities. Training should be applicable to the patient's activities/sport, so that a jumping athlete, for example, should have jumping incorporated in the program. Figure-of-eight running, bounding, jumping off boxes, jumping and turning, and other plyometric routines are particularly appropriate for the high performance athlete. However, the patient's VMO needs to be monitored at all times for timing and level of contraction relative to the VL.

The VMO plays an important stabilizing role for the PFJ, therefore endurance training is the ultimate goal.

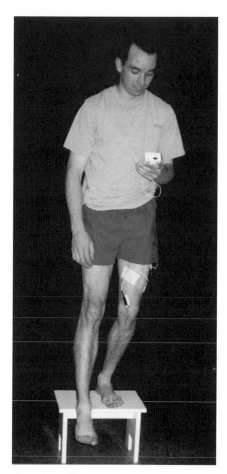

Figure 21.6   Stepping off a step with adequate pelvic control.

The number of repetitions performed by the patient at a training session will depend upon the onset of muscle fatigue. Initially, it is important to emphasize quality and not quantity, progressing to increase the number of repetitions before the onset of fatigue. Patients should be taught to recognize muscle fatigue or quivering, so that they do not train through the fatigue and risk exacerbating their symptoms.

IMPROVING LOWER LIMB MECHANICS

A stable pelvis minimizes unnecessary stress on the knee. Training of the gluteus medius (posterior fibers) will decrease hip internal rotation and the consequent valgus vector force that occurs at the knee. The posterior gluteus medius may be trained in weightbearing with the patient standing side-on to a wall (Fig. 21.7). The leg closest to the wall is flexed at the knee so that the foot is off the ground, and the hip is in a neutral position. All the weight should be on the slightly flexed weightbearing leg. The patient externally rotates the standing leg without moving the foot or the pelvis and at the same time pushes the other leg into the wall. If the patient is

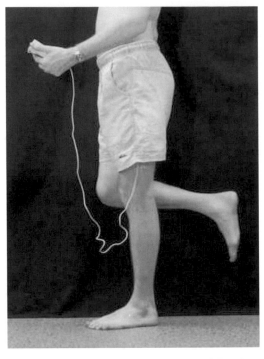

Figure 21.7 Training of the gluteus medius in weightbearing with the patient standing side-on to a wall. Note the use of EMG biofeedback.

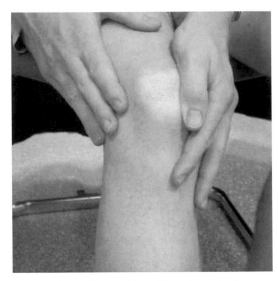

Figure 21.8 Patient self-stretching of the retinacular tissue.

doing this exercise correctly, a burning in the gluteus medius will be felt, especially if the contraction is sustained for at least 20 s. If the exercise is difficult for a patient to coordinate, then rubber tubing may be used around the ankles as the patient stands on the affected leg, while extending the other leg diagonally at 45°.

Some patients with marked internal femoral rotation may require stretching of anterior hip structures to increase available external rotation range. The patient lies prone with the hip to be stretched in an abducted, externally rotated and extended position, and with the foot of the externally rotated leg underneath the extended leg (Fig. 21.1). The therapist's hands hold the pelvis down. The patient is instructed to flatten the abducted and rotated hip (push the anterior superior iliac spine towards the plinth) and hold the stretch for 5 s. If the patient can achieve this position easily, an instruction is given to lift the knee of the externally rotated leg off the plinth.

OTHER

Stretching

Appropriate flexibility exercises must be included in the treatment regimen. The involved muscles may include the hamstrings, gastrocnemius, rectus femoris and tensor fascia lata/iliotibial band. Stretching tight lateral soft tissue structures may be achieved passively by therapist

mobilization of the lateral retinaculum and iliotibial band and by patient self-stretching of the retinacular tissue (Fig. 21.8).

Correcting abnormal foot pronation

Patients exhibiting prolonged pronation during mid-stance in gait may be shown how to train the supinators of their feet. This should improve the stability of the foot for push off and decrease the increased valgus vector force created at the knee by the abnormal foot pronation.

The position of training is mid-stance, the patient is instructed to lift the arch while keeping the great toe on the ground, and then to push the first metatarsal and great toe into the ground. The rationale behind this exercise is that, if the base of the first metatarsal is lifted using the tibialis posterior muscle, the line of action of the peroneus longus is improved. The peroneus longus can then efficiently act on the first metatarsal and improve the stability of the first ray in preparation for push off. If the patient is unable to keep the first metatarso-phalangeal joint on the ground when the arch is lifted, then the foot deformity is too large to correct with training alone and orthotics will be necessary to control the excessive pronation.

EFFICACY OF PHYSICAL THERAPY MANAGEMENT

Efficacy of physical therapy management is determined by well-controlled clinical trials. Similar to other musculoskeletal conditions, there are few trials that have evaluated the effectiveness of physical therapy for PFPS, and our research group has recently reviewed these trials (Crossley et al 2001a). Eight trials evaluated physical therapy, but none compared the intervention with a placebo control. This may reflect the ethical constraints of withholding treatment or difficulties in establishing an effective placebo for physical therapy treatment. Physical therapy interventions for PFPS are varied, but mostly focus on VMO retraining. Some trials utilize standard (open kinetic chain) (McMullen et al 1990, Thomee 1997) or isokinetic quadriceps strengthening (McMullen et al 1990, Stiene et al 1996). Other trials (Clark et al 2000, Eburne & Bannister 1996, Harrison et al 1999) include a McConnell based program. The results of these trials suggest that physical therapy may be effective in reducing the pain associated with PFPS.

There is inconsistency in the types of physical therapy interventions evaluated in these trials, making it difficult to recommend one physical therapy intervention relative to another. Five trials described an overall better response to treatment in the eccentric exercise group in all or some of the outcome measures (Clark et al 2000, Eburne & Bannister 1996, Harrison et al 1999, Stiene et al 1996, Witvrouw et al 2000b). This provides some evidence to support the use of eccentric exercises over alternative forms of quadriceps strengthening, but these result require further verification before they can be accepted.

Two of the most scientifically rigorous trials in this area essentially compared two physical therapy interventions with a group receiving education and advice (Clark et al 2000, Harrison et al 1999). Harrison et al (1999) investigated two physical therapy treatment options, one of which best reflects the protocol designed by McConnell (1986, 1996) while Clark et al (2000) compared four treatment groups: (1) eccentric quadriceps strengthening, (2) eccentric strengthening and patellar tape, (3) patellar tape and advice, (4) advice only. Despite similar methodology, these two trials reported contrasting results.

Clark et al (2000) found that proprioceptive muscle stretching and strengthening aspects of physical therapy have a beneficial effect at 3 months, sufficient to permit discharge from physical therapy. At the 12-month follow-up, the patients in the exercise group reported significantly less pain than those in the no-exercise group and were less likely to have severe knee pain.

In contrast, Harrison et al (1999) found that the patients in the McConnell-based program showed significant improvements in pain and function compared to a group who had supervised standardized quadriceps exercises, but did not differ from the group given a home standardized quadriceps exercise program only. However, the sample size was only sufficient to detect a large effect between the groups. The large dropout rate (up to 48%)

at 12 months may have affected the results at this time point, especially since a significantly greater number of patients in the intervention group who showed substantial improvement were lost to follow-up. The authors concluded that any of the treatments could provide long-term improvements in pain and function.

While the evidence indicates that physical therapy can reduce the pain associated with PFPS, there is inconclusive evidence to support the superiority of one physical therapy intervention compared with others. In general, the eccentric quadriceps strengthening program resulted in a better treatment response than other forms of strengthening, particularly for functional impairment measures.

We recently completed a randomized, double-blind, placebo controlled trial of a McConnell-based physical therapy program in 71 PFPS patients (Cowan et al 2001d, Crossley et al 2001b). Standardized treatments consisted of six treatments, once weekly for both the physical therapy and placebo groups. Sixty-seven (33 physical therapy; 34 placebo) subjects completed the trial. The physical therapy group demonstrated significantly better response to treatment and greater improvements in average pain, worst pain and functional activities (Fig. 21.9). Minor adverse reactions (mostly skin irritation) were reported in 30% of subjects causing them to cease taping for less than 2 days. Sixty-five subjects were included for EMG testing. At baseline, the EMG onset of VL occurred before that of VMO during a stair-stepping task. Following the 6-week treatment program, the physical therapy group demonstrated greater change in their EMG onset timing of VMO compared to VL (Fig. 21.10). This change resulted in the simultaneous onset of VMO and VL in the concentric phase of the stair-stepping task, and in the eccentric phase the onset of VMO actually

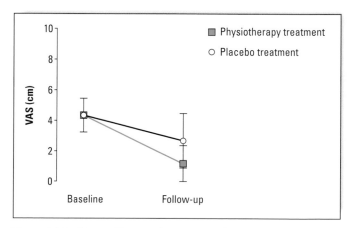

Figure 21.9 Mean difference in average pain in the preceding week for PFPS patients before and after physiotherapy and placebo treatment. Note that while the two groups are similar at baseline, at the completion of the 6-week treatment period, the physiotherapy treatment group demonstrates significantly greater decrease in pain than the placebo control group.

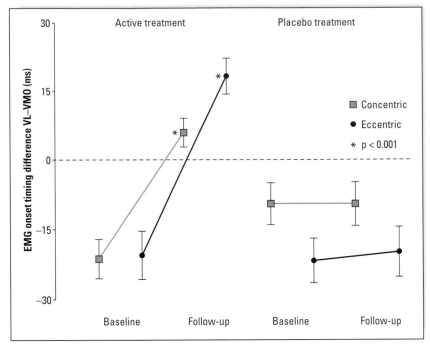

Figure 21.10 Mean difference in the EMG onsets of the VMO and VL for the PFPS in the concentric and eccentric phases of the stair-stepping task before and after physiotherapy or placebo treatment. Note that while the placebo group shows no difference (VL still precedes VMO after treatment) the physiotherapy group demonstrates a reversal in the onset timing deficit.

preceded VL. However, in the placebo group at the follow-up assessment, the onset of VL still occurred before that of VMO in both phases of the stair-stepping task group. This study demonstrates that a McConnell-based physical therapy program significantly improves pain and function and can alter EMG onset of VMO relative to VL compared with placebo treatment.

SUMMARY

It is unclear which structure is predominantly implicated as the pathological cause of pain associated with PFPS. Despite this, non-surgical treatment options have evolved, based on decreasing the load on the PFJ through improved patellar tracking and lower limb alignment. Patellar taping appears to improve quadriceps function (onset timing), torque, quadriceps moments and radiological patellar position. While it remains unclear as to how patellar taping affects the PFJ, sufficient evidence exists to suggest that patellar taping can provide short-term benefit for patients with PFPS.

Management of patellofemoral pain is no longer a conundrum if the therapist can determine the underlying causative factors and address these factors in treatment. It is imperative that the patient's symptoms are significantly reduced, which can often be achieved by patellar taping. Management should also include VMO retraining, gluteal control work and stretching tight lateral structures.

REFERENCES

Abernathy P J, Townsend P, Rose R et al 1978 Is chondromalacia patella a separate entity? Journal of Bone and Joint Surgery (Br) 60B:205–210

Aglietti P, Insall J N, Cerulli G 1983 Patellar pain and incongruence, I: measurement of incongruence. Clinical Orthopaedics and Related Research 176:217–224

Ahmed A, Burke D, Yu A 1983 In vitro measurement of static pressure distribution in synovial joints – Part II: retropatellar surface. Journal of Biomechanical Engineering 105:226–236

Ahmed A M, Burke D L, Hyder A 1987 Force analysis of the patellar mechanism. Journal of Orthopaedic Research 5:69–85

Almeida S A, Trone D W, Leone D M et al 1998 Gender differences in musculoskeletal injury rates: a function of symptom reporting. Medicine and Science in Sports and Exercise 31(12):1807–1812

Almeida S, Williams K M, Shaffer R A et al 1999 Epidemiological patterns of musculoskeletal injuries and physical training. Medicine and Science in Sports and Exercise 31(8):1176–1182

Arnoldi C C 1991 Patellar pain. Acta Orthopaedica Scandinavia 62(suppl 224):1–29

Arsenault A B, Falconer K A, Winter D A 1978 Diagonal-spiral versus cardinal patterns in the EMG activity of the knee extensors. Physiotherapy Canada 30(2):58–63

Baecke J A H, Burema J, Frijters J E R 1982 A short questionnaire for the measurement of habitual physical activity in epidemiological studies. American Journal of Clinical Nutrition 36:936–942

Baquie P, Brukner P 1997 Injuries presenting to an Australian sports medicine centre: a 12 month study. Clinical Journal of Sports Medicine 7:28–31

Basmajian J V, Harden T P, Regenos E M 1971 Integrated actions of the four heads of quadriceps femoris: an electromyographic study. Anatomical Record 172:15–20

Bennett J G, Stauber W T 1986 Evaluation and treatment of anterior knee pain using eccentric exercise. Medicine and Science in Sports and Exercise 18(5):526–530

Bierdert R, Stauffer E, Niklaus N F 1992 Occurence of free nerve endings in the soft tissue of the knee joint. A histologic investigation. American Journal of Sports Medicine 20(4):430–433

Bierdert R, Lobenhoffer P, Lattermann C et al 2000 Free nerve endings in the medial and posteromedial capsuloligamentous complexes: occurences and distribution. Knee Surgery, Sports Traumatology and Arthroscopy 8:68–72

Bockrath K, Wooden C, Worrell T et al 1993 Effects of patella taping on patella position and perceived pain. Medicine and Science in Sports and Exercise 25(9):989–992

Bose K, Kanagasuntheram R, Osman M B H 1980 Vastus medialis obliquus; an anatomic and physiologic study. Orthopedics 3:883–880

Boucher J P, King M A, Lefebvre R et al 1992 Quadriceps femoris muscle activity in patellofemoral pain syndrome. American Journal of Sports Medicine 20(5):527–532

Brownstein B A, Lamb R L, Mangine R E 1985 Quadriceps torque and integrated eletromyography. Journal of Orthopaedic and Sports Physical Therapy 6:309–314

Brukner P, Khan K 2001 Clinical sports medicine, 2nd edn. McGraw-Hill, Sydney

Bull A M J, Senavongse W W, Taylor A R et al 1998 The effect of the oblique portions of the vastus medialis and lateralis on patellar tracking. Proceedings of the 11th Conference of the ESB, Toulouse, France

Cerny K 1995 Vastus medialis oblique/vastus lateralis muscle activity ratios for selected exercises in persons with and without patellofemoral pain syndrome. Physical Therapy 75(8):672–682

Chew J T, Stewart N J, Hanssen A D et al 1997 Differences in patellar tracking and knee kinematics among three different total knee designs. Clinical Orthopaedics and Related Research 345:87–98

Clark D I, Downing N, Mitchell J et al 2000 Physiotherapy for anterior knee pain: a randomised controlled trial. Annals of the Rheumatic Diseases 59(9):700–704

Clement D B, Taunton J E, Smart G W et al 1981 A survey of overuse injuries. Physician and Sportsmedicine 9:47–58

Conlan T, Garth W P, Lemons J E 1993 Evaluation of the medial soft-tissue restraints of the extensor mechanism of the knee. Journal of Bone and Joint Surgery (Am) 75A:682–693

Conway A, Malone T, Conway P 1992 Patellar alignment/tracking alteration: effect on force output and perceived pain. Isokinetics and Exercise Science 2:9–17

Cowan S M 2002 Motor control of the vastii in patellofemoral pain syndrome. PhD Thesis. University of Melbourne, Australia

Cowan S M, Hodges P W, Bennell K L et al 2000 Anticipatory activity of vastus medialis obliquus delayed when subjects with patellofemoral pain syndrome complete a postural task. Proceedings of the 7th Scientific Conference of the International Federation of Orthopaedic Manipulative Therapists, Perth, Australia, The University of Western Australia

Cowan S M, Bennell K L, Hodges P W 2001a Therapeutic patellar taping changes the timing of vastii muscle activation in people with patellofemoral pain syndrome. Musculoskeletal Physiotherapy Australia, Adelaide, Australia

Cowan S M, Bennell K L, Hodges P W et al 2001b Delayed onset of electromyographic activity of vastus medialis obliquus relative to vastus lateralis in subjects with patellofemoral pain syndrome. Archives of Physical Medicine and Rehabilitation 82(2):183–189

Cowan S M, Hodges P W, Bennell K L 2001c Anticipatory activity of

vastus lateralis and vastus medialis obliquus occurs simultaneously in voluntary heel and toe raising. Physical Therapy in Sport 2(2):71–79

Cowan S M, Bennell K L, Crossley K M et al 2001d Physiotherapy treatment changes motor control of the vastii in patellofemoral pain syndrome (PFPS): a randomised, double-blind, placebo controlled trial. Medicine and Science in Sports and Exercise 33(5):S89

Crossley K M, Cowan S M, Bennell K L et al 2000 Patellar taping: is clinical success supported by scientific evidence? Manual Therapy 5(3):142–150

Crossley K, Bennell K, Green S et al 2001a A systematic review of physical interventions for patellofemoral pain syndrome. Clinical Journal of Sports Medicine 11(2):103–110

Crossley K M, Bennell K L, Cowan S M et al 2001b Efficacy of a physiotherapy treatment for patellofemoral pain syndrome: a randomized, double blind, placebo controlled trial. Medicine and Science in Sports and Exercise 33(5):S86

Cuddeford T, Williams A K, Medeiros J M 1996 Electromyographic activity of the vastus medialis oblique and vastus lateralis muscles during selected exercises. Journal of Manual and Manipulative Therapy 4(1):10–15

DeHaven K E, Lintner D M 1986 Athletic injuries: comparison by age, sport and gender. American Journal of Sports Medicine 14:218–224

Desio S M, Burks R T, Bachus K N 1998 Soft tissue restraints to lateral patellar translation in the human knee. American Journal of Sports Medicine 26(1):59–65

Devereaux M, Lachmann S 1984 Patellofemoral arthralgia in athletes attending a sports injury clinic. British Journal of Sports Medicine 18:18–21

Duri Z A, Aichroth P M, Dowd G 1996 The fat pad. Clinical observations. American Journal of Knee Surgery 9(2):55–66

Dye S F, Chew M H 1993 The use of scintigraphy to detect increased osseous metabolic activity about the knee. Journal of Bone and Joint Surgery (Am) 75A(9):1388–1406

Dye S F, Vaupel G L 1994 The pathophysiology of patellofemoral pain. Sports Medicine and Arthroscopy Review 2:203–210

Dye S F, Vaupel G L, Dye C C 1998 Conscious neurosensory mapping of the internal structures of the human knee without intraarticular anaesthesia. American Journal of Sports Medicine 26(6):773–777

Eburne J, Bannister G 1996 The McConnell regimen versus isometric quadriceps exercises in the management of anterior knee pain. A randomised prospective controlled trial. The Knee 3:151–153

Ernst G P, Kawaguchi J, Saliba E 1999 Effect of patellar taping on knee kinetics of patients with patellofemoral pain syndrome. Journal of Orthopaedic and Sports Physical Therapy 29(11):661–667

Farahmand F, Tahmasbi M N, Amis A A 1998 Lateral force-displacement behaviour of the human patella and its variation. Journal of Biomechanics 31(12):1147–1152

Fulkerson J, Hungerford D 1997 Disorders of the patellofemoral joint. Williams and Wilkins, Baltimore MD

Fulkerson J P, Gosling H R 1980 Anatomy of the knee joint lateral retinaculum. Clinical Orthopaedics and Related Research 153:183–188

Fulkerson J P, Shea K P 1990 Current concepts review: disorder of patellofemoral alignment. Journal of Bone and Joint Surgery (Am) 72A:1424–1429

Fulkerson J P, Tennant R, Jaivin J S et al 1985 Histological evidence of retinacular nerve injury associated with patellofemoral malalignment. Clinical Orthopaedics and Related Research 197:196–205

Gigante A, Pasquinellii F M, Palodini P et al 2001 The effects of patellar taping on patellofemoral incongruence: a computerised tomography study. American Journal of Sports Medicine 29(1):88–92

Gilleard W, McConnell J, Parsons D 1998 The effect of patellar taping on the onset of vastus medialis obliquus and vastus lateralis muscle activity in persons with patellofemoral pain. Physical Therapy 78(1):25–32

Goh J C H, Lee P Y C, Bose K 1995 A cadaver study of the function of the oblique part of vastus medialis. Journal of Bone and Joint Surgery (Br) 77B(2):225–231

Goodfellow J, Hungerford D S, Woods C 1976 Patello-femoral joint mechanics and pathology. 2. Chondromalacia patellae. Journal of

Bone and Joint Surgery (Br) 58B(3):291–299

Grabiner M D, Koh T J, Miller G F 1991 Fatigue rates of vastus medialis oblique and vastus lateralis during static and dynamic knee extension. Journal of Orthopaedic Research 9:391–397

Grabiner M D, Koh M A, Andrish J T 1992 Decreased excitation of vastus medialis oblique and vastus lateralis in patellofemoral pain. European Journal of Experimental Musculoskeletal Research 1:33–39

Grabiner M D, Koh T J, Draganich L F 1994 Neuromechanics of the patellofemoral joint. Medicine and Science in Sports and Exercise 26(1):10–21

Grelsamer R P, Klein J R 1998 The biomechanics of the patellofemoral joint. Journal of Orthopaedic and Sports Physical Therapy 28(5):286–297

Grelsamer R P, McConnell J 1998 The Patella. A team approach. Aspen Publishers, Gaithersburg MD

Gryzlo S M, Patek R M, Pink M et al 1994 Electromyographic analysis of knee rehabilitation exercises. Journal of Orthopaedic and Sports Physical Therapy 20:36–43

Handfield T, Kramer J 2000 Effect of McConnell taping on perceived pain and knee extensor torques during isokinetic exercise performed by patients with patellofemoral pain syndrome. Physiotherapy Canada Winter:39–44

Hanten W P, Schulthies S S 1990 Exercise effect on electromyographic activity of the vastus medialis oblique and the vastus lateralis. Physical Therapy 70:39–43

Harrison E L, Sheppard M S, McQuarrie A M 1999 A randomized controlled trial of physical therapy treatment programs in patellofemoral pain syndrome. Physiotherapy Canada Spring:93–106

Hautamaa P V, Fithian D C, Kaufman K R et al 1998 Medial soft tissue restraints in lateral patellar instability and repair. Clinical Orthopaedics and Related Research 349:174–182

Heegard J, Leyvraz P, van Kampen A et al 1994 Influence of soft structures on patellar three dimensional tracking. Clinical Orthopaedics and Related Research 299:235–243

Heir T, Glomsaker P 1996 Epidemiology of musculoskeletal injuries among Norwegian conscripts undergoing basic military training. Scandinavian Journal of Medicine and Science in Sports 6(3):186–191

Herrington L 2001 The effect of patellar taping on quadriceps peak torque and perceived pain: a preliminary study. Physical Therapy in Sport 2:23–28

Herrington L, Payton C J 1997 Effects of corrective taping of the patella on patients with patellofemoral pain. Physiotherapy 83(11):566–572

Hodges P, Richardson C A 1993 The influence of isometric hip adduction on quadriceps femoris activity. Scandinavian Journal of Rehabilitation Medicine 25:57–62

Hung Y-J, Gross M T 1999 Effect of foot position on electromyographic activity of the vastus medialis oblique and vastus lateralis during lower-extremity weight-bearing activities. Journal of Orthopaedic and Sports Physical Therapy 29(2):93–105

Hungerford D S, Barry M 1979 Biomechanics of the patellofemoral joint. Clinical Orthopaedics and Related Research 144:9–15

Insall J, Falvo K A, Wise D W 1976 Chondromalacia patellae: a prospective study. Journal of Bone and Joint Surgery (Am) 58A:1–8

Isear J A, Erickson J C, Worrell T W 1997 EMG analysis of lower extremity muscle recruitment patterns during an unloaded squat. Medicine and Science in Sports and Exercise 29(4):532–539

Jacobson K E, Flandry F C 1989 Diagnosis of anterior knee pain. Clinics in Sports Medicine 8(2):179–195

James S L, Bates B T, Osternig L R 1978 Injuries to runners. American Journal of Sports Medicine 6(2):40–50

Jones B H, Cowan D N, Tomlinson J R et al 1993 Epidemiology of injuries associated with physical training among young men in the army. Medicine and Science in Sports and Exercise 25(2):197–203

Kannus P, Aho H, Järvinen M et al 1987 Computerised recording of visits to an outpatient sports clinic. American Journal of Sports Medicine 15(1):79–85

Karst G M, Jewett P D 1993 Electromyographic analysis of exercises proposed for differential activation of medial and lateral quadriceps femoris muscle components. Physical Therapy 73:286–299

Karst G M, Willet G M 1995 Onset timing of electromyographic activity in the vastus medialis oblique and vastus lateralis muscles in subjects with and without patellofemoral pain syndrome. Physical Therapy 75(9):813–823

Karst G M, Willett G M 1997 Reflex response times of vastus medialis oblique and vastus lateralis in normal subjects and in subjects with patellofemoral pain. Letter to editor. Journal of Orthopaedic and Sports Physical Therapy 26(2):108–109

Kenna M 1991 The effect of patellofemoral joint taping on pain during activity. Paper presented at the Manipulative Physiotherapists Association of Australia 7th Biennial Conference, Blue Mountains, Australia

Kowal D M 1980 Nature and cause of injuries to women resulting from an endurance training program. American Journal of Sports Medicine 8(4):265–269

Kowall M G, Kolk G, Nuber G W et al 1996 Patellar taping in the treatment of patellofemoral pain. A prospective randomized study. American Journal of Sports Medicine 24(1):61–66

Lange G W, Hintermeister R A, Schlegel T et al 1996 Electromyographic and kinematic analysis of graded treadmill walking and the implications for knee rehabilitation. Journal of Orthopaedic and Sports Physical Therapy 23(5):294–301

Laprade J, Culham E, Brouwer B 1998 Comparison of five isometric exercises in the recruitment of the vastus medialis oblique in persons with and without patellofemoral pain syndrome. Journal of Orthopaedic and Sports Physical Therapy 27(3):197–204

Laurin C A, Levesque H P, Dussault R et al 1978 The abnormal lateral patellofemoral angle. Journal of Bone and Joint Surgery (Am) 60A(1):55–60

Leppala J, Kannus P, Natri A et al 1998 Bone mineral density in the chronic patellofemoral pain syndrome. Calcified Tissue International 62(6):548–553

LeVeau B F, Rogers C 1980 Selective training of the vastus medialis muscle using EMG biofeedback. Physical Therapy 60(11):1410–1415

Lieb F J, Perry J 1968 Quadriceps function. An anatomical and mechanical study. Journal of Bone and Joint Surgery (Am) 50A(8):1535–1548

Lieb F J, Perry J 1971 Quadriceps function: an electromyographic study under isometric conditions. Journal of Bone and Joint Surgery (Am) 53A:749–758

Lindberg U, Lysholm J, Gillquist J 1986 The correlation between arthroscopic findings and the patellofemoral pain syndrome. Arthroscopy 2:103–107

McConnell J 1986 The management of chondromalacia patellae: a long term solution. Australian Journal of Physiotherapy 32(4):215–223

McConnell J 1996 Management of patellofemoral problems. Manual Therapy 1:60–66

McFadyen B J, Winter D A 1988 An integrated biomechanics analysis of normal stair ascent and descent. Journal of Biomechanics 21(9):733–744

Macintyre J G, Taunton J E, Clement D B et al 1991 Running injuries: a clinical study of 4,173 cases. Clinical Journal of Sports Medicine 1:81–87

Mckay-Lyons M 1989 Low-load, prolonged stretching the treatment of elbow contractures secondary to head trauma. Physical Therapy 69:292

McMullen W, Roncarati A, Koval P 1990 Static and isokinetic treatments of chondromalacia patella: a comparative investigations. Journal of Orthopaedic and Sports Physical Therapy 12(6):256–266

Mariani P, Caruso I 1979 An electromyographic investigation of subluxation of the patella. Journal of Bone and Joint Surgery (Am) 61A:169–171

Matheson G O, Macintyre J G, Taunton J E et al 1989 Musculoskeletal injuries associated with physical activity in older ages. Medicine and Science in Sports and Exercise 21(4):370–385

Merchant A C, Mercer R L, Jacobson R H et al 1974 Roentgenographic analysis of patellofemoral congruence. Journal of Bone and Joint Surgery (Am) 56A:1391–1396

Milgrom C, Kerem E, Finestone A et al 1991 Patellofemoral pain caused by overactivity. A prospective study of risk factors in infantry recruits. Journal of Bone and Joint Surgery (Am) 73A(7):1041–1043

Miller J P, Sedory D, Croce R V 1997 Vastus medialis obliquus and vastus lateralis activity in patients with and without patellofemoral pain syndrome. Journal of Sport Rehabilitation 6:1–10

Mirzabeigi E, Jordan C, Gronley J K et al 1999 Isolation of the vastus medialis oblique muscle during exercise. American Journal of Sports Medicine 27(1):50–53

Moller B N, Moller-Larsen F, Frich L H 1989 Chondromalacia induced by patellar subluxation in the rabbit. Acta Orthopaedica Scandinavia 60:188–191

Morrish G M, Woledge R C 1997 A comparison of the activation of muscles moving the patella in normal subjects and in patients with chronic patellofemoral problems. Scandinavian Journal of Rehabilitation Medicine 29(1):43–48

Nagamine R, Otani T, White S E et al 1995 Patellar tracking measurements in the normal knee. Journal of Orthopaedic Research 13:95–96

Neptune R R, Wright I C, van den Bogert A J 2000 The influence of orthotic devices and vastus medialis strength and timing on patellofemoral loads during running. Clinical Biomechanics 15:611–618

Newberry W N, Zukosky D K, Haut R C 1997 Subfracture insult to a knee joint causes alterations in the bone and in the functional stiffness of overlying cartilage. Journal of Orthopaedic Research 15(3):450–455

Ng G Y F, Man V Y 1996 EMG analysis of vastus medialis obliquus and vastus lateralis during static knee extension with different hip and ankle positions. New Zealand Journal of Physiotherapy 4:7–10

Ohno O, Naito J, Iguchi T et al 1988 An electron microscopic study of early pathology in chondromalacia of the patella. Journal of Bone and Joint Surgery (Am) 70A(6):883–899

Outerbridge R E 1961 The etiology of chondromalacia patellae. Journal of Bone and Joint Surgery (Br) 43B:752–757

Outerbridge R, Dunlop J 1975 The problem of chondromalacia. Clinical Orthopaedics and Related Research 110:177–196

Pagliano J W, Jackson D W 1987 A clinical study of 3,000 long distance runners. Annals of Sports Medicine 3(2):88–91

Perez P L, Gossman M R, Lechner D et al 1995 Electromyographic temporal characteristics of the vastus medialis oblique and the vastus lateralis in women with and without patellofemoral pain. Paper presented at the12th International Congress of the World Confederation for Physical Therapy, Washington DC

Petschnig R, Baron R, Engel A et al 1991 Objectivation of the effects of knee problems on vastus medialis and vastus lateralis with EMG and dynamometry. Physical Medicine and Rehabilitation 2:50–54

Powers C M 2000a Patellar kinematics, Part I: the influence of vastus muscle activity in subjects with and without patellofemoral pain. Physical Therapy 80(10):956–964

Powers C M 2000b Patellar kinematics, Part II: the influence of the depth of the trochlear groove in subjects with and without patellofemoral pain. Physical Therapy 80(10):965–973

Powers C M, Landel R, Carpenter T et al 1995 The effects of patellar taping on loading characteristics in subjects with patellofemoral pain. Paper presented at the12th International Congress of the World Confederation for Physical Therapy, Washington DC

Powers C M, Landel R F, Perry J 1996 Timing and intensity of vastus muscle activity during functional activities in subjects with and without patellofemoral pain. Physical Therapy 76:946–955

Powers C M, Perry J, Hsu A et al 1997 Are patellofemoral pain and quadriceps femoris muscle torque associated with locomotor function? Physical Therapy 77(10):1063–1075

Powers C M, Shellock F G, Pfaff M 1998 Quantification of patellar tracking using kinematic resonance imaging. Journal of Magnetic Resonance Imaging 8:724–732

Radin E L, Parker H G, Pugh J W et al 1973 Response of joints to impact loading-III. Relationship between trabecular microfractures and cartilage degeneration. Journal of Biomechanics 6:51–57

Raimondo R A, Ahmad C S, Blankevoort L et al 1998 Patellar stabilization: a quantitative evaluation of the vastus medialis obliquus muscle. Orthopaedics 21(7):791–795

Reider B, Marshall J L, Koslin D et al 1981a The anterior aspect of the knee joint. Journal of Bone and Joint Surgery (Am) 63A:351–356

Reider B, Marshall J L, Ring B 1981b Patellar tracking. Clinical

Orthopaedics and Related Research 157:143–148

Reilly D T, Martens M 1972 Experimental analysis of the quadriceps muscle force and patellofemoral joint reaction forces for various activities. Acta Orthopedica Scandinavia 43:126–137

Reynolds L, Levin T, Medeiros J et al 1983 EMG activity of vastus medialis obliquus and vastus lateralis and their role in patella alignment. American Journal of Physical Medicine 62:61

Roberts J M 1989 The effect of taping on patellofemoral alignment – a radiological pilot study. Paper presented at the Manipulative Therapists Association of Australia Biennial Conference, Adelaide, Australia

Sakai N, Luo Z-P, Rand J A et al 2000 The influence of weakness in the vastus medialis oblique muscle on the patellofemoral joint: an in vitro biomechanical study. Clinical Biomechanics 15:335–339

Sanchis-Alfonso V, Rosello-Sastre E 2000 Immunohistochemical analysis for neural markers of the lateral retinaculum in patients with isolated symptomatic patellofemoral malalignment. American Journal of Sports Medicine 28(5):725–731

Sanchis-Alfonso V, Rossello-Sastre E, Monteagudo-Castro C et al 1998 Quantitative analysis of nerve changes in the lateral retinaculum in patients with isolated symptomatic patellofemoral malalignment. American Journal of Sports Medicine 26(5):703–709

Scharf W, Weinstable R, Othrner E 1985 Anatomical separation and clinical importance of two different parts of the vastus medialis muscle. Acta Anatomy 123:108–111

Schneider U, Wenz W, Breusch S J et al 2000 A new concept in the treatment of anterior knee pain: patellar hypertension syndrome. Orthopedics 23(6):581–586

Schutzer S F, Ramsby G R, Fulkerson J P 1986 Computed tomographic classification of patellofemoral pain patients. Orthopedic Clinics of North America 17(2):235–248

Schwellnus M P, Jordaan G, Noakes T D 1990 Prevention of common overuse injuries by the use of shock absorbing insoles. A prospective study. American Journal of Sports Medicine 18(6):636–641

Sheehan F T, Drace J E 1999 Quantitative MR measures of three-dimensional patellar kinematics as a research and diagnostic tool. Medicine and Science in Sports and Exercise 31(10):1399–1405

Sheehy P, Burdett R G, Irrgang J J et al 1998 An electromyographic study of vastus medialis oblique and vastus lateralis activity while ascending and descending steps. Journal of Orthopaedic and Sports Physical Therapy 27(9):423–429

Shwayhat A F, Linenger J M, Hofherr L K et al 1994 Profiles of exercise history and overuse injuries among United States Navy sea, air, and land (SEAL) recruits. American Journal of Sports Medicine 22(6):835–840

Signorile J F, Kacsik D, Perry A et al 1995 The effect of knee and foot position on the electromyographical activity of the superficial quadriceps. Journal of Orthopaedic and Sports Physical Therapy 22(1):2–9

Smith G P, Howe T E, Oldham J A et al 1995 Assessing quadriceps muscles recruitment order using rectified averages. Clinical Rehabilitation 9(1):40–46

Soderberg G, Cook T 1983 An electromyographic analysis of quadriceps femoris muscle setting and straight leg raise. Physical Therapy 63:1434–1438

Somes S, Worrell T W, Corey B et al 1997 Effects of patellar taping on patellar position in the open and closed kinetic chain: a preliminary study. Journal of Sports Rehabilitation 6:299–308

Souza D R, Gross M 1991 Comparison of vastus medialis obliquus: vastus lateralis muscle integrated electromyographic ratios between healthy subjects and patients with patellofemoral pain. Physical Therapy 71(4):310–320

Spencer J, Hayes K, Alexander I 1984 Knee joint effusion and quadriceps inhibition in man. Archives of Physical Medicine 65:171–177

Stiene H A, Brosky T, Reinking M F et al 1996 A comparison of closed kinetic chain and isokinetic joint isolation in patients with patellofemoral dysfunction. Journal of Orthopaedic and Sports Physical Therapy 24(3):136–141

Stokes M, Young A 1984 Investigations of quadriceps inhibition: implications for clinical practice. Physiotherapy 70(11):425–428

Taylor D, Dalton J, Seaber A 1990 Visco-elastic properties of muscle-tendon units. The biomechanical effect of stretching. American Journal of Sports Medicine 18:300

Terry G C, Hughston J C, Norwood L A 1986 The anatomy of the iliopatellar band and iliotibial tract. American Journal of Sports Medicine 14(1):39–45

Thiranagama R 1990 Nerve supply of the human vastus medialis muscle. Journal of Anatomy 170:193–198

Thomee R 1997 A comprehensive treatment approach for patellofemoral pain syndrome in young women. Physical Therapy 77(12):1690–1703

Thomee R, Renstrom P, Karlsson J et al 1995 Patellofemoral pain syndrome in young women. II. Muscle function in patients and healthy controls. Scandinavian Journal of Medicine and Science in Sports 5:245–251

Tobin S, Robinson G 2000 The effect of McConnell's vastus lateralis inhibition taping technique on vastus lateralis and vastus medialis obliquus activity. Physiotherapy 26(4):173–183

Tsirbas A, Paterson R S, Keene G C R 1991 Fat pad impingement; a missed cause of patello-femoral pain? Australian Journal of Science and Medicine in Sport 23(1):24–26

Vaatainen U, Lohmander L S, Thonar E et al 1998 Markers of cartilage and synovial metabolism in joint fluid and serum of patients with chondromalacia. Arthritis and Cartilage 6(2):115–124

van Kampen A, Huiskes R 1990 The three-dimensional tracking pattern of the human patella. Journal of Orthopaedic Research 8:372–382

Voight M, Weider D 1991 Comparitive reflex response times of the vastus medialis and the vastus lateralis in normal subjects with extensor mechanism dysfunction. American Journal of Sports Medicine 19(2):131–137

Wickiewicz T L, Roy R R, Powell P L et al 1983 Muscle architecture of the human lower limb. Clinical Orthopaedics and Related Research 179:275–283

Wild J J, Franklin T D, Woods G W 1982 Patellar pain and quadriceps rehabilitation: an EMG study. American Journal of Sports Medicine 10:12–15

Willett G M, Karst G M, Canney E M et al 1998 Lower limb EMG activity during selected stepping exercise. Journal of Sport Rehabilitation 7:102–111

Williams P L, Warrick R 1989 Gray's Anatomy. Churchill Livingstone, Edinburgh

Witonski D, Goraj B 1999 Patellar motion analyzed by kinematic and dynamic axial magnetic resonance. Archives of Orthopaedic and Trauma Surgery 119(1–2):46–49

Witonski D, Wagrowska-Danielewicz M 1999 Distribution of substance-P nerve fibers in the knee joint of patients with anterior knee pain. A preliminary report. Knee Surgery Traumatology and Arthroscopy 7:177–183

Witvrouw E, Delvaux K, Lysens R et al 1997 Reflex response times of vastus medialis oblique and vastus lateralis in normal subjects and in subjects with patellofemoral pain-response. Journal of Orthopaedic and Sports Physical Therapy 26(2):109–110

Witvrouw E, Lysens R, Bellemans J et al 2000a Intrinsic risk factors for the development of anterior knee pain in an athletic population. A two year prospective study. American Journal of Sports Medicine 28(4):480–489

Witvrouw E, Lysens R, Bellemans J et al 2000b Open versus closed kinetic chain exercises for patellofemoral pain syndrome. American Journal of Sports Medicine 28(5):687–694

Worrell T W, Ingersoll C D, Farr J 1994 Effect of patellar taping and bracing on patellar position: an MRI case study. Journal of Sport Rehabilitation 3:146–153

Worrell T, Ingersoll C D, Bockrath-Pugliese K et al 1998 Effect of patellar taping and bracing on patellar position as determined by MRI in patients with patellofemoral pain. Journal of Athletic Training 33(1):16–20

Zakaria D, Harburn K L, Kramer J F 1997 Preferential activation of the vastus medialis oblique, vastus lateralis, and hip adductor muscles during isometric exercises in females. Journal of Orthopaedic and Sports Physical Therapy 26(1):23–28

22

Leg

*Jack Taunton   Rob Lloyd-Smith
Christopher AM Johnston*

INTRODUCTION

Exercise-induced leg pain is a very common condition that presents a significant challenge to the athlete, coach, and medical team. Through adherence to useful nomenclature, careful history, physical examination, prudent investigation and related interpretation, and the institution of a planned comprehensive treatment program, most athletes can predictably return to their preferred activity. The causes of lower leg pain are extensive, however only the more common causes will be discussed in this chapter.

SPORT-SPECIFIC APPLIED ANATOMY

The tibia is the weightbearing bone and the fibula is for muscular support and attachment. There are four compartments in the leg:

1. The *anterior compartment* muscles are the tibialis anterior, extensor hallicus longus and extensor digitorum longus and brevis; all are innervated by the deep peroneal branch of the common peroneal nerve, and are ankle dorsiflexors.
2. The *lateral compartment* muscles are peroneus longus and brevis; both evert the foot, and both are innervated by the superficial branch of the common peroneal nerve.
   The *posterior compartment* of the leg has superficial and deep components.
3. The *superficial component* contains the triceps surae (the gastrocnemius and soleus muscles) and plantaris; all are innervated by the tibial nerve, and plantarflex the ankle. The popliteus is also in this compartment, and it unlocks the knee from full extension by internal rotation of the tibia on the femur.

419

4. The *deep posterior compartment* contains the tibialis posterior, flexor digitorum longus, and flexor hallicus longus; it is also innervated by the tibial nerve and plantarflexes the ankle.

A fifth compartment, located deep within the deep posterior compartment surrounding the posterior tibial muscle, has been described and implicated in exercise-induced leg pain (Detmer 1986, Rorabeck 1986).

COMMON SPORT-RELATED INJURIES

Stress fractures of the tibia, periostitis, and compartment syndrome comprise important conditions in the differential diagnosis of exercise-induced leg pain, and will be discussed in this section. That two or more of these specific entities can occur in an athlete presenting with leg pain is depicted in Figure 22.1.

TIBIAL STRESS FRACTURES

The tibia is a very common location for stress fractures, accounting for approximately 50% of all stress fractures (Hulkko & Orava 1987, Matheson et al 1987, McBryde 1965, Stanitski et al 1978, Sullivan et al 1984, Taunton et al 1981).

A stress fracture is an overuse injury to bone that occurs when the accumulation of microtrauma from repetitive loading (i.e. running) exceeds the ability of the body to lay down new bone. Bony deposition of new bone formation is more active 30 days after the onset of increased loading; however initially, resorption of bone is predominant, and stress fractures are more likely to occur during this period of bone porosity due to the decrease in

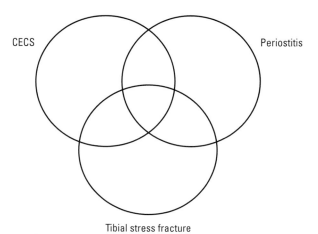

Tibial stress fracture

Figure 22.1 Interaction between stress fractures of the tibia, periostitis, and chronic exertional compartment syndrome (CECS) conditions causing shin pain. (Reproduced from Blackman 2000 with the permission of Lippincott Williams and Wilkins.)

bone resistance to strain (Beck 1998, Burr et al 1997, Li et al 1985).

Risk factors

Risk factors for the development of stress fractures have been studied. In female track and field athletes, lower bone density, history of menstrual disturbance, less lean mass in the lower limbs, lower fat diet, and leg length discrepancy were found to be of some predictive value (Bennell et al 1996). Female athletes who developed a stress fracture had a later age of menarche and fewer menses per year.

Intrinsic factors have been studied for an association with stress fractures of the tibia (Tsai-Fetlander et al 1996). These included anthropometry, range of motion, isokinetic plantar flexion muscle performance, and gait pattern. No intrinsic factors were associated with the development of stress fractures of the tibia. The only positive finding by Tsai-Fetlander et al (1996) was that the tibial stress fracture occurred in the push off/landing leg in nine of ten subjects.

Another study compared the tibial bone geometry, tibial bone mass, and ground reaction force parameter of runners who had sustained a tibial stress fracture with a control group who had not. The conclusion was that bone geometry played a role in stress fracture development and that male athletes with smaller bones in relation to body size are at greater risk of sustaining a tibial stress fracture (Crossley et al 1998). This supports studies from military recruits that show that bone geometry is related to stress fractures (Beck et al 1996).

In a study on military recruits, those who had poor physical fitness or lower levels of physical activity before entry into the military, had an increased risk of developing a stress fracture (Brodine et al 1999). Military recruits are clearly a different population with a different activity program from athletes.

History and clinical findings

The most suspicious diagnostic finding in the taking of a history for tibial stress fractures is the gradual, non-traumatic onset of a localized area of pain over anterior or medial tibial borders for tibial stress fractures, or lateral fibula for fibular stress fractures. If the athlete can point with a finger to an area of pain over bone, then this is a stress fracture until proven otherwise by negative bone scan. This does not mean that a more diffuse pain (greater than 5 cm) could not be due to a stress fracture, but the differential diagnosis has to be broadened to include periostitis and compartment syndrome. The usual location for tibial stress fracture is over the distal third medial tibial border. Also, more proximal medial tibia stress fractures tend to have a more diffuse pain pattern into the post medial calf, at times convincing the athlete that there is a muscle strain. Only an anatomically-directed physical examination, indicating that the area of maximal tenderness is over bone and not the medial gastrocnemius or soleus, with or without a positive bone scan at the proximal tibia, will change the athlete's mind.

Intrinsic (alignment, strength, flexibility, gender, history of previous injury) and extrinsic (training, footwear, terrain) factors are believed to be important in the development of stress fractures. Most of the extrinsic factors are discerned on history-taking. Since most stress fractures occur within 7–8 weeks of an increase in training frequency, duration, and/or intensity, this information must be extracted. It is notable that this encompasses the most porous phase of the bone remodeling cycle. The recurrence of pain with the reintroduction of activity after a period of decreased weightbearing can be of some help in the differentiation between various forms of exercise-induced leg pain. If the pain recurs immediately after several weeks or months off from weightbearing activity, it is more suggestive of periostitis or compartment syndrome and is less likely to be due to a stress fracture. If the pain recurs after several bouts of activity, it is suggestive of a stress fracture.

If the localized area of pain is over the anterior tibia or medial malleolus, then the clinical suspicion of the presence of a stress fracture should be heightened. Definitive diagnosis with a bone scan is important (Wilcox et al 1997), as a stress fracture at one of these sites is more prone to non-union, progressing to a completed fracture (Collier et al 1984). In these high-risk stress fractures, similar to femoral neck and navicular fractures, we would recommend a follow-up computed tomography (CT) scan to delineate the degree of fracture. Early diagnosis is imperative to reduce morbidity.

A past history of stress fractures is useful in pursuit of the determination of female athlete triad, repetitive training errors, and/or biomechanical issues.

Physical examination

The physical examination includes biomechanical assessment, pain response to the single leg hop (this may clarify the exact location of the pain), and strength and flexibility at the hip, knee and ankle. Palpation away from, and then over the area of maximal tenderness including muscle, tendon, and bone can help to ascertain the injured tissue. Neurovascular function should always be assessed. With a stress fracture, the hop test is generally positive. At times, hopping is not possible due to the pain or is guarded and limited. A vigorous hop test

that is negative makes the presence of a stress fracture unlikely, but a positive test is non-specific and can be due to other causes.

Treatment

Tibial stress fractures generally respond with a decrease in pain to: ice, physical therapy modalities, non-steroidal anti-inflammatory medications, non-weightbearing cardiovascular activity to maintain fitness, core and lower extremity strengthening/flexibility, optimizing footwear, and appropriate use of orthotics.

Based on the bowstring effect of the gastrocnemius–soleus complex on the tibia, there is the concern that strengthening and/or stretching this muscle complex will exacerbate the tibial strain and prolong healing, and they are therefore contraindicated (Beck 1998). Having said that, most rehabilitation programs for tibial stress fractures include flexibility and strengthening exercises in parallel with healing (Brukner 2000, Matheson et al 1987). Prospective clinical studies comparing the results of different treatment protocols on healing are required.

Once the injured leg is free of the awareness of pain for 10–14 days in activities of daily living, then the sport-specific activity can be gradually introduced (Table 22.1).

Stress fractures of the anterior tibial cortex may be evident as 'the dreaded black line' on X-ray. This is a horizontal cortical defect representing bony resorption and non-union at the stress fracture site. Bone scan may be negative in this setting. This fracture can be very slow to heal, therefore some suggest intramedullary nailing of the tibia, and drilling or scalloping out the bony cortex involving the fracture, or bone grafting, if there has not been healing by 4–6 months (Chang & Harris 1996). This approach can allow return to activity after 2 months (Brukner & Khan 2001). Stress fractures of the medial malleolus can also be slow to heal, prompting internal

Table 22.1 Program for gradual return to sport after tibial stress fractures

Day	Activity
1	Do 10% of a regular workout
3	Do 20% of a regular workout
5	Do 30% of a regular workout
7	Do 20% of a regular workout
9	Do 40% of a regular workout
11	Do 50% of a regular workout
13	Do 40% of a regular workout
15	Do 60% of a regular workout
17	Do 70% of a regular workout
19	Do 60% of a regular workout
21	Do 80% of a regular workout
23	Do 90% of a regular workout
25	Do 80% of a regular workout
27	Do 100% of a regular workout

On even days (i.e. 2, 4, 6, etc) crosstrain

fixation to hasten recovery if the X-ray shows a radiolucent line (Shelbourne et al 1988).

An alternative approach is a non-surgical trial with a modified load, long pneumatic leg brace (Aircast), and electrical stimulation for 10 h per day. If there has been no healing after 4–6 months, then surgery is pursued (Brukner 2000).

There have been a few studies on the use of a pneumatic leg brace in athletes with a stress fracture. These athletes demonstrated the ability to stay involved in their sports and also had a faster healing time compared to the non-brace group (DeLacerda 1981, Swenson et al 1997, Whitelaw et al 1991).

A promising adjuvant therapy to hasten stress fracture recovery is the use of electrical stimulation (Beck 1998, Benazzo et al 1995). This has been shown to be effective in traumatic non-union fractures and bone grafting (Scott & King 1994, Sharrard 1990, Wilber & Russell 1979).

When dealing with an entity that can cause significant disruption in sport, advances in non-surgical approaches that hasten healing are always welcome.

PERIOSTITIS

Periostitis is considered synonymous with medial tibial stress syndrome and inflammatory shin pain. This is characterized by gradual onset, with weightbearing-related diffuse medial or anterior border tibial pain near the junction of middle and distal third.

The etiology is uncertain and controversial. One proposal is that it is inflammation due to traction of muscle/fascial attachment along the periosteum (Batt 1995, Detmer 1986). The medial origin of the soleus and its fascia attach in the area (Michael & Holder 1985). The posterior tibial muscle has been implicated, but this would appear to be erroneous. The posterior tibial muscle origin is the upper two-thirds of the interosseous membrane, medial fibula, and lateral tibia, which is not the location of periostitis. A second proposal is that periostitis exists on a bone injury continuum with stress fracture being more severe and periostitis more mild (Beck 1998). This is supported by the entities being localized in the same area (the junction of the middle/distal third of the tibia), and being present in similar sports. According to this theory, activity results in abnormal bending of the tibia which stimulates resorption of bone and deposition of new bone on its periostial surface.

History

The history of periostitis involves a gradual onset of activity-related anterior or medial leg pain. It is frequent in the weightbearing sports of running, fitness class, soccer, basketball, rugby and ultimate frisbee. The pain worsens with sustained activities and settles with rest, although it can linger for days.

Treatment

Once the diagnosis is made, an appropriate treatment plan is instituted. This includes either the discontinuation of the weightbearing activity until the area is free of the awareness of pain, or a significant decrease of 50% of the duration/distance of the weightbearing activity on alternate days. If the latter approach results in an improvement of the pain, then this is continued until the athlete is free of the awareness of pain. If this does not result in an improvement, then the activity is discontinued. Otherwise, the treatment is similar to the stress fracture scenario with the addition of topical application of non-steroidal anti-inflammatory drugs and/or local phonophoresis or injection with corticosteroid. Also, electrical stimulation may be helpful in the more rapid healing of periostitis (Morris 1991).

If non-operative treatment fails, there is a surgical option involving a fasciotomy of the deep posterior compartment to release the fascial attachment onto the painful portion of the periosteum.

COMPARTMENT SYNDROME

Compartment syndrome is a condition occurring when the pressure within a muscle compartment exceeds the local arterial blood pressure with subsequent ischemia to muscle and nerve. There are four main compartments in the leg surrounded by a tough, inelastic fascial covering. Each compartment has a major nerve which can contribute to the clinical presentation: the deep peroneal nerve in the anterior compartment, the superficial peroneal nerve in the lateral compartment, the saphenous nerve in the superficial posterior compartment, and the tibial nerve in the deep posterior compartment (Fig. 22.2).

Compartment syndrome can present as an acute problem with rapid onset over several hours or as a chronic problem with the symptoms waxing and waning over months to years and often associated with exercise.

Acute compartment syndrome

Acute compartment syndrome most frequently occurs with traumatic tibial fractures, but also can occur with crush injuries, burns, drug overdoses, and exercise. With exercise, acute compartment syndrome usually occurs in the unconditioned individual performing strenuous exercise or in athletes with chronic exertional compartment syndrome who are exposed to a higher

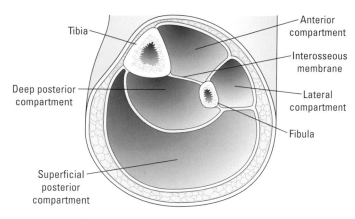

Figure 22.2   Compartments of the lower leg.

intensity and/or duration of exercise (Fehlandt & Micheli 1995, Leach et al 1967, Shrier 1991, Stollsteimer & Shelton 1997).

History and physical examination

As a result of history-taking, the salient features of acute compartment syndrome are significant: severe lower leg pain, swelling over the involved compartment, weakness such as foot drop or foot slapping for the anterior compartment, and numbness/tingling.

On examination, there is antalgic gait, severe pain on passive stretch of the muscles, poor active contraction, paresthenia/hypesthesia in the distribution of the involved nerve, and a possible impression of the presence of pain that is out of proportion to the physical findings.

Chronic exertional compartment syndrome

Chronic exertional compartment syndrome (CECS) has an uncertain etiology. It is normal for exercise to result in a 20% increase in compartment volume due to myofiber swelling and increased intracompartmental blood volume (Amendola & Rorabeck 1985). It has been suggested that the development of the abnormal increase in compartment pressure that characterizes compartment syndrome is due to: (1) the muscle hypertrophy that occurs with exercise (Amendola & Rorabeck 1985), (2) fascial hypertrophy becoming tight and unyielding from exercise (Amendola & Rorabeck 1985, Detmer 1986, Martens et al 1984), and (3) eccentric muscle contraction causing myofiber damage with release of protein-bound ions and an increase in osmotic pressures in the compartment (Edwards & Myerson 1996). The increase in compartment pressure causes ischemia due to: (1) the increase in osmotic pressure which results in increased capillary relaxation pressure, then decrease in blood flow

(Edwards & Myerson 1996); (2) arterial spasm, then decrease in arterial inflow (Matsen 1975); and/or (3) arteriolar or venous collapse due to transmural pressure (Raneman 1975). It is interesting that the best available techniques for detection of ischemia have been unsuccessful, although new infrared spectroscopy may show a decrease in muscle oxygenation (Amendola et al 1990, Blackman 2000, Breit et al 1997, Mohler et al 1997). The use of phosphofructose as a reflection of anaerobic metabolism, has demonstrated that phosphofructose within the muscle decreased after fasciotomy (Embrec 1996).

The anterior compartment is involved in 45% of CECS; the deep posterior in 40%; the lateral in 10%; and the superficial posterior in 5% (Edwards & Myerson 1996). Some have suggested that the anterior compartment is involved in 70–80% of CECS (Korkola & Amendola 2001). The posterior tibial compartment (the fifth compartment) involvement in CECS is rare.

History and physical findings

The characteristic symptoms of CECS include an achy, sharp or dull pain or tightness that comes on predictably with exercise, and settles within 30 min of rest. The symptoms are bilateral in 50–70% of athletes and tend to occur with running or repetitive stress sports. The athletes are usually young (less than 30 years old) (Edwards & Myerson 1996).

The physical examination is usually unremarkable. There may be the reproduction of characteristic symptoms with repetitive, manually resisted ankle movement, particularly for anterior CECS. Also, examining the athlete after sport participation that caused the symptoms may reveal swelling, tenderness, and weakness of the compartment, and hypesthesia to light touch of the involved nerve.

Treatment

The treatment of CECS is seemingly straightforward. Generally there is the impression that the only successful treatment is surgery (Howard et al 2000). There have been few reports of successful non-operative treatment of CECS (Hutchison & Ireland 1994). There may be some athletes with CECS who institute a conservative treatment program early in the disease process, settle their symptoms, and successfully return to their activities. They may not have had the condition long enough to prompt the compartment pressure measurements/fasciotomy path. The average duration of symptoms prior to diagnosis and fasciotomy can be 16 months for posterior CECS, and 6.8 months for anterior CECS (Schepsis et al 1993).

A conservative treatment program would address extrinsic factors of training, footwear and surface, and intrinsic factors of alignment (from leg length to foot function – pronation/supination), flexibility, and strength (core, hip, leg muscles).

The success rate of fasciotomy for anterior CECS is much higher (90% good to excellent) than for posterior CECS (50–65% good to excellent). This may reflect an inadequate release, a persistent soleus bridge, scarring over the fasciotomy defect, entrapment neuropathy in the scar, or incorrect diagnosis (Edwards & Myerson 1996, Howard et al 2000, Rorabek et al 1983, 1988, Schepsis et al 1993, Wiley et al 1987).

The postoperative treatment plan is assisted to full weightbearing active and passive leg exercise during the first week, cycling in the second week, strengthening through the 3rd and 4th weeks, running in the 5th and 6th weeks, speed/agility drills by the 8th week and back to sport for the 8th to 12th week (Edwards & Myerson 1996). Athletes with fasciotomy for posterior CECS often take longer to progress through the treatment plan.

LESS COMMON SPORT-RELATED INJURIES

NERVE ENTRAPMENT

Nerve entrapments commonly occur in the lower leg and diagnosis is often a challenge. Nerve entrapment injuries are often not immediately recognized. Symptoms depend on the function of the injured peripheral nerve. Injured motor nerves present more commonly with pain (even if they lack a sensory component) and weakness, and injured sensory nerves present with pain, numbness and/or tingling. Physical examination should identify any motor or sensory deficits. A lidocaine (lignocaine) injection test into the area of maximal tenderness can often facilitate muscle strength assessment if guarding is present. Abnormal reflexes are usually not found since a reflex is comprised of more than one nerve root. Light tapping over a nerve close to the skin surface that results in radiating tingling, numbness, or an electrical sensation can identify an entrapped nerve (a positive Tinel's sign). Nerve conduction studies conducted by a neurologist or physiatrist localize the nerve injury and provide a prognosis for recovery.

Common peroneal nerve

The common peroneal nerve, a branch of the sciatic nerve, passes through the lateral popliteal fossa, wraps around the head of the fibula and descends 10 cm before passing through the peroneus longus tendon. The nerve then divides into the deep and superficial peroneal nerve. The superficial peroneal nerve innervates the muscles of the lateral compartment (peroneus longus and brevis) as well as the skin of the dorsum of the foot. The deep peroneal nerve innervates the muscles of the anterior compartment (tibialis anterior, peroneus tertius, extensor digitorum longus, extensor hallucis longus, extensor digitorum brevis) and the skin of the first webspace.

The common peroneal nerve is more commonly injured than its superficial and deep branches. Injury can occur by traction, compression, laceration, and ischemia. Stretching of the common peroneal nerve occurs following ankle inversion injuries, major knee ligamentous injuries (anterior cruciate ligament, posterior cruciate ligament, and lateral collateral ligament injury), fractures or dislocations, and bungee jumping (Feinberg et al 1997).

Direct compression can be caused by isolated traumas to the proximal fibula. This may also cause posterolateral subluxation of the superior tibiofibular joint. This is often seen in contact sports via hockey pucks, soccer kicks, football helmets, and falls on a minimally flexed knee. Other more insidious causes are tight ski boots, ice skates, braces, and casts. An accessory ossicle in the lateral gastrocnemius muscle (fabella syndrome) and a tight fascial band at the edge of the peroneus longus muscle, which is most often symptomatic in runners, can compress the common peroneal nerve (Feinberg et al 1997).

Compartment syndromes are associated with compression of the superficial (lateral and occasionally anterior compartments) and deep peroneal (anterior compartment) nerve entrapments. Sensory function of the nerve is more commonly affected, though motor manifestations are possible in more extreme cases. Nerve injury of common peroneal tendon results in:

- Pain, numbness and/or tingling over the dorsum of the foot
- Weakness in the ankle dorsiflexors and evertors as well as toe extensors
- No change in ankle jerk reflex.

This is distinct from superficial peroneal nerve injury where there is only weakness of the ankle evertors and no sensory changes in the first webspace.

Tarsal tunnel syndrome

The tibial nerve, a continuation of the sciatic nerve, travels through the popliteal fossa into the posterior compartment of the leg and then resurfaces in the tarsal tunnel. The tarsal tunnel, which lies posterior to the medial malleolus, is formed by bones of the foot and roofed by the flexor retinaculum. Its contents include the posterior tibial nerve, artery and vein as well as the tendon sheaths of tibialis posterior, flexor digitorum longus and flexor hallucis longus. Beyond the tarsal tunnel, the tibial nerve branches further into the lateral plantar, medial plantar and calcaneal nerves, which supply sensation to the sole of the foot and innervate all intrinsic foot muscles.

Tibial nerve injuries are uncommon owing to protection by the calf muscles. Severe trauma such as tibial fractures and deep lacerations would be the most common injury scenario.

Reported mechanisms include:

- Compression by a synovial cyst, ganglion, or os trigonum (accessory ossicle of the posterior talus present in 10% of the population)
- Repetitive ankle flexion and extension that results in tenosynovitis of the adjacent tunnel occupants
- Fibrosis following ankle sprains
- Local trauma or overuse in individuals with excessive pronation (Lau & Daniels 1999).

The diagnosis of tarsal tunnel syndrome is common in runners and mountain climbers. Symptoms of tarsal tunnel nerve entrapment include:

- Pain, tingling and numbness over the sole of the foot which can be worsened with weightbearing
- Weakness of the intrinsic muscles of the foot which can result in a weak push-off phase of gait
- Clawing of the toes in longstanding injury.

Tarsal tunnel nerve entrapment is likely to be over-diagnosed since suspected clinical cases of tarsal tunnel syndrome often yield no abnormalities on nerve conduction studies (NCG) and electromyography (EMG).

Treatment of nerve injuries

The first step is to identify and correct contributing factors to the nerve injury. If inflammation is believed to contribute to the injury, treatment can include the use of oral anti-inflammatories or local corticosteroid injection from the treating physician. Footwear should be modified if it is too constrictive and orthotics may be prescribed if there is excessive pronation.

Decompressive surgery is indicated acutely in peroneal nerve sheath hematoma. It is also useful in cases resistant to conservative treatment, such as compartment syndromes, as well as impingement from osteophytes, accessory ossicles, ganglions, cysts, or soft tissue strictures.

If all contributing factors are corrected, time becomes the determining factor in recovery, provided the damage is not too extensive. Nerves regenerate at a rate of 1–7 mm per day.

TENDINOPATHY

Tendon disorders are easily diagnosed but treatment is a challenge. The majority of cases are seen in a setting of overuse and are a degenerative tendinopathy rather than inflammatory tendonitis. Tendon disease or tendinopathy is a spectrum of conditions:

- Tendinitis (inflammation of the tendon)
- Tenosynovitis or paratendinitis (inflammation of tissues surrounding tendon)
- Tendinosis (focal degenerative lesions of the tendon tissue)
- Partial rupture
- Complete rupture.

These pathologies can occur in isolation or in combination with each other. Leadbetter (1992) illustrated the association of pain and tissue damage in overuse tendinopathy (Fig. 22.3). References are provided for a more detailed explanation of the associated histopathological changes (Khan et al 1999, 2000, Kvist 1994).

There is a classification of symptom severity in tendinopathy: (1) pain after activity only; (2) pain at the start of activity that resolves but recurs after activity; (3) pain at start, during and after activity that limits full activity; and (4) pain with daily activities. Unfortunately, this classification does not provide any insight into prognosis.

Achilles tendon

Anatomy and risk factors

The Achilles tendon is made up of separate contributions from the gastrocnemius and soleus muscles. The Achilles tendon has a paratenon which is an elastic sleeve that allows freedom of movement of the tendon instead of a synovial sheath. Activities where Achilles tendinopathy is common include basketball, cycling, cross-country skiing, dancing, figure skating, and running.

More common risk factors are:

- Training errors: repetitive loading of a competitive athlete or the acute overload of a recreational athlete; higher weekly mileage, rapid increases in mileage, increased interval training, hard slippery training surfaces and a history of similar injury in the past 12 months are noted specially in runners
- Decreased calf muscle strength and flexibility
- Pes cavus feet due to the reduced shock absorption, and ankle dorsiflexion and pes planus which is a result of the wringing action on the tendon from the resultant overpronation

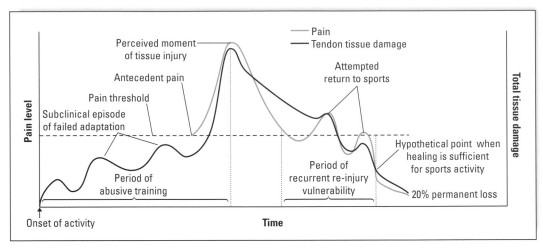

Figure 22.3 Illustration of pain and tissue damage in overuse tendinopathy. (Reproduced with permission from Leadbetter 1992.)

- Improper footwear
- Increasing age which is associated with a decrease in muscle strength and flexibility, as well as in tendon's vascular supply
- Male gender (Alfredson & Lorentzon 2000).

History and physical findings

The classification of Achilles tendinopathy and clinical findings are in Table 22.2. Individuals describe a history of heel pain that is the result of a defined episode. Usually, there is progressive worsening of symptom

Table 22.2 Classification of Achilles tendinopathy and clinical findings (reproduced from Brukner & Khan 1993 with the permission of McGraw Hill)

Classification	Pathology	History	Examination findings
Tendinitis	Local tissue edema Disruption of ground substance rather than damage to tendon fibers Focal degeneration of tendon fibers may develop	Gradual onset of symptoms Pain worse in morning Pain worse on commencing activity and some time after ceasing activity	Marked swelling Extending over several centimeters Thickening of site of pain extending a variable number of centimeters along tendon Decreased extensibility of tendon

Paratendinitis
  Acute
 	
  Chronic
	Acute inflammatory swelling within paratendon
	Chronic inflammation with fibrosis and scarring
		Sudden onset (e.g. pressure from shoes)
		Repeated trauma
			Swelling edema and crepitus in paratendon
			Firm scarred bands within paratendon

Focal degeneration	Granulomatous changes Loss of normal wavy alignment of collagen	Gradual onset of symptoms Significant pain	Local tenderness May have good function, little swelling
Partial tear	Variable size and site of tear Longitudinal or traverse tear Deep or superficial	Sudden onset of symptoms Pain often increases with activity	Local tenderness and swelling Palpable defect in tendon Pain on resisted plantarflexion (associated with paratendinitis)
Complete rupture	Complete rupture of tendon complex ?Related to degeneration ?Related to corticosteroid injection	Single incident Feel (hear) snap in tendon Immediate weakness and disability	Palpable (visible) defect in tendon when acute Thomson's test positive Some active plantarflexion may be possible
Mixed lesions	Combinations (e.g. paratendinitis and tendonitis or partial tear)	Combination of symptoms	Combination of signs makes diagnosis difficult

severity if it is left untreated. Complete Achilles tendon rupture is characterized by immediate pain that quickly resolves. Often, individuals hear a pop or snap and feel as though they have been kicked. Asymptomatic rupture has been noted to be as high as 30% in some case series and this can lead to a delay in diagnosis (Leppilahti & Orava 1998).

Physical examination helps to define the Achilles pathology. Paratendonitis can present with acute swelling and crepitation. As the condition becomes chronic, these findings are replaced by diffuse or local thickening of subcutaneous soft tissues. Tenderness is present on both sides of the tendon.

Insertional tendinopathy can be at the muscle–tendon or tendon–bone junctions. Proximally, diffuse tenderness is present more often in the medial portion of the gastrocnemius muscle. A defect can be palpated in the same area with partial muscle tears. Distally, a prominence at the posterosuperior aspect of calcaneus can contribute to the Achilles pathology. Bursitis can be either retrocalcaneal (between the insertion of the Achilles and the os calcis) or superficial (between the Achilles tendon insertion and the skin). This condition tends to elicit signs of inflammation (redness, swelling, and tenderness).

Tendinosis and partial tendon ruptures are often difficult to distinguish clinically from each other as they often coexist. Confirmation of these conditions is noted by the presence of nodules in the substance of the Achilles tendon.

The most commonly used signs of complete Achilles tendon rupture include significant swelling and bruising, as well as a palpable gap in the area of the Achilles tendon. Reduced or absent plantar flexion strength and absent plantar flexion following a squeeze of the calf muscle (Thompson's test) are almost universal.

Differential diagnosis

The differential diagnoses of Achilles tendon injuries are listed in Box 22.1.

Treatment

Conservative treatment is initially recommended for all Achilles tendinopathies with the exception of complete tendon ruptures, though this is not absolute. Conservative treatment typically consists of symptomatic relief and correction of etiological factors:

* *Activity modification.* Reduce the level (intensity or amount) of activity so that the individual experiences no symptoms. If necessary, the activity should be stopped and only non-aggravating sport-specific skills should be maintained. Cross-training with activities such as cycling, pool running, and swimming that do

Box 22.1 Differential diagnoses of Achilles tendon injuries (reproduced from Kvist 1994 with the permission of Adis Press International)

* Calcaneal apophysitis (Sever's disease)
* Posterior tibial stress syndrome, soleus syndrome (shin splints)
* Tenosynovitis or dislocation of the peroneal tendons
* Tenosynovitis of the plantar flexors of the foot (tibialis posterior, flexor hallucis longus, flexor digiti)
* Plantar fasciitis
* Stress fractures at the ankle region
* Tarsal tunnel syndrome (entrapment of medial calcaneal branch of posterior tibial nerve)
* Neuroma/neuritis of the sural nerve near the Achilles tendon
* Calcaneal periostitis (often post-traumatic bone bruise)
* Spontaneous rupture of the posterior tibial tendon muscle
* Tennis leg (medial gastrocnemius tear)
* Inflammation of ankle ligaments in the calcaneal insertion
* Bone anomalies (painful large os trigonum)
* Calf muscle and Achilles tendon anomalies: anomalous soleus muscle
* Post-traumatic pain syndromes in the ankle and leg (direct and indirect)
* Arthritic conditions (rheumatic arthritis, Rieter Syndrome, gout, ankylosing spondylitis, 'fibrositis')
* Tumors of the Achilles tendon (e.g. ossification, xanthomas)
* Systemic or local alterations in the tendon tissue (e.g. infections, vascular diseases, calcifying tendonitis)
* Diseases of the calcaneal bone (e.g. osteomyelitis, osteoid osteoma)

not cause the condition to flare up should be implemented. The duration of this phase is variable and graduated return to sports (see below) can be attempted when there are no longer any symptoms. Absolute rest is seldom needed and should be minimized.

* *Corticosteroid injections.* The effectiveness of this intervention is not well supported in the literature. It may contribute to tendon rupture though this cause and effect relationship is not fully supported.
* *Local treatment.* These interventions include cold, heat, massage, ultrasound, electrical stimulation, and laser therapy. They are commonly used, though they have not been well studied in controlled trials.
* *Non-steroidal anti-inflammatory drugs (NSAIDs).* These medications seem appropriate for flare-ups of inflammation but are not likely to be helpful in chronic painful tendinosis since the pain mediating mechanisms are not well understood.
* *Orthoses/Footwear.* Heel lifts and orthotics should be used to address concerns regarding tight calf muscles and excessive pronation, respectively. Individual consideration should be given in deciding the need for these orthoses and if they are needed, then to the amount of correction necessary. Appropriate shoes should be recommended for the individual's foot type. Gait studies can provide objective evidence to support orthotic prescription.

- *Stretching and strengthening.* Both stretching and eccentric strengthening have been advocated as the mainstay of treatment. A recent prospective study by Alfredson et al (1998) demonstrated significant improvement in patients with chronic mid-Achilles pain who had failed conservative treatment, including the above treatment options and physical therapy, and were awaiting surgery. The 12 week eccentric heel drop program (3 × 15 repetitions performed twice daily) for both the soleus (knee bent) and gastrocnemius (knee straight) muscles resulted in the resolution of pain, return to preinjury activity levels, and the avoidance of surgery. Despite the potential of symptom worsening in the first 2 weeks, the patient is advised to continue the program. Advancing the program with added weight in a backpack should take place when the exercise is pain-free. Niessen-Vertommen (1992) demonstrated the effectiveness of the eccentric heel drop as proposed by Curwin & Stanish (1984).
- *Lithotripsy extra-corporeal shock wave therapy.* This has recently been applied to the treatment of tendinopathies with promising preliminary results. The goal of treatment is to lessen pain and this may occur by the reduction of scar tissue; it also allows enhanced stretching and strengthening rehabilitation.
- *Return to sport.* A walk–run program is implemented when there are no longer any symptoms. After symptom-free running, sport-specific running drills are implemented. These drills include forward sprinting, backward sprinting, lateral cross-overs, zig-zag sprinting, and 90° turning (Fig. 22.4). Speed and distances should be sport specific (e.g. tennis drills that are performed on half the tennis court). When implementing this program, common errors that may result in non-resolution of the injury are: (1) accelerating the progress of a program which exceeds the ability of tissues to adapt, and (2) not backing down from pain, which is an indication of the body's inability to adapt to stresses placed on tissues.

Surgery is recommended for individuals who have not improved with conservative treatment. This happens in approximately 20–25% of patients initially diagnosed with Achilles tendinopathy. Achilles tendon ruptures are usually treated primarily by surgical intervention, though conservative treatment protocols are also used. In prospective studies with follow-up over several years, good to excellent results have been seen in approximately 80% of patients (Maffuli et al 1997, Rolf & Movin 1997). Outcome measures are needed to assess response to the various treatments proposed. Imaging studies are known to be inadequate in this capacity. The VISA Achilles tendon questionnaire (see Cook et al 2001) is a reliable and valid tool to assess the severity of Achilles tendinopathy (Khan et al 1998, Visentini et al 1998). Unlike imaging studies, this tool can be used as a clinical and research outcome measure in monitoring a patient's response to treatment (Fig. 22.5).

Tibialis tendons

Tibialis posterior

The tibialis posterior muscle acts to plantarflex the ankle, and invert the foot, which stabilizes the foot during gait. It is important to note that an accessory navicular bone that is secured to the medial side of the navicular bone by a non-osseus union is present in 5% of the population. It tends to be more prevalent in those with tibialis posterior tendinopathy.

The most common population with this condition is middle-aged or elderly women. Common risk factors include:

- Eversion ankle sprains
- Rheumatological diseases (most notably, lupus, gout, rheumatoid arthritis)
- Obesity (time and additional stress) (Schweitzer & Karasick 2000)
- Excessive pronation (Yeap et al 2001).

Activities commonly related to this condition include basketball, speed skating, and track running, especially on indoor tracks where tight banks exist.

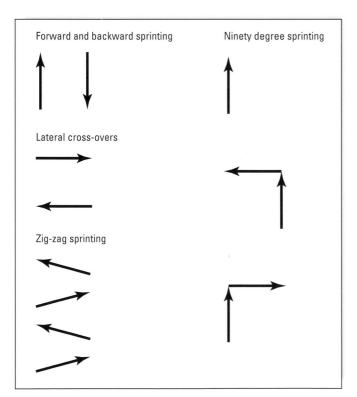

Figure 22.4 Return to sport running drills after Achilles tendinopathy.

1. For how many minutes can you sit pain free?

0 minutes | | | | | | | | | | | 100 minutes
           1 2 3 4 5 6 7 8 9 10

2. Do you have pain walking downstairs with a normal gait cycle?

Strong severe pain | | | | | | | | | | | No pain
           1 2 3 4 5 6 7 8 9 10

3. Do you have pain at the front of the knee with full active non-weightbearing knee extension?

Strong severe pain | | | | | | | | | | | No pain
           1 2 3 4 5 6 7 8 9 10

4. Do you have pain when doing a full weightbearing lunge?

Strong severe pain | | | | | | | | | | | No pain
           1 2 3 4 5 6 7 8 9 10

5. Do you have problems squatting?

Strong severe pain | | | | | | | | | | | No pain
           1 2 3 4 5 6 7 8 9 10

6. Do you have pain during or immediately after doing 10 single leg hops?

Strong severe pain | | | | | | | | | | | No pain
           1 2 3 4 5 6 7 8 9 10

7. Are you currently undertaking sport or other physical activity?

0	Not at all
4	Modified training ± modified competition
7	Full training ± competition but not at the same level as when symptoms began
10	Competing at the same or higher level as when symptoms began

8. Please complete **EITHER A, B, or C** in this question.
  • If you have **no pain** while undertaking sport, please complete Q8a only.
  • If you **have pain** while undertaking sport but it does not stop you from completing the activity, please complete Q8b only.
  • If you **have pain** that stops you from completing sporting activities, please complete Q8c only.

8a. If you have no pain while undertaking sport, for how long can you train/practice?

Nil	0–5 mins	6–10 mins	11–15 mins	> 15 mins
0	7	14	21	30

OR

8b. If you have some pain while undertaking sport, but it does not stop you from completing your training/practice, for how long can you train/practice?

Nil	0–5 mins	6–10 mins	11–15 mins	> 15 mins
0	4	10	14	21

OR

8c. If you have pain that stops you from completing your training/practice, for how long can you train/practice?

Nil	0–5 mins	6–10 mins	11–15 mins	> 15 mins
0	2	5	7	10

TOTAL VISA SCORE [ ]

Figure 22.5 VISA Achilles tendon questionnaire. (Reproduced with permission from Cook et al 2001.)

Presentation typically involves medial ankle pain that can radiate along the course of the tendon. Tendon rupture results in immediate pain, swelling, and disability. Examination findings can include pronated gait pattern, poor functional testing (single leg hop or heel raise) as compared to the uninjured side, and swelling and tenderness along the course of the tendon. Pain and weakness are seen on resisted inversion and pain can be experienced on passive eversion. The tibialis posterior tendon can gradually become insufficient and stretch out; this leads to excessive pronation and increased pes planus on that side. Physical findings include the inability to perform a single leg heel raise and the 'too many toes sign'. The latter is evident when the foot is viewed from the back, where one can see more toes beyond the posterior ankle/foot on the side with the weak tibialis posterior tendon. Tibialis posterior tendinopathy may coexist with tarsal tunnel syndrome due to pes planus.

Tibialis anterior

Tibialis anterior acts to dorsiflex the ankle, invert the foot, and stabilize the foot during gait. It is more commonly seen in sports with repeated dorsiflexion such as cross-country skiing or down hill running. Excessively tight footwear may also irritate the tendon. Pain is noted over the anterior ankle. Tenderness is localized over the tendon and pain is felt on resisted dorsiflexion and inversion. Swelling and crepitus may be noted.

Ultrasound (US) and magnetic resonance imaging (MRI) are helpful in confirming degenerative changes in the tibialis anterior and posterior tendons, including complete ruptures.

Treatment of tibialis tendinopathies

Conservative treatment for both tendinopathies should include relative rest, local treatment, and NSAIDs if they prove to be effective. Orthoses and motion control shoes should be considered in the case of tibialis posterior tendinopathy if pronation is present. Ankle stabilizer braces may be helpful in alleviating forces through the tendons. Loosening tight shoelaces or selecting less restrictive footwear may be helpful with treatment of tibialis anterior tendinopathy. The same principles as noted for Achilles tendinopathy should be used in eccentric strengthening of these tendons (ankle eversion drops for tibialis posterior and ankle plantarflexion drops for tibialis anterior). A period of immobilization in tibialis posterior tendinopathy may sometimes be suggested if symptomatic relief is not possible with the above regimen. Outcome of conservative treatment has not been assessed in the literature to date. Surgical treatment should be considered in cases of failed conservative treatment or acute rupture.

Peroneus longus and brevis tendons

The peroneal tendons originate from the lateral fibular shaft and travel posterior to the lateral malleolus. These muscles act together to plantarflex the ankle, and evert the foot, which stabilizes the foot during gait. Peroneal tendinopathy can often be associated with a secondary problem such as ankle instability, degenerative osteophytes, and tendon subluxation. Tears of the peroneus brevis tend to occur at the tip of the lateral malleolus whereas tears of the peroneus longus occur under the cuboid. Dislocation of the peroneal tendons can occur more commonly following recurrent ankle inversion injuries. These problems are more likely to occur in those who excessively supinate due to pes cavus.

Physical examination tends to reveal acute swelling and tenderness along the course of the tendon. Chronic swelling and tendon thickening may be seen.

Treatment of peroneal tendinopathies

Peroneal tendinopathies should initially be treated conservatively. Symptom relief should include relative rest, local treatment, and NSAIDs. If causative features include poor foot mechanics or ankle instability, orthoses and ankle stabilizer braces may be helpful. Eccentric strengthening is done using ankle inversion drops. Surgical treatment should be considered in cases of failed conservative treatment, peroneal subluxation/dislocation or acute rupture. Surgical outcomes are reported mainly for repair of tendon ruptures (Krause & Brodsky 1998, Sammarco 1995). Research needs to be done to assess the outcome of conservative treatment.

POPLITEAL ARTERY ENTRAPMENT SYNDROME

Popliteal artery entrapment syndrome (PAES) has become a more frequently diagnosed cause of exercise-induced lower limb symptoms, especially in young active males (Stager & Clement 1999). The syndrome's complex includes exercise-induced pain, cramping, claudication, and pain of the calf and/or feet. In addition, calf and or foot discoloration, coolness, paresthesia and numbness can occur. This is still an often overlooked diagnosis.

According to Murray et al (1991) the true incidence of PAES is not known. The etiology of the syndrome is based on the embryological development of the popliteal artery and musculature in the popliteal fossa, and according to the results of Stager (1997), can also be seen in association with chronic compartment syndromes of the lower extremity. Zund & Brunner (1995) reported that, in their 26 years of experience with the surgical management of PAES, up to 85% of the individuals diagnosed were males, with a mean age of 28 years. Interestingly, a study conducted by Stager (1997) showed that, of the 23 patients identified in the study, 18 were females (78%) and 5 were males (22%). The mean age was 24.9 years (range 14–41 years) but the females were younger at 22.3 years while the mean age of the males was 34.2 years. Stager (1997) believed that the male predominance in the literature might be due to the bulk of the earlier series being from the military which has high male predominance. In Vancouver (Stager 1997), an increasing female participation in fitness events has been seen. Twenty individuals had bilateral surgery (87%) and of these, 17 patients (85%) had bilateral symptoms, and 3 (15%) had unilateral symptoms. Collins et al (1989) found that up to 67% were bilateral.

Besides the possible variations in embryonic development of the gastrocnemius muscle and the popliteal artery, some have attributed the entrapment of the artery to be due to muscular hypertrophy as a result of exercise,

which compresses the artery between the muscle and the bone. This could occur with active plantarflexion or passive dorsiflexion of the foot. Other rare causes of popliteal artery compression have been large popliteal cysts and fibrous bands in the popliteal fossa.

Classification

There have been a number of different anatomical classifications of PAES. Most have now accepted the modified classification initially proposed by Delaney & Gonzalez (1971), along with a fifth type added by Rich et al (1979). This classification is presented in Figure 22.6.

In type I, the artery follows the classic abnormal route, looping medially and then beneath a normally positioned medial head of the gastrocnemius. In type II, the popliteal artery is in a normal position but is compressed by a more laterally positioned medial head of the gastrocnemius, which has originated from the intercondylar region rather than the medial epicondyle. With type III, the medial head of the gastrocnemius has an additional accessory musculotendinosis slip on its lateral

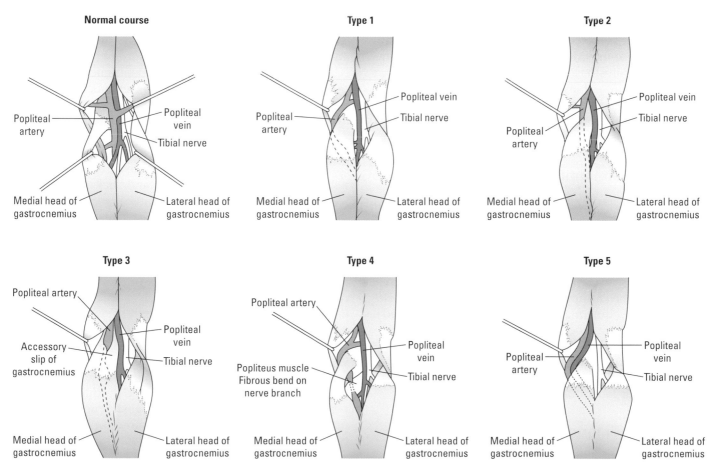

Figure 22.6   Classification of popliteal artery entrapment syndrome. (From Rich et al 1979 in Archives of Surgery 114: 1382, with the permission of the American Medical Association.)

side compressing the artery as it travels across it. In type IV, the popliteal artery is compressed as it passes beneath the popliteus muscle and medial head of the gastrocnemius and finally, with type V, both the popliteal artery and vein are compressed by a normally positioned medial head of the gastrocnemius. Not all anomalies seen at the time of surgery fit into this classification. In addition, the classification has been shown repetitively to have no bearing on clinical diagnosis, therapy or prognosis.

Signs and symptoms

The pathology is one of progressive repeated popliteal artery compressions, which ultimately damage the arterial wall, leading to aneurysm or premature localized atherosclerosis. In some individuals, there can be an acute ischemic presentation with sudden occlusion of the artery or thrombosis within an aneurysm. Most present with progressive exercise-induced leg pain. Murray et al (1991) reported that 90% of patients present with claudication (i.e. absence of pain at rest but calf pain at a fixed exercise level). They reported this to occur occasionally with fast walking, but not running, and believed it was due to the more prolonged gastrocnemius contraction in walking. In their series, 10% presented with signs and symptoms of either acute or chronic limb ischemia. These included coolness of the feet, discoloration of toes, paresthesis and numbness of the feet, and rarely, skin ulcers. Many were given an initial diagnosis of tibial stress pain and the concept of a serious vascular compromise was not considered until they were referred to our clinic after months of ongoing symptoms.

Physical examination

Often, no obvious abnormalities are identified at rest. On closer examination there is often a reduction in the pedal pulses with the ankle in passive dorsiflexion, and in active plantarflexion with the knee extended. In a more advanced case, a popliteal aneurysm may be identified as a pulsatile mass in the popliteal fossa. In the type V cases, the vein may be entrapped with the artery, and exercise-induced leg swelling may be seen. As mentioned already, ischemic changes are occasionally present with discoloration, coolness, and rarely, ischemic foot ulcers.

With a history of exercise-induced calf pain and any of the above signs, it is imperative to coordinate provocative vascular laboratory examination.

Differential diagnosis

The differential diagnosis of PAES is classified into (1) vascular, (2) local musculoskeletal and (3) central neurological etiologies as summarized by Stager (1997).

Treatment

Prior to the final diagnosis being established, patients with PAES have tried gastrocnemius–soleus stretching, and strength protocols and heel lifts, but to no avail. The treatment is ultimately surgical because of the progressive nature of the pathology, and should be done sooner rather than later, to prevent the progressive damage to the vascular wall of the artery and possible embolization. The goal of surgery is to release the compression and entrapment of the artery and to restore normal arterial flow with as normal an artery as possible.

GASTROCNEMIUS–SOLEUS STRAIN – ACUTE, OVERUSE, AND IN A SETTING OF DELAYED ONSET MUSCLE SORENESS (DOMS), AND CALF CONTUSIONS

Gastrocnemius–soleus strains are a very common cause of lower leg pain in sports. The gastrocnemius–soleus mechanism is one of the most commonly strained muscle units. The muscle strains occur in three settings: first, the acute strain as seen in court sports, soccer, football and basketball, occurs as a result of an explosive acceleration; in the second setting, repetitive overuse, one sees chronic overuse gastrocnemius–soleus strains in distance runners; and finally, with more acute exposure to unaccustomed eccentric exercise, the athlete can experience 3–5 days of calf pain as a result of delayed onset muscle soreness. Calf contusions are seen in sports that employ kicking and in those that utilize sticks, balls and pucks.

Gastrocnemius–soleus strains of the acute variety are seen in arenas involving explosive speed and jumping such as tennis, soccer, football and basketball. They occur with fatigue, lack of warm-up, and lack of flexibility. Strains of a chronic overuse nature are seen in the distance runner related to training errors, with sudden increases in volume or intensity, and are also associated with worn out shoes or changes from training shoes with good heel lift to racing flats or spikes. They occur in the face of deficiencies of strength or flexibility, and in changes of surfaces or terrain, such as soft sand running, increased road camber and hills.

The authors have just completed a retrospective analysis of 2002 running injuries seen over the past 2 years (Taunton et al 2002). Gastrocnemius–soleus overuse injuries were the 14th most common injury. The authors identified cases commonly seen in the athlete with the pes cavus foot and associated tight gastrocnemius–soleus unit and midfoot strike during marathon training. The typical case of delayed onset gastrocnemius soreness is seen on the day following a very hilly marathon or cross-country race, particularly in early season. Delayed onset muscle soreness (DOMS) can also be seen the day following unaccustomed skipping, high intensity aerobics, or dancing. Nasty gastrocnemius contusions are also seen in ice hockey when a player is struck by the puck or slashed by a stick on the back of the calf.

Signs and symptoms

Calf pain, local tenderness, swelling, bruising and loss of power are associated with an acute strain. These are graded into mild strains (grade I), partial tears (grade II) and complete tears (grade III). The differentiation of the grades can be confirmed by high resolution ultrasound (Anderson et al 1998). The chronic strain has pain that is more diffuse, has much less swelling, plus tightness in the gastrocnemius and/or soleus, and limited hop power and repetitive single leg heel raise power. Delayed onset muscle soreness is associated with diffuse tenderness in muscles that are tight and mildly swollen, and that have mild loss of function. Smith et al (1994) and Macintyre et al (1995) described DOMS as a feeling of discomfort that is predominantly at the myotendinous junction where connective tissue is most abundant. This occurs 1–2 days after exercise, peaking in intensity by day 3, and disappearing by day 5. Macintyre et al (1995) continued by describing it as a result of eccentric muscle activity which leads to mechanical and biochemical changes within the muscle, making it a 'gold standard' clinical model for muscle induced pain and inflammation. These changes, then, are responsible for the localized swelling, and reduction in range of motion and weakness. Babul (2001) has summarized the current cellular theories as proposed by a number of authors, including Appell et al (1992) and Armstrong (1984, 1990) (Fig. 22.7). The author went on to describe the role of cytokines and oxygen free radical formation leading to further inflammation in DOMS and muscle damage. Downhill injury has been a common initiator in many of the studies investigating DOMS.

Treatment

The classic treatment for the acute gastrocnemius–soleus strain is still pressure, ice and elevation. Pulsed US and interferential current reduce pain and swelling, along with muscle stimulation at a frequency of 2–3 HZ to provide a muscle twitch, not tetani, to create a muscle pump for lymphatic and venous drainage (Taunton et al 1996). This is very important in preventing a deep vein thrombosis in the setting of a calf strain or contusion. Using the principles of wound repair, Daley (1990) outlined, for grades I and II strains, treatment initiated with the principle of RICE (rest, ice, compression and elevation) and early weightbearing to tolerance during phase 1 of the healing cycle. Immediately postinjury, icing is accomplished over a damp elastic wrap for compression, with the leg elevated. This is continued in cycles of 20 min of icing over the next 24–72 h. A normal gait pattern is established with crutches first, with partial weightbearing to comfort, utilizing heel lifts in both shoes to reduce strain. To counteract the loss of the natural muscle pump action for circulation, external support with a compression tape is used. During this initial period, pain-free active foot and ankle motion is encouraged. After 24 h, regular ice massage and exercise is begun. One recommended treatment is to use ice massage for 30 s followed by active exercise for 2 min, progressing to 5 min with active dorsiflexion against an elastic tube or Theraband, then active plantarflexion. Active exercise then progresses to standing closed-kinetic chain exercises, which include partial weightbearing squats and lunges while still incorporating 2–5 cm heel lifts. The compression taping or elastic bandaging is

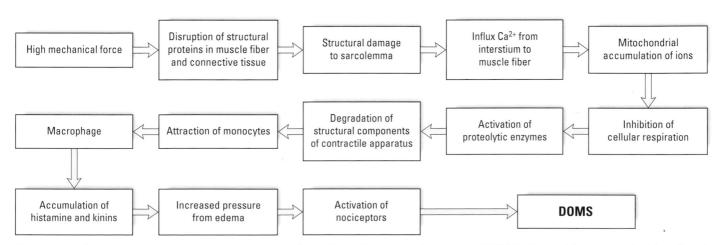

Figure 22.7 Sequence of events in fatiguing exercise leading to delayed onset muscle soreness (DOMS). (Adapted from the work of Appell et al 1992 and Armstong 1984.)

continued for 7–14 days. Dyson et al (1990) recommended pulsed US after the first 24 h to stimulate fibroblastic activity and collagen formation. Ebel (1965) recommended a combination of US muscle stimulation for initiating the muscle pump action. High voltage galvanic and interferential currents can be introduced in this phase to further reduce inflammation and pain and to add to the muscle pump for venous and lymphatic drainage. Phonophoresis using 10% hydrocortisone cream or 10% diclofenac cream can also be implemented.

Once the athlete is fully weightbearing, active exercise progresses to heel raises, followed by eccentric heel drop drills, initially using both heels, then as strength improves, single heel drops are introduced. Prior to this phase, massage and progressive stretching are added to the treatment plan. Cyriax (1981) has shown that friction massage followed by active exercise is often more effective in improving range of motion than passive stretching. As the athlete learns to tolerate the eccentric heel drops, then functional running drills are added. The athlete then progresses through short 20–30 m acceleration runs followed by 10–20 m backward runs, then crossover and cutting drills. Prior to the point of normal gait with full heel contact with the ground, cardiovascular fitness is maintained through pool running and cycling, leading to speed walking. When the athlete can tolerate 30 min of speed walking, a graduated walk/run program is introduced (Table 22.3).

For grade III gastrocnemius–soleus strains, especially at the musculotendinous junction, referral for surgical consideration is required. Conservative non-surgical treatment in a non-weightbearing functional cast or brace with heel lifts can be used, but full strength is seldom achieved and the chance of rerupture is greater than with surgical repairs. The athlete can be placed in a dorsal plaster non-weightbearing splint for the initial postoperative period of 10–14 days. The plaster splint is removed, the patient is placed in a walker boot with a 2.5 cm heel lift and starts immediate full weightbearing. The heel lift is composed of four wedges and one of these wedges is removed every 2 weeks until flat; this is usually at 8–10 weeks postoperatively. Once flat, the patient can then transit from a boot to a normal shoe. During the period of boot wear the patient begins an active physical therapy program consisting of active resisted range of motion exercise within a safe arc so as not to stretch the repair. In addition, gradual strengthening is also carried out with active dorsiflexion and minimal plantarflexion within a safe zone. Scar mobilization is also carried out during this early rehabilitation process. As strength improves, pool walking may begin as well as double leg toe raises with progression to single leg toe raises. By 3–4 months, patients should be walking with a normal gait. Once equal strength is achieved and endurance goals are reached, progression to a running program begins with return to explosive type sports at around 9–12 months postoperatively. Hyperbaric oxygen (HBO) therapy has become increasing popular in sports medicine (Babul 2001). Soft tissue treatment with HBO is effective by (1) reducing the local tissue hypoxia through the increase in partial pressure of oxygen, (2) reducing edema by vasoconstriction and decreasing blood flow to the injured area by hyperbaric compression and (3) by stimulation of fibroblastic processes, collagen synthesis and intracellular ATP production, promoting healing and also prevention of infection. HBO also promotes revascularization, epithelialization and angiogenesis, and capillary budding in tissue healing. Oriani et al (1987) were the first to recognize the use of HBO in sports-related injuries but it has been only recently that controlled double blind studies have been done (Staples & Clement 1996). Soolsma (1996) investigated the short-term recovery of grade II medial collateral ligament injuries of the knee and found more rapid recovery in the HBO treated group. From a clinical point of view, we have found that the regular use of HBO with professional National Hockey League and National Basketball Association players has been very effective in the early treatment of both muscle strains and contusions if utilized in the first 12–24 h. A single person chamber compressed to 2 ATA and the injured athlete breathing 100% oxygen is an example of treatment. The treatment lasts 60 min and is continued for the first 3–5 days, depending on the degree of tissue damage and swelling.

Table 22.3 Sample walk–run program for return to activity after gastrocnemius–soleus strains

Week	Monday	Wednesday	Friday
1	10 min walk	20 min walk	30 min walk
2	6× (4.5 min walk + 0.5 min run)	6× (4 min walk + 1 min run)	6× (3.5 min walk + 1.5 min run)
3	6× (3 min walk + 2 min run)	6× (2.5 min walk + 2.5 min run)	6× (2 min walk + 3 min run)
4	6× (1.5 min walk + 3.5 min run)	6× (1 min walk + 4 min run)	6× (0.5 min walk + 4.5 min run)
5	30 min run	30 min run	30 min run

The walk–run program is started after a patient has demonstrated the ability to walk 30 min consecutively without injury, 3 times per week on alternate days. The goal is to run pain-free 30 min 3 times per week. It involves a total activity period of 30 min structured into 6 sets of 5 min on alternate days. In each set, there is a combination of running and walking where the run component is increased after each session by 30 s.

Treatment of the chronic strain involves reduction of stress by pool running and cycling, reduction of inflammation with topical and oral NSAIDs and improvement of strength via eccentric exercises and stretching; then gradually, a return to weightbearing running on a walk–run basis.

DOMS has been improved with topical anti-inflammatory medication (Hasson et al 1992, Macintyre et al 1995) but stretching prior to exercise and icing have not been very successful in reducing DOMS (High et al 1989). Recently, Babul (2001) has shown that HBO was not effective in reducing DOMS. Previously, Staples et al (1999) conducted an animal and human study on a DOMS model and documented a reduction in the inflammatory marker myeloperoxidase in the animal model with HBO, and an enhanced recovery of eccentric strength, with no effect on pain.

Muscle contusion is treated in a similar manner to grade I and II muscle strains, initially with RICE followed by interferential current and muscle stimulation. Stretching, gentle massage and strength progression from concentric to eccentric heel drops is similar to that previously described. External muscle compression wraps are instituted immediately and continued for 5–7 days, followed by a neoprene sleeve as active exercise is initiated. HBO, if initiated immediately, is very effective in reducing the swelling with muscle contusions.

For all injuries to the calf, the criteria for the return to play are freedom from pain, full power and successful completion of functional sport-specific drills before active practice, then scrimmage and games.

Prevention

The goal of sports medicine is always prevention. In respect to acute calf strains, prevention includes avoidance of local muscle fatigue and dehydration leading to muscle cramps, then muscle strains, as the athlete attempts to run out the cramp in a game or race. Warm-up is essential in prevention of gastrocnemius–soleus strains with static stretching. In addition strength programs throughout the season are critical.

For chronic calf strains, prevention includes avoidance of training errors through not increasing running volume by more than 10% per week, running on a hard day/easy day basis, and avoiding hard training following races. Caution with hill training is also important with a slow introduction of volume and intensity on the hills, just as on the flat. Care with introduction of both uphill and downhill running is needed. Lower extremity strength programs and pre- and postexercise stretching for the runner are recommended, along with cross training on bikes or with pool running once or twice a week on recovery days. Proper shoe selection is also critical,

including choice of motion control shoe for the excessive pronator and curve lasted shoe for the pes cavus supinated foot (with added heel lift) (McKenzie et al 1985). Racing flats and spikes should incorporate heel lifts so that the transition from training to racing shoes is not as severe with regards to the track on gastrocnemius–soleus and Achilles tendon.

DOMS has been prevented, or the degree of damage reduced, with prior training and adaptation (Schwane et al 1983). Newham et al (1987) proposed a few theories for this protective effect of training. These include: (1) a change in pattern of motor unit recruitment, (2) specific muscle fiber adaptation becoming more resistant to fatigue and damaging effects of eccentric exercise, and (3) the first bouts of eccentric exercise causing damage and destruction to fibers at the end of their life cycle and time between exercise sessions allowing regeneration of a fiber population with a higher mechanical resistance. Byrnes et al (1985) and Nosaka et al (1991) reported that just a single bout of eccentric exercise can be sufficient enough to reduce markers of eccentric exercise induced muscle damage. This protective effect has been shown to last up to 9 and 10 weeks (Clarkson & Ebbeling 1988, Byrnes et al 1985, Nosaka et al 1991).

Calf contusions can be prevented by better protective equipment, incorporating not just the tibia but also the calf, in field hockey, soccer and hockey. As already discussed, many of the injuries in sports that involve sticks are a result of slashing, and hence proper enforcement of rules by the referee and education of the athlete as to severity of injury is imperative.

DEEP VEIN THROMBOSIS

Deep vein thrombosis (DVT) must be considered in individuals with increasing calf pain and swelling. The occurrence rate in healthy active individuals is very rare but thrombosis may occur with increased activity and has been described by Harvey (1978) as effort thrombosis. The major concern regarding thrombus formation in a vein is that of embolization resulting in pulmonary emboli. The risk of pulmonary emboli is significantly reduced with anticoagulation. Following DVT, venous insufficiency may occur and the venous stasis itself may be another uncommon cause of exertional leg pain in the older athlete. This can also be seen in incompetent veins with increased varicosities, which are improved with the use of support stockings.

Thromboembolic disorders have been recognized with increasing regularity over the past 2 decades. More and more vigilence in terms of identification has taken place because of the morbidity and mortality associated with deep vein thrombosis. As mentioned already, the major complication of DVT is that of pulmonary emboli. It is a major concern and complication in the postoperative state, particularly following trauma or surgery to the hip or pelvis or with individuals immobilized in bed for any period of time. In addition, ambulatory patients may also develop DVT. Pulmonary embolism is one of the most common causes of morbidity and mortality among the adult population and it is estimated that some 600 000 cases occur annually with a mortality of 10%. In addition to individuals who are not ambulatory and in the postsurgical or traumatic state, DVT and pulmonary emboli have been recognized as an important complication of pregnancy and oral contraceptive use (Speroff 1998). Speroff (1998) states further that the estimated risk of pulmonary emboli among women using oral contraceptives is three to four times greater than in non-users.

DVT occurs in a setting with platelet aggregation and further adhesion to the venous endothelium. Fibrin then forms around the platelets and allows the further entrapment of more platelets as well as red and white blood cells. This process causes the growth of a thrombus, which forms a head that slows the flow of blood in the vessel, and a tail that extends downstream. Venous thrombi form in areas of slower blood flow, particularly at valve pockets and venous sinuses. Virchow first described the triad of factors responsible for facilitating the formation of a blood clot: (1) an abnormal vessel wall, (2) blood stagnation (venous stasis) and (3) increased coagulation. Venous stasis occurs when blood remains confined by or in contact with the venous wall for longer periods of time than normal. In terms of intramuscular veins, the most prevalent area where DVT occurs is in the soleus plexus of veins. These larger valveless veins drain anteriorly and their emptying depends on the rate of arterial flow as well as the pressure gradient between the sinuses in the deeper veins to which they empty. These veins are primarily dependent on the calf muscle pump for emptying. The role of the calf pump here is to increase the pressure and rate of arterial flow. Calf vein thrombosis is seen particularly with prolonged rest due to inactivity of the calf muscle, allowing for an increase in the time that the blood pools in the lower extremity. Abnormalities of the vessel wall occur with changes in the venous intima caused by tissue injury. This results in chemotactic factors being released and diffusing across the venous wall and activating clotting factors. There is a resultant cascade of migration of leukocytes to the venous intima and adhesion and aggregation of the platelets. A thrombus 3–5 cm in length can be formed and becomes anchored to the vessel wall by fibrin strands. An additional theory describing vessel wall damage focuses on the role of stasis in sites at soleal veins and valve pockets. These areas are believed to be sites for platelet accumulation and activating clotting factors. These two theories can address both the role of stasis and the role of the venous intima in the process of thrombosus. States of increased coaguability have been well known to initiate a clotting sequence. This can occur with so called effort thrombosis and following fever and infection. It is also involved in the role of oral contraceptives in stimulating the coagulation cascade. Reduced levels of antithrombin 3, an anticoagulant found in the blood, were noted in women using oral contraceptives. Lower levels of antithrombin 3 may be necessary to begin the process of thrombosis (Strandness et al 1977, Stewart 1975).

Mackie & Webster (1981) described a marathon runner with gastrocnemius cramping in the final stages of a marathon. In the week after the marathon, this runner developed DVT in the calf. Williams & Williams (1994) described a case of DVT in a 65-year-old individual after a day of telemark skiing. The authors suggested that minor muscle trauma, dehydration and possibly an exercise-induced state might be the factors initiating clot formation in the otherwise healthy active athlete.

Signs and symptoms

Unfortunately, clinical signs are absent or unreliable in DVT with up to two-thirds of the cases of DVT being missed on examination. However, DVT of the lower leg intramuscular vein often presents with edema, localized warmth over the calf and a tight sensation or pain, particularly with walking or running. There may or may not be local deep tenderness and pain with forced dorsiflexion with positive Homan's sign. Some cases of DVT, uncomplicated by a pulmonary embolism, may be associated with fever or tachycardia. Pulmonary embolism, should it occur, is associated with shortness of breath and chest pain. Other symptoms can include hemoptysis, faintness, anxiety and light-headedness. Calf swelling is often present with DVT.

Differential diagnosis

The differential diagnosis of DVT is extensive and includes strains of the gastrocnemius–soleus complex, hematoma following contusion, a popliteal cyst from an intra-articular knee mechanism, compartment syndromes, popliteal artery entrapment and the post-thrombotic phlebitic syndrome.

Treatment

The treatment of DVT is aimed at the prevention of pulmonary emboli and starts with immediate hospitalization, followed by intravenous heparin administration. Heparin acts immediately to catalyze the cascade of clotting factors and is continued for at least

5–7 days. In addition, within the first 24 h, an oral anticoagulant of warfarin (coumadin) is also initiated to inhibit the synthesis of coagulant proteins. Hirsch et al (1996) emphasized the importance of a period of overlap between heparin and warfarin to ensure that the full effects of warfarin are exhibited. The oral anticoagulants should be continued for 3–6 months for a first occurrence patient. The reoccurrence rate is 4–7%. For the female, oral contraceptives should be stopped immediately upon diagnosis. When athletes are taking anticoagulants, they can continue non-contact endurance activities, gradually returning at a progressive increase in intensity, and being careful not to suffer any acute gastrocnemius–soleus strains. It should be obvious that individuals who are anticoagulated are not involved in contact sports. The level of anticoagulation with warfarin is monitored by the international normalized ratio (INR) with a level to be achieved between 2.02–3.00 for the INR therapeutic range. The INR should be monitored daily initially, then three times per week, and on a weekly basis thereafter. The INR can fluctuate with fever and other forms of stress and travel, so the level of warfarin (coumadin) needs to be adjusted accordingly.

Prevention

In the surgical setting, low dose heparin has been universally used as a means of reducing the likelihood of DVT. In addition, regular calf exercises to improve the calf muscle pump should be utilized in any situation of immobilization. Long car trips and flights are notorious for producing sufficient venous stasis to lead to the formation of a DVT. Regular stops with walking during a car trip, and regular walking and toe raises, either sitting or walking in the aisles on long flights are strongly recommended. In addition, in the postoperative setting, or in individuals with known varicose veins or previous venous stasis sigvarus, support stockings are recommended. In trauma to the calf with contusion or in the setting of gastrocnemius–soleus strains, early activation, calf support through taping, and increased exercise through pool running or cycling, are essential to prevent DVT. These situations are enhanced with the older athlete, as age has been identified as a risk factor for both DVT and pulmonary emboli. A family history of DVT should lead to a search for forms of contraception other than oral contraceptives. A recent report by Suissa et al (1997) reported an increased risk of venous thromboembolism with the use of the newer third generation of oral contraceptives than with the second generation agents. This was contradicted in a subsequent study by Farmer et al (1998) which showed no significant difference in the risk of venous thromboemboli between the users of second and third generation oral contra-

ceptives. Any family history of DVT should stimulate an analysis of the coagulation factors, particularly looking for reduced levels of antithrombin 3 and Factor V Leiden.

Due to the serious consequence of pulmonary embolism associated with DVT in known states of high risk, any athlete presenting with calf pain and swelling must be considered a potential case of DVT with appropriate investigation.

REFERRED AND SYSTEMIC CAUSES OF LOWER LEG PAIN

A discussion of exercised-induced lower leg pain would not be complete without a brief reference to referred and systemic causes. It goes without saying that practitioners should always be on the lookout for malignancy, both soft tissue and bony. This would be investigated by bone scan and followed up with a CT scan or MRI.

The neurogenic causes are most commonly seen with nerve entrapment by a lumbar disk, or possibly spinal stenosis, or the piriformis syndrome, which can be identified with CT or MRI of the lumbar spine, MRI of the gluteal-piriformis region, and nerve conduction and EMG studies. Other neurogenic causes of lower leg pain, aggravated by or initially presenting with the challenge of exercise, would be a peripheral neuropathy as seen with vitamin B_{12} or folate deficiency, diabetes, alcoholism or other toxins.

Vascular causes, besides PAES and DVT as previously discussed, would include, peripheral vascular disease with hyperlipidemia in the older athlete or Buerger's disease in the smoker. The authors have recently seen four cases of iliac or femoral artery stenosis from fibrous band entrapment or repetitive arterial compression in four high-level athletes. These were challenging to diagnose as they all presented with thigh fatigue and calf cramping and pain, only with high intensity exercise. Doppler studies at rest and traditional levels of exercise were normal and it was only at maximal effort that a high pitched femoral artery bruit was heard, and reduction in flow in the femoral triage was detected with Doppler and confirmed by angiography. Treatment included decompression of the surrounding soft tissue, and arterial repair.

More unusual causes of muscular pathology include myopathy and muscular dystrophies. The myopathy may be autoimmune in origin, or as in a case we investigated, involve dermatomyositis. The authors have treated cases of calf pain and fatigue with exercise that were confirmed on muscle biopsy to be a result of mitochondrial disease and red ragged muscle disease.

Calf cramping during exercise can also be seen with electrolyte disturbance combined with chronic diarrhea or dehydration in the endurance runner. Rarely, an endocrine disturbance may reduce calcium or potassium levels.

If the history, physical examination and initial investigations do not point to an obvious cause for exercise-related leg pain, then practitioners are forced to investigate further. Any exercise testing must be done at the level of exercise intensity necessary to produce the specific symptoms. Full laboratory investigation, appropriate imaging and neurovascular studies will lead to the appropriate diagnosis and then treatment can begin.

SUMMARY

This chapter shows the many and varied causes of leg pain for people involved in sport and exercise. It can be seen that leg injuries are incurred not only by high-level participants, but also those involved in what could be considered lower-level activity (e.g. walking, dancing, etc.). With the many potential contributing factors to leg injuries, differential diagnosis is imperative if the most appropriate form of management is to be chosen.

REFERENCES

Alfredson H, Lorentzon R 2000 Chronic Achilles tendinosis. Sports Medicine 29(2):135–146

Alfredson H, Pietila T, Jonsson P et al 1998 Heavy-load eccentric calf muscle training for chronic Achilles tendinosis. American Journal of Sports Medicine 26(3):360–366

Amendola A, Rorabeck C H 1985 Chronic exertional compartment syndrome. In: Welsh R P, Shephard R J et al (eds) Current therapy in sports medicine. BC Decker, Toronto

Amendola A, Rorabeck C H, Vellett D et al 1990 The use of magnetic resonance imaging in exertional compartment syndromes. American Journal of Sports Medicine 18:29–34

Anderson I, Read J, Steinweg J 1998 Atlas of imaging in sports medicine. McGraw-Hill, Sydney

Appell H J, Soares J M C, Durart J R 1992 Exercise, muscle damage and fatigue. Sports Medicine 13:108–115

Armstrong R B 1984 Mechanisms of exercise induced delayed onset muscle soreness: a brief review. Medicine and Science in Sport and Exercise 16:529–538

Armstrong R B 1990 Initial events in exercise induced muscular injury. Medicine and Science in Sport and Exercise 22:429–435

Babul S 2001 The effects of intermittent exposure to hyperbaric oxygen (HBO) for the treatment of a 'model' muscle injury utilizing spectroscopic and blood enzyme analysis. PhD Thesis, University of British Columbia, Canada

Batt M E 1995 Shin splints: a review of terminology. Clinical Journal of Sport Medicine 5:53–57

Beck B R 1998 Tibial stress injuries: an aetiological review for the purposes of guiding management. Sports Medicine 26:265–279

Beck T J, Ruff C B, Mourtada F A et al 1996 Dual energy x-ray absorptiometry derived structural geometry for stress fracture prediction in male U.S. Marine Corps recruits. Journal of Bone Mineral Research 11:645–653

Benazzo F, Mosconi M, Beccarisi G et al 1995 Use of capacitive coupled electric fields in stress fractures in athletes. Clinical Orthopaedics and Related Research 310:145–149

Bennell K L, Malcolm S A, Thomas S A et al 1996 Risk factors for stress fractures in track and field athletes. American Journal of Sports Medicine 24(6):810–818

Blackman P G 2000 A review of chronic exertional compartment syndrome in the lower leg. Medicine and Science in Sports and Exercise 32(3 suppl): S4–S10

Breit G A, Gross J H, Watenpaugh D E et al 1997 Near-infrared spectroscopy for monitoring of tissue oxygenation of exercising skeletal muscle in a chronic compartment syndrome model. Journal of Bone and Joint Surgery (Am) 79A:838–843

Brodine S K, Almeida S A, Shaffer R A et al 1999 Use of simple measures of physical activity to predict stress fractures in young men undergoing a rigorous physical training program. American Journal of Epidemiology 149:236–242

Brukner P 2000 Exercise-related lower leg pain: Bone. Medicine and Science in Sports and Exercise 32(suppl):515–526

Brukner P, Khan K 1993 Clinical sports medicine. McGraw-Hill, Sydney, p 430

Brukner P, Khan K 2001 Clinical sports medicine, 2nd edn. McGraw-Hill, Sydney

Burr D B, Forwood M R, Fyhrie D P et al 1997 Bone microdamage and skeletal fragility in osteoporotic and stress fractures. Journal of Bone Mineral Research 12:6–15

Byrnes W C, Clarkson P M, Spencer White J et al 1985 Delayed onset muscle soreness following repeated bouts of downhill running. Journal of Applied Physiology 59:710–715

Chang P S, Harris R M 1996 Intramedullary nailing for chronic tibial stress fractures. American Journal of Sports Medicine 24(5):688–692

Clarkson P M, Ebbeling C 1988 Investigation of serum creatine kinase variability after muscle damaging exercise. Clinical Science 75:257–261

Collier B D, Johnson R P, Carrera G F et al 1984 Scintigraphic diagnosis of stress-induced incomplete fractures of the proximal tibia. Journal of Trauma 24:156–160

Collins P S, McDonald P T, Lim R C 1989 Popliteal artery entrapment syndrome: an evolving syndrome. Journal of Vascular Surgery 10:484–490

Cook J L, Khan K M, Purdam C R 2001 Conservative treatment of patellar tendinopathy. Physical Therapy in Sport 2:54–65

Crossley K, Bennell K L, Wrigley T et al 1998 Ground reaction forces, bone characteristics, and tibial stress fracture in male runners. Medicine and Science in Sports and Exercise 31(8):1088–1093

Cyriax J A 1981 Clinical applications of massage. In: Basmajian J L (ed) Manipulation, traction and massage, 3rd edn. William Wilkins, Baltimore, MD

Curwin S L, Stanish W D 1984 Tendinitis: etiology and treatment. Heath, Lexington

Daley T J 1990 The repair phase of wound healing re-epithelialization and contraction. In: Kloth C L, McCulloch J M, Felder J A (eds) Wound healing: alternatives in management. FA Davis, Philadelphia, PA

DeLacerda F G 1981 A case study: application of ultrasound to determine a stress fracture of the fibula. Journal of Orthopaedic and Sports Physical Therapy 2:134

Delaney T A, Gonzalez L L 1971 Occlusion of the popliteal artery due to muscle entrapment. Surgery 69:97–101

Detmer D E 1986 Chronic shin splints. Sports Medicine 3:436–446

Dyson M, Biol C, Biol M I 1990 Role of ultrasound in wound healing. In: Kloth C L, McCulloch J M, Felder J A (eds) Wound healing: alternatives in management. FA Davis, Philadelphia, PA

Ebel A 1965 Exercise in vascular diseases. In: Licht D (ed) Therapeutic exercise, 2nd edn. E Licht, New Haven

Edwards P, Myerson M S 1996 Exertional compartment syndrome of the leg: steps for expedient return to activity. Physician and Sportsmedicine 24(4):31–46

Embrec M J 1996 Chronic compartment syndrome: an analysis at the cellular level. Thesis Faculty of Graduate Studies. The University of Western Ontario, Canada

Farmer R, Todd J, Lewis M et al 1998 The risk of venous

thromboembolism among German women using oral contraceptives: a data base study. Contraception 57:67–70

Fehlandt A, Micheli L 1995 Acute exertional anterior compartment syndrome in an adolescent female. Medicine and Science in Sports and Exercise 27:3–7

Feinberg J H, Nadler S F, Krivickas L S 1997 Peripheral nerve injuries in the athlete. Sports Medicine 24(6):385–408

Harvey J S 1978 Effort thrombosis in the lower extremity of a runner. American Journal of Sports Medicine 6:400–402

Hasson S M, Daniels J C, Divine J G et al 1992 Effect of ibuprofen use on muscle soreness, damage and performance: a preliminary investigation. Medicine and Science in Sport and Exercise 25:9–17

High D M, Hawley E T, Franks B D 1989 The effects of static stretching and warm-up on prevention of delayed-onset muscle soreness. Research Quarterly for Exercise and Sport 60(4):357–61

Hirsh D, Mikkola K, Marks P et al 1996 Pulmonary embolism and DVT during pregnancy and oral contraceptive use. Prevalence of factor V leidin. American Heart Journal 131:1145–1148

Howard J L, Mohtadi N G H, Wiley J P 2000 Evaluation of outcomes in patients following surgical treatment of chronic exertional compartment syndrome in the leg. Clinical Journal of Sport Medicine 10:176–184

Hulkko A, Orava, S 1987 Stress fractures in athletes. International Journal of Sports Medicine 8:221–116

Hutchison M R, Ireland M L 1994 Common compartment syndrome in athletes: treatment and rehabilitation. Sports Medicine 17:200–208

Khan K M, Cook J L, Taunton J E et al 2000 Overuse tendinosis, not tendonitis: part 1: a new paradigm for a difficult clinical problem. Physician and Sportsmedicine 28(5):38–48

Khan K M, Maffulli N, Coleman B D et al 1998 Patellar tendinopathy: some aspects of basic science and clinical management. British Journal of Sports Medicine 32:346–355

Khan K M, Cook J L, Bonar F et al 1999 Histopathology of common tendinopathies: update and implications for clinical management. Sports Medicine 27(6):393–408

Korkola M, Amendola A 2001 Exercise-induced leg pain: shifting through a broad differential. Physician and Sportsmedicine 29(6):35–50

Krause J O, Brodsky J W 1998 Peroneus brevis tendon tears: pathophysiology, surgical reconstruction, and clinical results. Foot and Ankle International 19(5):271–279

Kvist M 1994 Achilles tendon injury in athletes. Sports Medicine 18(3):173–201

Lau J T C, Daniels T R 1999 Tarsal tunnel syndrome: a review of the literature. Foot and Ankle International 20(3):201–209

Leach R E, Hammond G, Stryker W S 1967 Anterior tibial compartment syndrome. Acute and chronic. Journal of Bone and Joint Surgery (Am) 49A:451–462

Leadbetter W B 1992 Cell matrix response in tendon injury. Clinics in Sports Medicine 11:533–578

Leppilahti J, Orava S 1998 Total Achilles tendon rupture: a review. Sports Medicine 25(2):79–100

Li G, Zhang S, Chen G et al 1985 Radiographic and histologic analyses of stress fracture in rabbit tibias. American Journal of Sports Medicine 13:285–294

McBryde A M Jr 1965 Stress fractures in runners. Clinical Sports Medicine 4:737–752

Macintyre D L, Reid D W, McKenzie D C 1995 Delayed muscle soreness. The inflammatory response to muscle injury and its clinical implications. Sports Medicine 20:24–40

McKenzie D C, Clement D B, Taunton J E 1985 Running shoes, orthotics and injuries. Sports Medicine 21:334–344

Mackie J A, Webster M A 1981 Deep vein thrombosis in marathon runners. Physician and Sportsmedicine 9(5):91–98

Maffuli N, Testa V, Capasso G et al 1997 Results of percutaneous longitudinal tenotomy for Achilles tendinopathy in middle- and long-distance runners. American Journal of Sports Medicine 25(6):835–840

Martens M A, Backaert M, Vermont G et al 1984 Chronic leg pain in athletes due to a recurrent compartment syndrome. American Journal of Sports Medicine 12:148–151

Matheson G O, Clement D B, McKenzie D C et al 1987 Stress fractures in athletes: a study of 320 cases. American Journal of Sports Medicine 15(1):46–58

Matsen F A 1975 Compartment syndrome: a unified concept. Clinical Orthopaedics and Related Research 113:8–14

Michael R H, Holder L E 1985 The soleus syndrome. American Journal of Sports Medicine 13(2):87–94

Mohler L R, Styf J R, Pedowitz R A et al 1997 Intramuscular deoxygenation during exercise in patients who have chronic anterior compartment syndrome of the leg. Journal of Bone and Joint Surgery (Am) 79A:844–849

Morris R H 1991 Medial tibial syndrome: a treatment protocol using electric current. Chiropractic Sports Medicine 5:5–8

Murray A, Halliday M, Croft R 1991 Popliteal artery entrapment syndrome. British Journal of Surgery 78:1414–1419

Newham D J, Jones D A, Clarkson P M 1987 Repeated high force eccentric exercise: effects on muscle pain and damage. Journal of Applied Physiology 63:1381–1386

Niessen-Vertommen S L, Taunton J E, Clement D B et al 1992 The effect of eccentric versus concentric exercise in the management of Achilles tendonitis. Clinical Journal of Sport Medicine 2:109–113

Nosaka K, Clarkson P M, McGuiggin M E, et al 1991 Time course of muscle adaptation after high force eccentric exercise. European Journal of Applied Physiology and Occupational Physiology 63:70–76

Oriani G, Barnini C, Marroni G et al 1987 Hyperbaric oxygen therapy in treatment of various orthopaedic disorders. Minerva Medica 73:2983–2988

Raneman R S 1975 The anterior and the lateral compartmental syndrome of the leg due to intensive use of muscles. Clinical Orthopaedics and Related Research 113:69–80

Rich N M, Collins G J, McDonald P T et al 1979 Popliteal vascular entrapment: its increasing interest. Archives of Surgery 114:1377–1394

Rolf C, Movin T 1997 Etiology, histology, and outcome of surgery in Achillodynia. Foot and Ankle International 18(9):565–569

Rorabeck C H 1986 Exertional tibialis posterior compartment syndrome. Clinical Orthopaedics and Related Research 208:61–64

Rorabeck C H, Bourne R B, Fowler P J 1983 The surgical treatment of exertional compartment syndrome in athletes. Journal of Bone and Joint Surgery (Am) 65A:1245–1251

Rorabeck C H, Fowler P J, Nott L 1988 The results of fasciotomy in the management of chronic exertional compartment syndrome. American Journal of Sports Medicine 16:224–227

Sammarco G J 1995 Peroneus longus tendon tears: acute and chronic. 16(5):245–253

Schepsis A A, Martini D, Corbett M 1993 Surgical management of exertional compartment syndrome of the lower leg. American Journal of Sports Medicine 21:811–817

Schwane J A, Johnson S R, Vandenakher C B et al 1983 Delayed onset muscular soreness and plasma CPK and LDH activities after downhill running. Medicine and Science in Sport and Exercise 15:51–56

Schweitzer M E, Karasick D 2000 M R imaging of disorders of the posterior tibialis tendon. American Journal of Radiology 175:627–635

Scott G, King J B 1994 A prospective, double-blind trial of electrical capacitive coupling in the treatment of non-union of long bones. Journal of Bone and Joint Surgery (Am) 76A:820–826

Sharrard W J W 1990 A double-blind trial of pulsed electromagnetic fields for delayed union of tibial fractures. Journal of Bone and Joint Surgery (Am) 72A:347–355

Shelbourne K D, Fisher D A, Rettig A C et al 1988 Stress fractures of the medial malleolus. American Journal of Sports Medicine 16:60–63

Shrier 1991 Exercise-induced acute compartment syndrome: a case report. Clinical Journal of Sports Medicine 1:202–204

Smith L L, Fulmer M G, Holbert D et al 1994 The impact of a repeated bout of eccentric exercise on muscular strength, muscle soreness and creatine kinase. British Journal of Sports Medicine 28:267–270

Soolsma S 1996 The effects of intermittent hyperbaric oxygen on short term recovery from Grade II medial collateral ligament injuries. MSc Thesis University of British Columbia, Vancouver, Canada

Speroff L 1998 Oral contraceptives and arterial and venous thromboses: a clinicians formulation. American Journal of Obstetrics and Gynaecology 179:525–536

Stager A C 1997 Prognosis after popliteal artery entrapment syndrome surgery. MSc Thesis University of British Columbia, Canada

Stager A, Clement D 1999 Popliteal artery entrapment syndrome. Sports Medicine 28:61–70

Stanitski C L, McMaster J H, Scranton P E 1978 On the nature of stress fractures. American Journal of Sports Medicine 187:188–192

Staples J, Clement D 1996 Hyperbaric oxygen chambers and the treatment of sport injuries. Sports Medicine 22:219–227

Staples J R, Clement D B, Taunton J E et al 1999 Effects of hyperbaric oxygen on a human model of injury. American Journal of Sports Medicine 27:600–605

Stewart G A 1975 The role of the vessel wall in deep vein thrombosis. In: Nicolaides A N (ed) Thromboembolism. University Press, Baltimore, MD

Stollsteimer G T, Shelton W R 1997 Acute atraumatic compartment syndrome in an athlete: a case study. Journal of Athletic Training 32:248–250

Strandness D E, Ward K, Krugmire R Jr 1977 The present state of acute deep venous thrombosis. Surgical Gynaecology and Obstetrics 145:433–445

Suissa S, Blais L, SpitzerW et al 1997 First time use of new oral contraception. Contraceptives and the risk of venous thromboembolism Contraception 56:141–146

Sullivan D, Warren R F, Pavlov H et al 1984 Stress fractures in 51 runners. Clinical Orthopaedics and Related Research 187:188–192

Swenson R Jr, DeHaven K E, Sebastanelli W J et al 1997 The effect of pneumatic leg brace on return to play in athletes with tibial stress fractures. American Journal of Sports Medicine 25(3):322–328

Taunton J E, Clement D B, Webber D 1981 Lower extremity stress fractures in athletes. Physician and Sportsmedicine 9(1):77–86

Taunton J, Smith C, Magee D 1996 Leg, foot and ankle injuries. In:

Zachazewski J, Magee D, Quillen W (eds) Athletic injuries and rehabilitation. WB Saunders, Philadelphia, PA

Taunton J E, Ryan M, Clement D B et al 2002 A retrospective case control analysis of 2002 running injuries. Allan McGavin Sports Medicine Centre: 1998–2000. British Journal of Sports Medicine 36(2)95–101

Tsai-Fetlander L, Westblad P, Ekenman J et al 1996 A Study of intrinsic factors in patients with stress fractures of the tibia. Foot and Ankle International 17(8):477–482

Visentini P J, Khan K M, Cook J L et al 1998 The VISA score: an index of the severity of jumper's knee (patellar tendinosis). Journal of Science and Medicine in Sport 1:22–28

Whitelaw G P, Wetzler M J, Levy A S et al 1991 A pneumatic leg brace for the treatment of tibial stress fractures. Clinical Orthopaedics and Related Research 270:302–305

Wilber M C, Russell H L 1979 Central bioelectric augmentation in the healing of fractures. In: Brighton C T, Black J, Pollack S R (eds) Electrical properties of bone and cartilage. Experimental effects and clinical applications. Grune and Stratton, New York

Wilcox J R, Moniot A L, Green J P 1997 Bone scanning in the evaluation of exercise-related stress injuries. Radiology 123:699–703

Wiley J P, Doyle D L, Taunton J E 1987 A primary care perspective of chronic compartment syndrome of the leg. Physician and Sportsmedicine 15:111–120

Williams J S Jr, Williams J S Sr 1994 Deep vein thrombosis in a skier's leg. Did exertion contribute to clotting. Physician and Sportsmedicine 22(1):79–84

Yeap J S, Singh D, Birch R 2001 Tibialis posterior tendon dysfunction: a primary or secondary problem? Foot and Ankle International. 22(1):51–55

Zund G, Brunner U 1995 Surgical aspects of popliteal artery entrapment syndrome: 26 years of experience with 26 legs. Vasa 24:29–33

23

Foot and ankle

D S Blaise Williams III

INTRODUCTION

Ankle injuries are the most common acute injuries in the athletic population (Adamson & Cymet 1997, Lofvenberg et al 1995, Lynch & Renstom 1999). Lateral ankle injuries account for 15–25% of all sports injuries (Adamson & Cymet 1997). Because the foot is the contact with the ground, it is subjected to very high forces when the foot is in contact with the ground during sport activities. Overuse injuries are common at the foot and ankle complex as a result of the need to eccentrically control motion during landing activities. This chapter outlines the functional anatomy of the foot and ankle complex, gives a complete discussion of functional evaluation and describes current physical therapy approaches to treatment of common pathologies in the athletic population.

ARTHROLOGY

DISTAL TIBIOFIBULAR JOINT

The distal tibiofibular joint is the articulation between the inferior ends of the tibia and fibula. The joint is a syndesmotic fibrous joint and has little to no movement. The only motion that is available is a slight opening which accommodates the anterior portion of the talus during dorsiflexion. The convex surface of the fibula articulates with the concave surface of the tibia. A portion of the synovial membrane from the talocrural joint covers a small portion of the distal tibiofibular joint but does not encompass it. The primary connection between the distal tibia and fibula is a thickening of the interosseus membrane known as the interosseus ligament. The interosseus ligament is just superior to the anterior and posterior tibiofibular ligaments. These ligaments extend as far laterally as the malleolus on the fibula. The posterior tibiofibular ligament is much stronger than the anterior tibiofibular ligament and can create an avulsion fracture of the posterior tibia in severe ankle injuries. A great deal of the strength of the ankle joint is dependent on the stability provided by the distal tibiofibular joint.

TALOCRURAL JOINT

The talocrural joint is the articulation between the distal ends of the tibia and fibula (mortise) and the superior surface of the talus (trochlea). The joint is a diarthrodial or synovial joint and is classified as a hinge joint. This joint is typically referred to as the ankle joint. The joint allows for dorsiflexion and plantarflexion, which occurs with slight amounts of secondary plane motion. This is a result of the orientation of the talocrural joint axis, which essentially passes through the malleoli. In a static condition, this corresponds to approximately 20–30° of external rotation and 10° down and lateral in the frontal plane (Barnett & Napier 1952, Hicks 1953, Lundberg et al 1989). It is important to note that, in a dynamic condition, the axis of the joint changes its orientation as individuals move through the dorsiflexion/plantarflexion range of motion (Lundberg et al 1989) (Fig. 23.1). The concave surface of the mortise articulates with the convex surface of the talus when viewed in the sagittal plane. However, there is a slightly concave shape to the talus when viewed anteriorly. The joint is encompassed by a thin synovial membrane.

There are thickenings of the membrane medially and laterally, which provide the primary support at the ankle. Medially, the deltoid ligament is comprised of three separate parts named for their attachments (tibionavicular, posterior tibiotalar, and tibiocalcaneal). The deltoid ligament is thicker and stronger than the lateral ligaments. The lateral ligaments are separate from one another and are, again, named for their bony attach-

ments. The anterior talofibular ligament is the weakest and most often injured. The remaining two lateral ligaments, the calcaneofibular ligament and posterior talofibular ligament are stronger and injured less. The primary motions occurring at this joint are plantarflexion and dorsiflexion. The joint is most stable in dorsiflexion as the talus locks between the tibia and the fibula due to the larger anterior portion of the talus. The joint becomes less stable in the plantarflexed position as the smaller posterior surface of the talus moves forward allowing for more lateral movement of the talus within the mortise.

SUBTALAR JOINT

The subtalar joint is the articulation between the inferior surface of the talus and the superior surface of the calcaneus. The joint is a diarthrodial joint and is classified as a plane joint. This joint is often referred to as the 'keystone of the foot' because the subtalar joint transfers motion from the foot to the lower leg in closed kinetic chain situations. The joint allows for triplanar motion dominated by inversion and eversion. The axis for motion at the subtalar joint sits approximately 42° from horizontal in the sagittal plane and 16° laterally in the transverse plane. A significant amount of abduction and adduction is also present as a result of the orientation of the joint axis in the sagittal plane. Finally, a small amount of dorsiflexion and plantarflexion is possible at this joint, based on the orientation of the joint axis (Fig. 23.2). There are three articulations between the calcaneus and the talus. The large posterior talar facet on the calcaneus is convex and it articulates with the concave surface of the talus. The middle and anterior facets of the calcaneus have a concave orientation and an arthrokinematically function opposite to that of the posterior facet. The structure of the subtalar joint, therefore, acts to stabilize

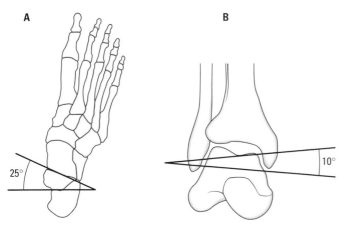

Figure 23.1A & B   Axis of the talocrural joint in the **A** transverse and **B** frontal planes.

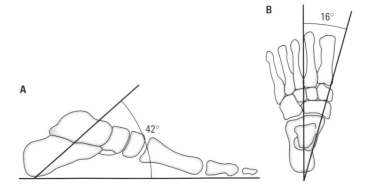

Figure 23.2 A&B   Axis of motion at the subtalar joint. **A** The lateral view demonstrates how almost equal amounts of frontal plane (inversion/eversion) and transverse plane (adduction/abduction) can occur about this joint. **B** The superior view shows the axis almost in line with the long axis of the foot, resulting in primarily frontal plane motion.

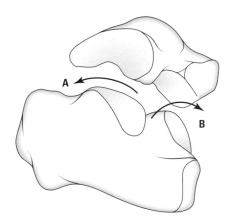

Figure 23.3   As the subtalar joint everts (in an open kinetic chain), the distal end of the calcaneus moves laterally. At the joint surfaces, the posterior facet glides medially while the anterior and medial facets glide laterally. This provides a screw-like mechanism that effectively locks the joint and provides stability even without the ligaments.

the joint dynamically (Fig. 23.3). The joint is further encompassed by its own capsule and is supported by the medial, lateral and posterior talocalcaneal ligaments. Additionally, the joint is supported anteriorly by the strong interosseus talocalcaneal ligament.

MIDTARSAL JOINT

The midtarsal joint is a complex articulation between four bones: the calcaneus, talus, navicular, and cuboid. The joint is a diarthrodial joint and is classified as a plane joint. There are two joint capsules: one surrounding the talus, calcaneus, and navicular, and one surrounding the lateral portion of the calcaneus and the cuboid. The joint is highly mobile and motion occurs about two primary joint axes: a longitudinal axis and an oblique axis. Inversion and eversion is the primary motion about the longitudinal axis while motion about the oblique axis is truly triplanar. The mobility of the midtarsal joint increases as the subtalar joint pronates and becomes less mobile as it supinates. The medial side of the joint is supported by the dorsal talonavicular ligament and more significantly by the plantar calcaneonavicular or spring ligament. The spring ligament plays an important role in maintaining the medial longitudinal arch of the foot. On the lateral side of the midtarsal joint, the long plantar ligament is most superficial and helps to support the calcaneocuboid articulation and to maintain the arches of the foot. The short plantar ligament is deep and only supports the calcaneocuboid articulation. Dorsolaterally, the bifurcate ligament supports the joint.

TARSOMETATARSAL JOINTS

The tarsometatarsal joints are the articulation between the cuboid, the three cuneiforms, and the five meta-

tarsals. The joints are diarthrodial and classified as plane joints. The three joint capsules are named for their positions in the foot: medial, intermediate, and lateral tarsometatarsal joints. The medial joint is the articulation between the medial cuneiform and the base of the first metatarsal and is the most mobile of the three tarsometatarsal joints. Motion occurs about a joint axis, which allows primarily for plantarflexion and dorsiflexion at the joint. The joints also abduct and invert with dorsiflexion. The most stable of the three tarsometatarsal joints is the intermediate joint. Due to the bony architecture, the second and third metatarsals create a rigid central pillar in the foot. The second and third metatarsals articulate with the three cuneiforms. The lateral tarsometatarsal joint is the articulation between the fourth and fifth metatarsals and the cuboid. A small amount of motion is available at this joint, primarily consisting of plantarflexion and dorsiflexion. All three joints are supported by the dorsal, plantar, and interosseus tarsometatarsal ligaments.

METATARSALPHALANGEAL JOINTS

The metatarsalphalangeal joints are articulations between the heads of the metatarsals and the bases of the proximal phalanges. Discussion in this section will be limited to the first metatarsalphalangeal joint as it is representative of the others, and the majority of published literature relates to this joint. The joint is a diarthrodial joint and is classified as a condyloid joint. The joint capsule surrounds the first metatarsal and the proximal phalanx. The medial and lateral sesamoid bones are extracapsular (Fig. 23.4). The joint allows for dorsiflexion and plantarflexion as well as abduction and adduction. The joint is supported medially and laterally by collateral ligaments and by a strong plantar ligament.

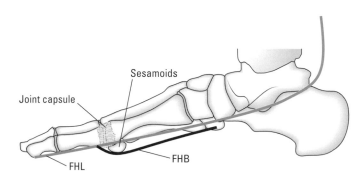

Figure 23.4   A synovial capsule encompasses the first metatarsalphalangeal joint while the sesamoid bones are outside the capsule. The sesamoids provide a greater moment arm for the flexor hallucis brevis (FHB) muscle and provide protection for the flexor hallucis longus (FHL) muscle, which passes between the sesamoids and the metatarsal head.

CALCANEAL FAT PAD

The plantar aspect of the heel is made up of connective and specialized fat tissue, which is between 10 and 20 mm in thickness (Whittle 1999). The pad is attached to the medial calcaneal tuberosity with the fat being divided into chambers. The heel pad acts to absorb between 47% and 66% of the shock when the plantar surface of the foot is in contact with the ground (Aerts et al 1995). Injuries and pain in the calcaneus are often attributed to decreased ability of the calcaneal fat pad to absorb shock. Injuries to the calcaneal fat pad are often the result of trauma to the area. Fortunately, due to the adequate blood supply, fat pad injuries often heal well with rest and anti-inflammatory intervention. Compressive heel cups may also provide support, and increase the resting thickness of the fat pad, allowing for compression without further damage to the tissue.

METATARSAL FAT PAD

A fat pad also protects the plantar aspect of the metatarsal heads. The pad is attached to the plantar fascia and the metatarsal heads themselves. The fat pad acts to absorb shock and provide lubrication when the plantar surface of the metatarsal heads is in contact with the ground. Injuries to the metatarsal are often attributed to atrophy or dislocation of the fat pad. However, recent evidence suggests that metatarsal fat pad atrophy is not associated with metatarsalgia (Waldecker 2001). Metatarsal fat pad injuries respond to treatment similar to that used for calcaneal fat pad injuries. Relieving the pressure on the metatarsal head with a metatarsal pad may also be an effective treatment.

EXTRINSIC MUSCLES

The primary plantarflexors of the ankle are the gastrocnemius and soleus, which are both innervated by the tibial nerve S1–S2. Several other muscles cross posterior to the malleoli and act as secondary plantar-flexors of the ankle. The tibialis posterior (tibial nerve L4–L5), flexor digitorum longus and flexor hallucis longus (both tibial S2–S3) are found on the medial side, while the peroneus longus and brevis (both superficial peroneal L5–S1) pass posterior to the lateral malleolus. Dorsiflexion is mainly provided by the tibialis anterior (deep peroneal L4–L5) and is supported by the extensor digitorum longus and extensor hallucis longus (both deep peroneal L5–S1). Inversion is provided by the posterior and anterior tibialis muscles. Eversion is accomplished by the peroneus longus and brevis muscles. Additionally, the medial longitudinal arch is supported externally by the anterior tibialis, posterior tibialis, and the peroneus longus.

INTRINSIC MUSCLES

There is little evidence to support the idea that the intrinsic muscles of the foot act as stabilizers of the arch during ambulation (Mann & Hagy 1979). Quantitative analyses (Kura et al 1997, Silver et al 1985) have revealed the potential for these muscles to produce force in the toes, especially for flexion. These conclusions are based on the structure and orientation of the intrinsic muscles of the foot and not upon electromyographic data. Therefore, it is difficult to clinically justify the training of these muscles (i.e. towel crunches) especially when there is no method of quantifying the progression of strength in these muscles.

EXAMINATION

A thorough history is especially important when evaluating the athlete with an injury of the foot and ankle. The therapist should ask the athlete if there have been any previous injuries to the lower extremities. Previous injuries to other lower extremity joints, even on the contralateral side, can provide crucial information for the possibility of the mechanical development of foot and ankle pathology. The mechanism of injury as described by the athlete can often provide enough information to determine the structure involved in the pathology. The therapist should ask the athlete to describe the exact location and the nature of the pain. Pain as it relates to time of day or activity level can also help determine the exact cause of injury development. Neuropathic pain, such as numbness, tingling, or burning into the foot may be related to an entrapment such as tarsal tunnel syndrome. The level of current and previous function should be determined first through history and then through physical examination.

Observation of patients in both static and dynamic conditions will give the therapist information about mechanical alignment, ability to move, and willingness to move. It is important to observe patients from anterior, posterior and side views in order to establish a complete picture of their posture as it relates to their pathology. When looking at the patient from the anterior and posterior views, comparisons should be made between sides for symmetry.

There are several structures that should be evaluated from the anterior view. The angle of gait refers to the amount of external rotation of the feet. This is approximately 5–18° in normal individuals (McGee 1992) (Fig. 23.5). The therapist should also observe symmetry between sides. The base of gait or base of support is how far apart the medial borders of the feet are during stance. A narrow or wide base of support can be a predictor of

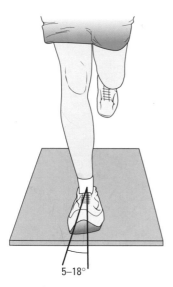

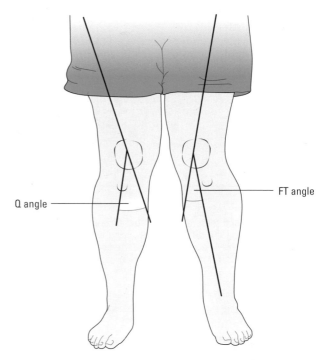

Figure 23.5   The angle of gait can be observed in standing, walking, or running. In the athlete, observing the angle of gait during running may give information that is more beneficial in identification of the pathology than the angle during standing or walking. The angle of gait most often decreases as the speed of locomotion is increased.

Figure 23.6   The Q-angle measures the alignment of the patella relative to the tibial tuberosity and the ASIS but gives no information about frontal plane knee joint alignment. The femoral tibial (FT) angle represents the angle formed between the long axis of the tibia and the long axis of the femur.

mechanical imbalances leading to pathology. Hallux position, whether neutral or valgus, can give some indication of dynamic function during gait. Midfoot position can be directly measured, preferably through an arch ratio (Saltzman et al 1995, Williams & McClay 2000) or can be visually assessed as normal, high or low (Giladi et al 1985). Symmetry should be observed in this measurement also. The patellar position (alta, baja, medial, lateral, internal or external rotation) should be assessed in the standing as well as supine positions. The Q angle may also be evaluated in conjunction with patellar position in order to further assess patellar position relative to the entire lower extremity (Fig. 23.6). The Q angle only assesses the relationship of the patella to the entire lower extremity. It does not evaluate knee joint valgus. Directly measuring the angle between the long axes of the femur and tibia will measure frontal plane knee joint orientation. Finally, the anterior superior iliac spine (ASIS) symmetry should be evaluated for possible differences in leg length.

Most of the information gained from observation from the side relates to range of motion and alignment issues. The resting knee angle should be evaluated for the presence of hyperextension or slight knee flexion. These could be related to changes in foot or ankle orientation. In the same way, resting hip angle may be increased or decreased. Pelvic tilt and lumbar position should also be evaluated. Changes in lumbar or pelvic orientation can relate to differences in muscle extensibility and have effects at the knee, tibia and subsequently the foot and ankle complex.

Many of the structures viewed from the posterior can help confirm observations made from the anterior. Tibial position, whether varum or valgum, helps give an indication of how much rearfoot (tibia relative to calcaneus) pronation may occur. Resting calcaneal stance position (RCSP) is the relationship of the calcaneus to the floor. Again, this measure alone may be important but it becomes more meaningful when compared to the tibial position. For instance, a rearfoot angle of 20° could be the result of 20° of calcaneal eversion and 0° of tibial angle, or of 10° of calcaneal eversion and 10° of tibial varum. The neutral calcaneal stance position (NCSP) is the relationship of the calcaneus to the floor with the joint held in a subtalar neutral position. The difference between this position and the RCSP provides a measurement of the motion of the subtalar joint (Fig. 23.7). Lateral toe sign is related to angle of gait and can be compared for symmetry and excessive external rotation. Typically, we would like to see only the 4th and 5th toes when they are viewed from behind. The popliteal fossa can also be viewed as a representation of internal or external rotation of the hips. This should be referenced to the patella. If the patella is neutral and the fossa is internally rotated then it is likely that the femur is internally rotated. However, if the patella is lateral and the fossa is neutral, the patella is likely to be laterally tracking. Posterior superior iliac spine and iliac crest symmetry are evaluated for

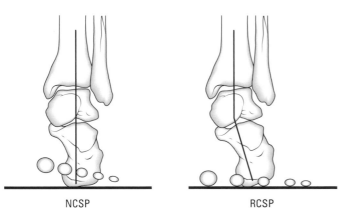

NCSP   RCSP

Figure 23.7   Subtalar joint motion can be assessed in the standing position by comparing the difference between the calcaneal position when the subtalar joint is placed in its neutral position (left) and when it is allowed to relax in normal weightbearing (right).

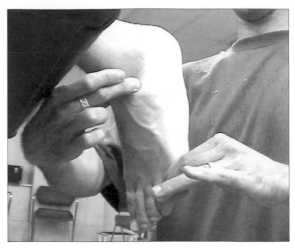

Figure 23.8   Subtalar neutral is obtained with the patient in the prone position and the foot hanging off the end of the table. The foot is in a relaxed to slightly plantarflexed position and the foot is moved from full inversion to full eversion with the outside hand holding just below the heads of the fourth and fifth metatarsals. The inside hand palpates the neck of the talus as it protrudes medially into the thumb and laterally into the index finger. When the pressure on the thumb and index finger are equal, the ankle is pushed toward dorsiflexion until slight resistance is felt. Forcing the ankle into dorsiflexion may change the natural alignment of the forefoot relative to the rearfoot.

innominate rotations or leg length discrepancies. Scapular asymmetry may indicate spinal curvatures or muscular imbalances.

NON-WEIGHTBEARING ASSESSMENT

Non-weightbearing evaluation of the foot and ankle begins in the prone position. The subtalar neutral position was first introduced by Root et al (1977) as a reference position for measuring motion at the ankle and subtalar joint. In order to accurately attain the neutral position of the subtalar joint, the hip should be held in a neutral (internal/external rotation) position. The calcaneus should then be bisected and marked with pen. The distal third of the tibia is also bisected. The calcaneus is then rocked between full inversion to full eversion until the talar heads are felt to be congruent beneath the thumb and index finger of the evaluating therapist (Fig. 23.8). This is the neutral position of the subtalar joint and it used as a reference point around which other measurements of the rearfoot are taken. Assessment of passive inversion and eversion allow the therapist to evaluate position as well as mobility of the subtalar joint. Forefoot orientation relative to the rearfoot can be measured with a goniometer projected up from the forefoot. Forefoot varus deformity is a medially facing position of the forefoot relative to the rearfoot. A varus position of the forefoot in subtalar neutral will result in compensatory pronation. Forefoot valgus is a lateral forefoot relative to the rearfoot and results in compensatory supination (Fig. 23.9). First ray orientation and mobility will dictate or be the result of pronation or supination. Fifth ray orientation and mobility should be assessed and evaluated for stress reactions. Lack of ankle dorsiflexion may lead to hypermobility in the midfoot and plantar fasciitis. The forefoot may also rest in an abducted or adducted position and lead to compensatory

pronation or supination, respectively. Muscle strength should be evaluated, especially of the peroneals and posterior tibialis. Functional strength must be evaluated through single leg standing tests or balance activities. Manual muscle testing may not be enough to determine functional strength.

In the supine position, leg length should be assessed. If there is an asymmetry, this may result in pronation on the longer side and supination on the shorter side during weightbearing. Leg length differences, whether functional or structural, can result in compensatory pronation or supination. The midtarsal joint axes (longitudinal and

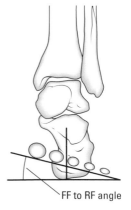

FF to RF angle

Figure 23.9   The forefoot (FF) to rearfoot (RF) alignment is measured with the athlete in the prone position and the subtalar joint in neutral. The measurement is the angle formed between the plane of the second through fifth metatarsal heads and the perpendicular to the calcaneal bisection. The axis of the goniometer should be placed laterally for a varus forefoot and medially for a valgus forefoot.

oblique) can be evaluated for mobility while holding the talocrural joint in dorsiflexion. First metatarsalphalangeal joint range of motion should be 70°. Hallux rigidus or hallux limitus can be the cause or the result of pronation during gait. The popliteal angle is the amount of available knee extension with the hip in 90° of flexion, and it assesses hamstring length. The Thomas test measures hip flexion range of motion. In the sidelying position, hip abduction and external rotation strength should be assessed. Ober's test measures iliotibial band extensibility. Again, these are important because changes at the hip will result in possible compensations at the foot and ankle.

Dynamically, the individual segments of the pelvis, thigh, lower leg and foot should be evaluated in the sagittal, frontal, and transverse planes. This can be difficult unless the segments are evaluated systematically. Athletes should be asked to walk or run on a treadmill if possible. For more thorough evaluation, a videotape can be made and viewed frame-by-frame. The motion should be evaluated either from the ground up, or from the pelvis down, and the segments should be compared for symmetry and normal motion. Evaluate the athlete both during the swing phase and stance phase. Segment and joint motion should be evaluated.

COMMON SPORT-RELATED INJURIES

LATERAL ANKLE SPRAIN

The lateral ankle sprain is one of the most common injuries sustained in sport and exercise activities. Lateral ligament injuries account for 15–25% of all sports injuries (Adamson & Cymet 1997). The most common mechanism of injury occurs with the ankle in a plantarflexed and inverted position. The anterior talofibular ligament (ATFL) has been found to be the weakest ligament in tensile strength when compared to other ligaments around the ankle (Pincivero et al 1993). Risk factors have been defined as intrinsic or extrinsic. Extrinsic factors include training errors, sport type, competition level, equipment, and environmental conditions. Intrinsic factors refer to structural malalignment, strength deficits, range of motion limitations, and ligamentous laxity. After the ATFL, the calcaneofibular ligament is the next most commonly injured, and the posterior talofibular ligament is the least often injured and the strongest.

The most common way of assessing a lateral ankle injury is by grading the sprain (Nicholas & Hershman 1986). A grade I sprain is microscopic tearing of the ligament with no loss of function. Grade II is partial disruption or stretching of the ligament with some loss of

function. Finally, grade III sprains involve a complete tear of the ligament with complete loss of function.

Management of lateral ankle sprains is usually conservative, especially when the sprain is grade I or II. Grade III ankle sprains can be treated surgically but research suggests that patients managed conservatively return to function faster than those managed surgically (Kaikkonen et al 1996). A positive anterior drawer or inversion stress test will indicate that the lateral structures are involved. The talar tilt tests inversion with the foot in a dorsiflexed position and is thought to test the calcaneofibular ligament.

The functional approach to ankle rehabilitation has been advocated by a number of researchers (Adamson & Cymet 1997, Clanton & Porter 1997, Lynch & Renstrom 1999, Molnar 1988, Seto & Brewster 1994). It is generally agreed that the acute or initial phase of rehabilitation should include management of effusion, pain control, and range of motion. The ankle should be placed in as much dorsiflexion as possible to keep the joint initially stable and to decrease capsular distension. During the first 3 weeks, the ankle should be protected from inversion to prevent formation of type III collagen, which leads to elongation of the ligament (Lynch & Renstrom 1999). Exercises should be focused in the sagittal plane. Regaining range of motion in all planes is important early on, to stimulate collagen type I formation as it responds best to tension (Buckwalter & Cooper 1987).

Once pain and effusion are managed, rehabilitation should focus on full return of full range of motion, weightbearing status and strength as tested with a manual muscle test. Elastic band or tubing exercises and modalities are common during this phase.

Functional strengthening and proprioception should be the focus of rehabilitation once the transition from open to closed kinetic chain exercises has begun. Activities in the weightbearing position have been shown to be of greater benefit to the patient in regaining functional stability of the joint (Stormont et al 1985). Exercises that induce motion in all planes are most likely to be of the highest benefit to the athlete.

Wobble boards and single leg standing tests have been used to increase proprioception and balance (Adamson & Cymet 1997, Clanton & Porter 1997, Lynch & Renstrom 1999, Molnar 1988, Seto & Brewster 1994). Balancing on the minitramp while throwing a ball both toward and away from the affected limb is a high-level functional activity (Fig. 23.10). Low load, high repetition tension exercises help most with healing of ligament while figure-of-eight runs, single leg hops, carioca crossovers, and shuttle runs train functional stability at the joint. Sport-specific tests should also be performed. It has been suggested that the return to function time is decreased with a progressive loading approach to rehabilitation

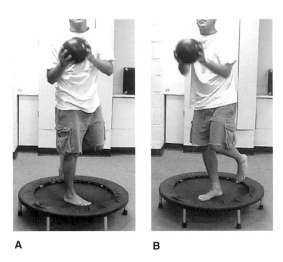

A   **B**

Figure 23.10   **A**: Catching the ball toward the side of the affected limb requires eccentric activity and control of the inverters and plantarflexors primarily. **B**: Eccentric control of the everters and dorsiflexors is required when the athlete is facing away from the affected side. All activities on the minitrampoline require balance and coactivation of the muscles around the ankle joint.

(Kern-Steiner et al 1999). Proprioceptive training is also found to be an important factor in ankle rehabilitation. Patients who have trained with wobble boards have shown increased proprioceptive ability and fewer recurrent ankle sprains (Hoffman & Payne 1995, Wester et al 1996). Additionally, balance and coordination training has been shown to decrease perceived ankle instability and to increase proprioception (Bernier & Perrin 1998, Rozzi et al 1999). Exercises that induce motion in all planes are most likely to be of the highest benefit to the athlete.

Shoe wear, bracing, and taping may also be important adjuncts to treatment of the lateral ankle sprain. Braces have been shown to reduce inversion velocity, while taping and high-top shoes have been shown to decrease the inversion moment when the ankle is placed in varying degrees of plantarflexion (Ottaviani et al 1995, Shapiro et al 1994a, Vaes et al 1998). Everter strength has been shown to be important in the decrease of the inversion moment during weightbearing activities (Ashton-Miller et al 1996).

HIGH ANKLE SPRAIN

A high ankle sprain is a sprain involving the distal tibiofibular syndesmosis and/or the anterior inferior tibiofibular ligament. This injury is much less common than a lateral ankle sprain and is often seen in conjunction with lateral ankle ligament injuries. The mechanism of injury at this joint is usually one of external rotation of the foot and internal rotation of the tibia. The recovery of the athlete with this type of injury is usually

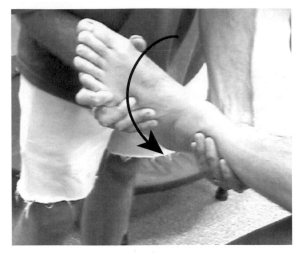

Figure 23.11   External rotation test will be positive in the individual with a high ankle sprain, as the abduction motion will act to separate the tibia and fibula, placing stress on the distal tibiofibular ligaments.

longer than that of an athlete with a lateral ligament injury (Boytim et al 1991).

Management of high ankle sprains is usually conservative as is the case with the lateral ankle sprain. Proper management of this injury begins with proper diagnosis of the sprain. Tenderness to palpation of the distal tibiofibular joint with associated effusion and ecchymosis is usually present. Dorsiflexion in a loaded condition will also be painful. The external rotation stress test (Fig. 23.11) and the tibiofibular compression tests (Fig. 23.12) may also be positive with high ankle sprains. The acute phase of rehabilitation should include management of effusion, pain control, and range of motion. While dorsiflexion is encouraged in the patient with lateral ankle sprain, dorsiflexion, even in an open chain, should be avoided early in order to keep the distal tibiofibular joint from separating. Gait training should

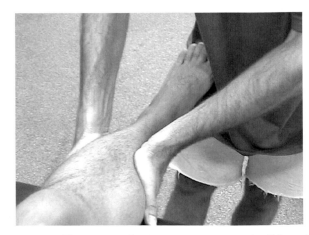

Figure 23.12   The compression test acts to separate the tibia and fibula and places stress on the injured ligaments at the distal tibiofibular joint.

progress only up to 50% weightbearing during this stage. Once the acute phase of rehabilitation is complete, full range of motion in an open chain, and progressive resistive exercises should be the focus. Weightbearing should still progress slowly as separation of the tibiofibular joint is still possible with dorsiflexion or foot external rotation in a closed chain. Taping or bracing may help advance weightbearing while limiting distal tibiofibular joint separation. Elastic band or tubing exercises in an open chain will help prepare for functional activities.

Transition to closed kinetic chain activities and return to function are the goals of the final stage of rehabilitation. Single leg standing exercises with a wedge under the heel (plantarflexion = 20°) has been suggested as a method of training proprioception and minimizing dorsiflexion stress (Brosky et al 1995). Wobble boards in a clockwise direction (for the right foot) will aid with normal foot progression during walking. Retrograde walking with slight elevation may help to decrease dorsiflexion stress on the joint. Minitramp, figure-of-eight runs, single leg hopping, carioca crossover, and shuttle run can be initiated toward the end of treatment. Proprioceptive training is also important in high ankle sprain rehabilitation. All of the above activities should be performed without pain or 'giving way'. If necessary, shoes, braces, and/or taping may be employed to provide stability.

SPRING LIGAMENT SPRAIN

The spring ligament runs from the sustentaculum tali on the medial side of the calcaneus to the navicular tuberosity. This injury is common in runners and is often seen in conjunction with posterior tibialis tendonitis or dysfunction. The mechanism of injury of this structure is usually traumatic, but can also be related to pronation. It is important to differentially diagnose this structure from the posterior tibialis tendon or peroneus longus tendon as they both insert on the navicular.

Management of spring ligament sprains is usually conservative and can be difficult if the true cause of the pathology is not determined. The injury is usually traumatic and the athlete will describe a hard landing on an uneven surface, which forces the forefoot into dorsiflexion or pronation. The patient will be tender directly over the spring ligament with deep palpation. Superficial palpation may not illicit complaints. The patient will likely have no pain with resisted plantarflexion when the rearfoot is neutral, everted, or inverted. Direct tension placed on the spring ligament through passive dorsiflexion of the midtarsal joint may also be painful. Finally, patients will usually complain of discomfort during single leg standing. These athletes often present with a pronated midfoot posture.

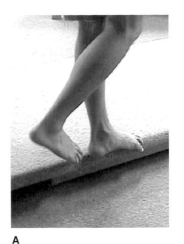 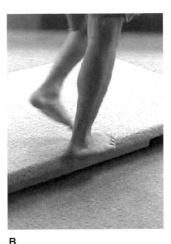

A **B**

Figure 23.13A & B   Walking on a balance beam or side of a step requires eccentric control of the (**A**) inverters or (**B**) everters.

The acute phase of rehabilitation should include management of any effusion and pain. Any activity that causes pain should be avoided and weightbearing status should be monitored. The patient may benefit from a short period of non-weightbearing if symptoms persist. Lack of motion is not an issue in these patients. In fact, these athletes usually present with an increased amount of midfoot motion and further treatment should focus on stabilization of the midfoot.

Once the acute phase of rehabilitation is complete, progressive resistive exercises should be the focus. Special attention should be paid to the strength of the anterior tibialis, posterior tibialis, and peroneus longus. Arch taping or foot orthoses may decrease tension to the structures supporting the medial longitudinal arch. Taping and orthotic management should focus on placing the forefoot in an adducted and plantarflexed position relative to the rearfoot.

Closed kinetic chain activities and return to full function are the goals of the final stage of rehabilitation. Activities that focus on the functional strength of the posterior tibialis and peroneus longus muscles should be included. Single leg standing on uneven surfaces or on the minitramp will aid in training these muscles. Balance beam activities focusing on eccentric control of pronation may also be beneficial (Fig. 23.13).

POSTERIOR TIBIALIS TENDONITIS

Posterior tibialis tendonitis is an overuse injury usually related to an inability to adequately control some aspect of pronation. Posterior tibialis tendonitis is the injury typically referred to as 'shin splints'. This injury is seen often in runners or in athletes whose sport requires a great deal of running. This is due to the need of the posterior tibialis to control pronation eccentrically during the loading phase of gait. This becomes especially demanding during running as the joint excursions, velocities, and forces are significantly increased (Mann & Hagy 1980). Posterior tibialis tendonitis may also result after the tendon has remained in a shortened position for a period of time, such as in an individual with a plantarflexed posture of the rearfoot or in an individual with a cavus medial longitudinal arch.

The patient will usually be tender just posterior to the medial malleolus and often tender on the posterior-medial distal third of the tibia. If the patient is especially painful along the tibia, the pathology should be differentially diagnosed from medial tibial stress syndrome (Mubarak et al 1982). Additionally, the presence of paresthesia or radicular pain in the foot may indicate the presence of tarsal tunnel syndrome. The patient with posterior tibialis tendonitis may also complain of pain with palpation over the navicular, pain with resisted plantarflexion and inversion, and pain with passive eversion and dorsiflexion. Passive dorsiflexion and eversion can be accomplished functionally with relaxed single leg stance. Management of posterior tibialis tendonitis can be challenging. Because the athlete must pronate, even during normal ambulation, decreasing stress on the tendon may be impossible without immobilization or casting. However, this is usually not a necessary measure.

The acute phase of rehabilitation should include management of pain and any swelling. Rest or complete cessation of activity appears to be the best treatment for the athlete in the acute stage. The athlete may still remain active during this stage through cross-training, as long as the activity does not increase the symptoms at the posterior tibialis tendon. Non-steroidal anti-inflammatory drugs (NSAIDs), ice, and other inflammation reducing modalities are also beneficial during this stage.

Passive range of motion for eversion and dorsiflexion should be the focus of the next stage of treatment. Regaining a normal resting length of the tendon is imperative in restoring the athlete to normal function. Although deterioration of pain and other symptoms should guide treatment, increasing passive range of motion is important, as decreased tendon length will likely be a main limiting factor to progress if not gained early. If increased pronation is a major mechanical problem leading to symptoms, this is a good time in the treatment to introduce some support to the medial longitudinal arch. Heel wedges or over-the-counter orthoses may help temporarily while custom-molded orthoses are being fabricated.

Closed kinetic chain activities and eccentric strengthening are the goals of the final stage of rehabilitation. Single leg standing toe raises with controlled lowering

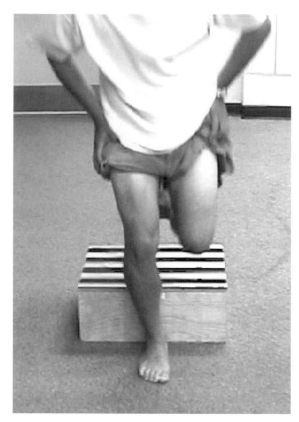

Figure 23.14 During controlled landing exercises, the athlete should be instructed to maintain the knee over the second toe of the foot. Restrictions on degrees and excursions of knee flexion can also be placed on the exercise.

eccentrically loads the posterior tibialis tendon in a functional situation. Wobble boards in both clockwise and counterclockwise directions provide training of multidirectional control of pronation and supination. Sidestepping and cariocas away from the effected side place increased eccentric demand on the posterior tibialis tendon. Finally, controlled landing activities from progressively increasing step heights train the athlete to control pronation during running, which is a landing activity (Fig. 23.14). Since posterior tibialis pathology is so often associated with pronation, external devices such as shoes or custom-molded orthoses may be necessary to control excess motion in the midfoot and rearfoot.

PERONEAL TENDONITIS

Peroneal tendonitis is a result of overuse of either the peroneus longus or peroneus brevis tendons. This injury is often seen in conjunction with lateral ankle sprains and may be the cause or the result of lateral ankle instability. Peroneal tendonitis differs in its mechanism of injury depending on whether the longus or the brevis is involved. Peroneus brevis involvement is more commonly associated with supinatory overuse as it is stressed in the inverted position of the foot and ankle. A slightly different mechanism is usually attributed to peroneus longus tendonitis. Like the brevis, the longus plantarflexes and everts the foot. However, the longus runs beneath the plantar surface of the foot to attach to the first metatarsal. Hypermobility of the first ray allows for excessive dorsiflexion, which forces the forefoot into pronation during weightbearing activities. Therefore, the inability to control pronation by the peroneus longus often results in tendonitis.

Tenderness to palpation distal and posterior to the lateral malleolus is most common in peroneal tendonitis (Mann & Coughlin 1993). The athlete may also be tender proximal to the malleolus and, depending on the structure involved, at the base of the first or fifth metatarsal. Regardless of the specific structure, the athlete will experience pain with resisted plantarflexion and eversion. Passive eversion and dorsiflexion will be painful for the brevis and most likely for the longus. Passive first metatarsal dorsiflexion will be painful if the longus is involved.

The acute phase of rehabilitation should include management of any swelling and pain. Taping or bracing may help prevent the tendon from further tension injury, especially if any instability or weakness is present. After the acute phase, passive range of motion and concentric resistive exercises should follow. Often, a muscle imbalance has developed, so stretching and strengthening antagonists such as the anterior and posterior tibialis muscles may be necessary, especially in the athlete with a cavus foot. Concentric training of first ray plantarflexion may also be beneficial. However, it is likely that the athlete with a hypermobile first ray will not be able to gain enough dynamic strength to control forefoot pronation, and orthoses or metatarsal support may be necessary.

Functional activities should complete the rehabilitation of athletes with peroneal tendonitis. Single leg standing exercises should be the focus in these patients, as they must regain eccentric control of frontal plane activities. This is especially important in athletes with associated lateral ankle sprains, as they will have decreased proprioceptive ability (Beckman & Buchanan 1995). Wobble boards and minitramp standing with a ball toss will help control eccentric supination or pronation. If instability or decreased proprioception remains toward the end of rehabilitation, taping or orthoses may be necessary in order for the athlete to return to play safely.

PLANTAR FASCIITIS

Plantar fasciitis is usually caused by progressive collagen degradation at the medial calcaneal tubercle. This injury is common in athletes in all sports, especially those involving running. However, dancers and gymnasts have some of the highest incidences of plantar fasciitis (Kamenski & Fu 1994, Weiss 1994). The mechanism of injury at this joint is usually one of overuse. The plantar fascia is placed on constant stretch and is often seen in the athlete with a pronated foot type. Athletes with supinated foot types are also prone to the development of plantar fasciitis where a short resting fascia is susceptible to any outside stretch placed on it. A tight gastrocnemius–soleus complex may also be present in individuals with plantar fasciitis (Marshall 1978) and seems to be commonly associated with the cavus foot (Franco 1987). Tenderness to palpation directly over the medial calcaneal tubercle is most common in these athletes, although some patients complain of pain along the entire plantar surface of the foot and into the fascial insertion at the metatarsal heads. Classic symptoms also include pain with the first few steps in the morning or during the first 5–10 min of running. The pain usually subsides with activity and increases after periods of rest. Athletes may also have increased symptoms when walking barefoot.

Management of plantar fasciitis can be difficult as the pathology is often described as self-limiting. The acute phase of rehabilitation focuses on pain management. Typical modalities at this point include ice massage, deep friction massage, and NSAIDs. Stretching and decreasing stress on the fascia should be the focus of the next phase of treatment. Stretching the gastrocnemius and soleus are important as they are proximally attached to the calcaneus and would increase tension on the fascia by means of this attachment. The athlete should be instructed to prevent stretch on the fascia itself especially in the pronated foot. Locking the foot into supination during stretching can be accomplished by placing a wedge or towel under the medial surface of the foot during wall stretches (Fig. 23.15). Stretching of the fascia in the supinated foot can be accomplished by deep friction massage or passive toe extension. Using a low dye taping technique may also relieve tension on the plantar fascia.

As always, functional weightbearing activities should be the focus of the final stage of rehabilitation. Training of extrinsic muscles, which support the medial longitudinal arch, is important to help take passive tension off the fascia. These muscles include the anterior and posterior tibialis muscles, as well as the peroneus longus. Although it is often suggested that the intrinsic muscles of the foot be trained (e.g. with towel crunches), there is little evidence to support that these muscles are even active in controlling foot posture (Mann & Hagy 1979). If increased midfoot mobility is present, a custom-molded orthotic may be necessary. Often a semirigid orthosis with good midfoot support can be helpful in the athlete with plantar fasciitis.

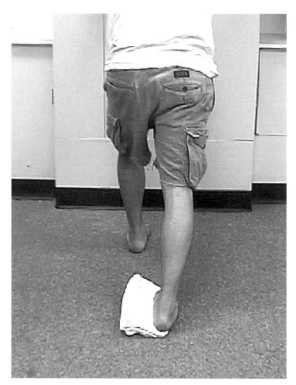

Figure 23.15 Placing a towel under the medial side of the foot places the subtalar joint in inversion and therefore locks the midtarsal joint, preventing it from pronating. The stretch is then focused on the posterior calf musculature without placing stress on the soft tissues of the arch.

SESAMOIDITIS

The sesamoid bones are embedded within the tendon of the flexor hallucis brevis. Sesamoiditis does not refer to the direct inflammation of the bones themselves but rather to the soft tissue surrounding the bones. Most individuals with sesamoid pain are those with a cavus foot. These individuals usually present with a rigid midfoot and forefoot and a plantarflexed first ray (Axe & Ray 1988). However, individuals who pronate and place excess force on the medial side of the first metatarsophalangeal (MTP) joint during push off are also susceptible to sesamoiditis. The pathology can result from repetitive trauma as described above or an acute incident of high impact (i.e. landing from a jump).

As the medial sesamoid is most often involved, radiographs may be inconclusive as to whether a fracture is present and contributing to symptoms. Tenderness to palpation over the involved sesamoid is most often present and may also present with a thickening or swelling of the tendinous sheath. The athlete will feel pain upon weightbearing especially with the shoes off. Passive or active dorsiflexion of the first MTP joint will be painful. Additionally, rising onto the toes will be painful or difficult for this patient.

The acute phase of rehabilitation should include pain control and decreasing first MTP dorsiflexion range of motion. Taping the joint in neutral or slight plantarflexion decreases stress on the tendons and weightbearing on the sesamoids. Additionally, plantarflexion of the first ray should be minimized as this imparts a relative dorsiflexion at the first MTP joint (Mann & Coughlin 1993). Therefore, a metatarsal pad placed just proximal to the first metatarsal head will limit plantarflexion of the first ray. Decreasing heel height, especially in women's shoes, will also decrease the amount of first MTP dorsiflexion.

Management of sesamoiditis is usually handled with orthoses or shoe inserts. Because the symptoms are often a result of a structural deviation, support of the first ray in either a supinated or pronated foot is important. A metatarsal pad under the first ray may be enough to support the medial column. However, in more severe cases, a full custom-molded orthotic device with significant medial midfoot support may be necessary. Cutouts in the orthosis under the first metatarsal head may also decrease pressure on the sesamoids (White 1996).

ACHILLES TENDONITIS

Achilles tendonitis is a common injury among athletes, especially those involved in sports which require constant eccentric loading of the posterior calf muscles (e.g. American football quarterbacks or basketball players). The tendon is especially susceptible to injury based on its reduced blood supply (Smart et al 1980) and the possible wringing effect of this tendon during pronation (Gross 1992). Older athletes may be more predisposed to this injury based on a further decreased blood supply and decreased extensibility of collagen.

Athletes usually feel pain with direct palpation over the Achilles tendon but not over the gastrocnemius or soleus muscles. The tendon may also feel fibrous upon palpation. The patient will likely feel pain with passive dorsiflexion and resisted plantarflexion of the talocrural joint. Going down steps or walking backwards will also increase symptoms.

The acute phase of rehabilitation should include management of effusion and pain control. Range of motion should be minimized or at least kept within a pain-free range of motion. A heel lift in the shoe will decrease passive dorsiflexion and the need for eccentric muscle activity during ambulation. Deep friction massage may also be beneficial, as soft tissue mobilization has been shown to aid in fibroblast formation during healing (Davidson et al 1997). Rest is also recommended to decrease stress on the tissue.

Once the acute phase of rehabilitation is complete, full range of motion in open chain and progressively resistive exercises should be the focus. Passive dorsiflexion range of motion will increase formation and alignment of collagen. Resistive exercises should begin with isometrics and advance to concentric exercises in an open chain. Eccentrics will be the final stage of strengthening as these exercises place the most tension on the tendon.

Closed kinetic chain activities and functional activities are the goals of the final stage of rehabilitation. Toe walking and single leg standing exercises with toe walking are functional activities with a strong eccentric component. Standing exercises on a wobble board will also help with muscle balance around the joints of the foot and ankle. Retrograde walking focusing on sagittal plane progression is important for specific eccentric training. Minitramp, figure-of-eight runs, single leg hopping, and carioca crossovers on the toes would be exercises utilized toward the end of treatment. Modification of shoewear (i.e. increasing heel height in the shoe) or orthotic management can be beneficial in these patients if intrinsic methods do not return the athlete to full function.

FRACTURES

Classification of ankle fractures can be difficult because of the large number of mechanisms for injuring the ankle. The most comprehensive system of classifying ankle injuries has been presented by Lauge-Hansen (1950). In general, he categorizes these fractures by the nature of the forces that cause the injury. For instance, a lateral malleolar fracture is most likely to be the result of a supinatory force.

Because of the large body of literature on ankle fractures, a general outline of postinjury rehabilitation will be discussed here. Fractures of the distal third of the lower leg are considered to be 'ankle' fractures and can involve the tibia, fibula, and talus. The mechanism of injury for the tibia and fibula is usually torsional while it is compressive for the talus.

The severity of the injury will dictate how rehabilitation will progress. Obviously, a simple fibular fracture in a 10-year-old boy will likely be easier to manage than a compound fracture with open reduction/internal fixation in an older person. Even so, the general guidelines for treatment should be the same. Most likely, as physical therapists, we will not see the athlete with the lower leg fracture until after the cast has been removed. However, if we are fortunate enough, early range of motion of adjacent joints should be implemented. Muscle setting and isometrics of muscles surrounding the area should begin as soon as pain allows. Cross-training with an upper body ergometer will help keep the athletes cardiovascular status high while the ankle is immobilized. Weightbearing should be encouraged as soon as possible to stimulate bone healing and regrowth.

Once the cast is removed, range of motion and strengthening should be the primary goals of rehabilitation. Full weightbearing should be achieved very soon after the removal of the cast. Strengthening should progress from concentrics to eccentrics and should not only focus on the previously immobilized muscles but also on the muscles of the adjacent joints. Full range of motion may not be an option after a surgical intervention where surgical hardware remains near the joint. Tendonitis is not an uncommon associated problem in the athlete with a recent fracture. Muscle atrophy and shortening contribute to the development of the pathology, especially once weightbearing activities begin. Passive range of motion and eccentric activities should continue through all stages of physical therapy treatment.

Jones fracture

The Jones fracture is a fracture involving the proximal portion of the fifth metatarsal just distal to the insertion of the peroneus brevis. This fracture is the most common fracture of the fifth metatarsal and should be differentiated from a Dancer's fracture or an avulsion fracture. Jones fractures have a high propensity for non-union and for this reason, are often managed with early surgical insertion of an intramedullary rod (Mindrebo et al 1993). Conservative management is most successful when a non-weightbearing cast is applied for up to 6 weeks.

Management of the Jones fracture after immobilization should follow a similar course to that of lower leg fractures. Since Jones fractures are often thought to be the result of increased stress to the fifth metatarsal, changing the alignment of the foot and therefore the forces, may help decrease the chances of future injury to the lateral side of the foot. Orthoses that redistribute the forces across the entire forefoot and away from the lateral side are an appropriate intervention in the athlete with a biomechanical dysfunction.

LESS COMMON INJURIES

SINUS TARSI SYNDROME

Sinus tarsi syndrome is a complicated problem that falls under the 'less common injuries' portion of this chapter, probably because it has been underdiagnosed. This injury is often referred to as a chronic ankle sprain or chronic lateral ankle pain (Brown 1960, O'Conner 1958, Taillard et al 1981). These athletes most commonly present with a significant pronated posture of the rearfoot. However, athletes with a supinated foot posture make up 20% of the individuals with sinus tarsi syndrome.

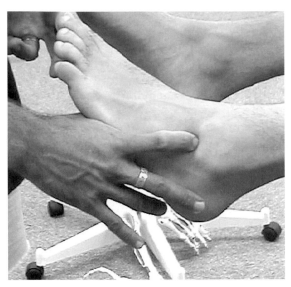

Figure 23.16 The sinus tarsus can be palpated just inferior and anterior to the lateral malleolus, inferior and slightly posterior to the anterior talofibular ligament, and superior and anterior to the peroneal tubercle on the lateral side of the foot.

Sinus tarsi syndrome is a result of repetitive trauma to the lateral articulation between the talus and calcaneus. An inflammatory response develops and may exacerbate to the point of compression within the entire sinus tarsus. Pain is most often felt on the lateral side just posterior to the anterior talofibular ligament. Athletes will complain of pain with forced eversion and palpation over the sinus tarsi laterally (Fig. 23.16). Swelling will likely be present laterally and may progress medially through the sinus tarsus.

The acute phase of rehabilitation should include management of effusion and pain control. Dorsiflexion and eversion should be avoided early in order to keep the subtalar joint separated on the lateral side. This can be accomplished with taping or an over-the-counter orthotic. Once the acute phase of rehabilitation is complete, a thorough biomechanical analysis should be employed to determine the source of the sinus tarsi syndrome. Supinatory patients are more difficult to manage but are also less common. Joint mobilizations to encourage pronation and midfoot mobility with plantarflexion stretching may be enough to decrease the lateral stress in these individuals.

Athletes with sinus tarsi syndrome who pronate should be managed in a way that will decrease the forces on the lateral side of the subtalar joint. Posterior tibialis dysfunction or weak plantarflexors may be contributing to the excessive pronation and can be rehabilitated with strengthening and functional activities. More than likely, these athletes will need to be managed extrinsically by maintaining the subtalar joint away from full eversion, thus decompressing the lateral joint space. This can be achieved with a standard orthotic or may require a more aggressive prescription of an inverted orthotics (Blake 1986).

LISFRANC DISLOCATION

A Lisfranc dislocation is a dislocation of any one or several of the tarsometatarsal joints. Dislocation without fracture at these joints usually occurs as a result of indirect trauma such as pronation of the rearfoot while the forefoot is plantarflexed and fixed to the ground (Shapiro et al 1994b). A dislocation, even if it is severe, will often reduce itself after an injury. This injury is much less common than a lateral ankle sprain and is often seen in conjunction with lateral ankle ligament injuries. The mechanism of injury at this joint is usually one of external rotation of the foot and internal rotation of the tibia. The recovery of the athlete with this type of injury is usually longer than that of an athlete with a lateral ligament injury

Depending on the severity of the dislocation, the patient may feel tenderness along the dorsal and plantar surface of the joints. Management of the Lisfranc dislocation is not difficult if all pathology has been recognized. There is often an associated fracture with a Lisfranc dislocation, which can significantly slow rehabilitation if it has gone undiagnosed. Care should be taken to begin physical therapy treatment only after fractures have begun to heal. Even without a fracture, internal fixation of the joint(s) is often necessary for stability after significant dislocation.

If swelling and pain are still present after injury, modalities and NSAIDs will help to reduce symptoms. Weightbearing should be monitored closely as the tarsometatarsal joint accepts a great deal of the force during weightbearing activities. Athletes with a Lisfranc injury will likely need good midfoot and forefoot support after physical therapy treatment. Additionally, shoes with firm soles and decreased toe break will help minimize mobility in the joint after injury.

SUMMARY

The ankle is the most commonly injured body part in sport and exercise. Due to the complex make-up of the foot and ankle, a thorough anatomical understanding is necessary in order to accurately diagnose and manage injuries in this region. Examination and assessment of foot and ankle injuries should consider all associated joints and soft tissue structures, and should incorporate functional and sport-specific tests. Management of foot and ankle injuries should consider the high-level demands placed on the foot and ankle in many sport and exercise activities.

REFERENCES

Adamson C, Cymet T 1997 Ankle sprains: evaluation, treatment, rehabilitation. Maryland Medical Journal 46:530–537

Aerts P, Ker R F, deClerq D et al 1995 The mechanical properties of the human heel pad: a paradox resolved. Journal of Biomechanics 28:1299–1308

Ashton-Miller J A, Ottaviani R A, Hutchinson C et al 1996 What best protects the inverted weightbearing ankle against further inversion? Evertor muscle strength compares favorably with shoe height, athletic tape, and three orthoses. American Journal of Sports Medicine 24:800–809

Axe M J, Ray R L 1988 Orthotic treatment of sesamoid pain. American Journal of Sports Medicine 16:411–416

Barnett C H, Napier J R 1952 The axis of rotation at the ankle joint in man: its influence upon the form of the talus and mobility of the fibula. Journal of Anatomy 86:1–9

Beckman S M, Buchanan T S 1995 Ankle inversion injury and hypermobility: effect on hip and ankle muscle electromyography onset latency. Archives of Physical Medicine and Rehabilitation 76:1138–1143

Bernier J N, Perrin D H 1998 Effect of coordination training on proprioception of the functionally unstable ankle. Journal of Orthopaedic and Sports Physical Therapy 27:264–275

Blake R L 1986 Inverted functional orthosis. Journal of the American Podiatric Medical Association 76:275–276

Boytim M J, Fischer D A, Neumann L 1991 Syndesmotic ankle sprains. American Journal of Sports Medicine 19:294–298

Brosky T, Nyland J, Nitz A et al 1995 The ankle ligaments: consideration of syndesmotic injury and implications for rehabilitation. Journal of Orthopaedic and Sports Physical Therapy 21:197–205

Brown, J F. 1960 The sinus tarsi syndrome. Clinical Orthopaedics and Related Research 18:231–233

Buckwalter J A, Cooper R R 1987 The cells and matrices of skeletal connective tissues. In: Albright J A, Brand R A (eds). The Scientific basis of orthopaedics. Appleton and Lange, Norwalk

Clanton T O, Porter D A 1997 Primary care of foot and ankle injuries in the athlete. Clinics in Sports Medicine 16:435–466

Davidson C J, Ganion L R, Gehlsen G M et al 1997 Rat tendon morphologic and functional changes resulting from soft tissue mobilization. Medicine and Science in Sports and Exercise 29:313–319

Franco A H 1987 Pes cavus and pes planus, analysis and treatment. Physical Therapy 67:688–694

Giladi M, Milgrom C, Stein M et al 1985 The low arch, a protective factor in stress fractures. Orthopedic Review 14:709–712

Gross M T 1992 Chronic tendonitis: pathomechanics of injury, factors affecting the healing response, and treatment. Journal of Orthopaedic and Sports Physical Therapy 16:248–261

Hicks J H 1953 Mechanics of the foot: joints. Journal of Anatomy 87:345–357

Hoffman M, Payne V G 1995 The effects of proprioceptive ankle disk training on healthy subjects. Journal of Orthopaedic and Sports Physical Therapy 21:90–93

Kaikkonen A, Kannus P, Järvinen M 1996 Surgery versus functional treatment in ankle ligament tears. A prospective study. Clinical Orthopedics 326:194–202

Kamenski R, Fu F H 1994 Dance and the Arts. In: Fu F H, Stone D A (eds). Sports injuries: mechanisms prevention treatment. Williams and Wilkins, Baltimore, MD

Kern-Steiner R, Washecheck H S, Kelsey D D 1999 Strategy of exercise prescription using an unloading technique for functional rehabilitation of an athlete with an inversion ankle sprain. Journal of Orthopaedic and Sports Physical Therapy 29:282–287

Kura H, Luo Z-P, Kitaoka H B et al 1997 Quantitative analysis of the intrinsic muscles of the foot. The Anatomical Record 249:143–151

Lauge-Hansen N 1950 Fractures of the ankle II. Combined experimental-surgical and experimental-roentgenological investigation. Archives of Surgery 60:957–972

Lofvenberg R, Karrholm J, Sudelin G et al 1995 Prolonged reaction time in patients with chronic lateral instability of the ankle. American Journal of Sports Medicine 23:414–417

Lundberg A, Svensson O K, Nemeth G et al 1989 The axis of rotation of the ankle joint. Journal of Bone and Joint Surgery (Br) 71-B:94–99

Lynch S A, Renstom A F H 1999 Treatment of acute lateral ankle ligament rupture in the athlete. Journal of Sports Medicine 21:61–71

McGee D J 1992 Orthopedic physical assessment, 2nd edn. WB Saunders, Philadelphia

Mann R A, Hagy J L 1979 The function of the toes in walking, jogging and running. Clinical Orthopaedics and Related Research 142:24–29

Mann R A, Hagy J 1980 Biomechanics of walking, running, and sprinting. American Journal of Sports Medicine 8:345–350

Mann R A, Coughlin M J 1993 Surgery of the foot and ankle, 6th edn. Mosby, St Louis, MO

Marshall R N 1978 Foot mechanics and joggers' injuries. New Zealand Medical Journal 88:288–290

Mindrebo N, Shelbourne K D, Van Meter C D, Rettig A C 1993 Outpatient percutaneous screw fixation of the acute Jones fracture. American Journal of Sports Medicine 21:720–723

Molnar M E 1988 Rehabilitation of the injured ankle. Clinics in Sports Medicine 7:193–204

Mubarak S J, Gould R N, Lee Y F et al 1982 The medial tibial stress syndrome. A cause of shin splints. American Journal of Sports Medicine 10:201–205

Nicholas J, Hershman E B 1986 The lower extremity and spine in sports medicine. CV Mosby, St. Louis, MO

O'Conner D 1958 Sinus tarsi syndrome. A clinical entity. Journal of Bone and Joint Surgery (Am) 40A:720–729

Ottaviani R A, Ashton-Miller J A, Kothari S U et al 1995 Basketball shoe height and the maximal muscular resistance to applied ankle inversion and eversion moments. American Journal of Sports Medicine 23:418–423

Pincivero D, Gieck J H, Saliba E N 1993 Rehabilitation of a lateral ankle sprain with cryokinetics and functional progressive exercise. Journal of Sport Rehabilitation 2:200–220

Root M L, Orien W P, Weed J H 1977 Normal and abnormal function of the foot. Clinical Biomechanics Corporation, Los Angeles, CA

Rozzi S L, Lephart S M, Sterner R et al 1999 Balance training for persons with functionally unstable ankles. Journal of Orthopaedic and Sports Physical Therapy 29:478–486

Saltzman C L, Nawoczenski D A, Talbot K D 1995 Measurement of the medial longitudinal arch. Archives of Physical Medicine and Rehabilitation 76:45–49

Seto J L, Brewster C E 1994 Treatment approaches following foot and ankle injury. Clinics in Sports Medicine 13:695–718

Shapiro M S, Kabo J M, Mitchell P W et al 1994a Ankle sprain prophylaxis: an analysis of the stabilizing effects of braces and tape. American Journal of Sports Medicine 22:78–82

Shapiro M S, Wascher D C, Finerman G A 1994b Rupture of Lisfranc's ligament in athletes. American Journal of Sports Medicine 22:687–691

Silver R L, de la Garza J, Rang M 1985 The myth of muscle balance. A study of relative strengths and excursions of normal muscles about the foot and ankle. Journal of Bone and Joint Surgery (Am) 67A:432–437

Smart G W, Taunton J E, Clement D B 1980 Achilles tendon disorders in runners: a review. Medicine and Science in Sports and Exercise 12:231–243

Stormont D M, Morrey B F, An K N et al 1985 Stability of the loaded ankle. Relation between articular restraint and primary and secondary static restraints. American Journal of Sports Medicine 13:295–300

Taillard W, Meyer J M, Garcia J et al 1981 The sinus tarsi syndrome. International Orthopedics 5:117–130

Vaes P H, Duquet W, Casteleyn P P et al 1998 Static and dynamic roentgenographic analysis of ankle stability in braced and nonbraced stable and functionally unstable ankles. American Journal of Sports Medicine 26:692–702

Waldecker U 2001 Plantar fat pad atrophy: a cause of metatarsalgia? Journal of Foot and Ankle Surgery 40:21–27

Weiss, J R 1994 Gymnastics. In: Fu F H, Stone D A (eds) Sports injuries: mechanisms prevention treatment. Williams and Wilkins, Baltimore, MD

Wester J U, Jespersen S M, Nielsen K D et al 1996 Wobble board training after partial sprains of the lateral ligaments of the ankle: a prospective randomized study. Journal of Orthopaedic and Sports Physical Therapy 23:332–336

White, S C 1996 Padding and taping techniques. In: Valmassey R L (ed). Clinical biomechanics of the lower extremities. Mosby, St. Louis, MO

Whittle M W 1999 Generation and attenuation of transient impulsive forces beneath the foot: a review. Gait and Posture 10:264–275

Williams D S, McClay I S 2000 Measurements used to characterize the foot and the medial longitudinal arch: reliability and validity. Physical Therapy 80:864–871

The role of sport and exercise physical therapies in active groups

24

Children and adolescents

*Elly Trepman   Lyle J Micheli
Lizanne M Backe*

INTRODUCTION

The popularity of organized sports activities for children and adolescents in recent years has been associated with an increased risk of musculoskeletal injury. Estimates are that 25 million children regularly engage in organized sports in the USA alone (Micheli et al 2000). The most rapid rise in organized sports participation is currently seen among high school girls and children younger than 10 years of age (Metzl 2000). Young athletes often begin their competitive careers as early as age 7 years and organized sports participation as early as age 4 years (Micheli et al 2000). Estimates are that youth sports-related injuries account for 3 million annual hospital emergency room visits and 5 million primary care/sports medicine clinic visits (Micheli et al 2000).

Twenty five percent to 30% of youth sports injuries occur in organized sports, and another 40% occur in unorganized sports (Micheli et al 2000). The remainder are categorized as recreational injuries.

In general, males are more commonly injured than females (Backx et al 1991, Kvist et al 1989, Zaricznyj et al 1980). However, with the recent rise in female sports participation (Warren & Shantha 2000) the numbers are becoming less disparate. The National Athletic Trainers' Association (NATA) high school injury data show that girls in soccer and softball have statistically significantly higher injury rates than boys in soccer and baseball, while rates in basketball are equal (Rice 2000). The peak incidence of sports injuries occurs between the ages of 16 and 19 years (Powell & Barber-Foss 2000).

One cause of sports injuries in the young is single impact macrotrauma, in which a single force exceeds the failure threshold of a tissue or bone. Injuries such as fractures, dislocations, ligament sprains, and musculotendinous strains occur in children and adolescents, but the nature of these injuries differs significantly from that in adults as a result of differences in musculoskeletal physiology. The majority of single impact injuries occur in organized sports activity (Backx et al 1989).

Participation in organized sports can also result in overuse injuries, which presently seem to be the most prevalent sports-related injury mechanisms (Micheli et al 2000). The stresses and strains on the musculoskeletal system resulting from sustained exercise, such as running or swimming, are usually below the threshold of macroscopic tissue failure, but may result in microscopic injury. The body may heal this microscopic injury, and also adapt by strengthening the musculoskeletal components in response to the applied stresses. For example, cortical thickening of the metatarsals, tibia, and femur in ballet dancers (Pelipenko 1973, Schneider et al 1974) is a result of many years of repetitive activity during childhood and adolescence. This 'musculoskeletal adaptation' may be analogous to the cardiopulmonary adaptation which occurs in response to aerobic exercise, but occurs more slowly and is more difficult to quantify. If the rate of repetitive microtrauma resulting from intensive training and competition in a single sport exceeds the rate of tissue healing or musculoskeletal adaptation, then clinical overuse injury occurs (Herring & Nilson 1987). The prevalence of overuse injuries may be underestimated in epidemiological studies in which a sports injury is defined as one which results in the need for first aid, medical treatment, or the filing of an accident report (Zaricznyj et al 1980).

RISK FACTORS

Etiological risk factors for sports injury in children have been identified and are helpful in diagnosis and treatment (Micheli et al 2000) (Box 24.1). Many youth sports coaches are well-meaning parents with little knowledge of youth sports, health, and injury. There is a growing national and international awareness of the need for youth sports education and credentialing, which currently occurs at variable levels in different sports, and that is predominantly voluntary. The preparticipation physical examination is an important precursor to sports participation (see Ch. 11). A standard examination and form has been created through the joint efforts of five medical academies/societies (Smith et al 1997). Such examinations elucidate existing problems as well as risk factors for potential injury. Primary care practitioners should include preparticipation physical examinations in the patient's regular check-up approximately 6 weeks prior to the commencement of the sport season. This allows for potential adequate rehabilitation of identified problems. Emphasis is on safe sports participation and not elimination.

Box 24.1 Risk factors for sports injury in children and adolescents

Lack of certified coach
Inadequate or no preparticipation physical examination
Training error
- abrupt increase in training
  - intensity
  - duration
  - frequency
- inadequate warm-up
- improper technique
- tired, injured, or inadequately rehabilitated
Musculotendinous imbalance
- strength
- flexibility
Anatomical malalignment/intrinsic structure
- lumbar hyperlordosis
- lower limb length discrepancy
- abnormal hip rotation
- patellar malalignment
- genu varum
- genu valgum
- pronated pes planus
- cavus foot
Footwear
- poor fit
- inadequate impact absorption
- excessive sole stiffness
- insufficient hindfoot support/heel counter
- arch support
- excessive wear
Playing surface characteristics
- poor shock absorption (e.g. concrete)
- poor resiliency
Genetics
- sex – cercival instability (e.g. Down syndrome)
Hormonal status
- delayed menarche
- amenorrhea
Growth
- prepubescent porus bone
- vulnerable growth cartilage
  - physis
  - articular cartilage
  - traction apophysis
- relative weakness of prepubescent growth plates
- decrease in flexibility during growth spurt
- abnormal development (e.g. diskoid lateral meniscus)
General
- poor nutrition/hydration
- psychological stress
- poor fitness (overall/sport-specific)
- size/weight differences among same age
- inclement weather
Activity-Specific Factors
- hyperextension of lumbar spine (gymnastics, dance)
- shoulder overuse (swimming, pitching)
- Little league elbow (pitching)
- wrist/distal radius overuse (gymnastics)
- lower extremity (running)
- 'spearing' (football)
- body checking (ice hockey)

Abrupt increase in training intensity, frequency, or duration may cause a greater rate of repetitive micro-trauma, exceeding that of either musculoskeletal adaptation or tissue healing (van Mechelen 1992). Therefore, overuse injuries are commonly seen during or after an intensive summer camp or off-season program in which the young athlete abruptly increases activity level in a single sport. Other training errors, such as inadequate warm-up, may result in injury such as muscle strains (Rodenburg 1994).

Previous injury and inadequate rehabilitation may result in altered mechanics of extremity use, placing greater demand on other, uninjured structures. For example, the pitcher who has shoulder pain with overhead delivery may compensate with a more horizontal ('sidearm') pitch, which may result in injury to the elbow (Albright et al 1978).

Musculotendinous imbalances and anatomical malalignment may accentuate the stresses on specific structures (Micheli & Fehlandt 1994). For example, young runners with genu valgum and tibia vara may develop patellofemoral stress syndrome, and dancers with excessive femoral anteversion may force the turnout at the knee or foot, resulting in strains of the medial knee and foot structures. Poor shoe or playing surface characteristics may aggravate repetitive stresses on the lower extremities, resulting in overuse injury. Softer running surfaces such as grass or dirt are more forgiving than concrete.

Underlying disease states or certain genetic compositions can increase the risk of both overuse and single impact injury. For example, cervical instability occasionally associated with Down or Morquio's syndrome may increase the risk of catastrophic sports injury in this population (Browner et al 1999). Limited hip motion secondary to previous Legg–Calvé–Perthes disease may result in increased stresses on other lower extremity structures during sports activity. Young females are at increased risk for anterior cruciate ligament (ACL) injuries compared to young males (Micheli et al 1999a). Hormonal imbalances, such as those seen with amenorrhea, increase a woman's risk for stress fracture (Warren & Shantha 2000). Changes with growth can increase the risk of specific injuries. This topic is addressed in the following section of this chapter.

Some general risk factors for sports injury include poor nutrition and hydration, psychological stress, poor overall or sport-specific fitness, and size and weight differences among same age athletes (Micheli & Jenkins 2001).

Injury patterns in different sports are directly related to sport-specific biomechanics. For example, acromio-clavicular sprains and separations are common in contact sports such as gridiron football, rugby, and hockey, as a result of lateral stresses on the upper torso. Gymnasts, figure skaters, and dancers frequently hyperextend the lumbar spine, and can develop symptomatic spondylolysis, which is a stress fracture of the pars interarticularis (Constantini & Warren 1994).

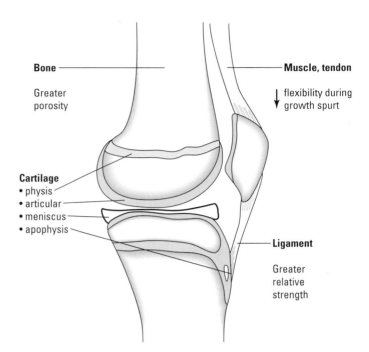

Figure 24.1 Factors related to musculoskeletal growth and development modulate sports injury patterns in children and adolescents.

GROWTH AND MATURATION

Injury patterns in the young athlete vary significantly from those in the adult because of several important differences in musculoskeletal structure and physiology (Fig. 24.1). Changes in bone and soft tissue structure during growth and maturation may result in age-dependent patterns of injury.

Bone tissue undergoes changes in mechanical properties during growth and maturation. The bones of the young child are more porous than those of adults, and may fail in compression; the buckle or torus metaphyseal compression fracture which commonly occurs in children, is not seen in adults (Rang 1983). An angulating force may cause a greenstick fracture, which consists of failure of the tension side and bending (plastic deformation) of the compression side. In adolescents, the hormonal responsiveness of bone is particularly important; female athletes with hypoestrogenism resulting from delayed menarche or amenorrhea have a greater incidence of stress fractures and scoliosis (Warren et al 1986).

The growth cartilage of the young athlete is another structure that can be injured, as in fractures of the growth plate (Larson & McMahan 1966, Salter & Harris 1963, Washer & Finerman 1994) (Fig. 24.2). The fracture pattern of the growth plate changes with age. For example, the Salter–Harris III fracture of the lateral part of the distal

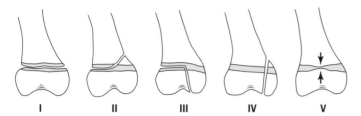

Figure 24.2   Salter–Harris classification of growth plate fractures.

tibia physis of the ankle ('juvenile Tillaux') occurs in a narrow age range (12–14 years), after closure of the middle and medial portion of the physis (Dias 1984, Kleiger & Mankin 1964). The evaluation of growth arrest after physeal injury may be facilitated with magnetic resonance imaging (MRI) (Havranek & Lizler 1991).

Joint problems specific to the young athlete include osteochondritis dissecans (OCD) (Stanitski 1994a) and diskoid lateral meniscus (Stanitski 1994b). OCD is a condition affecting subchondral bone which manifests as a pathological spectrum ranging from softening of the overlying cartilage with an intact articular surface to separation with loose bodies (Kocher et al 2001). Maldevelopment of the lateral meniscus of the knee may result in a diskoid lateral meniscus, which is a cause of occasional pain and snapping, and which often becomes symptomatic with childhood sports participation (Dickhaut & DeLee 1982).

The ligaments of children can be stronger than the growth plate at certain phases of growth, and excessive forces about joints may result in growth plate fracture (Rang 1983, Sanders et al 1980, Washer & Finerman 1994). However, ligament sprains and tears may be more common in children than previously believed. The growth plate is stronger before the onset of puberty (Bright et al 1974), and ligament tears have been documented in prepubescent children without injury to the growth plate (Bradley et al 1979, Clanton et al 1979, DeLee & Curtis 1983). Ligament tears have also been documented in adolescents (Lipscomb & Anderson 1986).

Joint laxity has been shown to decrease with increasing age during childhood (Cheng et al 1991). Furthermore, the adolescent growth spurt is associated with a loss of flexibility (Gurewitsch & O'Neill 1944). Some pediatric athletic injuries can result from increased tightness of the soft tissues or muscle imbalances during and after the pubescent growth period. Sport-specific adaptation in flexibility occurs in adolescents because of different biomechanical demands, such as shoulder flexibility changes observed in tennis players (Kibler & Safran 2000).

The traction apophyses, which consist of columns of growth cartilage that unite tendon to bone, can be subject to macroscopic avulsion or repetitive microscopic avul-

sions with secondary inflammation. These injuries, referred to as traction apophysitises, commonly occur at the tibial tubercle (Osgood–Schlatter disease), inferior patella (Sinding–Larsen–Johansson syndrome), calcaneus (Sever's disease), and iliac crest (Peck 1995). Musculotendinous tightness and associated loss of flexibility, as during a growth spurt, can cause or aggravate these conditions, and a directed flexibility program may alleviate the symptoms until growth is completed (Micheli 1987).

Rehabilitation of childhood injuries is often neglected. The younger athlete should be given the same consideration as the adult athlete. Physical therapy should be focused on attaining full range of motion and strength within 10% of the opposite extremity. Ultrasound is rarely used on the child over a growth plate due to concerns for physeal injury. High intensities of ultrasound to epiphyseal areas result in demineralization of bone, damage to epiphyseal plates, and retardation of long bone growth (Irrgang & Sawhney 1994). Current evidence indicates that both children and adolescents can increase muscular strength as a consequence of strength training. This increase in strength is largely related to the intensity and volume of loading and appears to be the result of increased neuromuscular activation and coordination, rather than muscle hypertrophy (Guy & Micheli 2001).

ACUTE INJURIES

SPINE

Acute spine injuries can be among the most serious of sports injuries since they can cause long-term disability or even death. Fortunately, these instances are rare. More common is the chronic back injury related to overuse, muscle weakness, and tightness, as well as spinal malalignments. Thorough evaluation is important for the diagnosis of these chronic conditions as well as the detection of the unusual tumor or infection.

Cervical spine

Acute neck injury in the young athlete must be treated with caution (Cantu 2000). A recent 5-year study utilizing the National Pediatric Trauma Registry revealed that 16% of pediatric cervical spine injuries were sports-related (Kokoska et al 2001). The four youth sports with the highest risk for head and spine injury are football, gymnastics, ice hockey, and wrestling (Proctor & Cantu 2000). However, rule changes, such as the prohibition of spearing in football, ball heading in young soccer players, and recreational usage of high school trampolines have been effective in reducing the rate of catastrophic neck injury (Proctor & Cantu 2000). Children with Klippel–Feil, Down, or Morquio's syndrome may have congenital anomalies or instability, and should be evaluated with lateral radiographs in flexion and extension prior to Special Olympics or other sports participation (Cantu 1988, Dawson & Smith 1979, Dyment 1989, Pueschel & Scola 1987).

When an acute neck injury occurs, the athlete should be removed from the event on a back board with the neck immobilized in the neutral position, utilizing a collar, sandbags, or rolled-up towel. Physical examination should include a detailed neurological examination. Evidence of head injury or facial trauma should raise the suspicion of an occult neck injury, particularly in the unconscious athlete. Radiographic evaluation should consist of plain anteroposterior, lateral, and oblique views of all seven cervical vertebrae, including an odontoid view. If pain is elicited with cervical flexion or extension, then lateral radiographs in flexion and extension may be obtained to assess ligamentous stability. MRI, computed tomography (CT) and bone scans may also be useful (Connolly 2001). Although ligament instability may occur, a physiological pseudosubluxation of C2 on C3 may be encountered in the young, and may be incorrectly identified as a sequela of trauma (Jackson et al 1995, Micheli & d'Hemecourt 1998).

If the cervical spine is stable, without evidence of fracture, ligament disruption, or neurological abnormalities, then initial treatment should consist of rest, a soft cervical collar, local ice and heat, and mild analgesics. As the pain and muscle spasm subside, progressive rehabilitation is started with gentle isometric exercises in the six directions of motion, followed by dynamic range of motion and strengthening exercises through the painless arc of motion in all directions (Micheli & Jenkins 1995).

Upper back and thoracic spine

Injury to the upper back and thoracic spine is relatively uncommon because the rib cage partially stabilizes and splints the thoracic spine from the sudden stresses of most sports (Schnebel 2000). Strains of the upper back and periscapular muscles may occur in lifting activities (d'Hemecourt et al 2000), and diagnosis is made by careful physical examination and radiographs to exclude the possibility of fracture. Vertebral body compression fracture can result from sudden flexion of the spine, as in a fall during an equestrian event, and may be demonstrated on radiographs with loss of vertebral body height. Treatment of a compression fracture is usually non-operative and includes initial rest, bracing, and subsequent rehabilitation to restore strength and range of motion, once stable bony union has been attained (d'Hemecourt et al 2000).

A common adolescent condition is Scheuermann's disease which consists of painful dorsal kyphosis ('roundbacking'), loss of anterior vertebral body height, and 'wedging' of the body as seen on the lateral radiograph. This condition may be an overuse syndrome, resulting from repetitive microfracture of the vertebral body end plates, and is often associated with tightness of the hamstrings, gluteals and lumbodorsal fascia (d'Hemecourt et al 2000). Treatment of Scheuermann's disease consists of progressive dorsal extension and lumbar exercises for strength and flexibility. Other postural concerns such as forward rounded shoulders and head thrust should be addressed with postural exercises and periscapular strengthening. If kyphosis is present (Cobb angle greater than 50°), extension bracing for 9–12 months has been shown to result in improvement of both pain and deformity (Ali et al 1999).

Low back injuries

The low back in the young athlete is susceptible to either single impact or overuse injury (d'Hemecourt et al 2000). The increase in tightness of the lumbodorsal fascia and quadriceps during the adolescent growth spurt (d'Hemecourt et al 2000) can cause a tight lumbar lordosis or swayback. Tight hamstrings may be associated with a relatively flat back. Tightness in these areas may increase susceptibility to injury (d'Hemecourt et al 2000). Therapy should focus on anterior and lateral thigh flexibility (the rectus femoris, iliotibial band, and quadriceps), strengthening of abdominal and perispinal muscles, and antilordotic exercises of the lumbar musculature (d'Hemecourt et al 2000).

Mechanical low back pain in children and adolescents is associated with increased lumbar lordosis, tight lumbodorsal fascia and hamstrings, and a lack of an anatomical lesion suggesting fracture, herniation, or narrowing of the spinal canal (Zetaruk 2000). This diagnosis should be made with caution in the young athlete, and only after other causes of low back pain, including infection or malignancy, have been excluded with appropriate radiographic and radioisotopic imaging studies. Historically, these children with mechanical low back pain complain of pain on extension maneuvers. The specific finding on examination is pain on provocative extension, similar to spondylolysis (Zetaruk 2000). However, no lesion of the posterior elements is identified with advanced imaging. It has been hypothesized that facet derangement is the origin of mechanical low back pain. This condition is often treated with a lumbar antilordotic exercise program, including low back and hamstring stretching and strengthening, as well as abdominal strengthening (Zetaruk 2000). For persistent mechanical low back pain, relief of symptoms may occur within several weeks utilizing an antilordotic brace. This brace may also be used during early return to sports activity (Micheli et al 1980).

Injury to the posterior spinal elements may occur in activities which involve repetitive lumbar hyper-extension, such as gymnastics, figure skating, or dance (d'Hemecourt et al 2000, Zetaruk 2000). Symptomatic spondylolysis is a stress fracture of the pars inter-articularis, which is often demonstrated on oblique radiographs of the lumbar spine. Stress reaction of the pars interarticularis can occur without changes being evident on plain radiography, and a single photon emission computer tomographic (SPECT) bone scan is usually necessary to confirm the diagnosis (d'Hemecourt et al 2000) (see Ch. 29). The pain associated with this condition is reproduced with lumbar hyperextension (d'Hemecourt et al 2000). Treatment includes a lumbar antilordotic strengthening and flexibility exercise program. This should consist of peripelvic and abdominal strengthening as well as postural alignment. Antilordotic bracing may result in resolution of symptoms and, in younger athletes, radiographic evidence of healing of the pars defect (as seen on CT scan) can be seen after 6 months (d'Hemecourt et al 2000). The athlete may be permitted to return to sports in the brace after 4–6 weeks of bracing if there is no pain on examination. The athlete with persistent symptoms and non-union at 4–6 months can be offered external electrical stimulation, or ultimately, spinal fusion (d'Hemecourt et al 2000).

Spondylolisthesis is the forward displacement of one vertebra over another, and is associated with bilateral pars defects (Fig. 24.3). This condition, which usually occurs at L5–S1 or L4–L5, is often asymptomatic, but severe displacement or progression may be indications for spinal fusion (d'Hemecourt et al 2000).

Repetitive flexion with axial loading to the lumbar spine may result in flexion injury to the low back (Yancey & Micheli 1994). This type of injury has been associated with gymnastics, running, football, weightlifting, basket-ball, soccer and tennis. Flexion injury can result in vertebral body or end-plate fracture, or intervertebral disk herniation (Yancey & Micheli 1994). Localized neurological symptoms and signs can be present with lateral disk herniation, as a result of specific nerve root impingement. However, a central disk bulge or hernia-tion without nerve root impingement can occur in the young athlete, resulting in localized low back pain and hamstring tightness (Zetaruk 2000). Diagnosis can be confirmed with MRI. Treatment for such conditions consists of an exercise program for abdominal and lumbar extension strengthening and posterior flexibility, being cautious not to increase radiculopathy (Zetaruk 2000). Occasionally, a low back brace may improve

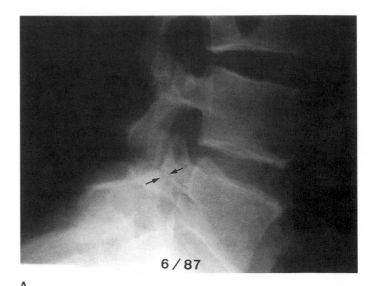

A

B

Figure 24.3A&B   Spondylolysis and spondylolisthesis in an adolescent female athlete. **A**: At the age of 14 years, this athlete developed low back pain with basketball activity. Spondylolysis at L5, without spondylolisthesis, was visible on the lateral radiograph. She was treated with a Boston brace, with resolution of her pain over several months. She subsequently had intermittent episodes of low back pain and occasionally used her brace during these periods. **B**: Two and a half years later, at the age of 16 years, she reinjured her back in a basketball incident. She complained of localized low back pain without radicular symptoms. Radiographs revealed bilateral L5 spondylolysis with grade I spondylolisthesis. She resumed use of the brace, with improvement of her pain.

symptoms by immobilizing the lumbar spine, and may allow early return-to-sports activity (Micheli et al 1980). For more recalcitrant cases, a series of epidural cortico-steroid injections to selective nerve roots may be helpful (d'Hemecourt et al 2000). Diskectomy is rarely required in the young athlete, but has been used when symptoms include progressive neurological involvement, bowel or bladder involvement, or pain unresponsive to non-operative treatment (Yancey & Micheli 1994).

The differential diagnosis of sciatica in children and adolescents is broad, and includes spinal problems such as disk herniation or tumor. Furthermore, sciatica can result from extraspinal causes such as piriformis syndrome, in which the sciatic nerve is compressed by a tight piriformis muscle or tendon near the insertion to the greater trochanter (Roos & Renstrom 1998). Proximal hamstring syndrome is another cause of sciatic nerve compression (Roos & Renstrom 1998). Scarring of an injured hamstring may cause the muscle and nerve to become adhered and, therefore, cause compression symptoms. Occasionally, long-standing spondylolysis may present with low back pain and L5 radiculopathy due to tethering of this nerve root by the hypertrophic pseudoarthosis tissue (Micheli & d'Hemecourt 1998).

Examination of the back in the young athlete should include an assessment for scoliosis or other spinal deformity. Preparticipation physical examination provides a screening opportunity for spinal conditions (Smith et al 1997). Persistent back pain in the child or adolescent may be a result of infection or tumor, and should never be attributed to a sports injury without thorough investigation (Fig 24.4).

In general, most back injuries in the young athlete can be resolved with physical therapy, activity modification and, occasionally, bracing for 3 to 6 months (Yancey & Micheli 1994).

HIP AND PELVIS

There are several sites about the hip and pelvis that are subject to overuse syndromes. However, it is imperative to always have a high index of suspicion for slipped capital femoral epiphysis in patients that present with either hip or knee pain.

Avulsion fractures

The hip and pelvis is a common site of avulsion fracture secondary to sudden muscle contraction, with seven different sites at risk (Waters & Millis 1988) (Table 24.1). Apophysitis may cause pain and limitation of activity, particularly during the adolescent growth spurt (Clancy & Foltz 1976, Pueschel & Scola 1987). The muscle groups involved are commonly treated with rest, ice, and a progressive strengthening and stretching exercise program (Metzmaker & Pappas 1985). Physical therapy includes stretching of the rectus femoris, iliotibial band, and sartorious. Neoprene shorts may be helpful during rehabilitation and in the early return-to-sports phase. While most of these avulsions are treated by first stage healing in situ, some do require operative fixation.

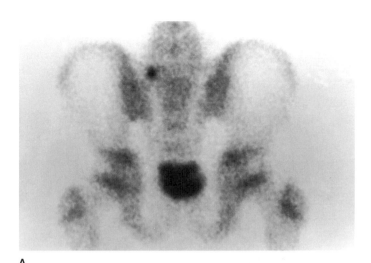

A

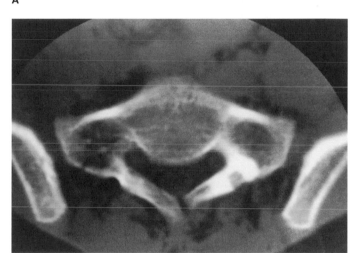

B

Figure 24.4A&B   Persistent low back pain may be a result of a pathological process independent of injury or mechanical factors. This 13-year-old boy complained of left low lumbar back pain and stiffness of several years duration, which became progressively worse during the previous year. Examination revealed an antalgic gait and dramatic tightness of the low back on forward bending. Although plain radiographs were normal, (**A**) technetium-99 bone scan and (**B**) computed tomography revealed an osteoid osteoma in the left arch of the S1 vertebra. After resection, the symptoms resolved completely.

Table 24.1   Apophyseal avulsion fracture sites about the hip/pelvis

Apophyseal avulsion fracture	Muscle involved
Anterior superior iliac spine	Sartorius
Ichial tuberosity	Hamstring
Lesser trochanter	Iliopsoas
Anterior inferior iliac spine	Rectus femoris
Iliac crest	External oblique abdominus
	Transverse abdominus
	Gluteus medius
	Tensor fascia lata
	Latissimus dorsi
	Gluteus maximus
Acetabular rim	
Symphysis pubis	Adductor insertion

Slipped capital femoral epiphysis

A high clinical index of suspicion of slipped capital femoral epiphysis (SCFE) should be maintained in the young adolescent who presents with complaints of hip or knee pain (Fig. 24.5). This problem may occur without any history of trauma. SCFE may be more common in physically active adolescents, and may contribute to the premature onset of osteoarthritis of the hip in later life (Carney et al 1991, Murray & Duncan 1971).

Risk factors for SCFE include obesity, puberty, hypothyroidism and tall thin individuals (Karlin 1995). Physical examination reveals limitation of internal rotation in flexion, and the diagnosis is confirmed by radiography. Treatment is operative and consists of pinning the slipped femoral neck to the femoral head. Physical therapy usually commences 4–6 weeks after surgery and consists of range of motion and strengthening exercises. Approximately 50% of cases of SCFE are seen bilaterally (Waters & Millis 1994) so contralateral hip pain should be evaluated urgently.

Fractures and dislocations

Fractures and dislocations of the hip are associated with high energy trauma, and can occur in sports activities such as football, motocross, and skiing (Fig. 24.6). Stress fractures of the femoral neck can be the result of repetitive microtrauma in runners or dancers, but are rare before the growth plate is closed (Karlin 1995, Pudda et al 1998). A SPECT bone scan or MRI may be necessary to make the diagnosis if plain radiographs are normal yet other symptoms indicate a stress reaction or stress fracture (Pirnay & Crielaard 2001).

Contusions

Thigh contusions occur from direct impact seen in such sports as ice hockey and soccer. Occasionally they are severe and cause significant thigh pain, swelling, and limitation of knee motion. The most commonly contused

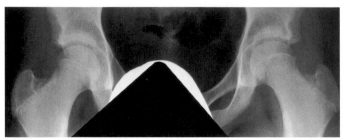

A

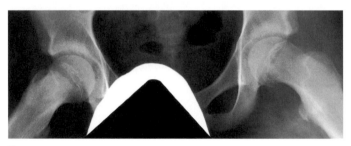

B

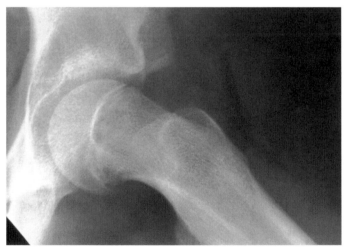

C

Figure 24.5A–C   Slipped capital femoral epiphysis. This 11-year-old female complained of diffuse left hip pain of three months duration, without any history of injury. Menarche was 2 months after onset of hip pain. Physical examination revealed a short, moderately overweight black female who walked with a left Trendelenberg limp, with the left lower extremity externally rotated at the hip. She had only 5° of left hip internal rotation in flexion, in contrast with 20° on the other side; external rotation in flexion was 80° on the left and 45° on the right. The anteroposterior radiograph (**A**) appeared normal; however, frog-lateral radiographs (**B** and **C**) revealed slipped capital femoral epiphysis. She underwent epiphysiodesis. A high clinical index of suspicion of this problem is important to avoid delay in diagnosis.

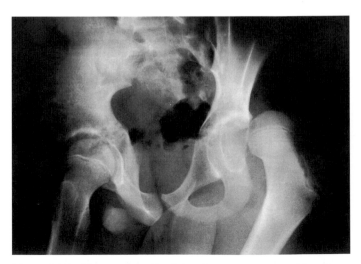

Figure 24.6   This posterior hip dislocation on an 11-year-old male occurred during vigorous football activity.

thigh sites are the anterior and antereolateral thigh (Javin & Fox 1995). Treatment normally consists of initial rest, ice, and gentle compression. Gentle progressive knee flexion is commenced early to disperse the hematoma. A strengthening and flexibility program may begin when the athlete is comfortable. Heat, warm water whirlpools and massage are avoided in the early rehabilitation of this injury to minimize muscular hemorrhage and swelling (Javin & Fox 1995). A severe thigh contusion may cause disability for over 1 year, particularly if it is complicated by the development of myositis ossificans or abscess (Gross 1994b). Myositis ossificans is a lesion of hypertrophic bone localized in soft tissue. Return to sports may be facilitated by the use of neoprene shorts which provide support and warmth to the injured tissues.

Hip pain or limp in the young athlete may be the first symptom or sign of Legg–Calvé–Perthes disease, slipped capital femoral epiphysis, infection, or a tumor such as osteosarcoma (Waters & Millis 1994). A coincident history of sports injury may delay the diagnosis of these conditions if thorough evaluation, including radiography, is not performed.

KNEE

The knee is a common site of single-impact and overuse injuries in the young athlete (Steiner & Grana 1988). The types of knee injuries that occur in the child and adolescent differ from those in the adult as a result of the different tissue characteristics associated with age and growth (Iobst & Stanitski 2000).

Patellofemoral pain

Patellofemoral pain is a frequent problem in the young athlete (Outerbridge & Micheli 1995). The symptoms are similar to that of chondromalacia patellae in adults. The usual presentation is a chief complaint of anterior knee pain that is aggravated by activities which increase patellofemoral pressure. Patients often note that stair climbing and sitting for prolonged periods are bothersome. However, the pathophysiology of patellofemoral pain in the young athlete differs from that in the adult because the articular surface is often normal on arthroscopic examination of the young athlete (Griffiths & Pinder 1981, Steiner & Grana 1988). The pain is believed to result from an increase in patellofemoral joint pressure associated with lateral malalignment (Outerbridge & Micheli 1995). This is often associated with tightness of the tensor fascia lata, rectus femoris and lateral retinaculum in conjunction with a weak vastus medialis (Outerbridge & Micheli 1995).

More than 80% of young athletes with patellofemoral pain improve with physical therapy (See Ch. 21). Therapy includes a static progressive resistance strengthening exercise program for the vastus medialis. Flexibility exercises for the quadriceps, hamstrings, and iliotibial band are also important. Activities which increase patellofemoral pressure should be minimized (Micheli & Jenkins 2001). McConnell taping or use of a tracking brace may be beneficial for the short term (Crossley et al 2001). If pain persists despite this program, lateral retinacular release with a medial thermal plication has been shown to be successful in relieving symptoms (Micheli 1999, Micheli & Stanitski 1981). Occasionally, medial realignment of the infrapatellar tendon insertion, with medial retinaculum plication and vastus medialis advancement, is indicated for refractory patellofemoral pain associated with malalignment or recurrent lateral patellar dislocation (Fondren et al 1985, Insall et al 1983). Custom orthotics should be considered for the athlete with malalignment or foot formation issues.

On occasion, anterior knee pain may progress to lateral subluxation of the patella. While therapy, orthotics, and a training modification are highly successful in treating patellofemoral stress syndrome, anterior knee pain with the onset of subluxation symptoms, usually associated with subluxation by radiographic criteria, suggests that therapy alone will be unsuccessful in relieving symptoms (Outerbridge & Micheli 1995). Surgical realignment of the extensor mechanism is usually necessary in such cases.

Traction apophysitis

The extensor mechanism of the knee in adolescents can be the site of traction apophysitis, such as Osgood–Schlatter disease (tibial tubercle) (Ogden & Southwick 1976) (Fig. 24.7) or Sinding–Larsen–Johansson syndrome (inferior pole of patella) (Fig. 24.8). These problems are associated with tightness of the extensor mechanism, demonstrated clinically with a positive Ely test, and may be exacerbated by jumping activities. Treatment consists of a program of pain-free quadriceps strengthening and stretching exercises (Micheli 1987). If knee flexion is minimized while strengthening, the load to the tibial tubercle will be effectively reduced. Thus, the cornerstone of rehabilitation remains static progressive resistance exercises (PRE), including straight leg raising, usually progressing with resistance. Cast treatment is rarely used now because immobilization may aggravate quadriceps weakness and tightness.

Osteochondritis dissecans

Osteochondritis dissecans (OCD) is another condition that may affect the knee of younger athletes (Fig. 24.9). The child or adolescent with OCD of the knee may complain of low-grade aching pain and intermittent

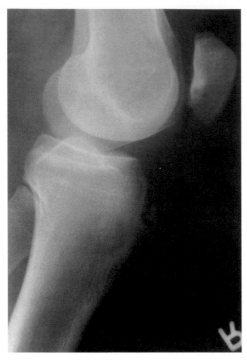

Figure 24.7 Osgood–Schlatter disease. This male developed persistent pain at the right tibial tubercle at the age of 10 years. This radiograph at 21 years of age revealed a non-union of the tibial tubercle apophysis. Fourteen years later, at the age of 35 years, the discomfort and radiographic appearance were unchanged.

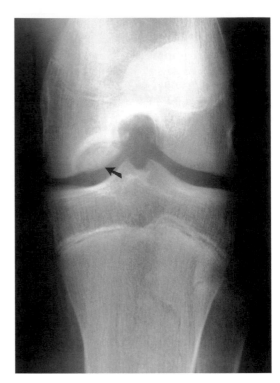

Figure 24.9 Osteochondritis dissecans of the medial femoral condyle in an adolescent. This lesion may be missed if a tunnel view is not obtained.

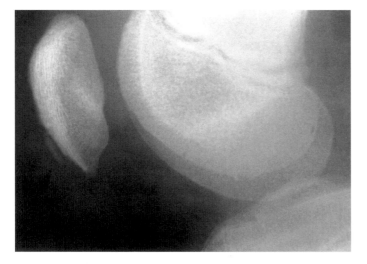

Figure 24.8 Sinding–Larsen–Johansson syndrome. This 9-year-old gymnast developed bilateral infrapatellar knee pain during a period of intensive springboard activity. Physical examination was remarkable for localized tenderness at the inferior pole of the patella, and radiography revealed evidence of Sinding–Larsen–Johansson traction apophysitis at the right knee. The symptoms resolved several weeks after starting a quadriceps flexibility program.

swelling. Locking may occur if the lesion is displaced. These lesions may be asymptomatic. Radiographs are usually diagnostic and a tunnel view should be obtained (Fig. 24.9). Treatment is controversial, and may vary depending on the presence of symptoms, age and skeletal maturity of the patient, and status of the lesion (loose or intact articular cartilage) (Kocher et al 2001). Relative rest alone may be the only treatment needed to attain healing. With advanced maturity, large lesion size or partial detachment, drilling of the lesion, with or without pinning in an attempt to revascularize the bony fragment and promote union to the underlying bony bed, may be indicated (Kocher et al 2001). In larger lesions, where the detached fragment has not been reimplanted and healed, cartilage transplant can be used (Kocher et al 2001).

If the lesion is loose and does not involve a major part of the weightbearing surface, it is occasionally excised. If OCD is diagnosed before skeletal maturity, and is left untreated, it is associated with a high incidence of subsequent osteoarthritis, especially if the defect is large or involves the lateral femoral condyle (Twyman et al 1991).

Meniscal injuries

Tears of the meniscus may occur in the young athlete in association with twisting injuries or ACL tears. MRI is valuable for diagnosis of such conditions and arthroscopy is useful in both diagnosis and treatment (Iobst & Stanitski 2000). Arthroscopic repair of peripheral tears of the meniscus may be feasible in specific instances (Iobst & Stanitski 2000). It is preferable to repair meniscal tears to preserve the protective articular cartilage. Postoperatively, these patients are partial weightbearing with a brace that limits their range of motion for 4 weeks. Athletes with simple partial meniscectomies may start exercises sooner and progress as tolerated.

Another meniscal problem of the young athlete is the diskoid lateral meniscus. These large, redundant lateral menisci may or may not have an intact posterior peripheral attachment. They tend to cause a prominent snapping sensation in the lateral compartment as the flexed knee is extended (Dickhaut & DeLee 1982) (Fig. 24.10). Treatment is operative and a more extensive meniscectomy may be required if the posterior horn is detached or additional tears are present (Aichroth et al 1991, Dickhaut & DeLee 1982, Steiner & Grana 1988).

Ligament injuries

The knee ligaments of the young athlete are relatively stronger than in adults, and the ACL in children is usually avulsed at the tibial spine rather than torn (Rang

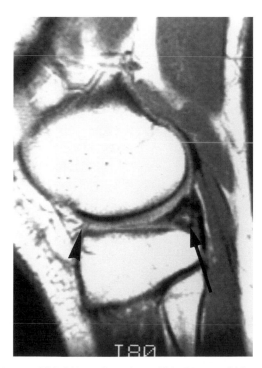

Figure 24.10 Diskoid lateral meniscus. This 15-year-old female had a 'clunking' sensation in the right knee from the age of 2 years, associated with pain. Physical examination revealed a loud, painful 'snap' during extension of the knee with valgus stress applied. MRI revealed a complex tear of the posterior horn of the lateral meniscus (large arrow), with absence of the anterior horn (arrowhead). Arthroscopic findings consisted of a large, complex tear of a diskoid lateral meniscus. The pain and snapping resolved after arthroscopic partial lateral meniscectomy.

1983). Nevertheless, ligament tears have been observed in prepubescent children (Bradley et al 1979, Clanton et al 1979, DeLee & Curtis 1983, Micheli et al 1999b), and ACL reconstruction may be indicated (Lipscomb & Anderson 1986, Micheli et al 1999b). The medial collateral ligament (MCL) may also be torn in children, as on occasion, stress radiographs can reveal MCL avulsion with physeal fracture of the distal femur or proximal tibia (Steiner & Grana 1988). Posterior cruciate ligament (PCL) injury is relatively rare in the young athlete (DeLee 1994, Mayer & Micheli 1979, Sanders et al 1980). Physical therapy for knee ligamentous rehabilitation consists of closed chain strengthening with progressive range of motion and weightbearing as indicated by tissue healing.

Young female athletes have a 2–8 times greater chance of tearing their ACL compared to young males (Micheli et al 1999b). The cause of this significantly increased risk is speculative. Much of the current research in this field has been focused on proper jumping and landing techniques for protection of injury (Hewett et al 2000, Micheli et al 1999a).

Fractures

Fractures about the knee in the young athlete have a high complication rate (Johnson 1998). The Salter–Harris II fracture of the distal femur is frequently followed by growth disturbance, particularly if displacement is present (Griffin & Briard 1998). Open reduction and internal fixation may be necessary to achieve an anatomical position, and the patient should be followed with radiographs, even after the fracture is healed, in order to detect growth disturbance early.

In the proximal tibia, collateral ligament insertion sites are distal to the physis. Therefore, varus and valgus stresses are usually transmitted to the metaphysis, and physeal fractures of the proximal tibia are rare (Burkhart & Peterson 1979). Nevertheless, proximal tibia growth plate fractures can occur from higher velocity trauma, or in association with avulsion of the tibial tubercle physis (Chow et al 1990). These fractures may be complicated by popliteal artery injury or compartment syndrome (Griffin & Briard 1998) (Fig. 24.11). Early treatment should include careful observation, and circumferential plaster should be avoided during the first few days following injury (Steiner & Grana 1988).

FOOT AND ANKLE

The foot and ankle are susceptible to injury in almost every sport. Foot and ankle problems are the second most common musculoskeletal problem facing primary care physicians in children under 10 years of age next to acute injury (Omey & Micheli 1999). Ankle sprains are the most

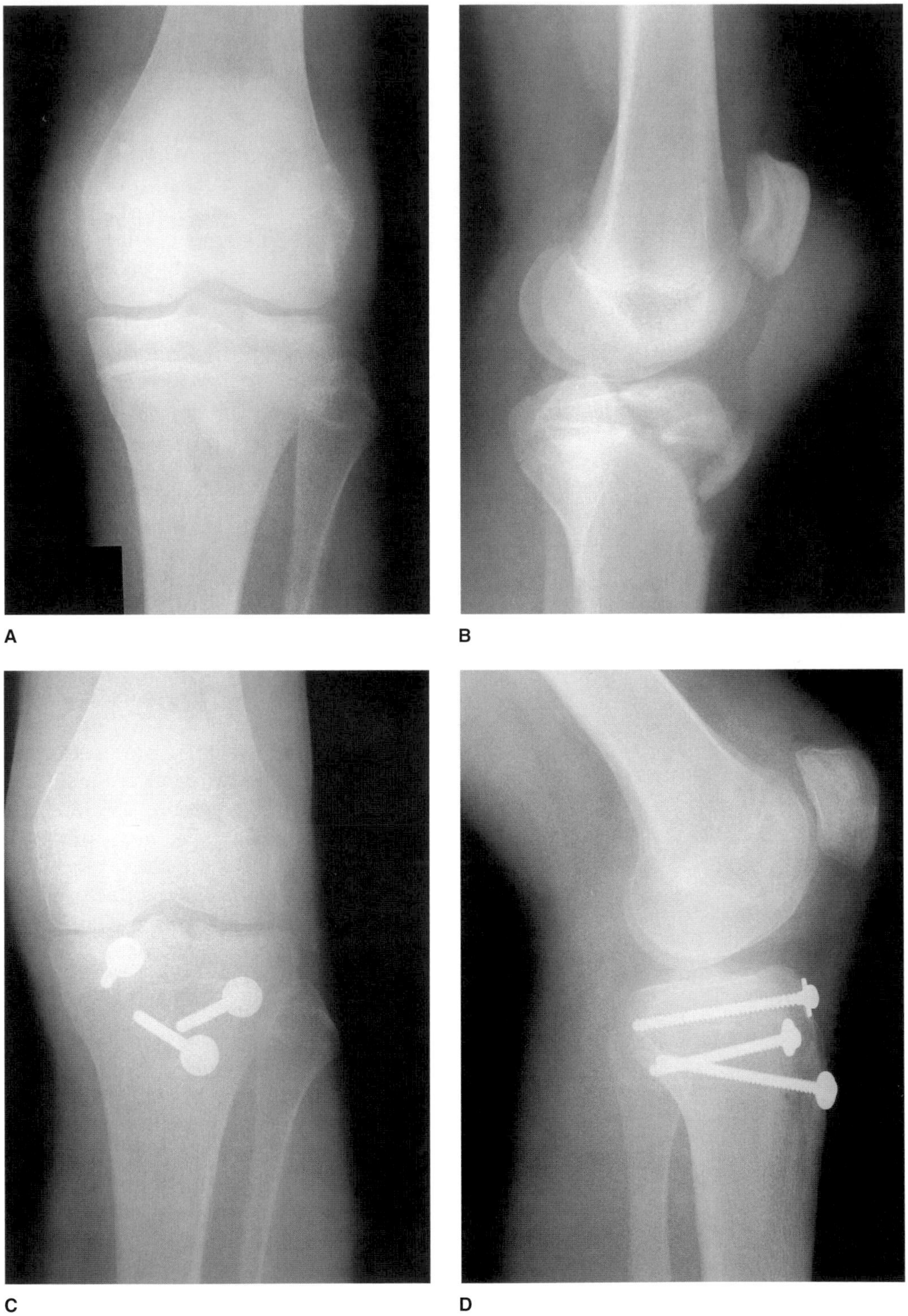

A

B

C

D

Figure 24.11A–D Avulsion of the tibial tubercle, with Salter IV fracture of the proximal tibia, in a 16-year-old male (**A** and **B**). An acute compartment syndrome developed several hours after injury, as a result of extensive bleeding into the compartments of the leg. Emergency fasciotomy, with open reduction and internal fixation, was performed. The fracture healed without sequelae (**C** and **D**).

commonly reported sports injury. Rehabilitation is crucial for the prevention of reinjury in most instances of foot or ankle injury.

Ligaments and associated injuries

Single impact injuries of the ankle in the young athlete are determined by the greater strength of ligaments relative to growth cartilage. In contrast to the adult, lateral ankle ligament sprains are unusual in the young. Inversion injuries more commonly cause a minimally displaced avulsion fracture or fracture of the distal fibular growth plate. Careful physical examination may localize the structure injured, with maximal point of tenderness at the ligaments, ligament origin, or growth plate. If a Salter–Harris I fracture of the distal fibula is present, radiographs may be normal except for some soft tissue swelling. Treatment of this kind of fracture consists of a short leg cast for 3–4 weeks, or longer if tenderness persists. The distal tibia may also sustain growth plate fractures, and these may be complicated by subsequent growth disturbance (Fig. 24.12) or degenerative change (Spiegel et al 1978, Taunton et al 1998).

Lateral ankle sprains are treated with initial rest, ice, compression and elevation. Painless active range of motion with avoidance of inversion should begin as early as possible. Protected motion and peroneal resistive strengthening exercises should follow. More severe ankle sprains may require short-term immobilization such as a walking boot or stirrup until the athlete is comfortable. Early rehabilitation, including tendoachilles stretching, dorsiflexion and eversion strengthening, and modalities are essential for prompt return to safe activity. Return to sports may be facilitated with braces which protect the lateral ligaments by preventing inversion, but allow dorsiflexion and plantarflexion (Stover 1980, Taunton et al 1998). Additionally, exercises to restore proprioception are usually essential for return to field or cutting sport play (Taunton et al 1998).

Peroneal tendon injuries

The peroneal tendons may subluxate or dislocate from the fibro-osseous tunnel inferior to the distal fibula. This problem is a result of either sudden supination of the dorsiflexed foot (Poll & Duijfjes 1984) or forced dorsiflexion and peroneal contraction with the foot everted (Micheli et al 1989). Acute injury is treated with closed repositioning of the tendons and cast immobilization in slight plantarflexion. However, residual laxity of the lateral retinaculum from acute injury or repetitive lateral sprains can predispose to recurrent peroneal tendon subluxation or dislocation as the retinaculum is relaxed by

hindfoot pronation and ankle dorsiflexion. Symptoms include pain and ankle instability. Recurrent, symptomatic dislocation is an indication for surgical reconstruction of the fibro-osseous groove (Micheli et al 1989, Poll & Duijfjes 1984).

Heel pain in younger athletes can be a result of calcaneal apophysitis (Sever's disease) (Micheli & Ireland 1987). This condition is a traction apophysitis of the calcaneal insertion of the tendo-Achilles. Physical examination reveals tenderness at this site. Radiographs should be obtained because acute fracture or stress fracture may also be a cause of heel pain in the child (Dowdy et al 1998). Calcaneal apophysitis may be caused or aggravated by tight Achilles tendon associated with the growth spurt, maltraining, and shoes with the heel lower than the toebox. Treatment includes a program of directed Achilles tendon stretching and dorsiflexion strengthening exercises (Sullivan 1994). Early symptomatic relief may be provided with improved shoe wear, heel cups, a temporary heel lift, intermittent ice, and anti-inflammatory medication (Sullivan 1994). Traction apophysitis may also occur at the base of the fifth metatarsal (Fig. 24.13).

Other foot and ankle injuries

Overuse injuries of the ankle and foot include stress fractures and tendinitis. Occasionally, a bone scan may be necessary to confirm the diagnosis of a stress fracture in the young athlete (Rosen et al 1982). Refer to Chapters 2, 5, and 23 for further details of such injuries.

The child or adolescent can develop foot or ankle pain from accessory ossicles (Sullivan 1994). The painful accessory navicular, associated with the insertion of the tibialis posterior tendon, can be aggravated by pronation and repetitive activity (Fig. 24.14). If pain relief is not achieved with orthotics, tibialis posterior stretching, and strengthening exercises, then short-term immobilization or, ultimately, excision of the accessory navicular may be indicated (Sella et al 1986).

Another common accessory ossicle is the os trigonum at the posterior aspect of the talus (Kadel et al 2000). This ossicle may cause posterior ankle pain as a result of impingement of the ossicle between the posterior tibia and calcaneus in activities such as dance and gymnastics, which involve repetitive pointing of the ankle and foot (Hamilton 1982, Kadel et al 2000). Excision is occasionally required.

Tarsal coalitions can also occur in young athletes. A tarsal coalition is a bony or fibrocartilaginous connection of two or more tarsal bones of unknown etiology. A coalition results from a failure of differentiation and segmentation of the primitive mesenchyme. A calcaneonavicular bar may be seen on the oblique radiograph of

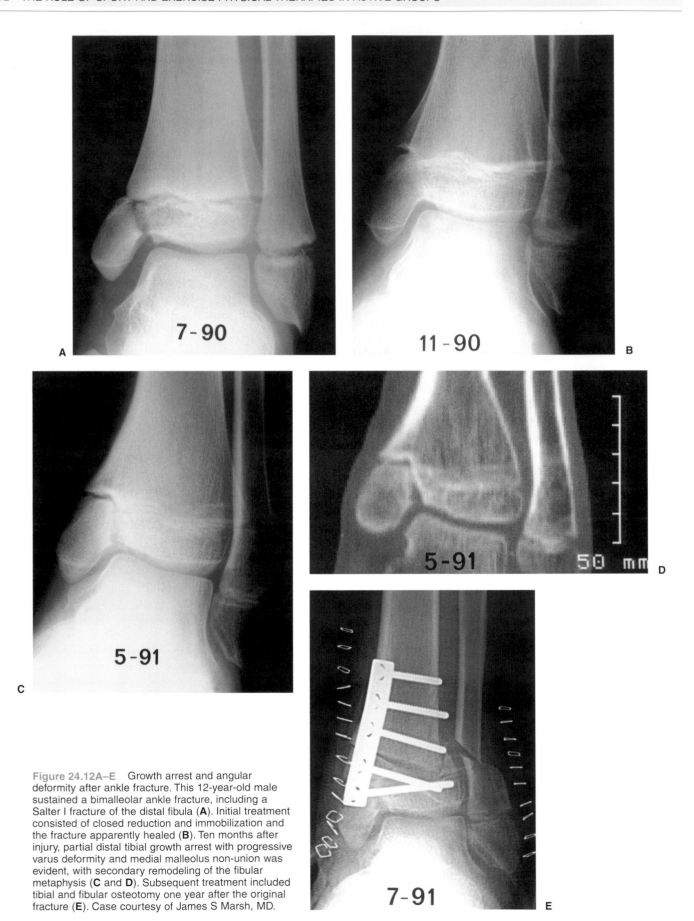

Figure 24.12A–E Growth arrest and angular deformity after ankle fracture. This 12-year-old male sustained a bimalleolar ankle fracture, including a Salter I fracture of the distal fibula (**A**). Initial treatment consisted of closed reduction and immobilization and the fracture apparently healed (**B**). Ten months after injury, partial distal tibial growth arrest with progressive varus deformity and medial malleolus non-union was evident, with secondary remodeling of the fibular metaphysis (**C** and **D**). Subsequent treatment included tibial and fibular osteotomy one year after the original fracture (**E**). Case courtesy of James S Marsh, MD.

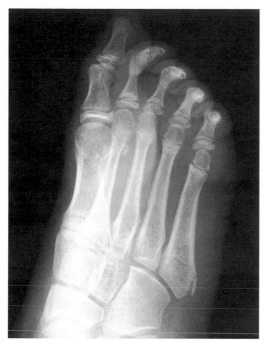

Figure 24.13   Traction apophysitis of the base of the fifth metatarsal. This 10-year-old female had gradually progressive pain at the base of the fifth metatarsal without any history of injury. Physical examination revealed hindfoot pronation, flexible flatfoot, and localized tenderness at the base of the fifth metatarsal. Treatment included peroneal stretching and metatarsal pads, and the pain resolved within 2 months.

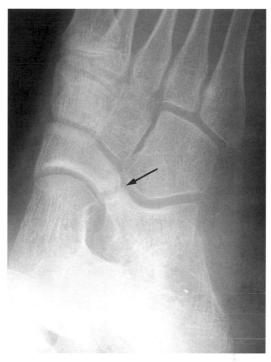

Figure 24.15   A calcaneonavicular coalition is often most clearly revealed in the oblique radiograph of the foot. This 14-year-old male had midfoot pain associated with this bar. Excision resulted in resolution of symptoms.

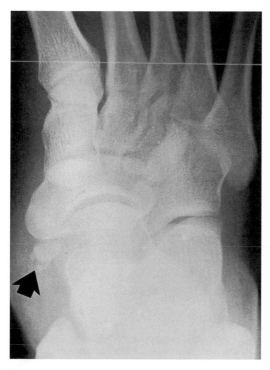

Figure 24.14   Painful accessory navicular in a skeletally mature aerobics dancer.

the foot (O'Neill & Micheli 1989) (Fig. 24.15). Talonavicular bars are also seen in this younger population. In the young athlete, excision of the bar may alleviate symptoms and improve function (O'Neill & Micheli 1989). The postoperative regimen usually includes a period of 2–4 weeks of immobilization to decrease inflammation and the chance of bone reformation. This is followed by systematic exercises to restore full range of motion and strength to the affected area.

SHOULDER AND SHOULDER GIRDLE

Sports activities which involve repetitive overhead use of the shoulder are common causes of problems of the shoulder region in the young athlete. These problems include fracture, instability, and subacromial impingement. The accuracy of diagnosis of glenohumeral and subacromial derangements has been improved with MRI and MRI arthrograms, as well as shoulder arthroscopy (Gross 1994a).

Fractures and dislocations

Proximal humerus stress fracture is common in throwing sports (Kocher et al 2000). 'Little league shoulder' is a stress fracture of the proximal humeral physis resulting from the cumulative effects of repetitive microtrauma secondary to vigorous pitching activity (Cahill et al 1974, Kocher et al 2000). Treatment consists of discontinuation of throwing activities for 6–8 weeks (Cahill et al 1974, Kocher et al 2000). Prevention of subsequent injury includes a vigorous preseason conditioning program, limits on the frequency of pitching during the subsequent year, and proper throwing mechanics. Control of the ball should be emphasized over speed (Kocher et al 2000).

Single-impact fracture of the proximal humerus physis in adolescents is usually a Salter–Harris II fracture, and remodeling may occur despite displacement. Treatment can include closed reduction and sling or spica cast. Operative treatment is rarely required (Rang 1983). Fracture of the base of the coracoid process is less common, and is also usually treated non-operatively (Fig. 24.16).

Glenohumeral dislocation is uncommon in the prepubescent, but may occur in the adolescent. Anterior dislocation is the most common type of instability, but posterior subluxation and dislocation can also occur (Kocher et al 2000, Norwood & Terry 1984, Samilson & Prieto 1983). In individuals with anterior shoulder instability requiring surgery, contralateral shoulder instability is more common if the initial dislocation occurred before the age of 15 years (O'Driscoll & Evans 1991). Therefore, bilateral shoulder conditioning programs are important.

Shoulder pain in the young swimmer or thrower can be a sign of anterior glenohumeral subluxation. These athletes may develop progressive anterior capsular laxity, reflected on examination by an increase in external rotation. Posterior capsule tightness can be associated with this problem, and treatment should include a posterior capsule stretching program in addition to anterior and internal rotation strengthening (Weldon & Richardson 2001). Multidirectional glenohumeral instability in the growing athlete is relatively rare, but may occur (Kocher et al 2000, Neer & Foster 1980). In contrast, physical signs of instability may be common in normal, asymptomatic adolescents, even in the absence of generalized joint laxity (Emery & Mullaji 1991).

In contrast to the adult, early detection of subluxation or multidirectional instability in the adolescent can often be successfully treated by physical therapy (Kocher et al 2000). In addition to treating the specific weakness or contracture of the glenohumeral joint and its musculature, great emphasis must be given to the restoration or enhancement of scapular stabilization with appropriate therapy (Weldon & Richardson 2001).

Impingement

Subacromial impingement problems are common in throwing athletes and swimmers, and include subacro-

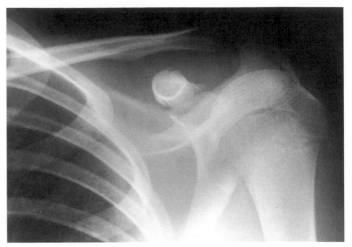

A

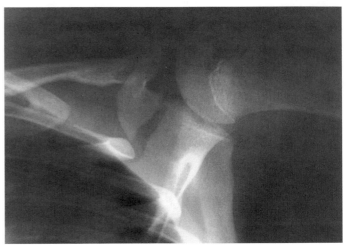

B

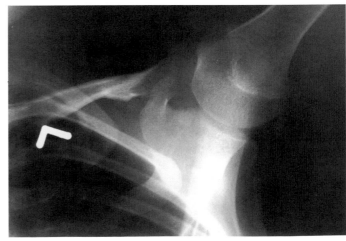

C

Figure 24.16A–C Fracture of the base of the coracoid. This 15-year-old male fell off a bicycle, landing on the posterior aspect of his shoulder. Maximal tenderness was at the coracoid process, and radiography (**A** and **B**) revealed a fracture of the base of the coracoid. Treatment included a sling and early motion, and the fracture healed without sequelae (**C**).

mial bursitis, rotator cuff tendinitis, and partial or full-thickness rotator cuff tears (Berkowitz et al 1998). Diagnosis has been improved with MRI. Arthroscopy can sometimes show associated glenohumeral derangements (Andrews & Gidumal 1987, Ireland & Andrews 1988). Physical therapy includes rotator cuff strengthening and periscapular strengthening for scapulothoracic stabilization, and stretching exercises, usually of the posterior glenohumeral capsule (Berkowitz et al 1998).

Other joints of the shoulder girdle

Acromioclavicular sprains and separations are less common in the prepubescent, but may occur in the adolescent in contact sports such as gridiron football, rugby, lacrosse, and hockey. Treatment is usually symptomatic, and open reduction is rarely required. Physical therapy consists of strengthening and acromioclavicular joint rotation exercises (Micheli & Jenkins 1995).

Sternoclavicular separation can also occur in contact sports, as a result of lateral stress on the upper torso. In the young athlete, this injury is usually an epiphyseal separation of the medial clavicle (Curtis 1994), because the physis does not fuse until the age of 23–25 years. With anterior displacement, the medial clavicle is prominent; posterior displacement of the medial clavicle may result in tracheal compression and dyspnea requiring emergency intervention. Treatment may be non-operative, but internal fixation is required in some cases (Curtis 1994).

Clavicle shaft fracture is common in the child, either from direct trauma (blow or fall) or indirect forces (fall on outstretched hand) (Curtis 1994). Treatment consists of a sling or figure-of-eight brace for comfort, and open reduction is rarely required. The parents should be instructed that the fracture callus may cause a prominent 'bump' because of the subcutaneous location of the bone.

ELBOW

Pediatric elbow injuries are common and patterns are related to age-related stage of elbow development and the sport-specific mechanism of injury (Kocher et al 2000).

Fractures

An acutely injured and swollen elbow in a child is an emergency which should be evaluated expeditiously. Some single-impact injuries, such as a displaced supracondylar fracture, may result in permanent disability or loss of the extremity because of neurovascular compromise.

At the scene of the accident, an initial neurovascular examination should be performed. The elbow should be immobilized in a position of comfort (usually in some extension), making sure that the radial pulse is not obliterated by either the splint or excessive elbow flexion. The extremity should be monitored for signs of ischemia resulting from arterial compression (loss of the pulse) or compartment syndrome (pain in the muscle compartment, which is aggravated by passive stretch of the muscles). If signs of vascular compromise persist despite removal of any potentially constricting bandages and extension of the elbow, then emergency arteriography or arterial exploration and forearm fasciotomy must be considered. Other fractures about the elbow in the young athlete may be less likely to cause vascular compromise than a displaced supracondylar fracture. Nevertheless, circumferential bandages or casts should be avoided in any acute elbow injury associated with swelling. Early range of motion is an essential component of elbow injury rehabilitation.

Throwing athletes, most commonly baseball pitchers, sustain single-impact and overuse injuries of the elbow as a result of valgus stresses (Kocher et al 2000). Avulsion of the medial collateral ligament from the medial epicondyle may occur secondary to throwing alone (Fig. 24.17), or may be associated with elbow dislocation sustained in contact sports (Ireland & Andrews 1988). Internal fixation of the medial epicondyle may be required to ensure anatomical reduction, in order to minimize subsequent laxity or instability, and may allow early protected motion to minimize stiffness (Ireland & Andrews 1988).

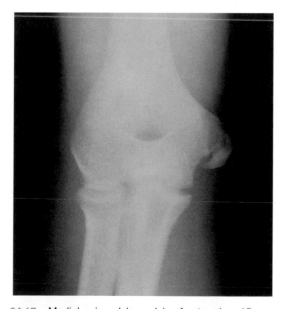

Figure 24.17 Medial epicondyle avulsion fracture in a 15-year-old Little league pitcher. The fracture was treated with open reduction and screw fixation because of the high demand on this elbow.

Overuse injuries

'Little league elbow' is a group of overuse injuries of the elbow joint resulting from repetitive lateral compression and medial traction secondary to valgus and sheering stresses on the elbow from pitching (Kocher et al 2000). The young pitcher complains of progressive medial or lateral elbow pain and tenderness over the medial epicondyle; pain increases with pitching and is relieved with rest. Little league elbow can be categorized into three disorders: medial epicondylitis, capitellar OCD, and premature arrest of the proximal radial physis. Young pitchers are subject to these injuries due to the presence of physeal tissue at the joint surface and medial epicondyle (Kocher et al 2000). As overtraining seems to be the common denominator for most of these injuries, young baseball players should limit their skilled throws (Kocher et al 2000) to 300 per week (Micheli & Jenkins 2001).

Medial epicondylitis can progress to a significant widening of the growth plate followed by fracture and displacement of the epicondyle (Kocher et al 2000). Treatment for the overuse injury to the medial epicondylar apophysis includes relative rest, followed by progressive strengthening exercises, as well as education regarding throwing mechanics (Kocher et al 2000). There is often an associated flexion contracture of the elbow with this overuse injury and therapy must be directed to address this abnormality. MCL tears may occur in adolescents, and may be difficult to diagnose (Ireland & Andrews 1988, Norwood et al 1981). Radiographs with valgus stress may reveal widening of the medial compartment, and arthrography can be helpful (Ireland & Andrews 1988). Primary surgical repair has been recommended in these high-demand athletes (Ireland & Andrews 1988).

Lateral elbow pain, catching, or locking, may be signs of OCD of the capitellum, which may be associated with loose bodies in the joint (Fig. 24.18). If detected early, this condition can improve with rest and strengthening exercises, and recurrence can be prevented by proper throwing mechanics (Albright et al 1978, Kocher et al 2000). However, occasionally this condition may require elbow arthroscopy or arthrotomy, with excision of loose bodies and curettage of the base of the lesion (McManama et al 1985). Premature arrest of the proximal radial physis can be seen in conjunction with the two other conditions of Little league elbow (Bradley 1994).

In children and adolescents, the elbow can also be injured in sports involving upper extremity weight-bearing. Gymnastic activity can result in fractures about the elbow, dislocations, and capitellar OCD (Bradley 1994, Priest & Weise 1981). Traction apophysitis of the triceps insertion to the olecranon can be caused by rapid

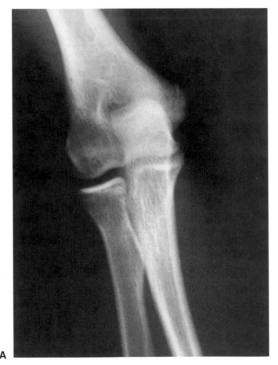
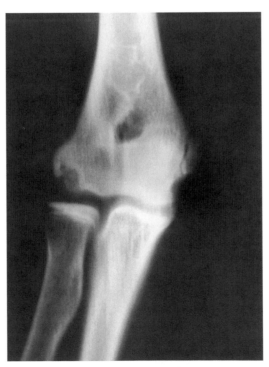

A   B

Figure 24.18A&B Osteochondritis dissecans of the capitellum, as demonstrated by (**A**) plain radiography and (**B**) tomography.

growth (Ireland & Andrews 1988, Micheli 1987). Also, medial and lateral epicondylitis can occur in the young athlete (Leach & Miller 1987, Renstrom 1998).

FOREARM, HAND AND WRIST

Hand and wrist injuries are common during athletic competition, accounting for up to 14% of all athletic injuries (McCue et al 1998). Typically, the hand is in front of the athlete and often absorbs the initial contact or repetitive stress. Injuries range from dislocations and fractures to overuse syndromes. Most injuries are treated in a non-operative fashion. Proper protection and appropriate rehabilitation are key to optimal healing (McCue et al 1998).

Fractures

Fractures of the distal radius vary in an age-related pattern which is determined by the changing mechanical properties of bone with age (Rang 1983). The younger child can sustain a minimally displaced metaphyseal buckle or torus fracture. Treatment consists of a short arm cast for 4 weeks. A greenstick forearm fracture may be associated with significant malrotation, and reduction is usually necessary, occasionally under anesthesia (Fig. 24.19). Adolescents can sustain Salter–Harris II

fractures through the distal radius growth plate with significant displacement (Fig. 24.20).

Evaluation of a forearm injury should include an examination of the entire extremity, and radiographs

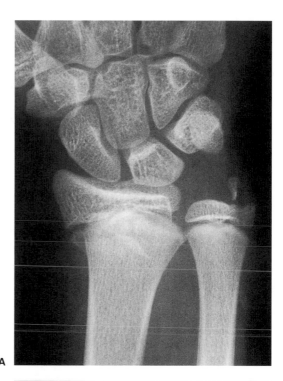

A

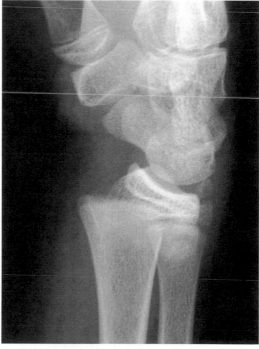

B

Figure 24.20A&B Anterior-posterior (**A**) and lateral (**B**) views of a Salter–Harris II fracture of the distal radius. This 13-year-old male fell on ice during a football activity, and landed on his outstretched hand. Closed reduction was performed after hematoma block, and the fracture healed without sequelae.

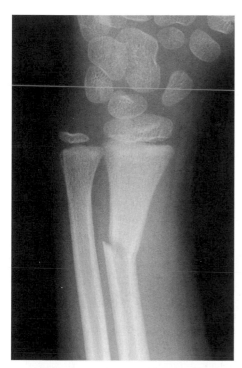

Figure 24.19 Greenstick fracture of the distal radius in a 6-year-old female who fell on her outstretched hand. The dorsal apex of the deformity resulted from pronation at the time of injury, and closed reduction required a supination maneuver.

should include both the elbow and wrist. Pain with forearm rotation can be a sign of injury. A Monteggia fracture is a fracture of the ulna shaft associated with a radial head dislocation, and the latter may be overlooked if the elbow is not included in the examination or radiographic studies. Neurovascular assessment is important as displaced fractures about the wrist can lead to median nerve injury.

Many gymnastic maneuvers require weightbearing on the upper extremities. Ground reaction forces put stresses on the wrist up to 2.37 times the gymnast's body weight in movements such as the back handspring (Zetaruk 2000). As a result of weightbearing on hyperdorsiflexed wrists, often with rotational forces, wrist injuries are common among young gymnasts (d'Hemecourt et al 2000). Salter–Harris type I microfractures of the growth plate are commonly incurred (Zetaruk 2000). Pain is usally localized to the dorsum of the radial aspect of the wrist. Treatment includes rest for 2–4 weeks, ice and anti-inflammatories. Severe cases require splinting. Flexibility and strength should be maintained during the rehabilitation phase while avoiding axial loading and torsion of the physis. Early recognition of pain and reduction of training may reduce the incidence of these types of fractures.

Fractures and other problems of the carpal bones are less common in the young athlete than in the adult (Kocher et al 2000, Simmons & Lovallo 1988). However, fractures of the digits are common in children and adolescents (Kocher et al 2000). An apparent dislocation or sprain of the finger in the child may actually be a fracture through the growth plate, and reduction must be performed with care to minimize further injury to the physis (Simmons & Lovallo 1988) (Figs 24.21 and 24.22).

SUMMARY

With the rise in youths participating in organized sports we have seen age- and sport-related injury patterns. Many youth injuries differ from adult injuries because of differing stages of physical development. Our aim is to recognize these risk factors, address them specifically through such modalities as education, physical therapy and protective devices, and therefore prevent initial or subsequent injury.

A knowledge of risk factors which predispose or contribute to musculoskeletal injury facilitates the clinical evaluation of the injured child and adolescent athlete (Box 24.1) (Micheli & Jenkins 1995). Awareness of injury patterns in specific sports may result in early diagnosis and treatment.

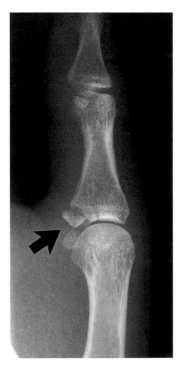

Figure 24.21 Avulsion fracture of the ulnar collateral ligament of the thumb metacarpophalangeal joint. This 15-year-old cheerleader fell on her thumb, with forceful thumb abduction. The Salter–Harris III ulnar collateral ligament avulsion fracture was treated with a thumb spica cast. Thumb stability was normal after the fracture had healed.

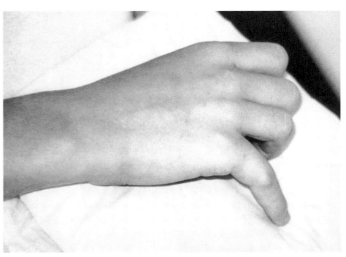

A

Figure 24.22A–C Salter–Harris II fracture of the base of the proximal phalanx. This 11-year-old male jammed his little finger against a baseball, with hyperextension of the digit. The abduction and supination deformity (**A**) was a result of a Salter–Harris II fracture of the base of the fifth proximal phalanx (**B** and **C**). Closed reduction was performed after hematoma block, and the fracture healed after 8 weeks of immobilization. It is important to correct the rotational deformity during the reduction, in order to prevent crossover with the ring finger during grasping activities.

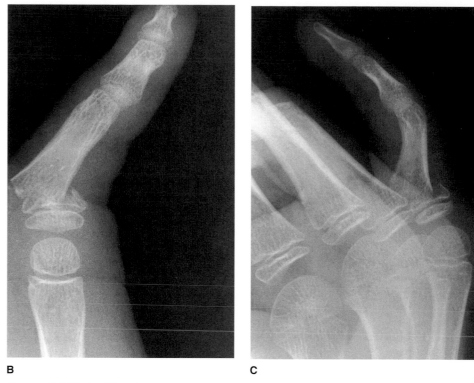

B

C

Figure 24.22A–C   *(Cont'd)*

Information based on risk factors can also be used in developing an approach to injury prevention (Faigenbaum 2000). Preparticipation clinical assessment of the young athlete can identify risk factors for injury in an individual (Micheli 1984, Rooks & Micheli 1988). Furthermore, based on the preparticipation evaluation, specific recommendations can be made for the improvement of physical characteristics such as strength and flexibility, which may increase safety and improve performance (Rooks & Micheli 1988). For example, the young gymnast with tightness of the lumbar spine and hamstrings may benefit from a directed low back and hamstring flexibility program, which could reduce the risk of spondylolysis.

The ability to improve certain physical characteristics in the prepubescent child (e.g. aerobic power, muscle strength, and anaerobic muscle power) has been documented in several studies (Bar-Or 1989, Faigenbaum 2000, Guy & Micheli 2001). Preseason conditioning, as well as the amount and content of practice sessions during a sports season, both appear to be correlated with a lower incidence of injury (Cahill & Griffith 1978, Ekstrand et al 1983, Smith et al 1997). Attention to sport-specific technique should also prevent injury in the young. For example, the young pitcher could reduce the risk of 'Little league elbow' by avoiding sidearm delivery (Albright et al 1978).

Protective equipment and rule changes can also reduce risk of injury. The use of bicycle helmets decreases the risk of head injury (Thompson et al 1989), and public health programs can increase the frequency of use of such equipment (DiGuiseppi et al 1989). Rule changes such as the banning of spearing in football, and the removal of trampolines from gymnastics programs, have resulted in a decreased incidence of cervical spine injury in these sports (Torg & Das 1985). The abolition of body checking in Pee Wee hockey could also reduce incidence of injury, particularly in leagues in which some players are twice as heavy as others (Roy et al 1989).

To minimize the risk of injury, young athletes should focus on developing muscle strength and endurance, cardiovascular fitness, and flexibility appropriate to their sport and level of physical development (NATA 2001). There is a growing interest in the research of young athletes, and with this focus, further gains in injury prevention and rehabilitation are anticipated.

REFERENCES

Aichroth P M, Patel D V, Marx C L 1991 Congenital discoid lateral meniscus in children. Journal of Bone and Joint Surgery 73B:932–936

Albright J A, Jokl P, Shaw R et al 1978 Clinical study of baseball pitchers: correlation of injury to the throwing arm with method of delivery. American Journal of Sports Medicine 6:15–21

Ali R M, Green D M, Patel T C 1999 Scheuermann's kyphosis. Current Opinion in Pediatrics 11(1):65–66

Andrews J R, Gidumal R H 1987 Shoulder arthroscopy in the throwing athlete: perspectives and prognosis. Clinics in Sports Medicine 6:565–571

Backx F J G, Erich W B M, Kemper A B A et al 1989 Sports injuries in school-aged children. An epidemiologic study. American Journal of Sports Medicine 17:234–240

Backx F J G, Beijer H J M, Bol E et al 1991 Injuries in high risk persons and high-risk sports. American Journal of Sports Medicine 19:124–130

Bar-Or, O 1989 Trainability of the prepubescent child. Physician and Sportsmedicine 17(5):65–82

Berkowitz M M, Bowen M K, Warren R F 1998 Injuries of the rotator cuff. In: Harries M, Williams C, Stanish W D et al (eds) Oxford textbook of sports medicine. Oxford University Press, Oxford

Bradley J P 1994 Upper extremity: elbow injuries in children and adolescents. In: Stanitski C L, DeLee J C, Drez D (eds) Pediatric and adolescent sports medicine. WB Saunders, Philadelphia

Bradley G W, Shives T C, Samuelson K M 1979 Ligament injuries in the knees of children. Journal of Bone and Joint Surgery 61A:588–591

Bright R W, Burstein A H, Elmore S M 1974 Epiphyseal-plate cartilage: a biomechanical and histological analysis of failure modes. Journal of Bone and Joint Surgery 56A:688–703

Browner B D, Jacobs L M, Poll A N (eds) 1999 American Academy of Orthopaedic Surgeons emergency care and transportation of the sick and injured, 7th edn. Jones and Bartlett, Sudbury, MA, p 682–713

Burkhart S S, Peterson H A 1979 Fractures of the proximal tibial epiphysis. Journal of Bone and Joint Surgery 61A:996–1002

Cahill B R, Griffith E H 1978 Effect of preseason conditioning on the incidence and severity of high school football knee injuries. American Journal of Sports Medicine 6:180–184

Cahill B R, Tullos H S, Fain R H 1974 Little league shoulder. Journal of Sports Medicine 2:150–153

Cantu R C 1988 Head and spine injuries in the young athlete. Clinics in Sports Medicine 7:459–472

Cantu R C 2000 Cervical spine injuries in the athlete. Seminars in Neurology 20(2):173–178

Carney B T, Weinstein S L, Noble J 1991 Long-term follow-up of slipped capital femoral epiphysis. Journal of Bone and Joint Surgery 73A:667–674

Cheng J C Y, Chan P S, Hui P W 1991 Joint laxity in children. Journal of Pediatric Orthopedics 11:752–756

Chow S P, Lam J J, Leong J C Y 1990 Fracture of the tibial tubercle in the adolescent. Journal of Bone and Joint Surgery 72B:231–234

Clancy W G, Foltz A S 1976 Iliac apophysitis and stress fractures in adolescent runners. American Journal of Sports Medicine 4:214–218

Clanton T O, DeLee J C, Sanders B et al 1979 Knee ligament injuries in children. Journal of Bone and Joint Surgery 61A:1195–1201

Connolly P J 2001 Physician decision making in return to play following cervical spine injury. Paper presented at the 68th Annual Meeting of the American Academy of Orthopaedic Surgeons.

Constantini N W, Warren M P 1994 Special problems of the female athlete. Bailliere's best practice and research. Clinical Rheumatology 8(1):199–219

Crossley K, Bennell K, Green S et al 2001 A systematic review of physical interventions for patellofemoral pain syndrome Clinical Journal of Sports Medicine 11(2):103–110

Curtis R J 1994 Skeletal injuries. In: Harries M, Williams C, Stanish W D et al (eds) Oxford textbook of sports medicine. Oxford University Press, Oxford

Dawson E G, Smith L 1979 Atlanto-axial subluxation in children due to vertebral anomalies. Journal of Bone and Joint Surgery 61A:582–587

d'Hemecourt P A, Gerbino P G, Micheli L J 2000 Back injuries in the young athlete. Clinics in Sports Medicine 19(4):663–679

DeLee J C 1994 Ligamentous injuries of the knee. In: Harries M, Williams C, Stanish W D et al (eds) Oxford textbook of sports medicine. Oxford University Press, Oxford

DeLee J C, Curtis R 1983 Anterior cruciate ligament insufficiency in children. Clinical Orthopaedics and Related Research 172:112–118

Dias L S 1984 Fractures of the tibia and fibula. In: Rockwood C A, Wilkins K E, King R E (eds) Fractures in children. JB Lippincott, Philadelphia

Dickhaut S C, DeLee J C 1982 The discoid lateral-meniscus syndrome. Journal of Bone and Joint Surgery 64A:1068–1073

DiGuiseppi C G, Rivara F P, Koepsell T D et al 1989 Bicycle helmet use by children. Evaluation of a community-wide helmet campaign. Journal of the American Medical Association 262:2256–2261

Dowdy P A, Miller M D, Fu F H 1998 Ankle and foot. In: Johnson R J, Lombardo J (eds) Current review of sports medicine, 2nd edn. Butterworth Heinemann, Philadelphia

Dyment P G 1989 Controversies in pediatric sports medicine. Physician and Sportsmedicine 17(7):57–76

Ekstrand J, Gillquist J, Moller M et al 1983 Incidence of soccer injuries and their relation to training and team success. American Journal Sports Medicine 11:63–67

Emery R J H, Mullaji A B 1991 Glenohumeral joint instability in normal adolescents. Journal of Bone and Joint Surgery 73B:406–408

Faigenbaum A D 2000 Strength training for children and adolescents. Clinics in Sports Medicine 19(4):593–619

Fondren F B, Goldner J L, Bassett F H 1985 Recurrent dislocation of the patella treated by the modified Roux-Goldthwait procedure. Journal of Bone and Joint Surgery 67A:993–1005

Griffin J R, Briard J L 1998 Fractures and dislocations. In: Harries M, Williams C, Stanish W D et al (eds) Oxford textbook of sports medicine. Oxford University Press, Oxford

Griffiths I D, Pinder I M 1981 Chondromalacia patellae: a clinical and arthroscopic study. Annals of the Rheumatic Diseases 40:617

Gross G W 1994a Imaging. In: Stanitski C L, DeLee J C, Drez D (eds) Pediatric and adolescent sports medicine. WB Saunders, Philadelphia

Gross R H 1994b Acute musculotendinous injuries. In: Stanitski C L, DeLee J C & Drez D (eds) Pediatric and adolescent sports medicine. WB Saunders, Philadelphia

Gurewitsch A D, O'Neill M A 1944 Flexibility of healthy children. Archives of Physical Therapy 25:216–221

Guy J A, Micheli L J 2001 Strength training for children and adolescents. Journal of the American Academy of Orthopaedic Surgeons 9(1):29–36

Hamilton W G 1982 Stenosing tenosynovitis of the flexor hallucis longus tendon and posterior impingement upon the os trigonum in ballet dancers. Foot and Ankle International 3:74–80

Havranek P, Lizler J 1991 Magnetic resonance imaging in the evaluation of partial growth arrest after physeal injuries in children. Journal of Bone and Joint Surgery 73A:1234–1241

Herring S A, Nilson K L 1987 Introduction to overuse injuries. Clinics in Sports Medicine 6:225–239

Hewett T E, Lindenfeld T N, Riccobene J V et al 2000 The effects of neuromuscular training on the incidence of knee injury in female athletes. A prospective study. American Journal of Sports Medicine 28(4):615–616

Insall J N, Aglietti P, Traino A J 1983 Patellar pain and incongruence II: clinical application. Clinical Orthopaedics and Related Research 176:225–232

Iobst C A, Stanitski C L 2000 Acute knee injuries. Clinics in Sports Medicine 19(4):621–635

Ireland M L, Andrews J R 1988 Shoulder and elbow injuries in the young athlete. Clinics in Sports Medicine 7:473–494

Irrgang J J, Sawhney R 1994 Rehabilitation for childhood and adolescent orthopaedic sports related injuries. In: Stanitski C L, DeLee J C, Drez D (eds) Pediatric and adolescent sports medicine. WB Saunders, Philadelphia

Jackson D W, Lowery W D, Ciullo J V 1995 Injuries of the spine. In: Nicholas J A, Hershman E B (eds) The lower extremity and spine in sports. Mosby, St. Louis

Javin J S, Fox J M 1995 Thigh injuries. In: Nicholas J A, Hershman E B (eds) The lower extremity and spine in sports medicine. Mosby, St. Louis

Johnson R J 1998 Acute knee injuries: an overview. In: Harries M, Williams C, Stanish W D et al (eds) Oxford textbook of sports medicine. Oxford University Press, Oxford

Kadel N, Micheli L J, Solomon R 2000 Os trigonum impingement syndrome in dancers. Journal of Dance Medicine and Science 4(3):1–4

Karlin L I 1995 Injuries to the hip and pelvis. In: Nicholas J A, Hershman E B (eds) The lower extremity and spine in sports edicine. Mosby, St. Louis

Kibler W B, Safran M R 2000 Musculoskeletal injuries in the young tennis player. Clinics in Sports Medicine 19(4):781–792

Kleiger B, Mankin H J 1964 Fracture of the lateral portion of the distal tibial epiphysis. Journal of Bone and Joint Surgery 46A:25–32

Kocher M S, Waters P M, Micheli L J 2000 Upper extremity injuries in the paediatric athlete. Sports Medicine 30(2):117–135

Kocher M S, Yaniv M, Adrignolo A A et al 2001 Functional and radiographic outcome of juvenile osteochondritis dissecans of the knee treated with antegrade arthroscopic drilling. American Journal of Sports Medicine 29(5):562–566

Kokoska E R, Keller M S, Rallo M C et al 2001 Characteristics of pediatric cervical spine injuries. Journal of Pediatric Surgery 36(1):100–105

Kvist M, Kujala U M, Heinonen O J et al 1989 Sports-related injuries in children. International Journal of Sports Medicine 10:81–86

Larson R L, McMahan R O 1966 The epiphyses and the childhood athlete. Journal of the American Medical Association 196:607–612

Leach R E, Miller J K 1987 Lateral and medial epicondylitis of the elbow. Clinics in Sports Medicine 6:259–272

Lipscomb A B, Anderson A F 1986 Tears of the anterior cruciate ligament in adolescents. Journal of Bone and Joint Surgery 68A:19–28

McCue F C, Dinsmore H H, Kowalk D L 1998 Athletic injuries to the hand and wrist. In: Johnson R J, Lombardo J (eds) Current review of sports medicine, 2nd edn. Butterworth Heinemann, Philadelphia

McManama G B, Micheli L J, Berry M V et al 1985 The surgical treatment of osteochondritis of the capitellum. American Journal of Sports Medicine 13:11–21

Mayer P J, Micheli L 1979 Avulsion of the femoral attachment of the posterior cruciate ligament in an eleven-year-old boy. Journal of Bone and Joint Surgery 61A:431–432

Metzl JD 2000 Sports medicine in pediatric practice: keeping pace with the changing times. Pediatric Annals 29(3):146–148

Metzmaker J N, Pappas A M 1985 Avulsion fractures of the pelvis. American Journal of Sports Medicine 13:349–358

Micheli L J 1984 Preparticipation evaluation for sports competition: musculoskeletal assessment of the young athlete. In: Kelley V C (ed) Practice of pediatrics. Harper and Row, Philadelphia

Micheli L J 1987 The traction apophysitises. Clinics in Sports Medicine 6:389–404

Micheli L J 1999 Pediatric lateral retinacular release with medial plication under arthroscopic control. Oratec Interventions Case Report K3

Micheli L J, Stanitski C L 1981 Lateral patellar retinacular release. American Journal of Sports Medicine 9:330–336

Micheli L J, Ireland M L 1987 Prevention and management of calcaneal apophysitis in children: an overuse syndrome. Journal of Pediatric Orthopedics 7:34–38

Micheli L J, Fehlandt A F 1994 Stress fractures. In: Letts R M (ed) Management of pediatric fractures. Churchill Livingstone, Edinburgh, p 973–987

Micheli L J, Jenkins M 1995 The sports medicine bible. Harper Perennial, New York

Micheli L J, d'Hemecourt P A 1998 Spine and chest wall. In: Johnson R J, Lombardo J (eds) Current review of sports medicine, 2nd edn. Butterworth Heinemann, Philadelphia

Micheli L J, Jenkins M 2001 The sports medicine bible for young athletes. Sourcebooks, Naperville, IL

Micheli L J, Hall J E, Miller M E 1980 Use of modified Boston brace for back injuries in athletes. American Journal of Sports Medicine 8:351–356

Micheli L J, Waters P M, Sanders D P 1989 Sliding fibular graft repair for chronic dislocation of the peroneal tendons. American Journal of Sports Medicine 17:68–71

Micheli L J, Metzl J D, DiCanzio J et al 1999a Anterior cruciate ligament reconstructive surgery in adolescent soccer and basketball players. Clinical Journal of Sports Medicine 9(3):138–141

Micheli L J, Rask B, Gerberg L 1999b Anterior cruciate ligament reconstruction in patients who are prepubescent. Clinical Orthopaedics and Related Research 364:40–47

Micheli L J, Glassman R, Klein M 2000 The prevention of sports injuries in children. Clinics in Sports Medicine 19(4):821–834

Murray R O, Duncan C 1971 Athletic activity in adolescence as an etiological factor in degenerative hip disease. Journal of Bone and Joint Surgery 53B:406–419

National Athletic Trainers' Association (NATA) 2001 NATA offers ways to minimize risk of injury in high school athletics. March 19

Neer C S, Foster C R 1980 Inferior capsular shift for involuntary inferior and multidirectional instability of the shoulder. Journal of Bone and Joint Surgery 62A:897–908

Norwood L A, Terry G C 1984 Shoulder posterior subluxation. American Journal of Sports Medicine 12:25–30

Norwood L A, Shook J A, Andrews J R 1981 Acute medial elbow ruptures. American Journal of Sports Medicine 9:16–19

O'Driscoll S W, Evans D C 1991 Contralateral shoulder instability following anterior repair. Journal of Bone and Joint Surgery 73B:941–946

Ogden J A, Southwick W O 1976 Osgood-Schlatter's disease and tibial tuberosity development. Clinical Orthopaedics and Related Research 116:180–189

Omey M L, Micheli L J 1999 Foot and ankle problems in the young athlete. Medicine and Science in Sports and Exercise 31:S470–476

O'Neill D B, Micheli L J 1989 Tarsal coalition: a followup of adolescent athletes. American Journal of Sports Medicine 17:544–549

Outerbridge A R, Micheli L J 1995 Overuse injuries in the young athlete. Clinics in Sports Medicine 14(3):503–516

Peck D M 1995 Apophyseal injuries in the young athlete. American Family Physian 51(8):1897–1898, 1981–1985

Pelipenko V I 1973 On peculiarities of the development of the foot skeleton in the pupils of a choreographic school. Archives of Anatomy Gistol Embryology 64:46–50

Pirnay L, Crielaard J M 2001 Stress fractures and sports. Review Medicale de Liege 56(5):369–374

Poll R G, Duijfjes F 1984 The treatment of recurrent dislocation of the peroneal tendons. Journal of Bone and Joint Surgery 66B:98–100

Powell J W, Barber-Foss K D 2000 Sex related injury patterns among selected high school sports. American Journal of Sports Medicine 28(3):385–391

Priest J D, Weise D J 1981 Elbow injury in women's gymnastics. American Journal of Sports Medicine 9:288–295

Proctor M R, Cantu R C 2000 Head and neck injuries in young athletes. Clinics in Sports Medicine 19(4):693–715

Pudda G C, Cerullo G, Selvanetti A et al 1998 Stress fractures. In: Harries M, Williams C, Stanish W D et al (eds) Oxford textbook of sports medicine. Oxford University Press, Oxford

Pueschel S M, Scola F H 1987 Atlantoaxial instability in individuals with Down syndrome: epidemiologic, radiographic, and clinical studies. Pediatrics 80:555–560

Rang M 1983 Children's fractures, 2nd edn. JB Lippincott, Philadelphia

Renstrom P A 1998 An introduction to chronic overuse injuries. In: Harries M, Williams C, Stanish W D et al (eds) Oxford textbook of sports medicine. Oxford University Press, Oxford

Rice S G 2000 Risks of injury during sports participation. In: Anderson S J, Sullivan J A 1994 (eds) Care of the young athlete. American Academy of Orthopaedics, Chicago

Rodenburg J B 1994 Warm-up, stretching and massage diminish harmful effects of eccentric exercise. International Journal of Sports Medicine 15:414–419

Rooks D S, Micheli L J 1988 Musculoskeletal assessment and training: the young athlete. Clinics in Sports Medicine 7:641–677

Roos H P, Renstrom P A 1998 Pain about the groin, hip and pelvis. In: Harries M, Williams C, Stanish W D et al (eds) Oxford textbook of sports medicine. Oxford University Press, Oxford

Rosen P R, Micheli L J, Treves S 1982 Early scintigraphic diagnosis of bone stress and fractures in athletic adolescents. Pediatrics 70(1):11–15

Roy M A, Bernard D, Roy B et al 1989 Body checking in Pee Wee hockey. Physician and Sportsmedicine 17(3):119–126

Salter R B, Harris W R 1963 Injuries involving the epiphyseal plate. Journal of Bone and Joint Surgery 45A:587–622

Samilson R L, Prieto V 1983 Posterior dislocation of the shoulder in athletes. Clinics in Sports Medicine 2:369–378

Sanders W E, Wilkins K E, Neidre A 1980 Acute insufficiency of the posterior cruciate ligament in children. Journal of Bone and Joint Surgery 62A:129–131

Schnebel B E 2000 Spine. In: Sullivan J A, Anderson S J (eds) Care of young athlete. AAOS & AAP, Oklahoma City

Schneider H J, King A Y, Bronson J L et al 1974 Stress injuries and developmental change of lower extremities in ballet dancers. Radiology 113:627–632

Sella E J, Lawson J P, Ogden J A 1986 The accessory navicular synchondrosis. Clinical Orthopaedics and Related Research 209:280–285

Simmons B P, Lovallo J L 1988 Hand and wrist injuries in children. Clinics in Sports Medicine 7:495–512

Smith D S, Kovan J R, Rich B S et al 1997 In: Preparticipation Physical Evaluation Task Force (eds) Preparticipation physical evaluation, 2nd edn. Monograph published by The Physician and Sportsmedicine, McGraw Hill, New York

Spiegel P G, Cooperman D R, Laros G S 1978 Epiphyseal fractures of the distal ends of the tibia and fibula. Journal of Bone and Joint Surgery 60A:1046–1050

Stanitski C L 1994a Osteochondritis dissecans of the knee. In: Stanitski C L, DeLee J C, Drez D(eds) Pediatric and adolescent sports medicine. WB Saunders, Philadelphia

Stanitski C L 1994b Meniscal lesions. In: Stanitski C L, DeLee J C, Drez D (eds) Pediatric and adolescent sports medicine. WB Saunders, Philadelphia

Steiner M E, Grana W A 1988 The young athlete's knee: recent advances. Clinics in Sports Medicine 7:527–546

Stover C N 1980 Air stirrup management of ankle injuries in the athlete. American Journal of Sports Medicine 8:360–365

Sullivan J A 1994 Ankle and foot injuries in the pediatric athlete. In: Stanitski C L, DeLee J C, Drez D(eds) Pediatric and adolescent sports medicine. WB Saunders, Philadelphia

Taunton J E, Robertson L S, Fricker P A 1998 Acute and overuse ankle injuries. In: Harries M, Williams C, Stanish W D et al (eds) Oxford textbook of sports medicine. Oxford University Press, Oxford

Thompson R S, Rivara F P, Thompson D C 1989 A case-control study of the effectiveness of bicycle safety helmets. New England Journal of Medicine 320:1361–1367

Torg J S, Das M 1985 Trampoline and minitrampoline injuries to the cervical spine. Clinics in Sports Medicine 4:45–60

Twyman R S, Desai K, Aichroth P M 1991 Osteochondritis dissecans of the knee. Journal of Bone and Joint Surgery 73B:461–464

van Mechelen W 1992 Running injuries: a review of the epidemiolgic literature. Sports Medicine 14:320–335

Warren M P, Shantha S 2000 The female athlete. Bailliere's best practice and research. Clinical Endocrinology and Metabolism 14(1):37–53

Warren M P, Brooks-Gunn J, Hamilton L H et al 1986 Scoliosis and fractures in young ballet dancers: relation to delayed menarche and secondary amenorrhea. New England Journal of Medicine 314:1348–1353

Washer D C, Finerman G A 1994 Physeal injuries in young athletes. In: Stanitski C L, DeLee J C, Drez D(eds) Pediatric and adolescent sports medicine. WB Saunders, Philadelphia

Waters P M, Millis M B 1988 Hip and pelvic injuries in the young athlete. Clinics in Sports Medicine 7(3):513–526

Waters P M, Millis M B 1994 Hip and pelvic injuries in the young athlete. In: Stanitski C L, DeLee J C, Drez D(eds) Pediatric and adolescent sports medicine. WB Saunders, Philadelphia

Weldon E J, Richardson A B 2001 Upper extremity overuse injuries in swimming, A discussion of swimmer's shoulder. Clinics in Sports Medicine 20(3):4230–4438

Yancey R A, Micheli L J 1994 Thoracolumbar spine injuries in pediatric sports. In: Stanitski C L, DeLee J C, Drez D(eds) Pediatric and adolescent sports medicine. WB Saunders, Philadelphia

Zaricznyj B, Shattuck L J M, Mast T A et al 1980 Sports-related injuries in school-aged children. American Journal of Sports Medicine 8:318–324

Zetaruk, M 2000 The young gymnast. Clinics in Sports Medicine 19(4):757–780

25

Older exercise participants

Jennifer Stevens   Domhnall MacAuley

INTRODUCTION

Aging is accompanied by inevitable deterioration of many physiological parameters. Research has sought to prevent the effects of aging and the decline that comes with increasing age. Joint crepitus, muscle atrophy, slowing down, failing eyesight, loss of hearing, and thinning hair and skin are a few examples of changes with aging.

From a physiological prime in the third decade of life, changes occur in almost every cell in the body including bones, muscle, and soft tissue. These cellular changes affect almost every function. We do not, of course, notice this gradual physiological decline unless we measure it. Athletes know when their performances slip: training becomes more difficult and they have to work harder to maintain their fitness. But most people are unaware of their declining fitness until it begins to affect their every day life. We can track the decline over years by measuring various physiological parameters, monitoring gross changes using X-ray and magnetic resonance imaging (MRI), and examining the changes at tissue level using microscopy and electron microscopy.

Although there is no single intervention able to prevent age-related deterioration in function, exercise, especially strength training, can help slow some of the inevitable decline (Mazzeo et al 1998). This chapter will outline the effect of age on tissue and function, its influence on physical fitness and wellbeing, and how physical activity may help delay some of the effects of aging.

PHYSIOLOGICAL EFFECTS OF AGING

Understanding the source of age-related declines in the neuromuscular system provides a basis for the goals of rehabilitation aimed at countering these changes. Many impairments in mobility stem from the cumulative effect of physiological changes in bone, muscle, articular cartilage, ligaments, and tendons, as well as alterations in the central and peripheral nervous system. By examining the physiological basis for age-related impairments, the mechanisms for successful interventions that slow the progression of age-related changes in the neuromuscular system can be better understood.

BONE AND ARTICULAR CARTILAGE

Bone is an active tissue with constant turnover that relies on a balance between bone resorption and bone formation. With increasing age, the balance between these two processes can shift, resulting in greater bone loss than formation. This progressive loss of bone mineral density, which occurs to a greater extent in women, leads to a disruption in the microarchitecture of the bone that makes bone more susceptible to fracture (American College of Sports Medicine 1995). On average, as people get older, they lose about 1% of bone per year after the age of 35 years (World Health Organization 1994). This is especially difficult for women where there is an increase in bone loss after the menopause of 2–3% per year that may lead to osteoporosis (World Health Organization 1994). Osteoporosis is defined as bone mass density that is ≥ 2.5 standard deviations below the mean bone density for young adults. Osteoporosis is a silent disease: bone loss often goes unnoticed until an individual experiences a compression fracture, most commonly in the vertebrae or the hips.

Prevention is essential to minimize the amount of bone loss that can occur in older adults, especially since bone loss is not often diagnosed until a fracture occurs (Siris et al 2001). Weightbearing exercise can help prevent or slow the age-related loss of bone mineral density, but exercise must be of sufficient intensity to load the musculoskeletal system adequately to promote an increase in bone mineral density (American College of Sports Medicine 1995).

Articular cartilage also changes with increasing age, and erosion and deformation of articular cartilage can result in osteoarthritis (Felson et al 2000). The primary role of articular cartilage is to protect the ends of bone from forces transmitted at the joints and to provide friction-free surfaces for joints to articulate. With increasing age, degenerative changes affect the ability of articular cartilage to perform this role. Changes in the chondrocytes, collagen fibers, and proteoglycans that comprise articular cartilage account for much of the deformation of articular cartilage. Progressive articular cartilage degeneration can eventually cause joint pain, swelling, and stiffness, and often profoundly impacts on function.

LIGAMENT AND TENDON

The majority of research examining age-related changes in connective tissue, such as ligaments and tendons, relies on animal models (Buckwalter 1997). The advantage of using animal models is that more precise measurements of connective tissue can be made, but the disadvantage is that assumptions are made that age-related changes in connective tissue are similar between animals and humans.

The compliance and flexibility of ligaments and tendons decreases with increasing age, such that connective tissue is less able to stretch with large loads. Collagen plays a large role in connective tissue changes because it provides much of the structure and tensile strength to connective tissue (Uitto 1986). With increasing age, collagen becomes more cross-linked, which results in greater stiffness of ligaments and tendons. Another major component of connective tissue is elastin, which allows tissue to stretch and react to loads (Uitto 1986). Structural and compositional changes in elastin also contribute to an increased stiffness in connective tissue. Decreased water content, secondary to a decrease in the proteoglycan content, adds to the loss of flexibility in the connective tissue of older adults (Buckwalter 1997). The overall result is that injuries of ligaments, tendons, and other soft tissues occur more easily because they lose the dynamic ability to respond to loads (Buckwalter 1997, Tipton et al 1975) when proper warm-up and stretching routines are not integrated with exercise programs. Regular exercise can mitigate the risk for injury by keeping soft tissue more supple and less susceptible to damage (Menard 1996).

MUSCLE

Aging is associated with a loss of muscle mass and muscle strength. Cross-sectional and longitudinal studies have documented the loss of muscle mass as a part of the normal aging process (Metter et al 1999). Muscle mass decreases at a rate of 1% per year in both men and women after the age of 60 years (Evans 1995, Lexell 1995). The changes in muscle mass are the result of a reduction in the total number of muscle fibers and a preferential atrophy of fast, type II muscle fibers, which results in slower muscle contractile properties.

Other age-related morphological changes in muscle include a decreased total number of motor units and a concurrent increased size of the remaining motor units (Porter et al 1995). Fewer motor units, now larger in size, compromise the precision of force control in older adults. Less precision may affect fine motor skills and may alter an older adult's response to unexpected perturbations.

NERVOUS SYSTEM

Changes in the peripheral and central nervous system affect nerve conduction velocity, sensory discrimination, muscle strength, and autonomic responses.

Peripheral nervous system

With aging, nerves undergo structural, functional, and biochemical changes (Verdu et al 2000). There is a loss of myelinated nerve fibers and a decrease in the size and myelin of the remaining myelinated fibers, both of which contribute to decreased nerve conduction velocities. Increasing age also decreases the ability of nerves to regenerate and reinnervate muscle after injury.

Central nervous system

Deficits in the ability of older adults to activate muscles fully (central activation) may contribute to age-related losses in strength. Some research has found that central activation deficits exist in healthy, older adults (Stevens et al 2001), while some studies have not found deficits (Connelly et al 1999). The majority of studies that have failed to find deficits in muscle activation have not used techniques that are sensitive enough to capture the presence of muscle activation deficits.

AGING AND BODY FUNCTION

STRENGTH

Muscle strength declines with age, although the decline in strength can be delayed by maintaining a physically active lifestyle or accelerated by illness or medication (Hurley & Roth 2000). In general, strength is maintained until the age of 45–50 years, after which, there is a subsequent pronounced decline. After the age of 50 years, muscular strength decreases at a rate of about 1.5–3.0% per year (Porter et al 1995, Vandervoort & McComas 1986). The loss of muscle strength with aging, however, is even greater than the loss of muscle mass. Muscle mass only decreases at the rate of 1% per year in both men and women after the age of 60 years (Evans 1995, Lexell 1995). The greater loss of strength than of muscle mass suggests that factors other than muscle mass (e.g. decreased central activation of muscle) must also account for some age-related muscle weakness (Stackhouse et al 2001, Stevens et al 2001).

Loss of strength may reach a critical level, below which there is a decline in function during tasks of daily living. If the physiological load remains the same but the amount of muscle mass is reduced, a larger percentage of the muscle will need to be recruited to perform a particular task (Chandler et al 1998). For example, an older adult might perceive that climbing a set of stairs is a harder task than it was 10 years ago. Even though individuals report being out of breath at the top of the stairs, their cardiovascular system may be taxed because of diminished lower extremity strength rather than a lack of endurance. Ascending a 6-inch step might require a greater percentage demand of each muscle group than would be required of a younger adult. As a result, it seems reasonable that older adults may report increasing difficulty with performing certain tasks.

Older muscle can be trained with high-intensity strength training programs, and although the inevitable decline in strength cannot be stopped, it is possible to slow the speed of progression and help maintain sufficient strength for daily living (Nadel & DiPietro 1995). Older adults have less muscle tissue, but the remaining muscle tissue responds well to training. Even adults aged 86–96 years had an average increase in quadriceps strength of 174% after 8 weeks of high-intensity strength training (Fiatarone et al 1990). The intensity of strength training was measured as a percentage of an individual's one Repetition Maximum (1 RM). A 1 RM is the maximum amount of weight an individual can lift once, while maintaining proper technique (Evans 1999). In Evans' study, subjects performed 3 sets of 8 repetitions at 50% of their 1 RM for the first week of exercise. By the end of the second week, the intensity was increased to 80% of the 1 RM. The 1 RM was remeasured every 2 weeks and weights for strength training were adjusted accordingly.

A similar study in adults, aged 72–98 years, found that strength training of the hip and knee extensors resulted in an average strength gain of 113% (Fiatarone et al 1994). Strength training was performed at 80% of the 1 RM, 3 times a week for 10 weeks. Lower extremity strength gains translated to improved gait velocities and stair-climbing power.

ENDURANCE

There are inevitable changes in endurance capacity with increasing age. Changes in endurance capacity can be attributed to changes in both the cardiovascular system and in muscle energetics.

Cardiovascular system

Cardiovascular fitness, as measured by maximal oxygen consumption (VO_2 max), declines with age. Even in elite athletes, an individual decline in cardiovascular fitness with age is evident (Ashworth et al 1994, Brooks et al 1994, Evans & Meredith 1989). On average, VO_2 max decreases 4–5.5 ml/min/kg/decade in older men and 2–3.5 ml/min/kg/decade in older women, which translates to around a 12–13% decrease per decade (Holloszy & Kohrt 1995). Even active, lean older adults have a 9% decrease in VO_2 max/decade and master athletes (who maintain a very vigorous activity level) have a 5% decrease in VO_2 max/decade (Kohrt et al 1991).

The age-related declines in cardiovascular function (Bouvier et al 2001) occur largely because of a decrease in heart rate (HR), although other changes in the cardiovascular system contribute as well. Maximal HR can be calculated using the following formula: HR max = 220 – age.

This formula only provides a crude calculation of maximal HR because recent evidence indicates that it may underestimate maximal HR by ~10 bpm (Guccione 2000). Regardless of the exact decrement in HR, if HR decreases and the size of the chambers of the heart remain the same, there has to be a reduction in the maximum flow (cardiac output). In fact, cardiac output has been shown to decrease by 2–30% (Menard 1996). Reduced cardiac output limits endurance capacity because the older heart has to work harder in response to a given workload (Astrand & Rodahl 1977).

Other age-related changes in the cardiovascular system include an increase in the total peripheral vascular resistance (McArdle et al 1994). This occurs largely because of a decrease in arterial wall elasticity and an increase in the accumulation of fatty deposits on the vessel walls. The result is higher blood pressure with increasing age.

Age-related changes in hormone regulation may also affect cardiovascular performance, in particular, the HR (Guccione 2000). The release of adrenaline (epinephrine) and noradrenaline (norepinephrine) is less during exercise in older adults compared to younger adults. Changes in the release of these catecholamines may, in part, explain the decreases in HR with increasing age. Additional age-related changes to the cardiovascular system may affect endurance, but the majority of evidence indicates that the reduction in pump efficiency (i.e. HR) is arguably the most important (McArdle et al 1994).

Although regular exercise cannot completely counter all the changes in the cardiovascular system with increasing age, there is ample evidence to suggest that exercise attenuates the progression of some of the age-related changes. In particular, older adults still retain the ability to increase VO_2 max with prolonged endurance exercise to the same extent as younger adults (Mazzeo et al 1998).

Muscle endurance

There is less consensus regarding changes in muscle energetic pathways, but it appears that muscle endurance in older, healthy muscle is comparable to that of younger muscle (Guccione 2000, Stevens et al 2001). When healthy, older adults participate in voluntary and electrically-elicited isokinetic or isometric fatigue protocols, there are no differences in the rate of fatigue compared to younger adults (Stevens et al 2001) (Fig. 25.1). Although the absolute strength of older adults is less, the rate of fatigue is comparable to that of younger adults. Most of these studies have been performed in healthy adults, so it is possible that the findings may not be generalized to all older adult populations.

FLEXIBILITY

Soft tissues require greater effort with increasing age to maintain the same degree of mobility and flexibility that is present in younger adults (Buckwalter 1997), yet there are few studies that have explored interventions to improve flexibility in older adults (Mazzeo et al 1998). The small number of studies that have focused on improving flexibility with exercise are somewhat inconclusive because they have not systematically determined a dose–response relationship for flexibility training (Mazzeo et al 1998). Yet there is no question that older adults would benefit from increased flexibility; the question is how to effectively increase flexibility. Most studies have indirectly focused on flexibility by enrolling older adults in regular exercise programs and monitoring changes in range of motion (Mazzeo 1998). At least from these studies, we can conclude that exercise offers one possibility for increasing flexibility in older adults, but more research is necessary to design interventions specifically intended to improve flexibility.

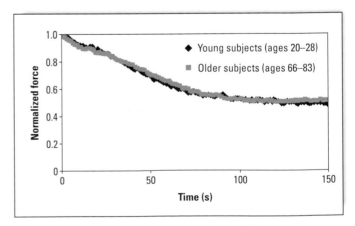

Figure 25.1 Quadriceps femoris muscle fatigability during an electrically-elicited fatigue test (n = 20 young, 20 older adults). Torque values are expressed as a percentage of each individual's initial torque. Younger and older adults had a similar degree of quadriceps muscle fatigue.

MOBILITY AND BALANCE

Balance is impaired with increasing age secondary to a variety of changes in strength and postural control. Increasing age is accompanied by changes in the vestibular ocular reflex, increased joint stiffness, decreased tissue flexibility, increased static sway, a greater number of steps necessary to respond to a perturbation, and an increased cocontraction of antagonist muscle groups (Guccione 2000). In addition, older adults have slower postural responses (20–30 ms delay), which may be caused by a slower processing of sensory information, combined with a decrease in nerve conduction velocity (Studenski et al 1991).

The combination of these sensorimotor changes and decreased muscle strength predisposes older adults to an increased risk of falling. In fact, falls are a major cause of morbidity and mortality in adults over the age of 65 years and often result in hospitalization (Rose & Maffulli 1999). Even falls that do not lead to injury have profound consequences because as little as one fall may encourage an older adult to avoid situations that may increase the risk of falling. Yet, decreasing the exposure to falls does not necessarily result in fewer falls (Gregg et al 2000). In fact, the tendency for older adults to avoid activities that put them at risk perpetuates the inability to respond appropriately to an impending fall. Consequently, a fear of falling may promote social isolation and greater dependence.

One of the most devastating consequences of falling is a hip fracture, which almost always necessitates hospitalization. Research indicates that a 50-year-old Caucasian female has a 17% risk of sustaining a hip fracture during her remaining lifetime (Rose & Maffulli 1999). After the age of 50 years, the risk of sustaining a hip fracture has been estimated to double every 5 years. By the age of 90, 1 in 4 women and 1 in 8 men will have had a hip fracture (Rose & Maffulli 1999). A third of patients who sustain a hip fracture die within a year of the fracture (Rose & Maffulli 1999). Of patients who live past the first year, only 66% return home after a hip fracture (Rose & Maffulli 1999). Unfortunately, the total number of hip fractures in older adults is increasing each year because of a growing proportion of older adults in the population (Rose & Maffulli 1999).

In addition to the sensorimotor changes that impair balance in older adults, other factors also partially account for the incidence of falls each year. Muscle weakness, especially of the knee and ankle, is significantly related to recurrent falls in older adults. (Whipple et al 1987). In addition, medications that cause sedation or affect vestibular function can result in dizziness and potentially a fall. Environmental factors can also contribute to an increased risk of falling because environmental hazards, like carpets, increase this risk (Allegrante et al 1991).

Prevention has been shown to be the most important factor in reducing the incidence of falls. In addition to carefully monitoring medication use, physical activity plays a very important role in decreasing fall risk (Gregg et al 2000). O'Loughlin et al (1993) suggested that those who remain active can maintain balance, flexibility, reflexes, muscle strength, coordination and appropriate reaction times required to avoid imbalance. Paradoxically, physical activity increases exposure to falls, and yet physical activity is related to a decreased risk of falls.

Exercise interventions for older adults often involve a multifaceted approach that makes it difficult to identify the specific components of each program that contribute to a decreased fall risk. Nevertheless, there is evidence that exercise interventions that incorporate balance and lower extremity strength training appear to be most effective in decreasing the risk of falls (Gregg et al 2000). In a major US study (Province et al 1995), older people who took part in an exercise intervention were 10% less likely to fall. People who followed an individualized exercise program that included resistance, flexibility, and balance training, reduced their risk of falling. The greatest benefit was found with exercise programs that had a balance retraining component and, in particular, those that included Tai Chi (discussed later in this chapter) (Wolfson et al 1996).

Other studies have also shown positive results for reducing fall risk with exercise programs. Tinetti and colleagues demonstrated that patients who participated in an intervention with medication monitoring, patient education, and exercise prescription had 31% fewer falls than with those who did not receive the intervention (Tinetti et al 1994). Similarly, a randomized controlled trial of home-based strength and balance retraining in women aged 80 years and older showed a comparable reduction in falls rate (Campbell et al 1997).

EPIDEMIOLOGICAL STUDIES OF PHYSICAL ACTIVITY IN OLDER ADULTS

Epidemiological studies around the world give us some indication of the levels of physical fitness of the general population. It is difficult to make direct comparisons because studies use different instruments and criteria, but some general observations can be made. The American College of Sports Medicine (ACSM), in their Position Stand on exercise and physical activity for older adults (Mazzeo et al 1998), emphasized how participation in a regular exercise program is an effective means of reducing some of the functional decline associated with aging. Only 10% of those over the age of 65 years, however, engage in vigorous activity in the USA (Elward & Larson 1992). Studies from the UK also showed that a large proportion of older adults are relatively inactive, and more importantly, have poor physical fitness (Allied Dunbar National Fitness Survey Level 1992, MacAuley et al 1994). Comparative data from Australia shows a similar pattern to that of the UK and US studies; a national cardiovascular risk factor study in 1991 classified 32% of respondents as inactive, 54% as moderately active and 15% as aerobic (Bauman & Owen 1991). A further study by the same group, showed that those who were inactive were more likely to be older, less well educated, and to have lower incomes (Owen & Bauman 1992). In a more recent study, Booth et al (2000) found that more males than females in Australia were physically active and that physical activity participation was related to age. Specifically, a greater proportion of those aged 65–69 were active than those aged 60–64 or 70 or older. The factors most associated with being active were high self-efficacy, regular participation in exercise with friends and family, finding footpaths safe for walking, and access to local facilities (Booth et al 2000).

BENEFITS OF EXERCISE THROUGHOUT THE AGING PROCESS

In light of the plethora of changes in physical functioning associated with aging, exercise becomes increasingly important with advancing age. The effects of exercise on strength, balance, and endurance are key factors in reducing falls, minimizing ill health, and maintaining independence (Gill et al 1995). When physical activity is promoted to those in their older years, it is often done so as to improve physical fitness in order to maintain functional independence (Wagner 1997) or to enhance already existing levels of athletic performance. The main objectives of exercise for older adults are to improve strength, agility, and cardiovascular fitness by promoting physiological adaptations to exercise (Guccione 2000, Mazzeo et al 1998).

If physical fitness can be maintained, even if we do not prolong life, we may theoretically delay 'dependency'. Delaying and shortening the time period of illness and dependency is an interesting concept that has been called the 'compression of morbidity' (Fries 1998, Vita et al 1998). Similarly, the Medical Research Council Topic Review on the elderly uses the term 'Healthy Active Life Expectancy' (HALE) with the emphasis on extending the active period within one's life rather than the actual duration of life (Medical Research Council 1994).

Strength training in older adults has a myriad of benefits, aside from the most obvious one: increasing muscle strength. Strength training improves insulin action, increases bone density, helps maintain metabolically active tissue mass, decreases blood pressure, reduces body fat, decreases pain from arthritis, increases

levels of physical activity, improves the quality of sleep, enhances functional performance, and decreases the risk of falls (Brill et al 1995, Mazzeo et al 1998). Being older, inactive, or unfit is not a contraindication to strength training and age is no barrier (Fiatarone et al 1990).

Endurance training enhances cardiovascular function. In particular, aerobic exercise promotes an increase in VO_2 max and cardiac output (McArdle et al 1994). The degree of increase depends on the baseline level of fitness and the intensity of training. Endurance exercise is also associated with lower blood pressure, improved plasma lipoprotein profiles, and decreased overall percentage of body fat. Endurance training especially benefits individuals with poor glucose tolerance or insulin sensitivity, as aerobic exercise improves both (Borghouts & Keizer 2000, Ryan 2000).

Balance training improves postural stability and decreases the risk of falls (Maffulli et al 2001, Province et al 1995). Balance training also reduces the fear of falling, which encourages older adults to increase their physical activity levels (Wolf et al 1996). Tai Chi has recently become one of the most popular and effective means of enhancing balance.

Physical activity also has a positive effect on psychological wellbeing in older adults. Physical activity improves depression in older adults, although the mechanism for the improvements is not yet understood (Butler et al 1998, Tsutsumi et al 1997). In a randomized clinical trial involving progressive resistance strength training, 14 of 16 initially depressed individuals were no longer clinically depressed at the end of a 10-week strength training program. Interestingly, the intensity of strength training was related to the degree of improvement in depression scores. Tsutsumi et al (1997) also found strength training programs improved psychological status. Training was performed three times a week for 12 weeks and included either high (75–85% 1 RM) or low intensity (55–65% 1 RM) strength training. For both training intensities, there were improvements in mood, anxiety, and perceived confidence for physical capability, compared to controls. Interestingly, there were no improvements in cognitive function, which is consistent with a variety of studies that question whether exercise can effectively impact on the cognitive status of older adults (Mazzeo et al 1998).

GUIDELINES FOR EXERCISE

ASSESSING RISKS OF EXERCISE PARTICIPATION IN OLDER ADULTS

As people get older, they are more likely to suffer from chronic medical conditions where vigorous exercise requires more supervision (Guccione 2000, Mazzeo et al 1998). Although the contraindications for exercise and the warning signs to cease exercising are the same for younger and older adults (Boxes 25.1 and 25.2), the likelihood of experiencing health-related problems during exercise increases with advancing age. All older adults should seek medical advice before commencing an exercise program, but whether they need to undergo extensive pre-exercise testing is more controversial. The American College of Sports Medicine (Evans 1999) recommends an exercise stress test for anyone over the age of 50 years who wants to initiate a vigorous exercise program, and anyone who has a history of ischemic heart disease, angina, diabetes, or hypertension. Others contend that adults over the age of 50 years who do not have significant cardiovascular disease risk factors may not necessitate a stress test. In fact, among 14 studies that used high-intensity strength training programs for older adults, only three included exercise stress tests in the prescreening (American Geriatrics Society Panel on Exercise and Osteoarthritis 2001). Alternatives to physician-supervised stress tests may be appropriate for many relatively healthy older adults who wish to initiate an exercise program (Evans 1999). Evans (1999) proposed

a weightlifting stress test where patients perform 3 sets of 8 repetitions at around 80% 1 RM. Meanwhile, electrocardiographic (ECG) and blood pressure measurements are used to gauge responses to exercise.

There are aspects of a medical history that may indicate risks of falling and particular care needed for physical activity participation. For example, if a patient lost consciousness on a previous fall, they may have an underlying medical condition (Puisieux et al 2000). Prescribed drugs should be reviewed, and lying and standing blood pressure measured. Simple tests of balance and muscle strength can be important but a history of previous falls is consistently the strongest risk factor for further falls (Bloem et al 2001).

Increased risks with exercise and medications

Older adults have a two- to three-fold greater risk of experiencing an adverse drug reaction than younger adults (Nolan & O'Malley 1988). Older adults not only ingest a larger number of drugs, but they also have an altered response to drugs (Naranjo et al 1995, Tsujimoto et al 1989) and this can therefore affect exercise tolerance. Medications can affect older adults differently than younger adults because of changes in drug distribution to tissues, drug metabolism, and drug excretion (Guccione 2000, Naranjo et al 1995). Those taking medication should consult their physician, particularly those taking medication for hypertension, diabetes, or any heart condition.

Some medication used for blood pressure regulation and cardiac disease management can adversely affect activity tolerance (Brukner & Khan 2001, Guccione 2000) (Table 25.1). With congestive heart failure, medications are frequently used to increase the strength of myocardial contraction (e.g. digitalis and beta blockers). With both hypertension and congestive heart failure, medications are used to decrease fluid volume and vascular resistance (e.g. ACE inhibitors and diuretics). Each of these medications can alter responses to exercise (Guccione 2000). For example, one effect of beta blockers is to reduce resting HR and stabilize the HR, which interferes with the normal HR response to exercise. This means that patients taking beta blockers may have more difficulty with exercise and may fatigue easily. Those taking beta blockers should be aware that HR will no longer be an adequate guide to exercise intensity, and that perceived exertion is a more relevant indication of intensity than HR (Table 25.1). Patients with cardiac conditions may also be taking diuretics to reduce fluid volume in order to decrease cardiac workload. Usually, diuretics do not affect exercise tolerance unless there is significantly altered fluid and electrolyte balance. Warning signs

---

Box 25.1 Contraindications to exercise in older adults

Absolute contraindications
• Acute myocardial infarction
• Unstable angina
• Uncontrolled arrhythmias
• Third degree heart block
• Acute congestive heart failure

Relative contraindications
• Uncontrolled blood pressure
• Cardiomyopathy
• Valvular heart disease
• Uncontrolled metabolic disease

Box 25.2 Warning signs to stop exercise in older adults

• Chest pain – always stop exercise with chest pain. Heart-related chest pain is usually described as a tightness or weight in the central chest, often radiating to the neck or left arm. If in doubt, stop exercising and seek help
• Palpitations – if the heart rate is excessive or irregular
• Feeling of weakness, pale, clammy, fainting
• Dizziness or light-headedness – this may simply be due to exercise intensity, but if there is an associated risk of falling, cease exercise
• Other reasons to stop exercising include sickness, nausea, vomiting, becoming short of breath or wheezy

Table 25.1 Possible drug side-effects with exercise

Drug	Primary intended use	Possible side-effects with exercise
Cardiovascular drugs		
Beta blockers	↓ HR	Hypotension Greater fatigue HR is not a good indicator of exercise intensity
Digitalis	↑ contraction force of heart	Cardiac arrhythmias, gastrointestinal symptoms, confusion, sedation, and blurred vision with digitalis toxicity
ACE inhibitors	↓ BP	Hypotension
Diuretics	↓ fluid volume	Hypotension Confusion, mood changes, weakness, and fatigue with extreme fluid and electrolyte imbalance
Psychotropic drugs		
Sedative-hypnotic	Improve sleep	Drowsiness, sluggishness
Anti-anxiety	↓ anxiety without sedation	None
Antidepressants	Treat depression	Possible sedation and confusion
Antipsychotics	Normalize behavior and treat mental illness	Possible sedation Possible onset of extrapyramidal symptoms
Drugs for pain and inflammation		
Glucocorticoids	Reduce inflammation	With prolonged use: 1. Ligament or tendon rupture 2. Muscle strain 3. Osteoporotic bone fracture
Non-opiate analgesics (NSAIDs and acetominophen)	Reduce pain and inflammation	Minimal side-effects with exercise
Opiate analgesics	Reduce severe pain	Sedation Mood changes Gastrointestinal problems
Drugs for diabetes		
Insulin or hypoglycemic drugs	Control blood sugar levels	Headaches, dizziness, confusion, sweating, fatigue, or nausea from hypoglycemia

include confusion, mood changes, weakness, and fatigue. In these situations, electrolyte balance should be carefully monitored. ACE inhibitors decrease cardiac workload because they decrease peripheral vascular resistance by interfering with the formation of angiotensin II, a vasoconstrictor. One of the most important side-effects of many drugs used to improve cardiovascular performance is postural hypotension, especially when standing suddenly or initiating exercise.

Psychotropic drugs have been associated with a greater risk of falling in a growing number of studies (Campbell et al 1999, Leipzig et al 1999, Schwab et al 2000). These medications include agents that affect mood, behavior, or cognition and can be described as sedative-hypnotic agents, antianxiety agents, antidepressants, or antipsychotics (Guccione 2000, Leipzig et al 1999, Naranjo et al 1995) (Table 25.1). All of these drugs can alter alertness and perceptions and contribute to an increased risk of falls. In particular, the sedative-hypnotic agents that are often used to treat sleep disorders can be the most dangerous for falling (Guccione 2000). They produce drowsiness and sluggishness in the morning, which can predispose an individual to a greater risk of

falling, especially with exercise. For this reason, individuals taking sedative-hypnotic agents should exercise in the afternoon when they are alert. Antidepressants can also be associated with sedation and even confusion, as can antianxiety and antipsychotic drugs, although not as often (Guccione 2000, Leipzig et al 1999).

Medication for pain and inflammation remains a focal point of research because of the growing number of older adults who are afflicted with arthritis. There are three classes of drugs used to treat pain and inflammation: opioid analgesics, non-opioid analgesics, and glucocorticoids (Fine 2001, Guccione 2000) (Table 25.1). Opioid analgesics are narcotics that are used to treat severe pain (Fine 2001). Adverse side-effects that can affect exercise include sedation, mood changes, and gastrointestinal problems. Non-opioid analgesics include non-steroidal antiinflammatory drugs (NSAIDs) and acetaminophen and do not typically interfere with exercise, but rather, enhance the ability of individuals to carry out an exercise program. The development of a recent class of NSAIDs (cox 2 inhibitors) has vastly decreased the incidence of gastrointestinal problems and increased the safety of long-term use of NSAIDs to treat arthritic pain (Bell &

Schnitzner 2001). Finally, glucocorticoids are steroids that effectively reduce inflammation, but they do so at the expense of catabolic effects on the body. Prolonged use of glucocorticoids contributes to a gradual breakdown of bones, ligaments, tendons, skin, and muscle. This is especially important during exercise because an individual may have a greater risk of rupturing a tendon or ligament, developing a muscle strain, or suffering from an osteoporotic fracture.

Older adults with non-insulin dependent diabetes mellitus (type II) may take hypoglycemic drugs or insulin to control blood sugar levels (Rosenstock 2001) (Table 25.1). Sometimes, these drugs may cause blood glucose levels to drop too much, resulting in hypoglycemia. Warning signs include headaches, dizziness, confusion, fatigue, nausea, and sweating. Hypoglycemia is most likely to manifest itself when older adults increase their activity level or initiate exercise programs without adjusting their medication.

GENERAL EXERCISE GUIDANCE FOR THE OLDER PERSON

In general, exercise-training principles are the same in older and younger athletes (Evans 1999, Mazzeo et al 1998). The most effective training involves structured, goal-directed exercise regimens. It is important to establish why an older person wishes to exercise and what level of exercise they seek to advance towards, in order to design an exercise program to meet their needs. Some older adults may have decided to become active and attend a specific exercise class and others may already be active, but seek to improve their peak physical performance. Other older adults may have participated in athletic activities throughout their lives, but now find it increasingly difficult to maintain their previous level of physical performance. With all older adults, it is important to discuss the importance of strength, balance, and cardiovascular fitness, with evidence for why each is essential for minimizing long-term health problems. Although information should be presented in a way that will not intimidate older adults who may have just begun to think about exercise, follow-up discussions should soon be aimed at increasing the intensity of exercise.

Routinely, older adults underestimate their exercise capacity for fear of injury from excessively increasing the intensity of exercise. Patient education regarding the proven safety of higher-intensity levels of physical activity, after proper warm-up and stretching, is imperative (Fig. 25.2). Warm-up should include a low-intensity activity that slowly increases the HR (Guccione 2000). For example, activities such as walking and swimming should begin with a slower-paced warm-up, with a gradual increase in the intensity of activity during

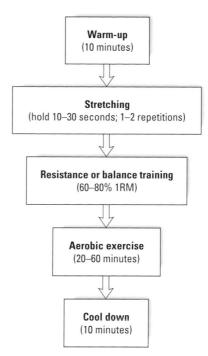

Figure 25.2   Recommended exercise progression.

the first 5–10 min of exercise. Once the tissues and joints have been warmed-up, stretching should be initiated. Stretching should avoid ballistic or jerky movements that can cause injury. Instead, each stretch should be performed to the point of mild discomfort, but not pain, and held for 10–30 s (Pollock et al 1998). Each stretch should be performed at least twice. Older adult athletes may have been able to skip warm-ups and stretching when they were younger, but tissue changes with advancing age necessitate the inclusion of proper warm-up and stretching in order to minimize injury. A cool-down phase at the end of an exercise session is equally important because if one stops exercising suddenly, there may be a sudden drop in blood pressure, or arrhythmia, with dizziness, fainting and a fall (Mazzeo et al 1998).

Many older adults are able to successfully engage in higher-level athletic activities, such as running, tennis, or skiing without significant limitations (Maffulli et al 2001). Many of these individuals have been active all their lives, but now require modification of existing exercise programs to continue to engage in high-level athletic activities. Cross-training is one such modification that offers advantages because it reduces the risk of overuse injury, prevents boredom, and conditions a greater variety of muscles (Guccione 2000). Individuals who have pain with high-level activities, such as running or tennis, may find that swimming offers some relief by minimizing joint impact. A program that alternates between swimming and walking or tennis offers an ideal combination because of the preservation of bone density with weightbearing exercise, while minimizing repeated stress to lower extremity joints (O'Grady et al 2000).

Compliance with exercise programs can be increased by encouraging older adults to join a local fitness center where they can interact with other adults who are engaged in comparable activities. By making exercise a social activity, older adults are much more likely to continue to exercise (Kirkby et al 1999). Alternatively, a spouse or 'exercise buddy' can be equally effective in encouraging compliance with a regular exercise program.

STRENGTH TRAINING PRINCIPLES

A common misconception regarding the intensity of strength training with older adults is that the training intensity should be less than that used for younger adults, especially for frail older adults. In fact, a growing body of literature advocates the use of high-intensity strength training (above 60% of the 1 RM), 3 times a week, for active older adults, as well as frail older adults (Brill et al 1995, Evans 1999, Fiatarone et al 1990) (Box 25.3). Injury with high-intensity strength training is not common, and several studies have demonstrated that high-intensity strength training can be performed safely when adequate warm-up and stretching are incorporated into an exercise program (Brill et al 1995, Evans 1999, Fiatarone et al 1990). Exercise with elastic bands or tubing, light weights, light manual resistance, or against body weight is not likely to result in strength gains for the majority of older adults. For example, asking a healthy older adult to perform a sitting knee extension exercise with a 5 lb cuff weight is not likely to overload the quadriceps muscle sufficiently to promote hypertrophy of the muscle.

With any high-intensity strength training program, some muscle soreness is inevitable (McArdle et al 1994). Patients must be informed that they should expect muscle soreness 24–48 h after exercise, especially when initiating new exercises. Compliance with any exercise program is related to an understanding of what to expect, and unexplained muscle soreness may discourage older adults from complying with their prescribed exercise regimen.

If time does not permit measurement of an individual's 1 RM, a general rule of thumb can be substituted to facilitate adequate overload of muscle: at the end of each set of 8–12 repetitions of an exercise (maintaining proper form), an individual should feel fatigued to the point they cannot perform another repetition (Mazzeo et al 1998). At least 1 min of rest should separate each set of 8–10 repetitions. Ideally, 2 to 3 sets of each exercise should be performed (Fig. 25.3).

ENDURANCE TRAINING PRINCIPLES

Aerobic exercise should follow strength and balance training (Mazzeo et al 1998) and can include activities such as walking, bicycling, swimming, dancing, rowing,

---

Box 25.3 Resistance training exercise guidelines for older adults

Goal:	Increase muscle strength
Frequency:	3 days per week
Intensity:	60–80% of 1 RM[a]
Sets/Repetitions:	3 sets of 8 to 12 repetitions[b]
Rest between sets:	60 s

[a] Weight should produce fatigue by the last repetition in each set. 1 RM is the greatest amount of weight that can be lifted one time with proper form. If an individual's 1 RM was 10 lb with biceps curls, then exercise should be initiated with 6 lb (60% of 1 RM) and progressed to 8 lb within the first week of strength training.

[b] More than 12 repetitions will not increase strength, but rather endurance. If an individual can perform more than 12 repetitions, the weight should be increased if increasing muscle strength is the goal.

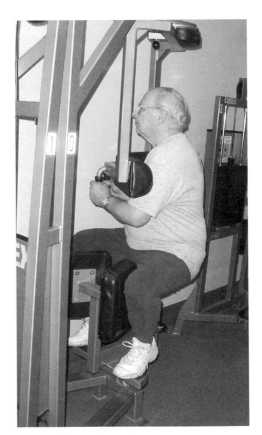

Figure 25.3 High-intensity strength training has been shown to be safe and effective for older adults.

Box 25.4 Aerobic exercise guidelines for older adults

Goal:	Increase cardiovascular fitness
Frequency:	3–5 days per week
Mode:	Walking, cycling, swimming, rowing, dancing
Duration:	20–60 min
Intensity:	55–65% of HR max

Table 25.2 Relationships among methods of quantifying exercise intensity during endurance exercise

Relative intensity			
HR max	VO$_2$ max	Rating of perceived exertion	Classification of intensity
<35%	<30%	<10	Very light
35–59%	30–49%	10–11	Light
60–79%	50–74%	12–13	Somewhat hard
80–89%	75–84%	14–16	Hard
>89%	>84%	>16	Very hard

and playing tennis. Aerobic exercise should be performed 3–5 days per week for 20–60 min each day, at an intensity of 55–65% of the estimated maximum HR (Mazzeo et al 1998) (Box 25.4). This is a level of exercise that should leave an individual slightly out of breath, but still able to carry on a conversation. Another means of quantifying exercise intensity is with a rating of perceived exertion (RPE), which correlates well with exercise HRs and work rates (Guccione 2000) (Table 25.2). The RPE is also known as the Borg scale and it allows individuals to subjectively rate their level of exertion with exercise. It is especially useful for individuals who cannot depend on HR monitoring, secondary to a heart transplant or medications that artificially control HR (Guccione 2000).

BALANCE TRAINING – TAI CHI

In recent years, Tai Chi has been shown to be an effective, low-cost means of improving balance and functional status in older adults (Province et al 1995, Wolf et al 1996). When combined with a strength training program, it offers tremendous benefits for older adults of various levels of physical health (Wolfson et al 1996). Tai Chi is a martial art that developed in China and it combines a series of postures and slow movements with deep breathing and meditation. It has been shown to improve balance, to lower blood pressure, and to give older adults an overall sense of wellbeing (Mazzeo et al 1998). A study conducted by Wolf et al (1996) found that older people taking part in a 15-week Tai Chi program reduced their risk of multiple falls by 47.5%. Subjects also had a

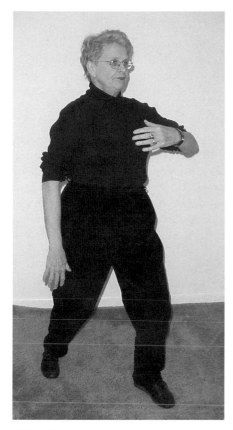

Figure 25.4 Tai Chi has become an increasingly popular form of balance training for older adults.

reduction in their fear of falling with Tai Chi (Wolf et al 1996).

Tai Chi conditions individuals to move more slowly through an enhanced body awareness, which is one of the biggest reasons why it may successfully reduce fall risk in older adults (Fig. 25.4). The movements of Tai Chi are less jarring than those of a low-impact exercise class, so patients with arthritis may benefit tremendously from Tai Chi. Tai Chi classes can be found at health clubs, martial arts schools, hospitals, and community centers. Video instruction is also available, but hands-on instruction is invaluable for maximizing the potential of Tai Chi.

EXERCISE AND CHRONIC ILLNESS

Patients with chronic illness often avoid exercise for fear of making their condition worse or overexerting themselves, yet these patients are the ones that stand to benefit most from a regular exercise program. Chronic illness is not a contraindication to exercise when adequate attention is provided for the medical management of each medical condition in response to exercise (Mazzeo et al 1998).

CARDIAC DISEASE

Exercise is not contraindicated in cardiac disease, but rather, exercise is an integral part of both primary and secondary prevention of future cardiac problems (Ades 1999, Lavie & Milani 1996). Patients with a previous myocardial infarction, cardiac failure, valve disease, irregular heart rhythm, or angina can benefit from exercise (Ades 1999, Lavie & Milani 1996). The decision to exercise is often precipitated by a cardiac event. Most patients now undergo an exercise stress test before they leave the hospital, following a myocardial infarction, and are given guidance on the appropriate level of exercise. Many hospitals have exercise classes as part of their cardiac rehabilitation programs where the focus is on low-intensity mobility exercises, progressing to more intense endurance type activity.

Exercise intensity may be restricted by angina, but those with angina may exercise within the limits of their symptoms (DeGroot et al 1998). For some, this may mean walking only short distances on level ground, but most individuals should be able to engage in regular exercise. Antiangina medication, usually in the form of a spray or sublingual medication, should be used in advance of exercise and patients should carry their medication with them while exercising.

HYPERTENSION

Aerobic and resistance training are not only safe for individuals with high blood pressure, they also help reduce resting systolic and diastolic blood pressure (Dickey & Janick 2001, Ehsani 2001, Hurley & Roth 2000). Although some health professionals are reluctant to prescribe resistance training for individuals with elevated blood pressure, when a proper technique is used, strength training does not result in substantial increases in systolic blood pressure (Evans 1999). In particular, patients should be cautioned not to hold their breath during any phase of weight-training. Patients should be instructed to inhale before lifting a weight, exhale when lifting the weight, and inhale as they lower the weight (Evans 1999). Even moderate aerobic activity that helps to control blood pressure can be an important part of medical management of hypertension (Ehsani 2001, Hurley & Roth 2000).

DIABETES MELLITUS

Exercise is particularly indicated for the medical management of non-insulin dependent diabetes mellitus because exercise can increase insulin sensitivity and improve glucose tolerance (Katz & Lowenthal 1994). Diabetic patients initiating an exercise program should pay particular attention to their glucose balance because exercise increases the utilization of glucose (Rosenstock 2001). If an individual with diabetes exercises without understanding the need to increase glucose intake, or reduce insulin, they may experience hypoglycemia (Rosenstock 2001). Patients who inject insulin should be especially careful about injection sites. If they inject insulin into a muscle, blood flow will increase with exercise, giving more rapid insulin absorption and hypoglycemia.

Foot care is also very important in diabetic patients who exercise (Springett 2000). If there is neurological impairment, there may be some loss of sensation in the feet so that patients may be unaware of blisters, or skin irritation and cause damage to their feet. There may be impairment of the circulation to both large blood vessels and, more importantly, the microcirculation which inhibits tissue repair and recovery (Rosenstock 2001). Prevention is essential, so it is very important that all diabetic patients are educated regarding proper monitoring of feet for signs of irritation or skin breakdown.

ARTHRITIS

There is growing evidence that patients with osteoarthritis can achieve the same health benefits with exercise as healthy, older adults (Mazzeo et al 1998, O'Grady et al 2000), yet patients with advanced osteoarthritis should seek medical advice before initiating an unsupervised exercise program. Many older adults with osteoarthritis are afraid to exercise for fear of exacerbating their arthritis, yet randomized clinical trials have found that exercise training does not exacerbate pain or accelerate disease progression (American Geriatrics Society Panel on Exercise and Osteoarthritis 2001). In fact, exercise improves mobility, reduces pain, and improves function in patients with arthritis (Fisher et al 1991). Although exercise may not actually slow the pathological disease process of osteoarthritis, many benefits are still conferred with exercise in arthritic patients (O'Grady et al 2000). Exercise may increase muscle strength and decrease the stress at arthritic joints, which may explain the decreased arthritic pain and improved function in arthritic patients who initiate an exercise program. In addition, weight loss from regular exercise also decreases the stress at lower extremity joints afflicted with arthritis. Of course, the same general health benefits of exercise seen in healthy, older adults are also conferred to patients with arthritis.

An exercise program for patients with osteoarthritis should emphasize options that minimize excessive compression of arthritic joints, while promoting strength gains and endurance (O'Grady et al 2000). Such activities include, but are not limited to, bicycling, swimming, dance, water aerobics, walking, Tai Chi, and rowing. Cross-training is advocated in any older adult population, but in particular, patients with arthritis benefit the most from alternating different forms of exercise in order to vary the compressive forces across their joints. The intensity and mode of exercise should be determined by how much pain they feel with the activity.

Exercise prescription for resistance training requires creativity for patients with arthritis. Patients with arthritis may not be able to perform resistance training at the same intensities as non-arthritic patients, if severe joint pain limits them, but every attempt should be made to experiment with various resistance exercises to find those that allow patients to maximize their strength gains (O'Grady et al 2000). For example, patients may have knee pain with a closed chain, leg press activity performed at 60% of their 1 RM, but when they perform an open chain sitting knee extension exercise, they may be able to surpass 60% of their 1 RM and achieve higher training intensities. Alternatively, patients may be able to perform exercises pain-free throughout their entire range of motion, but strength gains can still be achieved with exercise through partial ranges of motion (Evans 1999).

Patient education is essential for compliance with any long-term exercise program (O'Grady et al 2000). Patients with arthritis should be aware that physical performance and arthritic symptoms may vary from day to day. They should also understand that the warning signs for excessive exercise include joint pain for more than 1–2 h after exercise, swelling, and excessive fatigue. Patients should limit their exercise if their joints become acutely inflamed, until the inflammation returns to baseline. Exercise may be most comfortable in the afternoon, as morning stiffness and pain are common features of osteoarthritis.

In addition to resistance and aerobic exercise, arthritic patients should understand the importance of stretching and joint mobilization to maintain their range of motion, since the persistent joint swelling and stiffness that accompany arthritis can lead to a progressive loss of joint range of motion (O'Grady et al 2000). Treatment aimed at restoring joint range of motion should begin in conjunction with resistance and aerobic exercise programs.

PERIPHERAL VASCULAR DISEASE

Exercise has been shown to be of value in people with peripheral vascular disease (Ciaccia 1993, Tan et al 2000). Long-standing atherosclerosis may result in narrowing of the main arteries, and in particular those providing blood supply to the lower limbs. When exercise raises the oxygen needs of the muscle, but the arteries are unable to supply sufficient oxygen-rich blood, muscles become painful. With rest, the muscles recover. This occurs most often in the calf muscles and can cause problems when someone undertakes an exercise program (Creager 2001). Evidence exists that exercise itself can help in this condition (Tan et al 2000). With exercise there may be minor changes in the blood vessels, but more importantly, the muscles become more efficient and patients can tolerate a greater level of exercise (Tan et al 2000). Those with peripheral vascular disease are encouraged to exercise but within the level of comfort. For example, it is better to walk slowly for a longer distance than to set off too fast and have to stop because of muscle pain.

OSTEOPOROSIS

Older women should be especially aware of the risks associated with osteoporosis (see Chs 5 and 26). Depending on the severity of the osteoporosis, many individuals with osteoporosis can still engage in high-intensity strength training. Extreme care must be taken to perform all exercises with proper postural alignment to minimize the risk of fractures. In particular, individuals should avoid exercises that put excess pressure on the spine (Hertel & Trahiotis 2001). Some individuals may have such severe osteoporosis that even daily activities put them at risk for fracture, which makes strength training contraindicated with severe osteoporosis.

Weightbearing exercise plays an important role in increasing bone mass. Even brisk walking for 30 min a day, 3 times a week, has been found to increase bone density in older women (Hatori et al 1993). Other studies have shown that combining strength training and aerobic exercise also increases bone density in older women (Chow et al 1987).

SUMMARY

Exercise mitigates the physical deterioration that occurs with increasing age, yet many older adults engage in little to no physical activity. As a growing proportion of our population consists of older adults, more attention must be directed towards encouraging older adults to exercise regularly to prevent many health-related problems.

Exercise programs must combine strength, endurance, and balance training to optimally protect older adults from developing functional deficits. A common misconception is that exercise interventions for older adults should be performed at lower intensities. Until recently, high-intensity strength training was often avoided, for fear of injury. Now, research indicates it is one of the most important parts of an exercise program. Numerous studies have safely carried out high-intensity strength training programs with even the oldest of adults, and have produced substantial strength gains. Not only does strength training improve muscle strength, it also decreases risk of falling and improves functional performance.

Exercise is one of the most effective ways to reduce the chances of falling, which is a major cause of morbidity in older adults. Exercise that improves balance and coordination (e.g. Tai Chi) has received increasing popularity, as increasing evidence indicates that the health benefits from Tai Chi are numerous. Although more recent attention has been focused on strength and balance training, the cardiovascular benefits of regular aerobic exercise cannot be overlooked.

Older adults with chronic medical conditions often avoid exercise, yet these adults are the most likely to benefit from a regular exercise program. Health professionals must educate all older adults regarding the importance of exercise and attempt to counter the perception that certain patient populations should avoid exercise.

REFERENCES

Ades P A 1999 Introduction – the elderly in cardiac rehabilitation. American Journal of Geriatric Cardiology 8(2):61–62

Allegrante J P, MacKenzie C R, Robbins L et al 1991 Hip fracture in older persons. Does self-efficacy-based intervention have a role in rehabilitation? Arthritis Care and Research 4(1):39–47

Allied Dunbar National Fitness Survey 1992 Activity and Health Research. Health Education Authority and The Sports Council, London

American College of Sports Medicine 1995 ACSM position stand on osteoporosis and exercise. Medicine and Science in Sports and Exercise 27(4):i–vii

American Geriatrics Society Panel on Exercise and Osteoarthritis 2001 Exercise prescription for older adults with osteoarthritis pain: consensus practice recommendations. A supplement to the AGS Clinical Practice Guidelines on the management of chronic pain in older adults. Journal of the American Geriatric Society 49(6):808–823

Ashworth J B, Reuben D V, Benton L A 1994 Functional profiles of healthy elder persons. Age and Ageing 23:34

Astrand P-O, Rodahl K 1977 Textbook of work physiology. McGraw Hill, New York

Bauman A, Owen N 1991 Habitual physical activity and cardiovascular risk factors. Medical Journal of Australia 154(1):22–28

Bell G M, Schnitzer T J 2001 Cox-2 inhibitors and other nonsteroidal anti-inflammatory drugs in the treatment of pain in the elderly. Clinics in Geriatric Medicine 17(3):489–502

Bloem B R, Boers I, Cramer M et al 2001 Falls in the elderly. I. Identification of risk factors. Wiener Klinische Wochenschrift 113(10):352–362

Booth M L, Owen N, Bauman A et al 2000 Social-cognitive and perceived environment influences associated with physical activity in older Australians. Preventive Medicine 31(1):15–22

Borghouts L B, Keizer H A 2000 Exercise and insulin sensitivity: a review. International Journal of Sports Medicine 21(1):1–12.

Bouvier F, Saltin B, Nejat M et al 2001 Left ventricular function and perfusion in elderly endurance athletes. Medicine and Science in Sports and Exercise 33(5):735–740

Brill P A, Drimmer A M, Morgan L A et al 1995 The feasibility of conducting strength and flexibility programs for elderly nursing home residents with dementia. Gerontologist 35(2):263–266

Brooks S V, Larsson L, Woledge R et al 1994 Impairments in the structure and function of skeletal muscle with aging. Medicine and Science in Sports and Exercise 26:s27

Brukner P, Khan K 2001 Clinical sports medicine, 2nd edn. McGraw Hill, Sydney, p 702–703

Buckwalter J A 1997 Maintaining and restoring mobility in middle and old age: the importance of the soft tissues. Instructional Course Lectures 46:459–469

Butler R N, Davis R, Lewis C B et al 1998 Physical fitness: benefits of exercise for the older patient. 2. Geriatrics 53(10):46, 49–52, 61–62

Campbell A J, Robertson M C, Gardner M M et al 1997 Randomised controlled trial of a general practice program of home based exercise to prevent falls in elderly women. British Medical Journal 315:1065–1069

Campbell A J, Robertson M C, Gardner M M et al 1999 Psychotropic medication withdrawal and a home-based exercise program to prevent falls: a randomised controlled trial. Journal of the American Geriatric Society 47(7):850–853

Chandler J M, Duncan P W, Kochersberger G et al 1998 Is lower extremity strength gain associated with improvement in physical performance and disability in frail, community-dwelling elders? Archives of Physical Medicine and Rehabilitation 79:24–30

Chow R, Harrison J E, Notarius C 1987 Effect of two randomized exercise programs on bone mass of healthy postmenopausal women. British Medical Journal 295:1441–1444

Ciaccia J M 1993 Benefits of a structured peripheral arterial vascular rehabilitation program. Journal of Vascular Nursing 11(1):1–4

Connelly D M, Rice C L, Roos M R et al 1999 Motor unit firing rates and contractile properties in tibialis anterior of young and old men. Journal of Applied Physiology 87(2):843–852

Creager M A 2001 Medical management of peripheral arterial disease. Cardiology in Review 9(4):238–245

DeGroot D W, Quinn T J, Kertzer R et al 1998 Circuit weight training in cardiac patients: determining optimal workloads for safety and energy expenditure. Journal of Cardiopulmonary Rehabilitation 18(2):145–152

Dickey R A, Janick J J 2001 Lifestyle modifications in the prevention and treatment of hypertension. Endocrine Practice 7(5):392–399

Ehsani A A 2001 Exercise in patients with hypertension. American Journal of Geriatric Cardiology 10(5):253–259, 273

Elward K, Larson E B 1992 Benefits of exercise for older adults: a review of existing evidence and current recommendations for the general population. Clinics in Geriatric Medicine 8:35–50

Evans W J 1995 What is sarcopenia? Journal of Gerontology SOA (Special issue): S8

Evans W J 1999 Exercise training guidelines for the elderly. Medicine and Science in Sports and Exercise 31(1):12–17

Evans A, Meredith B 1989 Exercise and nutrition in the elderly. In: Munro H N, Danford D E (eds) Nutrition, aging and the elderly. Plenum Press, New York

Felson D T, Lawrence R C, Dieppe P A et al 2000 Osteoarthristis: new insights. Part 1: the disease and its risk factors. Annals of Internal Medicine 133(8):635–646

Fiatarone M A, Marks E C, Ryan N D et al 1990 High intensity strength training in nonagenarians: effects on skeletal muscle. Journal of the American Medical Association 263(22):3029–3034

Fiatarone M A, O'Neill E F, Ryan N D et al 1994 Exercise training and nutritional supplementation for physical frailty in very elderly people. New England Journal of Medicine 330:1769–1775

Fine P G 2001 Opioid analgesic drugs in older people. Clinics in Geriatric Medicine 7(3):479–487

Fisher N M, Pendergast D R, Gresham G E et al 1991 Muscle rehabilitation: its effect of muscular and functional performance of patients with knee osteoarthritis. Archives of Physical Medicine and Rehabilitation 72(6):367–374

Fries J P 1998 Reducing cumulative lifetime disability: the compression of morbidity. British Journal of Sports Medicine 32(3):193

Gill T M, Williams C S, Tinetti M E 1995 Assessing risk for the onset of functional dependence among older adults: the role of physical performance. Journal of the American Geriatric Society 43:603–609

Gregg E W, Pereira M A, Caspersen C J 2000 Physical activity, falls, and fractures among older adults: a review of the epidemiologic evidence. Journal of the American Geriatric Society 48(8):883–893

Guccione A A 2000 Geriatric physical therapy, 2nd edn. Mosby, St. Louis

Hatori M, Hasegawa A, Adachi H et al 1993 The effects of walking at the anaerobic threshold level on vertebral bone loss in postmenopausal women. Calcified Tissue International 52:411–414

Hertel K L, Trahiotis M G 2001 Exercise in the prevention and treatment of osteoporosis. Nursing Clinics of North America 36(3):441–453

Holloszy J O, Kohrt W M 1995 Exercise. In: Masoro E J (ed) Handbook of physiology – aging. University Press, Oxford

Hurley B F, Roth S 2000 Strength training in the elderly: effects of risk factors for age-related diseases. Sports Medicine 30(4):249–268

Katz M S, Lowenthal D T 1994 Influences of age and exercise on glucose metabolism: implications for management of older diabetics. Southern Medical Journal 87(5):S70–73.

Kirkby R J, Kolt G S, Habel K et al 1999 Exercise in older women: motives for participation. Australian Psychologist 34(2):122–127

Kohrt W M, Malley M T, Coggan A R et al 1991 Effects of gender, age, and fitness level on response of VO$_2$max to training in 60–71 year olds. Journal of Applied Physiology 71(5):2004–2011

Lavie C J, Milani R V 1996 Effects of nonpharmacologic therapy with cardiac rehabilitation and exercise training in patients with low levels of high-density lipoprotein cholesterol. American Journal of Cardiology 78(11):1286–1289

Leipzig R M, Cumming R G, Tinetti M E 1999 Drugs and falls in older people: a systematic review and meta-analysis: I. Psychotropic drugs. Journal of the American Geriatric Society 47:30–39

Lexell J 1995 Human aging, muscle mass, and fiber type composition. Journal of Gerontology. Series A 50A (special issue):11–16

MacAuley D, McCrum E E, Stott G et al 1994 The Northern Ireland Health and Activity Survey. Her Majesty's Stationery Office, London

McArdle W D, Katch F I, Katch V L 1994 Essentials of exercise physiology. Lea and Febiger, Philadelphia, PA

Maffulli N, Chan K M, Macdonald R et al 2001 Sports medicine for specific ages and abilities. Churchill Livingstone, Edinburgh

Mazzeo R S, Cavanagh P, Evans W J et al 1998 American College of Sports Medicine Position Stand: exercise and physical activity for older adults. Medicine and Science in Sports and Exercise 30(6):992–1008

Medical Research Council 1994 The Health of the UK's elderly people. Medical Research Council, London

Menard D 1996 The aging athlete. In: Harries M, Williams C, Stanish W D et al Oxford textbook of sports medicine. Oxford University Press, Oxford

Metter E J, Lynch N, Conwit R et al 1999 Muscle quality and age: cross-sectional and longitudinal comparisons. The Journals of Gerontology. Series A, Biological Sciences and Medical Sciences 54(5):B207–218

Nadel E R, DiPietro L 1995 Effects of physical activity on functional ability in older people: translating basic science findings into practical knowledge. Medicine and Science in Sports and Exercise 25:s36

Naranjo C A, Herrmann N, Mittmann N et al 1995 Recent advances in geriatric psychopharmacology. Drugs and Aging 7(3):184–202

Nolan L, O'Malley K 1988 Prescribing for the elderly. Part I: sensitivity of the elderly to adverse drug reactions. Journal of the American Geriatric Society 36(2):142–149

O'Grady M, Fletcher J, Ortiz S 2000 Therapeutic and physical fitness exercise prescription for older adults with joint disease. Rheumatic Disease Clinics of North America 26(3):617–646

O'Loughlin J L, Robitaille Y, Boivin J F et al 1993 Incidence and risk factors for falls and injurious falls among the community dwelling elderly. American Journal of Epidemiology 137:342–354

Owen N, Bauman A 1992 The descriptive epidemiology of a sedentary lifestyle in adult Australians. International Journal of Epidemiology 21(2):305–310

Pollock M L, Gaesser G A, Butcher J D et al 1998 The recommended quantity and quality of exercise for developing and maintaining cardiorespiratory and muscular fitness, and flexibility in healthy adults. Medicine and Science in Sports and Exercise 30(6):975–991

Porter M M, Vandervoort A A, Lexell J 1995 Aging of human muscle: structure, function and adaptability. Scandinavian Journal of Medicine and Science in Sports 5:129–142

Province M A, Hadley E C, Hornbrook M C et al 1995 The effects of exercise on falls in elderly patients. A pre planned meta-analysis of the FICSIT trials. Journal of the American Medical Association 273(17):1341–1347

Puisieux F, Bulckaen H, Fauchais A L et al 2000 Ambulatory blood pressure monitoring and postprandial hypotension in elderly persons with falls or syncopes. The Journals of Gerontology. Series A, Biological Sciences and Medical Sciences 55(9):M535–540

Rose S, Maffulli N 1999 Hip fractures. An epidemiological review. Bulletin (Hospital for Joint Diseases) 58(4):197–201

Rosenstock J 2001 Management of type 2 diabetes mellitus in the elderly: special considerations. Drugs and Aging 18(1):31–44

Ryan A S 2000 Insulin resistance with aging: effects of diet and exercise. Sports Medicine 30(5):327–346

Schwab M, Roder F, Aleker T et al 2000 Psychotropic drug use, falls and hip fracture in the elderly. Aging (Milano) 12(3):234–239

Siris E S, Miller P D, Barrett-Connor E et al 2001 Identification and fracture outcomes of undiagnosed low bone mineral density in postmenopausal women: results from the national osteoporosis risk assessment. Journal of the American Medical Association. 286(22):2815–2822

Springett K 2000 Foot ulceration in diabetic patients. Nursing Standard 14(26):65–68,70–71

Stackhouse S K, Stevens J E, Pearce K M et al 2001 Maximum voluntary activation in fresh and fatigued muscle of young and elder individuals. Physical Therapy 81(5):1102–1109

Stevens J E, Binder-Macleod S, Snyder-Mackler L 2001 Characterization of the human quadriceps muscle in active elders. Archives of Physical Medicine and Rehabilitation. 82(7):973–978

Studenski S A, Duncan P W, Chandler J M 1991 Postural responses and effector factors in persons with unexplained falls: results and methodologic issues. Journal of the American Geriatric Society 39:229–234

Tan K H, De Cossart L, Edwards P R 2000 Exercise training and peripheral vascular disease. British Journal of Surgery 87(5):553–562

Tinetti M E, Baker D I, McAvay G et al 1994 A multifactorial intervention to reduce the risk of falling among elderly people living in the community. New England Journal of Medicine 331:821–827

Tipton C M, Mathes R D, Maynard J A et al 1975 The influence of physical activity on ligaments and tendons. Medicine and Science in Sports and Exercise 7:165–175

Tsujimoto G, Hashimoto K, Hoffman B B 1989 Pharmacokinetic and pharmacodynamic principles of drug therapy in old age. International Journal of Clinical Pharmacology, Therapy, and Toxicology 27(1):13–26

Tsutsumi T, Don B M, Zaichkowsky L D et al 1997 Physical fitness and psychological benefits of strength training in community dwelling older adults. Applied Human Science 16(6):257–266

Uitto J 1986 Connective tissue biochemistry of the aging dermis. Age-related alterations in collagen and elastin. Dermatologic Clinics 4(3):433–446

Vandervoort M, McComas A J 1986 Contractile changes in opposing muscles of the human ankle joint with aging. Journal of Applied Physiology 61:361–367

Verdu E, Ceballos D, Vilches J J et al 2000 Influence of aging on peripheral nerve function and regeneration. Journal of the Peripheral Nervous System 5(4):191–208

Vita A J, Terry R B, Hubert H B et al 1998 Aging, health risks and cumulative disability. New England Journal of Medicine 338(15):1035–1041

Wagner E H 1997 The effect of strength and endurance training on gait, balance, fall risk and health services use in community living adults. Journal of Gerontology 52(4):M218–224

Whipple R, Wolfson L, Amerman P 1987 The relationship of knee and ankle weakness to falls in nursing home residents. An isokinetic study. Journal of the American Geriatric Society 35:13–20

Wolf S L, Barnhart H X, Kutner N G et al 1996 Reducing frailty and falls in older persons: an investigation of Tai Chi and computerized balance training. Atlanta FICSIT Group. Frailty and Injuries: Cooperative Studies of Intervention Techniques. Journal of the American Geriatric Society 44(5):489–497

Wolfson L, Whipple R, Derby C 1996 Balance and strength training in older adults: intervention gains and Tai Chi maintenance. Journal of the American Geriatric Society 44:498–506

World Health Organization 1994 Assessment of fracture risk and its application to screening for osteoporosis. Technical Services Report 843. World Health Organization, Geneva

26

The active female

Amanda Weiss

INTRODUCTION

The role of women in sport has changed dramatically over the last century. Forbidden from participation in the first modern Olympic Games in 1896, women made up 42% of the competitors at the 2000 Games in Sydney, and, for the first time in Olympic history, women competed in the same number of team sports as did their male counterparts.

Historically, women were discouraged from participation in physical activity for fear that exertion would harm the reproductive system and because it was not felt to be feminine (Lutter 1994).

More recently, the growing realization of the significant health and social benefits that sport and exercise has for girls and women has led physicians, physical therapists, and parents to encourage girls to participate in sports. Girls who play sport are less likely to become pregnant during their adolescent years, smoke, or experience depression than their non-athletic counterparts (Aaron et al 1996, Colton & Gore 1991, Women's Sports Foundation Report 1998). Furthermore, females involved in sports participation are more likely to graduate from high school and college (NCAA 1997, Wilson Report 1989).

As the number of girls and women participating in sport rises, it becomes increasingly important to understand the health effects and benefits that exercise has for women (Fig. 26.1).

ANATOMICAL AND PHYSIOLOGICAL CONSIDERATIONS FOR ATHLETIC WOMEN

HEIGHT AND WEIGHT

Females are, in general, both shorter and lighter than males. For example, mature women are 13 cm shorter

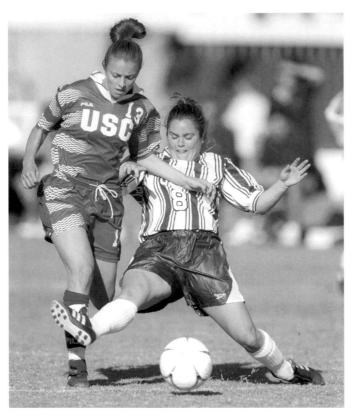

Figure 26.1 Female soccer players. (Reproduced with the permission of UCLA Athletic Department.)

and 18–22 kg lighter than men (Ebben & Jensen 1998). Women also have a larger surface area to mass ratio than men (Wells 1985). When exercising in a warm dry environment, this may offer an advantage for women; however, it may also allow for increased heat loss during exercise in a cold environment (Sanborn & Jankowski 1994).

BODY COMPOSITION

On average, women have 8–10% more body fat than men (Sanborn & Jankowski 1994). This higher proportion of body fat could be disadvantageous for women during weightbearing activities (O'Toole & Douglas 1994). Excess fat increases the energy cost of activities like running, cycling and cross-country skiing (Fahey 1994). Contrary to this, however, increased body fat can enhance swimming performance since it adds buoyancy that raises female swimmers out of the water and decreases drag (Mirkin 1994, Sanborn & Jankowski 1994).

MUSCLE TISSUE

Until the onset of puberty, girls exhibit about 90% of the muscular strength of boys. By the age of 15–16 years, girls

have 75% of the strength of boys and mature women have about 67% of the strength of men (Beim & Stone 1995, Komi 1992, Sanborn & Jankowski 1994). These strength differences are more pronounced for upper body strength than lower body strength (Stone et al 2001, Wells 1985). Despite these strength differences, the muscle composition of men and women is similar, with each having the same relative proportion of fast and slow twitch fibers (Cureton et al 1988).

With resistance training, women have similar relative gains in strength to men (Cureton et al 1988). Strength training can offer significant health and performance benefits for women. For example, when added to aerobic training activities, resistance training has been shown to improve aerobic capacity beyond that found with aerobic training alone (Kraemer et al 2001). This combination of activities can also decrease the percentage of body fat and improve work economy, both of which may enhance performance (Ebben & Jensen 1998, Hoff et al 1999, Stone et al 2001, Wilmore 1983). Since connective tissue strength is enhanced with resistance training, such exercise could help prevent injury during other activities (Ebben & Jensen 1998, Fleck & Falkel 1986, Lehnhard et al 1996, Stone et al 2001). Resistance training can also lead to increased bone density at the sites of mechanical loading, improving overall bone health (Ayalon et al 1987, Ebben & Jensen 1998, Marcus et al 1992, Snow-Harter et al 1992). Improvements in strength have been shown to reduce the physiological stresses encountered during daily activities that require strength, allowing trained women to perform such activities more easily (Ebben & Jensen 1998, Stone et al 2001). Finally, aside from physiological changes, women who participate in strength training have also reported an improvement in self-esteem and confidence (Ebben & Jensen 1998).

Investigators have also demonstrated that women tend to demonstrate less muscle tightness than men. There is significant disagreement in the literature, however, about whether or not this increased flexibility can help prevent injury. A recent review of 18 studies found that strong evidence was lacking to support the idea that injury rate is influenced by degree of flexibility in athletes.

AEROBIC PERFORMANCE

Maximal aerobic power is measured as VO_2max. VO_2max is considered to be the best measure of an athlete's cardiovascular fitness (Wells 1985). Before puberty, boys and girls have similar VO_2max. After puberty, however, women have 40–60% lower VO_2max than men (Eisenmann et al 2001, Sparling 1980). When VO_2max is expressed relative to body mass, the difference is decreased to 20–30% (Eisenmann et al 2001, Sparling 1980). Furthermore, when VO_2max is expressed relative to fat free mass, the difference is reduced to only 8–10% (Sady & Freedson 1984). Thus, body composition (specifically the amount of fat-free mass) is important in explaining much of the difference in VO$_2$max between genders. This means that the higher fat content of females will place them at a disadvantage in weightbearing aerobic activities where VO$_2$max plays an important role in performance (Berg 1984). In an early study, Cureton & Sparling (1980) simulated the effect of the increased body fat load with which women exercise by having a group of men exercise with external weights. This decreased the men's VO$_2$max and the differences in VO$_2$max between men and women were reduced to insignificant levels. This further illustrates the importance that the increased body fat found in women plays in the maximal aerobic power attainable by female athletes.

Differences in oxygen transport and oxygen carrying capacity also help to explain the gender difference in VO$_2$max. Cardiac output, stroke volume, blood volume, hemoglobin and hematocrit all contribute to an individual's ability to transport oxygen to the body. Women have both smaller heart and stroke volumes than men, resulting in lower maximal cardiac outputs (Sanborn & Jankowski 1994). Women also have lower blood volumes and concentrations of hemoglobin and hematocrit than men, which limits their oxygen carrying capacity (Green et al 1999, Sanborn & Jankowski 1994, Wiebe et al 1998).

ANAEROBIC POWER

Anaerobic activities are those performed at a high intensity for a short duration. Lactic acid is produced during the anaerobic breakdown of glucose and glycogen (Wells 1985). Lactic acid concentrations reflect the degree of anaerobic metabolism occurring (Nattiv 2001). The concentrations of lactic acid found in the blood during anaerobic activities are determined by lactic acid production from anaerobic breakdown of glucose and glycogen, and lactic acid removal from oxidation (Wells 1985). The lactate threshold is defined as the level of exercise needed to produce blood lactate levels above 4 mM (Wells 1985). Exercise beyond the lactate threshold is difficult, secondary to fatigue (Wells 1985).

In females, the lactate threshold is reached at a lower absolute workload than in males (Helgerud 1994, Wells 1985). These differences in lactate threshold between men and women, however, are insignificant when expressed as a percentage of VO$_2$max (Helgerud 1994, Wells 1985). Also, when comparing well-trained athletes, there is less absolute difference in anaerobic threshold between men and women. Thus, the difference in anaerobic threshold between men and women is less than initially believed (Serresse et al 1989).

HEAT TOLERANCE

The findings of several investigations suggested that women were less tolerant of heat stress than men (Shephard 2000, Wells 1985). However, in these studies, the female subjects were not as physically fit as the males (Griffin 1994, Wells 1985). When men and women exercise at the same relative intensity, it has been shown that they tolerate heat equally well (Stephenson & Kolka 1993, Wells 1985). In temperatures higher than body temperature, women may be at a small disadvantage compared to men, since their higher surface to mass ratio will allow women to gain heat by convection faster than men (Shephard 2000, Wells 1985).

The more current literature indicates that level of fitness and acclimatization are more important than gender in terms of heat tolerance (Shephard 2000, Wells 1985). Women acclimatize to exercise in warm environments as well as men (Nunneley 1979).

SKELETAL CONSIDERATIONS

Women have a different lower extremity alignment to men. For example, their wider pelvis and increased femoral anteversion result in higher Q angles in women. Although increased Q angles have been implicated as a predisposing factor for patellofemoral pain, a clear consensus on the importance of the Q angle in patellofemoral pain has not been established (Baker & Juhn 2000). The role of the Q angle has been questioned because Q angle values have not been found to vary significantly between symptomatic and asymptomatic subjects. Also, there are wide variations in Q angles with significant overlap between values found in men and women (Baker & Juhn 2000). See Chapter 21 for a complete discussion of patellofemoral pain.

Women have also been found to have a narrower femoral notch, increased genu valgum and external tibial torsion compared to men (Ireland 1994) (Fig. 26.2). The importance of these factors in terms of predisposition to injury, however, has not been established.

ORAL CONTRACEPTIVE USE AND PERFORMANCE

Athletes often choose to use oral contraceptive pills (OCP) to prevent pregnancy, regulate menstrual cycles, or decrease premenstrual symptoms. Since use by athletes is rising, interest in the potential effect of OCP on performance has increased (Bennell et al 1999).

Some beneficial effects have been noted. Since OCP use can decrease menstrual blood loss significantly, the risk of iron deficiency anemia is decreased for women using

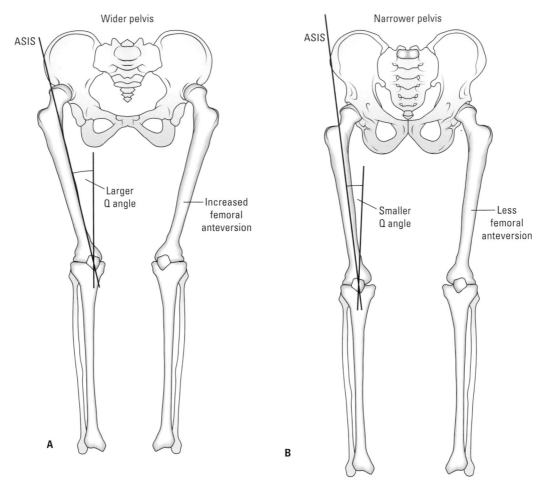

Figure 26.2A&B Women (**A**) have a different lower extremity alignment from men (**B**). A wider pelvis and increased femoral anteversion result in increased Q angles in women compared with men.

OCP (Bennell et al 1999). As iron deficiency anemia, and possibly even decreased iron stores, have been shown to adversely affect performance, this is an important benefit (Friedmann et al 2001, Hinton et al 2000, Nattiv 2001). Also, the OCP allows athletes to manipulate their menstrual cycle around competition.

Some investigators have found that OCP use has negative effects on VO_2max. Daggett et al (1983) found an 11% decrease in VO_2max with OCP use. After discontinuation of OCP, VO_2max returned to previous levels. In a prospective study of trained women, Notelovitz et al (1987) found a 7% decrease in VO_2max in the group using OCP, while controls demonstrated a slight increase in VO_2max over the study period. Again, VO_2max returned to normal with discontinuation of the OCP.

Other investigators have failed to demonstrate any change in VO_2max with OCP use. Bryner et al (1996) investigated 10 women randomly assigned to low dose OCP or placebo and found no difference in VO_2max, endurance or performance on a maximal treadmill test between the groups. Another study compared women taking low dose OCP with women taking placebo and found that, despite a small decrease in VO_2max in the OCP group, no differences in aerobic endurance or anaerobic capacity were evident (Frankovich & Lebrun 2000). Thus, the effects of OCP use on VO_2max and aerobic performance are not clear.

In one study on anaerobic performance and OCP use, no difference was found in maximal anaerobic performance between women using monophasic OCP and eumenorrheic women not using OCP (Giacomoni et al 2000).

MENSTRUAL CYCLE PHASE AND PERFORMANCE

The potential effects that the cyclical endogenous hormonal variations associated with the menstrual cycle may have on performance have been a topic of great interest for female athletes. The increased level of progesterone during the luteal phase of the menstrual cycle has been associated with increased minute ventilation at rest and with increased hypoxic and hypercapnic respiratory drives (Dombovy et al 1987, Jurkowski et al 1978). This has led to speculation that performance may be decreased during the luteal phase (Dombovy et al 1987).

Some investigators have found changes in athletic performance with different menstrual phases. Nicklas et al (1989) and Jurkowski et al (1978) studied trained women and found small but significant improvements in endurance during the luteal phase. Contrary to this, Williams & Krahenbuhl (1997) found that running economy during the luteal phase was decreased at 85% VO_2max, but not at 55% VO_2max. Lebrun et al (1995) found a small, statistically insignificant, decrease in VO_2max during the luteal phase. No significant differences in aerobic endurance or maximum minute ventilation were noted, despite the change in VO_2max. Furthermore, Schoene et al (1981) found that untrained women had significant decreases in maximal exercise performance during the luteal phase.

Many other investigators have failed to demonstrate any difference in performance during the phases of the menstrual cycle. In a study of eight untrained women, Dombovy et al (1987) failed to demonstrate any difference in VO_2max, perceived exertion, or maximal workload during the luteal or follicular phase. De Souza et al (1990) included amenorrheic and eumenorrheic athletes in their investigation of the effects of menstrual phase and amenorrhea on exercise performance. No differences were found between early follicular and midluteal phases, or among amenorrheic and eumenorrheic athletes for VO_2max, maximum minute ventilation, maximum heart rate, or perceived exertion (De Souza et al 1990). More recently, Beidleman et al (1999) investigated the effects of menstrual cycle phase on minute ventilation and physical performance at altitude and at sea level. Neither of these factors were affected by menstrual cycle phase at sea level or high altitude (Beidleman et al 1999).

Giacomoni et al (2000) and Lebrun et al (1995) investigated the influence of menstrual cycle phase on anaerobic performance and found that no significant changes in anaerobic performance occurred during different menstrual cycle phases. Thus, some variation exists in the literature concerning the effects of menstrual cycle phase on performance. However, it does not seem that menstrual cycle phase can be consistently related to alterations in aerobic or anaerobic exercise performance in athletic women.

THE FEMALE ATHLETE TRIAD

The female athlete triad consists of three interrelated components: disordered eating, amenorrhea, and osteoporosis (Nattiv et al 1994). These components are intimately associated in etiology, pathogenesis, and health consequences (American College of Sports Medicine 1997). The female athlete may adopt disordered eating patterns as she strives to lose weight in order to achieve the thin appearance or low body weight deemed necessary for excellence in her sport. These disordered eating patterns can then lead to menstrual dysfunction and osteoporosis (Nattiv et al 1994). Athletes involved in sports that emphasize leanness for the purposes of appearance (e.g. ballet), performance (e.g. rhythmic gymastics), or inclusion in a specific weight class (e.g. rowing) are at increased risk for development of the triad (Sundgot-Borgen 1993a). This includes sports such as gymnastics, long distance running and crew. However, it is important to remember that the triad can affect athletes involved in any sport (Sundgot-Borgen 1993a).

DISORDERED EATING

Most athletes with disordered eating do not meet the criteria for anorexia nervosa or bulimia nervosa. Severe restriction of food intake and an intense fear of gaining weight are characteristics of anorexia nervosa. (Box 26.1). Bulimia nervosa is characterized by binge eating followed by purging to prevent weight gain. (Box 26.2).

The fact that many athletes do not meet the strict criteria for anorexia or bulimia nervosa, but still have significant problems associated with disordered eating, has led some authors to propose a classification of dis-

---

Box 26.1   Diagnostic criteria for anorexia nervosa (Data from American Psychiatric Association 1994:544–545)

1. Refusal to maintain body weight at or above a minimally normal weight for age and height (e.g. weight loss leading to maintenance of body weight less than 85% of that expected; or failure to make expected weight gain during period of growth, leading to body weight less than 85% of that expected).

2. Intense fear of gaining weight or becoming fat, even though underweight.

3. Disturbance in the way in which one's body weight or shape is experienced; undue influence of body weight or shape on self-evaluation, or denial of the seriousness of the current low body weight.

4. In postmenarcheal females, amenorrhea (i.e. the absence of at least three consecutive menstrual cycles). A woman is considered to have amenorrhea if her periods occur only following hormone (e.g. estrogen) administration.

Specifiy type:
Restriction type: the person has not regularly engaged in binge eating or purging behavior (self-induced vomiting or the misuse of laxatives, diuretics, or enemas) during the current episode of anorexia nervosa.

Binge eating/purging type: the person has regularly engaged in binge eating or purging behavior during the current episode of anorexia nervosa.

Box 26.2 Diagnostic criteria for bulimia nervosa (Data from American Psychiatric Association 1994:549–550)

1. Recurrent episodes of binge eating. An episode of binge eating is characterized by both of the following:
   a. eating in a discrete period of time (e.g. within any 2-h period), an amount of food that is definitely larger than most people would eat during a similar period of time and under similar circumstances
   b. a sense of lack of control over eating during the episode (e.g. a feeling that one cannot stop eating or control what or how much one is eating).
2. Recurrent, inappropriate compensatory behavior in order to prevent weight gain, such as self-induced vomiting; misuse of laxatives, diuretics, enemas, or other medications; fasting; or excessive exercise.
3. The binge eating and inappropriate compensatory behaviors both occur, on average, at least twice a week for 3 months.
4. Self-evaluation is unduly influenced by body shape and weight.
5. The disturbance does not occur exclusively during episodes of anorexia nervosa.

Specify type:
Purging Type: during the current episode of bulimia nervosa, the person has regularly engaged in self-induced vomiting or the misuse of laxatives, diuretics or enemas.

Non-purging Type: during the current episode of bulimia nervosa, the person has used other inappropriate compensatory behaviors, such as fasting or excessive exercise, but has not regularly engaged in self-induced vomiting or the misuse of laxatives, diuretics, or enemas.

Box 26.3 Criteria for anorexia athletica (Data from Sundgot-Borgen 1993a: 3:29–40)

Absolute criteria (all must be present)
1. Weight loss: >5% of expected body weight
2. Gastrointestinal complaints
3. Absence of medical illness or affective disorder explaining the weight reduction
4. Excessive fear of becoming obese
5. Restriction of food (<1200Kcal/day)

Relative criteria (one or more must be met)
1. Delayed puberty: lack of menstruation at age 16 (primary amenorrhea)
2. Menstrual dysfunction: primary amenorrhea, secondary amenorrhea or oligomenorrhea
3. Distorted body image
4. Use of purging methods: self-induced vomiting, laxatives, and diuretics
5. Bingeing
6. Compulsive exercise

Box 26.4 Criteria for eating disorders not otherwise specified (EDNOS) (Data from American Psychiatric Association 1994: 550)

1. For females, all of the criteria for anorexia nervosa are met except that the individual has regular menses.
2. All of the criteria for anorexia nervosa are met except that, despite significant weight loss, the individual's current weight is in the normal range.
3. All of the criteria for bulimia nervosa are met except that the binge eating and inappropriate compensatory mechanisms occur at a frequency of less than twice a week or for a duration of less than 3 months.
4. The regular use of inappropriate compensatory behavior by an individual of normal body weight after eating small amounts of food (e.g. self-induced vomiting after the consumption of two cookies).
5. Repeatedly chewing and spitting out, but not swallowing, large amounts of food.
6. Binge eating disorder: recurrent episodes of binge eating in the absence of the regular use of inappropriate compensatory behaviors characteristic of bulimia nervosa.

---

ordered eating called anorexia athletica. Criteria for this disorder were originally set by Pugliese et al (1983) and were modified by Sundgot-Borgen (1993a) (Box 26.3).

The Diagnostic and Statistical Manual of Mental Disorders-IV (DSM-IV) (American Psychiatric Association 1994) also acknowledges that this issue exists and has a category of eating disorders not otherwise specified (EDNOS), which includes disorders that do not meet the criteria for anorexia or bulimia nervosa. Some athletes with anorexia athletica meet the criteria for EDNOS (Box 26.4).

The reported prevalence of disordered eating among athletes varies among studies from 10–62% (Dummer et al 1987, Marshall & Harber 1996, O'Connor et al 1995, Rosen et al 1986, Sundgot-Borgen 1993a, Sundgot-Borgen & Corbin 1987, Taub & Blinde 1992, Warren et al 1990, Weight & Noakes 1987). An explanation for the large variance in reported prevalence lies in the different methods used to collect data, definitions used to define disordered eating, and athletic populations included in each of the studies. While athletes competing in sports that emphasize leanness are believed to be at increased risk for disordered eating and the female athlete triad, athletes involved in any sport can be affected (Fig. 26.3).

Most investigators used surveys, including the Eating Disorders Inventory (EDI) and Eating Attitudes Test (EAT), to assess an athlete's risk for disordered eating behaviors. The EDI (Garner et al 1983, 1984), EDI-2, an updated version of the EDI (Garner 1991), and EAT (Garner & Garfinkel 1979) are standardized measures that have been tested for reliability and validity in the general population, but not in athletes. They are intended for use as screening, not diagnostic, tools (Garner et al 1998). Scores on these tests have been correlated with disordered eating in athletes (O'Connor et al 1995, Sundgot-Borgen 1993a).

The use of surveys alone to assess risk for disordered eating is problematic. Sundgot-Borgen (1993a) demonstrated that significant under-reporting of disordered

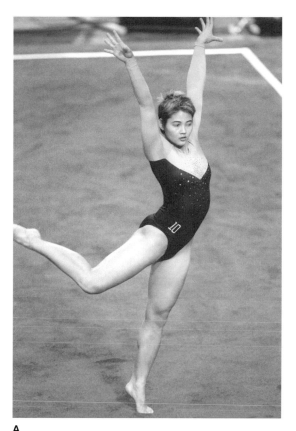

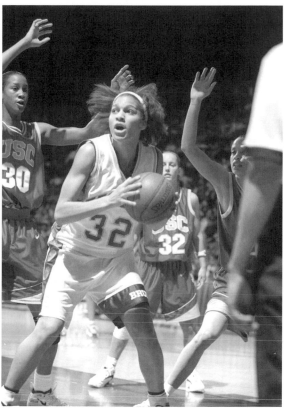

A   B

Figure 26.3A&B   While athletes competing in sports that emphasize leanness (e.g. gymnastics) (**A**) are believed to be at increased risk for disordered eating and the female athlete triad, athletes involved in any sport (e.g. basketball) (**B**) can be affected. (Reproduced with the permission of UCLA Athletic Department.)

eating symptoms occurred when only screening question-naires were used, compared to when surveys were combined with clinical interviews and physical examinations as assessment tools. Also, O'Connor et al (1995) showed that athletes can fake the EDI-2. A study by Wilmore (1991) further highlights the problems with using self-report questionnaires to assess disordered eating. None of the respondents to the EAT in this study were determined to be at risk for disordered eating; however, in the ensuing 2 years, 18% of the respondents entered treatment for eating disorders.

Elite athletes and athletes involved in sports that emphasize leanness are at increased risk for disordered eating. Sundgot-Borgen (1993a) found that elite athletes in all sport groups were at increased risk for disordered eating compared to controls. Also, the prevalence of disordered eating was significantly higher in sports that emphasized leanness (esthetic, weight dependent, and endurance sports) in comparison to other sports (technical and ball game sports) and controls.

Prevalence estimates for the use of pathogenic weight control techniques or preoccupation with weight in the college athlete, range from 0–62% (Dummer et al 1987,

Johnson et al 1999, O'Connor et al 1995, Rosen & Hough 1986, Sundgot-Borgen & Corbin 1987, Warren et al 1990). As in elite athletes, college women participating in sports that emphasize leanness are at increased risk for preoccupation with weight and use of pathogenic weight control techniques (Sundgot-Borgen & Corbin 1987, Warren et al 1990). Some investigators have, however, found that college athletes are not at increased risk for disordered eating compared to controls (Ashley et al 1996, O'Connor et al 1995, Sundgot-Borgen & Corbin 1987, Warren et al 1990).

Studies of eating disorders in high school athletes are limited. The prevalence of the use of pathogenic weight control techniques by high school female athletes is estimated to be between 15–25% (Dummer et al 1987, Rhea 1999). However, in studies that included a control group, an increased risk for disordered eating among female athletes was not found (Fulkerson et al 1999, Rhea 1999, Taub & Blinde 1992). In fact, female athletes have been found to have higher self-efficacy and self-esteem compared to controls, which might actually provide a protective effect against the development of disordered eating behaviors (Fulkerson et al 1999, Rhea 1999).

Many triggers for the onset of disordered eating in athletes have been identified (Rosen et al 1986, Sundgot-Borgen 1994). Rosen & Hough (1986) found that 75% of gymnasts who were told by coaches that they were overweight resorted to pathogenic weight control techniques to lose weight. Sundgot-Borgen (1994) found that prolonged periods of dieting, weight fluctuations, coaching changes, injury, and casual comments made about weight by coaches, parents and friends, were the most common reasons given by athletes for the development of disordered eating. Personal stressors including leaving home, problems in a relationship, family trouble, death of a significant other, and sexual abuse, were also identified as triggers. Beginning sport-specific training at a younger age was identified as another risk factor (Sundot-Borgon 1994).

Disordered eating and pathogenic weight loss can lead to serious medical complications for athletes. The changes in fluids and electrolytes that accompany purging and starvation behaviors can lead to dehydration, electrolyte abnormalities, hypotension, and cardiac dysrrythmias (Becker et al 1999, Palla & Litt 1988, Pomeroy & Mitchell 1992). Clearly, these sequelae pose a particular risk to the competitive athlete. Boxes 26.5 and 26.6 provide a more complete list of medical complications associated with disordered eating.

Disordered eating may also have detrimental effects on athletic performance, such as decreased endurance, strength, and coordination (Fogelholm 1994, Webster et al 1990). Webster et al (1990) demonstrated decreased VO_2max, upper body strength, and coordination in athletes who had rapid weight loss due to the accompanying dehydration. Gradual weight loss has also been associated with decreased VO_2max in some studies (Fogelholm et al 1993).

Evaluation of the athlete with disordered eating includes measurement of serum electrolytes and glucose, and a complete blood investigation. Also, since arrhythmias and prolonged Q–T intervals can be found in athletes with disordered eating, an electrocardiogram should be obtained.

Usually, athletes with disordered eating can be effectively treated as outpatients. Inpatient management should, however, be considered in patients who have cardiac arrhythmias, electrolyte disturbances, weight loss to 75% expected body weight, suicidal ideation, or a history of rapid weight loss (Becker et al 1999).

Proper treatment of disordered eating requires recognition of the problem, identification and resolution of psychosocial precipitants, and establishment of healthy eating patterns (Becker et al 1999). When caring for athletes with disordered eating, physicians usually act as part of a multidisciplinary team (Nattiv et al 1994). The role of the team physician is to assure that the athlete's medical condition is stable and to coordinate care. A nutritionist provides nutritional guidance and a psychologist or psychiatrist should address the psychosocial issues using individual, group, and family therapy as needed (Becker et al 1999, Johnson 1994). Sundgot-Borgen & Sundgot-Schnieder (2001), highlighted the importance of the psychiatric component of treatment in a recent study. They found that cognitive behavioral therapy was more effective than nutrition counseling or no counseling in reducing the pursuit of thinness and use of pathogenic weight control techniques. Nutritional counseling was more helpful than no treatment. Coaches, physical therapists, and athletic trainers can often help identify athletes with signs of disordered eating and facilitate treatment, since they have the most contact with the athletes.

Box 26.6 Laboratory findings in disordered eating

EKG abnormalities
Prolonged QTc

Electrolyte abnormalities
Hypokalemia
Hypoglycemia

Hematological abnormalities
Anemia
Leukopenia
Thrombocytopenia

Box 26.5 Symptoms and physical examination findings in disordered eating

Head and neck
Face edema
Enlargement of parotid glands
Erosion of dental enamel

Heart
Bradycardia
Hypotension
Arrhythmia

Gastrointestinal
Constipation
Esophagitis
Rectal prolapse

Skin
Dry skin
Lanugo
Carotenemia
Russel's Sign: callused knuckles from scraping teeth with induced vomiting

Thermoregulation
Hypothermia
Cold intolerance

Pharmacotherapy is not usually indicated in the initial stages of treatment for anorexia nervosa, but fluoxetine may stabilize the patient during the recovery period once 85% of expected weight has been reached (Becker et al 1999). Fluoxetine, desipramine, and imipramine have all been used in the treatment of bulimia (Becker et al 1999).

AMENORRHEA

The prevalence of amenorrhea in the athletic woman has been reported to range from 1–66% (Johnson et al 1999, Loucks & Horvath 1985, Otis 1992, Sundgot-Borgen & Corbin 1987, Sundgot-Borgen & Larsen 1993). The prevalence in the general population is estimated to be 2–5% (Bachmann & Kemmann 1982, Loucks & Horvath 1985).

Secondary amenorrhea is defined as the cessation of menstrual periods for three or more consecutive menstrual cycles in a woman who has achieved menarche (Shangold et al 1990). A spectrum of menstrual disorders occur in the female athlete. Hypoestrogenic amenorrhea is at one end of the spectrum and periods of oligomenorrhea are at an intermediate point (Nattiv 2001). Oligomenorrhea is defined as infrequent menstrual cycles that are greater than 35 days in length (Loucks & Horvath 1985, Nattiv 2001). Ovulatory and luteal dysfunction also occur in athletes. Athletes with these disorders may remain unrecognized since they can continue to have cycles at normal intervals, making it difficult to estimate the prevalence of these conditions (Bullen et al 1985, Loucks et al 1989). Luteal phase dysfunction is manifested by a shortened luteal phase with inadequate progesterone production (Shangold et al 1990).

Primary amenorrhea or delayed menarche is defined as the absence of menses by the age of 16 years (Loucks & Horvath 1985). While sports participation has been associated with delayed menarche in girls, a causal relationship has not been established (Loucks 1990, Malina et al 1994).

Investigators have shown that menstrual history and dysfunction are significant predictors for decreased bone mineral density (BMD) (Cann et al 1988, Drinkwater et al 1990, Grimston et al 1990, Myburgh et al 1993, Wolman et al 1990). Amenorrheic and oligomenorrheic athletes have decreased BMD compared to their eumenorrheic peers (Cann et al 1984, Drinkwater et al 1984, Marcus et al 1985). Also, some evidence suggests that athletes with luteal phase dysfunction may also be at increased risk for low bone density (Drinkwater et al 1990).

Loss of bone mineral density can have serious health consequences for the female athlete. Lower peak bone mineral density in the athlete with menstrual dysfunction can predispose her to osteoporosis and fractures later in life (Drinkwater et al 1990, Snow-Harter 1994) (Figs 26.4, 26.5). Also, amenorrhea and low bone density

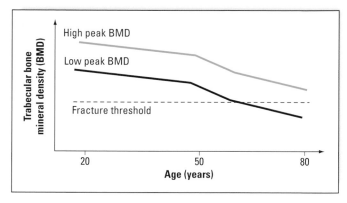

Figure 26.4   The individual who enters adulthood with a higher peak bone mass may lose similar amounts of bone to an individual with lower peak bone mass, but may still remain above a critical fracture threshold. (Reproduced with permission from Snow-Harter 1994.)

have been identified as risk factors for stress fractures in young athletes, which are not only a serious medical issue, but can have consequences for the athlete's performance (Bennell et al 1995, 1996, Lloyd et al 1986, Myburgh et al 1990). Drinkwater et al (1990) demonstrated a linear relationship between degree of menstrual dysfunction and degree of bone loss.

The normal menstrual cycle is characterized by pulsatile secretion of gonadotrophin releasing hormone (GnRH) from the hypothalamus. GnRH stimulates the pulsatile release of luteinizing hormone (LH) and follicle stimulating hormone (FSH) from the pituitary gland. FSH stimulates the granulosa cell to produce estrogen, which promotes proliferation of the endometrium during the follicular phase. LH stimulates the corpus luteum

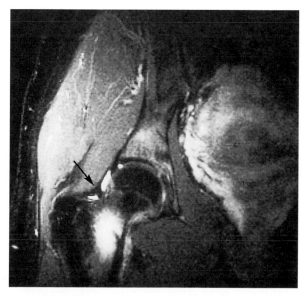

Figure 26.5   MRI demonstrating a stress fracture of the femoral neck in an amenorrheic athlete.

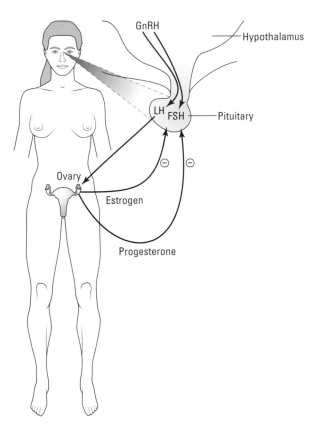

Figure 26.6 Basic physiology of the menstrual cycle. Pulsatile release of GnRH from the hypothalamus stimulates the release of FSH and LH from the pituitary. LH and FSH stimulate the release of estrogen and progesterone in the ovaries.

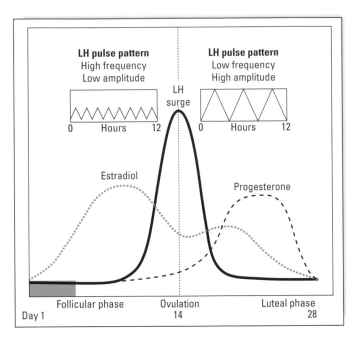

Figure 26.7 Patterns of hormone secretion across the normal menstrual cycle. An LH surge occurs at the time of ovulation and marks the division between the follicular phase (days 1–14) and the luteal phase (days 15–28). LH pulse pattern also changes across the menstrual cycle; pulse frequency decreases from the follicular phase (~ 65- to 80-min intervals) to the luteal phase (~ 185- to 200-min intervals), whereas pulse amplitude increases from the follicular phase (~ 5 mIU/mL) to the luteal phase (~ 12 mIU/mL)

to produce progesterone, which stimulates the endometrium to mature into a secretory lining suitable for implantation of the fertilized egg (Fig. 26.6).

The pulse pattern of LH secretion varies with the phases of the menstrual cycle (Harber 2000). During the follicular phase, LH is secreted in a low amplitude, high frequency fashion (Harber 2000). At ovulation, a surge of LH occurs. Finally, during the luteal phase, LH is released in a high amplitude, low frequency pattern (Harber 2000) (Fig. 26.7).

In athletes with menstrual dysfunction, the normal monthly phasic changes in LH do not occur (Loucks et al 1989, 1994, Veldhuis et al 1985, Williams et al 1995). LH patterns in amenorrheic athletes demonstrate a decreased frequency of pulses and variable interpulse intervals (Loucks et al 1989). Athletes with luteal phase dysfunction have LH patterns characterized by reduced frequency of pulses and increased pulse amplitude (Loucks et al 1989). These changes in LH pattern are due to alterations in the hypothalamic pituitary ovarian axis, with reduced GnRH release (Loucks et al 1989, Veldhuis et al 1985). Thus, exercise-associated amenorrhea is hypothalamic in origin (Fig. 26.8).

While many mechanisms for the disruption of normal menstrual function have been proposed, the energy availability hypothesis is the most widely accepted. This hypothesis states that insufficient energy availability, defined as the difference between dietary caloric intake and energy expenditure from exercise, is responsible for alterations in menstrual function. The observation that athletes, both amenorrheic and cyclic, take in fewer calories than expected for their level of activity without a resultant decrease in body weight, provided the initial evidence for this hypothesis (Drinkwater et al 1984, Loucks et al 1989, Marcus et al 1985, Myerson et al 1991).

Bullen et al (1985) demonstrated that increasing energy expenditure in untrained eumenorrheic women by the introduction of a strenuous exercise routine, could lead to a reversible disruption in normal menstrual cycle. Further investigations have revealed that exercise alone will not disrupt LH pulsatility; a failure to replace the increased energy expenditure with increased dietary intake and a resultant energy imbalance must also occur (Loucks et al 1998, Williams et al 1995).

Amenorrheic athletes have endocrine signs of energy deficiency, which support the energy drain hypothesis (Loucks et al 1989, 1998). Low levels of serum triiodothyronine (T_3) are found in amenorrheic athletes but

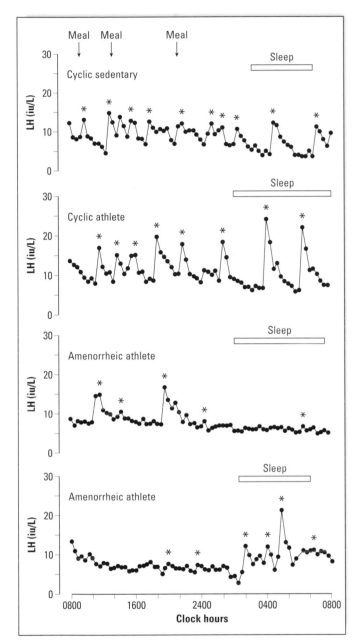

Figure 26.8 LH pulsatility in cyclic athletes and controls compared to amenorrheic athletes. In amenorrheic athletes, a range of pulse patterns with decreased frequency and variable interpulse intervals are found. (Reproduced with permission from Loucks A B, Mortola J F, Girton L, Yen S S 1989 Alterations in the hypothalamic–pituitary–ovarian and the hypothalamic–pituitary–adrenal axes in athletic women. Journal of Clinical Endocrinology and Metabolism 68: 402–411, © The Endocrine Society.)

not in athletes with regular menses (Loucks 1992b, Loucks & Heath 1994).

Zanker & Swaine (1998b) attempted to demonstrate the relationship between estradiol concentration ·and multiple indices of energy balance in young female distance runners. They found that estradiol concentrations were more strongly related to calculated energy

imbalance, T_3, and insulin-like growth factor (IGF) than to body mass index or body fat (Zanker & Swaine 1998c). As expected, T_3 and IGF were closely related to energy balance. Specifically, T_3 and IGF were more highly correlated with energy intake than energy expenditure. These relationships between estradiol and energy imbalance further support the idea that reproductive dysfunction in female athletes is associated with an energy deficit (Zanker & Swaine 1998c).

Recently, investigators have attempted to identify the specific metabolic signal that leads to the disruption of normal hypothalamic GnRH release in response to decreased energy availability. Evidence suggests that leptin, a protein product of the obesity gene, may be the metabolic signal that integrates nutritional status and reproductive function (Laughlin & Yen 1997). Also, receptors for leptin are found in both the hypothalamus and ovary (Laughlin & Yen 1997). Leptin levels are correlated with the percentage of body fat and they decrease with weight loss. In amenorrheic athletes, the normal diurnal variation of leptin is absent (Considine et al 1996, Laughlin & Yen 1997). Also, in the study by Laughlin & Yen (1997), compared to controls, both amenorrheic and athletes within a normal cycle had lower 24 h leptin levels. Finally, Hilton & Loucks (2000) demonstrated that exercise must be associated with low energy availability in order for changes in diurnal pattern of leptin to occur. These findings highlight the connection between leptin and energy availability, diet, and reproductive function in the athlete.

Prevention plays an important role in the management of the female athlete triad. It has been found that providing education about the female athlete triad to coaches and athletes leads to decreases in the prevalence of eating disorders.

Initial evaluation of the amenorrheic athlete usually includes a pregnancy test, thyroid studies, and FSH and prolactin level tests. If polycystic ovarian syndrome is suspected or features of androgen excess are noted on examination for LH, free testosterone and dihydroepiandosterone sulfate levels should be obtained.

The main goal in the treatment of exercise-associated amenorrhea is to restore normal menstrual patterns and to prevent associated osteoporosis. Successful return of menses in the amenorrheic athlete should occur if the existing energy imbalance is treated. Hilton & Loucks (2000) demonstrated that an improvement in nutritional status will lead to return of normal LH patterns, even with continued exercise. In a case study of a 19-year-old amenorrheic track athlete, Dueck et al (1996) demonstrated that a 15-week program of diet supplementation combined with a moderate decrease in training frequency (1 day/week) led to weight gain, increased body fat, increased LH levels, and eventual return of menses.

Of note is that the athlete reported a dramatic improvement in performance with the adjustment in energy balance. More recently, similar results were obtained with this intervention in four other amenorrheic athletes (Kopp-Woodroffe et al 1999).

Treatment of the decreased BMD found in amenorrheic athletes is a challenging issue. As these athletes are often found to have inadequate calcium and vitamin D intake (Sundgot-Borgen 1993b, Kirchner et al 1995), appropriate supplementation should be provided. Also, athletes with stress fractures have been found to have lower calcium intakes than athletes without stress fractures (Myburgh et al 1990). Drinkwater et al (1993) observed an increase in tibial BMD in amenorrheic athletes taking supplemental calcium compared to those not taking supplemental calcium. Another study demonstrated a positive linear correlation between dietary calcium and spinal trabecular bone density (Wolman et al 1990). The recommended calcium intake for athletes with menstrual dysfunction is 1200–1500 mg/day and the recommended intake for vitamin D is 400–800 IU/day.

The usefulness of estrogen replacement, whether in the form of the OCP or as estrogen replacement therapy (ERT), in the treatment of menstrual dysfunction and decreased BMD in young amenorrheic athletes is a controversial issue. Prospective data involving the effects of estrogen on bone density in young athletes with menstrual disturbances is quite limited. Several cross-section investigations have demonstrated an association between estrogen use and increased bone density. Lloyd et al (1986) and Myburgh et al (1990) found that athletes without stress fractures were more likely to have used the OCP. In another retrospective study, Cumming (1996) found that amenorrheic athletes using estrogen replacement had significantly higher BMD at the lumbar spine and femoral neck compared to amenorrheic controls who received no therapy.

In a randomized controlled trial study of amenorrheic women, Hergenroeder et al (1997) found significant increases in BMD at the lumbar spine and in the total body in amenorrheic subjects taking the OCP in comparison to controls using medroxyprogesterone or placebo. Athletes with amenorrhea were included in this study, but the study group was not composed entirely of athletes. In another study following 52 women with amenorrhea of various etiologies, Gulekli et al (1994) found a significant increase in bone mass with the use of various types of estrogen therapy. Of note was that the authors found that weight gain was more effective than any type of estrogen therapy in increasing BMD. Haenggi et al (1994) also found a small positive effect on BMD with OCP treatment.

Some prospective studies have found that estrogen replacement had either no effect or a negative effect on BMD. In a study of 40 women with hypothalamic amenorrhea, Warren et al (1994) found no difference in BMD in the spine, wrist or foot in women treated with estrogen compared to non-treated controls. However, in three subjects who gained weight during the study period, a significant increase in BMD was noted. Polatti et al (1995) followed 200 healthy women who were either receiving the OCP or no estrogen therapy and found that the group of women who were not taking the OCP had a significant increase in BMD over the study period, while those taking the OCP did not. This led them to suggest that OCP use may prevent peak bone mass in healthy young women (Polatti et al 1995). In another prospective study, Klibanski et al (1995) evaluated the effects of estrogen therapy on anorexic women with amenorrhea. The group treated with estrogen did not show significant improvement in BMD compared to controls. However, women in the control group who had weight gain and spontaneous resumption of menses did have a significant increase in BMD compared to other subjects.

The mixed findings in these studies suggest that estrogen deficiency may not be the only, or even the most important etiology, for the loss of BMD in amenorrheic athletes. The energy deficit associated with amenorrhea in athletes might play a role in decreased BMD (Zanker & Swaine 1998b).

Cyclic medroxyprogesterone has also been studied as a treatment for decreased BMD in active women with menstrual dysfunction. Prior et al (1994) found that treatment with cyclic medroxyprogesterone led to significant increases in bone density in active women with menstrual disturbances. Hergenroeder et al (1997), however, did not demonstrate an improvement in BMD with medroxyprogesterone therapy.

OSTEOPOROSIS

Osteoporosis has been defined as a disease characterized by low bone mass, microarchitectural deterioration of bone tissue leading to enhanced skeletal fragility, and an increased risk for fracture (Consensus Development Conference 1991) (also see Ch. 5). The World Health Organization (WHO) developed diagnostic criteria for osteoporosis in postmenopausal women, based on bone density measurements, however, criteria using bone density have not been established for young women (Box 26.7).

The osteoporosis found in female athletes with menstrual dysfunction has been attributed to the hypo-estrogenic state that accompanies hypothalamic amenorrhea (Drinkwater et al 1984, Marcus et al 1985, Loucks et al 1992a). Support for this conclusion comes from the documentation of the causal relationship between hypo-estrogenemia and osteoporosis in postmenopausal women. In postmenopausal women, loss of BMD is associated with increased bone turnover and exaggerated bone resorption, demonstrated by evidence from measurement of serum markers of bone turnover (Delmas 1992).

In amenorrheic runners, however, Zanker & Swaine (1998a) demonstrated that bone turnover is actually decreased. They measured serum markers of bone formation in amenorrheic athletes and found evidence of decreased bone formation. The different patterns of bone turnover between amenorrheic runners and postmenopausal women led Zanker & Swaine (1998a) to propose that hypoestrogenemia is not the sole factor responsible for the decreased BMD found in amenorrheic athletes. They suggested that the negative energy balance found in amenorrheic athletes plays a significant role in decreased BMD (Loucks 1990, Loucks & Callister 1993, Zanker & Swaine 1998b). The fact that estrogen replacement did not lead to improvement in BMD in some studies supports the idea that hypoestrogenemia may not be the only factor responsible for loss of bone density in these athletes.

The prognosis for the young amenorrheic athlete with osteoporosis is guarded. With weight gain and the return of normal menses, these athletes do have a significant increase in BMD. However, in comparison to cyclic controls, previously amenorrheic athletes continue to have significantly lower BMD even after weight gain (Drinkwater et al 1986, Herzog et al 1993, Iketani et al 1995, Jonnavithula et al 1993, Keen & Drinkwater 1997, Rigotti et al 1991). Thus, the loss of bone density in amenorrheic athletes may be partially irreversible.

If osteoporosis is suspected in an athlete, dual energy X-ray absorptiometric scan (DXA) is useful for evaluating BMD. If the athlete is found to be osteopenic or osteoporotic, bone markers can be measured. Urine N-telopeptide is used to assess bone resorption and serum osteocalcin to assess bone formation (Nattiv 2001).

The treatment of decreased BMD with the OCP in amenorrheic athletes is discussed above. Other pharmacological modalities may be useful in the treatment of osteoporosis in young athletes. Drinkwater et al (1993) found that miacilin nasal spray had a positive effect on BMD in the proximal femur and spine in amenorrheic athletes. Other medicines used to treat osteoporosis in postmenopausal woman including bisphosphonates and selective estrogen receptor modulators have not been well studied and have not been approved for use in young amenorrheic athletes. A more indepth discussion of osteoporosis can be found in Chapter 5.

BONE HEALTH

The factors that determine bone mass in postmenopausal women are peak bone mass and age-related bone loss (Nichols et al 2000). Maximizing peak bone mass and minimizing age-related bone loss will decrease the risk for osteoporosis and fragility fractures.

Bone mass gains during childhood are important for the attainment of an optimal peak bone mass. The maximum rate of bone formation occurs between the ages of 10–14 years and peak bone mass is attained between the ages of 20–30 years (Bonjour et al 1991, Sabatier et al 1996). By the end of adolescence, almost 90% of adult bone mass has been obtained (Sabatier et al 1996). Genetics, participation in weightbearing activities, and diet all influence bone mass in children (Pollitzer & Anderson 1989, Ruiz et al 1995, Slemenda et al 1991).

Bone loss in adult women is most rapid in the 3–4 years following menopause. The marked hypoestrogenemia associated with this time period is felt to be the cause of this bone loss, and it can be prevented with estrogen replacement (Ettinger et al 1985, Prestwood et al 1994). Evidence indicates that increased bone turnover and resorption is occurring during this phase of rapid bone loss (Delmas 1992). After this period of rapid bone loss, a phase of gradual bone loss takes over.

Strategies to minimize adult bone loss include optimizing nutrition, pharmacotherapy, and exercise programs. Calcium supplementation may slow bone loss in women after the first 5 years of menopause (Dawson-Hughes et al 1990); and, in combination with estrogen replacement or vitamin D, calcium supplementation may help increase BMD in postmenopausal women (Nichols et al 2000). Estrogen replacement therapy has been proven to increase BMD and to decrease risk for fracture in post-menopausal women (Ettinger et al 1985, Nichols et al 2000). However, all women may not experience improvement in BMD with estrogen replacement (Nichols et al 2000, Stevenson et al 1993).

Calcitonin is another medication that has been shown to increase BMD and to decrease fracture risk. Other, newer classes of drugs for the treatment of osteoporosis include bisphosphonates and selective estrogen receptor modulators.

While the results of exercise intervention are variable, resistance exercise and high impact training do seem to lead to site-specific increases in bone mass at the areas of greatest stress (Bassey et al 1998, Dook et al 1997, Drinkwater 1996, Friedlander 1995, Pruitt et al 1992, Simikin et al 1987, Taaffe et al 1995). Mature women with a history of participation in high impact sports, (e.g. basketball) and medium impact sports (e.g. running) exihibit greater bone density than those who had a history of participation in low impact sports (e.g. swimming) or who were non-athletic (Dook et al 1997). Children and adolescents participating in significant impact loading activites have been found to have higher levels of bone density than children in non-impact activies (Grimston et al 1993, Taaffe et al 1995). In a randomized controlled trial, Snow-Harter et al (1992) found that young women who did weight training or jogging had significantly greater gains in lumbar BMD than controls over an 8-month study period. Creighton et al (2001) used markers of bone formation to demonstrate that athletes participating in high-impact sports had more bone formation than those in non-impact sports. The high-impact sports athletes also had increased BMD. Premenopausal women may have larger BMD responses to impact activities than postmenopausal women, although postmenopausal women have been shown to have some increases in BMD with impact and resistance exercise (Bassey et al 1998, Maddalozzo & Snow 2000).

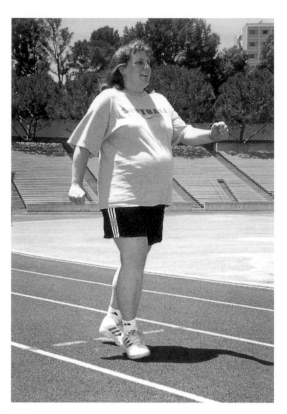

Figure 26.9 As the number of women participating in regular exercise rises, more women are continuing to exercise during pregnancy. (Reproduced with permission of Suzanne Hecht.)

PREGNANCY AND EXERCISE

Exercise has become an essential part of life for many women. That a large proportion of women wish to continue a regular exercise routine during pregnancy, raises questions about the safety of exercise during pregnancy (Fig. 26.9).

PHYSIOLOGICAL CONSIDERATIONS AND THEORETICAL CONCERNS

It has been suggested that physiological responses to exercise in pregnant woman could lead to poor pregnancy outcomes, including abortion, fetal malformations, poor fetal growth, fetal injury, and premature labor. There are concerns that exercise and pregnancy-induced changes in hemodynamics, body temperature, circulating stress hormones, caloric expenditure, and the musculoskeletal system could lead to poor maternal or fetal outcomes (Clapp 2000, Clapp & Rizik 1992). Fortunately, most of these concerns have not been validated in the literature. In the following section, each of these areas of theoretical concern will be addressed.

Hemodynamics

The hemodynamic responses to exercise, especially alterations in splanchnic blood flow, have raised concern that adequate uterine blood flow may not be maintained during exercise. Decreased uterine blood flow could decrease oxygen and nutrient availability to the fetus, inhibiting growth and development (Clapp 1994). Also, there is a concern that decreased myometrial oxygen delivery to the uterus could stimulate uterine contractions, leading to premature labor and delivery (Clapp 2000). In non-pregnant women, weightbearing exercise causes splanchnic flow to decrease to 40–50% of normal resting levels (Clapp 1994). Fortunately, the cardiovascular changes associated with both pregnancy and regular exercise offer protection against large decreases in splanchnic flow during exercise. A 40–50% increase in blood volume typically occurs during pregnancy (Capeless & Clapp 1989, Clapp 2000, Pivarnik et al 1992). In exercising pregnant women, this increase may be as much as 35% more than in sedentary controls (Hale & Milne 1996, Pivarnik et al 1993, 1994). In addition, trained pregnant women have significantly higher cardiac outputs than their sedentary counterparts (Clapp 2000, Pivarnik et al 1993). These changes in the cardiovascular system result in decreases in splanchnic flow with exercise that are 20–30% less in trained pregnant women than in sedentary controls (Clapp 2000). Ultrasound studies have been performed to assess uteroplacental blood flow before and after exercise in pregnant women. These studies have yielded mixed results, some showing no difference in uteroplacental blood flow with exercise, and others showing decreased uterine circulation with exercise (Baumann et al 1989, Rauramo & Forss 1988). Definitive evidence of decreased uteroplacental flow during exercise in pregnant women is not available. Results similar to splanchnic flow have been obtained with assessment of umbilical artery flow during exercise (Baumann et al 1989, Veille et al 1989, Veille 1996).

In order to assess fetal distress with maternal exercise, some studies have monitored fetal heart rate before and immediately after exercise. The results are mixed, but even in studies where changes in fetal heart rate are documented, the changes are transient and no prolonged adverse fetal effects have been documented as a result, indicating that adequate blood flow to the fetus is maintained (Carpenter et al 1988, Clapp 1985, Clapp et al 1992, Collings et al 1983, Hall & Kaufmann 1987, Hauth et al 1982, O'Neill 1996, Veille 1996).

Body temperature

The increased body temperatures associated with exercise have led to concerns about the potential for fetal malformations. In women who are not pregnant, body temperature can be elevated above 39.2°C with exercise, a level felt to have teratogenic potential (American College of Obstetrics and Gynecology 1994). Studies indicating an increase in neural tube defects due to hot tub use by pregnant women added to these concerns (Milunsky et al 1992). Both pregnancy and regular exercise improve heat dissipation, which helps prevent increased body temperatures during exercise (Clapp et al 1987). Clapp (1991) demonstrated that, during pregnancy, maternal body temperature decreased by 0.3°C in the first trimester, and continued to decrease 0.1°C each month until the 37th week. Also, trained pregnant woman demonstrate an even better ability to dissipate heat than untrained pregnant women (Clapp 1990, 1994, Clapp et al 1987). Several investigators have measured the rectal temperatures of trained pregnant women during exercise and found that the body temperatures of these women do reach levels felt to have teratogenic potential (Clapp et al 1987, O'Neill 1996). Finally, prospective studies involving women who exercise during pregnancy have failed to demonstrate an increased risk for congenital anomalies or early pregnancy loss, compared to controls (Clapp 1989, Clapp & Dickstein 1984).

Caloric expenditure

As glucose is the main fetal substrate, there is concern that glucose use by exercising muscles might limit fetal substrate availability. It has been shown that maternal blood glucose levels do fall during exercise (Clapp 1991, Clapp et al 1987, Soultanakis et al 1996). In spite of this, investigations of fetal growth have provided mixed results, most showing no difference in the growth of fetuses of exercising women compared to sedentary women (Bell et al 1995, Clapp 1990, 2000, Clapp & Dickstein 1984, Clapp & Little 1995, Clapp et al 1992, Collings et al 1983, Hall & Kaufmann 1987, Hatch et al 1993, Jackson et al 1995, Klebanoff et al 1990, Lokey et al 1991, Sternfeld et al 1995). Compensatory mechanisms to improve substrate delivery to the fetus may develop in the exercising pregnant woman, including increased placental size and increased glucose delivery after bouts of exercise (Clapp 2000, Clapp et al 1992, Jackson et al 1995). Also, since exercise performance tends to decrease late in pregnancy, the amount of glucose used by working muscles is limited during this time (Clapp et al 1987).

While women who continue to exercise during pregnancy do tend to gain less weight than sedentary women, their level of weight gain does fall within acceptable ranges (Clapp & Little 1995). Women who continue to exercise during pregnancy may require increased energy intake in order to achieve appropriate weight gains during pregnancy.

Stress hormones

Exercise leads to a stress response with increased levels of catecholamines (Artal et al 1981, Bonds & Delivoria-Papadopoulos 1985). Noradrenaline (norepinephrine) has been shown to increase strength and frequency of contractions, leading to concerns that exercise might lead to uterine contractions (Artal et al 1981). Subjectively, some women note contractions during exercise. However, assessment with tocodynamometry immediately after exercise has not demonstrated that increased uterine activity occurs with exercise (Veille et al 1985).

Musculoskeletal

There is concern that the increases in maternal weight, changes in center of gravity, and increased ligamentous laxity associated with pregnancy may cause maternal injury with exercise during pregnancy (Clapp et al 1992, Clapp 1994). Despite these changes, very few maternal injuries have been associated with exercise during pregnancy (Clapp 2000). This may be due to the decrease in performance that occurs late in pregnancy when weight is highest and ligamentous laxity is most profound (Clapp 1990, 2000, Clapp et al 1987).

Maternal effects

The effects of exercise during pregnancy on pregnancy length, course of labor, and symptoms of pregnancy have all been investigated (Clapp & Dickstein 1984, Clapp 1990, Hall & Kaufmann 1987, Hatch et al 1993, Kulpa et al 1986). Exercise during pregnancy has been associated with many beneficial effects for the mother.

Exercise has been related to a decrease in some of the symptoms associated with pregnancy. Women who exercise during pregnancy have fewer complaints of low back pain and other musculoskeletal complaints than sedentary women (Hall & Kaufmann 1987, Kihlstrand et al 1999, Sternfeld et al 1995). Also, pregnant women who continue to exercise report improved self image and fewer depressive symptoms, both during pregnancy and the postpartum period, compared to those who do not (Hall & Kaufmann 1987, Sternfeld et al 1995).

Exercise has not been associated with increased risk of premature delivery (Clapp 1990, Clapp & Dickstein 1984, Hatch et al 1993, Kulpa et al 1986, Lokey et al 1991, Sternfeld et al 1995). However, Clapp (1990) found that exercising women tend to deliver about 1 week earlier than women who do not exercise, an effect that the women in the study found to be beneficial.

Investigations examining the effects of maternal exercise on the course of labor have produced inconsistent results (Clapp 1990, Collings et al 1983, Hall & Kaufmann 1987, Kardel & Kase 1998, Kulpa et al 1986, Lokey et al 1991). While most studies suggest that maternal exercise has no effect on the course of labor, some have demonstrated a shorter active phase and second stage of labor in exercising women (Clapp 1990, Kulpa et al 1986). Finally, some investigators have found that women who exercise during pregnancy have a lower incidence of operative deliveries and episiotomies (Clapp 1990, Hall & Kaufmann 1987, Kulpa et al 1986, Sternfeld et al 1995).

It has been suggested that the increased blood volume gained by women who exercise during pregnancy may offer some protection in the event of a hemorrhage during delivery (Clapp 2000). Also, exercise during pregnancy may protect against problems with loss of bladder control, both in the immediate postpartum period and 1 year after delivery (Clapp 2000).

Finally, women who continue to exercise during and after pregnancy may return to their prepregnancy weight faster than sedentary women, since they have lower overall weight gain and subcutaneous fat deposition (Clapp 2000). However, during lactation, exercise does not increase the rate of weight loss without concomitant caloric restriction (Clapp 2000, 2001, Clapp & Little 1995, Dewey 1998). Despite concerns to the contrary, exercise, dieting, and gradual weight loss in the postpartum period do not seem to adversely affect lactation or infant growth (Dewey 1998, Lovelady et al 2000, McCrory et al 1999).

Fetal effects

Studies investigating the effects of maternal exercise on birth weight are numerous and have provided mixed results. Most investigators have found no difference in birth weight of offspring born to exercising mothers compared to sedentary controls, but some have found either increased or decreased weight in the offspring of exercising mothers (Bell et al 1995, Clapp 1990, 1996, 2000, Clapp & Dickstein 1984, Clapp & Little 1995, Clapp et al 1992, Clapp et al 1998, Collings et al 1983, Hall & Kaufmann 1987, Hatch et al 1993, Jackson et al 1995, Klebanoff et al 1990, Kulpa et al 1986, Lokey et al 1991, Sternfeld et al 1995). The level of exercise performance may influence birth weight. Studies involving women who participated in low intensity, non-weightbearing exercise routines tend to show either no change or a slight increase in birth weight (Bell et al 1995, Clapp 2000, Clapp et al 1992, Collings et al 1983, Hall & Kaufmann 1987, Hatch et al 1993, Jackson et al 1995, Klebanoff et al 1990, Kulpa et al 1986, Lokey et al 1991, Sternfeld et al 1995). It has been hypothesized that the increased birth weight observed in these infants may be due to alterations in placental growth and blood flow induced by exercise (Clapp 1990, 2000, Clapp et al 1992, Hatch et al 1993, Jackson et al 1995). High intensity exercise may be associated with a decrease in birth weight, especially if maternal weight gain is limited (Bell et al 1995, Clapp 1990, 1996, Clapp & Dickstein 1984, Clapp & Little 1995, Clapp et al 1998). Clapp (1990) found that the decreased birth weight in these infants could be attributed to lower fat mass and slightly decreased gestational age. Little or no change has been demonstrated in head circumference, length, or lean body mass in infants born to exercising vs. sedentary mothers (Clapp 1990).

During labor, infants of mothers who exercised during pregnancy show fewer signs of distress (Clapp 1990). They have a decreased incidence of meconium stained amniotic fluid and abnormal fetal heart rate patterns (Clapp 1990). APGAR scores of infants born to exercising mothers are similar to or higher than those of infants born to sedentary mothers (Clapp 1990, Kardel & Kase 1998, Lokey et al 1991, Sternfeld et al 1995).

Finally, maternal exercise during pregnancy may have an effect on newborn activity level and later development. During the early postnatal period, Clapp et al (1999) found that infants born to exercising mothers are more alert and more able to quieten themselves after exposure to stimuli than infants born to sedentary mothers. This may be the result of learned fetal responses to intermittent arousal stimulus produced by maternal exercise during gestation (Clapp et al 1999). Later in development, Clapp et al (1998) demonstrated that children of mothers who exercised during pregnancy had slightly better motor skills at 1 year of age. Further, at 5 years of age, they were leaner and performed better on standardized tests of intelligence than controls (Clapp 1996).

Placental effects

Maternal exercise has been shown to have effects on placental growth and composition (Clapp 2000, Clapp et al 1992, Jackson et al 1995). Ultrasound studies indicate that women who exercise during pregnancy have larger placentas (Clapp 2000, Clapp et al 1992). Jackson et al (1995) found that sustained exercise during pregnancy led to changes in placental composition and enhanced villous growth. These changes may increase placental perfusion and improve transport of nutrients and oxygen in the placentas of exercising women, enhancing fetal substrate availability during the periods of decreased uterine blood flow associated with exercise.

GUIDELINES FOR EXERCISE DURING PREGNANCY

Current data suggests that healthy women with an uncomplicated pregnancy may safely continue or begin a regular exercise program during pregnancy (Clapp 2000). Maternal symptoms should dictate the intensity of exercise (ACOG 1994, Hartmann & Bung 1999). Certain positions and types of sports should be avoided. For example, the supine position should be avoided as it may lead to decreased cardiac output (ACOG 1994). Also, activities which may cause abdominal trauma, like the martial arts and some ball sports, should be avoided (Hartmann & Bung 1999).

Contraindications to exercise during pregnancy include premature rupture of membranes, uterine bleeding, preterm labor and incompetent cervix (ACOG 1994, Hartmann & Bung 1999).

SUMMARY

As more women become active participants in sports and exercise, it becomes increasingly important to understand the health effects of such involvement. There are many health benefits associated with regular exercise in women. Sports participation can lead to improvements in strength, heat tolerance, and aerobic and anaerobic performance in women. Regular exercise can also improve the physical and psychological symptoms associated with pregnancy. Also, regular weightbearing exercise may improve bone density and overall bone health.

Despite these many benefits, female athletes participating at the elite level or in sports that emphasize leanness, are at particular risk for disordered eating and the female athlete triad. Since this can have important consequences for the female athlete's overall health, and bone health in particular, medical professionals and coaches should be aware of these issues. Athletes with signs of disordered eating or amenorrhea should be referred to a physician for a complete evaluation.

Finally, available evidence suggests that regular exercise is not only safe during pregnancy, but can offer important benefits for both mother and child. Exercise during pregnancy has not been associated with premature delivery, retardation of fetal growth, or problems with lactation. Women who exercise during pregnancy have fewer musculoskeletal complaints and depressive symptoms associated with pregnancy. Children born to exercising mothers demonstrate fewer signs of distress during labor and are more alert in the early postnatal period.

REFERENCES

Aaron D J, Dearwater S R, Anderson R et al 1996 Physical activity and the initiation of high risk activities in adolescents. Medicine and Science in Sports and Exercise 27:1639–1645

American College of Obstetrics and Gynecology (ACOG) 1994 Technical Bulletin Number 189. Washington, DC, ACOG Press

American College of Sports Medicine 1997 The female athlete triad. Medicine and Science in Sports and Exercise 26:i–ix

American Psychiatric Associaton 1994 Diagnostic and statistical manual of mental disorders, 4th edn (DSM-IV). American Psychiatric Association, Washingtion, DC

Artal R, Platt L D, Sperling M et al 1981 Maternal cardiovascular and metabolic responses in normal pregnancy. American Journal of Obstetrics and Gynecology 140:123–127

Ashley C D, Smith J F, Robinson J B et al 1996 Disordered eating in female collegiate athletes and collegiate females in an advanced program of study: a preliminary investigation. International Journal of Sports Nutrition 6:391–401

Ayalon J, Simkin A, Leichter I, et al 1987 Dynamic bone loading exercises for post menopausal women: effect on the density of the distal radius. Archives of Physical Medicine and Rehabilitation 68:280–283

Bachmann G A, Kemmann E 1982 Prevalence of oligomenorrhea and amenorrhea in a college population. American Journal of Obstetrics and Gynecology 144:98–102

Baker M M, Juhn M S 2000 Patellofemoral pain syndrome in the female athlete. Clinics in Sports Medicine 19:315–329

Bassey E J, Rothwell M C, Littlewood J J et al 1998 Pre- and postmenopausal women have different bone mineral density responses to the same high-impact exercise. Journal of Bone and Mineral Research 13:1805–1813

Baumann H, Hutch A, Huch R 1989 Doppler sonographic evaluation exercise-induced blood flow velocity and changes in fetal, uteroplacental and large maternal vessels in pregnant women. Journal of Perinatal Medicine 17:279–287

Becker A E, Grinspoon S K, Klibanski A et al 1999 Eating disorders. The New England Journal of Medicine 340:1092–1098

Beidleman B A, Rock P B, Muza S R et al 1999 Exercise V_E and physical performance at altitude are not affected by menstrual cycle phase. Journal of Applied Physiology 86:1519–1526

Beim G, Stone D A 1995 Issues in the female athlete. Sports Medicine 26:443–451

Bell R J, Palma S M, Lumley J M 1995 The effect of vigorous exercise during pregnancy on birth-weight. Australia and New Zealand Journal of Obstetrics and Gynecology 35:46–51

Bennell K L, Malcolm S A, Thomas S A et al 1995 Risk factors for stress fractures in female track-and-field athletes: a retrospective analysis. Clinical Journal of Sports Medicine 5:229–235

Bennell K L, Malcolm S A, Thomas S A 1996 Risk factors for stress fractures in track and field athletes: a twelve-month prospective study. American Journal of Sports Medicine 24:810–818

Bennell K, White S, Crossley K 1999 The oral contraceptive pill: a revolution for sportswomen? British Journal of Sports Medicine 33:231–238

Berg K 1984 Aerobic function in female athletes. Clinics in Sports Medicine 3:779–789

Bonds D R, Delivoria-Papadopoulos M 1985 Exercise during pregnancy – potential fetal and placental metabolic effects. Annals in Clinical and Laboratory Science 15:91–99

Bonjour J P, Theintz G, Buchs B et al 1991 Critical years and stages of puberty for spinal and femoral bone mass accumulation during adolescence. Journal of Clinical Endocrinology and Metabolism 73:555–563

Bryner R W, Toffle R C, Ullrich I H et al 1996 Effect of low dose oral contraceptives on exercise performance. British Journal of Sports Medicine 30:30–36

Bullen B A, Skrinar G S, Beitins I Z et al 1985 Induction of menstrual disorders by strenuous exercise in untrained women. The New England Journal of Medicine 312:1349–1353

Cann C E, Martin M C, Genant H K et al 1984 Decreased spinal mineral content in amenorrheic women. Journal of the American Medical Association 251:626–629

Cann C E, Cavanaugh D J, Schnurpfiel K et al 1988 Menstrual history is the primary determinant of the trabecular bone density in women. Medicine and Science in Sports and Exercise 20:S59

Capeless E L, Clapp J F 1989 Cardiovascular changes in early phase of pregnancy. American Journal of Obstetrics and Gynecology 161:1449–1453

Carpenter M W, Saddy S P, Hoegsberg B 1988 Fetal heart rate response to maternal exertion. Journal of the American Medical Association 259:3006–3009

Clapp J F 1985 Fetal heart rate response to running in midpregnancy and late pregnancy. American Journal of Obstetrics and Gynecology 153:251–252

Clapp J F 1989 The effects of maternal exercise on early pregnancy outcome. American Journal of Obstetrics and Gynecology 161:1453–1457

Clapp J F 1990 The course of labor after endurance exercise during pregnancy. American Journal of Obstetrics and Gynecology 163:1799–1805

Clapp J F 1991 The changing thermal response to endurance exercise during pregnancy. American Journal of Obstetrics and Gynecology 165:1684–1689

Clapp J F 1994 A clinical approach to exercise during pregnancy. Clinics in Sports Medicine 13:443–458

Clapp J F 1996 Morphometric and neurodevelopmental outcome at age five years of the offspring of women who continued to exercise regularly throughout pregnancy. Journal of Pediatrics 129:856–863

Clapp J F 2000 Exercise during pregnancy: a clinical update. Clinics in Sports Medicine 19:273–286

Clapp J F 2001 Exercise during pregnancy and lactation. In: Garret W E, Lester G E, McGowan J et al (eds) Women's health in sports and exercise. American Academy of Orthopaedic Surgeons, Maryland

Clapp J F, Dickstein S 1984 Endurance exercise and pregnancy outcome. Medicine and Science in Sports and Exercise 16:556–562

Clapp J F, Rizk K H 1992 Effect of recreational exercise on midtrimester placental growth. American Journal of Obstetrics and Gynecology 167:1518–1521

Clapp J F, Little K D 1995 Effect of recreational exercise on pregnancy weight gain and subcutaneous fat deposition. Medicine and Science in Sports and Exercise 27:170–177

Clapp J F, Wesley M, Sleamaker R H 1987 Thermoregulatory and metabolic responses to jogging prior to and during pregnancy. Medicine and Science in Sports and Exercise 19:124–130

Clapp J F, Rokey R, Treadway J L et al 1992 Exercise in pregnancy. Medicine and Science in Sports and Exercise 24:S294–S300

Clapp J F, Simonian S, Lopez B et al 1998 The one-year morphometric and neurodevelopmental outcome of the offspring of women who continued to exercise regularly throughout pregnancy. American Journal of Obstetrics and Gynecology 178:594–599

Clapp J F, Lopez B, Harcar-Sevcik R 1999 Neonatal behavioral profile of the offspring of women who continued to exercise regularly throughout pregnancy. American Journal of Obstetrics and Gynecology 180:91–94

Collings C A, Curet L B, Mullin J P 1983 Maternal and fetal responses to a maternal aerobic exercise program. American Journal of Obstetrics and Gynecology 145:702–707

Colton, Gore 1991 Risk, resiliency, and resistance: current research on adolescent girls. Ms. Foundation. New York, NY

Consensus Development Conference 1991 Prophylaxis and treatment of osteoporosis. American Journal of Medicine 90:107–110

Considine R V, Sinha M K, Heiman M L 1996 Serum immunoreactive-leptin concentrations in normal-weight and obese humans. The New England Journal of Medicine 334:292–295

Creighton D L, Morgan A L, Boardley D et al 2001 Weight-bearing exercise and markers of bone turnover in female athletes. Journal of Applied Physiology 90:565–570

Cumming D C 1996 Exercise-associated amenorrhea, low bone density and estrogen replacement therapy. Archives of Internal Medicine 156:2193–2195

Cureton K J, Sparling P B 1980 Distance running performance and metabolic responses to running in men and women with excess weight experimentally equated. Medicine and Science in Sports and Exercise 12:288–294

Cureton K J, Collins M A, Hill D W et al 1988 Muscle hypertrophy in men and women. Medicine and Science in Sports and Exercise 20:338–344

Daggett A, Davis B, Boobis L 1983 Physiological and biochemical responses to exercise following oral contraceptive use [abstract]. Medicine and Science in Sports and Exercise 15:174

Dawson-Hughes B, Harris S S, Krall E A et al 1990 A controlled trial of the effect of calcium supplementation on bone density in postmenopausal women. New England Journal of Medicine 323:878–883

Delmas P D 1992 Clinical use of biochemical markers of bone remodeling in osteoporosis. Bone 13:S17–S21

De Souza M J, Maguire M S, Rubin K R et al 1990 Effects of menstrual phase and amenorrhea on exercise performance in runners. Medicine and Science in Sports and Exercise 22:575–580

Dewey K G 1998 Effects of maternal caloric restriction and exercise during lactation. Journal of Nutrition 128:S386–S389

Dombovy M L, Bonekat H W, Williams T J et al 1987 Exercise performance and ventilatory response in the menstrual cycle. Medicine and Science in Sports and Exercise 19:111–117

Dook J E, Henderson N K, Price R I 1997 Exercise and bone mineral density in mature female athletes. Medicine and Science in Sports and Exercise 29:291–296

Drinkwater B L 1996 Exercise and bones lessons learned from female athletes. American Journal of Sports Medicine 24:S33–S35

Drinkwater B L, Nilson D, Chesnut C H et al 1984 Bone mineral content of amenorrheic and eumenorrheic athletes. The New England Journal of Medicine 311:277–281

Drinkwater B L, Nilson K, Ott S et al 1986 Bone mineral density after resumption of menses in amenorrheic athletes. Journal of the American Medical Association 256:380–382

Drinkwater B L, Bruemner B, Chesnut C H 1990 Menstrual history as a determinant of current bone density in young athletes. Journal of the American Medical Association 263:545–548

Drinkwater B L, Healy N L, Rencken M L et al 1993 Effectiveness of nasal calcitonin in preventing bone loss in young amenorrheic women [abstract]. Journal of Bone and Mineral Research 8:S264

Dueck C A, Matt K S, Manore M M et al 1996 Treatment of athletic amenorrhea with a diet and training intervention program. International Journal of Sports Nutrition. 6:24–40

Dummer G M, Rosen L W, Heusner W W et al 1987 Pathogenic weight-control behaviors of young competitive swimmers. The Physician and Sportsmedicine 15:75–78

Ebben W P, Jensen R L 1998 Strength training for women debunking myths that block opportunity. The Physician and Sportsmedicine 26:86–97

Eisenmann J C, Pivarnik J M, Malina R M 2001 Scaling peak VO₂ to body mass in young male and female distance runners. Journal of Applied Physiology 90:2172–2180

Ettinger B F, Genant H K, Cann C E 1985 Long term estrogen replacement therapy prevents bone loss and fractures. Annals of Internal Medicine 102:319–324

Fahey T D 1994 Endurance training. In: Shangold M M, Mirkin G (eds) Women and exercise: physiology and sports medicine, 2nd edn. FA Davis, Philadelphia, p. 73–88

Fleck S J, Falkel J E 1986 Value of resistance training for the reduction of sports injuries. Sports Medicine 3:61–68

Fogelholm M 1994 Effects of bodyweight reduction on sports performance. Sports Medicine 18:249–267

Fogelholm G M, Koskinen R, Laakso J et al 1993 Gradual and rapid weight loss: effects on nutrition and performance in male athletes. Medicine and Science in Sports and Exercise 25:371–377

Frankovich R J, Lebrun C M 2000 Menstrual cycle, contraception and performance. Clinics in Sports Medicine 19:251–271

Friedlander A L 1995 Two-year program of aerobics and weight training increases bone mineral density in young women. Journal of Bone and Mineral Research 10:574–585

Friedmann B, Weller E, Mairbaurl H et al 2001 Effects of iron repletion on blood volume and performance capacity in young athletes. Medicine and Science in Sports and Exercise 33:741–746

Fulkerson J A, Keel P K, Leon G R et al 1999 Eating-disordered behaviors and personality characteristics of high school athletes and nonathletes. International Journal of Eating Disorders 26:73–79

Garner D M 1991 The Eating Disorders Inventory-2. Psychological Assessment Resourses. Odessa, Florida

Garner D M, Garfinkel P E 1979 An index of symptoms of anorexia nervosa. Psychological Medicine 2:273–279

Garner D M, Olmstead M P, Polivy J 1983 Development and validation of a multidimensional eating disorder inventory for anorexia and bulimia. International Journal of Eating Disorders 2:15–34

Garner D M, Olmstead M P, Polivy J 1984 Manual of eating disorder inventory EDI. Psychological Assessment Resources. Odessa, Florida

Garner D M, Rosen L W, Barry D 1998 Eating disorders among athletes: research and recommendations. Sport Psychiatry 7:839–857

Giacomoni M, Bernard T, Gavarry O et al 2000 Influence of the menstrual cycle phase and menstrual symptoms on maximal anaerobic performance. Medicine and Science in Sports and Exercise 32:486–492

Green H J, Carter S, Grant S et al 1999 Vascular volumes and hematology in male and female runners and cyclists. European Journal of Applied Physiology and Occupational Physiology 79:244–250

Griffin L Y 1994 The female athlete In: DeLee J C, Drez D Jr (eds) Orthopedic sports medicine principles and practices. W B Saunders, Philadelphia, p 356–373

Grimston S K, Sanborn C F, Miller P D et al 1990 The application of historical data for evaluation of osteopenia in female runners: The menstrual index. Clinical Sports Medicine 2:108–118

Grimston S K, Willows N D, Hanley D A 1993 Mechanical loading regime and its relationship to bone mineral density in children. Medicine and Science in Sport and Exercise 25:1203–1210

Gulekli B, Davies M C, Jacobs H S 1994 Effect of treatment on established osteoporosis in young women with amenorrhea. Clinical Endocrinology 41:275–281

Haenggi W, Casez J P, Birkhaeuser M H et al 1994 Bone mineral density in young women with long-standing amenorrhea: limited effect of hormone replacement therapy ethinylestradiol and desogestrel. Osteoporosis International 4:99–103

Hale R W, Milne L 1996 The elite athlete and exercise in pregnancy. Seminars in Perinatology 20:277–284

Hall D C, Kaufmann D A 1987 Effects of aerobic and strength conditioning on pregnancy outcomes. American Journal of Obstetrics and Gynecology 157:1199–1203

Harber V J 2000 Menstrual dysfunction in athletes: an energetic challenge. Exercise and Sport Sciences Reviews 28:19–22

Hartman S, Bung P 1999 Physical exercise during pregnancy: physiological considerations and recommendations. Journal of Perinatal Medicine 27:204–215

Hauth J C, Gilstrap H C, Widmer K 1982 Fetal heart rate reactivity before and after maternal jogging during the third trimester. American Journal of Obstetrics and Gynecology 142:545–547

Hatch M, Shu X O, McLean D E et al 1993 Maternal exercise during pregnancy, physical fitness and fetal growth. American Journal of Epidemiology 137:1105–1114

Helgerud J 1994 Maximal oxygen uptake, anaerobic threshold and running economy in women and men with similar performances level in marathons. European Journal of Applied Physiology and Occupational Physiology 68:155–161

Hergenroeder A C, Smith E O, Shyailo R et al 1997 Bone mineral changes in young women with hypothalamic amenorrhea treated with oral contraceptives, medroxyprogesterone, or placebo over 12 months. American Journal of Obstetrics and Gynecology 176:1017–1025

Herzog W, Minne H, Deter C et al 1993 Outcome of bone mineral density in anorexia nervosa patients 11.7 years after first admission. Journal of Bone and Mineral Research 8:597–605

Hilton L K, Loucks A B 2000 Low energy availability, not exercise stress, suppresses the diurnal rhythm of leptin healthy young women. Endocrinology and Metabolism 278:E43–E49

Hinton P S, Giordano C, Brownlie T et al 2000 Iron supplementation improves endurance after training in iron-depleted, nonanemic women. Journal of Applied Physiology 88:1103–1111

Hoff J, Helegerud J, Wisloff U 1999 Maximal strength training improves work economy in trained female cross-country skiers. Medicine and Science in Sports and Exercise 31:807–877

Iketani T, Kiriike N, Nakanishi S et al 1995 Effects of weight gain and resumption of menses on reduced bone density in patients with anorexia nervosa. Biological Psychiatry 37:521–527

Ireland M L 1994 Special concerns of the female athlete. In: Fu F H, Stone D A (eds) Sports injuries: mechanism, prevention, and treatment, 2nd edn. Williams and Wilkins, Baltimore

Jackson M R, Gott P, Lye S J et al 1995 The effects of maternal aerobic exercise on human placental development: placental volumetric composition and surface areas. Placenta 16:179–191

Johnson M D 1994 Disordered eating in active and athletic women. Clinics in Sports Medicine 13:355–369

Johnson C, Powers P S, Dick R 1999 Athletes and eating disorders: the national collegiate athletic association study. International Journal of Eating Disorders 26:179–188

Jonnavithula S, Warren M P, Fox R P et al 1993 Bone density is compromised in amenorrheic women despite return of menses: a 2-year study. Obstetrics and Gynecology 81:669–674

Jurkowski J E, Jones N I, Walker C et al 1978 Ovarian hormonal responses to exercise. Journal of Applied Physiology 44:109–114

Kardel K R, Kase T 1998 Training in pregnant women: effects on fetal development and birth. American Journal of Obstetrics and Gynecology 178:280–286

Keen A D, Drinkwater B L 1997 Irreversible bone loss in former amenorrheic athletes. Osteoporosis International 4:311–315

Kihlstrand M, Steman B, Nilsson S et al 1999 Water-gymnastics reduced the intensity of back/low back pain in pregnant women. Acta Obstetricia et Gynecologica Scandinavia 78:180–185

Kirchner E M, Lewis R D, O'Connor P J 1995 Bone mineral density and dietary intake of female college gymnasts. Medicine and Science in Sports and Exercise 27:543–549

Klebanoff M A, Shiono P H, Carey J C 1990 The effect of physical activity during pregnancy on preterm delivery and birth weight. American Journal of Obstetrics and Gynecology 163:1450–1456

Klibanski A, Biller B M, Schoenfeld D A et al 1995 The effects of estrogen administration on trabecular bone loss in young women with anorexia nervosa. Journal of Clinical Endrocrinology and Metabolism 80:898–904

Komi P V (ed) 1992 Strength and power in sport. Blackwell Scientific Publication, Oxford, England

Kopp-Woodroffe S A, Manore M M, Dueck C A et al 1999 Energy and nutrient status of amenorrheic athletes participating in a diet and exercise training intervention program. International Journal of Sport Nutrition 9:70–88

Kraemer W J, Keuning M, Ratamess N A et al 2001 Resistance training combined with bench-step aerobics enhances women's health profile. Medicine and Science in Sports and Exercise 33:259–269

Kulpa P J, White B M, Visscher R 1986 Aerobic exercise in pregnancy. American Journal of Obstetrics and Gynecology 156:1395–1403

Laughlin G A, Yen S S 1997 Hypoleptinemia in women athletes: absence of a diurnal rhythm with amenorrhea. Journal of Clinical Endocrinology and Metabolism 82:318–321

Lebrun C M, McKenzie D C, Prior J C et al 1995 Effects of menstrual cycle phase on athletic performance. Medicine and Science in Sports and Exercise 27:437–444

Lehnhard R A, Lehnard H R, Young R et al 1996 Monitoring injuries on a college soccer team: the effect of strength training. Journal of Strength and Conditioning Research 10:115–119

Lloyd T, Triantafyllou S J, Baker E R et al 1986 Women athletes with menstrual irregularity have increased musculoskeletal injuries. Medicine and Science in Sports and Exercise 18:374–379

Lokey E A, Tran Z V, Wells C L et al 1991 Effects of physical exercise on pregnancy outcomes: a meta-analytic review. Medicine and Science in Sports and Exercise 23:1234–1239

Loucks A B 1990 Effects of exercise training on the menstrual cycle: existence and mechanisms. Medicine and Science in Sports and Exercise 22:275–280

Loucks A B, Horvath S M 1985 Athletic amenorrhea: a review. Medicine and Science in Sports and Exercise 17:56–72

Loucks A B, Callister R 1993 Induction and prevention of low-T_3 syndrome in exercising women. American Journal of Physiology 264:R924–R930

Loucks A B, Heath E M 1994 Induction of low-T_3 syndrome in exercising women occurs at a threshold of energy availability. American Journal of Physiology 35:R817–R823

Loucks A B, Mortola J F, Girton L et al 1989 Alterations in the hypothalamic-pituitary-ovarian and the hypothalamic-pituitary-adrenal axes in athletic women. Journal of Clinical Endocrinology and Metabolism 68:402–411

Loucks A B, Vaitukaitis J, Cameron J L et al 1992a The reproductive system and exercise in women. Medicine and Science in Sports and Exercise 24:S288–S292

Loucks A B, Laughlin G A, Mortola J F et al 1992b Hypothalamic-pituitary-thyroidal function in eumenorrheic and amenorrheic athletes. Journal of Clinical Endocrinology and Metabolism 75:514–518

Loucks A B, Heath E M, Law T et al 1994 Dietary restriction reduces luteinizing hormone pulse frequency during waking hours and increases LH pulse amplitude during sleep in young menstruating women. Journal of Clinical Endocrinology and Metabolism 78:910–915

Loucks A B, Verdun M, Heath E M 1998 Low energy availability, not stress of exercise, alters LH pulsatility in exercising women. Journal of Applied Physiology 84:37–46

Lovelady C A, Garner K E, Moreno K L et al 2000 The effect of weight loss in overweight, lactating women on the growth of their infants. New England Journal of Medicine 17:449–453

Lutter J M 1994 History of women in sports: societal issues. Clinics in Sports Medicine 13:263–279

McCrory M A, Nommsen-Rivers L A, Mole P A et al 1999 Randomized trial of the short-term effects of dieting compared with dieting plus aerobic exercise on lactation performance. American Journal of Clinical Nutrition 69:959–967

Maddalozzo G F, Snow C M 2000 High intensity resistance training:

effects on bone in older men and women. Calcified Tissue International 66:399–404

Malina R M, Ryan R C, Bonci C M 1994 Age at menarche in athletes and their mothers and sisters. Annals of Human Biology 21:417–422

Marcus R, Cann C, Madvig P et al 1985 Menstrual function and bone mass in elite women distance runners. Annals of Internal Medicine 102:158–163

Marcus R T, Drinkwater B, Dalsky G et al 1992 Osteoporosis and exercise in women. Medicine and Science in Sports and Exercise 24:S301–S307

Marshall J D, Harber V J 1996 Body dissatisfaction and drive for thinness in high performance: field hockey athletes. International Journal of Sports Medicine 17:541–544

Milunsky A, Ulcickas M, Rothman K J et al 1992 Maternal heat exposure and neural tube defects. Journal of the American Medical Society 268:882–885

Mirkin G 1994 Nutrition for Sports. In: Shangold M, Mirkin G (eds) Women and exercise physiology and sports medicine, 2nd edn. F A Davis, Philadelphia

Myburgh K H, Hutchins J, Gataar A B et al 1990 Low bone density is an etiologic factor for stress fractures in athletes. Annals of Internal Medicine 113:754–759

Myburgh K H, Bachrach L K, Lewis B et al 1993 Low bone mineral density at axial and appendicular sites in amenorrheic athletes. Medicine and Science in Sports and Exercise 25:1197–1202

Myerson M, Gutin B, Warren M P 1991 Resting metabolic rate and energy balance in amenorrheic and eumenorrheic runners. Medicine and Science in Sports and Exercise 23:15–22

Nattiv A 2001 The female athlete triad. In: Garrett W E, Lester G E, McGowan J et al (eds) Women's health in sports and exercise. American Academy of Orthopaedic Surgeons, Laurel, MD

Nattiv A, Agostini R, Drinkwater B et al 1994 The female athlete triad. The inter-relatedness of disordered eating, amenorrhea and osteoporosis. Clinics in Sports Medicine 13:405–418

Nattiv A, Arendt E A, Hecht S S 2001 The female athlete. In: Garrett W E, Kirkendall D T, Squire D L (eds) Principles and practice of primary care sports medicine. Lippincott Williams and Wilkins, Philadelphia

National Collegiate Athletic Association 1997 NCAA Division I Graduation Rates Report 1997. National Collegiate Athletic Association, Indianapolis, Indiana

Nichols D L, Bonnick S L, Sandborn C F 2000 Bone health and osteoporosis. Clinics in Sports Medicine 19:233–249

Nicklas B J, Hackney A C, Sharp R L 1989 The menstrual cycle and exercise: performance, muscle glycogen, and substrate responses. International Journal of Sports Medicine 10:264–269

Notelovitz M, Zauner C, McKenzie L et al 1987 The effect of low-dose oral contraceptives on cardiorespiratory function, coagulation, and lipids in exercising young women: a preliminary report. American Journal of Obstetrics and Gynecology 156:591–598

Nunneley S A 1979 Physiological responses of women to thermal stress: a review. Medicine and Science in Sports and Exercise 10:250–255

O'Connor P J, Lewis R D, Kirchner E M 1995 Eating disorder symptoms in female college gymnasts. Medicine and Science in Sports and Exercise 27:550–555

O'Neill M E 1996 Maternal rectal temperature and fetal heart rate responses to upright cycling in late pregnancy. British Journal of Sports Medicine 30:32–35

O'Toole M L, Douglas P S 1994 Fitness: definition and development. In: Shangold M, Mirkin G (eds) Women and exercise. Physiology and sports medicine, 2nd edn. FA Davis, Philadelphia

Otis C L 1992 Exercise-associated amenorrhea. Clinics in Sports Medicine 11:351–362

Palla B, Litt I F 1988 Medical complications of eating disorders in adolescents. Pediatrics 81:631–623

Pivarnik J M, Marichal C J, Spillman T et al 1992 Menstrual cycle phase affects temperature regulation during endurance exercise. Journal of Applied Physiology 72:543–548

Pivarnik J M, Ayres N A, Mauer M B et al 1993 Effects of maternal aerobic fitness on cardiorespiratory responses to exercise. Medicine and Science in Sports and Exercise 25:993–998

Pivarnik J M, Mauer M B, Ayres N A et al 1994 Effects of chronic exercise on blood volume expansion and hematologic indices during pregnancy. Obstetrics and Gynecology 83:265–269

Polatti F, Perotti F, Filippa N et al 1995 Bone mass and long-term monophasic oral contraceptive treatment in young women. Contraception 51:221–224

Pollitzer W S, Anderson J B 1989 Ethnic and genetic differences in bone mass: a review with a hereditary versus environmental perspective. American Journal of Clinical Nutrition 50:1244–1259

Pomeroy C, Mitchell J E 1992 Medical issues in the eating disorders. In: Brownell K D, Rodin J, Wilmor J H (eds) Eating, body weight and performance in athletes. Disorders in modern society. Lea and Febiger, Philadelphia

Prestwood K M, Pilbeam C C, Burleson J A et al 1994 The short term effects of conjugated estrogen on bone turnover in older women. Journal of Clinical Endocrinology and Metabolism 79:366–371

Prior J C, Vigna Y M, Barr S I et al 1994 Cyclic medroxyprogesterone treatment increases bone density: a controlled trial in active women with menstrual cycle disturbances. The American Journal of Medicine 96:521–530

Pruitt L A, Jackson R D, Bartels R L 1992 Weight training effects on bone mineral density in early postmenopausal women. Journal of Bone and Mineral Research 7:179–185

Pugliese M T, Lipshitz F, Grad G et al 1983 Fear of obesity: a cause of short stature and delayed puberty. The New England Journal of Medicine 309:513–518

Quirk J E, Sinning W E 1982 Anaerobic and aerobic responses of males and female to rope skipping. Medicine and Science in Sports and Exercise 14:26–29

Rauramo J, Forss M 1988 Effect of exercise on maternal hemodynamics and placental blood flow in healthy women. Acta Obstetricia et Gynecologica Scandinavia 67:21–25

Rhea D J 1999 Eating disorder behavior of ethnically diverse urban female adolescent athletes and non-athletes. Journal of Adolescence 22:379–388

Rigotti N A, Neer R M, Skates S J et al 1991 The clinical course of osteoporosis in anorexia nervosa: a longitudinal study of cortical bone mass. Journal of the American Medical Association 265:1133–1138

Rosen L W, Hough D O 1986 Pathogenic weight-control behavior of female college gymnasts. The Physician and Sportsmedicine. 16:141–144

Rosen L W, McKeag D B, Hough D O et al 1986 Pathogenic weight-control behavior in female athletes. The Physician and Sportsmedicine 14:79–86

Ruiz J C, Mandel C, Garabedian M 1995 Influence of spontaneous calcium intake and physical exercise on the vertebral and femoral bone mineral density of children and adolescents. Journal of Bone and Mineral Research 10:675–682

Sabatier J P, Guaydier-Souquieres G, Laroche D et al 1996 Bone mineral acquisition during adolescence and early adulthood: a study in 574 healthy females 10–24 years of age. Osteoporosis International 6:141–148

Sady S P, Freedson P S 1984 Body composition and structural comparisons of female and male athletes. Clinics in Sports Medicine 3:755–777

Sanborn C F, Jankowski C M 1994 Physiologic considerations for women in sport. Clinics in Sports Medicine 13:315–327

Schoene R B, Robertson H T, Pierson D J et al 1981 Respiratory drives and exercise in menstrual cycles of athletic and nonathletic women. Journal of Applied Physiology 50:1300–1305

Serresse O, Ama P F, Simoneau J A et al 1989 Anaerobic performances of sedentary and trained subjects. Canadian Journal of Sport Science 14:46–52

Shangold M, Rebar R, Wetz A C et al 1990 Evaluation and management of menstrual dysfunction in athletes. Journal of the American Medical Association 263:1665–1669

Shephard R J 2000 Exercise and training in women, part I: influence of gender on exercise and training responses. Canadian Journal of Applied Physiology 25:19–34

Simikin A, Ayalon J, Leichter I 1987 Increased trabecular bone density due to bone loading exercises in postmenopausal osteoporotic women. Calcified Tissue International 40:59–63

Slemenda C, Christian J, Williams C 1991 Genetic determinants of bone mass in adult women: a reevaluation of the twin model and the potential importance of gene interaction on heritability estimates. Journal of Bone and Mineral Research 6:561–567

Snow-Harter C M 1994 Bone health and prevention of osteoporosis in active and athletic women. Clinics in Sports Medicine 13:389–404

Snow-Harter C, Bouxsein ML, Lewis BT et al 1992 Effects of resistance and endurance exercise on bone mineral status of young women: a randomized exercise intervention trial. Journal of Bone and Mineral Research 7:761–769

Soultanakis H N, Artal R, Wiswell R A 1996 Prolonged exercise in pregnancy: glucose homeostasis, ventilatory and cardiovascular responses. Seminars in Perinatology 20:315–327

Sparling P B 1980 A meta-analysis of studies comparing maximal oxygen uptake in men and women. Research Quarterly for Exercise and Sport 51:542–552

Stephenson L A, Kolka M A 1993 Hemoregulation in women. Exercise and Sport Science Review 21:231–262

Sternfeld B, Quesenberry C P, Eskenazi B et al 1995 Exercise during pregnancy and pregnancy outcome. Medicine and Science in Sports and Exercise 27:634–640

Stevenson J C, Hillard T C, Lees B et al 1993 Postmenopausal bone loss: does HRT always work? International Jounal of Infertility and Menopausal Study 28 (suppl): 88–91

Stone M H, Triplett-McBride T, Stone M E 2001 Strength training for women: intensity, volume and exercise selection factors. In: Garrett W E, Lester G E, McGowan J et al (eds) Women's health in sports and exercise. American Academy of Orthopaedic Surgeons, Laurel, MD

Sundgot-Borgen J 1993a Prevalence of eating disorders in elite female athletes. International Journal of Sport Nutrition 3:29–40

Sundgot-Borgen J 1993b Nutrient intake of female elite athletes suffering from eating disorder. International Journal of Sport Nutrition 3:431–442

Sundgot-Borgen J 1994 Risk and trigger factors for the development of eating disorders in female elite athletes. Medicine and Science in Sports and Exercise 26:414–419

Sundgot-Borgen J, Corbin C B 1987 Eating disorders among female athletes. The Physician and Sportsmedicine 15:89–95

Sundgot-Borgen J, Larsen S 1993 Preoccupation with weight and menstrual function in female elite athletes. Scandinavian Journal of Medicine and Science in Sports and Exercise 3:156–163

Sundgot-Borgen J, Klungland M 1998 The female athlete triad and the effect of preventive work. Medicine and Science in Sports and Exercise 30:S181

Sundgot-Borgen J, Sundgot-Schneider L 2001 The long term effect of CBT and nutritional counseling in treating bulimic elite athletes: a randomized controlled study. Medicine and Science in Sports and Exercise 33:S97

Taaffe D R, Snow-Harter C, Connolly D A et al 1995 Differential effects of swimming versus weight-bearing activity on bone mineral status of eumenorrheic athletes. Journal of Bone and Mineral Research 10:586–593

Taub D E, Blinde E M 1992 Eating disorders among adolescent female athletes: influence of athletic participation and sport team membership. Adolescence 27:832–848

Veille J C 1996 Maternal and fetal cardiovascular response to exercise during pregnancy. Seminars in Perinatology 20:250–262

Veille J C, Hohimer A R, Burry K et al 1985 The effect of exercise on uterine activity in the last eight weeks of pregnancy. American Journal of Obstetrics and Gynecology 151:727–730

Veille J C, Bacevice A E, Wilson B et al 1989 Umbilical artery waveform during bicycle exercise in normal pregnancy. Obstetrics and Gynecology 73:957–960

Veldhuis J D, Evans W S, Demers L M et al 1985 Altered neuroendocrine regulation of gonadotropin secretion in women distance runners. Journal of Clinical Endocrinology and Metabolism 61:557–563

Warren B J, Stanton A L, Blessing D L 1990 Disordered eating patterns in competitive female athletes. International Journal of Eating Disorders 9:565–569

Warren M P, Fox R P, DeRogatis A J et al 1994 Osteopenia in

hypothalamic amenorrhea: a 3 year longitudinal study [abstract]. Program of the Endocrine Society Annual Meeting, Anaheim, California

Webster S, Rutt R, Weltman A 1990 Physiological effects of a weight loss regimen practiced by college wrestlers. Medicine and Science in Sports and Exercise 22:229–234

Weight L M, Noakes T D 1987 Is running an analog of anorexia?: a survey of the incidence of eating disorders in female distance runners. Medicine and Science in Sports and Exercise 19:213–217

Wells C 1985 Physiologic differences and similarities. In: Wells C (ed) Women, sports and performance: a physiological perspective. Human Kinetics, Champaign, IL, p 19–34

Wiebe C G, Gledhill N, Warburtion D E et al 1998 Exercise cardiac function in endurance-trained males versus females. Clinical Journal of Sports Medicine 8:272–279

Williams T J, Krahenbuhl G S 1997 Menstrual cycle phase and running economy. Medicine and Science in Sports and Exercise 29:1609–1618

Williams N I, Young J C, McArthur J W et al 1995 Strenuous exercise with caloric restriction: effect on luteinizing hormone secretion. Medicine and Science in Sports and Exercise 27:1390–1398

Wilmore J H 1983 Body composition in sport and exercise: directions for future research. Medicine and Science in Sports and Exercise 15:21–31

Wilmore J H 1991 Eating and weight disorders in the female athlete. International Journal of Sport Nutrition 1:104–117

Wilson Report 1989 Moms, dads, daughters and sports. Women's Sports Foundation. East Meadow, NY

Wolman R L, Clark P, NcNally E et al 1990 Menstrual state and exercise as determinants of spinal trabecular bone density in female athletes. British Journal of Sports Medicine 301:516–518

Women's Sports Foundation Report 1998 Sport and teen pregnancy. Womens Sport Foundation. East Meadow, NY

Zanker C L, Swaine I L 1998a Bone turnover in amenorrhoeic and eumenorrhoeic women distance runners. Scandinavian Journal of Medicine Science and Sports 8:20–26

Zanker C L, Swaine I L 1998b Relation between bone turnover, oestradiol, and energy balance in women distance runners. British Journal of Sports Medicine 32:167–171

Zanker C L, Swaine I L 1998c The relationship between serum oestradiol concentration and energy balance in young women distance runners. International Journal of Sports Medicine 19:104–108

27

Athletes with disability

Zoë Hudson   Amy Brown

INTRODUCTION

The history of sport and disability lies in the field of medical rehabilitation. Dr Ludwig Guttmann is generally recognized as one of the main pioneers and is known as 'the father of disabled sport'. As a neurosurgeon at Stoke Mandeville hospital in the UK towards the end of the Second World War, he saw that sport had a valuable role to play in the rehabilitation of physically disabled service men, and specifically those with spinal cord related injuries who were confined to wheelchairs. In 1948, the first 'games' took place at Stoke Mandeville and by 1960 the first Paralympic Games were held in Rome following the Olympic Games. Since Seoul in 1988, the Paralympics have always been held in the same place as the Olympic Games, with the athletes using the same venues and competition sites. Since 1960 there has been an exponential rise in both the number of countries and the number of athletes competing. At the Sydney 2000 Paralympic Games there were 4000 competitors representing 123 countries (Searle 2000). This increase reflects the growing interest and participation of people with a disability in sport. This growth has developed, in part, through an increased public awareness and participation in physical activity and recreational sports. At the same time, a myriad of sports organizations now exist that provide information, coordination, and support for people with all levels of physical and mental impairment who wish to participate in sporting activity.

The International Paralympic Committee reported that over 500 million people worldwide are affected by disabilities (Sydney Paralympic Organizing Committee 2000). The Paralympic Games are a good reflection of the progression and development of sport and disability. The significance of the Paralympic Games for disabled-bodied athletes, so-called because they are parallel to the Olympic Games, is similar to that of the Olympic Games to the able-bodied. Competition at the 1996 Games involved 17 events, 14 of which were conducted under the same rules as their Olympic counterparts. The majority of these contests were seen in the same stadiums and venues. The Paralympic athletes shared parallel stories of dedication, sacrifice, past failure or injury and, at times, controversy in arriving at the elite level of their sport. For this reason, this chapter will describe sport and disability in the context of elite athletes at the Paralympic Games. This is not intended to diminish other events such as the Special Olympics, which is a large international sporting organization for people with learning disabilities. There are many thousands of disabled-bodied athletes competing at the non-elite level and it is due to the lack of available literature that they are not covered in this chapter.

BENEFITS OF EXERCISE FOR PEOPLE WITH DISABILITY

The physiological and psychological benefits of exercise for those with and without disability have been well documented (Durstine et al 2000). Physical benefits of exercise include improved cardiopulmonary function, strength, muscle coordination, and balance. In some cases, functional ability of the disabled may improve through physical training; for example, gait quality and speed improved with strength training in a study of those with spastic cerebral palsy (Damiano & Abel 1998). Preliminary findings of the effect of an aerobic training program on lower extremity amputee subjects suggested a decrease in the metabolic cost of ambulation (Ward & Meyers 1995). A strength and flexibility training program has been shown to decrease the prevalence of shoulder pain in long-time wheelchair users (Curtis et al 1999b). The physically active disabled population may also enjoy decreased comorbidities such as diabetes, heart disease and obesity (Rimmer 1999). Psychologically, too, exercise can enhance mood, self-confidence, and self-esteem (Shephard 1991). Labronici et al (2000) studied the effects of sport participation over a 2-year period and found that the sport group showed higher levels of vigor, lower levels of depression, and improved social integration. Improved community integration that included satisfaction with leisure activities, social contacts, and relationships with partners was reported in wheelchair athletes, in comparison to predisability levels of function (Pluym et al 1997). However, along with the benefits of exercise, there is also an inherent risk of injury. Injury patterns in athletes with disability have been shown to be similar to their able-bodied counterparts, but the location of injuries appears to be disability and sport dependent (Ferrara & Peterson 2000). Much of the data collected to

date have been facilitated by increasing numbers of participants at competition and records kept of those seeking medical attention. Some predictable patterns of injury related to sport, disability, or adaptive equipment were identified in the 1996 Summer Paralympic Games (Nyland et al 2000.) The injury experience for the disabled ski athlete was also found to be similar to the able-bodied athlete in terms of extremity involvement and total injury history (Ferrara et al 1992). A further study by Laskowski & Murtaugh (1992) found disabled skiers incur less severe injuries than the able-bodied. Much information has also been gained by self-report of injury and retrospective study. One such valuable source was the Athletes with Disabilities Injury Registry that detailed risk and severity of injury to disabled athletes from 1990 to 1992 (Ferrara & Buckley 1996). Management of medical problems specific to the physically challenged athlete is also a consideration (Dec et al 2000). This chapter will describe the different sports and disabilities and how different impairments are classified.

SPORTS

There are five main categories of disability with respect to sport: visual impairment, cerebral palsy, intellectual disability, amputees, and wheelchair athletes. Each disability or impairment has its own organization for registration, governing rules, and regulation of sporting events at the local, regional, and national levels of competition (Table 27.1). The United States Olympic Committee (USOC) and International Paralympic Committee (IPC) oversee sanctioned events for Paralympic qualification. The International Olympic Committee (IOC) is the top of this organizational structure presiding over both the USOC and the IPC at all Olympic sanctioned international sporting events.

Table 27.1 Disability associations in the USA and internationally

Disability	National organization	International organization
Amputee	Disability Sports USA	International Sport Organization for the Disabled
Cerebral palsy	US Cerebral Palsy Athletic Association	Cerebral Palsy Sport and Recreation Association
Intellectual disability	Special Olympics[a]	International Sports Federation for People with Intellectual Disability
Visual impairment	US Association of Blind Athletes	International Blind Sport Association
Wheelchair sport	Wheelchair Sports USA	International Stoke Mandeville Wheelchair Sport Federation

[a] Not under the auspices of the International Paralympic Committee

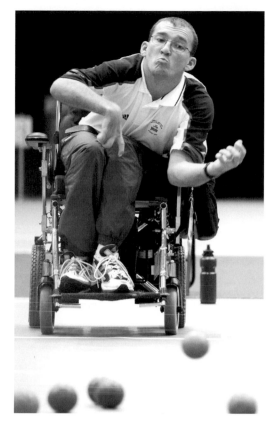

Figure 27.1 Boccia player. (Reproduced with permission of © Allsport, UK Ltd.)

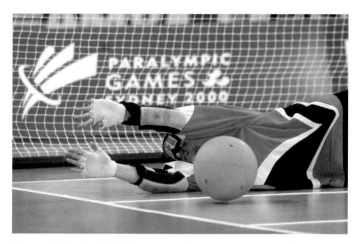

Figure 27.2 Goalball player attempting to block the ball. (Reproduced with permission of © Allsport, UK Ltd.)

Box 27.1 Medal sports at the most recent Summer and Winter Paralympic Games	
Summer Olympic sports	
Archery	Swimming
Athletics	Table tennis
Basketball	Tennis
Wheelchair dance	Volleyball
Equestrian	Boccia[a]
Fencing	Goalball[a]
Judo	Wheelchair Basketball[a]
Powerlifting	Wheelchair Rugby[a]
Sailing	Wheelchair Fencing[a]
Shooting	Wheelchair Tennis[a]
Winter Olympic sports	
Cross-country skiing	
Ice sledge race	
Ice sledge hockey	
Alpine ski racing	
Biathlon	
[a] Unique to Paralympic Games	

Disabled athletes participate in a variety of sports that can either be described as the same as or a modified version of the able-bodied counterpart, or as a disability-specific sport. Boccia, for example, is a disability-specific sport. It has been adapted from boules or petanques, and is played by people with cerebral palsy using a wheelchair during competition. It is a game of precision whereby the athlete attempts to throw leather balls as close to the jack as possible, down a long, narrow playing field (Fig. 27.1). Boccia can be played in an individual or team format.

Goalball is a sport designed to be played by athletes with a visual impairment. Two teams of six players compete, with only three from each team allowed on the court at any one time. The aim is to score by getting the ball over the opponent's goal line; the athletes defend their goal line by trying to block the ball using their body (Fig. 27.2). The ball has a bell inside and can only be thrown underarm. The players need to concentrate on the sound from the ball, therefore requiring all spectators to be silent.

While these are two examples of disability-specific sports, most sports are the same as, or adapted from, able-bodied sport (Fig. 27.3). Box 27.1 shows the sports that are currently sanctioned at Paralympic competition.

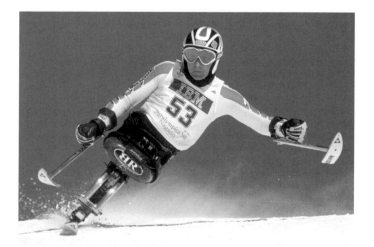

Figure 27.3 Alpine skiing at the Winter Paralympic Games. (Reproduced with permission of © Allsport, UK Ltd.)

This list has continued to evolve and does not reflect the numerous other sporting events or recreational activities that are available to the disabled athlete at the local and regional level. Although no exhibition sports were included at the Sydney 2000 Paralympic Games, increasing participation in yachting and wheelchair rugby was the force behind the move to include these competitions in Sydney after they were non-medal events in Atlanta 1996. With this trend, the addition of more sports may be anticipated in future Paralympic Games.

CLASSIFICATION FOR COMPETITION

It is often hard for a layperson to comprehend the complex classification system within the various disabled-bodied competitions. The purpose of any classification system is an attempt to create parity in competition, and to this effect, it is no different to classification systems that exist in able-bodied sport, such as different weight categories in boxing. Classification in disability sport has traditionally been structured by the disability. However, in several sports, a change of emphasis is developing away from the medical disability towards the athlete's level of function. Each sport has a different classification structure. Sports that utilize a functional classification system commonly have a classification team that conducts examinations on the athletes. A classification team may typically include a physician, physical therapist or athletic trainer, and a sports technician. Range of motion, strength, balance, and motor coordination are evaluated and assigned a point value in phase one of the evaluation. The second phase is actual assessment of sport performance with point values assigned for biomechanics and sport-specific abilities. The sum of these points is used to determine classification. Most athletes with cerebral palsy are typically classified by this manner, although again, it is sport dependent. The medical model is typically utilized for classification of amputee athletes, the visually impaired, and those with spinal lesions. Readers are referred to www.paralympic.org for a complete account of classification systems for disabled-bodied sports. Tables 27.2 and 27.3 illustrate the differences between the classification structures in track and field, and swimming respectively.

For track and field classification, the letters 'T', 'F', or 'P' indicate whether the event is on the track, field, or pentathlon. These letters will precede class numbers in the classification system. In swimming, the prefix 'S' is used for backstroke, butterfly, and freestyle, 'SB' for breaststroke, and 'SM' for the individual medley. Therefore, a swimmer with no light perception at all in either eye, and who is competing in the 200 m individual

Table 27.2 Classification for athletes competing in track and field events

Class	Description
11–13	Different levels of visual impairment
20	Learning disability
33–38	Athletes with cerebral palsy (with and without wheelchairs)
42–46	Ambulant athletes with different levels of amputation and other disabilities
51–58	Wheelchair athletes with different levels of spinal cord injury and amputations

Table 27.3 Classification for athletes competing in swimming events

Class	Description
1–10	Wheelchair athletes, amputees and those with cerebral palsy
11–13	Different levels of visual impairment
14	Learning disability

medley, will race in class 200 m SM11. In classes 1 to 10, the higher the class number, the greater the degree of functional ability.

Team sports such as wheelchair basketball and wheelchair rugby operate on a points system, whereby each player is given a points rating according to their level of physical function. For example, an athlete with a lower spinal lesion who has better trunk control and upper limb function would have a higher rating than someone with a higher lesion and less function. In wheelchair basketball, the points range from 1 (the lowest) to 4.5, and a team is not allowed more than 14 points between the five players on court at any one time.

The classification process has often come under criticism, partly due to the subjectivity in the functional classification process. While the functional process seeks to create an equal ground for competition, there has been concern that training effects may be confused with functional ability. In this system, those athletes who may have improved through training alone may be penalized if they 'over-perform' during testing and be reclassified to compete against athletes with lesser disability. Athletes can be classified many times during their sporting career, and it is not unusual to move up or down a class. It has been suggested that classification could be exploited by athletes wishing to gain an unfair advantage, and that this is the disability sports equivalent of doping (Firth 1999). The lengths that some athletes go to achieve success has been illustrated by the Spanish team who won the gold medal in the intellectual disability basketball game at the Sydney 2000 Paralympic Games. It was subsequently discovered that there were members in the team who were not at all intellectually disabled.

ATHLETES WITH CEREBRAL PALSY

Cerebral Palsy (CP) is the term used to refer to a non-progressive group of brain disorders resulting from a lesion or developmental abnormality in fetal life or early infancy. CP is characterized by altered muscle tone, adaptive length changes in muscles, poor coordination and control of movement, and in some cases, skeletal deformity (Shepherd 1995). Disorders of movement are typically differentiated and classified clinically in terms of tone and involuntary movement. There are five main descriptors:

* *Spastic:* involving tight muscles and limited range of motion
* *Athetoid:* involving slow writhing and purposeless movement
* *Hypotonic:* having low tone of extremities and/or poor trunk control
* *Ataxic:* involving balance and gait deficits
* *Mixed lesions:* involving multiple factors as above.

CP can be further classified depending on the part of the body involved, using terms such as monoplegia, diplegia, triplegia, hemiplegia, paraplegia, or quadriplegia. CP can also be associated with cognitive deficits, deafness, visual impairment, dysphagia, seizures, speech, and communication disorders. According to the degree of impairment, athletes may be ambulant or wheelchair dependent.

The physiological benefits of exercise and CP have been well documented. Hutzler et al (1998) showed a 65% increase in the baseline vital capacity of children with CP who embarked on a 6-month exercise program that included swimming, in comparison to an increase of 23% in the control group. Energy consumption is higher in CP athletes and is dependent on the extent of impairment. Duffy et al (1996) examined the energy expenditure in ambulant children with and without CP. The rate of oxygen consumption was significantly higher in those with CP, and higher in those with diplegia as opposed to hemiplegia. Duffy and colleagues attributed abnormal equilibrium reactions to the increased expenditure in those with diplegia. Use of orthoses or appropriate bracing for those with spastic CP may help to lower ambulatory energy expense (Maltais et al 2001). Cocontraction of lower extremity muscle groups has also been implicated as a significant factor in increased energy cost in gait of those with spastic CP (Unnithan et al 1996). Due consideration, therefore, must be made to the intensity of training programs and recovery times needed for an athlete with CP. As the motor impairment is the result of an alteration of the descending pathways, the concept of trying to alter movement patterns in terms of training and technique is contentious. It was previously believed that strengthening programs may create increased negative tone in those with spasticity. Recent research on children with either spastic diplegia or hemiplegia demonstrated that strength programs improved both motor function and gait quality in this group (Damiano & Abel 1998). Massage is commonly used in practice both before and after sporting activity for able-bodied athletes. Theoretically, massage can have either an excitatory or an inhibitory effect on muscle tone. Therefore athletes with CP must be cautious with the utilization of massage in the training program, especially if the athlete is reliant on tone for sport performance. Massage has been advocated in those with hypotonic muscles, but contraindicated in spastics and athetoids (Levitt 1982). There have been some anecdotal reports of the benefits of massage for athletes with CP (Clews 1995, Stewart 2000), but otherwise there is a paucity of research in the available literature. As with able-bodied athletes, it is important that the inclusion of massage in an athlete's schedule has been explored in training and not just introduced at a competition when it may be more readily available.

Maintaining flexibility is important for those with spasticity, and proprioceptive neuromuscular facilitation techniques can be employed by the therapist to address the muscle groups affected. As with massage, this may also affect the tone that the athlete relies on for stability and function, and thus the effect of stretching techniques must be assessed on an individual basis. The physical therapist also needs to consider the positioning of these athletes during assessment and treatment, from both a safety and tone aspect. Narrow portable treatment couches may be unsafe, and in the prone position lying may increase tone and therefore be inappropriate.

In competition, CP athletes are susceptible to a wide variety of injury. At the 1996 Summer Paralympic Games, CP athletes were treated most frequently for soft tissue injuries or muscle strains of the low back, lower extremities, foot, and ankle (Nyland et al 2000). Those who compete in wheelchairs sustain injuries common to all wheelchair athletes, largely to the upper extremities. Standing athletes are harder to pattern, largely because CP athletes are the least homogeneous group. For those athletes who use ankle-foot orthoses or other orthoses, special attention should be paid to skin for signs of redness or breakdown. Some athletes who compete in standing events utilize crutches; these should be appropriately padded to avoid friction and pressure injury.

ATHLETES WITH LEARNING DISABILITIES

Athletes with learning disabilities may or may not present the physical therapist with any different physical problems from those of able-bodied athletes. For many individuals, the physiological potential is independent of the mental deficit. However, in some conditions such as Down syndrome and other forms of mental disability, the maximal heart rate is lower and may impact on training programs (Fernhall et al 2001). Target heart rate during intense training should be adjusted appropriately. Exercise has been shown to have some positive effects on both gait and bone metabolism in people with profound mental disability (Lancioni et al 2000). The physical therapist must understand the limitations of cognitive impairment and have realistic expectations both of physical and mental ability. Management must be tailored to account for the cognitive impairments that may exist. If dysarthria or expressive deficits exist, the therapist should allow appropriate time for the athlete to communicate. Signboards, gesture, or written communication may be utilized. Second party communication by the athlete's family or assistant should be utilized only as necessary to avoid miscommunications with the athlete. Athletes with learning disabilities may have difficulties understanding injury processes and explanations for the rationale behind therapeutic interventions. Problems with retention and recollection are often exhibited. The physical therapist on subsequent treatments should repeat an explanation for an intervention that was given at the initial instigation. Reiteration is very important with this group of athletes to facilitate comprehension and understanding. For example, in order to ensure adequate hydration during training and competition, checks may need to be made that all athletes have their own water bottles. The athletes may also need to be reminded to consume fluid at regular intervals. Prophylactic exercise based programs, such as core stability work or rehabilitation programs postinjury, may need to be formally supervised to ensure compliance and correct technique.

To be eligible to compete in the Paralympic Games, an athlete with learning disabilities has to meet minimum disability criteria, which in accordance with the World Health Organization (WHO) definition is determined by:

• An IQ score below 70
• Limitations in regular skills areas (e.g. communication, self care, social skills, etc.)
• Onset of learning disability before the age of 18 years.

ATHLETES WITH VISUAL IMPAIRMENT

Athletes with visual impairment are normally classified under one of three categories from B1 to B3 according to the International Blind Sports Association (IBSA) (Table 27.4).

Table 27.4 Classification of visually impaired athletes (International Blind Sport Association)

Class	Description
B1	No light perception at all in either eye, or may have some light perception but an inability to recognize the shape of a hand at any distance or in any direction
B2	Can recognize the shape of a hand, and has the ability to perceive clearly up to 2/60. The visual field is less than 5°
B3	Can recognize the shape of a hand, and has the ability to perceive clearly from 2/60 to 6/60. The visual field more than 5° and less than 20°

The effect of visual impairment and musculoskeletal dysfunction is an area that to date has been poorly researched. In competition, visually impaired athletes have been found to have higher numbers of lower extremity injuries (Ferrara 2000), which are often attributed to an increased risk of accidents and inadvertent collisions. Further investigation may also implicate gait mechanics as a possible factor for increased incidence of lower extremity injury. Compared to those with sighted gait, the visually impaired demonstrate shorter stride length, slower walking speed, and longer stance phase (Nakamura 1997). When attention is diverted to another task, gait quality may be significantly and potentially negatively altered (Ramsey et al 1999). These factors have the potential to create a higher incidence in overuse type injuries in the lower extremities.

Cervicothoracic complaints were also commonly reported by visually impaired athletes during the 1996 Summer Paralympic Games (Nyland et al 2000). This was suggested to be related to higher velocity injuries such as falls or rapid direction changes. However, the nature of visually impaired gait adaptation may also predispose this population to increased cervicothoracic stresses. Many visually impaired people find the use of a long cane helpful in daily mobility and obstacle avoidance. Long cane users were found to lack normal intersegmental movement of the neck, trunk and shoulder during gait (Mount et al 2001). This could lead to an increase in posture-related spinal problems, especially at the cervical and lumbar levels. Morioka & Maeda (1998) studied the effect of cane-transmitted vibration to the hand and upper extremity and determined that potentially detrimental effects may exist. Athletes with visual impairment who use the assistance of a cane or guide dog have the inherent potential to become overdeveloped on the side that the cane or dog is used. This could be problematic in a sport that relies on limb symmetry. For example, if a freestyle swimmer has muscle imbalance in the upper limb, this could manifest itself in an unequal arm pull, resulting in a less efficient stroke. Conversely, those who do not use a cane or the assistance of a guide dog, may adopt a kyphotic or poorer posture, and flex much more at the neck in order to judge the ground for distance.

A common strategy for those with tunnel vision or significant loss of peripheral vision is a 'scanning' approach that utilizes the central visual field for obstacle detection. The adaptation is typically seen as a persistent movement of the cervical spine, which consists of rotation usually, and some degree of side-bending. This constant, repeated movement has the potential to lead to cervical dysfunction. Those who rely on vision from one eye only, may develop abnormal cervical alignment. The resultant effects on the rest of their postural alignment could potentially lead to upper limb overload and neuromusculoskeletal dysfunction.

The protocol for the use of guides during competition is sport and Games specific. In some sports, such as tandem cycling and alpine skiing, a guide is necessary. Track and field events also utilize sighted pilots. In these events, every effort should be made to appropriately match the athlete gait and pace with that of the pilot to maximize potential and prevent injury.

AMPUTEE ATHLETES

Limb deficiency in the amputee athlete category may be of a congenital or traumatic origin. It occurs more commonly in the lower than upper limb, and the athlete may need to compete with a prosthesis in certain sports such as athletics (sprinting), standing volleyball, and cycling. In other sports such as swimming, a prosthesis is not necessary. Classification of the athlete is dependent on the use of prostheses, wheelchair, or other adaptive equipment during competition, as well as the location and extent of the amputation(s) (Webster et al 2001). For those athletes who compete with a prosthesis, the development of strong, lightweight materials (carbon fiber, titanium, and Kevlar), using advanced technology and design, have all contributed to the potential for increased levels of performance.

There are many considerations for the type and design of a prosthesis for athletic use. For example, the socket design, fit, and interface are of paramount importance for the amputee runner. The use of interface materials such as silicone liners, gel liners, or hypobaric socks provides added padding and helps to absorb and disperse potentially damaging pressure and shear forces (Webster et al 2001). For transfemoral amputees, a flexible inner liner may be used to decrease the weight of the prosthesis and to accommodate the changing shape of the thigh during muscular contraction. For an above knee amputee, an ultra-lightweight pylon is usually used to connect the knee unit to the foot. Several options may enhance function, but at the same time, add expense and weight to the prosthesis. Torque absorbers, placed between the knee and the pylon, can absorb rotational forces and thus reduce shear at the socket/residual limb interface. This allows a certain amount of twisting between the foot and the knee (Huang et al 2001). The advent of high-profile elastic-response-type feet are now the choice of those athletes involved in sprinting sports (Fig. 27.4).

Cycling is a very popular sport for amputee athletes, and the design considerations differ greatly from the running athlete. Athletes with a limb deficiency above the midtransfemoral level will not usually use a prosthesis as they cannot gain sufficient power to drive the pedal. Those who do use a prosthesis can have a problem keeping the foot component on the pedal. To counteract this, the component can be locked onto the pedal, although this raises injury potential in the event of falls or collisions.

Upper limb prostheses are also highly specialized and can be designed for those involved in throwing, swinging, or catching sports. There are many devices available for holding hockey sticks, rackets, golf clubs, bowling balls, fishing rods, baseball bats, and ski poles (Webster et al 2001).

With such a vast array of different components and materials, other considerations such as the location of the limb deficiency, the demand of the sport, and the expectation of the athlete, mean that the prosthetist must work closely with the athlete, physical therapist, and coach through all phases of the assessment, design, fitting, and follow-up to ensure the optimal outcome.

The main problems encountered by amputee athletes are:

- Skin breakdown
- The consequence of limb asymmetry
- Component failure.

Skin breakdown at the socket/residual limb interface is common (Levy 1995). Shear forces and abnormal pressures on the residual limb within the prosthesis can contribute to skin breakdown. Silicon liners and total contact sockets have been found to considerably decrease pressure related pain, however, they have also been associated with increased problems with dermatitis secondary to increased perspiration, residual moisture and folliculitis (Hachisuka et al 2001). Skin irritation and pain can result in decreased tolerance to prosthesis use and subsequent loss of training days for the amputee athlete. Some considerations in the design of the prosthesis to reduce the forces at this interface, and therefore decrease the risk of skin breakdown, have already been discussed. Athletes may encounter

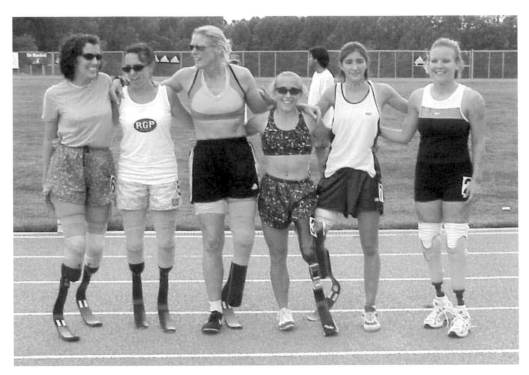

Figure 27.4 Examples of high-profile elastic-response type feet (athletes on the left). (Reproduced with permission of Ossur/Flex-Foot, Aliso Viejo, CA.)

problems with adapting to a new prosthesis and training may have to be modified or reduced in order to overcome this. A tight socket will impede vascular performance. Problems may also develop as a prosthesis or socket wears out and a loose-fitting socket will cause areas of friction. The stump is very sensitive to overload, which can cause stump soreness. Sweating during activity can lead to pressure sores and stump breakdown. The therapist must be aware of the causes and implications, and regular inspection of the stump is recommended. This is particularly important when the athlete is more vulnerable, such as after training and during competition.

Limb asymmetry can cause its unique set of problems. For example, in order for an athlete with an above-knee amputation to swim in a straight line, there may be a need to pull more with the contralateral upper limb, thereby creating muscle imbalance and musculoskeletal problems as a consequence. This could cause a dilemma for the physical therapist who may not want to address the imbalance, but concentrate on injury prevention strategies on the side that is prone to overload.

Energy expenditure during gait is increased in lower limb amputees, dependent on the level of amputation (Waters et al 1976), and therefore, they are likely to fatigue more quickly compared to an able-bodied athlete on a comparable training program. The sound limb on a unilateral below-knee amputee or above-knee amputee

may also experience increased work load and moments of force resulting in potential for overuse type injuries (Czerniecki et al 1996, Czerniecki & Gitter 1992, Serroussi et al 1996). Data from a recent Paralympic Games indicated that sound side lower extremity injuries were common in the running athlete. Measured moments of the amputated side hip and reattached musculature were also significantly increased in ambulation and running gait of both transtibial and transfemoral subjects with possible implications for overuse injury (Jaegers et al 1996, Buckley 1999). Different weights of the prosthesis do impact on the work capacity and kinematics of both the sound and amputated sides. Attempts to match limb weight of the sound side with the weight of the prosthesis actually worsened the energy expense of gait and created a larger differential in limb loads (Mattes et al 2000). The lighter prosthesis (50% of the sound side) decreased energy expenditure and limb load suggesting that anatomical recreation is not the biomechanical advantage. Rehabilitation of a prosthetic-sided injury using the rest, ice, compression, elevation (RICE) principles are difficult to apply for the amputee athlete, for whom the loss of use of the prosthesis means the loss of functional mobility. Alerting the prosthetist to any area of concern may not only prevent days lost from training but also avoid the frustration of altered mobility and ability to carry out normal daily activities.

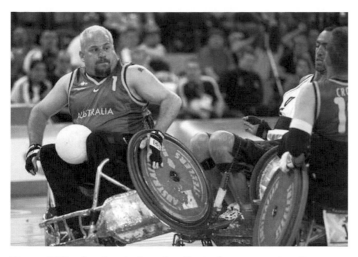

Figure 27.5   Quad rugby in action, illustrating upper extremity weightbearing demands. (Reproduced with permission of www.quadrugby.com and photographer Dariyoosh Hariri.)

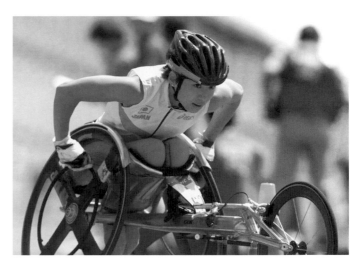

Figure 27.6   A track-racing wheelchair. The athlete is wearing extensive hand protection. (Reproduced with permission of © Allsport, UK Ltd.)

WHEELCHAIR ATHLETES

Athletes competing in the wheelchair category are most often associated with those who have a spinal cord injury (SCI), but they also include those with spina bifida, postpoliomyelitis, and limb deficiency. Wheelchair athletes compete in a wide variety of sports, the most popular being track and field, basketball, and swimming. However, there is a vast array of other sports, such as archery, table tennis, tennis, rugby, sailing, and winter sports, to name but a few.

Wheelchair designs have changed dramatically over the last 20 years, and just as prostheses have become sport-specific for athletes with limb deficiency, so too have wheelchairs. For example, the design of a chair used in basketball or quad rugby (Fig. 27.5) has demands for high maneuverability, and rapid acceleration and deceleration that differ greatly from the design of a chair used in track racing (Fig. 27.6).

Most chairs will be further adapted in accordance with the athlete's degree of trunk control. The biomechanical efficiency of wheelchair propulsion has been studied in order to maximize performance and reduce the risk of injury (Vanlandewijck et al 2001). It is not surprising that upper limb injuries predominate in this group of athletes (Ferrara & Peterson 2000). Common injuries include soft tissue injuries (33%), blisters (18%), and skin lacerations and abrasions (17%), and 5% reported symptoms of hand weakness or numbness (Curtis & Dillon 1985). Repetitive and forceful hand movements and pressure of the heel of the hand on the push rim of the chair may contribute to peripheral nerve entrapments. Burnham & Steadward (1994) reported a 23% incidence of peripheral nerve entrapment in wheelchair athletes. The median nerve at the carpal tunnel was most frequently affected, followed by the ulnar nerve at the wrist and forearm. Gloves and tape are often used to try and prevent the onset of symptoms (Fig. 27.6).

A high incidence of shoulder pain has also been reported in wheelchair athletes. In a study of 46 female wheelchair basketball players, only 14% reported shoulder pain prior to using a wheelchair (Curtis & Black 1999). This incidence rose to 72% since using a chair, with 52% reporting current symptoms. Furthermore, in another recent study, the prevalence and intensity of shoulder pain was reported as significantly higher in subjects with tetraplegia than in subjects with paraplegia (Curtis et al 1999a). However, these findings must be considered in light of the fact that they are based on self reporting and/or retrospective questionnaires. Webborn & Turner (2000) also found that shoulder symptoms were the most common presentation in the British squad before and during the Atlanta Paralympic Games in 1996. On clinical assessment, however, cervicothoracic dysfunction was by far the most common source, and accounted for 59% of those reporting shoulder symptoms. Wheelchair athletes who are involved with overhead activities such as tennis, basketball, and field throwing sports are more likely to incur shoulder pathology than those who are not. Wheelchair propulsion alone does not necessitate sufficient levels of abduction to give rise to symptoms such as impingement (Fig. 27.7). The additive stressors of the sport are compounded by the use of the upper extremities for activities of daily living, weightbearing in transfers, and daily mobility.

Despite careful consideration of seating needs, poor flexed sitting posture is common in wheelchair users. In

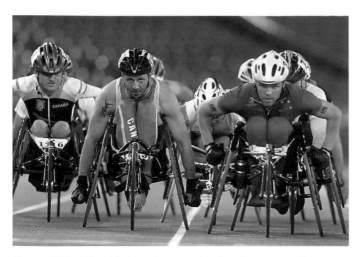

Figure 27.7 Wheelchair track racers showing the amount of shoulder abduction required during different phases of the propulsion technique. (Reproduced with permission of © Allsport, UK Ltd.)

addition, during sports such as track racing, athletes adopt a flexed posture in order to achieve greater speed and to improve aerodynamics (Fig. 27.7). This position will force the cervical spine into protraction and stress the cervicothoracic junction. If wheelchair athletes present with pain in the shoulder area (C5 dermatome), it is important to determine the origin of the symptoms. Preventative measures may be identified in screening programs, and postural re-education implemented. Due to the repetitive nature and overload of wheelchair propulsion and transfers, these athletes are prone to muscle imbalance with a tendency to develop overactive latissimus dorsi, trapezius, and pectoralis major muscles. Any imbalance/flexibility issues should also be incorporated into the athlete's training program. Testament to such an approach was seen in a 6-month exercise protocol, which was effective in decreasing the intensity of shoulder pain in wheelchair users during functional activities in a randomized controlled study (Curtis et al 1999b). The protocol involved five shoulder exercises that were performed daily over the 6-month period. Two exercises involved stretching the anterior structures, whilst the other three addressed muscle strengthening of the posterior structures.

While upper extremity complaints are the most commonly reported in the wheelchair athlete, the potential for lower extremity injury is especially high in contact or collision sports such as rugby and basketball. Athletes with sensory deficits may not be aware of the injury. Additionally, drag injuries to the lower extremity may occur if the leg is displaced off a footrest after contact or collision. Asensory areas should be appropriately protected and checked for signs of abrasions or contusions after training or competition. Lack of protec-

tive sensation also puts the wheelchair user at risk of developing abnormal pressures over weightbearing surfaces, which if left untreated, could lead to ulceration and potential infection. Pressure injuries should be avoided with appropriate seating systems, cushioning and frequent weight shifting (Minkel 2000).

Wheelchair athletes are also more prone to other medical conditions. Autonomic dysreflexia (ADR) is a potentially dangerous condition that can affect anyone with a SCI at the T6 level or above (Ericksson 1980). It can result from a variety of noxious stimuli, which in turn, trigger sympathetic hyperactivity. Patients usually present with elevated blood pressure and bradycardia due to stimulation of the cranial nerve X (vagus) below the level of the injury. The body's attempt to reduce blood pressure causes vasodilation above the level of injury. The common signs and symptoms of autonomic dysreflexia are shown in Box 27.2. This condition must be properly assessed and treated quickly and efficiently at the earliest signs or symptoms to prevent a potentially life-threatening crisis (Ericksson 1980). The elevated blood pressure is of most concern, and the blood pressure will drop with the removal of the stimulus. If the stimulus is not removed immediately, seizures, stroke and death can occur (Ericksson 1980). ADR is commonly triggered by an obstructed bowel or bladder (Ericksson 1980).

There have been reports of athletes self-inflicting ADR in order to elevate the blood pressure and enhance performance. This is a doping method unique to disability sport and is known as 'boosting' (Webborn 1999). Boosting may be achieved by using cutaneous, visceral, or proprioceptive stimuli below the level of the cord lesion or by consuming large quantities of fluids with a clamped catheter drain. Boosting is considered a widespread and effective practice by wheelchair athletes, with improvements in mean race time reported to be as much as 9.7% (Burnham et al 1994). It is a dangerous practice that has been banned by the International Paralympic Committee. No athlete exhibiting signs of ADR is allowed to participate in competition.

Box 27.2 Common signs and symptoms of autonomic dysreflexia

- A sudden and significant increase in both systolic and diastolic blood pressure
- Pounding headache
- Profuse sweating above the level of the lesion
- Goose bumps above the level of the lesion
- Blurred vision
- Nasal congestion

OTHER GENERAL ISSUES

Several general issues that relate to athletes with disability are important for physical therapists to be aware of. These include environmental considerations, drugs and doping, and travel issues.

ENVIRONMENTAL ISSUES

A change of climate, whether related to temperature, humidity, or altitude will pose problems for any athlete. For example, the selection of Atlanta for the Olympic and Paralympic Games in 1996, where the average temperature in August was 85°F and there was 60% humidity (Webborn 1996), posed problems for able- and disabled-bodied athletes alike. However, athletes with SCI are particularly vulnerable because their normal thermoregulation is affected. SCI above the level of T1 will compromise the parasympathetic nervous system, affecting the circulating blood volume and sweat production. As a result, quadriplegics do not perspire below the site of the lesion and therefore cannot effectively cool the body. In effect, such athletes have a decreased functional surface area by which to control thermoregulation. These athletes are equally at risk from heat and cold-related conditions. Progressively higher levels of paraplegics were also found to have higher body core temperatures during comparable exercise in a hot environment due to lack of perspiration below the level of the lesion (Yamasaki et al 2001). Thermoregulation in temperatures below 50°F is also compromised in those with SCI lesions above T1 who lack circulatory shunting, reflexive shivering, or goosebump production. Winter sport participants should have adequate clothing and access to indoor shelter in these conditions.

The same principles regarding fluids and rehydration apply for disabled-bodied athletes as for able-bodied athletes in both hot and cold weather environments. All athletes should be encouraged to maintain fluid intake. Intellectually impaired athletes may need particular attention in this area. Monitoring of athlete weight during intense training may be an effective way to track fluid replacement. In hot conditions, additional water should be sprayed frequently on the skin for the cooling effect of evaporation. The Atlanta Games found the utilization of misting booths for athletes particularly helpful. Water bottles are typically mounted onto wheelchairs. Athletes who are catheterized typically utilize a collection bag strapped to the leg. Because of the added weight of the filling bag, some athletes may defer taking on water to prevent competing with the filling bag or the interruption of draining the bag close to start of competition. This practice may predispose them to dehydration

and the subsequent effects this has on performance. Athletes with SCI are also particularly vulnerable to the harmful effects of sun exposure. Circulatory changes and decreased sensory input put this population at greater risk, and therefore, the appropriate preventative precautions of adequate sun block and shaded shelters are recommended. Certain medications have the potential to affect thermoregulatory ability and some magnify the effect of sun exposure. Athletes should be advised when the medications may alter typical body response and take appropriate precautions with their training program.

Change of setting can have a great impact on both visually impaired athletes and those dependent on wheelchairs. For those dependent on wheelchairs, there are issues of access to accommodation, such as width of doors, and space in the bedroom to maneuver the wheelchair. Sport chairs, particularly, can have cambered wheels that exceed normal doorway frames or entries. The terrain to be covered, access to the training and competition venues, and transport, etc. all need to be considered; for example, the Paralympic Village in the Sydney 2000 Paralympic Games was built on a fairly steep bank that was quite difficult for wheelchair athletes to negotiate. A regular bus service ensured that the athletes could avoid this difficulty.

A change of setting for athletes with visual impairment can also be very disorienting. For those with low vision, different lighting at the competition venue may impact on their visual acuity (Kuyk et al 1996) and subsequently their performance. The use of a guide may help the athlete make the transition into the new setting, both in the competition arena and in residents' accommodation. As discussed above, these athletes are more vulnerable to inadvertent collisions and avoidance of injury is a priority.

DRUGS AND DOPING

As the level of competition rises, so does the potential for an athlete to attempt to utilize means to gain the competitive edge that is not provided by training alone. Use of ergogenic aids and doping are not exclusive to able-bodied sports. At the 2000 Sydney Paralympics there were several incidences of positive drug tests indicating a rise in prevalence nearing that of the able-bodied counterparts.

The list of prohibited classes of substances and prohibited methods of doping for disabled-bodied athletes are the same as for their able-bodied counterparts. In testing for drugs and doping, the primary difference between able- and disabled-bodied athletes is the fact that more disabled-bodied athletes may be on medication for underlying medical conditions. For example, 10% of the British swimming team at the European Championships in 1995 had some form of epilepsy (Webborn 1996).

Exemptions allowing the use of drugs on the list for medical purposes can be sought by medical certification.

An official attending with any athlete who is to be drug tested must be familiar with the procedures and regulations (see Ch. 28). The main difference in procedures for the disabled, rather than able-bodied sport, is for athletes who are catheterized. Their leg bags must be emptied prior to testing and a fresh specimen obtained.

In terms of cheating for advantage, trying to deceive the classification procedure may be perceived, at present, as an easier route than taking performance enhancing drugs. As classification systems develop further, this may change.

TRAVEL ISSUES

Since the advent of the Americans with Disabilities Act, and similar legislation in other countries, accessibility for the disabled has been the buzzword for all businesses, including the travel and tourism industry. Transportation difficulties have previously deterred the disabled from enjoying recreational travel. Today, there exist no less than 50 organizations that facilitate disabled travel worldwide (see www.routesinternational.com). The Air Carrier Access Act, implemented in 1986, stipulates that no airline may discriminate against persons with disabilities. The airline must supply an appropriate van or shuttle ground service, aircraft stowing procedures for power or specialized wheelchairs, collapsible boarding chairs, and an appropriate environment to allow for safe boarding. Advance notice to the airline is necessary to detail all specific needs. Arrangements may need to be made in advance to accommodate some assistive devices, special seating or boarding assistance. However, even the most careful of planning can succumb to unexpected airline schedule changes or delays. This may present itself as the accessible aircraft being unavailable at the scheduled time. While able-bodied travelers are not inconvenienced by traveling on another aircraft, the disabled traveler may be in for significant delays. The disabled traveler may not be able to be rerouted onto non-jet planes or those that need to be boarded by stairwell rather than jetwalks. For travel delay reasons, the disabled flyer may be wise to carry on all medications as well as all pertinent emergency contact information, physicians' names, and numbers.

Hotel accommodation also needs to be carefully researched in advance of booking. The advent of the Americans with Disabilities Act has prompted numerous changes in building codes to accommodate the needs of the disabled, however, compliance is still an issue even in healthcare facilities (Sanchez et al 2000). 'Handicapped accessible' can encompass a very broad range of descriptors, or include only the minimum to meet legal requirements. Other countries may have different regulations regarding building codes for accessibility. Obtaining a complete description of shower facilities, grab bars, lowered sink measurements, raised toilet seats, doorway widths, closet facilities, and other facility accommodations, may avoid potential pitfalls. The facility may need to know some information regarding wheelchair dimensions, and weight or type of tires to further determine barriers to accessibility. Cambered chairs, as frequently used in wheelchair sports, add width and may be a consideration in planning for both hotel accommodation and ground transport. Hotel facilities may also need advance notice to accommodate guide dogs or assistive pets.

Another consideration during travel is special dietary needs. When planning the trip, the disabled athlete will want to ensure that at all stages during the travel process, appropriate nutrition is available, making advance plans as necessary. Delays in travel should also be anticipated and supplies planned ahead for this. Water consumption in some countries is not advised and careful planning is needed to avoid inadvertent ingestion during bathing, tooth brushing or use of water for cooling in hot weather competition. Medications, as discussed above, should be carried on the person or assistant at all times. A physician-issued card may be necessary to allow travel with syringes, and also in the case of metal implants that may set off airport and other security metal detectors; carrying of these documents can prevent untimely delays in travel.

Travel for the able-bodied can be wrought with frustration, but even more consideration and planning are required for the disabled traveler to minimize travel difficulties. Careful planning can eliminate unnecessary inconveniences and lessen the effects of problems from typical travel woes.

SUMMARY

This chapter illustrates many of the considerations of therapy in disabled sport, and provides a description of the scope of the needs of athletes with disability. From the social and psychological benefits to the health-enhancing aspects of exercise, the physical therapist can have an important role in helping the athlete minimize days lost from training or activity. With the steady rise of participants in disabled sports, physical therapists will need increased awareness of rehabilitation considerations and will need to be able to identify potential risks inherent in this population. Few therapists or facilities work regularly with the disabled athlete, making expertise in the field a rarity. However, with knowledge of disability-specific issues, the therapist can provide the highest standard of care to the athlete. In addition, the therapist has a role of promoting sport and exercise to all disabled patients who may not be aware of the opportunities that exist. Referring patients to the appropriate sport association or club may be paramount to any therapy otherwise provided. Further research is needed in all aspects of disabled sport to advance the role of therapy, injury prevention, and rehabilitation. Some topics, such as athlete classification, are expected to continue to evolve. Ever advancing biotechnology, as seen in prosthetics and wheelchair design, may also influence therapy considerations. Increasing visibility of disabled competition, local through international, will result in a rise of disabled sport participants. Physical therapists will have an ever-increasing role in education, health promotion, and rehabilitation of this population.

Acknowledgements

Thanks go to Chris Holmes MBE, nine times Paralympic gold medalist, and member of the British swimming team for his help in the preparation of this chapter.

REFERENCES

Buckley J G 1999 Sprint kinematics of athletes with lower limb amputations. Archives of Physical Medicine and Rehabilitation 80(5):501–508

Burnham R S, Steadward R D 1994 Upper extremity peripheral nerve entrapments among wheelchair athletes: prevalence, location, and risk factors. Archives of Physical Medicine and Rehabilitation 75:519–524

Burnham R, Wheeler G, Bhambhani Y et al 1994 Intentional induction of autonomic dysreflexia among quadriplegic athletes for performance enhancement: efficacy, safety and mechanism of action. Clinical Journal of Sports Medicine 4:1–10

Clews W 1995 Cerebral palsied athletes: massage benefits. Sport Health 13(4):22–23

Curtis K A, Dillon D A 1985 Survey of wheelchair athletic injuries: common patterns and prevention. Paraplegia 23:170–175

Curtis K A, Black K 1999 Shoulder pain in female wheelchair basketball players. Journal of Orthopaedic and Sports Physical Therapy 29:225–231

Curtis K A, Drysdale G A, Lanza R D et al 1999a Shoulder pain in wheelchair users with tetraplegia and paraplegia. Archives of Physical Medicine and Rehabilitation 80:453–457

Curtis K A, Tyner T M, Zachary L et al 1999b Effect of a standard exercise protocol on shoulder pain in long-term wheelchair users. Spinal Cord 37:421–429

Czerniecki J M, Gitter A 1992 Insights into amputee running. A muscle work analysis. American Journal of Physical Medicine and Rehabilitation 71(4):209–218

Czerniecki J M, Gitter A J, Beck J C 1996 Energy transfer mechanisms as a compensatory strategy in below knee amputee runners. Journal of Biomechanics 29(6):717–722

Damiano D L, Abel M F 1998 Functional outcomes of strength training in spastic cerebral palsy. Archives of Physical Medicine and Rehabilitation 79(2):119–125

Dec K L, Sparrow K J, McKeag D B 2000 The physically-challenged athlete: medical issues and assessment. Sports Medicine 29(4):245–258

Duffy C M, Hill A E, Cosgrove A P et al 1996 Energy consumption in children with spina bifida and cerebral palsy: a comparative study. Developmental Medicine and Child Neurology 38(3):238–243

Durstine J L, Painter P, Franklin B A et al 2000 Physical activity for the chronically ill and disabled. Sports Medicine 30:207–219

Ericksson R P 1980 Autonomic hyperreflexia: pathophysiology and medical management. Archives of Physical Medicine and Rehabilitation 61:431–440

Fernhall B, McCubbin J A, Pitetti K H et al 2001 Prediction of maximal heart rate in individuals with mental retardation. Medicine and Science in Sports and Exercise 33(10):1655–1660

Ferrara M S, Buckley W E 1996 Athletes with Disabilities Injury Registry. Adapted Physical Activity Quarterly 13:50–60

Ferrara M S, Peterson C L 2000 Injuries to athletes with disabilities: identifying injury patterns. Sports Medicine 30:137–143

Ferrara M S, Buckley W E, Messner D G et al 1992 The injury experience and training history of the competitive skier with a disability. American Journal of Sports Medicine 20(1):55–60

Ferrara M S, Palutsis G R, Snouse S et al 2000 A longitudinal study of injuries to athletes with disabilities. International Journal of Sports Medicine 21(3):221–224

Firth F Y 1999 Seeking misclassification: 'doping' in disability sport. British Journal of Sports Medicine 33:152

Hachisuka K, Nakamura T, Ohmine S et al 2001 Hygiene problems of residual limb and silicone liners in transtibial amputees wearing the total surface bearing socket. Archives of Physical Medicine and Rehabilitation 82(9):1286–1290

Huang M E, Levy C E, Webster J B 2001 Acquired limb deficiencies. 3. Prosthetic components, prescriptions, and indications. Archives of Physical Medicine and Rehabilitation 82:S17–S24

Hutzler Y, Chacham A, Bergman U et al 1998 Effects of a movement and swimming program on vital capacity and water orientation skills of children with cerebral palsy. Developmental Medicine and Child Neurology 40:176–181

Jaegers S M, Arendzen J H, de Jongh H J 1996 An electromyographic study of the hip muscles of transfemoral amputees in walking. Clinical Orthopedics 328:119–128

Kuyk T, Elliott J L, Biehl J et al 1996 Environmental variables and mobility performance in adults with low vision. Journal of the American Optometric Association 67(7):403–409

Labronici R H, Cunha M C, Oliveira A D et al 2000 [Sport as integration factor of the physically handicapped in our society] Arquivos de Neuro-psiquiatria 58(4):1092–1099

Lancioni G E, Gigante A, O'Reilly M F et al 2000 Indoor travel and simple tasks as physical exercise for people with profound multiple disabilities. Perceptual and Motor Skills 91(1):211–216

Laskowski E R, Murtaugh P A 1992 Snow skiing injuries in physically disabled skiers. American Journal of Sports Medicine 20(5):553–557

Levitt S 1982 Outline of treatment approaches. In: Levitt S (ed) Treatment of cerebral palsy and motor delay. Blackwell Scientific, Oxford

Levy S W 1995 Amputees: skin problems and prostheses. Cutis 55(5):297–301

Lyon C C, Kulkarni J, Zimerson E et al 2000 Skin disorders in amputees. Journal of the American Academy of Dermatology 42(3):501–507

Maltais D, Bar-Or O, Galea V et al 2001 Use of orthoses lowers the O_2 cost of walking in children with spastic cerebral palsy. Medicine and Science in Sports and Exercise 33(2):320–325

Mattes S J, Martin P E, Royer T D 2000 Walking symmetry and energy cost in persons with unilateral transtibial amputations: matching prosthetic and intact limb inertial properties. Archives of Physical Medicine and Rehabilitation 81(5):561–568

Minkel J L 2000 Seating and mobility considerations for people with spinal cord injury. Physical Therapy 80(7):701–709

Morioka M, Maeda S 1998 Measurement of hand-transmitted vibration of tapping the long cane for visually handicapped people in Japan. Industrial Health 36(2):179–190

Mount J, Howard P D, Dalla Palu A L et al 2001 Postures and repetitive movements during use of a long cane by individuals with visual impairment. Journal of Orthopaedic and Sports Physical Therapy 31(7):375–383

Nakamura T 1997 Quantitative analysis of gait in the visually impaired. Disability and Rehabilitation 19(5):194–197

Nyland J, Snouse S L, Anderson M et al 2000 Soft tissue injuries to USA paralympians at the 1996 summer games. Archives of Physical Medicine and Rehabilitation 81(3):368–373

Pluym S M, Keur T J, Gerritsen J et al 1997 Community integration of wheelchair-bound athletes: A comparison before and after onset of disability. Clinical Rehabilitation 11(3):227–235

Ramsey V K, Blasch B B, Kita A et al 1999 A biomechanical evaluation of visually impaired persons' gait a long-cane mechanics. Journal of Rehabilitation Research and Development 36(4):323–332

Rimmer J H 1999 Health promotion for persons with disabilities: the emerging shift from disability prevention of secondary conditions. Physical Therapy 79:495–502

Sanchez J, Byfield G, Brown T T et al 2000 Perceived accessibility versus actual physical accessibility of healthcare facilities. Rehabilitation Nursing 25(1):6–9

Searle C 2000 The golden games. The British Paralympic Association Official Games Report: Sydney 2000. The British Paralympic Association, Croydon

Seroussi R E, Gitter A, Czerniecki J M et al 1996 Mechanical work adaptations of above knee amputee ambulation. Archives of Physical Medicine and Rehabilitation 77(11):1209–1214

Shephard R J 1991 Benefits of sport and physical activity for the disabled: implications for the individual and for society. Scandinavian Journal of Rehabilitation Medicine 23:51–59

Shepherd R B 1995 Cerebral palsy. In: Shepherd R B (ed) Physiotherapy in paediatrics. Butterworth Heineman, Oxford

Stewart K 2000 Massage for children with cerebral palsy. Nursing Times 96:50–51

Sydney Paralympic Organizing Committee 2000 Sydney 2000 Paralympic Games Official Programme. News Custom Publishing, Southbank, Victoria

Unnithan V B, Dowling J J, Frost G et al 1996 Role of cocontraction in the O_2 cost of walking in children with cerebral palsy. Medicine and Science in Sports and Exercise 28(12):1498–1504

Ward K H, Meyers M C 1995 Exercise performance of lower-extremity amputees. Sports Medicine 20(4):207–214

Waters R L, Perry J, Antomelli D et al 1976 Energy cost of walking of amputees: influence of level of amputation. Journal of Bone and Joint Surgery (Am) 58A:42–46

Vanlandewijck Y, Theisen D, Daly D 2001 Wheelchair propulsion biomechanics: Implications for wheelchair sports. Sports Medicine 31:339–367

Webborn A D 1996 Heat-related problems for the Paralympic Games, Atlanta 1996. British Journal of Therapy and Rehabilitation 3:429–434

Webborn A D 1999 'Boosting' performance in disability sport. British Journal of Sports Medicine 33:74–75

Webborn A D J, Turner H M 2000 The aeitiology of shoulder pain in elite Paralympic wheelchair athletes – the shoulder or cervical spine. Proceedings from the 5th International Paralympic Committee Scientific Congress, Sydney, Australia

Webster J B, Levy C E, Bryant P R et al 2001 Sports and recreation for persons with limb deficiency. Archives of Physical Medicine and Rehabilitation 82:S38–S44

Yamasaki M, Kim K T, Choi S W et al 2001 Characteristics of body heat balance of paraplegics during exercise in a hot environment. Journal of Physiological Anthropology and Applied Human Science 20(4):227–232

Medical considerations for rehabilitation practitioners in sport and exercise settings

---

SECTION CONTENTS

28

Pharmacological agents in sport and exercise

Andrew Garnham

INTRODUCTION

Modern medicine to a large degree is dependent on a wide armamentarium of drugs for a great diversity of conditions. Medicine in relation to sport is no exception, with the misuse of drugs, in particular, having assumed a very prominent role. Clinical treatment of sporting injury and sport-associated illness has relied upon a much narrower range of agents, but is not without controversy.

This chapter explores both the drugs commonly used in the treatment of sport and exercise injury, and drugs that are used to achieve unfair advantage. The rationale for use, benefits and side-effects of each of these two distinct, but not entirely separate, classes of drugs are detailed. While the use of the great majority of these agents is restricted to physicians, it is important for all working in the field of sports injury to have an understanding of them. Legal considerations regarding drug prescription, regulation of drug use in sport, and drug testing are essential knowledge for any practitioner working with athletes.

While reading this chapter, it should be acknowledged that the laws and regulations regarding the prescription and use of pharmacological agents differ between countries.

THERAPEUTIC AGENTS

A range of pharmacological agents have been used in the treatment of sport and exercise injuries. Some of the better known include nonsteroidal anti-inflammatory drugs (NSAIDs), corticosteroids, analgesics, rubefacients, and thrombolytic agents. While there is a great deal of information on NSAIDs and corticosteroids in the rheumatology literature, in particular, there is a relative paucity of sound evidence-based material on the benefits or otherwise of these agents in the treatment of sports injury (Leadbetter 1995, Stanley & Weaver 1998, Weiler 1992). The majority of studies have focussed on the anti-inflammatory effects of these medications in acute injuries. Particularly conspicuous, is a lack of evidence of both an inflammatory process, and a therapeutic response to anti-inflammatory agents in chronic and overuse sports injuries. Analgesia probably plays a larger part in favorable outcomes than has been generally recognized.

Recently, hyperbaric oxygen therapy and novel anti-arthritic drugs have also been used for the management of sports injuries, but are yet to find an established place in mainstream injury management. In the future, agents such as bone and tendon growth factors and their analogs will become more readily available, and may take on an increasingly important role in the management of chronic and overuse injuries in particular.

THE INFLAMMATORY PROCESS

The cardinal features of tissue inflammation are pain (dolor), heat (calor), redness (rubor), swelling (tumor), and inevitable loss of function (functio laesa). These features are particularly evident in rheumatological conditions, such as inflammatory arthritis, with gout being the classical example of acute inflammatory effects. The patient with gouty arthritis is grateful for the swift and often complete relief that anti-inflammatory medications bring. In chronic inflammatory diseases, such as rheumatoid arthritis, the valuable role of anti-inflammatory medications is well established. However, when an athlete sustains an injury, loss of function, pain, and to a lesser extent, swelling, are generally the symptoms most important to them, rather than heat or redness. It has been assumed that these changes are the deleterious effects of the inflammatory process, and therefore, reversal of inflammation should expedite recovery. This assumption is founded on very limited and largely anecdotal evidence. Whenever anti-inflammatory medication is proposed for treatment of an injury, consideration must be given to both the potential benefits and deleterious effects of the drug.

When tissue is injured, a well-ordered sequence of events follow, extending over 48–72 h in the acute phase, but spanning weeks to months before healing is complete. The three components of the inflammatory process are: first, the acute vascular inflammatory phase; second, the repair and regeneration phase; and third, the maturation phase. Features of the initial vascular inflammatory phase are dilatation of blood vessels (with an increase in blood flow and vascular permeability), exudation of fluids (including plasma proteins), activation and release of immunologically active mediators,

activation of humoral response mechanisms, and leukocyte migration to the inflammatory focus (Leadbetter 1995).

As part of these processes, a range of chemicals is produced at the site of injury. At the outset, vascular injury results in the liberation of vasoactive amines, anaphylatoxins, and kinins. Neutrophil activation results in the production of oxygen-free radicals that attack the phospholipases of cell membranes, leading to breakdown of the cell wall and the generation of arachidonic acid metabolites, including various prostaglandins (Leadbetter 1995). This process is shown in Figure 28.1, along with the sites at which anti-inflammatory medications inhibit the process.

During repair and regeneration, which is the second phase of the inflammatory process, cellular debris is removed by macrophages, vessels regenerate, and collagen synthesis begins. Fibroblasts and macrophages are the dominant infiltrating cells at this stage.

The third phase of the inflammatory process involves the maturation of collagen. Forces applied to the tissue influence cross-linkages and orientation of collagen fibers, affecting the ultimate tensile strength of the healed tissue (Best & Garrett 1994).

Medications can have an influence at any of the three phases of inflammation. Pain and swelling in the first phase, mediated in part by prostaglandins, is inhibited by the use of anti-inflammatory medications (Almekinders et al 1995, Stanley & Weaver 1998). These medications

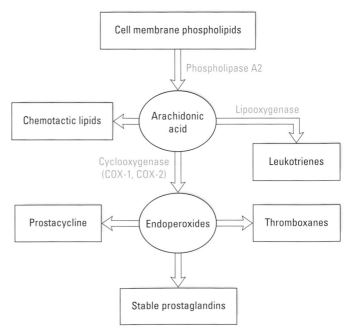

Figure 28.1 Arachidonic acid metabolism and the influences of corticosteroids and NSAIDs. Corticosteroids inhibit phospholipase A2. NSAIDs inhibit cyclooxygenase. Some NSAIDs also inhibit lipooxygenase.

may then interfere with the repair process of the second phase by impairing DNA synthesis (Almekinders 1993, Almekinders et al 1995). Finally, relief of muscle pain and spasm, mediated by analgesic medication, can facilitate the rehabilitation process as tissue remodeling and maturation proceeds, as well as enhancing protein synthesis (Almekinders et al 1995, Mazanec 1998). Most research attention has been centered on the influence of NSAIDs and corticosteroids on these processes. There is clear evidence that part of the process is impaired, while other parts are enhanced by these drugs, with no major change in tissue healing overall. Whether the ultimate outcome is influenced positively or negatively remains uncertain, and is the subject of continuing investigation (Almekinders et al 1995, Best & Garrett 1994, Leadbetter 1995).

NON-STEROIDAL ANTI-INFLAMMATORY DRUGS (NSAIDs)

NSAIDs have been widely used, both in prescription and over-the-counter forms, for virtually all types of musculoskeletal injury. They are widely promoted for the relief of spinal and joint pain. However, it is only in the last decade that their place in sports injury treatment has been scrutinized. There remains much to be learned in this respect, and these drugs should certainly not be regarded as an injury panacea.

Clinical effects of NSAIDs in sports injury

Many recent studies have investigated the benefits of NSAIDs in the treatment of sports injury. From critical reviews of such investigations (Ogilvie-Harris & Gilbart 1995, Weiler 1992) it has been shown that athletes with acute injuries (typically ankle sprains) who are treated with NSAIDs return to sport slightly more quickly, and with lower levels of pain, than control groups. However, these studies show little difference in terms of overall outcome where swelling and functional capacity are concerned. It has not been possible to determine whether the tissue healing process has been enhanced or impaired through the use of NSAIDs (Ogilvie-Harris & Gilbart 1995, Slatyer et al 1997, Stanley & Weaver 1998, Weiler 1992). NSAIDs, when used prophylactically, have been shown to be effective in reducing parameters associated with delayed onset muscle soreness, such as pain, power, swelling, and creatine kinase levels (Dudley et al 1997, Hasson et al 1993, O'Grady et al 2000, Sayers et al 2001). However, these findings cannot be translated to most clinical situations, as the experimental model is not typical of sporting injuries for which NSAIDs are commonly used. Most studies involving the use of NSAIDs on ligamentous injury have been methodologically flawed

by limitations in injury classification, use of other concurrent therapy modalities, poor randomization, and lack of true control groups (Weiler 1992). It can be concluded that individual athlete circumstances are the major determining factor in choosing to employ NSAIDs following injury; for example, a desire to return to sport quickly would encourage their use. Pain, leading to impaired rehabilitative capability is also an indication, although other analgesics may be just as effective. In light of these theoretical concerns regarding whether NSAIDs impair the repair, regeneration, and remodeling processes, they should probably only be used for short periods.

Choice of NSAID

There is no evidence to suggest that any one NSAID is more effective in the treatment of sports injury (Ogilvie-Harris & Gilbart 1995, Weiler 1992) than another. As seen in Table 28.1, NSAIDs belong to a range of quite different chemical classes, but this has little effect on their clinical usefulness. NSAIDs that inhibit lipooxygenase in addition to cyclooxygenase (diclofenac, indometacin and ketoprofen) are arguably more potent, but this contention is not well supported by clinical evidence (Sayers et al 2001). The relative degree of inhibition of cyclooxygenase-1 and cyclooxygenase-2 by different agents may affect the extent of central and peripheral

Table 28.1 Commonly used NSAIDs in the management of sport and exercise injuries

Class	Sub class	Generic drug name
Carboxylic acids	Acetic acids	Diclofenac Etodolac Indometacin Sulindac Tolmetin
	Fenamates	Meclofenamic acid Mefanamic acid
	Propionic acids	Fenoprofen Flurbiprofen Ibuprofen Ketoprofen Naproxen Oxaprozin Tiaprofenic acid
	Salicylates	Aspirin Diflunisal Salsalate Sulfasalazine
Enolic acids	Oxicams	Piroxicam Tenoxicam
	Pyrazoles	Celecoxib Ketorolac Phenylbutazone
	Furanones	Rofecoxib

action, and therefore potency. However, clinical evidence for this proposed effect is again lacking in the literature.

Factors determining the choice of an NSAID include side-effect profile, relative cost, onset of action, and duration of action. The dosage form (i.e. tablet, capsule, suspension, or suppository) may be important to some patients. Dosage frequency, which can vary between one and four times daily, should be considered. In the treatment of acute injury, an NSAID with a rapid onset of action is probably most suitable. For patients less likely to remember their medication, a longer acting, once daily form may be better suited. Patients should always be reminded to take NSAIDs immediately after meals, and never on an empty stomach, to minimize direct gastric irritation. However, it should be borne in mind that many gastric side-effects are systemic in nature, and are not prevented by taking the medication with food. Ketorolac, while particularly potent, is only indicated for postoperative pain relief, and not for the treatment of sports injury.

In general, a practitioner will become familiar with several different NSAIDs, and prescribe on the basis of their personal experience. Although many NSAIDs are packaged to allow about 4 weeks supply at normal dosages, it should be explained to patients that this is not a defined course of treatment, and that if no benefit is apparent after 1 week, there is probably no reason to continue the medication. If one NSAID is not having the desired benefit, there is no evidence to suggest that changing to another agent is worthwhile, assuming the initial dosage was adequate. In acute sprains of mild to moderate severity, 3–7 days of use is probably optimal to facilitate recovery (Mazanec 1998, Weiler 1992). In chronic conditions, such as degenerative joint disease in active patients, NSAIDs can be used as required to control symptoms, where the condition itself is unlikely to be modified. For example, NSAIDs may be used for a day or so before and after a weekly sporting activity to minimize pain and potential drug side-effects, and to optimize function and enjoyment.

Selective cyclooxygenase-2 (COX-2) inhibitors (celecoxib and rofecoxib) have been major advances in NSAID technology. Cyclooxygenase-1 (COX-1) is the constitutional isoenzyme primarily responsible for the production of prostaglandins that regulate normal physiological functions, such as gastric cytoprotection, renal parenchymal function, and platelet activity. COX-2 is an inducible isoenzyme primarily responsible for the production of prostaglandins that regulate pain, inflammation, and fever. Most of the anti-inflammatory benefits of NSAIDs appear to be the result of COX-2 inhibition (Stanley & Weaver 1998). As many of the side-effects of NSAIDs are associated with COX-1 inhibition, selective COX-2 inhibitors should have a more favorable side-effect profile, while still maintaining efficacy. This benefit is borne out in a significant reduction in peptic ulceration and minimal effect on platelet aggregation (Drew 2001). However, gastrointestinal side-effects do still occur with the selective COX-2 inhibitors, and they may also have prothrombotic effects (Drew 2001). Efficacy appears to be similar to established NSAIDs. Greater expense, and lack of long-term experience of side-effects are the main barriers to more widespread use.

Side-effects of NSAIDs

A large number of side-effects of NSAIDs have been recorded. Gastrointestinal side-effects are common. However, the great majority of side-effects are infrequent, and details are readily available in pharmacology texts (e.g. Hardman & Limbird 2001, Goldman & Bennett, 2000). The use of NSAIDs in pregnancy and lactation is relatively contraindicated. All NSAIDs have been shown to produce a low incidence of teratogenic effects in animal studies, and all are excreted in breast milk. A history of previous side-effects with use, or allergy to NSAIDs, including aspirin, should always be sought before prescription. Substitution of a different NSAID may prove satisfactory, but should only be undertaken with great caution.

Major side-effects of NSAIDs include the following (Hardman & Limbird 2001):

- Gastrointestinal disturbance, including indigestion, epigastric pain, gastroesophageal reflux, nausea, diarrhea and constipation
- Peptic ulceration, with a risk of bleeding, which may be occult in nature and lead to anemia
- Renal dysfunction, including sodium retention with consequent fluid retention and renal failure
- Impaired platelet aggregation, leading to prolongation of bleeding time. This effect may persist for days, or even weeks after cessation of the medication
- Precipitation of asthma
- Rash
- Headache
- Tiredness
- Interaction with other drugs, particularly anticoagulants and antihypertensives.

Gastrointestinal symptoms may occur in as many as 25% of patients treated with NSAIDs (Hardman & Limbird 2001, Leadbetter 1995). Serious complications such as peptic ulceration are most likely to occur with long-term use, and in the elderly (Hardman & Limbird 2001). However, peptic ulcer should be considered in any patient using NSAIDs who has persistent or severe gastrointestinal symptoms. Generally, patients who suffer symptoms should be advised to cease the medication, as long-term use is most often not required in the treatment of sports injury. If necessary, a different NSAID may not cause symptoms. Various anti-ulcer drugs can be used in combination with NSAIDs to minimize symptoms, but this approach should only be necessary in the presence of chronic disease that is unresponsive to other therapy. Interaction with alcohol is a side-effect concern often raised by athletes who are prescribed NSAIDs. No significant interaction occurs, but athletes should be reminded that both agents can cause gastrointestinal disturbance, and are best not combined. Alcohol consumption soon after injury should be avoided in any case, due to its vasodilatory effects.

The risk of bleeding at the injury site following administration of NSAIDs is a concern often raised in relation to the timing of commencement of dosage. NSAIDs should not precipitate bleeding once clotting has occurred. The standard measures of rest, ice, compression, and elevation (RICE) should be commenced as soon as possible following any traumatic injury, and bleeding at the site should then cease within minutes. Therefore, it should be reasonable to commence NSAIDs as soon as 1 hour after initial treatment. However, there is no evidence to suggest when is the most suitable time. It should be remembered that many athletes might already be taking NSAIDs at the time of injury, or in the days beforehand. In this situation, extra effort should be made to minimize bleeding.

Topical NSAIDs

A number of well-known NSAIDs are available in topical forms such as creams, gels, slow release patches, and sprays. Their use as topical agents has two major potential advantages over systemic forms. Firstly, side-effects, especially gastrointestinal, should be reduced. Secondly, the patient may gain additional therapeutic benefit by the method of administration, such as massage or phonophoresis. Topical NSAIDs are probably most useful for conditions affecting relatively superficial structures, as their depth of penetration is limited at normal dosage levels, and probably extends to 3–4 cm (Burnham et al 1998). Blood concentrations of less than 10% of those achieved with oral medications have been demonstrated with topical agents (Stanley & Weaver 1998). Topical agents have been shown to be effective in reducing pain in acute and chronic sporting injuries (Burnham et al 1998, Stanley & Weaver 1998). Despite the lack of objective evidence of their benefit in sports injuries, anecdotally, they are effective, particularly in joint synovitis. Large doses applied over extensive areas of skin can lead to significant systemic absorption, and consequently to the potential side-effects associated with oral NSAIDs. Prolonged use of topical NSAIDs is associated with a significant incidence of skin irritation,

and some patients develop rashes early in the use of the products (Burnham et al 1998). Use beyond 10–14 days should be avoided, as should application to broken skin.

CORTICOSTEROIDS

Corticosteroids (referred to as glucocorticosteroids in doping literature), especially in injected forms, are the most notorious drugs commonly used in the treatment of sports injury. Reports of almost immediate and complete relief of pain lead to exaggerated expectations of benefit in some athletes. Other athletes avoid corticosteroids at all costs, fearing permanent tissue damage, long-term systemic illness, and severe pain with injection. The truth lies between these two extremes, with corticosteroids certainly having an important and useful place in clinical sports medicine. The potent anti-inflammatory action of corticosteroids is a result of their inhibition of the chemical chain of inflammation almost at its beginning (Fig. 28.1). The inhibition of leukocyte migration to the site of injury is an important distinction between effects of corticosteroids and NSAIDs. This effect is the main reason for the immunosuppression associated with corticosteroid use. Corticosteroids are also important membrane stabilizers, reducing enzyme release from cells (Leadbetter 1995, Stanley & Weaver 1998). By their action, corticosteroids must have some analgesic properties, but the extent of this uncertain. Athletes often regard corticosteroid injections as painkillers, but this is primarily the effect of the accompanying local anesthetic. The effects of corticosteroids extend well beyond controlling inflammation, and facets of their action remain to be elucidated.

A major concern with the use of corticosteroids is their known inhibition of collagen synthesis and fibroblast proliferation in healing tissue (Best & Garrett 1994, Leadbetter 1995, Stanley & Weaver 1998). These factors lead to concerns about impaired healing and possibly an increased predisposition to new or further injury. The majority of evidence leading to concern is derived from animal models, often in isolated cell cultures, and extrapolation of findings to human sporting injuries must be undertaken with caution (Leadbetter 1995, Stanley & Weaver 1998). Clinical studies of the benefits and hazards of corticosteroid injections are often poorly controlled and rely on subjective and anecdotal evidence (Leadbetter 1995, Read 1999, Shrier et al 1996). Well-controlled clinical studies are hampered by the difficulty in recruiting sufficient numbers of patients with similar conditions where corticosteroid injection is appropriate. However, some conclusions can be drawn. Corticosteroids are most effective early in the course of inflammatory conditions such as bursitis, tenosynovitis, paratenonitis, and joint synovitis. While they are used in conditions such as epicondylitis, tendinopathies, osteoarthritis, spinal facet joint pain, and active trigger points, there is no sound evidence that the benefit is more than temporary symptom relief. Nevertheless, anecdotally, reports have indicated that excellent responses are sometimes achieved in these conditions, while other patients with seemingly similar pathology gain no benefit from corticosteroid injection.

The most important determinant in electing to use a corticosteroid injection is a thorough and accurate anatomical and pathological diagnosis. A considered decision can then be made in regard to risks and benefits. As level of knowledge and personal experience of the physician tend to strongly influence decision making, the incidence of corticosteroid use in practice varies greatly. The physician must be confident that the affected structure can be well localized and injected without risk to neurovascular structures and other sensitive tissues. Also, there must be no signs of local infection. Following injection, the area must be rested, or at least excessive load avoided, for a suitable period of time, usually between 2–14 days. The athlete must understand that even if there is very good initial symptom relief following injection, all aspects of rehabilitation such as stretching, strengthening, and technique modification must still be carried out diligently. Too often, injection is seen as a quick fix or short cut to return to sport, only to fail when the condition recurs and rehabilitation has been neglected. It is accepted practice to avoid injecting the same site of injury more than three times (Stanley & Weaver 1998). Likewise, repeated injections at intervals of less than several weeks are discouraged (Stanley & Weaver 1998). These practices are based on extrapolations of evidence from animal tissue studies, with minimal human clinical basis. Nevertheless, these are sound practices in that the need for repeated injection may imply an inaccurate diagnosis, inadequate treatment in other respects, or simply an attempt to ignore a very strong message to reduce activity. Of important consideration is that corticosteroid injections must be notified in competition, and prior permission obtained from the sporting organization if any doubt exists about regulations.

Side-effects of corticosteroid injections are relatively uncommon. Infection of the injection site must be avoided by good sterile technique. Local subcutaneous atrophy and skin pigmentation or depigmentation can be avoided by ensuring that the injection is more deeply placed. However, in superficial conditions the patient must be warned of this risk. Pain associated with injection can be minimized by the accompanying use of local anesthetic, a narrow gauge needle, and good injection technique (Leadbetter 1995). Postinjection flare of symptoms sometimes occurs, but usually settles within a day or so, and patients should be advised of this risk, and analgesics recommended where necessary. Postinjection flare is said to have been more common in the past when less soluble corticosteroids were used (Leadbetter 1995). In diabetic patients, a short-term rise in blood glucose is likely, but systemic effects are otherwise rare (Leadbetter 1995).

Tendon rupture is the most widely-known side-effect of corticosteroid injection, but it is in fact rare. Reviews of reported postinjection ruptures confirm that the association of injection with rupture is anecdotal, and no direct relationship is usually present (Leadbetter 1995, Shrier et al 1996). It is well accepted that intratendinous injection should be avoided (Leadbetter 1995, Shrier et al 1996). Even if the corticosteroid does not affect tendon structure, the needle tip may lacerate the tendon. If there is any risk of complete or partial tendon rupture being present, this should be established by imaging studies, and injection avoided. The only common exception to this rule is pre-existing rotator cuff tear, where symptoms may be largely the result of coexisting bursitis and impingement. It is likely that tendon rupture is the natural outcome of some conditions, and injection is an incidental and unsuccessful attempt to relieve the symptoms of an inevitable tendon failure. Injection around intact tendons appears to be accompanied by minimal risk of tendon rupture (Leadbetter 1995, Read 1999). Spontaneous rupture of the Achilles tendon, which is sometimes bilateral, is a well-recognized result of the use of oral corticosteroids (Shrier et al 1996). However, this again may often be an expression of the attrition of diseased tendon, as severe inflammatory disorders are usually the indication for this therapy. Nevertheless, all patients should be warned that a small risk of tendon rupture exists, and a suitable period of reduced activity should be advised.

Long-term articular cartilage damage is a further important concern with respect to the use of corticosteroids. Again, most studies are based on animal models, and clinical evidence is limited (Leadbetter 1995). The use of intra-articular injections should be restricted along the same lines as soft tissue injections, with injections into weightbearing joints, and areas of known articular cartilage injury, being treated with particular caution.

Oral corticosteroids are occasionally used in the management of recalcitrant inflammatory conditions, or in situations where injection may not be physically feasible such as around the pelvis, and in areas close to nerves and arteries. This therapy, however, is not used widely enough in the treatment of sports injury to evaluate its efficacy. Courses of oral corticosteroids should last no longer than 10 days, and should preferably use a tapering dosage regimen to minimize side-effects. Potent oral agents such as dexamethasone should be avoided, as high doses have led to avascular necrosis of the hip (Hardman &

Limbird 2001). Common side-effects include gastro-intestinal disturbance, altered fluid balance, and insomnia (Hardman & Limbird 2001). Oral corticosteroids are banned in sport, and specific permission must be sought for their use, and only then outside of competition.

Iontophoresis has been used as an alternative to injection to administer corticosteroids. While possibly useful in those afraid of needles, advantages of this technique are otherwise unclear. Penetration of the agent to the site of injury must be reduced, and systemic absorption increased relative to injection. Short-term pain relief has been demonstrated, but convincing benefits are otherwise lacking (Gudeman et al 1997).

RUBIFACIENTS AND OTHER TOPICAL AGENTS

Heat rubs and liniments, collectively referred to as rubifacients, are one of the oldest forms of sports injury treatment. Their ingredients usually include methyl salicylate and a variety of plant derived essential oils, such as menthol, thymol, camphor, capsaicin, and eucalyptus oil, and often a 'secret or unidentified unique' ingredient. They act by encouraging blood flow to the area, and may have a topical analgesic effect. They have been widely used to warm up tight and sore muscles. As a result of their direct warming effect on the skin, and their often pungent aroma, these agents are popular with some athletes. As their depth of penetration is limited, they do not take the place of the normal warming up processes of activity and stretching, but may be a useful adjunct. Evidence to demonstrate therapeutic benefits is lacking. Allergic reactions can occur, but the most common side-effect is the severe burning that can be experienced if applied to broken skin or sensitive areas such as mucous membranes and the eyes. The hands should always be washed thoroughly after applying rubifacients. Olive oil is helpful in displacing these agents from sensitive skin. Experience indicates that rubifacients should never be used simultaneously with heat packs, as subcutaneous necrosis has been reported from excessive tissue heating.

Various anticoagulant and hemolytic topical agents have been employed for the treatment of contusions and muscle strains. In theory, assistance with the removal of blood from tissues is probably beneficial, however, convincing evidence of this benefit is not available, and it is often suggested that the massage used for application of these agents is possibly their greatest virtue.

ANALGESICS

Pain is a prominent feature of many sporting injuries and its relief is essential to recovery and return to function.

The role of NSAIDs in this process has been discussed above, and it may well be that analgesia is the major clinical benefit of these drugs. There is no questioning the benefit of relief of pain following traumatic injury, in assisting early mobilization and progression to rehabilitation. In severe injury, such as fracture where further competition is impossible, injected analgesics such as pethidine and morphine should not be withheld for fear of drug testing or addiction. In less severe injury, where analgesia is used to permit continuing participation, serious consideration must be given to the possibility of the athlete sustaining further harm.

Widely used analgesics such as aspirin, paracetamol (acetaminophen), and codeine are used in standard dosage regimens to relieve the pain of sports injury. These drugs are permitted for use both in and out of competition. Patients should understand that it is good practice to make use of a regular dosage of a relatively mild but safe analgesic such as paracetamol, in order to control pain levels. Practices such as withholding pain relief, or trying to demonstrate a high pain tolerance, are counterproductive, and lead to a greater risk of side-effects when more potent agents become necessary.

In chronic pain, agents such as tricyclic antidepressants have a beneficial pain modifying effect (Mazanec 1998). However, these circumstances require the involvement of a physician experienced in pain management, and fall beyond the normal scope of sports injury therapy.

HYPERBARIC OXYGEN

Hyperbaric oxygen therapy is well established as a treatment for a range of medical conditions including various soft tissue injuries. Consequently, it has been assumed that it may be beneficial for the treatment of sports injuries, in particular traumatic soft tissue and joint injuries. This possibility has been embraced by the manufacturers of hyperbaric oxygen equipment, and enthusiastically supported by some athletes in anecdotal reports. These circumstances have resulted in a widespread perception that hyperbaric oxygen therapy is a well-established and effective treatment for sports injury. However, this perception is not supported by sound evidence (see Ch. 13) (Babul & Rhodes 2000).

Hyperbaric oxygen therapy involves the inspiration of 100% oxygen at pressures greater than the ambient barometric pressure at sea level (1 atmosphere). Pressures of between 2 and 3 atmospheres are commonly used. Hyperbaric oxygen can offset local hypoxia by increasing the partial pressure of oxygen in the tissues, which in turn promotes healing and helps to prevent infection. Vasoconstriction results in the reduction of edema, and blood flow is also reduced by the direct compression of increased atmospheric pressure (Babul & Rhodes 2000).

Hyperbaric oxygen is the primary treatment modality for decompression sickness and air embolism associated with underwater diving, and carbon monoxide poisoning. It has also been shown to accelerate the healing process in burns, crush injuries, acute compartment syndromes, and osteomyelitis (Babul & Rhodes 2000). These benefits are thought to derive from both the direct pressure effect and the physiological benefit of increased oxygen availability, resulting in both improved wound healing and enhanced tissue survival (Babul & Rhodes 2000). Consequently, logic suggests that many traumatic sports injuries such as muscle tears should benefit. However, the known benefits occur in situations of severe soft tissue damage and hypoxia, and measurable improvements may not occur in lesser degrees of damage. Experimental human models of delayed onset muscle soreness, induced by eccentric exercise, have failed to show improvement on parameters of soft tissue swelling, isometric strength, and creatine kinase levels when treated with hyperbaric oxygen (Harrison et al 2001, Mekjavic et al 2000). Also, no beneficial effect was seen in a study of traumatic ankle sprains (Borromeo et al 1997).

Anecdotally, hyperbaric oxygen therapy does have a pronounced, but possibly temporary effect in reducing joint effusions. This is probably a direct compression benefit, and is not related to any improvement in the underlying pathology. Further studies are being carried out, particularly using animal models for bone cartilage and tendon healing, and it may be possible to demonstrate benefits in the future. Hyperbaric oxygen therapy requires expensive equipment and close supervision by a physician. It is a very expensive and time intensive form of treatment. It cannot be widely recommended at present, but its future place in the treatment of sports injuries remains to be determined.

OTHER ANTIARTHRITIC AGENTS

Glucosamine and chondroitin sulfate have become popular as treatments for chronic joint conditions, in particular arthritis. Both agents have been promoted as natural treatments for arthritis, being derived from shellfish and sharks respectively. Increasing evidence suggests that they are useful in the treatment of mild to moderate arthritis (Bellamy & Lybrand 2001). They do not appear to be of benefit in more severe arthritic conditions (Bellamy & Lybrand 2001). It is proposed that both glucosamine and chondroitin sulfate assist the regeneration of articular cartilage (Bellamy & Lybrand 2001). Both products are readily available without prescription, and appear to be relatively free of side-effects, but with the proviso that patients allergic to seafood should avoid them. Glucosamine may affect glucose regulation in diabetics (Drew 2001). Anecdotally,

their use has been proposed for the treatment of intervertebral disk injuries and other soft tissue injury but convincing evidence of any benefits is not yet available.

Hyaluronic acid is a natural constituent of several human tissues, including synovial fluid, the skin, and joint cartilage. Osteoarthritis is associated with the breakdown of hyaluronic acid, resulting in increased susceptibility of the articular cartilage to injury. Hyaluronic acid in injectable form is available as a palliative treatment for osteoarthritis, particularly of major joints, such as the knee. It is effective in producing symptom relief, but side-effects, such as subsequent joint effusion, are not uncommon. It is an expensive form of treatment, and it has not found widespread patient and physician acceptance.

MUSCLE RELAXANTS

Muscle relaxant agents are sometimes used in addition to NSAIDs and analgesics for acute musculoskeletal injuries such as muscle strains, particularly when the paraspinal muscles are affected. All muscle relaxant agents rely on a central neurological mechanism to modulate stretch reflexes (Mazanec 1998). All muscle relaxants also have a sedative effect, which may account in part for their efficacy (Mazanec 1998). It has not been demonstrated that they are any more effective than analgesics in relieving muscle spasm (Mazanec 1998). Also, it is doubtful that muscle relaxant medications are any more effective than various physical methods such as stretching, heat packs, and massage. They may have a short-term role following acute injury.

The use of muscle relaxants is controlled in some sports that require high levels of skill and balance, such as gymnastics, archery, and equestrian events. Their effects in terms of prolonged reaction time, reduced balance, and sedation make them potentially dangerous (Henderson 1998).

ANTIBIOTICS AND ANTIVIRAL AGENTS

Although antibiotics are widely used in the community for the treatment of bacterial infections, there are many concerns about their inappropriate use for non-bacterial or minor infections. Concerns center on the increased risk of bacterial resistance, and the side-effects suffered by many patients. Nevertheless, in active bacterial infection, antibiotics remain extremely valuable. In their need for treatment of infection, athletes are no different to other members of the community. However, athletes often blame subsequent poor performances on the fact that they are taking antibiotics. Consequently, many athletes are reluctant to make use of antibiotics when they are indicated, because they believe that they may produce fatigue, or other symptoms of impaired performance. There is no evidence to support this contention and the athlete should always be reminded that it is the illness that is causing the impaired performance, rather than the medication. Notwithstanding, side-effects such as gastro-intestinal upset and skin reaction are quite common with antibiotic use and would certainly have a negative effect on performance. Whenever antibiotics are required, isolation of the athlete from other team members should always be considered. Prior to prescription of antibiotics, athletes should always be closely questioned about the possibility of allergic reaction. The type of infection, cost, availability, and dosage regimen of the drug concerned dictates choice of antibiotic. In athletes, compliance issues are of particular importance, especially with regard to training and travel requirements.

Antibiotics are sometimes used prophylactically for the prevention of traveler's diarrhea (Brukner & Khan 2001, Goldman & Bennett 2000). Local conditions and safe sources of food and water should always be ascertained prior to travel. The choice to use antibiotics for prevention of traveler's diarrhea will be determined by previous experience, knowledge of the local conditions, and a consideration of the potential benefits in regards to competition vs. the possibility of athletes suffering side-effects.

Some antibiotics such as ciprofloxacin and related quinolones have been associated with impaired fibroblast metabolism and consequent tendon rupture (Williams et al 2000). It has been proposed that these antibiotics effectively produce a toxic tendinopathy (Williams et al 2000). This effect may persist for several weeks after cessation of the drug. Further research is required to determine the extent of this problem.

Antiviral agents are becoming increasingly available for a variety of infections. Specific antivirals are useful for the treatment of common skin conditions such as herpes simplex and herpes zoster infections. These infections are particularly relevant in sports that require close skin contact, such as wrestling. It is advisable that, along with specific treatment, athletes with active infections be isolated from competition. Antiviral agents have been proposed as prophylaxis for common upper respiratory viral infections in athletes subject to major physical stress, such as severe training and overseas travel for major competition. This therapy is expensive, and demonstrated efficacy and acceptance have not yet been achieved.

ORAL CONTRACEPTIVES

Oral contraceptives are widely used by females for contraception, but also for regulation of the menstrual cycle, and relief of premenstrual and menstrual symptoms. In amenorrheic and oligoamenorrheic athletes, oral contraceptives also provide benefit in improving bone density when this is reduced (Bennell et al 1999). Oral contraceptives are permitted in all forms of competition. They are effective in regulating the menstrual cycle, which is of particular benefit to female athletes who find that premenstrual or menstrual symptoms impair their training and competition. It is possible by manipulation of dosage to delay or miss a period altogether without deleterious effects. This is often of particular importance in traveling to major events. Oral contraceptives generally reduce the amount of menstrual blood loss (Bennell et al 1999), which is of benefit in those who tend to suffer from iron depletion.

The effects of the oral contraceptive on performance have been studied quite extensively, but no firm conclusions have been drawn. Some studies (e.g. Bennell et al 1999, Quadagno 2000) have suggested that oral contraceptives may result in a small reduction in maximal oxygen uptake but this does not appear to be borne out in competitive performance. Weight gain is popularly attributed to the oral contraceptive but this is not supported by a number of studies. Any weight gain that occurs when a female athlete commences the oral contraceptive is more likely to be the result of lifestyle and dietary modifications, rather than any true physiological effect of the medication. This is particularly the case with low dose formulations that are now available (Bennell et al 1999).

The menstrual cycle has been associated with increased risk of soft tissue injury, such as ligamentous tears (Bennell et al 1999). Concerns have also been raised about the potentially increased risk of stress fracture in amenorrheic and oligoamenorrheic athletes, where estrogen levels are low (Bennell et al 1999). In both soft tissue injury and stress fracture, the possibility that the oral contraceptive may offer a protective effect is appealing. However, convincing evidence of this is not available (Bennell et al 1999).

From a practical point of view, the oral contraceptive certainly offers benefits for many female athletes. Many different preparations are available, allowing choices that optimize convenience of dosage and that minimize side-effects. A practitioner experienced in the needs of female athletes should be able to offer an oral contraceptive most suited to the individual's needs.

ASTHMA MEDICATIONS

Asthma is a common condition in the community, and is similarly common in athletes. Exercise-induced asthma is especially prevalent in the athletic population (Langdeau & Boulet 2001). Several reasons have been put forward for this. Firstly, many asthmatic children are encouraged to take up sport, especially swimming, in order to help control their respiratory symptoms. Swimming however may cause problems because of exposure to high chlorine levels in poorly ventilated pools (Langdeau & Boulet 2001). Secondly, intensive exercise, particularly in endurance sports, may expose symptoms that would otherwise go unnoticed in less active people. Thirdly, there are some concerns that exercise-induced asthma is over-diagnosed in athletes, when other conditions may be the cause of their respiratory symptoms. Finally, it has been suggested and observed clinically that some athletes make use of asthma medications, even though they do not suffer asthma, in the hope that they will provide some ergogenic benefit.

Bacterial and viral illnesses, allergens, pollutants, smoking, and exercise may provoke asthmatic symptoms (Langdeau & Boulet 2001, Smith & LaBotz 1998). Asthma is also intrinsic in some people with no specific provocative stimuli. In the case of exercise-induced asthma, the relative hyperventilation of exercise prevents the upper airways from adequately warming and humidifying the inhaled air. This results in an influx of cool dry air, which then results in a cascade of events, leading to airways inflammation and bronchoconstriction (Langdeau & Boulet 2001, Smith & LaBotz 1998). This is particularly relevant when the ambient conditions are cold and dry, and especially so in alpine sports. Training and competition in a polluted environment may also contribute to symptoms. Successful asthma therapy is reliant upon the control of the longer-term inflammation of airways and reversal of the short-term bronchoconstriction that results in the well-recognized symptoms of breathlessness often associated with wheezing and coughing.

Asthma medications fall into two major categories: preventer and reliever medications. Fundamental to successful asthma treatment is the prevention of symptoms. Many athletes tend to rely on reliever medications only, which is likely to result in suboptimal respiratory function. Any athlete who frequently requires use of reliever medication during training or competition should have their asthma management plan reviewed by a physician. Preventer medications commonly used as inhaled agents in athletes include sodium cromoglycate, nedocromil sodium, and corticosteroids. Common reliever medications are beta-2 agonists, which in longer acting forms, can also be used as preventive medications. Other agents include leukotriene antagonists, oral corticosteroids, and theophylline.

Sodium cromoglycate and nedocromil sodium both act by stabilization of the cell membranes of mast cells, which release a number of the mediators causing asthma (Smith & LaBotz 1998). They appear to be particularly beneficial in exercise-induced asthma, and are administered on a regular daily basis. They should be used shortly before exercise, and they act for several hours afterwards. Such agents are of no benefit in relieving acute symptoms. Both drugs are relatively free of side-effects and are permitted for use in competition without restriction.

Inhaled corticosteroids are the mainstay of preventive treatment in moderate to severe asthma, whether exercise-induced or not. They are effective in reducing both the inflammation of airways and bronchial hyper-reactivity (Langdeau & Boulet 2001, Smith & LaBotz 1998). They are only effective on a preventive basis, and are generally not useful in an acute attack. Inhaled corticosteroids are administered on a regular daily basis, and can be taken without regard to the timing of exercise. Side-effects are minimal. At the dosages normally used by athletes, systemic corticosteroid side-effects are most unlikely to occur. Other preventer and reliever medications can be used in combination with inhaled corticosteroids. They are permitted for use in competition, but some sporting federations may require notification of their use.

Beta-2 agonists have been widely used for the relief of asthma symptoms. Short-acting inhaled beta-2 agonists induce bronchodilation within minutes, and also have some impact on the mediators released by mast cells (Smith & LaBotz 1998). A positive response to beta-2 agonists is a simple tool for the diagnosis of exercise-induced asthma, and can be used for ongoing treatment in milder cases. However, any symptoms not readily controlled by pre-exercise use of an inhaled beta-2 agonist demand review by a physician, and the likely institution of effective preventer medications. Long-term use of beta-2 agonists, both in short- and long-acting forms, leads to a level of tolerance to these medications, and may ultimately reduce respiratory performance (Brukner & Khan 2001, Smith & LaBotz 1998). Common side-effects of short-acting beta-2 agonists are tachycardia and skeletal muscle tremor (Hardman & Limbird 2001). Tolerance to these side-effects usually develops in regular users. Longer acting beta-2 agonists such as salmeterol have become increasingly widely used, but similar concerns about their long-term effect on respiratory performance remain.

Beta-2 agonists in both short- and long-acting form are classified as both stimulants and anabolic agents in the Olympic Movement anti-doping code. However, the use of some beta-2 agonists is permitted with specific notification (see later in this chapter). Since 2001, permission to use inhaled beta-2 agonists requires the submission of clinical and laboratory findings confirming the diagnosis of asthma. A range of appropriate tests is available (Brukner & Khan 2001). Inhaled beta-2 agonists have not been shown to have any ergogenic effect in non-asthmatic athletes (Morton et al 1996, Smith & LaBotz 1998). However, inhaled and injectable forms of beta-2 agonists, which are not widely available, have been shown to have an anabolic effect, and are hence banned (Van Baak et al 2000).

Leukotrienes are potent agents given in oral form for asthma management. They are generally reserved for use by severe asthmatics, and will most often be prescribed by a respiratory specialist. Theophylline was once a frequent preventive asthma medication taken in oral form. Its use has declined, but it maintains a place in the management of severe asthma, in combination with other drugs. It has no specific role in the management of exercise-induced asthma.

Oral and intravenous corticosteroids are very effective at relieving severe episodes of asthma (Hardman & Limbird 2001); however, these medications are banned in sport competition. They may, however, occasionally be essential to the management of severely asthmatic athletes. In these circumstances, the relevant national sporting federation should be contacted, as special provision for treatment may be possible, under the supervision of an independent respiratory specialist.

LEGAL CONSIDERATIONS

Many drugs are restricted by law, and can only be prescribed by physicians, and dispensed by physicians and pharmacists. A few minor exceptions exist in relation to specific medications used in dentistry, podiatry, and other areas. The prescription or dispensing of restricted medications by other practitioners is specifically prohibited, to avoid dangers to the patient. Physicians and pharmacists receive extensive training in pharmacology, and have a good understanding of the effects, side-effects, contraindications, and interactions of a wide range of drugs. Other practitioners, in general, do not have this training.

Many medications, such as simple analgesics and some NSAIDs are available for over-the-counter purchase in pharmacies, supermarkets, and convenience stores. The recommendation and dispensing of these medications by practitioners other than physicians and pharmacists is often not clearly spelled out by the law. Whilst these drugs are generally safer than prescription only medication, risks of side-effects, interaction, and allergy remain, and it is good practice to avoid recommendation of any form of medication without the specific advice of a trained practitioner.

PERFORMANCE-ENHANCING DRUGS

HISTORICAL PERSPECTIVE OF PERFORMANCE-ENHANCING DRUGS IN SPORT

Drugs have been used in the hope of enhancing performance ever since the recording of organized sporting competitions began (Verroken 1996). One of the better known classes of performance-enhancing drugs, anabolic steroids, was first developed in 1927 and is first known to have been used at the Olympic Games by Russian weightlifters in 1952. There is, however, some suggestion that they may have been used as early as 1936. At that time, no regulations controlling use, and no effective detection measures, were in place. In 1960, the death of a Danish cyclist in the team time trial event at the Rome Olympics was associated with the use of amphetamines. In 1967, champion British cyclist Tom Simpson died during the Tour de France whilst the event was being covered on television. His death was attributed to heat exhaustion and amphetamines, traces of which were found in his jersey pockets. An increasing tide of public concern resulted in the formation of the International Olympic Committee Medical Commission in 1967, and performance-enhancing drugs were banned in Olympic competition. Soon after, a drug-testing program was introduced, initially testing only for stimulants and narcotics. Controls were introduced at the 1968 Olympics, and at that event and every subsequent Olympic Games, a number of athletes have tested positive for various drugs and suffered the consequences. With each Olympic Games since 1968 there have been revelations of new drugs being used, and allegations made that many more athletes are using drugs than the number detected. Testing procedures have been continually refined. Out of competition testing was first introduced in 1987. The issue of drugs in sport was brought into sharp international focus in 1988 after Ben Johnson was stripped of his gold medal in the 100 m sprint following a positive test for anabolic steroids. Several countries undertook inquiries into the issue of drugs in sport, and more stringent testing and regulations were introduced. Increasingly stringent controls have been put in place subsequently. The year 2001 saw the advent of a universal regulation and testing program under the auspices of the International Olympic Committee (IOC) and the World Anti-Doping Agency (WADA).

New challenges continue to arise in the battle against drug use in sport. The use of synthetic forms of various hormones, which are almost indistinguishable from the natural products, has presented a major challenge in both drug detection and regulation. New technology will continue to produce new drugs and the requirement for ever more sophisticated testing technology. There is some hope that there will be fewer and fewer avenues by which performance may be enhanced with drugs, and that the battle may then be won. However, gene therapy may generate a whole new range of testing and legislative challenges.

The IOC Medical Commission, working in conjunction with WADA, is the peak body in establishing anti-doping regulations. The Olympic Movement anti-doping code is the prototype for anti-drug regulations used by all sporting federations. Variations do occur in relation to the specific circumstances of each sport, and these also vary from country to country. However, an objective of WADA is to make basic regulations universal to all sports and countries.

OLYMPIC MOVEMENT ANTI-DOPING CODE

Prohibited classes of substances and prohibited methods are published under the auspices of the Olympic Movement Anti-Doping Code. This code is subject to continual review and update and is best accessed through the IOC website. Its current details are as follows:

I. *Prohibited classes of substances*
   A. Stimulants
   B. Narcotics
   C. Anabolic agents
   D. Diuretics
   E. Peptide hormones, mimetics and analogs.

II. *Prohibited methods*

III. *Classes of prohibited substances in certain circumstances*
   A. Alcohol
   B. Cannabinoids
   C. Local anesthetics
   D. Glucocorticosteroids
   E. Beta blockers

IV. *Out-of-competition testing*

Within the code, examples of prohibited substances are given in each class but it is made clear that no list is exhaustive, and any drug that is deemed to fall within a specific class may be considered banned. Each of these major categories and classes will be considered in turn.

I. Prohibited classes of substances

All substances that fall within this category are banned in all Olympic competition.

A. Stimulants

Historically, stimulants have been the most widely-abused drugs. Well-established detection methods are in place, but athletes continue to test positive for stimulants at each Olympic Games. Various stimulants are widely used in society, both for their stimulant effect (e.g. caffeine) and for other benefits (e.g. the bronchodilating effect of beta-2 agonists and decongestant effects of sympathomimetics such as pseudoephedrine). More potent stimulants such as strychnine and cocaine have been used for many years, and continue to be abused. All stimulants act on the central nervous system and, in so doing, increase alertness and reduce tiredness (George 1996a). They also improve concentration, which is beneficial in many precision events (George 1996a). In theory at least, they may help athletes achieve maximal explosive power, and may also help endurance athletes avoid the normal sensation of fatigue. In everyday life, there is abundant empirical evidence that commonly used stimulants (e.g. caffeine) help overcome tiredness and may improve concentration. However, there is no convincing experimental evidence to show that improvements can be achieved in the concentration, power generation, or endurance of a well-prepared athlete attempting optimal performance. They may be of benefit in prolonged events, but evidence for this is lacking. Caffeine has been shown to have some ergogenic benefit, but probably for reasons other than its stimulant effect.

As a result of the widespread use of stimulant drugs in society, outside of sporting competition, a number of specific provisions in regard to their use have been made. For caffeine, the definition of a positive test is a concentration in urine greater than 12 µg/mL. As much as 1000 mg of caffeine needs to be consumed within 2–3 hours to achieve this level.

Approximate caffeine levels in various readily available substances are shown in Table 28.2. Individuals vary in their absorption rate and response to caffeine. At a urinary concentration of 12 µg/mL, side-effects such as tremor and a diuretic effect would most often be intolerable (George 1996a). Guarana, a popular herbal stimulant, is chemically closely related to caffeine, but is more potent, and is likely to result in positive tests if overused.

Sympathomimetic drugs such as pseudoephedrine and phenylpropanolamine are frequently used as decongestants to counteract the symptoms of upper respiratory infections. They are most often taken as oral tablets and capsules, but also can be used as nasal drops and inhalers. A positive test for these drugs is defined as a concentration in urine greater than 25 µg/mL. This level will generally only be achieved where the drugs have been used in high dosage or on the day of competition.

Table 28.2   Caffeine levels of common products

Substance		Caffeine content (mg)
Instant coffee	250 ml	100
Brewed coffee	250 ml	200
Tea	250 ml	30–60
Coca-Cola	375 ml	65
Diet Coke	375 ml	65
Pepsi	375 ml	45
Chocolate	50 g	30
Tablets and suppositories		100–500

Usage at recommended dosages, ceasing 3 or more days before competition, should not lead to a positive result. Common side-effects of these drugs are tremor, tachycardia, headache, and occasionally acute hypertension (George 1996a, Henderson 1998). Whilst widely used as nasal decongestants, their use for more than 7 days can often result in a paradoxical exacerbation of nasal symptoms. Pseudoephedrine and phenylpropanolamine are contained in a wide variety of combination preparations for relief of upper respiratory symptoms and other conditions. The trade names for these medications vary greatly from country to country, and a brand that is permissible for sport in one country may not be in another. Also, under the one well-known trade name, a number of different formulations may be marketed. To avoid inadvertent doping, packaging must be examined with great care, and if any doubt remains, expert advice should be sought, or the medication avoided altogether.

Beta-2 agonist drugs used for the prevention and treatment of asthma and exercise-induced asthma (e.g. salbutamol, salmeterol, terbutaline and formoterol [eformoterol]) are classified as stimulants and may only be used in inhaled form with prior written notification. This must be provided by a respiratory physician or team physician confirming that the athlete suffers asthma and/or exercise-induced asthma. At the Olympic Games, an independent medical panel will assess athletes who request permission to use inhaled beta-2 agonists.

Many so-called social and recreational drugs such as amphetamines, cocaine, and ecstasy are potent stimulants, and will result in positive drug tests, even though there has been no intention to gain a performance enhancing benefit.

B. Narcotics

Narcotics are well known and widely used in medicine as potent analgesic agents. There is no evidence that they produce performance-enhancing effects as such, however, there are concerns that pre-existing injury and illness may be exacerbated by the use of painkillers during continued participation. Common side-effects of the use of narcotics are drowsiness, constipation, nausea, and vomiting. Allergic reactions to these drugs are also quite common (Verroken 1996).

Morphine, methadone, pethidine and diamorphine (heroin) are not permitted. However, as very effective analgesics, their use should not be withheld in situations of severe traumatic injury, where continued participation is clearly impossible.

Widely used narcotic analgesics of mild to moderate potency are permitted for use in training and competition. These permitted drugs are codeine, dextromethorphan, dextropropoxyphene, dihydrocodeine, diphenoxylate, ethylmorphine, pholcodine, propoxyphene, and tramadol.

C. Anabolic agents

1. Anabolic androgenic steroids:
   a. Synthetic anabolic androgenic steroids
   b. Naturally occurring anabolic androgenic steroids
2. Beta-2 agonists.

Anabolic androgenic steroids (AAS) are all close chemical relations of testosterone, the principal anabolic and androgenic hormone in males, which is also found in lesser concentrations in females. The testes, adrenal glands, and ovaries normally produce testosterone. All of these drugs, whether synthetic or natural have a combination of both anabolic (bodybuilding) and androgenic (masculinizing) effects. The relative proportion and potency of the anabolic and androgenic effect tends to determine the side-effect profile of each drug, and also their usefulness for abusers. Major side-effects of AAS are listed in Table 28.3.

Technology to detect the use of AAS has become increasingly sophisticated, and the recent use of all synthetic forms in competition should be readily detected. Evidence of use months before competition can also be obtained from metabolic profiles (Bowers 1998). These techniques rely on the detection of metabolic breakdown products of the synthetic hormones being present in the urine. The proportions of these products can then determine that AAS have been used, even though the specific drug may not be detected.

The major challenge in the fight against the use of AAS is the use of testosterone and related naturally occurring steroids, such as androstenediol, androstenedione, norandrostenedione, and dehydroepiandrosterone (DHEA), all of which are naturally occurring in varying levels. All of these AAS, except testosterone, have a very weak anabolic effect, and have doubtful (if any) direct benefit in enhancing performance. However, norandrostenedione, which is naturally occurring and also contained in some food supplements, is metabolized to nandrolone, which in high doses, is well known as a potent synthetic

Table 28.3 Major side-effects of anabolic androgenic steroids

System	Effects
Musculoskeletal	Tendon rupture Premature closure of epiphyses
Endocrine – Males	Testicular atrophy Decreased or nil sperm production Prostatic hypertrophy Prostatic carcinoma Reduced hormone production Gynecomastia
Endocrine – Females	Masculinization – male pattern hair growth and baldness Breast tissue reduction Voice changes Clitoral hypertrophy Menstrual irregularity
Hepatic	Abnormal liver enzyme function Hepatic carcinoma Jaundice
Cardiovascular	Coronary artery disease Altered lipid profile Hypertension Clotting problems
Renal	Renal tumors Impaired renal function
Central nervous system	Psychosis Aggression Altered libido
Skin	Acne Striae

AAS (Bowers 1998). Detection of these drugs currently relies upon variations in the testosterone: epitestosterone ratio, epitestosterone being an inactive isomer of testosterone produced naturally. The normal ratio is subject to variation in some circumstances, and so confirmation of positive test results can be difficult. Athletes have exploited uncertainties relating to testosterone:epitestosterone ratios to avoid suspension following positive tests.

AAS such as norandrostenedione and DHEA may be contained in readily available food supplements, and even in trace amounts, can result in positive tests. Extreme caution in the use of supplements must be taken. The potential for contamination of food supplements has been used as a means to avoid suspension following positive tests for these drugs.

The performance-enhancing benefits of AAS were debated for many years. Many clinical trials (George 1996b, Sturmi & Diorio 1998) failed to show the expected performance benefits in terms of strength gains, with or without the presence of changes in muscle bulk. However, it is well recognized that the doses used by athletes have been many times greater than the recommended doses for various medical conditions. Consequently, ethical constraints have prevented the depth of study

necessary to fully delineate the performance benefits of AAS. Anecdotally, there is abundant evidence that great improvements in strength and muscle bulk can be achieved. It is now generally accepted that AAS can increase muscle protein synthesis and block the catabolic effects of glucocorticosteroids (George 1996b, Sturmi & Diorio 1998). In order to be effective, the drugs must be used in collaboration with an intensive training program and a high quality diet (George 1996b, Sturmi & Diorio 1998).

AAS abuse has been most closely linked with power sports such as throwing events, weightlifting, power lifting, wrestling, and sprinting. However, their benefits can be translated to a wide variety of sports, as many athletes will benefit from measurable gains in strength and speed. AAS are also reputed to enhance recovery and improve endurance (George 1996b, Sturmi & Diorio 1998). There is little evidence to support this, but on a theoretical basis it is plausible. While the common perception of an AAS abuser is of an extremely powerfully built athlete, dosage regimen can be tailored to suit even lightly built athletes in endurance sports, in the hope that specific strength and recovery can be enhanced, without the penalty of weight gain. In prolonged events, AAS could help counter both the catabolic effects of sustained exercise and the lack of appetite for the large amounts of food required (Sturmi & Diorio 1998).

The abuse of AAS has been associated with a wide variety of well-recognized side-effects. Many of the well-known side-effects are reversible on cessation of the drugs, but there is significant concern about a number of long-term, potentially fatal, side-effects. Some of the major side-effects are detailed in Table 28.3.

Trade in AAS is either severely restricted or prohibited in most countries. Consequently, the majority of these drugs are obtained illegally and their exact identity and purity must be questioned. Abuse of AAS in activities outside organized competitive sport is widespread, for potential improvement in strength and appearance. The use of injectable forms of AAS raises additional concerns with regard to the potential for infectious disease transmission via the sharing of needles.

Beta-2 agonists have been used for many years for the treatment of asthma, but their potential anabolic effect has only been recognized relatively recently (Van Baak et al 2000). They have been widely used in animal production to produce rapid gains in muscle bulk. All beta-2 agonists in oral and injectable form are banned in competitive sport. Inhaled salbutamol, salmeterol, terbutaline and formoterol (eformoterol) are, however, permitted. For salbutamol, the definition of a positive test under the anabolic agent category is a concentration in urine greater than 1000 ng/mL, which could not normally be achieved by the use of the inhaled medication. Salbutamol is reported to be a stimulant if the urinary concentration exceeds 100 ng/L.

D. Diuretics

A wide range of diuretic drugs has been used to increase urinary output. This has two potential benefits to the athlete. Firstly, body weight can be suddenly reduced in order to make weight for sports where specific categories are applied (e.g. weightlifting, lightweight rowing, and all fighting sports). Secondly, a large output of very dilute urine makes the presence of other drugs difficult to detect. In this context, diuretics are often used as a masking agent. For making weight, diuretics are often combined with other potentially dangerous practices such as the use of saunas and severe restriction of food and fluids.

Abuse of diuretics can lead to severe dehydration, cramps, fall in blood pressure, and electrolyte and metabolic disturbances (Verroken 1996). Fatal events are possible. To extend the dangers, the technique of rapidly infusing large volumes of intravenous fluids to regain weight rapidly following diuresis, has been an accepted practice in some sports.

E. Peptide hormones, mimetics, and analogs

Prohibited substances in Class E include the following examples and their analogs and mimetics:

1. Chorionic Gonadotrophin (hCG) prohibited in males only
2. Pituitary and synthetic gonadotrophins (LH) prohibited in males only
3. Corticotrophins (ACTH, tetracosactide)
4. Growth hormone (hGH)
5. Insulin like growth factor (IGF-1) and all the respective releasing factors and their analogs relating to the above
6. Erythropoietin (EPO)
7. Insulin is permitted only to treat athletes with certified insulin-dependent diabetes. Written certification of insulin-dependent diabetes must be obtained from an endocrinologist or team physician.

The presence of an abnormal concentration of an endogenous hormone in Class E or its diagnostic marker(s) in the urine of a competitor constitutes an offence, unless it has been proven to be due to a physiological or pathological condition.

Each of the above substances is a naturally occurring human hormone which has a wide variety of metabolic influences. All of these hormones can now be synthesized, and have specific uses in medical practice for a variety of disease conditions; the best known in this respect being insulin for diabetes. Once peptide hormones have been synthesized, active components of the molecules can then be identified, and synthesized as mimetic drugs. Analogs are close chemical relations of the naturally occurring hormones, which have undergone minor chemical modification, resulting in similar effects, increased potency, or a longer or shorter duration of action. This potential to continue producing a wide range of drugs with actions similar to the naturally occurring hormones is the reason for the broad definition of drugs within this class.

These Class E drugs have presented a major challenge to drug testing authorities. It can be very difficult, if not impossible, to distinguish the natural hormone level from doping. In some cases breakthroughs have been made because of minor chemical differences between the natural hormone and synthetic drug. Concurrent blood and urine testing expedites detection of abuse, but further research is necessary before testing can be widely applied and results upheld.

II. Prohibited methods

The following procedures are prohibited:

1. Blood doping: the administration of blood, red blood cells, and/or related products to an athlete, which may be preceded by withdrawal of blood from the athlete, who continues to train in such a blood-depleted state.
2. The administration of artificial oxygen carriers or plasma expanders.
3. Pharmacological, chemical, and physical manipulation.

Blood doping has effectively been replaced by the abuse of recombinant erythropoietin. Artificial oxygen carriers are only in the early stages of development in clinical medicine, but nevertheless have been utilized by athletes for doping purposes. Pharmacological, chemical, and physical manipulation relate to the practices of diluting, adulterating, and substituting urine when a sample is presented for testing. As blood testing becomes more widespread, similar measures are being attempted to disguise the presence of doping agents.

III. Classes of prohibited substances in certain circumstances

A. Alcohol

The dangerous effects of alcohol on judgement and motor control are well recognized in the operation of machinery, especially motor vehicles. Similar risks apply in many sports, particularly those involving high speed, and it is up to the rules of the relevant sporting federation to decide whether alcohol should be banned in competition for the safety of all participants.

B. Cannabinoids (marijuana, hashish)

As for alcohol, judgement and motor control may be impaired with the use of cannabinoids and it is the responsibility of the relevant sports federation to determine the need for a ban.

C. Local anesthetics

These are permitted in the form of local and intra-articular injection, only when medically justified. Notification of administration may be necessary, depending on the rules of the sporting authority. The use of epinephrine (adrenaline) in combination with local anesthetic is permitted, but cocaine is not permitted in any circumstances.

D. Glucocorticosteroids (clinically referred to as corticosteroids)

Systemic use, whether by oral, rectal, intramuscular, or intravenous administration, is prohibited. When medically necessary, local and intra-articular injections of glucocorticosteroids are permitted but prior notification may be required. Inhaled agents for asthma and nasal conditions, and topical agents for skin conditions are permitted.

E. Beta blockers

These drugs act as membrane stabilizers, slowing the heart rate and reducing muscle tremor (Henderson 1998, Reilly 1996). They are useful in precision sports such as archery, shooting, biathlon, ski jumping, and luge, and are prohibited by the relevant sporting authority where they may be of benefit.

IV. Out-of-competition testing

Unless specifically requested by the responsible authority, out-of-competition testing is directed solely at prohibited substances in classes I.C. (anabolic agents), I.D. (diuretics), I.E. (peptide hormones, mimetics and analogs), and II (prohibited methods).

Stimulants are the main class of prohibited drugs that are likely to be used outside competition, most often for upper respiratory illnesses, and will not be tested for. Athletes and team staff must, however, be aware of the use of these drugs, and ensure that they are ceased at least 3 days before competition.

There are circumstances where a prohibited substance may be therapeutically necessary for the treatment of uncommon conditions. In this situation, most countries have established a specialist panel to review such circumstances. If a prohibited substance is to be permitted, it must be demonstrated that health would be impaired if the substance was not available, and that there is no therapeutic alternative. The condition and dosage must be monitored by an independent specialist physician.

DRUG TESTING

In the past, there has been a wide range of drug testing procedures utilized by different countries and sporting organizations. This has often led to allegations of inadequate or unfair testing protocols. With the advent of the WADA, a major goal has been the undertaking of universal testing practices.

An athlete may be selected for testing at any time outside competition, at the conclusion of an event, or during the course of a multiple day event. Athletes may be selected in competition on the basis of their finishing place or randomly. Where an athlete or event is the subject of rumor, selection may be specifically targeted.

It is advisable for team medical staff to be familiar with drug testing protocols, by personally observing the testing process. Staff can then attend with team members who may be chosen for testing, to ensure that all processes are carried out correctly, and that the athlete fully understands all aspects of testing. There is usually provision for the accompanying person to countersign all paperwork as the athlete's representative. As testing protocols can vary between different sports and countries, it is important to ensure that all steps are clearly understood, and that language interpretation is available when necessary. Normally the representative will be permitted to observe all aspects of the testing process, except the actual passing of urine. When athletes are selected for testing, they are permitted to first complete all necessary victory ceremonies and media commitments. They may also complete a warm-down, change their clothing, and undertake any necessary medical care, prior to presenting at the drug testing facility; however, all of these activities should take place under the direct observation of the chaperone acting for the drug testing authority. Competition testing must always involve the first urine passed after completion of the event.

Essential components of any testing process are the following:

- The athlete must be formally notified in writing of selection for testing.
- The drug testing room must be clearly identified, private, and secure.

29

Medical imaging of injury

Douglas Mintz

INTRODUCTION

Imaging of musculoskeletal injury requires a detailed knowledge of the normal anatomy of the body along with the changes that reflect the pathophysiology of injury. There are many ways to image an injury, and the method chosen depends on the information required. Types of imaging vary in cost, availability, use of radiation, comfort for the patient, expertise required of the performer of the examination, and expertise required of the interpreter of the examination. If clinicians understand both the disease processes and the imaging options, they will be able to use the least expensive and least invasive test that will answer the appropriate clinical question.

IMAGING MODALITIES AND TECHNIQUES

PLAIN FILM

Conventional radiographs are relatively inexpensive, widely available, and provide a good starting point for imaging evaluation. Radiographs provide excellent bony, but not very good soft tissue detail. Despite their utility, they do involve a low dose of radiation. Therefore, if many radiographs are to be obtained over time (e.g. following scoliosis) protective lead shields should be used to cover the breasts and gonads (Andersen et al 1982, Butler et al 1986, Nash et al 1979). The usual procedure involves obtaining at least two views of a body part (preferably orthogonal), with additional views, such as oblique views, stress views, or special views, added as necessary (Harris et al 1993). Specific X-ray positions have been developed to better assess the ankle mortise, the carpal tunnel, the calcaneus, the subtalar joints, and even the sesamoid bones at the base of the first metatarsal

(Pavlov et al 1999). For example, the Harris heel view is used to evaluate the calcaneus. The carpal tunnel view is used to look for bony spurs that may contribute to carpal tunnel syndrome and to look for fractures of the hamate or pisiform bone. Using the principle that to evaluate a structure radiographically it should be visible, unencumbered by overlapping structures, and in two orthogonal views, radiologists and clinicians have developed appropriate projections over the years. Some bear the name of the inventor (e.g. Broden's view of the subtalar joint, Grashey's view of the glenohumeral joint, Judet's views of the acetabulum), while others are descriptive (e.g. the inlet and outlet views of the pelvis, and the sesamoid view of the great toe).

X-rays are created by passing an electrical current through an X-ray tube, which can be aimed so that the X-rays go into the body (Curry et al 1990). Some of the X-rays are absorbed and those that pass through the body expose a film or detector on the other side of the patient from the tube. More modern techniques produce a digital image rather than an image on film.

Several methods of adding information to the routine radiograph using X-rays include fluoroscopy, tomography, arthrography, and myelography.

Fluoroscopy

In fluoroscopy, continuous radiographic images are obtained and viewed on a monitor enabling a clinician or radiologist to see what is happening while it occurs. This technique is useful to guide procedures such as facet and nerve root injections and to perform arthrograms where real-time examination of contrast injections is useful. Information can also be recorded, either digitally or with video, to show controlled motion as a cine loop. Whereas this technique is commonly used for other reasons, such as to evaluate patients' swallowing mechanisms or the stucture of the gastrointestinal tract, it can be useful in the evaluation of carpal bones (Mathoulin et al 1990, Werber et al 1990) for suspected midcarpal instability. It can also be useful when performing an arthrogram, to facilitate the tracking of contrast. For example, if a radiocarpal joint injection is performed, and contrast extends into the midcarpal compartment, there is a tear of either the scapholunate or lunotriquetral ligament. If a video was taken at the time of the injection, it might be possible to better follow the course of the contrast and identify the exact location of the tear.

Tomography

Tomography is a technique that puts one level plane or depth in focus. By moving that plane up or down, you can see one level of a structure, bone or soft tissue, in focus, and the rest out of focus (Fig. 29.1). The level in focus is moved up or down systematically to evaluate the structure in question. This is achieved by moving the X-ray tube and the plate simultaneously so that only one area remains in focus. The patterns of motion can be simple (linear tomography) or complex (e.g. hypocycloidal) depending on the details required. Tomography is useful in assessing for articular step-off in intra-articular fractures and also in looking for fractures that might otherwise be obscured by adjacent bone (e.g. odontoid fractures or pars interarticularis fractures). Plain tomography has, for the most part, been replaced by computed tomography (CT), and so much so that there are few complex tomogram machines that remain in practice.

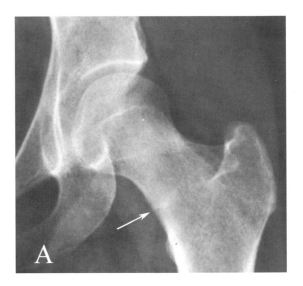

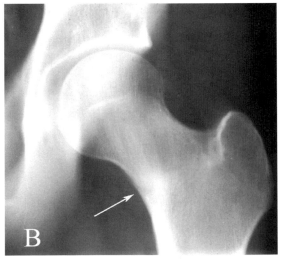

Figure 29.1A&B **A** Frontal view of the left hip demonstrating stress fracture of the medial femoral neck (arrow). **B** Tomogram of the same fracture (arrow). Note that the fracture is better seen on the tomogram.

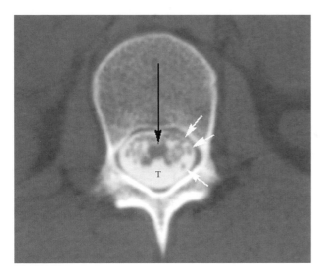

Figure 29.2 Axial CT image at the L1 level after the subarachnoid administration of iodinated contrast for a myelogram. Note the CSF in the thecal sac (T) is dense from the contrast. The large arrow is on the conus medullaris. The short arrows point to the individual nerve roots of the cauda equina, outlined by contrast.

Myelography/arthrography

Myelography is a procedure in which contrast is injected into the subarachnoid space and then examined with radiographs and with CT scans (Fig. 29.2). This can be achieved in the cervical, thoracic or lumbar spine. The injection is performed with a thin needle in the lower lumbar or upper thoracic spine in such a way as to limit the risk of contacting the spinal cord. Myelography was formerly the mainstay of imaging of the spine for soft tissue abnormalities such as disk herniations. The technique has been largely replaced, however, by magnetic resonance imaging (MRI), although myelograms are still used as a preoperative tool.

When performing a myelogram, as much information as possible should be obtained from the examination. For example, when assessing the lumbar spine, images of the patient's spine in flexion and extension should be obtained. These images can be used both to evaluate stability and to look at the effect of the motion on the degree of any stenosis or impingement that is present.

Arthrograms, in which contrast is injected into a joint, was once the most common approach to imaging the shoulder for rotator cuff tear, the knee for meniscal tear, and the wrist for evaluation of the triangular fibrocartilage (Fig. 29.3). These techniques have been largely replaced by MRI and ultrasound. Arthrography is still used for patients who are unable to undergo MRI in evaluation of the knee meniscus, for injecting or aspirating a joint (e.g. the hip or shoulder), and for therapeutic or diagnostic purposes.

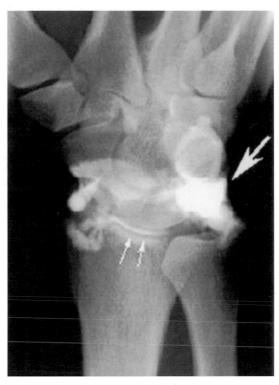

Figure 29.3 Arthrogram of the wrist. The contrast is white and outlines the radiocarpal joint (small arrows) and collects in the pisiform bursa (large arrow).

NUCLEAR MEDICINE

Nuclear medicine is the field of radiology in which radioactive agents, called radionuclides, are injected into the body and subsequently imaged using radiation detectors placed over the body. Radionuclides are bioactive substrates allowing nuclear medicine to evaluate physiological properties.

Bone scan

In nuclear medicine, there are many procedures used to image the body. The procedure that is most common in evaluating injuries is the bone scan, whereby the patient is injected with radioactive technetium-labeled diphosphonate which distributes itself to metabolically active bone. There are three potential phases to imaging. Phase 1 (the vascular phase) involves imaging the patient immediately, while the substance is in the artery. Phase 2 (the blood pool phase), involves imaging when the radionuclide is starting to perfuse the soft tissues. Phase 3 is the imaging of the bone after the radionuclide has left the soft tissues and been concentrated into the bone. This occurs 2 h after injection and the patient is imaged under a radiation counter to produce the image (Fig. 29.4). This should be done with the detector close to the body and after the radionuclide has left the soft tissue and become

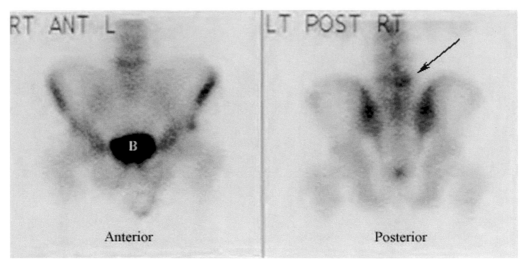

Figure 29.4   Bone scan with anterior and posterior views with faint increased uptake in the right lower lumbar region. The bladder (B) contains concentrated radionuclide.

more conspicuous in the bone. Since the bone scanning agent is excreted in the urine, it gets concentrated in the bladder, so that the bladder becomes black on the images (Fig. 29.4). This image of the bladder can obscure the sacrum thereby requiring patients to empty their bladders before being scanned.

Bone scans are very sensitive, but not very specific. The lack of specificity means that the clinical setting is very important. In a runner, a stress fracture can be seen on bone scan before it is demonstrated on X-ray. The same appearance, in a different location or clinical setting, however, may represent an infection, arthritis, or a bone tumor (Levin et al 1967). Another use of bone scan is to identify fractures of the pars interarticularis and to evaluate healing as a function of radionuclide uptake (Anderson et al 2000). Cross-sectional images can be obtained using single photon emission computed tomography (SPECT) (Fig. 29.5), where the detector passes around the body, as in regular CT, but much more slowly. MRI has also been used for this purpose (Standaert et al 2000).

Bone densitometry

Several methods are available to measure the density of bone. Bone density is correlated to bone mineral content to evaluate for osteopenia/osteoporosis. Statistical comparisons are made to the young healthy general population (T-values) and age-matched controls (Z-values). Osteopenia is defined as having a bone density of 1 standard deviation below the mean and osteoporosis is defined as 2.5 standard deviations below the mean (see Chs 5 and 26).

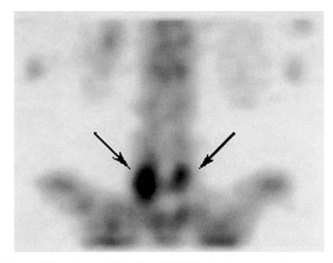

Figure 29.5   Coronal slice from SPECT of the bone scan in Fig. 29.4, with more conspicuous uptake, seen on the right more than left. The finding indicates pars fractures, more active on the right. These are seen in the CT scan of Fig. 29.10.

Bone density can be determined using many imaging modalities, including X-ray, MRI, CT, and ultrasound. In general, radiographs are not sensitive enough to bone loss to be useful for evaluating bone density. It is said that 30–50% of the bone mineralization from a given bone must be lost before the finding is evident on radiograph (Greenspan 2000, Resnick 1996). The most commonly used method (which is inexpensive, convenient, has a low radiation dose, and is reproducible) of measuring bone densitometry is dual emission X-ray absorptometry (DEXA). DEXA quantitatively compares absorption of X-ray beams of two different energies. This test is

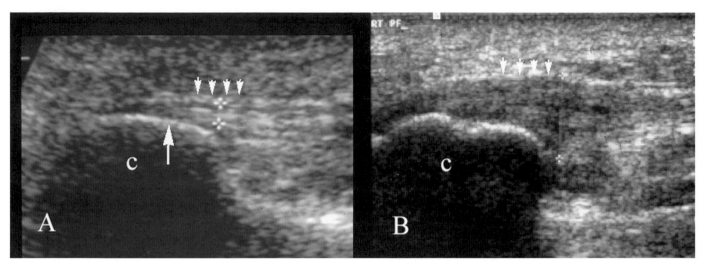

Figure 29.6A & B   Ultrasound images comparing normal plantar fascia (**A**) with plantar fasciitis (**B**). The plantar fascia (small arrowheads) is normally a thin echogenic structure arising from the calcaneus (c). Note the white line (big arrow) indicating the reflective cortical surface of the calcaneus. In **B**, the plantar fascia is markedly thickened (calipers) and has decreased echogenicity.

performed on different parts of the body, including the spine, hip, and wrist. It is useful in identifying and following osteopenia or osteoporosis (Faulkner 2001). In the young injured population, DEXA is used in the presence of stress fractures to identify a more important underlying problem such as osteoporosis and malnutrition (see Ch. 5 for a further account of the use of DEXA).

ULTRASOUND

Ultrasound is an excellent tool to image musculoskeletal injury. Diagnostic ultrasound uses lower energy than the therapeutic ultrasound (discussed in Ch. 13). Ultrasound scans invoke principles of transmission and reflection of sound waves, as in sonar, to obtain a cross-sectional image of an area. Modern ultrasound uses high frequency transducers to get high level detail in evaluation of the soft tissues, particularly superficially (Fig. 29.6) Ultrasound studies are user dependent, meaning that the practitioner who holds the ultrasound probe (or transducer) must be able to manipulate it to an appropriate position to obtain good specific images. It is the operator who, to a great extent, performs the evaluation, and the person who is evaluating the study (if not the operator), is dependent upon the operator to identify and produce good images of the pathology.

In order to create an ultrasound image, there must be an 'acoustic window', which is an area that does not reflect sound waves and allows them to be transmitted. The internal structures of the knee, such as the cruciate ligaments, are therefore not amenable to ultrasound, nor are the deep structures of the other joints. Imaging of the shoulder and acetabular labra is possible, but limited

in its extent, as is the evaluation of the menisci of the knee. Ultrasound does not image into bone because bone reflects most of the sound waves (Fig. 29.6 and 29.7). Therefore only the surface of a bone can be seen and nothing underneath the surface. Cortical breaks, such as in fractures, can be seen, as can spikes of bone (osteophytes) arising from normally smooth surfaces (Fig. 29.7) (Hubner et al 2000, Patten et al 1992).

Ultrasound is of great benefit for evaluation of superficial tendons such as in the foot, ankle, and wrist (Fig. 29.8), as well as the tendons and ligaments around the shoulder, elbow, and knee. Ultrasound has the advantage of being a real-time modality so that an ultrasonographer can manipulate patients and discuss their symptoms with them while the study is being performed

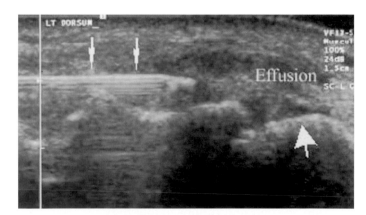

Figure 29.7   Ultrasound image of a metatarsalphalangeal joint injection. Note the needle (thin arrows) within the joint effusion. The cortex of bone is a white line because it reflects the sound waves (fat arrow).

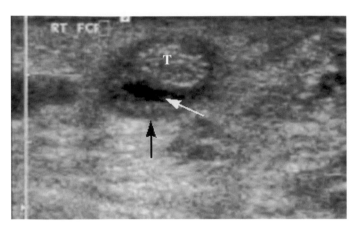

Figure 29.8 Ultrasound image of the flexor carpi radialis (T) in cross section. There is tenosynovitis with fluid in the tendon sheath (white arrow) and thickening of the tendon sheath itself (black arrow). Note the osteophytes on the dorsal surface of the joint.

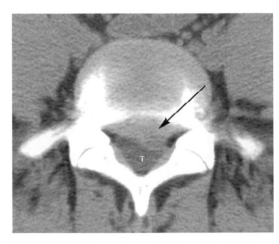

Figure 29.9 Axial CT image demonstrating moderately large left-sided disk herniation at L5–S1 (arrow), pressing on the thecal sac (T).

and apply force and pressure to further elicit patient symptoms. Since it can be a dynamic, ultrasound can also directly diagnose impingement in the shoulder, observing the supraspinatus tendon bunching up at the coracoacromial arch with abduction (Read & Perko 1998).

Musculoskeletal ultrasound is less commonly used in the USA than in other regions of the developed world. This is in part related to the ready availability of MRI in the USA and to a preference for MRI over ultrasound because it is easier to appreciate anatomical structures on MRI.

COMPUTED TOMOGRAPHY

Computed tomography (CT) is an X-ray technique that uses ionizing radiation. Higher doses than with conventional radiography are absorbed (in the order of 1–2 rads in modern imaging) by the body part being imaged. CT shows very clear bony detail but not as good soft tissue contrast. The images are obtained by a rotating X-ray tube circling a patient who is lying on a radiolucent table. Detectors can either be fixed around the torus (the housing of the X-ray hole) or can rotate opposite the tube. As the patient goes through the middle of the torus, images of cross-sections of the body part in the transverse plane are obtained. These sections can be reformatted so that they can be viewed in any plane. Newer generations of CT scanners exist which comprise multiple detectors, making scans quite fast, so that scans can now take a matter of seconds, rather than minutes. CT is more available than MRI in most clinical settings (many emergency departments have CT scanners), is less expensive and there are no contraindications to the study.

In trauma, CT is a good screening test for internal organ injury (Harris & Harris 1999). For the musculo-skeletal system, fractures can usually be screened for, and

evaluated by radiograph. CT is used for further evaluation such as for inadequate or suspicious radiographs of the cervical spine. Due to the excellent bony detail afforded by CT, it is used for evaluating complex intra-articular fractures, such as those of the tibial plateau, wrist, and acetabulum. Another structure amenable to CT examination is the spine, where myelographic and non-myelographic CT is excellent for evaluating disk disease, particularly in the lumbar spine (Fig. 29.9). Some advocate using CT for evaluating the pars interarticularis for potential lysis (Congeni et al 1997) (Fig. 29.10).

MAGNETIC RESONANCE IMAGING

Magnetic resonance imaging (MRI) is the best overall test for imaging sport-related injury. Its excellent soft tissue contrast and multiplanar capabilities make it useful for evaluation of all of the anatomical structures, including articular cartilage (Fig. 29.11), bone, the myotendinous unit (Fig. 29.12), and ligamentous structures (Fig. 29.13). MRI has sensitivity to fracture and bone contusion, creating typical signal characteristics in the bone. MRI, therefore, gives the most information about a structure, and after plain film, is the most common test to evaluate injury.

MRI uses a strong magnet and radiofrequency pulses to obtain its image: patients go into a magnetic field (about 25 000 times stronger than the earth's) and their bodies' hydrogen ions are aligned in the magnetic field. The hydrogen ions are deflected by radiofrequency waves and the signal generated is used to create an image. The behavior of the ions is dependent on their local environment, and different substances produce different signal strengths and frequencies. The behavior of the hydrogen ions is also dependent on the strength of the magnetic field, thereby allowing characteristics of

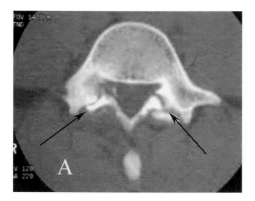
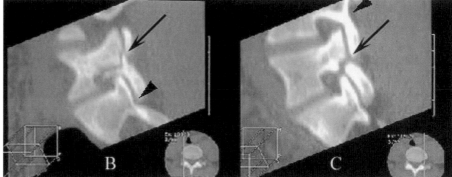

Figure 29.10A–C   Axial (**A**) and reformatted (**B** = left, **C** = right) demonstrating bilateral pars fractures at L5. The pars interarticularis of L4 (right) and S1 (left) are intact.

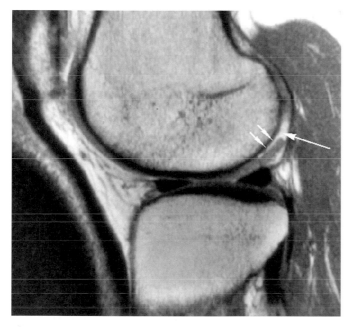

Figure 29.11   Sagittal MR image demonstrating a focal full-thickness defect in the articular cartilage of the lateral femoral condyle (long arrow), creating a flap (short arrows).

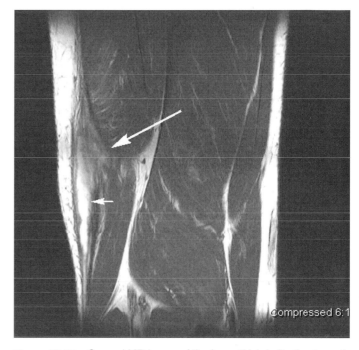

Figure 29.12   Coronal MR image of the lower thigh indicating tear of the long head of the biceps femoris (long arrow) with adjacent hematoma (short arrow), which was drained under ultrasound guidance.

tissue to be exploited using different techniques. Ions other than hydrogen can be used for imaging (most often sodium), however, since there is such a high concentration of hydrogen in the body, it is easier to use. MRI is dependent on a strong and homogeneous magnetic field. It is dangerous to bring loose ferromagnetic substances (e.g. wheelchairs, oxygen canisters, tools) near the magnetic field because they can be pulled into the magnet, however, immobile metal objects, such as orthopedic instrumentation are safe. Imaging ferromagnetic substances is challenging since they distort the field and thus the image. To some extent, the radiologist can compensate for instrumentation (White et al 2000).

There are contraindications to the use of MRI (Table 29.1). Patients with pacemakers are not allowed near the

magnet due to possible inactivation of the pacemaker. Patients with cerebral aneurysm clips, due to the risk of the clip moving, are imaged only if a non-ferromagnetic clip is used, and then only at the discretion of the radiologist. Likewise, patients with stents and other intravascular devices should not be put in the MRI magnet for at least 6 weeks after placement of such devices, which gives a chance for the device to be secured by the body's fibrous tissue. Spinal cord and nerve stimulators are not permitted in the magnet due to the risk of causing stimulation/damage to the nerves (Shellock 1999, Shellock et al 1993). MRI safety is an important issue. Patients should be screened and if questions arise, they

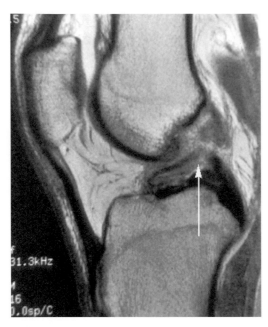

Figure 29.13 Sagittal MR image demonstrating acute proximal anterior cruciate ligament tear (arrow).

Table 29.1 Contraindications to magnetic resonance imaging (MRI)

Absolute	Relative
Pacemaker	Claustrophobia
Aneurysm clip	Pregnancy
Implanted nerve stimulator	Tremor
Implanted tissue expander	Metal worker (ocular foreign body)

should be answered before a patient gets close to the magnet (Sawyer-Glover & Shellock 2000).

Knowledge of some of the terms used in MRI is important. These include spin echo, fast (turbo) spin echo, gradient echo, and STIR (short tau inversion recovery). These are all types of pulse sequences used in obtaining images. In a magnetic field, hydrogen ions have their own magnetic dipole and line up facing either toward or away from the direction of the field, which is along the z-axis using Cartesian coordinates. A greater number of hydrogen ions line up toward the field and these are the ions used in MRI. Using radiofrequency pulses, the ions that are lined up are perturbed into the x–y plane. This puts them into higher energy states, so that they want to go back to the z-axis. When they realign, they release energy in the form of radiofrequency waves. A receiver listens for these waves, which are then used to create the MRI image. While the ions are going back to line up along the z-axis, they disperse in the x–y plane. This dispersion reduces the strength of signal so, before listening, another radiofrequency pulse refocuses or realigns the ions in the x–y plane. This sequence of events is called spin echo imaging. If multiple refocusing pulses

are used for each perturbing pulse, it is called fast (turbo) spin echo imaging. Gradient echo imaging does not use a refocusing pulse. A STIR sequence is different in that it uses different sequences of perturbing pulses that are timed to be able to take advantage of the protons' characteristic behaviors and remove the signal from the protons in molecules of fat.

T1 and T2 are terms that describe characteristics of a tissue. T1 (presented as a number) is defined as 63% of the length of the time it takes for a proton that is perturbed into the x–y plane to line up with the magnet. T2 (also presented as a number) is defined as the length of time it takes for a proton in the x–y plane to disperse in that plane. MRI pulse sequences can accentuate T1 characteristics of a tissue or T2 characteristics of a tissue. These are called T1- and T2-weighted sequences, respectively. Fat has a lot of signal on T1-weighted sequences and is, therefore, 'bright' or white on T1-weighted images. Fluid has high signal on T2-weighted images and is, therefore, 'bright' on T2-weighted images.

Images can be manipulated to exclude signal from fat. Fat suppression techniques include STIR and frequency-selective fat suppression. Every study should include at least one plane which has fat suppression (Fig. 29.17). Suppressing the fat on an image, or making it dark, makes pathology more conspicuous and allows detection of minor injuries such as bone contusions, which would otherwise be difficult to recognize (Mirowitz et al 1994).

There is variation in the way MRIs are obtained. There are differences in hardware, such as magnet strength and coil design, as well as differences in software. On any given system, there are many variables that can be manipulated to obtain an image. The degrees to which imaging centers, hospitals, or radiologists optimize these variables for particular studies are considerably different, based on individual preference, bias, and expertise. For example, to image the glenoid labrum of the shoulder, some radiologists feel that it is necessary to inject contrast into the joint (MR arthrography) (Beltran et al 1997). Others believe that this is unnecessary and distorts the anatomy, limiting evaluation of other structures (Connell & Potter 1999, Connell et al 1999b). Sample imaging protocols are provided in Table 29.2.

TYPES OF INJURIES

Due to the many imaging modalities available and the redundancy of the information that can be obtained through these methods, deciding on the appropriate imaging study for a particular injury can be confusing. There are criteria for imaging developed by the American College of Radiology (2000), but the best way to determine

Table 29.2 MRI protocols (These parameters are courtesy of Dr Hollis Potter, Hospital for Special Surgery, New York. Reproduced with permission from Mintz 2000.

Body part	Plane	Sequence	TR/TE	Matrix	FOV (cm)	ETL	Slice Thickness (mm)	NEX	Bandwidth (kHz)	Reason
Knee Linear or phased array extremity coil	Sagittal	FSE	3500–4000/ 34 (Ef)	512×256–384	16	8	3.5	2	32	Cruciate ligaments, femorotibial and trochlear articular cartilage, quadriceps mechanism
	Sagittal	FSE, fat suppressed	3500–4000/ 40 (Ef)	256×224	16	8	3.5–4.0	2	20	Makes bone (and other) pathology more conspicuous, e.g. bone bruises
	Coronal	FSE	4000–4500/ 34 (Ef)	512×256–384	11–13	8	3.5	2	32	Collateral ligaments, meniscal bodies, femorotibial cartilages
	Axial	FSE	4500/34 (Ef)	512×256–384	14	10	3.5	2	32	Patellofemoral cartilage, retinacula, quadriceps mechanism
	Sagittal	FSE	2300/13 (Ef)	256×224	16	4–5	3.0	2	20	Menisci
Shoulder Medical Advances shoulder phased array coil	Coronal/ oblique (along supra-spinatus)	FSE	4000/3 (Ef)	512×384	16	10	3.0	2	32	Rotator cuff, bursa, A-C joint, glenohumeral joint cartilage, superior labrum
	Coronal/ oblique (along supra-spinatus)	FSE, fat suppressed	3000/60 (Ef)	256×224	16	8	3.0	2	20	Makes pathology more conspicuous Confirms cuff tears
	Sagittal/ oblique (perpendicular to coronal oblique)	FSE	4000/30 (Ef)	512×224	16	8	4.0	2	31	Global comparison of rotator cuff muscles. Biceps origin, A-C joint, axillary nerves
	Axial	FSE	4000/34 (Ef)	512×256	15–16	8	3.5	2	32	Labrocapsular complex, biceps, subscapularis, glenohumeral joint cartilage, suprascapular nerve
	Axial (optional)	FSE	2300/15 (Ef)	256×224	14	5	3.0	2	20	Evaluate labrum
Ankle Linear extremity coil with ankle in neutral position, at 90 degrees	Sagittal	FSE	4000/32 (Ef)	512×384	14–16	8	3.0	2	32	Tibiotalar, midfoot, subtalar articular cartilage, sinus tarsi, Achilles tendon, plantar fascia
	Sagittal	Fast inversion recovery	5300/17 (Ef) TI= 150ms	256×192	14–16	N/A	3	2	32	Makes pathology more conspicuous Bony edema such as stress fractures, arthrosis
	Coronal/ oblique parallel to talonavicular joint	FSE	4000/32 (Ef)	512×384	13	8	4.0	2	32	Tendons, deltoid and calcaneofibular ligaments, hindfoot articular cartilages
	Axial	FSE	4500/34 (Ef)	512×256–288	13	10	3.5–4.0	2	32	Tendons, lateral ligaments, spring and bifurcate ligaments, Achilles tendon, cartilage in gutters
Wrist Coil and bandwidth	Axial	FSE	4500/34 (Ef)	512×256	8	10	3.0–4.0	2	32	Carpal tunnel, extensor tendons, dorsal capsule, neurovascular bundles, DRUJ
	Coronal	FSE	4000–4500/ 34 (Ef)	512×256–384	8–9	8–10	2.0	3	32	Intrinsic and extrinsic ligaments, triangular fibrocartilage complex, articular cartilage
	Sagittal	FSE	4000/34 (Ef)	512×288–384	9	10	2.5–3.0	3	32	Alignment, articular cartilage, short radiolunate ligament
	Coronal	3-D volume gradient echo	40/20 10 degree flip angle	256×256	8	N/A	1.0, 28 slices	2	16	Intrinsic and extrinsic ligaments, triangular fibrocartilage complex
	Coronal	Fast inversion recovery	4200/16 TI=150ms	256×192	9	N/A	2.5–3.0	3	16	Makes pathology more conspicuous, especially bony pathology
Elbow Extended, supinated, at side of body 5″ curved shoulder coil	Coronal	FSE	3500–4000/ 34 (Ef)	512×256–384	11–13	6–8	3.0–3.5	2	32	Collateral ligaments, flexor/pronator and extensor origins, articular cartilage
	Axial	FSE	3000– 4000/ 34 (Ef)	512×256–384	11–12	8	3.5–4.0	2	32	Neurovascular structures, biceps and brachialis insertions
	Sagittal	FSE	3500–4000/ 34 (Ef)	512×256	12–13	6–8	3.5–4.0	2	32	Alignment, triceps insertion, posterior capsule, loose bodies
	Coronal	2D gradient echo*	400–450/20 45° flip angle	256×192–256	11–13	N/A	1.6–1.8	2	15	Collateral ligaments, flexor/pronator and extensor origins

* Volume acquisition if not using high speed gradient system
FOV= field of view; ETL= echo train length; Ef= effective; FSE= fast spin echo; TI= time to inversion.

the appropriate test is to discuss the clinical situation with an experienced radiologiist. Some guidelines for specific injuries are included in Table 29.3. There is not so much a correct or incorrect way to use imaging to assist diagnosis, as methods that people are more or less comfortable and experienced with. Open communication between the practitioner and radiologist is important to obtain appropriate studies and helps the radiologist to specifically address the clinical problem and target the examination.

The different types of tissues that make up the neuro-musculoskeletal system are discussed in Chapters 2–6.

The differences of tissue character mean that each tissue type cannot be imaged in the same way, and the challenges created by having to image different types of tissue create one of the more interesting aspects of musculoskeletal radiology. Most imaging techniques define anatomy: abnormal anatomy indicates pathology. This is true except in nuclear medicine, where physiological characteristics of tissue are imaged. In bone scans, the injected agent goes to the metabolically active bone and the differences in activity are reflected on the scan. In an X-ray or MRI, we know what the normal anatomy is. For example, bones should have well-defined cortical

Table 29.3   Choice of imaging modality

Body part	Suspected problem	First examination	Second examination	Comments
Any	Stress fracture	X-ray	MRI or bone scan	Stress fractures can be readily identified on both MRI and bone scan. MRI has the advantage of better defining the extent of the fracture. If X-ray is positive, further imaging is usually not required
Back pain	Pars fracture, pedicle stress fracture, disk herniation, facet arthrosis or synovitis, sacroiliitis	X-ray	MRI	X-ray can identify some pathologies, obviating the need for further testing. Whereas CT scan is good for pars defects and disk herniations, MRI gives more information without ionizing radiation. Bone scan can be useful for active pars defects but does not look for other etiologies of pain
Shoulder pain (older patient)	Rotator cuff tear, bursitis, arthrosis, fracture	X-ray	MRI or ultrasound	To evaluate the tendons of the rotator cuff and biceps, MRI and ultrasound are both useful and accurate
Shoulder pain (young patient)	Rotator cuff tear, labral or capsular pathology, cartilage abnormality, fracture	X-ray	MRI	In younger patients, MRI can evaluate pathologies such as the labral capsular complex and articular cartilage, as well as the bone marrow, that can not be seen on ultrasound
Elbow pain	Fracture, tendon/ ligament injury, osteochondritis dissecans, overuse syndromes	X-ray	MRI or ultrasound	Medial and lateral epicondylitis can be evaluated with both ultrasound and MRI
Wrist/finger pain	Ligament tears, ganglion, fracture, tendon pathologies	X-ray	MRI or ultrasound	In trauma, avulsion fractures can define tendon or ligament pathology on plain X-ray. Further evaluation of the superficial structures can be done with ultrasound. The deeper structures require MRI for evaluation. Deeper structures include the bony abnormalities. Bone scan and CT can be used to identify occult fractures but provide less information than MRI
Knee pain	Meniscal tear, ligament tear, cartilage injury, tendon abnormality, synovitis, fracture	X-ray	MRI	Ultrasound can be useful for looking at superficial structures around the knee such as the patellar tendon or collateral ligaments. To look at the deeper structures, including the menisci, articular cartilage, and cruciate ligaments, MRI is necessary
Ankle pain	Fracture, ligament tears, tendon pathologies, impingement syndromes, nerve pathologies, Achilles tendon and plantar fascia problems	X-ray	MRI or ultrasound	For superficial pathologies such as tenosynovitis or tendon degeneration or tear, ultrasound is a good test. For a global picture including cartilage, ligament, tendons, and bone, MRI is a better test. Plantar fascia and Achilles tendon pathologies are excellently seen on ultrasound, which can also guide injections
Compartment syndrome		Compartment pressures		Exertional compartment syndrome is still evaluated using compartment pressures before and after exercise. Whereas there is a role for other modalities these are best used in centers experienced with them
Focal pain	Muscle injury, tendon injury, fascial injury, mass, stress fracture, ganglion cyst	MRI or ultrasound		For a general evaluation, MRI is easier to evaluate many structures in a region, however ultrasound has the advantage of direct interaction with the patient and real time scanning. The choice relies upon clinicians' judgement and radiologists' experience

lines. When we see a break in this line (e.g. as in a fracture), we identify the pattern as being abnormal anatomy. The recognition of abnormality comes only with an appreciation of normal anatomy. Radiologists learn what is normal through repetition. Non-radiologists are encouraged to do the same by examining all imaging studies that deal with their patients.

BONE

A bone can be evaluated in all imaging modalities, from the fracture seen on radiographs, to the contusional pattern seen on MRI. Even ultrasound, which does not penetrate bone, is able to image the cortex and to detect occult greater tuberosity fractures when looking at the rotator cuff (Patten et al 1992). The primary modality for the imaging of bone injury is the conventional radiograph. As mentioned earlier in this chapter, radiographs are very specific, but not as sensitive as other modalities. They are, however, the primary method for diagnosing and following fractures. Radiographs also continue to be the best test to evaluate most bone tumors (Greenspan 2000).

The clearest images of bone are obtained by CT scan, where the windows can be created to accentuate the differences in density between bone and the surrounding soft tissues. Tomographic capabilities allow sections as thin as 1 mm and can define some ultrastructural bone characteristics (Buchman et al 1998). On MRI, bone gives a similar signal intensity to fat, because of the fat in bone marrow. Abnormalities become low signal on T1-weighted images, making them stand out. Fat suppression techniques make MRI an ideal modality for identifying stress fractures or stress injuries by making them more conspicuous (high signal) than the adjacent bone. The resolution of MRI is similar to that of CT, although thinner images can be obtained routinely in CT. Bone scans provide a sensitive method for looking for global bone injury or tumor, since the whole body can be imaged at the same sitting without additional radiation. Bone scans, however, are dependent on bone being metabolically active and pathology being more active than normal bone. Since they are less expensive than MRI, and almost as sensitive, bone scans can be used to confirm a diagnosis, such as stress fracture (Fig. 29.14), for which there is a high clinical suspicion – a situation where a positive result (increased activity) will not yield ambiguous interpretation.

MYOTENDINOUS UNIT

The myotendinous unit comprises the muscle, myotendinous junction, and the tendon itself, and is best imaged with MRI and ultrasound. When imaging

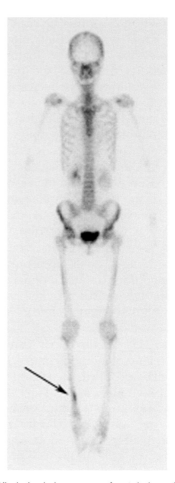

Figure 29.14 Whole body bone scan, frontal view, demonstrating increased uptake in the medial aspect of the right distal tibia (arrow).

muscle, ideally one looks at three things: muscle size and composition, to look for atrophy and fatty infiltration from early disuse or chronic injury; structure, where damage to the structure is the result of direct or indirect injury; and indirect signs of ultrastructural abnormalities, such as denervation or inflammation (myositis). CT, more readily than radiograph, demonstrates gross differences in muscle size or fat infiltration, thus defining atrophy. To evaluate structural abnormalities, except the indirect sign of contour abnormality from mass or hematoma, MRI and ultrasound prove better tools than CT (Berquist 1992). Nuclear medicine does not have a strong role in imaging of myotendinous injuries. Contrast tenography, where contrast is injected into the tendon sheath and radiographs are obtained, is rarely used currently.

Both ultrasound and MRI are able to evaluate muscle tendon junction, tendon, and insertion of tendon onto bone (van Holsbeeck & Introcaso 2001). On ultrasound, muscle abnormality is evidenced by loss of the normal architecture of the muscle and loss of the normal echo texture. Inflammation can often be seen using Doppler techniques to identify increased blood flow (van Holsbeeck & Introcaso 2001). The anatomical structure can be examined for size, and the presence of fatty infiltration can be determined by increased echogenicity. The structure can be examined along its course in a dynamic setting, and the muscle tendon junction can be carefully examined for tear. In tendons surrounded by a sheath, the first sign of pathology is fluid in the sheath (tenosynovitis). Tendinopathy is evidenced by thickening of a tendon, a loss in the normal increased echogenicity, as well as loss of the normal fibrillar architecture (van Holsbeeck & Introcaso 2001). Chronic tendinopathy can lead to calcifications within the tendon. (Fornage 1995). Tendon tear is seen as discontinuity of the tendon. Common areas imaged with ultrasound include the tendons of the shoulder (rotator cuff and biceps), wrist, and elbow. In the lower extremity, the hamstring origin and the foot and ankle tendons are easy to demonstrate using ultrasound imagery.

In the USA, MRI is the most common imaging modality used for myotendinous injury. It is possible to define muscle size and intrinsic abnormal signal, either from denervation, injury, or myositis. Injuries to the muscle, tendon, or muscle–tendon junction are directly visualized, as are potential secondary hematomas (Fig. 29.12). Only relatively few injuries to the myotendinous unit require imaging. In the case of tear, if surgical repair is considered, imaging is useful to delineate the anatomy. Tears of the tendinous insertions onto bone are more amenable to surgical repair than are the more common muscle–tendon junction injuries (Connell et al 1999a). Identification, in acute injures, of muscle hematomas is also useful, as these can be drained, both to reduce pain and to decrease the chance of developing myositis ossificans (Arrington & Miller 1995). Injuries that are refractory to non-operative management may be imaged to exclude partial tendon tears that might be more amenable to operative treatment.

In the tendon itself, tendinosis is evidenced by loss of the normal homogenous low signal of the tendon. Normally, a tendon on MRI is a homogeneously low signal structure because of the immobility of the protons in a tendon's regular structure. When a tendon degenerates (tendinosis), it becomes thicker and higher in signal. Tears and partial tears are defined by partial or complete discontinuity of the tendon. Tenosynovitis is evidenced by fluid in the tendon sheath in both MRI and ultrasound. There can be thickening of the tendon sheath and the entity of the calcific tendonitis can be identified on radiographs where a small focus of calcification is seen in the tendinous insertion (Fig. 29.15). This calcification is less conspicuous on MRI but visible and evident on ultrasound by the reflective interface of the calcification.

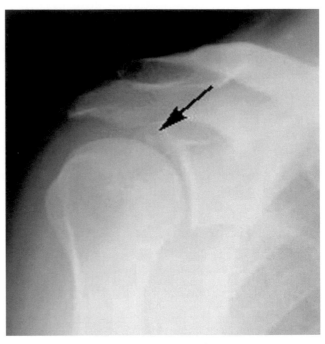

Figure 29.15 Frontal radiograph of the right shoulder demonstrating calcification at the origin of the long head of the biceps off the glenoid indicating calcific tendinitis (arrow).

An entity that involves the muscles but is not an injury per se is exertional compartment syndrome. Various methods have been used to document the entity, most reliably, compartment pressure measurements before and after exercise. Imaging methods have looked at two aspects of such diagnosis: blood flow, done with nuclear medicine studies and ultrasound (Edwards et al 1999); and morphological changes using MRI immediately after exercise (Yao et al 1994). The type of study is difficult to perform due to issues of timing. It is necessary to have a treadmill set up next to the MRI scanner for appropriate procedures of this nature.

LIGAMENTS

Ligaments have the same imaging characteristics as tendons, and where an acoustic window is available, ultrasound can be used to evaluate them. MRI is the mainstay of evaluation of ligaments, although ultrasound can be used for the collateral ligaments in the knee and for the talofibular ligaments of the ankle. In the imaging of ligaments on MRI, frank discontinuity is not always evident. Thus, tears of ligaments (e.g. anterior talofibular ligament) are evidenced as thickening and diffuse high signal, rather than discontinuity. These 'tears' correspond to what may clinically be called a sprain. MRI is accurate in evaluating the integrity of ligaments such as the anterior cruciate ligament (Cotten et al 2000, Ha et al 1998).

CARTILAGE

The imaging of articular cartilage is an area of great interest. Articular cartilage injury can be difficult to diagnose by physical examination and is important to the outcome of a joint injury. Formerly, arthrography was used to image articular cartilage. Irregularity of the surface or lack of space between cartilage and bone indicated abnormality. More recently, CT arthrography has been used. Currently, however, MRI is the study of choice for evaluating articular cartilage (Fig. 29.11). Ultrasound can evaluate cartilage, but is limited in its ability to visualize both joint services of a given joint. The techniques used in MRI for evaluating cartilage differ. Some radiologists use gradient echo techniques, others use fast spin echo imaging (Disler 1997, Disler et al 2000, McCauley & Disler 2001, Potter et al 1998), and some radiologists make no effort to evaluate articular cartilage. Cartilage is graded by a modified Outerbridge grading scale for articular cartilage, with I indicating softening, II being fibrillation less than 50% of the cartilage thickness, III being fibrillation or fissuring greater than 50% of the cartilage thickness, and IV being a full-thickness defect (Outerbridge 1961).

Fibrocartilage, such as the menisci of the knee and the labrum of the hip, can best be seen with MRI (Resnick & Kang 1997), with arthrography as the second choice. Patterns and location of meniscal injury can be defined on MRI and can explain symptoms of pain or locking (Green 2001, Resnick & Kang 1997).

NERVE

Clinicians can augment information gained by electro-physiological tests on peripheral nerves, with images from cross-sectional imaging modalities. Nerve injuries include avulsion of a root from the spinal cord, traumatic laceration, traction injuries, and secondary inflammation from an adjacent mass or adjacent inflamed soft tissue (e.g. hamstring tendinosis causing radicular symptoms). An example of this is an osteochondroma causing a mass effect or lesions in closed spaces like ganglia in the carpal or tarsal tunnel. High-resolution imaging can define the nerve fascicles and the nerve can be traced on sequential axial images or seen in longitudinal images taken. The named nerves of the extremities can be seen with high-quality cross-sectional imaging, extending to the peripheral and even to the digital nerves of the hands and feet (van Holsbeeck & Introcaso 2001). Secondary findings of nerve abnormality (e.g. denervation of muscle) can be apparent as high T2 signal on MRI. Often the goal of imaging peripheral nerves is to exclude treatable pathologies, such as masses that can be treated to reduce nerve entrapment syndromes (Resnick & Kang 1997).

SPECIFIC DISEASE ENTITIES AND INJURIES

There are certain specific injuries or entities that warrant further discussion in a chapter of this nature. In the clinical setting, certain injuries are suspected and imaging is used to confirm those suspicions and to exclude a more sinister cause of patients' symptoms. For example, in a runner with posteromedial tibial pain, the diagnosis of a stress fracture may be clinically apparent. It may still be prudent, however, to obtain a radiograph to exclude the presence of neoplasm in this region with pathological fracture.

STRESS FRACTURES

The imaging of stress fractures should begin with a radiograph (Fig. 29.16). If this is normal, a repeated radiograph after 1 week may start to show periosteal reaction, associated with fracture (Berquist 1992). More accurate and more acute information can be sought with a nuclear medicine bone scan (Fig. 29.14) or MRI, as radiographs can miss stress fractures, especially those involving primarily trabecular bone (Berquist 1992). MRI is particularly useful in the hip to guide the need for operative intervention. If a compression-side (medial) stress fracture is present and partial, the decision may be made to treat the patient non-operatively, with close clinical follow-up (Fig. 29.17). The major concern for stress fractures is that they not go on to become complete fractures that might require more aggressive treatment.

HEAD AND NECK INJURIES

Head and neck injuries are of major clinical concern, especially when there is loss of consciousness or neurological symptoms (Feinberg 2000, Proctor & Cantu 2000). Imaging is usually not required for these injuries, but if a reparable nerve avulsion is a clinical consideration, MRI or CT myelogram can confirm or refute this diagnosis (Carvalho et al 1997). In contact sports, concussions are common, and even after brief loss of consciousness, imaging of the head is usually not required (Sturmi et al 1998) (see Ch. 30 for an account of such injuries). If the clinical suspicion of a subdural or epidural hematoma is present, a CT scan of the brain is a useful method of excluding this diagnosis. MRI of the brain can also be performed but close monitoring of patients in MRI is more difficult.

For severe cervical spine injuries where instability or fracture is suspected, radiographs should be obtained, including the C7–T1 junction on the lateral view. Flexion and extension views can be obtained to look for

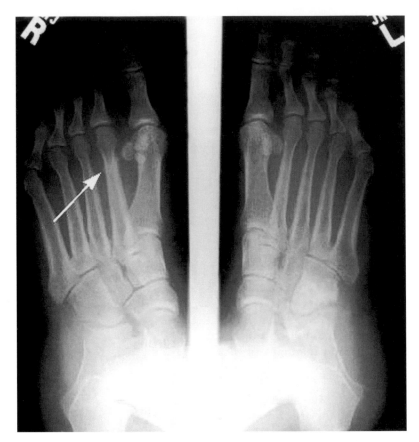

Figure 29.16 Oblique radiograph of both feet demonstrating a stress fracture of the right second metatarsal (arrow). There is callus forming. Incidental note is made of a bipartite medial sesamoid on the right.

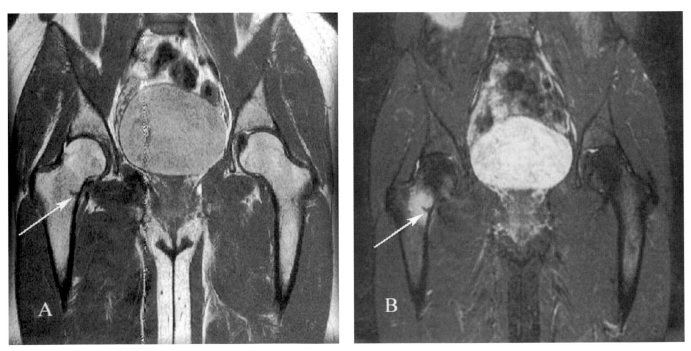

Figure 29.17A & B Coronal MRI of the hip in a woman runner demonstrating right medial femoral neck fracture as indicated by the low-signal line extending part of the way through the bone (**A** and **B**). Note the surrounding reactive signal on the fat-suppressed image (**B**).

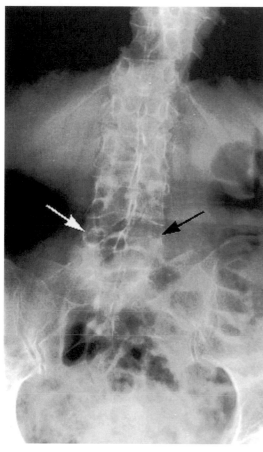

Figure 29.18 Frontal view of the spine in a patient with congenital absence of the left L5 pedicle (black arrow). There is a normal pedicle on the right, seen with its normal circular appearance (white arrow).

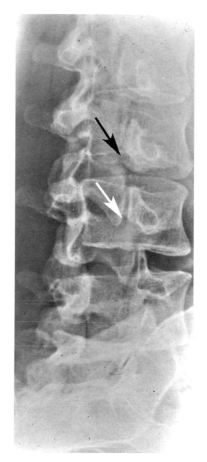

Figure 29.19 –Oblique view of the lumbar spine demonstrating a defect in the pars interarticularis of L3 (black arrow). The pars interarticularis at L4 is intact (white arrow).

ligamentous stability (Graber & Kathol 1999). In contact sports, fractures of the posterior spinous process of the lower cervical/upper thoracic spine (clay shoveler's fracture) are not uncommon (see Ch. 14).

LUMBAR SPINE

Pars defects

The technique used for imaging the lumbar spine is dependent upon the suspected pathology. Congenital anomalies can be excluded with frontal and lateral radiographs (Fig. 29.18) and often defects in pars interarticularis can be excluded by examining the neck of the 'Scottie dog' on oblique views (Fig. 29.19). The activity of the pars defect can be evaluated with a bone scan (Fig. 29.5) or MRI. CT evaluation can also define the fractures (Fig. 29.10). The presence of a stress injury to the pars or stress fracture of the pedicle can mimick a pars fracture and can be identified on cross-sectional imaging techniques (MRI and CT scan) (Standaert & Herring 2000).

Diskogenic disease

The imaging of suspected diskogenic disease should not be undertaken until symptoms have persisted for 6 weeks or longer, with the patient having failed non-operative treatments (Deyo et al 1990). Additional indications for the imaging of suspected diskogenic disease are provided in Box 29.1. If imaging is required, unless there is a contraindication, MRI is the study of choice. The second choice would be a CT scan. CT myelography makes the non-invasive CT scan more invasive by

---

Box 29.1 Indications for imaging the lumbar spine

Initial complaint (X-rays to exclude congenital anomalies)
Worsening deficit
Suspicion of infection
Suspicion of tumor
Prolonged symptoms
Preprocedure

requiring subarachnoid contrast injection. The studies are evaluated for acute and chronic abnormalities. In addition to looking for disk herniations, the study is evaluated for degenerative disk disease, facet arthrosis, fractures, masses, and paraspinal disease that may mimick disk disease (Cacayorin & Kieffer 1991).

Pediatric injuries

Pediatric injuries merit separate discussion. The injuries that children and younger adolescents incur are slightly different from those of adults and may be missed without special attention to them. In the developing body, tendons and ligaments are sometimes stronger than the bone at their insertion sites (Green 2001). Therefore, bony avulsions are more common (Green 2001). Examples of this phenomena include the extensor tendon of a mallet finger or an avulsion of the tibial spine at the footprint of the anterior cruciate ligament.

In children, the physes are open; indeed, some physes do not fuse until the late teens or early 20s (e.g. iliac apophysis, medial clavicle). Physeal injuries should be identified and treated to prevent early fusion and subsequent growth disturbance (Fig. 29.20). For example, a slipped capital femoral epiphysis is usually pinned to prevent further deformity and subsequent arthrosis. Long bone fractures in children can be very subtle (torus

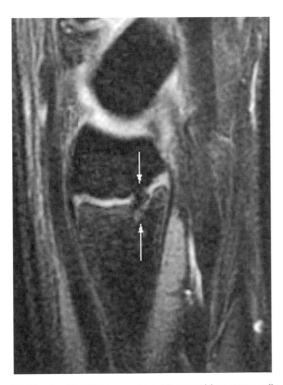

Figure 29.20 Sagittal MR image in a 15 year-old soccer goalie showing a bony bar (arrows) crossing the normal physis.

fractures). Indeed, children's bones can 'bend' rather than break (plastic deformity). It is important to maintain a high index of suspicion for pediatric injuries and to look for secondary signs of injury on radiographs, such as joint effusion and soft tissue swelling. Obtaining additional views, obtaining additional tests, or repeating radiographs for persistent symptoms may bring to light a fracture that was previously overlooked (Harris et al 1993).

CONGENITAL/DEVELOPMENTAL MIMICS OF INJURIES

There are several clinical mimics of injury (entities that can lead to pain or discomfort). These include congenital anomalies such as tarsal coalition (Greenspan 2000), which causes ankle pain while walking on uneven surfaces, and transitional lumbosacral junctions which have been thought to be a cause of pain themselves and that are associated with disk herniations. (Castellvi et al 1984). These entities can be identified radiographically and are among the reasons for obtaining radiographs in patients with persistent symptoms.

Other entities are radiographic mimics of disease. These tend to be developmental, are present in the pediatric population, and can be symptomatic. It is important to be able to identify these entities so as not to be inappropriately aggressive in treatment. Therefore, if a radiographic appearance does not fit the clinical situation, treat the patient, not the radiograph. Keats (1996) provides an excellent coverage of these mimics. They include the normal appearance of an epiphysis mimicking fracture, and a category of diseases (the osteochondroses), all of which have eponyms. Köhler's disease (tarsal navicular), Legg–Calvé–Perthes disease (proximal femoral apophysis), Blount's disease (medial proximal tibial apophysis), Osgood–Schlatter's disease (tibial tubercle), and Freiberg's infraction (2nd or 3rd metatarsal head) (Fig. 29.21) all have characteristic appearances. These lesions may be symptomatic and resolve (as with Köhler's) or go on to cause deformity that requires treatment (e.g. valgus osteotomy for Blount's). Breck (1971), in his atlas of osteochondrosis, describes 41 named osteochondroses. A few of the more common osteochondroses are listed in Table 29.4.

Other developmental conditions, such as unfused apophyses or accessory ossicles, can also cause symptoms. These include os acromiale (Ryu et al 1999, Salamon 1999), accessory navicular (Resnick & Kang 1997), and os trigonum (Jones et al 1999). Although these are not examples of injuries themselves, they do appear during the radiological work-up of injury. It is important to be aware of these entities and the potential for symptoms.

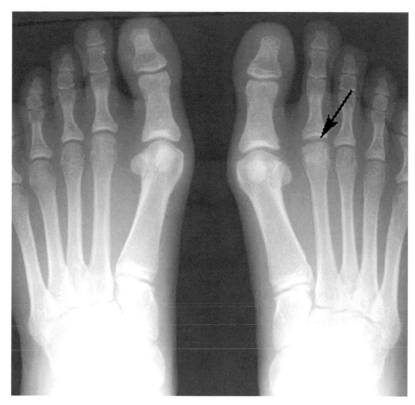

Figure 29.21 Frontal radiograph of the feet in a teenager demonstrating Freiberg's infraction, or osteonecrosis of the second metatarsal head (black arrow). Note the flattening and sclerosis.

Table 29.4 Examples of common osteochondroses (Reproduced with permission from Resnick & Kang 1997).

Osteochondroses	Common age (years)	Site
Köhler's disease	3–7	Tarsal navicular
Legg–Calvé–Perthes disease	4–8	Femoral head
Panner's disease	5–10	Capitellum
Blount's disease	8–15	Tibial plateau
Sinding–Larsen–Johansson syndrome	10–14	Inferior patellar pole
Osgood–Schlatter disease	11–15	Tibial tuberosity
Scheuermann's disease	13–17	Thoracic spine
Freiberg's infraction	13–18	2nd or 3rd metatarsal

COMPLICATIONS

It is important to be aware of the complications of injuries. For bone, the many complications include non-union of a fracture, osteonecrosis, early arthrosis and, in the case of ostechondral impaction, osteochondritis dissecans (Rogers 1992).

Osteochondritis dissecans is an osteochondral fracture that occurs in typical locations (Resnick & Kang 1997). It is most frequently seen in the ankle on the medial talar dome and in the knee at the lateral aspect of the medial femoral condyle (Fig. 29.22) (Cassidy & Petty 2001). It is less often seen on the capitellum and the medial patellar facet. The disorder is believed to be post-traumatic, occurring after one or more traumatic events (Cassidy & Petty 2001). The importance of recognizing osteochondritis dissecans is to explain a patient's symptoms, and because the lesion can become dislodged and present as a foreign body. The role of imaging of this condition is to identify the lesion (commonly done with X-ray) and to evaluate the overlying articular surface, with the goal of surgically intervening if the articular surface is damaged or if the lesion appears loose (De Smet et al 1990a, De Smet et al 1990b). If the lesion is not displaced, loosening is evidenced by fluid extending into the interface between the fragment and native bone (as seen by imaging with MRI or athrographic techniques).

Another complication of injury is osteonecrosis, a condition that can effect fractures, especially in the talus, scaphoid, and the humeral and femoral heads (Rogers 1992). The blood supply for these bones is tenuous (Greenspan 2000). Osteonecrosis is suspected when pain persists, and can be a cause for non-union (Rogers 1992). The early radiographic sign for this condition is an area of sclerosis or lucency. The necrotic area can progress to

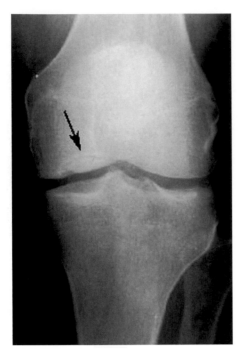

Figure 29.22 Frontal radiograph of the left knee demonstrating osteochondritis dissecans in the typical location (arrow).

the point of collapse and eventual arthrosis (Mazières 1994). Bone scan and MRI can detect osteonecrosis before it is visible on radiograph (Resnick & Kang 1997). The finding on radiograph, termed Hawkins sign in the talus, is the presence of relative osteoporosis. The osteoporosis indicates that the vasculature is intact and normal healing is occurring (Hawkins 1970). If the blood supply was cut off, the bone would remain dense since normal remodeling could not occur.

THERAPEUTICS

In addition to its role in diagnosis, imaging also plays an important role in guiding therapeutics.

INJECTION GUIDANCE

Image-guided injections can be performed using CT, fluoroscopy, and ultrasound. The advantage of using image guidance is that one knows exactly where the injected material is going (e.g. into a joint, tendon sheath, bursa, cyst, neuroma, or nerve root sleeve). Despite clinicians' comfort with performing injections without image guidance, the injections are not as accurate in position as one would hope (Partington & Broome 1998). Joint injections can be diagnostic or therapeutic. A joint can be injected with anesthesia and steroid (Fig. 29.7).

The anesthesia can determine if a known pathology (such as labral tear of the hip, or subtalar arthrosis) is the cause of a patient's symptoms. If the injection relieves symptoms, the pathology is likely to be intra-articular. The steroid may relieve symptoms for a longer time. Tenosynovitis can be treated in a similar way. The injection of saline can be used to distend the shoulder capsule as a treatment for adhesive capsulitis (Rizk et al 1994). Nerve roots and facet and sacroiliac joints can be injected under CT or fluoroscopic guidance (Dussault et al 2000, Murtagh 1988). Morton's neuromas can be injected under ultrasound (Sofka et al 2001). The advantage of ultrasound is that the operator can directly see the needle and what is being injected as it is injected. Unlike fluoroscopically-guided injections, there is no ionizing radiation involved. In using fluoroscopy, one injects contrast and watches its distribution, while injecting. Thereafter, if the distribution is appropriate, the anesthesia/steroid are injected, being careful not to move the needle. Radiofrequency ablations of osteoid osteomas can also be performed percutaneously using image guidance (Rosenthal 1997), as can bone and soft tissue biopsies (Ghelman 1998, van Holsbeeck & Introcaso 2001).

ULTRASOUND THERAPY

Ultrasound, in the guise of extracorporeal shock wave therapy, is available for treating plantar fasciitis (Maier et al 2000, Ogden et al 2001) and calcific tendonitis. (Chaudhry 1999, Ebenbichler et al 1999) This, however, does not involve actual imaging.

FUTURE DEVELOPMENTS

This short section aims to outline the many potential developments and applications of imaging. Radiology is driven by the need to answer clinical questions and is supported by new technology. Technology will continue to advance and as this happens, two things will be likely to occur: the imaging tools that we have now will improve, and new imaging tools will be developed.

The increase in computer speed and memory capacity has boosted the speed of all cross-sectional imaging modalities and will continue to allow higher resolution imaging. Tube designs in CT, probe designs in ultrasound, and coil designs in MRI are constantly improving.

Magnet improvements have enhanced the comfort and strength of MR machines, allowing only the body part being imaged to be enclosed. New pulse sequences in MRI allow better tissue characterization, such as the T2 mapping techniques of articular cartilage, meaning that detailed information regarding the structure/composition of cartilage is available to assess for injury and repair.

In ultrasound, three-dimensional representation and extended field-of-view imaging allow better representation of the images for easier understanding. Techniques for evaluating the presence and degree of blood flow have become quite sensitive and quantification of blood flow is on the horizon. In nuclear medicine, new radionuclides have recently allowed more accurate evaluation of intravascular thrombi. Antibody tagged agents may foster new agents for nuclear medicine. New contrast agents for ultrasound and MRI are being looked at, in order to improve our ability to perform angiography.

Radiographic manipulation has improved with digital imaging techniques, and it is possible with new film–screen combinations to obtain increasingly better images. Computer screens are replacing X-ray film. In some fields, such as mammography and chest radiography, computers can assist in the evaluation of the images, in order to limit human error. Lastly, the burgeoning field of computer-assisted surgery has image-driven aspects.

It is hard to predict new imaging tools. Infra-red imaging has been used in vivo for skin and muscle and in vitro for bone and articular cartilage (Kuboki et al 2001, Ou-Yang et al 2001). This general field is called solid state spectroscopy.

SUMMARY

When imaging is required for a musculoskeletal injury, there are many relevant options available. One must remember the importance of an appropriate history and dedicated physical examination. Imaging should be used only when appropriate and when it will affect patient care. When imaging is deemed necessary, the images should be interpreted in concert with the patient's presentation to guide appropriate therapy. Attention to detail is required in performing and interpreting the studies, with an understanding of the patterns of disease and the musculoskeletal disease processes.

REFERENCES

American College of Radiology 2000 ACR Appropriateness Criteria 2000. Radiology 215 Suppl:1–1511

Andersen P E Jr, Andersen P E, van der Kooy P 1982 Dose reduction in radiography of the spine in scoliosis. Acta Radiology Diagnostica 23(3A):251–253

Anderson K, Sarwark J F, Conway J J et al 2000 Quantitative assessment with SPECT imaging of stress injuries of the pars interarticularis and response to bracing. Journal of Pediatric Orthopedics 20(1):28–33

Arrington E D, Miller M D 1995 Skeletal muscle injuries. Orthopaedic Clinics of North America 26(3):411–422

Beltran J, Rosenberg Z S, Chandnani V P 1997 Glenohumeral instability: evaluation with MR arthrography. Radiographics 17(3):657–673

Berquist T H 1992 Imaging of sports injuries. Aspen Publishers, Gaithersburg

Breck L W 1971 An atlas of the osteochondroses. Charles C Thomas, Springfield

Buchman S R, Sherick D G, Goulet R W et al 1998 Use of microcomputed tomography scanning as a new technique for the evaluation of membranous bone. Journal of Craniofacial Surgery 9(1):48–54

Butler P F, Thomas A W, Thompson W E et al 1986 Simple methods to reduce patient exposure during scoliosis radiography. Radiologic Technology 57(5):411–417

Cacayorin E D, Kieffer S A 1991 The herniated intervertebral disc. In: Taveras J M, Ferrucci J T (eds) Radiology: diagnosis – imaging – intervention. v3: 105 Lippinncott-Raven, Philadelphia

Carvalho G A, Nikkhah G, Matthies C et al 1997 Diagnosis of root avulsions in traumatic brachial plexus injuries: value of computerized tomography myelography and magnetic resonance imaging. Journal of Neurosurgery 86(1):69–76

Cassidy J T, Petty R E 2001 Pediatric rheumatology, 4th edn. WB Saunders Company, Philadelphia

Castellvi A E, Goldstein L A, Chan D P 1984 Lumbosacral transitional vertebrae and their relationship with lumbar extradural defects. Spine 9(5):493–495

Chaudhry H J 1999 Ultrasound therapy for calcific tendinitis of the shoulder. New England Journal of Medicine 341(16):1237

Congeni J, McCulloch J, Swanson K 1997 Lumbar spondylolysis. A study of natural progression in athletes. American Journal of Sports Medicine 25(2):248–253

Connell D A, Potter H G 1999 Magnetic resonance evaluation of the labral capsular ligamentous complex: a pictorial review. Australasian Radiology 43(4):419–426

Connell D A, Potter H G, Sherman M F et al 1999a Injuries of the pectoralis major muscle: evaluation with MR imaging. Radiology 210(3):785–791

Connell D A, Potter H G, Wickiewicz T L et al 1999b Noncontrast magnetic resonance imaging of superior labral lesions. 102 cases confirmed at arthroscopic surgery. American Journal of Sports Medicine 27(2):208–213

Cotten A, Delfaut E, Demondion X et al 2000 MR imaging of the knee at 0.2 and 1.5 T: correlation with surgery. American Journal of Roentgenology 174(4):1093–1097

Curry T, Dowdey J, Murry R 1990 Christensen's physics of diagnostic radiology, 4th edn. Lea and Febiger, Philadelphia

De Smet A A, Fisher D R, Burnstein M I et al 1990a Value of MR imaging in staging osteochondral lesions of the talus (osteochondritis dissecans): results in 14 patients. American Journal of Roentgenology 154(3):555–558

De Smet A A, Fisher D R, Graf B K et al 1990b Osteochondritis dissecans of the knee: value of MR imaging in determining lesion stability and the presence of articular cartilage defects. American Journal of Roentgenology 155(3):549–553

Deyo R A, Loeser J D, Bigos S J 1990 Herniated lumbar intervertebral disk. Annals of Internal Medicine 112(8):598–603

Disler D G 1997 Fat-suppressed three-dimensional spoiled gradient-recalled MR imaging: assessment of articular and physeal hyaline cartilage. American Journal of Roentgenology 169(4):1117–1123

Disler D G, Recht M P, McCauley T R 2000 MR imaging of articular cartilage. Skeletal Radiology 29(7):367–377

Dussault R G, Kaplan P A, Anderson M W 2000 Fluoroscopy-guided sacroiliac joint injections. Radiology 214(1):273–277

Ebenbichler G R, Erdogmus C B, Resch K L et al 1999 Ultrasound therapy for calcific tendonitis of the shoulder. New England Journal of Medicine 340(20):1533–1538

Edwards P D, Miles K A, Owens S J et al 1999 A new non-invasive test for the detection of compartment syndromes. Nuclear Medicine Communications 20(3):215–218

Faulkner K G 2001 Update on bone density measurement. Rheumatic Diseases Clinics of North America 27(1):81–99

Feinberg J H 2000 Burners and stingers. Physical Medicine and Rehabilitation Clinics of North America 11(4):771–784

Fornage B D 1995 Musculoskeletal ultrasound. Churchill Livingstone, New York

Ghelman B 1998 Biopsies of the musculoskeletal system. Radiologic Clinics of North America 36(3):567–580

Graber M A, Kathol M 1999 Cervical spine radiographs in the trauma patient. American Family Physician 59(2):331–342

Green W B 2001 Essentials of musculoskeletal care, 2nd edn. American Academy of Orthopaedic Surgeons, Rosemont

Greenspan A 2000 Orthopedic radiology: a practical approach, 3rd edn. Lippincott Williams and Wilkins, Philadelphia

Ha T P, Li K C, Beaulieu C F et al 1998 Anterior cruciate ligament injury: fast spin-echo MR imaging with arthroscopic correlation in 217 examinations. American Journal of Roentgenology 170(5):1215–1219

Harris J H, Harris W H 1999 The radiology of emergency medicine, 4th edn. Williams and Wilkins, Philadelphia

Harris J H, Harris W H, Novelline R A 1993 The radiology of emergency medicine, 3rd edn. Williams and Wilkins, Baltimore

Hawkins L G 1970 Fractures of the neck of the talus. Journal of Bone and Joint Surgery (Am) 52(5):991–1002

Hubner U, Schlicht W, Outzen S et al 2000 Ultrasound in the diagnosis of fractures in children. Journal of Bone and Joint Surgery (Br) 82(8):1170–1173

Jones D M, Saltzman C L, El-Khoury G 1999 The diagnosis of the os trigonum syndrome with a fluoroscopically controlled injection of local anesthetic. Iowa Orthopaedic Journal 19:122–126

Keats T E 1996 Atlas of normal roentgen varients that may simulate disease, 6th edn. Mosby, St. Louis

Kuboki T, Suzuki K, Maekawa K et al 2001 Correlation of the near-infrared spectroscopy signals with signal intensity in T(2)-weighted magnetic resonance imaging of the human masseter muscle. Archives of Oral Biology 46(8):721–727

Levin D C, Blazena M E, Levina E 1967 Fatigue fractures of of the shaft of the femur: simulation of a malignant tumor. Radiology 89:883–885

McCauley T R, Disler D G 2001 Magnetic resonance imaging of articular cartilage of the knee. Journal of the American Academy of Orthopaedic Surgeons 9(1):2–8

Maier M, Steinborn M, Schmitz C et al 2000 Extracorporeal shock wave application for chronic plantar fasciitis associated with heel spurs: prediction of outcome by magnetic resonance imaging. Journal of Rheumatology 27(10):2455–2462

Matholin C, Saffar P, Roukoz S 1990 [Lunar-triquetral instability]. Annales de Chirurgie de la Main et du Membre Superieur 9(1):22–28

Mazières B 1994 Osteonecrosis. In: Klippel J H, Dieppe P A (eds) Rheumatology. Mosby, St. Louis

Mintz D N 2000 Imaging of sports injuries. Physical Medicine and Rehabilitation Clinics of North America 11(2):435–469

Mirowitz S A, Apicella P, Reinus W R et al 1994 MR imaging of bone marrow lesions: relative conspicuousness on T1-weighted, fat-suppressed T2-weighted, and STIR images. American Journal of Roentgenology 162(1):215–21

Murtagh F R 1988 Computed tomography and fluoroscopy guided anesthesia and steroid injection in facet syndrome. Spine 13(6):686–689

Nash C L Jr, Gregg E C, Brown R H et al 1979 Risks of exposure to X-rays in patients undergoing long-term treatment for scoliosis. Journal of Bone and Joint Surgery 61(3):371–374

Ogden J A, Alvarez R, Levitt R et al 2001 Shock wave therapy for chronic proximal plantar fasciitis. Clinical Orthopaedics and Related Research 387:47–59

Outerbridge R 1961 The etiology of chondromalacia patellae. Journal of Bone and Joint Surgery (Br) 43:752–757

Ou-Yang H, Paschalis E P, Mayo W E et al 2001 Infrared microscopic imaging of bone: spatial distribution of $CO_3(2-)$. Journal of Bone and Mineral Research 16(5):893–900

Partington P F, Broome G H 1998 Diagnostic injection around the shoulder: hit and miss? A cadaveric study of injection accuracy. Journal of Shoulder and Elbow Surgery 7(2):147–150

Patten R M, Mack L A, Wang K Y et al 1992 Nondisplaced fractures of the greater tuberosity of the humerus: sonographic detection. Radiology 182(1):201–204

Pavlov H, Burke M, Giesa M et al 1999 Orthopaedist's guide to plain film imaging. Thieme, New York

Potter H G, Linklater J M, Allen A A et al 1998 Magnetic resonance imaging of articular cartilage in the knee. An evaluation with use of fast-spin-echo imaging. Journal of Bone and Joint Surgery 80(9):1276–1284

Proctor M R, Cantu R C 2000 Head and neck injuries in young athletes. Clinics in Sports Medicine 19(4):693–715

Read J W, Perko M 1998 Shoulder ultrasound: diagnostic accuracy for impingement syndrome, rotator cuff tear, and biceps tendon pathology. Journal of Shoulder and Elbow Surgery 7(3):264–271

Resnick D 1996 Bone and joint imaging, 2nd edn. WB Saunders Company, Philadelphia

Resnick D, Kang H 1997 Internal derangements of joints: emphasis on MR imaging, WB Saunders, Philadelphia

Rizk T E, Gavant M L, Pinals R S 1994 Treatment of adhesive capsulitis (frozen shoulder) with arthrographic capsular distension and rupture. Archives of Physical Medicine and Rehabilitation 75(7):803–807

Rogers L F 1992 Radiology of skeletal trauma, 2nd edn. Churchill Livingstone, New York

Rosenthal D I 1997 Percutaneous radiofrequency treatment of osteoid osteomas. Seminars in Musculoskeletal Radiology 1(2):265–272

Ryu R K, Fan R S, Dunbar W H 1999 The treatment of symptomatic os acromiale. Orthopedics 22(3):325–328

Salamon P B 1999 The treatment of symptomatic os acromiale. Journal of Bone and Joint Surgery 81(8):1198

Sawyer-Glover A M, Shellock F G 2000 Pre-MRI procedure screening: recommendations and safety considerations for biomedical implants and devices. Journal of Magnetic Resonance Imaging 12(1):92–106

Shellock F G 1999 Pocket guide to MR procedures and metallic objects: update 1999. Lippincott Williams and Wilkins, Philadelphia

Shellock F G, Morisoli S, Kanal E 1993 MR procedures and biomedical implants, materials, and devices: 1993 update. Radiology 189(2):587–599

Sofka C M, Collins A J, Adler R S 2001 Use of ultrasonographic guidance in interventional musculoskeletal procedures: a review from a single institution. Journal of Ultrasound in Medicine 20(1):21–26

Standaert C J, Herring S A 2000 Spondylolysis: a critical review. British Journal of Sports Medicine 34(6):415–422

Standaert C J, Herring S A, Halpern B et al 2000 Spondylolysis. Physical Medicine and Rehabilitation Clinics of North America 11(4):785–803

Sturmi J E, Smith C, Lombardo J A 1998 Mild brain trauma in sports. Diagnosis and treatment guidelines. Sports Medicine 25(6):351–358

van Holsbeeck M T, Introcaso J H 2001 Musculoskeletal ultrasound, 2nd edn. Mosby, St. Louis

Werber K D, Wuttge-Hannig A, Hannig C 1990 [Cinematography, a new diagnostic procedure in evaluation of the injured painful wrist joint]. Langenbecks Archiv fur Chirurgie. Supplement II. Verhandlungen der Deutschen Gesellschaft fur Chirurgie 727–729

White L M, Kim J K, Mehta M et al 2000 Complications of total hip arthroplasty: MR imaging-initial experience. Radiology 215(1):254–262

Yao L, Dungan D, Seeger L L 1994 MR imaging of tibial collateral ligament injury: comparison with clinical examination. Skeletal Radiology 23(7):521–524

30

Medical issues in sport and exercise

Bruce Hamilton

INTRODUCTION

With the increasing number of individuals involved in both competitive and recreational sport and exercise activities, it is imperative that medical and healthcare personnel involved in sports medicine have an understanding of the impact that common medical conditions have on such participation, and the impact of exercise on common medical conditions. While professional sports codes may have a physician at their disposal, at most sporting events the most medically qualified person is the physical therapist or athletic trainer. While well prepared to manage musculoskeletal injuries, those involved in the physical therapies often lack the understanding and preparation for the management of common medical problems. This has become of increasing importance now that physical therapists are primary contact practitioners in many countries around the world.

In recent years, authors have concentrated entire volumes on medical subspecialties within sports medicine, and it is beyond the scope of this chapter to comprehensively cover all topics in this area. The following chapter aims to provide an up-to-date outline of the presentation and management of common medical conditions, which a medical practitioner, physical therapist or athletic trainer involved in sports medicine may encounter.

ASTHMA

Asthma is a common condition affecting up to 10% of the population and is associated with a high morbidity (McFadden 1991). It is characterized by intermittent wheeze, shortness of breath, chest tightness, and persistent cough. Pathophysiologically, asthma is considered a chronic inflammatory condition resulting in a reversible airways obstruction (Asthma Management Handbook 2002). People with asthma fall into one of three categories: atopic, classical, and exercise-induced asthma. Atopic asthma is characterized by seasonal variations in symptom severity. It is associated with both the presence of antigens in the environment, and a history of atopy (Tang et al 1996). By contrast, classical asthma involves perennial symptoms. For example, the airways in classical asthma display persistent low-grade inflammation, with intermittent, severe exacerbations (Crimi et al 2001). Exercise-induced asthma (EIA) however, is characterized by symptoms during or after exercise, and while up to 80% of true asthmatics will suffer symptoms of EIA, it may also occur in otherwise healthy individuals (Storms 1999). This review will focus on EIA.

EIA is the term used to describe the transient narrowing of the airways that follows vigorous exercise of 6–8 min duration (Anderson & Holzer 2000, Spooner et al 2000). EIA may result in symptoms such as stomach pains and nausea, in addition to the classic asthma symptoms of shortness of breath, wheeze, cough, and chest tightness. EIA has been shown to limit endurance and prolong recovery from exercise (Spooner et al 2000). EIA is now recognized as being very common, occurring in up to 23% of Olympic athletes (Wilber et al 2000). Exercising in cold, dry air, with a high minute ventilation is considered to be most provocative, and subsequently, participants in winter sports have a higher incidence than their summer counterparts (Rundell et al 2000). EIA is provoked more by continuous than intermittent exercise, and exercising in polluted or allergen-filled air will also increase its incidence (Beck 1999, Gavett & Koren 2001). As a result, EIA is very common in sports such as running, cross-country skiing, and ice skating (Provost-Craig et al 1996, Weiler & Ryan 2000, Wilber et al 2000). In the general population, EIA is often unrecognized, untreated, and may significantly impair performance (Spooner et al 2000, Storms 1999).

Airway function in mild to moderate asthmatics varies depending on the nature of the exercise. With constant load exercise, there is an initial period of mild bronchodilation, followed by bronchoconstriction after 15–20 min of exercise, lasting for the duration of the exercise. By contrast, incremental exercise results in progressive bronchoconstriction, while variable intensity exercise results in relative bronchodilation during higher exercise intensity, and bronchoconstriction at lower intensities (Beck 1999). In non-asthmatic individuals, the airways bronchodilate during exercise or undergo a mild bronchoconstriction. Following the induction of bronchoconstriction secondary to exercise and subsequent recovery, there is a variable period of reduced airway responsiveness, known as a 'refractory period'. This has been found to last up to 2 h (Anderson & Holzer 2000, Beck 1999). In addition, a second drop in airway function may occur 6–8 h following exercise and this is thought to be secondary to an increase in inflammatory cell activity following the initial antigenic (exercise) challenge (Beck 1999).

Two classic hypotheses attempt to explain the transient bronchospasm associated with exercise. The thermal hypothesis, first proposed in 1979 (Anderson & Daviskas 2000, Deal et al 1979), suggests that it is the airway cooling and rapid rewarming following exercise that is responsible for the bronchoconstriction. This theory, however, has largely been discredited (Anderson & Daviskas 2000). By contrast, evidence supporting the osmotic hypothesis (Fig. 30.1), which suggests that dehydration and subsequent increases in osmolarity may precipitate EIA, is mounting (Anderson & Daviskas 2000, Anderson & Holzer 2000).

DIAGNOSIS OF EXERCISE-INDUCED ASTHMA (EIA)

There are several ways in which a diagnosis of EIA may be made, depending on the resources that are available.

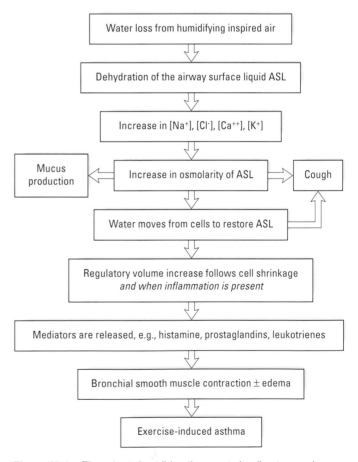

Figure 30.1 Flow chart describing the events leading to cough, mucus production and exercise-induced asthma. (Reproduced with permission from Anderson & Holzer 2000)

The simplest means is a clinical trial with an inhaled bronchodilator. With a history consistent with asthma, an improvement in both symptoms and peak expiratory flow rate (PEFR) of approximately 15% following the inhalation of bronchodilator therapy provides a presumptive diagnosis (Fields & Reimer 1997). The use of an exercise challenge is similarly practical. Classically, this involves exercising at an intensity just below anaerobic threshold for 10–12 min, with PEFR measurements being taken pre-exercise and 1, 3, 6, 10 and 15 min following exercise. A positive test for EIA is most frequently defined as a >10% fall in forced expiratory volume in 1 s (FEV1) or PEFR (Anderson & Holzer 2000). However, it has recently been suggested that the lower limit for the fall in FEV1 and PEFR for normal, elite, cold weather athletes may be 6.4% and 12% respectively (Rundell et al 2000). The benefits of PEFR and field-testing (Fig. 30.2) are the relatively inexpensive cost and ease of administration, and in addition, it has been found that laboratory testing may underestimate EIA in cold weather athletes (Rundell et al 2000).

Testing for EIA using either the hyperventilation of dry air containing 4.9% carbon dioxide, or hyperosmolar saline aerosols, has a very high sensitivity for EIA, but requires more specialized and expensive equipment. The use of pharmacological agents for EIA testing,

such as methacholine and histamine, has recently been questioned, as elite athletes have been found to show increased bronchial reactivity to such agents (Anderson & Holzer 2000, Helenius et al 1998). As a result, positive responses to histamine and methacholine challenges may not imply EIA is present, and similarly negative responses do not negate its presence (Anderson & Holzer 2000). Similarly, it has recently been shown that increasing the exercise load from 85% to 95% of maximum doubled the reduction in FEV1 (Carlsen et al 2000).

MANAGEMENT OF EIA

The management of EIA is multi-faceted. All people with EIA should be provided with an asthma action plan, which outlines the steps to be taken should their breathing deteriorate. Education of the athlete is mandatory and should be ongoing (Fields & Reimer 1997, Storms 1999). Regular assessment of pulmonary function will allow an athlete and coach to objectively assess the relationship of lung function to performance. Environmental manipulation, such as running with a mask in cool air, using a humidifier when training indoors, nose breathing, maintaining hydration, and avoiding exercise in polluted air can assist in minimizing the extent of EIA (Fields & Reimer 1997, Storms 1999). Similarly, the induction of a refractory phase, by using a slower, longer warm-up is proposed, to reduce the impact of EIA (Storms 1999). Recently, however, the ability of athletes to utilize this refractory period effectively has been questioned (Rundell et al 2000).

Historically, EIA has been managed with beta 2-agonists, taken either once or twice, 15–30 min prior to exercise (Storms 1999). Long-acting beta 2-agonists have also been found to be beneficial, should a prolonged duration of coverage be required (Kemp et al 1994, Storms 1999). It is important to note, that the International Olympic Committee (IOC) has restrictions on the use of some beta 2-agonists, requiring formal notification of dose and indications, and has banned several beta 2-agonists as a result of reported ergogenic effects (see Ch. 28). Hence, care needs to be taken when prescribing for athletes with EIA.

A comprehensive metaanalysis has recently illustrated the role of mast cell stabilizing agents in reducing both the duration and severity of EIA (Spooner et al 2000). Similarly, recent work has suggested a role for leukotriene receptor antagonists in the management of EIA (Edelman et al 2000). Inhaled corticosteroids should continue to be used to minimize airway inflammation, in the management of classical asthma and refractory EIA (Edelman et al 2000, Thien 1999).

A preferred approach to pharmacological management of uncomplicated EIA is the use of a beta 2-agonist

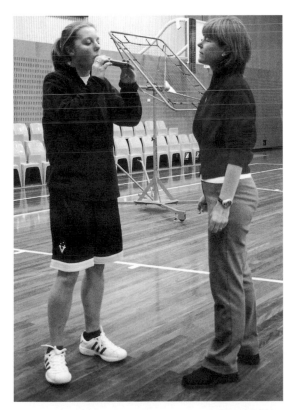

Figure 30.2 Field testing of an athlete with Peak Expiratory Flow Rate.

inhaler 30 min prior to exercise, followed by a mast cell stabilizer 15 min later. Treatment failure with this method may be the result of a number of factors including drug dosage, empty canisters, and drug inhalation technique. With continued failure to respond to treatment, misdiagnosis and possible secondary gain should be considered.

Treatment of the acute, severe asthma attack 'on the field', where an individual is clearly in distress, involves the administration of bronchodilator therapy (e.g. salbutamol) and the immediate transportation to a medical facility. If a nebulizer or oxygen is available then they should be utilized. Similarly, spacer devices can assist in the delivery of inhaled medications. The preferred method of transportation is in an ambulance (Thomas 2001).

EPILEPSY

Epilepsy is a neurological disorder characterized by recurrent seizure activity (Sirven & Varrato 1999). A seizure is an abnormal electrical discharge within the cortical and subcortical neurons of the brain, which may or may not result in convulsive activity (Spiegel & Gates 1997). While true epilepsy may affect up to 3% of the population, up to 10% of the population will experience a single seizure in their lifetime (Spiegel & Gates 1997). Of all people who experience epilepsy, most are diagnosed before the age of 30 years (Cantu 1998a). Most cases of epilepsy are idiopathic, but it can also result from cerebrovascular accidents, central nervous system infections, neoplasms, metabolic derangements, birth trauma, or anatomical abnormalities such as in Sturge–Weber syndrome (Gates and Spiegel 1993, Sirven & Varrato 1999).

DIAGNOSIS OF EPILEPSY

Up to 25% of patients referred to neurologists with a tentative diagnosis of epilepsy have other causes for their brief, sudden loss of consciousness and muscle tone (syncope) (Williams & Bernhardt 1995), and the most useful diagnostic tool to avoid misdiagnosis is an accurate history (McLaughlin 1999). Seizures that occur only while sitting or standing are more likely to be syncopal in origin (McLaughlin 1999). Brief stiffening of the body may occur in syncope, but can usually be differentiated from epilepsy by its brief duration (usually only a few seconds). Prior to a syncopal episode, a patient may have faintness or dizziness, while in epilepsy the first symptom may be an aura, which is actually the commencement of the seizure. While an aura is often

difficult to describe, it will usually be similar on each occasion (McLaughlin 1999). The presence of drowsiness, headache, and fatigue following an epileptic seizure are common. Other than in the immediate postictal phase, examination of a patient with epilepsy is usually normal (McLaughlin 1999). However, as the differential diagnosis for seizures includes cardiogenic and vasovagal syncope, transient ischemic attacks, metabolic disturbances, and psychological causes, a full physical examination is required.

If epilepsy is suspected, then an electroencephalogram (EEG) should be performed. Ideally, this should be performed as close to the seizure as possible, but despite this, the EEG may still be normal in up to 50% of subsequently diagnosed sufferers. In addition, up to 15% of sufferers may always have a normal EEG. Magnetic resonance imaging (MRI), single photon emission computerised tomography (SPECT) and positron emission tomography (PET) scans are all used to localize the focus of epileptic seizures (McLaughlin 1999).

Seizures are classified on the basis of their external manifestations, but can also be differentiated on the basis of their EEG findings. Table 30.1 illustrates a current classification system for epilepsy.

GENERAL MANAGEMENT OF EPILEPSY

Management of epilepsy is predominantly pharmacological, with up to 80% of individuals able to be controlled on a single drug. A number of drug classes are

Table 30.1 Classification of seizure type (data from McLaughlin 1999 and van Linschoten et al 1990)

Type of seizure	Category	Sub-category
1. Partial (focal, localized) seizure	Simple partial (no altered level of consciousness)	With motor signs (e.g. limb twitching) With somatosensory hallucinations (e.g. taste or smell sensations) With autonomic signs and symptoms With psychic symptoms
	Complex partial (altered level of consciousness)	Simple followed by impairment of consciousness With impaired consciousness from the onset
	Partial evolving to generalized	
2. Generalized (convulsive or non-convulsive seizure)	Absence Atypical absence Myoclonic Clonic Tonic Tonic clonic Atonic	
3. Unclassified seizure		

used to control epilepsy. The most common include sodium channel blockers (e.g. phenytoin, carbemazepine), gamma-aminobutyric acid (GABA) release stimulators (e.g. valproic acid), and more recently, the GABA analogs (vigabatrin, gabapentin) (Quinn et al 2001). Many of the drugs, however, have drowsiness and visual disturbances as potential side-effects and these must be considered prior to making exercise recommendations. Exercise has not been found to influence the efficacy of antiepileptic medication (Cantu 1998a).

EXERCISE AND EPILEPSY

In considering the relationship between exercise and epilepsy, it is important to consider both the effect of epilepsy on exercise and the effect of exercise on epilepsy. It has been found that during exercise there is a reduction in seizure frequency (Nakken et al 1997), but that immediately following exercise cessation, an increased risk of seizure activity is present (Nakken 1999, van Linschoten et al 1990). It has been postulated that this is a result of the increased concentration of gamma-aminobutyric acid (GABA) during exercise, which may suppress electrical activity in the brain (Cantu 1998a). Also, a reduction in blood pH levels following exercise could account for an increased risk of seizure immediately following activity (Sirven & Varrato 1999).

If epilepsy is well controlled with medication, it should have no effect on an athlete's performance (van Linschoten et al 1990). However, during the postictal phase (which may last up to a few days) performance may be affected by fatigue, and impaired alertness, balance, and coordination (Spiegel & Gates 1997). Similarly, anticonvulsant medication may impair cognition, vision, concentration and coordination, all of which are important in exercise and sport performance. While exercise has not been found to significantly affect serum levels of antiepileptic medications, any abrupt change in body weight or composition as a result of training may alter the distribution of medications. Subsequently, serum levels of medications should be monitored carefully (Nakken et al 1990).

It is clear that the cardiovascular and psychosocial benefits of exercise outweigh its risks in people experiencing epilepsy. Athletes who are seizure-free and who are well controlled on medication, have few contraindications to sport (Sirven & Varrato 1999). Similarly, there is little evidence that repeated minor head trauma will induce seizure activity (Sirven & Varrato 1999, van Linschoten et al 1990). However, some activities are associated with unacceptable risk to both the individual and other participants should a seizure occur, and as a result, are contraindicated for people with epilepsy. Sports that are absolutely contraindicated with epilepsy

include rock climbing, scuba diving, flying, hang gliding, parachuting, shooting, archery, and boxing. Sports that are relatively contraindicated include swimming and water sports, cross-country skiing, back packing, cycling, skating, horse riding, gymnastics, motor sports, and many contact sports (Cantu 1998a, Fallon 1997, Sirven & Varrato 1999, van Linschoten et al 1990). In addition, there are a number of physiological states, commonly encountered in competitive sport, which may precipitate seizure activity (e.g. fatigue, sleep deprivation, hypoxia, hyponatremia, hyperthermia, hypoglycemia) (Sirven & Varrato 1999, Speigel & Gates 1997, van Linschoten et al 1990). For example, participation in high altitude activities could result in hypoxia and subsequently increase the risk of seizures (Sirven & Varrato 1999). While there is little evidence that exercise-induced physiological changes will necessarily precipitate seizures (Speigel & Gates 1997), caution is recommended when advising athletes with epilepsy regarding their participation in sports which induce extreme physiological states (van Linschoten et al 1990). Common sense should always prevail and the potential risk to the both the individual and others should a seizure occur, should be carefully assessed (Cantu 1998a).

MANAGEMENT OF EPILEPTIC SEIZURES

Management of a seizure should follow basic first-aid guidelines. An area should be cleared so the patient does not harm themselves, but do not move the patient unless they are at risk of harming themselves. Do not place objects in the patient's mouth, or try to restrain a convulsing individual (Sirven & Varrato 1999). Attempts should be made to protect the airway, while being careful to avoid damaging the cervical spine. Any medical bracelets should be looked for, and professional assistance be sought should the convulsion not resolve rapidly. Following seizure cessation, ensure pulse and breathing are present. If absent, immediately begin cardiopulmonary resuscitation and enlist medical assistance (Sirven & Varrato 1999). All seizures require medical review, and first time convulsions require assessment by a neurologist. The decision to return to activity following a seizure requires individualized assessment (Spiegel & Gates 1997).

HEAD AND NECK INJURIES IN SPORT

One of the most anxious situations for the physician, physical therapist, or athletic trainer to be faced with, is the athlete with a head or neck injury. Assessment is often difficult, time is pressured, and the consequences of inappropriate initial management of even a minor injury can be devastating (Newcombe et al 1994, Warren & Bailes 1998a). While catastrophic head and neck injuries are rare, mild head and neck injuries are common, accounting for, for example, between 14% and 37% of injuries in elite level football in Australia (Seward et al 1993a). It is important that physicians, physical therapists, and athletic trainers have a clear understanding of their role in the management of both severe and mild head and neck injury.

CONCUSSION

Concussion is defined as 'a clinical syndrome characterized by immediate and transient post-traumatic impairment of neural function, such as alteration of consciousness, disturbance of vision and/or equilibrium' (Johnston et al 2000). Concussion is a significant problem with up to 300 000 episodes per year in contact sport in the USA (Johnston et al 2000) and up to 3.9 per 1000 player hours in Australian Football (McIntosh et al 2000, Newcombe et al 1994, Seward et al 1993a). McIntosh et al (2000), in a study of rugby union and rugby league players, found that 97% of cases of concussion were the result of direct contact. Most head impacts were caused in a tackle situation and involve collision with the upper body or upper limb of an opponent.

Diagnosis and assessment of concussion

Concussion may cause a variety of symptoms, but one must be aware that loss of consciousness (LOC) is not a prerequisite for diagnosis. While concussive symptoms may include LOC, memory problems, headache, nausea, poor coordination, dizziness, double/blurred vision, and confusion, the only pathognomonic symptom of concussion is memory disturbance (Maddocks et al 1995, McCrory 1999). There are several approaches that have been taken in the assessment and diagnosis of concussion. An athlete suffering concussion may have a blank stare, delayed verbal responses, and slowed actions (Warren & Bailes 1998a). Maddocks et al (1995) found that asking a series of questions aimed at evaluating recent memory were more sensitive than long-term recall in the diagnosis of concussion. Examples of these questions are:

- At which ground are we?
- Which quarter is it?
- How far into the quarter is it – the first, middle, or last 10 minutes?
- Which side scored last?
- Which team did we play last week?
- Did we win last week?

Typically, the assessment of the severity of concussion has involved measurement of the duration of post-

traumatic amnesia and loss of consciousness (Cantu 1998c, Moeller 1996). The validity of this approach has recently been questioned, as these systems are not based on any scientific evidence (Johnston et al 2000, McCrory 1999).

On-field assessment of concussion involves first-aid (Fig. 30.3), followed by careful review for associated injuries, such as to the cervical spine. Should cervical spine injuries be suspected, neck immobilization and transport on a suitable spinal frame should be expedited (Warren & Bailes 1998a). In an unconscious patient, a spinal injury should be assumed to be present until proven otherwise (Newcombe et al 1994). Once a patient has been stabilized and removed from the field of play, assessment should continue in the quiet of the dressing room. Full history and neurological examination, including serial assessment of recent memory function should be performed. If a player has any symptoms or signs of concussion, then that player should not be allowed to return to play, should not be left alone, and should be reviewed serially by medical personnel (Johnston et al 2000). The rationale for not allowing an immediate return to play is based on an observed reduction in information processing and

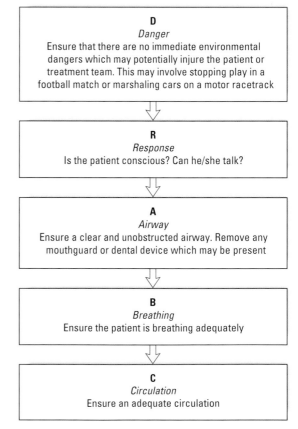

D
Danger
Ensure that there are no immediate environmental dangers which may potentially injure the patient or treatment team. This may involve stopping play in a football match or marshaling cars on a motor racetrack

R
Response
Is the patient conscious? Can he/she talk?

A
Airway
Ensure a clear and unobstructed airway. Remove any mouthguard or dental device which may be present

B
Breathing
Ensure the patient is breathing adequately

C
Circulation
Ensure an adequate circulation

Figure 30.3 Guide to the initial management of concussion. (Reproduced from McCrory P R 1997 Were you knocked out? A team physician's approach to initial concussion management. Medicine and Science in Sport and Exercise 29:S207–212, with the permission of Lippincott Williams and Wilkins.)

reaction times following head injury, which can predispose an individual to further injury.

In children and adolescents, there may also be an increased risk of diffuse brain swelling, known as second impact syndrome (SIS) (Cantu 1998b). More recent literature, however, has suggested that in the past, the risk of SIS following concussion has been overemphasized (McCrory 1999, McCrory 2001b, McCrory & Bercovic 1998a). Indications for urgent referral following concussive incidents include signs of a cervical spine fracture, focal neurology, prolonged LOC or confusion, convulsive movements, or a significant medical history (e.g. hemophilia) (McCrory 1997). Discharge home should only be allowed under the supervision of a mature adult, with instructions on how to manage any deterioration in symptoms.

Returning to play after concussion

Return-to-play guidelines following concussion is an area shrouded in controversy. The most recognized return-to-play guidelines are based on injury severity grading systems (Cantu 1998c, Johnston et al 2000, McCrory 1999, Moeller 1996); however, many of these systems are not based on sound scientific research (McCrory 1997). Mandatory exclusion criteria, based on a particular grade of injury, are inherently dangerous in that they may lead to under-reporting of concussive events. Furthermore, such criteria could allow a premature return to play. The approach of choice is that based upon neuropsychological testing in conjunction with symptom assessment (McCrory 1997). In the days following a concussive incident, regular symptom assessment and examination should be performed. Examination should include a digit symbol substitution test (DSST), which should be compared with a preseason baseline assessment. The DSST is a simple neuropsychological test which is thought to reflect information processing and psychomotor speed, as well as visual short-term memory. It involves the copying of symbols and matching them with numbers over a 90 s period (Grindel et al 2001). On return of the DSST to baseline levels and with no symptoms at rest, the athlete is allowed to perform light aerobic exercise. If this is managed without any symptoms, the following day the athlete should perform non-contact drills, finally returning to contact training, prior to being allowed to return to play (Johnston et al 2000, McCrory 1997). Persistence, or deterioration of symptoms warrants further investigation by a neurologist or sports physician.

Prevention of concussion

In recent years there has been an increase in the use of headgear and mouthguards with a view to preventing concussive head injury. McIntosh et al (2000) found that the average head impact energy causing concussion in 97 subjects was 56 joules, and that the impact attenuation ability of foam headgear was lost above an impact energy of 20 joules (McIntosh & McCrory 2000). This suggests that the commercially available headgear was unlikely to reduce the risk of concussion. Interestingly, it has been shown that players wearing headgear perceived increased levels of safety and hence had an ability to tackle harder (Finch et al 2001). It could be that headgear alters on-field behavior, and subsequently increases the risk of injury.

A further device historically thought to decrease the risk of concussion is the mouthguard (Hickey et al 1967, Kerr 1986). However, while mouthguards do offer protection against dental injury, there is only limited evidence that they offer any protective effect against concussion (McCrory 2001a). Prevention of concussion and other head injury is best achieved by education and enforcement of appropriate rules preventing dangerous play, with severe penalties for breach of these rules (Johnston et al 2000, Johnston et al 2001, McCrory & Berkovic 1998b, Newcombe et al 1994).

CERVICAL SPINE INJURY IN SPORT

Serious spinal cord injuries continue to occur in contact sport despite progressive law and attitude changes (Rotem et al 1998). Such injuries have a significant impact on both individuals' lives and community resources. While conditions such as spinal canal stenosis may predispose to cervical spine injury, the role of screening for such conditions, and their relative risk for spinal cord injury continue to be debated (Cantu 1997, Torg & Glasgow 1991, Torg & Ramsey-Emrhein 1997).

Assessment of cervical spine injuries

Assessment of the patient with a suspected cervical spine injury on the field is difficult, and brief guidelines only follow, which need to be viewed in the context of differing clinical situations. The primary aim of the initial management is to prevent any further neurological insult (Warren & Bailes 1998b), and in order to achieve this, it is recommended that physical therapists, athletic trainers, and medical personnel practice the use of cervical collars and stretcher carrying prior to the commencement of the sports season (Warren & Bailes 1998b).

Often the symptoms and signs of cervical injury are subtle and a high index of clinical suspicion is required. Observation of the mechanism of injury is critical, as this will increase one's index of suspicion (Newcombe et al 1994). This is particularly so if the mechanism was either hyperflexion or hyperextension associated with axial loading or rotation (McLatchie & Lloyd-Parry 1997, Warren & Bailes 1998b). As outlined earlier, the unconscious patient is assumed to have a cervical spine injury and should be treated as such (Newcombe et al 1994). If breathing is absent, log roll the patient into a supine position, remove the mouthpiece or facemask, and begin cardiopulmonary resuscitation immediately (Warren & Bailes 1998b). Following management of the airway, the head and neck should be immobilized and the patient stabilized prior to any further movement.

More commonly, however, the patient is conscious and the initial on-ground assessment should involve airway, breathing, and circulation considerations. Questions such as 'Do you feel pain?', 'Can you move your arms/legs?', and 'Are you feeling any tingling?' can assist in localizing difficulties (McLatchie & Lloyd-Parry 1997). The presence of pain may assist in localizing an injury to the cervical spine, and the presence of neurological symptoms implies the involvement of the spinal cord (Newcombe et al 1994). Neurological deficits in both the arms and legs is an especially concerning sign of spinal cord injury (Warren & Bailes 1998b).

If a cervical spine injury is suspected, the patient should immediately be prevented from attempting to move, the airway should be secured and a semirigid collar applied as soon as is practical (Newcombe et al 1994). However, if the patient has no peripheral symptoms, palpation of the cervical spine should be undertaken with the patient lying still. The location of tenderness should be carefully noted. Mild paraspinal or interspinous tenderness is common. Tenderness over the spinous process or higher cervical vertebrae should arouse suspicion. It is the author's practice that if there is no pain and no neurological symptoms, the athlete may be allowed to sit up slowly whereby a further assessment of concussion and the cervical spine should be performed. A natural response of athletes will often, at this point, be to 'test out their range of motion' and this should be discouraged. Slow, controlled, active range of motion may, however, be allowed and if there is a full, pain-free range of cervical motion, with minimal tenderness, no peripheral neurological symptoms or signs, and no signs of concussion then the athlete, if willing and confident, may continue. If there is any doubt, a conservative approach is recommended (Newcombe et al 1994). By contrast, painful limitation of range of movement necessitates immobilization and removal from the field of play. Immobilization involves use of a semirigid collar and a spinal board. It is essential that these are available at every sports ground where contact sport is played (Newcombe et al 1994). When using a stretcher or spinal board, one person should carry each corner and the leader should control the patient's head (Warren & Bailes 1998b). Prior to transfer to hospital, it is important to ensure that the airway and breathing are stable, the entire spine is immobilized, and a full neurological assessment is carried out and documented (Newcombe et al 1994, Warren & Bailes 1998b). In the event of a significant injury, the game should be ceased until the patient is in a stable condition to be moved. This may require an ambulance or helicopter entering the ground, as unnecessary transfers should be avoided.

CARDIAC CONDITIONS IN SPORT AND EXERCISE

SUDDEN CARDIAC DEATH

Sudden cardiac death (SCD) is defined as 'a witnessed or unwitnessed natural death resulting from sudden cardiac arrest occurring within 6 hours of a previously normal state of health' (Basilico 1999). Cardiac deaths account for the majority of sudden non-traumatic deaths among athletes and while considered a relatively rare occurrence, the death of a young, apparently healthy sportsperson results in considerable societal concern (Jensen-Urstad 1995). The prevalence of SCD in young athletes is estimated to be in the range of 1:100 000 to 1:300 000, and in older athletes from 1:15 000 to 1:50 000 (Maron et al 1998).

It is now well recognized that the risk factors for SCD differ for athletes either younger or older than 30 years of age (Futterman & Myerburg 1998, Maron et al 1996b). In young athletes, the most common causes of SCD are hypertrophic obstructive cardiomyopathy (36%), coronary artery anomalies (19%), increased cardiac mass (10%), ruptured aorta (5%), and tunneled coronary artery (5%) (Maron et al 1996b).

Hypertrophic obstructive cardiomyopathy (HOCM) is typically considered the most common cause of SCD in athletes under the age of 35 years (Maron et al 1996b, Shephard 1996). HOCM is an autosomal dominant inherited condition with variable penetrance, and has a prevalence of approximately 1:500 individuals (Maron et al 1994). Pathophysiologically, there is disruption of the cardiac sarcomere, with disorganization of the left ventricle and a subsequent ventricular outflow obstruction resulting in an increased risk of myocardial ischemia (Maron et al 1994). While the exact criteria for its diagnosis are still debated (Shephard 1996), it is recognized that the echocardiogram is the most reliable diagnostic tool. By comparison, in athletes over the age of 30 years, coronary artery disease accounts for over 92% of cases of SCD (Jensen-Urstad 1995). More recently, inherited arrhythmias such as Brugada syndrome have been implicated in SCD (Link et al 2001).

Given the low incidence of SCD in young asymptomatic athletes, the value of routine screening has been questioned (Fuller et al 1997, Jensen-Urstad 1995). Fuller et al (1997) predicted the sensitivity of electrocardiogram (ECG) screening to be in the range of 60–70%, compared to history taking, auscultation, and inspection, which may be as low as 3%.

The American Heart Association guidelines for preparticipation screening recommend a complete personal and family history, as well as a physical examination, prior to being eligible to participate in organized sports in high school and college (Maron et al 1996b). Recommended items for inclusion in the history and examination are as follows. The history should consider previous symptoms of chest pain, such as syncope, shortness of breath, and fatigue, and also family history of premature death, cardiovascular disability, or conditions such as Marfan's syndrome, long QT syndrome, or dilated cardiomyopathy. Also, past detection of heart murmur or increased systolic blood pressure should be ascertained. The examination should include lying and standing auscultation to identify heart murmurs, palpation of femoral pulses to exclude aortic coarctation, recognition of stigmata of Marfan's syndrome, and sitting brachial blood pressure. It is further recommended that each subsequent year in which athletic participation continues, an interim history and blood pressure be obtained (Maron et al 1998). Clearly, any abnormalities detected on either history or examination, should be further investigated by a suitably qualified cardiologist prior to sports participation being recommended.

THE ATHLETE'S HEART

The concept of 'the athlete's heart' refers to the structural and functional adaptations that the heart undergoes in response to exercise. First described in the late 19th century in relation to cross-country skiers (see Urhausen & Kindermann 1999), it has subsequently been recognized as a physiological adaptation to stresses placed upon the cardiovascular system (Holly et al 1998, Mills et al 1997).

Endurance training subjects an athlete's heart to a volume overload stress. The result of this is an increased intracavity dimension involving all four chambers of the heart, with a concomitant increase in cardiac mass, known as eccentric hypertrophy (Pelliccia et al 1991). In addition, vagal tone increases and β-adrenergic receptiveness decreases, resulting in a bradycardia (Holly et al 1998, Huston et al 1985, Stolt et al 1997). As a result of these adaptations, endurance trained athletes have characteristic ECG findings (Holly et al 1998, Stolt et al 1997) (Box 30.1). By comparison, strength training results in increased ventricular wall thickness, with little change

Box 30.1 ECG findings in an endurance trained athlete that may be considered normal

Secondary to vagotonia
- Sinus bradycardia
- Sinus arrythmia
- Junctional escape beats
- AV conduction blocks (first degree, second degree Mobitz type one)

Secondary to cardiac mass
- Increased QRS voltage (S-V1 + R-V5 > 35 mm)
- Prominent u waves
- Intraventricular delays (right bundle branch block, left anterior fascicle block)
- Early repolarization (upward displaced ST segment)
- Long QT Interval (normalizes when corrected for rate)

in chamber volume, known as concentric hypertrophy (Pelliccia et al 1991). This is thought to result from an increase in afterload, as a result of vascular compression caused by the static muscular contraction.

It is important to distinguish physiological ventricular hypertrophy from pathological cardiomyopathy. As has been noted above, HOCM is considered to be the leading cause of SCD among young athletes, and the distinction between the two entities often creates a diagnostic dilemma. Figure 30.4 illustrates the relationship between the two entities. With deconditioning, many of the ECG findings of the athlete's heart will resolve, and with exercise testing, any suspected abnormalities should disappear (Basilico 1999). Should exercise testing induce atypical cardiovascular changes, pathological conditions should be considered.

In summary, cardiac conditions are the leading cause of sudden death in otherwise fit individuals participating in exercise. Careful preparticipation screening (see Ch. 11), combined with an awareness of normal cardiac variations found in an athlete, and an understanding of the demands of different sports, can assist in reducing the risk of sudden death.

DIABETES MELLITUS

Diabetes mellitus is a major cause of death and disability in the USA (Albright et al 2000). It is a disease characterized by chronic hyperglycemia, due to defects in either insulin secretion, insulin action, or a combination of the two. Diabetes has two major subgroups. Type I diabetes results from a deficiency of endogenous insulin, and is common in childhood and adolescence. Management is predominantly pharmacological, with exogenous insulin replacement (Pierce 1999). Type II diabetes

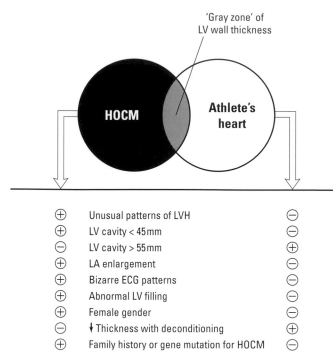

'Gray zone' of
LV wall thickness

⊕ Unusual patterns of LVH	⊖
⊕ LV cavity < 45 mm	⊖
⊖ LV cavity > 55 mm	⊕
⊕ LA enlargement	⊖
⊕ Bizarre ECG patterns	⊖
⊕ Abnormal LV filling	⊖
⊕ Female gender	⊖
⊖ ↓ Thickness with deconditioning	⊕
⊕ Family history or gene mutation for HOCM	⊖

Figure 30.4 Relationship between physiological hypertrophy and hypertrophic obstructive cardiomyopathy (HOCM). LVH = left ventricular hypertrophy; LV = left ventricle; LA = left atrium; ECG = electrocardiogram. (Reproduced from Maron B J, Pelliccia A, Spirito P 1995 Cardiac disease in young trained athletes. Insights into methods for distinguishing athlete's heart from structural heart disease, with particular emphasis on hypertrophic cardiomyopathy. Circulation 91:1596–1601.)

accounts for up to 90% of cases, with an incidence of approximately 3–5% in the Western world. Type II diabetes has a strong genetic basis and is primarily the result of reduced end organ sensitivity to insulin. This type of diabetes is managed with a combination of dietary manipulation, exercise, and often oral hypoglycemics (Colman et al 1999).

Diabetes may present with excessive urine losses, nocturnal urination, dehydration, and increased thirst, as a result of elevated blood glucose levels. Weight loss, blurred vision and recurrent infections are also common presentations (Gale 1990). Ketoacidotic or hyperosmolar coma may result from severely elevated blood glucose levels (Funk & Feingold 1995). There are several chronic complications of diabetes. Microvascular disease, resulting in both a retinopathy and nephropathy, as well as macrovascular diseases such as atherosclerosis, hypertension, and hypertriglyceridemia are very common (Pierce 1999). Neuropathy involving either single or multiple peripheral nerves, as well as the autonomic nervous system, results in a high morbidity (Pierce 1999). Foot ulcers, secondary to both neuropathic and microvascular disease, are also common, as are infections resulting from both vascular disease and defective white cell

function (Albright et al 2000). Cataracts are also frequently observed, as a result of sorbitol accumulation in the lens of the eye.

In 1999, the Australian Diabetes Society released new diagnostic criteria with a view to increasing the sensitivity of diabetes screening (Colman et al 1999). By detecting type II diabetes earlier, it is anticipated that many of the chronic complications may be avoided.

It is well recognized that regular aerobic exercise results in improved lipoprotein profile, blood pressure, and cardiovascular fitness (Agurs-Collins et al 1997, Diabetes Control and Complications Trial Research Group 1993, Pan et al 1997). As macrovascular disease is one of the major causes of morbidity and mortality in diabetes, exercise is believed to be of significant benefit (Zinman et al 1997). In addition, regular exercise has been shown to reduce an individual's insulin requirements, and the psychosocial benefits of exercise for the adolescent are invaluable (Zinman et al 1997). With particular regard to type II diabetes, the potential benefits of exercise are substantial. An abundance of literature has recently summarized the potential metabolic benefits of aerobic exercise in type II diabetes (Albright et al 2000, Eriksson 1999, Zinman et al 1997). These benefits include reduced blood glucose levels, improved insulin sensitivity, improved cardiovascular fitness, lowered blood pressure, improved lipid profile, improved body weight, and improved stress management abilities and self-esteem. Additionally, there is increasing evidence that exercise may prevent or delay the onset of type II diabetes (Pan et al 1997, Zinman et al 1997).

EXERCISE AND THE DIABETIC

Individuals with type I diabetes, with no chronic complications and good blood glucose control, are able to perform in most forms and levels of sport and exercise (Zinman et al 1997). An exception to this, however, is scuba diving (Hazel 1994), which as a result of its unpredictable nature and dependence on a buddy system, make it an inappropriate activity for people with this condition (Gorman 1993). It is important that prior to the commencement of any exercise program, a full examination is performed. Particular attention must be paid to the cardiovascular, ocular, and neurological systems, as well as to the feet. It is recommended that individuals over the age of 35 years, or with a 15-year history of diabetes, undergo either a resting or exercise ECG to exclude any underlying, silent, coronary artery disease (Zinman et al 1997). Baseline levels of renal function, glucose control, and lipids should be performed (Eriksson 1999). Irregularities in the examination or investigative findings may alter the suitability of various exercise programs, and this requires individualized assessment (Zinman et al 1997).

Upon the initiation of an exercise program, it needs to be emphasized to the individual that the regular monitoring and subsequent adjustment of the therapeutic regimen is critical for ongoing safe participation (Zinman et al 1997). The education of, and understanding by the individual, family, and training partners is fundamental to the success of an exercise program in this group of people.

Hypoglycemia is a common complication both during and up to 14 h after exercise, and needs to be ably recognized by both the individual and their training partners (Hernandez et al 2000). Common features of hypoglycemia include symptoms and signs secondary to both catecholamine release and central nervous system dysfunction. Sweating, shakiness, anxiety, palpitations, weakness, tremor, hunger, faintness, and tachycardia can all occur secondary to catecholamine release. Confusion, irritability, headaches, abnormal behavior, weakness, diplopia, inappropriate affect, motor incoordination, convulsion, and coma can occur secondary to central nervous system dysfunction. The risks of both hyperglycemia and hypoglycemia can be minimized with alterations in both the insulin regimen and carbohydrate intake, based on pre-exercise blood glucose levels. Guidelines for the manipulation of insulin dosage and carbohydrate intake are shown in Table 30.2. Exercise intensity and duration are the key variables to consider.

The keeping of an accurate exercise diary is critical in allowing an individual to assess responses to varying exercise intensities and insulin regimens (Fig. 30.5). It is recommended that blood glucose measurements be made immediately before, during, and after exercise in order to observe individual responses to differing regimens. It should be remembered that subcutaneous injections of insulin will be more rapidly absorbed from working muscles, and therefore, injections into active limbs should be avoided (Koivisto & Felig 1978).

The maintenance of hydration with glucose containing fluids, and having carbohydrate rich foods available both during and following exercise, will prevent intra-exercise, postexercise, and nocturnal hypoglycemia (Hernandez et al 2000, Zinman et al 1997). Low glycemic index (GI) foods prior to exercise, combined with high GI foods during exercise has been found to optimize a diabetic's blood glucose profile (Perlstein et al 1997). A 5–10 min low intensity warm-up and warm-down should be included in each exercise session in order to gradually prepare the cardiovascular, metabolic, and musculoskeletal systems (Zinman et al 1997). To prevent podiatric complications, appropriate footwear and socks should be worn. Any blisters or foot discomfort should be addressed rapidly, in order to prevent any progressive complications (e.g. foot ulcers) (Zinman et al 1997). The wearing of a diabetes identification bracelet,

Table 30.2 Guidelines for carbohydrate and insulin requirements before exercise (reproduced from Perlstein et al 1997 with the permission of the International Diabetes Institute, Australia)

Blood glucose levels before exercise	Exercise	Approximate amount of carbohydrate to eat prior to exercise[a]
< 6 mmol/L	Short duration (30–45 min), low/moderate intensity (e.g. walking, aerobic dance)	25 g
	Short duration (30–45 min), high intensity (e.g. sprints, weight lifting)	25 g
	Moderate duration (60 min), moderate intensity, (e.g. cycling, basketball, tennis, swimming)	25–50 g
	Long duration (> 75 min), low to moderate intensity/intermittent (e.g. marathon, triathlon, soccer, football)	50 g
6–10 mmol/L	Short duration (30–45 min), low/moderate intensity	0 g
	Short duration (30–45 min), high intensity	0 g
	Moderate duration (60 min), moderate intensity	0–25 g
	Long duration (> 75 min), low to moderate intensity	25–50 g
10–15 mmol/L	Short duration (30–45 min), low/moderate intensity	0 g
	Short duration (30–45 min), high intensity	0 g
	Moderate duration (60 min), moderate intensity	0 g
	Long duration (>75 min), low to moderate intensity	0–25 g
> 15 mmol/L, ketones absent	The effect of any exercise may be to raise blood glucose levels if there is not enough circulating insulin present. Knowing whether blood glucose levels were rising or falling in the few hours prior to exercise may help. If blood glucose levels are falling, exercise can be undertaken	
> 15 mmol/L, ketones present	Rest and take some short acting insulin and delay exercise until blood glucose levels are under better control	

[a] Individuals have different responses to physical activity and food. The above recommendations are a guide and it is advisable for individuals to discuss these with a dietitian, diabetes nurse educator and/or doctor before undertaking any changes.

COMPETITIVE ATHLETES

	Exercise					Blood glucose (Time)					Insulin dose (Time)				Food/Fluid			Weight		Comments, e.g., cold weather, heart rate, injuries
Date	Time	Type	Min	Intensity	Density (km)						7am	12md	6pm	11pm	Pre	During	Post	Pre	Post	
Mon 3/3											10H	8H	8H	12P						
Tue 4/3	6pm	Cycle	90	H	45	7am 6	12md 5.5	6pm 8.5	8pm 9.9	11pm 7.5	10	8	5	10	Jam sandwich 500mL water	1L dilute cordial, 1 banana	500mL sports drink and dinner	76kg	75kg	
Wed 5/3																				
Thur 6/3	6pm	Cycle	80	H	40	7am 5	12md 7.8	6pm 13.0	8pm 7.4	11pm 6.0	10	8	6	10	1 glass juice, 500mL water	1L dilute cordial	1 can cola and dinner	–	–	Snack pre-bed: 1 cup milk and 2 raisin toast
Fri 7/3																				
Sat 8/3	10am	Cycle	150	M	75	7am 5	10am 10.0	12:30pm 3.5	3pm 7.0	11pm 8.0	6	6	7	11	1/2L water, 2 bananas	2L dilute cordial, 10 dried apricots	See comments	75.5kg	75.0kg	Hypo 12:30pm after cycle. Ate jelly beans and lunch straight away. Felt fine
Sun 9/3											10	8	8	12						

Distance this week: 160 km

Cumulative distance: 1574 km for 2002

Codes : Intensity: E – Easy
M – Moderate
H – Hard

Notes:

Figure 30.5 Example of a training diary for a diabetic individual.

and not training alone are simple but important recommendations.

When exercising with type II diabetes, the risk of exercise-induced hypogylcemia is reduced (Eriksson 1999). If the diabetes is being managed with diet control alone, then dietary manipulation prior to exercise may suffice. When requiring oral hypoglycemic medication, the dose may need to be reduced or withheld, and the timing of drug administration may need to be altered (Albright et al 2000). An individual's response to differing regimens should be closely monitored. In order to achieve health improvements, it is recommended that individuals with type II diabetes exercise 3–5 times per week, at a low to moderate intensity (Constance & Clure 1996). Duration should begin at 10–15 min, gradually increasing to approximately 60 min as tolerated (Albright et al 2000). Both aerobic and resistance training are recognized to offer significant benefits (Albright et al 2000).

The most frequent complication that diabetics experience during exercise is a hypoglycemic episode. While this can be avoided with regular monitoring, the ability of both the individuals and their training partners to recognize early signs and symptoms is vital. Should symptoms become apparent, the consumption of high GI foods, and glucose containing fluid is the most appropriate initial management. Should symptoms persist or progress, then medical advice should be sought.

In summary, it is well recognized that the benefits of exercise in diabetics outweigh the risks. With regular monitoring and by following the basic principles carefully, the risks associated with exercise may be minimized.

THE TIRED ATHLETE

While fatigue is a common reaction to hard and persistent training, ongoing fatigue that is not responsive to recovery warrants attention. There are a multitude of medical conditions that may result in prolonged tiredness. The most common causes in the highly trained athlete include overtraining syndrome, infections, sleep disturbance, and dietary imbalances (Table 30.3) (Brukner 1996). Most significantly, underlying medical conditions can be eliminated with a concise medical history and examination; however, in the absence of any overt medical condition a more comprehensive history will be required. Critical features to elucidate in the history from the athlete include nature of the fatigue (constant, sleepiness, post-training, during training), associated recent illnesses, volume and intensity of training (including any modifications), amount of recovery time following sessions, dietary intake (carbohydrate, protein, and fat, and relationship to training), fluid intake, quality and quantity of sleep, and extracurricular psychosocial stresses.

Routine first line investigations for fatigued athletes may include full blood profile, electrolytes, renal and liver function tests, iron studies, and urinalysis. Further investigations to consider include viral serology, vitamin and mineral status, thyroid function tests, glucose tests, and creatine kinase assessment. If indicated, a chest radiograph or lung spirometry should be considered (Brukner 1996).

Table 30.3 Possible causes of recalcitrant fatigue in the athlete (reproduced from Brukner P. The tired athlete. Table 1: Causes of persistent tiredness in athletes. Aus Fam Physician 1996; 25(8):1285, with the permission of Australian Family Physician. Text copyright to Australian Family Physician. Permission to reproduce must be sought from the publisher, the Royal Australian College of General Practitioners).

Common causes	Less common causes	Causes not to be missed
Overtraining syndrome	Dehydration	Malignant disease
Viral illness	Exercise-induced asthma	Cardiac problems
URTI	Mg, Zn or B_{12} deficiency	Bacterial endocarditis
Infectious mononucleosis	Postviral fatigue syndrome	Cardiac failure
Inadequate carbohydrate intake	Allergic disorders	Diabetes
Depletion of iron stores	Jet-lag	Hypothyroidism
Inadequate protein intake	Anemia	Renal failure
Insufficient sleep	Psychological stress	Neuromuscular disorders
	Anxiety	Infection
	Depression	Hepatitis A, B, C
	Medications	HIV
	Beta-blockers	Malaria
	Anxiolytics	Eating disorders
	Antihistamines	Anorexia
		Bulimia
		Pregnancy
		Postconcussive syndrome

OVERTRAINING SYNDROME

With adequate recovery from training, the body will adapt to increased demands (Wilmore & Costill 1994). A common principle in athletic training involves stressing the body as a stimulus for adaptation, which is known as progressive overload training (Wilmore & Costill 1994). However, if the recovery period is inadequate for the volume and intensity of training undertaken, then an athlete can experience an increase in fatigue and a reduction in performance. This temporary deterioration is known as overreaching (Smith 2000). While overreaching can usually be reversed with a few days of adequate recovery, if athletes fail to recognize this phenomenon and modify their training appropriately, then an overtraining syndrome may develop (Fry et al 1991, Hedelin et al 2000).

The overtraining syndrome is characterized by a vast number of symptoms that can be categorized as physiological, psychological, immunological, and biochemical (Fry et al 1991) (Box 30.2). The most common presenting symptoms of overtraining are fatigue, reduced performance, sleep disturbance, muscle soreness, recurrent injury, and infection (Costill et al 1988, Fry et al 1991, Fry

---

Box 30.2 Symptoms of overtraining syndrome (reproduced from Fry et al 1991 with the permission of Adis International Ltd.)

Physiological/performance
- Decreased performance
- Inability to meet previously attained performance standards/criteria
- Recovery prolonged
- Reduced toleration of loading
- Decreased muscular strength
- Decreased maximum work capacity
- Loss of coordination
- Decreased efficiency/decreased amplitude of movement
- Reappearance of mistakes already corrected
- Reduced capacity of differentiation and correcting technical faults
- Increased difference between lying and standing heart rate
- Abnormal T wave pattern in ECG
- Heart discomfort on slight exertion
- Changes in blood pressure
- Changes in heart rate at rest, exercise and recovery
- Increased frequency of respiration
- Perfuse respiration
- Decreased body fat
- Increased oxygen consumption at submaximal workloads
- Increased ventilation and heart rate at submaximal workloads
- Shift of the lactate curve towards the x-axis
- Decreased evening postworkout weight
- Elevated basal metabolic rate
- Chronic fatigue
- Insomnia with and without night sweats
- Feels thirsty
- Anorexia nervosa
- Loss of appetite
- Bulimia
- Amenorrhea/oligomenorrhea
- Headaches
- Nausea
- Increased aches and pains
- Gastrointestinal disturbances
- Muscle soreness/tenderness
- Tendinostic complaints
- Periosteal complaints
- Muscle damage
- Elevated C-reactive protein
- Rhabdomyolysis

Psychological/information processing
- Feeling of depression
- General apathy
- Decreased self-esteem/worsening feeling of self
- Emotional instability
- Difficulty in concentrating at work and training
- Sensitive to environmental and emotional stress
- Fear of competition
- Changes in personality
- Decreased ability to narrow concentration
- Increased internal and external distractability
- Decreased capacity to deal with large amounts of information
- Gives up when the going gets tough

Immunological
- Increased susceptibility to and severity of illness/colds/allergies
- Flu-like illnesses
- Unconfirmed glandular fever
- Minor scratches heal slowly
- Swelling of lymph glands
- One-day colds
- Decreased functional activity of neutrophils
- Decreased total lymphocyte counts
- Reduced response to mitogens
- Increased blood eosinophil count
- Decreased proportion of null (non-T, non-B lymphocytes)
- Bacterial infection
- Reactivation of herpes viral infection
- Significant variations in CD4:CD8 lymphocytes

Biochemical
- Negative nitrogen balance
- Hypothalamic dysfunction
- Flat glucose tolerance curves
- Depressed muscle glycogen concentration
- Decreased bone mineral content
- Delayed menarche
- Decreased hemoglobin
- Decreased serum iron
- Decreased serum ferritin
- Lowered TIBC
- Mineral depletion (Zn, Co, Al, Mn, Se, Cu, etc)
- Increased urea concentrations
- Elevated cortisol levels
- Elevated ketosteroids in urine
- Low free testosterone
- Increased serum hormone binding globulin
- Decreased ratio of free testosterone to cortisol of more than 30%
- Increased uric acid production

et al 1994, Morgan et al 1987, Morgan et al 1988, Nieman 1995). Unlike the overreached athlete, the overtrained athlete may take many months to recover (Hedelin et al 2000). There are several theories as to the etiology of the overtraining syndrome. These include autonomic nervous system dysfunction (Lehmann et al 1998), glutamine depletion (Kingsbury et al 1998, Smith & Norris 2000), tryptophan depletion (Smith 2000), and glycogen depletion (Snyder 1998). Smith (2000) recently attempted to integrate the existing theories into a single paradigm, proposing that the inflammatory cytokines released in response to normal training may be responsible for inducing each of the features observed in the overtraining syndrome. While the proposal is very attractive, it requires further consideration prior to being universally accepted.

If overtraining syndrome is suspected, the monitoring of testosterone, cortisol, creatine phosphokinase, and immunological markers such as complement levels can assist in the monitoring of the athlete's progress, but cannot be used to provide a firm diagnosis (Brukner 1996).

Initial management of the overtrained athlete involves exclusion of other possible causes of fatigue, and the recognition of the condition by both athlete and coach. Prolonged rest from training is the most important aspect of treatment, with return to training being gradual, progressive, and guided by symptoms. Monitoring of morning heart rate may provide a simple guide to recovery from training, with an elevation of more than 6 beats per min considered to be significant (Brukner & Khan 1993). Concurrently, issues such as injuries, nutrition, training program, and psychosocial stresses should be addressed. Full recovery may take weeks to months (Hedelin et al 2000).

Prevention of overtraining syndrome requires that training programs be carefully constructed so that they incorporate the correct balance between load and recovery (Kuipers & Keizer 1988). As individuals respond differently to the same training load, and have differing professional and private stresses and pressures which can all impact upon the response to training (Kuipers & Keizer 1988), the individualization of training regimens, which take into account not only the training itself, but also environmental, psychological, and social factors, is necessary to maximize the benefits of training (Pyne et al 2000a). Education of coaches and athletes about over-training syndrome is the most significant step in prevention. Strategies such as periodization, cross-training, psychological skills training, dietary assistance, environmental manipulation, regular medical review, and the use of regenerative techniques such as massage and hydrotherapy may all assist in the prevention of overtraining (Brukner 1996, Pyne et al 2000a).

TRAVEL MEDICINE FOR THE INTERNATIONAL ATHLETE

The ease of modern air travel has enabled athletes to travel to competitions throughout the world with relative ease. In many situations, athletes may be accompanied by a team physician, but more often, the physical therapist or sports trainer will be the only travelling medical team member. There are three important phases in the provision of care for the travelling athlete: pretravel, travel, and on location care (Young et al 1998).

Prior to travelling, it is important that the responsible medical officer be fully aware of any medical issues facing individual athletes and staff. A comprehensive history and examination should be performed prior to departure.

VACCINATIONS

It is important that a detailed travel itinerary is available in order to accurately plan for vaccinations (Young et al 1998). One of the major difficulties facing the medical practitioner is the short notice of impending travel often provided, making appropriate scheduling of vaccinations difficult. Athletes should therefore, keep an accurate vaccination schedule in their training diary. Vaccinations which should be considered as mandatory include tetanus, diptheria, measles, mumps, poliomyelitis, and rubella. Those that should be considered on a more individualized basis (dependent on the nature of the sport, ages, and location being visited) include hepatitis A, hepatitis B, influenza, malaria, typhoid, Japanese encephalitis, cholera, rabies, meningococcus, and yellow fever. It is important that all athletes have received their basic childhood vaccinations. It is also recommended that all travelling athletes be vaccinated against hepatitis A, and for those involved in contact sports, hepatitis B should be considered (Young et al 1998). The ever-changing distribution of diseases and disease vectors, as well as the increasing availability of international travel, ensures that the vaccination requirements of travel continue to change (WHO 2001). It is important that an up-to-date vaccination schedule is consulted prior to travel.

ISSUES WITH AIR TRAVEL

Circadian rhythms are the body's daily rhythms that are synchronized to the day/night cycle. These rhythms control the body's physiological and psychological systems. Many components of sports performance such as flexibility, power output, and muscle strength have been shown to vary with the time of day as a result of the circadian rhythm (Atkinson & Reilly 1996). Flights across time zones can result in desynchronization of circadian rhythms, leading to circadian dysrhythmia or 'jet-lag'. Jet-lag is more pronounced when travelling over a greater number of time zones, and when travelling eastwards (Reilly et al 2001). Symptoms of jet-lag include disrupted sleep, gastrointestinal distress, headaches and general malaise. While anecdotally it would appear that jet-lag may impair performance, methodological difficulties have meant that the scientific substantiation of jet-lag impairing performance is lacking (Youngstedt & O'Connor 1999). It is estimated that it takes one day to readjust to the new environment, for each time zone crossed (Loat & Rhodes 1989, Reilly et al 2001).

Jet-lag symptoms can be reduced with a number of simple strategies. In preparation for travel, adjusting one's sleeping pattern to the arrival time zone a few days prior to departure, can reduce symptoms on arrival (Loat & Rhodes 1989). Sleeping well on the night prior to departure, minimizing time spent in transit with appropriate flight scheduling, and adjusting watches to the destination local time on boarding will also aid the traveller (Loat & Roades 1989, Young et al 1998). Either regular short sleep episodes or attempting to establish a new sleep–wake cycle, in synchronization with the destination local time are both recommended, but need to be individualized (Young et al 1998). Use of relaxation techniques, ear plugs, and eye shields may also assist in sleeping during and after the flight, by minimizing visual and auditory distractions (Young et al 1998). It has been suggested that following westward and eastward flights, competition be arranged in the morning and evenings respectively, in order to optimize performance, by taking advantage of the circadian delay. Other means of minimizing jet-lag include avoiding alcohol, regularly mobilizing in the aircraft cabin, and maintaining fluid and food intake. There is some suggestion that eating a high protein breakfast and a low protein/high carbo-hydrate dinner following a time zone change, may assist in resynchronization (Loat & Rhodes 1989).

The use of short-acting hypnotic medication or melatonin are considered useful in achieving sleep and assisting in establishing a new circadian rhythm. Melatonin is a peptide secreted by the pineal gland, which helps to induce sleep as the eyes register dusk (Waterhouse et al 1998). While it has been shown to reduce the subjective symptoms of jet-lag when taken before and after air travel (Herxheimer & Petrie 2001, Petrie et al 1993), it must be used carefully in order not to further upset the body's circadian rhythm (Reilly et al 1998). Reilly et al (2001) recently showed no benefit of using low dose temazepam on recovery from jet-lag, following a westerly flight over five time zones. As a result of the unpredictable individual effects, and the potential for prolonged drowsiness, the British Olympic Association Medical Committee advises against the use of hypnotics or melatonin in international travel (Reilly et al 1998). Under no circumstances should hypnotic medication or melatonin be used for the first time prior to a major competition.

On arrival, the risk of infection from oral-fecal contamination or insect vectors needs to be evaluated. If the water supply is suspected of being contaminated, then only sealed, bottled water should be used for drinking and teeth washing. Similarly, salads or other foods washed in tap water, as well as ice cubes should be avoided. If concerns regarding the water supply are expressed, the general rule of 'cook it, peel it or leave it alone,' should be applied. Drink bottles should be regularly cleaned, with bottled water, especially if sports drinks are being used. A brush should be taken for this purpose. Mosquitoes transmit parasites such as in malaria, as well as arboviruses causing dengue fever, yellow fever and Japanese encephalitis (Bell et al 1995). As it is known that the Anopheline mosquito carrying malaria and the Aedes mosquito carrying dengue fever bite during the dusk and daylight hours respectively, it is possible to take preventive measures, such as the use of light-colored, long-sleeved clothing, insect repellents, and nets for sleeping in, which are recommended in high risk areas. Anti-malarial prophylactic medication requirements vary depending on the location and duration of stay, as well as an individual's medical history, and should be discussed with a medical practitioner prior to departure.

Hot and humid climates place thermal demands on athletes, who require time to adapt. Acclimatization to heat may take up to 2 weeks, and until achieved, may impair performance. If travelling to a particularly hot environment, it is recommended that at least 2 weeks be allowed for optimal acclimatization prior to competing. Training volume and intensity should be reduced on arrival, with a gradual increase over 2 weeks; it should also initially be performed during the coolest part of the day, with a progressive introduction to the hotter parts of the day. (Young et al 1998). Fluid intake should be increased during rest and activity and both body weight and urine volume can be used to monitor fluid replace-ment. Light-colored, loose fitting clothing and sunblock should be worn, in order to minimize the risks of heat illness, and maximize the likelihood of successful performance. If travelling from sea level to compete at altitude, a similar period of acclimatization may be required. The alternative is to travel and compete within 24 h of arrival.

INFECTIONS IN ATHLETES

Infectious conditions are common both in athletes and non-athletes. Upper respiratory tract, chest and generalized viral infections are the most common presentation to an elite sports medicine center (Fricker 1997). It has recently been shown that even a mild respiratory infection within 6 weeks of a major competition can have a significant impact on the competition outcome (Pyne et al 2000b). For this reason, it is important that athletes and support staff have an understanding of those infections to which athletes may be particularly susceptible.

UPPER RESPIRATORY TRACT INFECTIONS

While recent research suggests that elite athletes may be at no greater risk of upper respiratory tract infections (URTI) than the general public (Fricker et al 2000), there is mounting evidence that transient alterations in the bodies immune system as a result of intensive training, may predispose some athletes to infection (Gleeson 2000). While URTIs are commonly either viral or bacterial in origin, up to 80% are considered to be viral. Causative agents include the adenovirus, coxsackie virus, rhinovirus, coronavirus and others. Sore throat, conjunctivitis, headache, hoarseness, malaise and fever are the most common presenting symptoms. Management of the viral URTI is predominantly symptomatic and includes: lozenges, paracetamol to control fevers, fluids to maintain hydration and relative rest. There is some evidence that zinc may reduce the duration of symptoms (Mossad et al 1996), and it is the author's practice to use a short course of vitamin C. One must be cautious, however, of the interaction between vitamin C and the oral contraceptive.

Epstein-Barr Virus (EBV), the causative agent in glandular fever (infectious mononucleosis) in the young athlete, often presents with a thick exudative pharyngitis, lymphadenopathy, fever and malaise. Serology will allow confirmation of an acute infection and treatment is then supportive. EBV can result in a number of significant complications, including splenomegaly, which needs to be excluded before return to contact sport is permitted. Should splenomegaly be detected, clinically or on ultrasound investigation, contact sport is contraindicated for 4 weeks, or until the swelling is reduced, in order to prevent the theoretical risk of rupture (Young 1999).

Bacterial infections will commonly have an exudative tonsillitis and cervical lymphadenopathy, and should be treated with appropriate antibiotics. In severe infections, when intravenous antibiotics are required, antibiotic enhancing medications such as probenecid are often used. It is important to recognize that this is an International Olympic Committee (IOC) banned medication. Similarly, many over-the-counter decongestants and mucolytics contain IOC banned substances and caution needs to be exercised when prescribing.

Return-to-sport guidelines should be individualized. General principles are that if the illness is limited to the head, then it is acceptable to continue with moderate training, until symptoms have resolved. However, if there are generalized symptoms of fever, tachycardia, malaise, lymphadenopathy and fatigue, then all training should cease until symptoms have disappeared (Nieman 1993, Young 1998). The aim of this is to minimize the risk of complications such as myocarditis and postviral fatigue which may complicate an otherwise simple respiratory infection. Should fatigue persist following a URTI, it is recommended that exercise be very gradually resumed with light aerobic exercise at an intensity less than 65% of maximum heart rate. Subsequently, the frequency, duration and finally the intensity of exercise may be sequentially and gradually increased (Young 1999).

BLOOD BORNE PATHOGENS

The transmission of blood borne viruses such as human immunodeficiency virus (HIV), hepatitis B (HBV) and hepatitis C (HCV) have been a major concern to sports people and support staff in recent years. Despite the high degree of public concern, there has only been one reported case of HIV transmission as a result of a sporting injury (Torre et al 1990), and even this case is considered dubious (Mast et al 1995). Similarly, there are limited examples of hepatitis B transmission as a result of sports participation (AMSSM & AASM 1995, Kashiwagi et al 1982). Transmission in the sporting arena is most likely to occur when two open wounds are opposed, allowing direct contact between the blood of seropositive and seronegative individuals. Despite a relatively high incidence of bleeding wounds being documented in professional football of varying codes (Brown et al 1995, Seward et al 1993b), the risk of HIV transmission has been estimated to be less than 1 per 85 million game contacts (Brown et al 1995). There are no known cases of HIV being transmitted via sweat or saliva (Feller & Flanigan 1997). Similarly, there is no evidence for increased transmission of hepatitis B in Australian Football players (Siebert et al 1995). Indeed, it is thought that off-the-field behavior of athletes may place them at greater risk of infection transmission, than bleeding episodes on the field (Feller & Flanigan 1997, Rich et al 1998). In 1995, the American Medical Society for Sports Medicine and the American Academy of Sports Medicine, in a joint position statement, outlined some specific preventative measures (AMSSM & ACSM 1995) (Box 30.3). It is vital that medical practitioners and sports trainers are proactive in ensuring that sporting clubs with which they work employ these recommendations, in order to minimize the risk of transmission of blood borne pathogens.

Box 30.3 Specific measures to prevent the transmission of blood borne pathogens (Data from the American Medical Society for Sports Medicine and the American Academy of Sports Medicine (AMSSM & AASM 1995), with the permission of the American Journal of Sports Medicine)

- Pre-event dressing of all open wounds with occlusive dressings.
- Use of gloves, disinfectant, bleach, antiseptic, for washing/cleaning surfaces and clothing.
- Receptacles for contaminated clothing, bandages, dressing, needles, must be available on the side of the field of play and in the dressing rooms.
- Removal of players from play if active bleeding is present.
- Control of bleeding, covering of wound with occlusive dressing and change of blood stained clothing prior to return to play.
- Wearing of adequate, appropriate protective equipment by players.
- Athlete education and empowerment with responsibility to report wounds.
- Caregiver precautions including the using and changing of gloves between contacts.
- Covering of minor cuts and abrasions while on the field.
- Airway devices should be available for use in case of life threatening emergencies.
- Contaminated areas (e.g. mats) should be wiped down immediately and disinfected with bleach. The area should be dry before being re-used.
- Postevent, wounds should be reviewed and redressed.
- Soiled clothing and towels should be washed separately.
- All personnel involved in coaching and support of a team should be trained in basic first-aid.

CUTANEOUS INFECTIONS

Herpes simplex virus (HSV) is a commonly transmitted cutaneous infection in contact sports (Mast & Goodman 1997, Stacey & Atkins 2000). Transmission occurs via direct contact between infectious lesions or secretions, and broken skin. It is estimated that up to 15% of the population may be excreting HSV at any given time. HSV lesions are painful vesicles that rapidly increase in number and ulcerate. Oral and topical antiviral agents are now available to treat HSV, however once infected, the virus may remain deactivated in the sensory nerve ganglion, awaiting an opportunity to reappear. Players with active herpetic lesions should be prohibited from returning to play until the lesions are fully resolved (Stacey & Atkins 2000).

Streptococcal and staphylococcal bacterial outbreaks in sports teams, have also been reported (Mast & Goodman 1997, Stacey & Atkins 2000). Direct contact with a discharging skin lesion or contact with an asymptomatic nasal carrier may result in vesicular, bullous or pustular skin lesions. Athletes in contact sports with bacterial skin lesions, which cannot be adequately covered, should be prohibited from play.

The warm, moist environment of the feet and groin, combined with constant friction in these areas predisposes athletes to fungal infections. These can be transmitted by direct contact or via infected skin scales in dressing rooms. Use of topical antifungal medication and using footwear in communal showers will help prevent the transmission of foot infections.

SUMMARY

Unlike many common musculoskeletal problems encountered by physical therapists and physicians, medical problems in the sporting environment often create a great deal of anxiety. This chapter provides a detailed account of a select number of significant medical issues commonly encountered by a team medical or paramedical officer. A common theme throughout all the sections of this chapter has been 'if in doubt, refer on'. It is the author's opinion that no-one has ever had a sleepless night over, or had to defend, a decision to seek another opinion. Indeed, the over-riding principle we should follow is 'first do no harm'.

Asthma attacks, epileptic seizures, concussive episodes, and spinal cord injuries are all acute, serious conditions that physical therapists and athletic trainers can expect to encounter while working with a sporting team. The background and management of these conditions has been outlined in detail, but the initial management is very similar in each. The principles of safety, airways, breathing, and circulation, followed by stabilization and transportation to an appropriate referral center are universal to these conditions. Thus, it is important that attendants are knowledgeable in cardiopulmonary resuscitation. Similarly, the nearest hospital to the sporting venue, and emergency phone numbers are mandatory knowledge.

Diabetes is a condition associated with a huge morbidity. Exercise has been shown to benefit the diabetic in a number of ways. With adequate preparation and support there is no reason why a diabetic athlete cannot compete at the top level in any number of sports. As medical professionals we should endeavor to expedite this through our association with sporting bodies.

Overtraining is a condition which is much easier to prevent than to treat, and early recognition is critical in its management. The medical professional working with a team can play a pivotal role in preventing the development of this condition. The transmission of infection within the sporting environment is an area of increasing concern in the community. It is the responsibility of sporting organizations to provide a safe environment for athletes, and it is the role of the medical and paramedical professional to ensure that recommendations are instigated.

REFERENCES

Agurs-Collins T D, Kumanyika S K, Ten Have T R et al 1997 A randomized controlled trial of weight reduction and exercise for diabetes management in older African-American subjects. Diabetes Care 20:1503–1511

Albright A, Franz M, Hornsby G et al 2000 American College of Sports Medicine position stand. Exercise and type 2 diabetes. Medicine and Science in Sport and Exercise 32:1345–1360

AMSSM, AASM 1995 Human immunodeficiency virus (HIV) and other blood-borne pathogens in sports. Joint position statement. The American Medical Society for Sports Medicine (AMSSM) and the American Academy of Sports Medicine (AASM). American Journal of Sports Medicine 23:510–514

Anderson S, Daviskas E 2000 The mechanism of exercise-induced asthma is … Journal of Allergy and Clinical Immunology 106:453–459

Anderson S D, Holzer K 2000 Exercise-induced asthma: is it the right diagnosis in elite athletes? Journal of Allergy and Clinical Immunology 106:419–428

Asthma Management Handbook 2002 National Asthma Council of Australia

Atkinson G, Reilly T 1996 Circadian variation in sports performance. Sports Medicine 21:292–312

Basilico F C 1999 Cardiovascular disease in athletes. American Journal of Sports Medicine 27:108–121

Beck K C 1999 Control of airway function during and after exercise in asthmatics. Medicine and Science in Sport and Exercise 31:S4–S11

Bell D, Gilks C, Molyneux M et al 1995 Lecture notes on tropical medicine, 4th edn. Blackwell Sciences Ltd, Oxford, UK

Brown L S Jr, Drotman D P, Chu A et al 1995 Bleeding injuries in professional football: estimating the risk for HIV transmission. Annals of Internal Medicine 122:273–274

Brukner P 1996 Sports medicine. The tired athlete. Australian Family Physician 25:1283–1288

Brukner P, Khan K 1993 Clinical sports medicine, 1st edn. McGraw Hill Book Company, Roseville, NSW

Cantu R 1997 Stingers, transient quadriplegia, and cervical spinal stenosis: return to play criteria. Medicine and Science in Sport and Exercise 29:S233–S235

Cantu R C 1998a Epilepsy and athletics. Clinical Sports Medicine 17:61–69

Cantu R C 1998b Second-impact syndrome. Clinical Journal of Sports Medicine 17:37–44

Cantu R C 1998c Return to play guidelines after a head injury. Clinics in Sports Medicine 17:45–60

Carlsen K H, Engh G, Mork M 2000 Exercise-induced bronchoconstriction depends on exercise load. Respiratory Medicine 94:750–755

Colman P G, Thomas D W, Zimmet P Z et al 1999 New classification and criteria for diagnosis of diabetes mellitus. Position Statement from the Australian Diabetes Society, New Zealand Society for the Study of Diabetes, Royal College of Pathologists of Australasia and Australasian Association of Clinical Biochemists. The Medical Journal of Australia 170:375–378

Constance A, Clure C 1996 Diabetes and exercise. A Guide for health professionals, vol. 2001, UP Diabetes Outreach Network. www.diabetesliving.com/manage/aguide.htm

Costill D L, Flynn M G, Kirwan J P et al 1988 Effects of repeated days of intensified training on muscle glycogen and swimming performance. Medicine and Science in Sport and Exercise 20:249–254.

Crimi E, Milanese M, Oddera S et al 2001 Inflammatory and mechanical factors of allergen-induced bronchoconstriction in mild asthma and rhinitis. Journal of Applied Physiology 91:1029–1034

Deal E C Jr, McFadden E R Jr, Ingram R H Jr et al 1979 Esophageal temperature during exercise in asthmatic and nonasthmatic subjects. Journal of Applied Physiology 46:484–490

Diabetes Control and Complications Trial Research Group 1993 The effect of intensive treatment of diabetes on the development and progression of long-term complications in insulin-dependent diabetes mellitus. New England Journal of Medicine 329:977–986

Edelman J M, Turpin J A, Bronsky E A et al 2000 Oral montelukast compared with inhaled salmeterol to prevent exercise-induced bronchoconstriction. A randomized, double-blind trial. Exercise Study Group. Annals of Internal Medicine 132:97–104

Eriksson J G 1999 Exercise and the treatment of type 2 diabetes mellitus. An update. Sports Medicine 27:381–391

Fallon K 1997 Neurology. In: Fields K, Fricker P (eds) Medical problems in athletes. Blackwell Science, Boston, MA

Feller A, Flanigan T P 1997 HIV-infected competitive athletes. What are the risks? What precautions should be taken? Journal of General Internal Medicine 12:243–246

Fields K, Reimer C 1997 Pulmonary problems in athletes. In: K Fields, P Fricker (eds) Medical problems in athletes. Blackwell Science, Boston, MA

Finch C F, McIntosh A S, McCrory P 2001 What do under 15 year old schoolboy rugby union players think about protective headgear? British Journal of Sports Medicine 35:89–94

Fricker P 1997 Infectious problems in athletes: an overview. In: Fields K, Fricker P (eds) Medical problems in athletes. Blackwell Science, Boston MA

Fricker P, Gleeson M, Flanagan A et al 2000 A clinical snapshot: do elite swimmers experience more upper respiratory illness than nonathletes? Clinical Exercise Physiology 2:155–158

Fry R W, Morton A R, Keast D 1991 Overtraining in athletes. An update. Sports Medicine 12:32–65

Fry R W, Grove J R, Morton A R et al 1994 Psychological and immunological correlates of acute overtraining. British Journal of Sports Medicine 28:241–246

Fuller C M, McNulty C M, Spring D A et al 1997 Prospective screening of 5,615 high school athletes for risk of sudden cardiac death. Medicine and Science in Sport and Exercise 29:1131–1138

Funk J, Feingold K 1995 Disorders of the endocrine pancreas. In: McPhee S, Lingappa V, Ganong W et al (eds), Pathophysiology of disease. An introduction to clinical medicine. Appleton and Lange, Stamford

Futterman L G, Myerburg R 1998 Sudden death in athletes: an update. Sports Medicine 26:335–350

Gale E 1990 Diabetes mellitus and other disorders of metabolism. In: Kumar P J, Clark M L (eds), Clinical medicine, Baillière Tindall, London

Gates J R, Spiegel R H 1993 Epilepsy, sports and exercise. Sports Medicine 15:1–5

Gavett S H, Koren H S 2001 The role of particulate matter in exacerbation of atopic asthma. International Archives of Allergy and Immunology 124:109–112

Gleeson M 2000 Mucosal immunity and respiratory illness in elite athletes. International Journal of Sports Medicine 21:S33–S43

Gorman D 1993 Fitness for diving. In: Gorman D (ed), Diving and hyperbaric medicine – course notes. Royal Adelaide Hospital Hyperbaric Medicine Unit, Adelaide

Grindel S H, Lovell M R, Collins M W 2001 The assessment of sport-related concussion: the evidence behind neuropsychological testing and management. Clinical Journal of Sports Medicine 11:134–143.

Hancock K 2001 Management issues in adult asthma. Australian Family Physician 30(2):114–119

Hazel J 1994 Australian Diabetes Society position statements: scuba diving. Australian Diabetes Society, Sydney, Australia

Hedelin R, Kentta G, Wiklund U et al 2000 Short-term overtraining: effects on performance, circulatory responses, and heart rate variability. Medicine and Science in Sport and Exercise 32:1480–1484

Helenius I J, Tikkanen H O, Sarna S et al 1998 Asthma and increased bronchial responsiveness in elite athletes: atopy and sport event as risk factors. Journal of Allergy and Clinical Immunology 101:646–652

Hernandez J M, Moccia T, Fluckey J D et al 2000 Fluid snacks to help persons with type 1 diabetes avoid late onset postexercise hypoglycemia. Medicine and Science in Sport and Exercise 32:904–910

Herxheimer A, Petrie K J 2001 Melatonin for preventing and treating jet lag (Cochrane Review). Cochrane Database Syst Rev 1:CD001520

Hickey J C, Morris A L, Carlson L D et al 1967 The relation of mouth protectors to cranial pressure and deformation. Journal of the American Dental Association 74:735–740

Holly R G, Shaffrath J D, Amsterdam E A 1998 Electrocardiographic alterations associated with the hearts of athletes. Sports Medicine 25:139–148

Huston T P, Puffer J C, Rodney W M 1985 The athletic heart syndrome. New England Journal of Medicine 313:24–32

Jensen-Urstad M 1995 Sudden death and physical activity in athletes and nonathletes. Scandinavian Journal of Medicine and Science in Sports 5:279–284

Johnston K, Barootes B, Barwitzki G et al 2000 Guidelines for assessment and management of sport-related concussion. Canadian Academy of Sport Medicine Concussion Committee. Clinical Journal of Sport Medicine 10:209–211

Johnston K M, McCrory P, Mohtadi N G et al 2001 Evidence-based review of sport-related concussion: clinical science. Clinical Journal of Sports Medicine 11:150–159

Kashiwagi S, Hayashi J, Ikematsu H et al 1982 An outbreak of hepatitis B in members of a high school sumo wrestling club. Journal of the American Medical Association 248:213–214

Kemp J P, Dockhorn R J, Busse W W et al 1994 Prolonged effect of inhaled salmeterol against exercise-induced bronchospasm. American Journal of Respiratory and Critical Care Medicine 150:1612–1615

Kerr I L 1986 Mouth guards for the prevention of injuries in contact sports. Sports Medicine 3:415–427

Kingsbury K J, Kay L, Hjelm M 1998 Contrasting plasma free amino acid patterns in elite athletes: association with fatigue and infection. British Journal of Sports Medicine 32:25–32.

Koivisto V A, Felig P 1978 Effects of leg exercise on insulin absorption in diabetic patients. New England Journal of Medicine 298:79–83

Kuipers H, Keizer H A 1988 Overtraining in elite athletes. Review and directions for the future. Sports Medicine 6:79–92

Lehmann M, Foster C, Dickhuth H H et al 1998 Autonomic imbalance hypothesis and overtraining syndrome. Medicine and Science in Sport and Exercise 30:1140–1145

Link M S, Wang P J, Estes N A 2001 Ventricular arrhythmias in the athlete. Current Opinions in Cardiology 16:30–39

Loat C E, Rhodes E C 1989 Jet-lag and human performance. Sports Medicine 8:226–238

McCrory P R 1997 Were you knocked out? A team physician's approach to initial concussion management. Medicine and Science in Sport and Exercise 29:S207–212

McCrory P 1999 The eighth wonder of the world: the mythology of concussion management. British Journal of Sports Medicine 33:136–137

McCrory P 2001a Do mouthguards prevent concussion? British Journal of Sports Medicine 35:81–82

McCrory P 2001b Does second impact syndrome exist? Clinical Journal of Sports Medicine 11:144–149

McCrory P R, Berkovic S F 1998a Second impact syndrome. Neurology 50:677–683

McCrory P R, Berkovic S F 1998b Concussive convulsions. Incidence in sport and treatment recommendations. Sports Medicine 25:131–136

McFadden E 1991 Asthma. In: Wilson J, Braunwald E, Isselbacher K et al (eds), Harrison's principles of internal medicine, vol. 2. McGraw Hill, New York

McIntosh A S, McCrory P 2000 Impact energy attenuation performance of football headgear. British Journal of Sports Medicine 34:337–341

McIntosh A S, McCrory P, Comerford J 2000 The dynamics of concussive head impacts in rugby and Australian rules football. Medicine and Science in Sport and Exercise 32:1980–1984

McLatchie G, Lloyd-Parry J 1997 Injuries to the neck and spine. Sports Exercise and Injury 3:183–190

McLaughlin D 1999 Epilepsy: key management issues. Australian Family Physician 28:889–896

Maddocks D L, Dicker G D, Saling M M 1995 The assessment of orientation following concussion in athletes. Clinical Journal of Sport Medicine 5:32–35

Maron B J, Mitchell J H 1994 Revised eligibility recommendations for competitive athletes with cardiovascular abnormalities. Journal of the American College of Cardiology 24:848–850

Maron B J, Isner J M, McKenna W J 1994 26th Bethesda conference: recommendations for determining eligibility for competition in athletes with cardiovascular abnormalities. Task Force 3: hypertrophic cardiomyopathy, myocarditis and other myopericardial diseases and mitral valve prolapse. Medicine and Science in Sport and Exercise 26:S261–267

Maron B J, Pelliccia A, Spirito P 1995 Cardiac disease in young trained athletes. Insights into methods for distinguishing athlete's heart from structural heart disease, with particular emphasis on hypertrophic cardiomyopathy. Circulation 91:1596–1601

Maron B J, Shirani J, Poliac L C et al 1996a Sudden death in young competitive athletes. Clinical, demographic, and pathological profiles. Journal of the American Medical Association 276:199–204

Maron B J, Thompson P D, Puffer J C et al 1996b Cardiovascular preparticipation screening of competitive athletes. A statement for health professionals from the Sudden Death Committee (clinical cardiology) and Congenital Cardiac Defects Committee (cardiovascular disease in the young), American Heart Association. Circulation 94:850–856

Maron B J, Thompson P D, Puffer J C et al 1998 Cardiovascular preparticipation screening of competitive athletes: addendum: an addendum to a statement for health professionals from the Sudden Death Committee (Council on Clinical Cardiology) and the Congenital Cardiac Defects Committee (Council on Cardiovascular Disease in the Young), American Heart Association. Circulation 97:2294

Mast E E, Goodman R A 1997 Prevention of infectious disease transmission in sports. Sports Medicine 24:1–7

Mast E E, Goodman R A, Bond W W et al 1995 Transmission of blood-borne pathogens during sports: risk and prevention. Annals of Internal Medicine 122:283–285

Mills J D, Moore G E, Thompson P D 1997 The athlete's heart. Clinical Journal of Sports Medicine 16:725–737

Moeller J 1996 Contraindications to athletic participation: cardiac, respiratory, and central nervous system conditions. The Physician and Sportsmedicine 24:47–49, 53–54, 55–58

Morgan W P, Brown D R, Raglin J S et al 1987 Psychological monitoring of overtraining and staleness. British Journal of Sports Medicine 21:107–114

Morgan W P, Costill D L, Flynn M G et al 1988 Mood disturbance following increased training in swimmers. Medicine and Science in Sport and Exercise 20:408–414

Mossad S B, Macknin M L, Medendorp S V et al 1996 Zinc gluconate lozenges for treating the common cold. A randomized, double-blind, placebo-controlled study. Annals of Internal Medicine 125:81–88

Nakken K O 1999 Physical exercise in outpatients with epilepsy. Epilepsia 40:643–651

Nakken K O, Bjorholt P G, Johannessen S I et al 1990 Effect of physical training on aerobic capacity, seizure occurrence, and serum level of antiepileptic drugs in adults with epilepsy. Epilepsia 31:88–94

Nakken, K, Loyning A, Loyning T et al 1997 Does physical exercise influence the occurrence of epileptiform EEG discharges in children. Epilepsia 38(3):279–284

Newcombe R, Reid R, Smethills R et al 1994 Football injuries of the head and neck. National Health and Medical Research Council, Australian Government Publishing Service, Canberra

Nieman D 1993 Exercise and upper respiratory tract infection. Sports Medicine, Training and Rehabilitation 4:1–14

Nieman D C 1995 Upper respiratory tract infections and exercise. Thorax 50:1229–1231

Pan X R, Li G W, Hu Y H et al 1997 Effects of diet and exercise in preventing NIDDM in people with impaired glucose tolerance. The Da Qing IGT and Diabetes Study. Diabetes Care 20:537–544

Pelliccia A, Maron B J, Spataro A et al 1991 The upper limit of physiologic cardiac hypertrophy in highly trained elite athletes. New England Journal of Medicine 324:295–301

Perlstein R, McConell K, Hagger V 1997 Off to a flying start … insulin dependent diabetes and exercise. Everything you need to know. International Diabetes Institute, Caulfield, Victoria

Petrie K, Dawson A G, Thompson L et al 1993 A double-blind trial of melatonin as a treatment for jet lag in international cabin crew. Biological Psychiatry 33:526–530

Pierce NS 1999 Diabetes and exercise. British Journal of Sports Medicine 33:161–173

Provost-Craig M A, Arbour K S, Sestili D C et al 1996 The incidence of exercise-induced bronchospasm in competitive figure skaters. Journal of Asthma 33:67–71

Pyne D B, Gleeson M, McDonald W A et al 2000a Training strategies to maintain immunocompetence in athletes. International Journal of Sports Medicine 21:S51–S60

Pyne D B, McDonald W A, Gleeson M et al 2000b Mucosal immunity, respiratory illness, and competitive performance in elite swimmers. Medicine and Science in Sports and Exercise 33:348–353

Quinn D, Markus, R, Day R 2001 Antiepileptic therapy. Current Therapeutics 39(7):23–39

Reilly T, Maughan R, Budgett R 1998 Melatonin: a position statement of the British Olympic Association. British Journal of Sports Medicine 32:99–100

Reilly T, Atkinson G, Budgett R 2001 Effect of low-dose temazepam on physiological variables and performance tests following a westerly flight across five time zones. International Journal of Sports Medicine 22:166–174

Rich J D, Dickinson B P, Merriman N A et al 1998 Hepatitis C virus infection related to anabolic-androgenic steroid injection in a recreational weight lifter. American Journal of Gastroenterology 93:1598

Rotem T, Lawson J S, Wilson S F et al 1998 Severe cervical spinal cord injuries related to rugby union and league football in New South Wales, 1984–1996. Medical Journal of Australia 168:379–381

Rundell K W, Wilber R L, Szmedra L et al 2000 Exercise-induced asthma screening of elite athletes: field versus laboratory exercise challenge. Medicine and Science in Sport and Exercise 32:309–316

Seward H G, Orchard J W, Hazard H et al 1993a Football injuries in Australia at the elite level. Medical Journal of Australia 159:298–301

Seward H G, Orchard J W, Hazard H et al 1993b Frequency of bleeding in football. Medical Journal of Australia 159:353

Shephard R J 1996 The athlete's heart: is big beautiful? British Journal of Sports Medicine 30:5–10

Siebert D J, Lindschau P B, Burrell C J 1995 Lack of evidence for significant hepatitis B transmission in Australian Rules footballers. Medical Journal of Australia 162:312–313

Sirven J, Varrato J 1999 Physical activity and epilepsy. What are the rules? The Physician and Sportsmedicine 27:63–64, 67–70

Smith D J, Norris S R 2000 Changes in glutamine and glutamate concentrations for tracking training tolerance. Medicine and Science in Sport and Exercise 32:684–689

Smith L L 2000 Cytokine hypothesis of overtraining: a physiological adaptation to excessive stress? Medicine and Science in Sport and Exercise 32:317–331

Snyder A C 1998 Overtraining and glycogen depletion hypothesis. Medicine and Science in Sport and Exercise 30:1146–1150

Spiegel R, Gates J 1997 Epilepsy. In: Wikgren S (ed), ACSM's exercise management for persons with chronic diseases and disabilities. Human Kinetics, Champaign, IL

Spooner C, Rowe B H, Saunders L D 2000 Nedocromil sodium in the treatment of exercise-induced asthma: A meta-analysis. European Respiratory Journal 16:30–37

Stacey A, Atkins B 2000 Infectious diseases in rugby players: incidence, treatment and prevention. Sports Medicine 29:211–220

Stolt A, Kujala U M, Karjalainen J et al 1997 Electrocardiographic findings in female endurance athletes. Clinical Journal of Sports Medicine 7:85–859

Storms W 1999 Exercise-induced asthma: diagnosis and treatment for the recreational or elite athlete. Medicine and Science in Sport and Exercise 31:S33–S38

Tang C, Rolland I M, Ward C et al 1996 Seasonal comparison of cytokine profiles in atopic asthmatics and atopic non-asthmatics. American Journal of Respiratory and Critical Care Medicine 154:1615–1622

Thien F C 1999 Leukotriene receptor antagonist drugs for asthma. Medical Journal of Australia 171:378–381

Thomas P 2001 Acute asthma. The management in the community. Australian Family Physician 30(2):100–105

Torg J, Glasgow S 1991 Criteria for return to contact activities following cervical spine injury. Clinical Journal of Sport Medicine 1:12–26

Torg J, Ramsey-Emrhein J 1997 Suggested management guidelines for participation in collision activities with congenital, developmental, or postinjury lesions involving the cervical spine. Medicine and Science in Sport and Exercise 29:S256–S272

Torre D, Sampietro C, Ferraro G et al 1990 Transmission of HIV-1 infection via sports injury. Lancet 335:1105

Urhausen A, Kindermann W 1999 Sports-specific adaptations and differentiation of the athlete's heart. Sports Medicine 28:237–244

van Linschoten R, Backx F J, Mulder O G et al 1990 Epilepsy and sports. Sports Medicine 10:9–19.

Warren W, Bailes J 1998a On field evaluation of athletic head injuries. Clinics in Sports Medicine 17(1):13–26

Warren W, Bailes J 1998b On field evaluation of athletic neck injury. Clinics in Sports Medicine 17(1):99–110

Waterhouse J, Reilly T, Atkinson G 1998 Melatonin and jet lag. British Journal of Sports Medicine 32:98–99

Weiler J M, Ryan E J 3rd 2000 Asthma in United States Olympic athletes who participated in the 1998 Olympic winter games. Journal of Allergy and Clinical Immunology 106:267–271

WHO 2001 International Travel and Health. Vaccination requirements and health advice, World Health Organization, Geneva

Wilber R L, Rundell K W, Szmedra L et al 2000 Incidence of exercise-induced bronchospasm in Olympic winter sport athletes. Medicine and Science in Sport and Exercise 32:732–737

Williams C C, Bernhardt D T 1995 Syncope in athletes. Sports Medicine 19(3):223–234

Wilmore J, Costill D 1994 Physiology of sport and exercise, 1st edn. Human Kinetics, Champaign, IL

Young M 1998 What athletes often ask. Should I train when I have a cold and if not when can I return? British Journal of Sports Medicine 32:84

Young M 1999 How I treat: return to sport after post-viral fatigue. British Journal of Sports Medicine 33:173

Young M, Fricker P, Maughan R et al 1998 The traveling athlete: issues relating to the Commonwealth Games, Malaysia, 1998. Clinical Journal of Sports Medicine 8:130–135

Youngstedt S D, O'Connor P J 1999 The influence of air travel on athletic performance. Sports Medicine 28:197–207

Zinman B, Ruderman N, Campaigne B et al 1997 American College of Sports Medicine and American Diabetes Association joint position statement. Diabetes mellitus and exercise. Medicine and Science in Sport and Exercise 29:i–vi

Index

*Note: Page numbers in **bold** refer to figures and tables.*
This index is in letter-by-letter order whereby spaces and hyphens between words are ignored in the alphabetization, e.g. football precedes foot injuries.

Abbreviations used in this index include: